Davis's Comprehensive Handbook of Laboratory and Diagnostic Tests— with Nursing Implications

Davis's Comprehensive Handbook of Laboratory and Diagnostic Tests— with Nursing Implications

Second Edition

Anne M. Van Leeuwen, MA, BS, MT (ASCP)
Todd R. Kranpitz, MS, BS, ARRT (R) (N),
  NM (NMTCB), ASCP (N)
Lynette S. Smith, FNP-BC, MSN, RN, MLT (ASCP)

F. A. DAVIS COMPANY • PHILADELPHIA

F. A. Davis Company
1915 Arch Street
Philadelphia, PA 19103
www.fadavis.com

Printed in the United States of America

Last digit indicates print number: 10 9 8 7 6 5

Acquisitions Editor: Lisa B. Deitch
Project Editor: Ilysa H. Richman
Art and Design Manager: Carolyn O'Brien

As new scientific information becomes available through basic and clinical research, recommended treatments and drug therapies undergo changes. The authors and publisher have done everything possible to make this book accurate, up to date, and in accord with accepted standards at the time of publication. The authors, editors, and publisher are not responsible for errors or omissions or for consequences from application of the book, and make no warranty, expressed or implied, in regard to the contents of the book. Any practice described in this book should be applied by the reader in accordance with professional standards of care used in regard to the unique circumstances that may apply in each situation. The reader is advised always to check product information (package inserts) for changes and new information regarding dose and contraindications before administering any drug. Caution is especially urged when using new or infrequently ordered drugs.

Library of Congress Cataloging-in-Publication Data

Van Leeuwen, Anne M.
  Davis's comprehensive handbook of laboratory and diagnostic tests : with nursing implications / Anne M. Van Leeuwen, Todd R. Kranpitz, Lynette Smith.— 2nd ed.
    p. ; cm.
  Rev. ed. of: Davis's comprehensive handbook of laboratory and diagnostic tests / Zoanne Burgess Schnell, Anne M. Van Leeuwen, Todd R. Kranpitz. c2003.
  Includes bibliographical references and index.
  ISBN 10: 0-8036-1464-0   ISBN 13: 978-0-8036-1464-2
  1. Diagnosis, Laboratory—Handbooks, manuals, etc. 2. Nursing—Handbooks, manuals, etc.
  [DNLM: 1. Laboratory Techniques and Procedures—Handbooks. 2. Laboratory Techniques and Procedures—Nurses' Instruction. 3. Nursing Diagnosis—methods. 4. Diagnostic Techniques and Procedures—Handbooks. 5. Diagnostic Techniques and Procedures—Nurses' Instruction. QY 39 V217d 2006] I. Title: Comprehensive handbook of laboratory and diagnostic tests. II. Kranpitz, Todd R. III. Smith, Lynette. IV. Schnell, Zoanne Burgess. Davis's comprehensive handbook of laboratory and diagnostic tests. V. Title.
  RB38.2.S37 2006
  616.07′5—dc22

                                        2005053757

DEDICATION

Inspiration springs from Passion.... Passion is born from unconstrained love, commitment, and a vision no one else can own. Thank you Lynda, Mom & Dad, Adele, Gram, Regina & Mark, Helen & Ricky, Todd, Kent & Cathy, JT, Bev, Cathy, Ev, Ruth, and Lois...I am truly blessed by your friendship, love, and support. A huge hug for my daughters, Sarah and Margaret—I love you very much. To my puppies, Maggie and Tayor, for their endless and unconditional love. With appreciation and in recognition of Stacey for her assistance with this edition. My thanks and welcome to Lynette for her contributions to this second edition; I look forward to our continued collaboration. Very special thanks to Lisa Deitch, Acquisitions Editor, for her friendship, excellent direction, and unwavering encouragement.

Anne M. Van Leeuwen, MA, BS, MT (ASCP)
Chief Technologist
Highlands Regional Medical Center
Sebring, Florida

To my wife, Mindy, for her never ending support, and my son, Jake, for his demonstration of commitment to a goal. I could not have done this book without them. To my coauthors, for their dedication, endless commitment, and organizational skills. To Lisa Deitch, for her continued faith in us, and support.

Todd R. Kranpitz, MS, BS, ARRT (R) (N), NM (NMTCB), ASCP (N)
Director of Imaging Services
King's Daughters Medical Center
Ashland, Kentucky

To my husband, Steve, whose unconditional love, support, and encouragement holds me steadfast in all my endeavors. To my sons, Eric and Michael, for their wisdom and humor beyond their ages, you rock my world. To Anne, Todd, and Lisa, humble thanks for taking this novice writer under your wings and believing in what I had to offer for this edition. I look forward to future editions with this great team. And lastly, I wish to thank Dr. Mary Bennett for her years of friendship and look forward to our continual mentoring of minds in years to come.

Lynette S. Smith, FNP-BC, MSN, RN, MLT (ASCP)
Family Nurse Practitioner
Office of Lynette Smith FNP
Clinton, Indiana
Adjunct Faculty, Family Nurse Practitioner Program
College of Nursing, Indiana State University
Terre Haute, Indiana

ABOUT THIS BOOK

Laboratory and diagnostic studies are essential components of a complete patient assessment. Examined in conjunction with an individual's history and physical examination, laboratory and diagnostic data provide clues about health status. Nurses are increasingly expected to integrate an understanding of laboratory and diagnostic procedures and expected outcomes in assessment, planning, implementation, and evaluation of nursing care. The data help develop and support nursing diagnoses, interventions, and outcomes.

Nurses may interface with laboratory and diagnostic testing on several levels, including:

- Interacting with patients and families of patients undergoing diagnostic tests or procedures, and providing pretest, intratest, and post-test information and support
- Maintaining quality control to prevent or eliminate problems that may interfere with the accuracy and reliability of test results
- Ensuring completion of testing in a timely and accurate manner
- Collaborating with other health care professionals in interpreting findings as they relate to planning and implementing total patient care
- Communicating significant alterations in test outcomes to other appropriate health care team members
- Coordinating interdisciplinary efforts

Whether the nurse's role at each level is direct or indirect, the underlying responsibility to the patient, family, and community remains the same.

This book is a reference for nurses, nursing students, and other health care professionals. It is useful as a clinical tool as well as a supportive text to supplement clinical courses. It guides the nurse in planning what needs to be assessed, monitored, treated, and taught regarding pretest requirements, intratest procedures, and post-test care. It can be used by nursing students at all levels as a textbook in theory classes, integrating laboratory and diagnostic data as one aspect of nursing care; by practicing nurses, to update information; and in clinical settings as a quick reference. Designed for use in academic and clinical settings, *Davis's Comprehensive Handbook of Laboratory and Diagnostic Procedures—with Nursing Implications* provides the user with a comprehensive reference that allows easy access to information about laboratory and diagnostic tests and procedures. A general overview of how all the tests and procedures included in this book relate to body systems can be found in tables at the end of the monographs. All tests and procedures are listed in alphabetical order by their complete name, allowing the user to locate information quickly without having to place tests in a specific category or body system. Each monograph is presented in a consistent format for easy identification of specific information at a glance. The following information is provided for each laboratory and diagnostic test:

- *Test Name* for each monograph is given as a commonly used designation, and all test monographs in the book are organized in alphabetical order by name.
- *Synonyms/Acronyms* for each test are listed where appropriate.
- *Specimen Type* includes the amount of specimen usually collected and, where appropriate, the type of collection tube or container commonly recommended. Specimen requirements vary from laboratory to laboratory. The amount of specimen collected is usually more than what is minimally required so that additional specimen is available, if needed, for repeat testing (quality control failure, dilutions, or confirmation of unexpected results). In the case of diagnostic tests, the *type of test* procedure (e.g., nuclear medicine, x-ray) is given.
- *Reference Values* for each monograph include age-specific and gender-specific variations, when indicated. It is important to give consideration to the normal variation of laboratory values over the life span and across cultures; sometimes what might be considered an abnormal value in one circumstance is actually what is expected in another. Reference values for laboratory tests are given in conventional and standard international (SI) units. The factor used to convert conventional to SI units is also given. Because laboratory values can vary by method, each laboratory reference range is listed along with the associated methodology.
- *Description & Rationale* of the study's purpose and insight into how and why the test results can affect health are included.
- *Indications* are a list of what the test is used for in terms of assessment, evaluation, monitoring, screening, identifying, or assisting in the diagnosis of a clinical condition.
- *Results* present a list of conditions in which values may be increased or decreased and, in some cases, an explanation of variations that may be encountered.
- *Critical Values,* or findings that may be life-threatening or for which particular concern may be indicated, are given along with age span considerations where applicable. This section also includes signs and symptoms associated with a critical value as well as possible nursing interventions.
- *Interfering Factors* are substances or circumstances that may influence the results of the test, rendering the results invalid or unreliable. Knowledge of interfering factors is an important aspect of quality assurance and includes pharmaceuticals, foods, natural and additive therapies, timing of test in relation to other tests or procedures, collection site, handling of specimen, and underlying patient conditions.
- *Nursing Implications and Procedure* provides an outline of pretest, intratest, and post-test concerns.
- *Pretest* section addresses the need to:

- Obtain pertinent clinical, laboratory, dietary, and therapeutic history of the patient, especially as it pertains to comparison of previous test results, preparation for the test, and identification of potentially interfering factors.
- Understand the interrelationship between various body systems. In this section, the reader is informed of the body systems that may be involved in the study of interest and is referred to system tables where related studies are alphabetically cross-referenced.
- Explain the requirements and restrictions related to the procedure as well as what to expect; provide the education necessary for the patient to be properly informed.
- Anticipate and allay patient concerns or anxieties.
- Provide for patient safety.
- *Intratest* section can be used in a quality control assessment by the nurse or as a guide to the nurse who may be called on to participate in specimen collection or perform preparatory procedures and gives:
  - Specific directions for specimen collection and test performance.
  - Important information such as patient sensation and expected duration of the procedure.
  - Precautions to be taken by the nurse and patient.
- *Post-test* section provides guidelines regarding:
  - Specific monitoring and therapeutic measures that should be performed after the procedure (e.g., maintaining bed rest, obtaining vital signs to compare with baseline values, signs and symptoms of complications).
  - Specific instructions for the patient and family, such as when to resume usual diet, medications, and activity.
  - General nutritional guidelines related to excess or deficit as well as common food sources for dietary replacement.
  - Indications for interventions from public health representatives or for special counseling related to test outcomes.
  - Indications for follow-up testing that may be required within specific time frames.
  - Related tests for consideration and evaluation, an alphabetical listing of related laboratory and/or diagnostic tests that is intended to provoke a deeper and broader investigation of multiple pieces of information; the tests provide related data that, when combined, can form a more complete picture of health or illness.

Color and icons have been used to facilitate locating critical information at a glance. The nursing process is evident throughout the laboratory and diagnostic monographs. Within each phase of the testing procedure, the nurse has certain potential roles and responsibilities. These should be evident in reading each monograph.

Information provided in the appendices includes a summary of specimen collection procedures and materials, describing specific tube tops used for various blood tests and their recommended order of draw; a summary chart of transfusion reactions, their signs and symptoms, associated laboratory findings, and potential nursing interventions; an introduction to CLIA with an explanantion of the different levels of testing complexity; a summary chart that details suggested approaches to persons at various developmental stages to assist the provider in facilitating cooperation and understanding; a list of some of the herbs and nutraceuticals that have been associated with adverse clinical reactions or have been associated with drug interactions related to the affected body system; and guidelines for Standard and Universal Precautions.

Finally, additional supportive materials are provided for the instructor and student in an *Instructor's Guide*. Presentations and case studies with emphasis on laboratory and diagnostic test–related information and nursing implications have been developed for selected conditions and body systems. Open-ended and NCLEX-type, multiple-choice questions are provided as well as suggested critical thinking activities. This supplemental material will aid the instructor in integrating laboratory and diagnostic materials in assessment and clinical courses and provide examples of activities to enhance student learning.

PREFACE

*L*aboratory and diagnostic testing. The words themselves often conjure up cold and impersonal images of needles, specimens lined up in collection containers, and high-tech electronic equipment. But they do not stand alone. They are tied to, bound with, and tell of health or disease in the blood and tissue of a person. Laboratory and diagnostic studies augment the health care provider's assessment of the quality of an individual's physical being. Test results guide the plans and interventions geared toward strengthening life's quality and endurance. Beyond the pounding noise of the MRI, the cold steel of the x-ray table, the sting of the needle, the invasive collection of fluids and tissue, and the probing and inspection is the gathering of evidence that supports the health care provider's ability to discern the course of a disease and the progression of its treatment. Laboratory and diagnostic data must be viewed with thought and compassion, however, as well as with microscopes and machines. We must remember that behind the specimen and test result is the person from whom it came, a person who is someone's son, daughter, mother, father, husband, wife, friend.

This book is written to help health care providers in their understanding and interpretation of laboratory and diagnostic procedures and their outcomes. Just as important, it is dedicated to all health care professionals who experience the wonders in the science of laboratory and diagnostic testing, performed and interpreted in a caring and efficient manner.

CONSULTANTS

Connie J. Frisch, RN, MA
Nursing Instructor
Central Lakes College
Brainerd, Minnesota

Mary K. Gerepka, MS, APRN, BC
Instructor
Mountainside Hospital School of Nursing
Montclair, New Jersey

Peggy L. Hawkins, RN, MSN, PHD, BC
Professor of Nursing, Nursing Programs
   Director
College of Saint Mary
Omaha, Nebraska

Beth Langlois, RN, MSN, APRN, BC
CCU and Heart Failure Center Coordinator
Overlook Hospital, Atlantic Health System
Summit, New Jersey

Deborah Little, MSN, RN, CCRN, CNRN,
   APRN, BC
Faculty Instructor
Mountainside Hospital School of Nursing
Montclair, New Jersey

Brooke C. Martin, RN, MSN, CNM,
   ARNP
Associate Professor Practical Nursing Program
Ivy Tech State College
Indianapolis, Indiana

Patricia A. Parsons RN, MSN, MS
Director of Associate Degree Nursing
   Program
Riverland Community College
Austin, Minnesota

CONTENTS

ACETYLCHOLINE RECEPTOR ANTIBODY

SYNONYM/ACRONYM: AChR.

SPECIMEN: Serum (1 mL) collected in a red-top tube.

REFERENCE VALUE: (Method: Radioimmunoassay) Less than 0.03 nmol/L.

DESCRIPTION & RATIONALE: Normally when impulses travel down a nerve, the nerve ending releases a neurotransmitter called acetylcholine. Acetylcholine binds to receptor sites in the neuromuscular junction, which eventually results in muscle contraction. When present, acetylcholine receptor (AChR) antibodies block acetylcholine from binding to receptor sites on the muscle membrane. AChR antibodies also destroy acetylcholine receptor sites, interfering with neuromuscular transmission and causing muscle weakness. Antibodies to AChR sites are present in 90% of patients with generalized myasthenia gravis (MG) and in 55% to 70% of patients who either have ocular forms of MG or are in remission. MG is an acquired autoimmune disorder that can occur at any age. It seems to strike women between the ages of 20 and 40 years; men appear to be affected later in life than women. It can affect any voluntary muscle, but muscles that control eye, eyelid, and facial movement and swallowing are most frequently affected. Antibodies may not be detected in the first six to twelve months, after the first appearance of symptoms. MG is the most common complication associated with thymoma. The relationship between the thymus gland and MG is not completely understood. It is believed that miscommunication in the thymus gland directed at developing immune cells may trigger the development of autoantibodies responsible for MG. Remission after thymectomy is associated with a progressive decrease in antibody level. Other markers used in the study of MG include muscle AChR binding antibodies, muscle AChR blocking antibodies, muscle AChR modulating antibodies, striational antibodies, thyroglobulin, HLA-B8, and HLA-DR3. These antibodies are often undetectable in the early stages of MG. ∎

INDICATIONS:
• Confirm the presence, but not the severity, of MG
• Monitor the effectiveness of immunosuppressive therapy for MG
• Monitor the remission stage of MG

RESULT

Increased in:
• Generalized MG
• Thymoma associated with MG

Decreased in: Post-thymectomy

CRITICAL VALUES: N/A

INTERFERING FACTORS:

- Drugs that may increase AChR levels include penicillamine.

- Biologic false-positive results may be associated with amyotrophic lateral sclerosis, autoimmune hepatitis, patients who have had a bone marrow transplant, Eaton-Lambert myasthenic syndrome, first-degree relatives of patients with MG (rare), thymoma with no evidence of MG, primary biliary cirrhosis, encephalomyeloneuropathies associated with carcinoma of the lung, and elderly patients prone to autoimmune disorders.

- Immunosuppressive therapy is the recommended treatment for MG; prior immunosuppressive drug administration may result in negative test results.

- Recent radioactive scans or radiation within 1 week of the test can interfere with test results when radioimmunoassay is the test method.

- Inability of the patient to cooperate or remain still during the procedure because of age, significant pain, or mental status may interfere with the test results.

Nursing Implications and Procedure • • • • • • • • • • •

Pretest:

> Inform the patient that the test is used to identify antibodies responsible for decreased neuromuscular transmission and associated muscle weakness.

> Obtain a history of the patient's complaints, including a list of known allergens (especially allergies or sensitivities to latex) and any prior complications with general anesthesia, and inform the appropriate health care practitioner accordingly.

> Obtain a history of the patient's musculoskeletal system and results of previously performed laboratory tests, surgical procedures, and other diagnostic procedures. For related tests, refer to the Musculoskeletal System table.

> Note any recent procedures that can interfere with test results.

> Obtain a list of the medications the patient is taking, especially immunosuppressive drugs or prednisone. Include herbs, nutritional supplements, and nutraceuticals. The requesting health care practitioner and laboratory should be advised if the patient regularly uses these products so that their effects can be taken into consideration when reviewing results.

> Review the procedure with the patient. Inform the patient that specimen collection takes approximately 5 to 10 minutes. Address concerns about pain related to the procedure. Explain to the patient that there may be some discomfort during the venipuncture.

> There are no food, fluid, or medication restrictions unless by medical direction.

Intratest:

> If the patient has a history of severe allergic reaction to latex, care should be taken to avoid the use of equipment containing latex.

> Instruct the patient to cooperate fully and to follow directions. Direct the patient to breathe normally and to avoid unnecessary movement.

> Observe standard precautions, and follow the general guidelines in Appendix A. Positively identify the patient, and label the appropriate tubes with the corresponding patient demographics, date, and time of collection. Perform a venipuncture; collect the specimen in a 5-mL red-top tube.

> Remove the needle, place gauze over the puncture site and apply gentle pressure to stop bleeding. Observe venipuncture site for bleed-

ing or hematoma formation. Apply paper tape to hold gauze in place or replace with adhesive bandage.

➤ Promptly transport the specimen to the laboratory for processing and analysis.

➤ The results are recorded manually or in a computerized system for recall and postprocedure interpretation by the appropriate health care practitioner.

Post-test:

➤ A written report of the examination will be sent to the requesting health care practitioner, who will discuss the results with the patient.

➤ Recognize anxiety related to test results, and be supportive of impaired activity related to lack of neuromuscular control, perceived loss of independence, and fear of shortened life expectancy. Discuss the implications of positive test results on the patient's lifestyle. It is important to note that a diagnosis of MG should be based on positive results from two different diagnostic tests. These tests include AChR antibody assay, edrophonium test, repetitive nerve stimulation, and single-fiber electromyography. Evaluate test results in relationship to a future general anesthesia. Provide teaching and information regarding the clinical implications of the test results as appropriate. Educate the patient regarding access to counseling services. Provide contact information, if desired, for the Myasthenia Gravis Foundation of America (*http://www. myasthenia.org*) and Muscular Dystrophy Association (*http://www. mdausa.org*).

➤ Reinforce information given by the patient's health care provider regarding further testing, treatment, or referral to another health care provider. Answer any questions or address any concerns voiced by the patient or family.

➤ Depending on the results of this procedure, additional testing may be performed to evaluate or monitor progression of the disease process and determine the need for a change in therapy. If a diagnosis of MG is made, a computed tomography scan of the chest should be performed to rule out thymoma. Evaluate test results in relation to the patient's symptoms and other tests performed.

Related laboratory tests:

➤ Related laboratory tests include antinuclear antibodies, antithyroglobulin and antithyroid peroxidase antibodies, myoglobin, rheumatoid factor, thyroid-stimulating hormone, and thyroxine.

ACID PHOSPHATASE, PROSTATIC

· ·

SYNONYMS/ACRONYM: Prostatic acid phosphatase, *o*-phosphoric monoester phosphohydrolase, AcP.

SPECIMEN: Serum (1 mL) collected in a red-top tube.

A swab with vaginal secretions may be submitted in the appropriate transfer container. Other material such as clothing may be submitted for analysis. Consult the laboratory or emergency services department for the proper specimen collection instructions and containers.

REFERENCE VALUE: (Method: Spectrophotometric)

Conventional & SI Units
Less than 2.5 ng/mL

DESCRIPTION & RATIONALE: Acid phosphatases are enzymes found in many tissues, including the prostate gland, bone, spleen, liver, and kidney, as well as in red blood cells and platelets. Seminal fluid also contains high concentrations of acid phosphatase, and detection of this enzyme in vaginal swabs or from other physical evidence is used to investigate rape. Acid phosphatase activity is highest in the prostate gland; however, prostatic acid phosphatase (AcP) levels are not significantly increased in the early stages of prostatic cancer, so this test is not recommended as a screening tool. Prostate-specific antigen has replaced AcP for the staging of carcinoma of the prostate and diagnosis of metastatic adenocarcinoma of the prostate. ∎

INDICATIONS:
- Assist in the investigation of sexual assault and rape.

- Assist with differential diagnosis of other disorders associated with elevated AcP of nonprostatic origin.

- Evaluate the effectiveness of treatment for prostatic cancer (recurrence after prostatectomy). Levels decrease with effective treatment. Rising levels are associated with a poor prognosis.

- Investigate or evaluate an enlarged prostate gland, especially if prostatic carcinoma is suspected.

RESULT

Increased in:
- Acute myelogenous leukemia
- After prostate surgery or biopsy
- Benign prostatic hypertrophy
- Gaucher's disease
- Liver disease
- Metastatic bone cancer
- Niemann-Pick disease
- Paget's disease
- Prostatic cancer
- Prostatic infarct
- Prostatitis
- Sickle cell crisis
- Thrombocytosis

Decreased in: N/A

CRITICAL VALUES: N/A

INTERFERING FACTORS:
- Drugs that may increase AcP levels include androgens (females), and clofibrate.

- Drugs that may decrease AcP levels include alcohol, ketoconazole, buserelin and leuprolide.

- There is growing evidence that rectal palpation does not cause elevated AcP. However, increases can occur due to prostatic needle biopsy, cytoscopy, prostatic infarction either by undergoing catheterization or the presence of an indwelling catheter, and rupture of a prostatic cyst (rare).

- Specimens should be drawn in the morning because AcP exhibits diurnal variation.

- Hemolysis interferes with the test methodology.

Nursing Implications and Procedure ● ● ● ● ● ● ● ● ● ● ● ●

Pretest:

➤ Inform the patient that the test is primarily used to assist in monitoring treatment for prostate cancer.

➤ Obtain a history of the patient's complaints, especially alterations in urinary elimination. Obtain a list of known allergens, especially allergies or sensitivities to latex, and inform the appropriate health care practitioner accordingly.

➤ Obtain a history of the patient's genitourinary, immune, and reproductive systems and results of previously performed laboratory tests, surgical procedures, and other diagnostic procedures. For related laboratory tests, refer to the Genitourinary, Immune, and Reproductive System tables.

➤ Note any recent procedures that can interfere with test results.

➤ Obtain a list of the medications the patient is taking, including herbs, nutritional supplements, and nutraceuticals. The requesting health care practitioner and laboratory should be advised if the patient regularly uses these products so that their effects can be taken into consideration when reviewing results.

➤ Review the procedure with the patient. Inform the patient that specimen collection takes approximately 5 to 10 minutes. Address concerns about pain related to the procedure. Explain to the patient that there may be some discomfort during the venipuncture.

➤ There are no food, fluid, or medication restrictions unless by medical direction.

Intratest:

➤ If the patient has a history of severe allergic reaction to latex, care should be taken to avoid the use of equipment containing latex.

➤ Instruct the patient to cooperate fully and to follow directions. Direct the patient to breathe normally and to avoid unnecessary movement.

➤ Observe standard precautions, and follow the general guidelines in Appendix A. Positively identify the patient, and label the appropriate tubes with the corresponding patient demographics, date, and time of collection. Perform a venipuncture; collect the specimen in a 5-mL red-top tube.

➤ Remove the needle, place gauze over the puncture site and apply gentle pressure to stop bleeding. Observe venipuncture site for bleeding or hematoma formation. Apply paper tape over gauze or replace with adhesive bandage.

➤ Promptly transport the specimen to the laboratory for processing and analysis. AcP is very labile. Immediate seperation from blood cells and freezing of the serum stabilizes AcP.

➤ The results are recorded manually or in a computerized system for recall and postprocedure interpretation by the appropriate health care practitioner.

Post-test:

➤ A written report of the examination will be sent to the requesting health

care practitioner, who will discuss the results with the patient.

➤ *Social and cultural considerations:* Recognize anxiety related to test results, and offer support. Provide teaching and disease information, as appropriate. Counsel the male patient, as appropriate, that sexual dysfunction related to altered body function, drugs, or radiation may occur. Educate the patient regarding counseling services, as appropriate.

➤ *Social and cultural considerations:* Offer support, as appropriate, to patients who may be the victim of rape or sexual assault. Educate the patient regarding access to counseling services. Provide a nonjudgmental, nonthreatening atmosphere for discussing the risks of sexually transmitted diseases. Discuss problems the patient may experience (e.g.,

guilt, depression, anger) as a victim of rape or sexual assault.

➤ Reinforce information given by the patient's health care provider regarding further testing, treatment, or referral to another health care provider. Answer any questions or address any concerns voiced by the patient or family.

➤ Depending on the results of this procedure, additional testing may be performed to evaluate or monitor progression of the disease process and determine the need for a change in therapy. Evaluate test results in relation to the patient's symptoms and other tests performed.

Related laboratory tests:

➤ Related laboratory tests include prostate biopsy, prostate-specific antigen, and semen analysis.

ADRENAL GLAND SCAN

SYNONYM/ACRONYM: Adrenal scintiscan.

AREA OF APPLICATION: Adrenal gland.

CONTRAST: Intravenous radioactive NP-59 (iodomethyl-19-norcholesterol) or metaiodobenzylguanidine (MIBG).

DESCRIPTION & RATIONALE: This nuclear medicine study evaluates function of the adrenal glands. The secretory function of the adrenal glands is controlled primarily by the anterior pituitary, which produces adrenocorticotropic hormone (ACTH). ACTH stimulates the adrenal cortex to produce cortisone and secrete aldosterone. Adrenal imaging is most useful in differentiation of hyperplasia versus adenoma in primary aldosteronism when computed tomography (CT) and magnetic resonance imaging (MRI) findings are equivocal. High concentrations of cholesterol (the precursor in the synthesis of adrenocorticosteroids, including aldosterone) are stored in the adrenal cortex. This allows the radionuclide, which attaches to the cholesterol, to be used in identifying pathology in the secretory function of the adrenal cortex. The uptake of the radionuclide occurs gradually over time; imaging is performed within 24 to 48 hours of injection of the radionuclide dose and continued daily for 3 to 5 days. Imaging reveals increased uptake, unilateral or bilateral uptake, or absence of uptake in the detection of pathologic processes. Following prescanning treatment with corticosteroids, suppression studies can be done to differentiate the presence of tumor from hyperplasia of the glands. ■

INDICATIONS:
- Aid in the diagnosis of Cushing's syndrome and aldosteronism
- Aid in the diagnosis of gland tissue destruction caused by infection, infarction, neoplasm, or suppression
- Aid in locating adrenergic tumors
- Determine adrenal suppressibility with prescan administration of corticosteroid to diagnose and localize adrenal adenoma, aldosteronomas, androgen excess, and low-renin hypertension
- Differentiate between asymmetric hyperplasia and asymmetry from aldosteronism with dexamethasone suppression test

RESULT

Normal Findings:
- No evidence of tumors, infection, infarction, or suppression
- Normal bilateral uptake of radionuclide and secretory function of adrenal cortex
- Normal salivary glands and urinary bladder; vague shape of the liver and spleen sometimes seen

Abnormal Findings:
- Adrenal gland suppression
- Adrenal infarction

- Adrenal tumor
- Hyperplasia
- Infection
- Pheochromocytoma

INTERFERING FACTORS

This procedure is contraindicated for:
- Patients who are pregnant or suspected of being pregnant, unless the potential benefits of the procedure far outweigh the risks to the fetus and mother.

Factors that may impair clear imaging:
- Inability of the patient to cooperate or remain still during the procedure because of age, significant pain, or mental status
- Retained barium from a previous radiologic procedure
- Obesity, because patients may exceed the weight limit for the equipment
- Incorrect positioning of the patient, which may produce poor visualization of the area to be examined

Other considerations:
- Improper injection of the radionuclide may allow the tracer to seep deep into the muscle tissue, producing erroneous hot spots.
- Consultation with a physician should occur before the procedure for radiation safety concerns regarding younger patients or patients who are lactating.
- Risks associated with radiologic overexposure can result from frequent x-ray procedures. Personnel in the room with the patient should wear a protective lead apron, stand behind a shield, or leave the area while the examination is being done. Badges that reveal the level of exposure to radiation should be worn by persons working in the area where the examination is being done.

Nursing Implications and Procedure

➤ Inform the patient that the procedure detects adrenal gland function.

➤ Obtain a history of the patient's complaints and symptoms, including a list of known allergens.

➤ Obtain a history of results of previously performed diagnostic procedures, surgical procedures, and laboratory tests. All adrenal blood tests should be done before doing this test. For related tests, refer to the Endocrine System table.

➤ Record the date of last menstrual period and determine the possibility of pregnancy in perimenopausal women.

➤ Obtain a list of the patient's current medications.

➤ Review the procedure with the patient. Address concerns about pain related to the procedure. Explain to the patient that some pain may be experienced during the test, and there may be moments of discomfort. Inform the patient that the procedure is performed in a nuclear medicine department, usually by a nuclear medicine technologist with support staff, and takes approximately 60 minutes to 120 minutes each day. Inform the patient the test usually involves a prolonged scanning schedule over a period of days.

➤ Administer saturated solution of potassium iodide (SSKI) 24 hours before the study to prevent thyroid uptake of the free radioactive iodine.

➤ *Sensitivity to cultural and social issues,* as well as concern for modesty, is important in providing psychological support before, during, and after the procedure.

➤ There are no food, fluid, or medication restrictions unless by medical direction.

➤ Instruct the patient to remove dentures, jewelry (including watches), hairpins, credit cards, and other metallic objects.

➤ *Make sure a written and informed consent has been signed prior to the procedure and before administering any medications.*

➤ Ensure that the patient has removed jewelry, dentures, all external metallic objects, and the like prior to the procedure.

➤ Have emergency equipment readily available.

➤ Patients are given a gown, robe, and foot coverings to wear and instructed to void prior to the procedure.

➤ Insert an intravenous line, and inject the radionuclide intravenously on day 1; images are taken on days 1, 2, and 3. Imaging is done from the urinary bladder to the base of the skull to scan for a primary tumor. Each image takes 20 minutes, and total imaging time is 1 to 2 hours per day.

➤ Instruct the patient to cooperate fully and to follow directions. Instruct the patient to remain still throughout the procedure because movement produces unreliable results.

➤ Observe standard precautions, and follow the general guidelines in Appendix A.

➤ The images are recorded on film or stored electronically for recall and postprocedure interpretation by a health care practitioner specializing in this branch of medicine.

➤ Unless contraindicated, advise patient to drink increased amounts of fluids for 24 to 48 hours to eliminate the radionuclide from the body. Tell the patient that radionuclide is eliminated from the body within 24 to 48 hours.

➤ No other radionuclide tests should be scheduled for 24 to 48 hours after this procedure.

➤ Instruct the patient in the care and assessment of the injection site; observe for bleeding, hematoma formation, and inflammation.

- If a woman who is breast-feeding must have a nuclear scan, she should not breast-feed the infant until the radionuclide has been eliminated. This could take as long as 3 days. She should be instructed to express the milk and discard it during the 3-day period to prevent cessation of milk production.

- Instruct the patient to immediately flush the toilet and to meticulously wash hands with soap and water after each voiding for 48 hours after the procedure.

- Instruct all caregivers to wear gloves when discarding urine for 48 hours after the procedure. Wash gloved hands with soap and water before removing gloves. Then wash ungloved hands after the gloves are removed.

- A written report of the examination will be completed by a health care practitioner specializing in this branch of medicine. The report will be sent to the requesting health care practitioner, who will discuss the results with the patient.

- Reinforce information given by the patient's health care provider regarding further testing, treatment, or referral to another health care provider. Advise the patient that SSKI (120 mg/day) will be administered for 10 days after the injection of the radionuclide. Answer any questions or address any concerns voiced by the patient or family.

- Depending on the results of this procedure, additional testing may be needed to evaluate or monitor progression of the disease process and determine the need for a change in therapy. Evaluate test results in relation to the patient's symptoms and other tests performed.

Related diagnostic tests:

- Computed tomography of the abdomen and magnetic resonance imaging of the abdomen.

ADRENOCORTICOTROPIC HORMONE (AND CHALLENGE TESTS)

Synonym/Acronym: Corticotropin, ACTH.

Specimen: Plasma (2 mL) from lavender-top (EDTA) tube for adrenocorticotropic hormone (ACTH), and serum (1 mL) from a red-top tube for cortisol. Collect specimens in a prechilled heparinized plastic syringe, and carefully transfer into collection containers by gentle injection to avoid hemolysis. Alternatively, specimens can be collected in prechilled lavender- and red-top tubes. Tiger- and green-top (heparin) tubes are also acceptable for cortisol, but take care to use the same type of collection container for serial measurements. Immediately transport specimen tightly capped and in an ice slurry to the laboratory. The specimens should be immediately processed. Plasma for ACTH analysis should be transferred to a plastic container.

Procedure	Medication Administered, Adult Dosage	Recommended Collection Times
ACTH stimulation, rapid test	1 μg (low-dose protocol) cosyntropin IM	3 cortisol levels: baseline immediately before bolus, 30 min after bolus, and 60 min after bolus
Corticotropin-releasing hormone (CRH) stimulation	IV dose of 1 μg/kg ovine CRH at 9 a.m. or 8 p.m.	8 cortisol and 8 ACTH levels: baseline collected 15 min before injection, 0 minutes before injection, and then 5, 15, 30, 60, 120, and 180 min after injection
Dexamethasone suppression (overnight)	Oral dose of 1 mg dexamethasone (Decadron) at 11 p.m.	Collect cortisol at 8 a.m. on the morning after the dexamethasone dose
Metyrapone stimulation (overnight)	Oral dose of 30 mg/kg metyrapone with snack at midnight	Collect cortisol and ACTH at 8 a.m. on the morning after the metyrapone dose

IM = intramuscular, IV = intravenous.

REFERENCE VALUE: (Method: Immunoradiometric assay)

ACTH

Age	Conventional Units	SI Units (Conventional Units × 0.22)
Cord blood	50–570 pg/mL	11–125 pmol/L
Newborn	10–185 pg/mL	2–41 pmol/L
Adult supine specimen collected in morning	9–52 pg/mL	2–11 pmol/L
Women on oral contraceptives	5–29 pg/mL	1–6 pmol/L

ACTH Challenge Tests

ACTH (Cosyntropin) Stimulated, Rapid Test	Conventional Units	SI Units (Conversion Factor × 27.6)
Baseline	Cortisol greater than 5 μg/dL	Greater than 138 nmol/L
30- or 60-min response	Cortisol 18–20 μg/dL or incremental increase of 7 μg/dL over baseline value	496–552 nmol/L

Corticotropin-Releasing Hormone Stimulated	Conventional Units	SI Units (Conventional Units × 27.6)
	Cortisol 10 a.m. 13 μg/dL or 9 p.m. 17 μg/dL	359 nmol/L or 470 nmol/L
	ACTH 9:30 a.m. 80 pg/ml or 8:30 p.m. 29pg/ml	17.6 pmol/L or 6.4 pmol/L

Dexamethasone Suppressed Overnight Test	Conventional Units	SI Units (Conventional Units × 27.6)
	Cortisol less than 3 μg/dL next day	Less than 83 nmol/L

Metyrapone Stimulated Overnight Test	Conventional Units	SI Units (Conventional Units × 0.22)
	ACTH greater than 75 pg/mL	Greater than 16.5 pmol/L
	Cortisol less than 3 μg/dL next day	Less than 83 nmol/L

DESCRIPTION & RATIONALE:

Hypothalamic-releasing factor stimulates the release of adrenocorticotropin hormone (ACTH) from the anterior pituitary gland. This hormone stimulates adrenal cortex secretion of glucocorticoids, androgens, and, to a lesser degree, mineralocorticoids. Angiotensin II is the other primary adrenal cortex stimulant. Cortisol is the major glucocorticoid secreted by the adrenal cortex. ACTH and cortisol test results are evaluated together because normally a change in one causes a change in the other. ACTH secretion is stimulated by insulin, metyrapone, and vasopressin. It is decreased by dexamethasone. Cortisol excess from any source is termed *Cushing syndrome.* Cortisol excess resulting from ACTH excess produced by the pituitary is termed *Cushing disease.* ACTH levels exhibit a diurnal variation, peaking between 6 and 8 a.m. and reaching the lowest point between 6 and 11 p.m. Evening levels are generally one-half to two-thirds lower than morning levels. Cortisol levels also vary diurnally, with the lowest values occurring during the morning hours and peak levels occurring in the evening. ▪

INDICATIONS:

• Determine adequacy of replacement therapy in congenital adrenal hyperplasia

- Determine adrenocortical dysfunction
- Differentiate between increased ACTH release with decreased cortisol levels and decreased ACTH release with increased cortisol levels

RESULT:

ACTH Result:

Because ACTH and cortisol secretion exhibits diurnal variation with values being highest in the morning, a lack of change in values from morning to evening is clinically significant. Decreased concentrations of hormones secreted by the pituitary gland and its target organs are observed in hypopituitarism. In primary adrenal insufficiency (Addison's disease) due to adrenal gland destruction by tumor, infectious process, or immune reaction, ACTH levels are elevated while cortisol levels are decreased. Both ACTH and cortisol levels are decreased in secondary adrenal insufficiency (i.e., secondary to pituitary insufficiency). Excess ACTH can be produced ectopically by various lung cancers such as oat cell carcinoma and large-cell carcinoma of the lung and by benign bronchial carcinoid tumor.

Challenge Tests and Results:

The *ACTH (cosyntropin) stimulated rapid test* directly evaluates adrenal gland function and indirectly evaluates pituitary gland and hypothalmus function. Cosyntropin is a synthetic form of ACTH. A baseline cortisol level is collected before the injection of cosyntropin. Specimens are subsequently collected at 30- and 60-minute intervals. If the adrenal glands function normally, cortisol levels rise significantly after administration of cosyntropin.

The *CRH stimulation test* works as well as the dexamethasone suppression test (DST) in distinguishing Cushing's disease from conditions in which ACTH is secreted ectopically (e.g., tumors not located in the pituitary gland that secrete ACTH). Patients with pituitary tumors tend to respond to CRH stimulation, whereas those with ectopic tumors do not. Patients with adrenal insufficiency demonstrate one of three patterns depending on the underlying cause:

- Primary adrenal insufficiency—high baseline ACTH (in response to intravenous [IV] ACTH) and low cortisol levels pre- and post-IV ACTH.
- Secondary adrenal insufficiency (pituitary)—low baseline ACTH that does not respond to ACTH stimulation. Cortisol levels do not increase after stimulation.
- Tertiary adrenal insufficiency (hypothalmic)—low baseline ACTH with an exaggerated and prolonged response to stimulation. Cortisol levels usually do not reach 20 μg/dL.

The *DST* is useful in differentiating the causes of increased cortisol levels. Dexamethasone is a synthetic glucocorticoid that is 64 times more potent than cortisol. It works by negative feedback. It suppresses the release of ACTH in patients with a normal hypothalamus. A cortisol level less than 3.0 μg/dL usually excludes Cushing's syndrome. With the DST, a baseline morning cortisol level is collected, and the patient is given a 1-mg dose of dexamethasone at bedtime. A second specimen is collected the following morning. If cortisol levels have not been suppressed, adrenal adenoma is suspected. The DST also produces abnormal results in the presence of certain psychiatric illnesses (e.g., endogenous depression).

The *metyrapone stimulation test* is used to distinguish corticotropin-dependent causes (pituitary Cushing's disease and ectopic Cushing's disease) from corticotropin-independent causes (e.g., carcinoma of the lung or thyroid) of increased cortisol levels. Metyrapone inhibits the conversion of 11-deoxycortisol to cortisol. Cortisol levels should decrease to less than 3 μg/dL if normal pituitary stimulation by ACTH occurs after an oral dose of metyrapone. Specimen collection and administration of the medication are performed as with the overnight dexamethasone test.

ACTH Increased in:
- Addison's disease (primary adrenocortical hypofunction)
- Carcinoid syndrome
- Congenital adrenal hyperplasia
- Cushing's disease (pituitary dependent)
- Depression
- Ectopic ACTH-producing tumors
- Lung cancer
- Menstruation
- Nelson's syndrome (ACTH-producing pituitary tumors)
- Non–insulin-dependent diabetes
- Pregnancy
- Sepsis
- Septic shock
- Stress

ACTH Decreased in:
- Adrenal adenoma
- Adrenal cancer
- Adrenal cortical hyperfunction
- Glucocorticoid excess (in Cushing patients with primary adrenocortical tumor)
- Hemochromatosis
- Hypopituitarism
- Major depressive order
- Secondary adrenocortical insufficiency

CRITICAL VALUES: N/A

INTERFERING FACTORS:
- Drugs that may increase ACTH levels include aminoglutethimide, amphetamines, calcium gluconate, estrogens, insulin, levodopa, metoclopramide, metyrapone, mifepristone (RU 486), pyrogens, spironolactone, and vasopressin.
- Drugs that may decrease ACTH levels include adrenal corticosteroids, dexamethasone, ethanol, and lithium carbonate.
- Test results are affected by the time the test is done because ACTH levels vary diurnally, with the highest values occurring between 6 and 8 a.m. and the lowest values occurring at night. Samples should be collected at the same time of day, between 6 and 8 a.m.
- Excessive physical activity can produce elevated levels.
- Recent radioactive scans or radiation within 1 week before the test can interfere with test results when immunoradiometric assay is the test method.
- ⚠ The metyrapone stimulation test is contraindicated in patients with suspected adrenal insufficiency.
- ⚠ Metyrapone may cause gastrointestinal distress and/or confusion. Administer oral dose of metyrapone with milk and snack.
- ⚠ Rapid clearance of metyrapone, resulting in falsely increased cortisol levels, may occur if the patient is taking drugs that enhance steroid metabolism (e.g., phenytoin, rifampin, phenobarbital, mitotane, and corticosteroids). The primary care practitioner should be consulted prior to a metyrapone stimulation test regarding a decision to withhold these medications.

Nursing Implications and Procedure • • • • • • • • • • •

➤ Inform the patient that the test is used to assess for pituitary hormone deficiency.

➤ Obtain a history of the patient's complaints, including a list of known allergens (especially allergies or sensitivities to latex), and inform the appropriate health care practitioner accordingly.

➤ Weigh patient and report weight to lab for 30 mg/kg dosing of metyrapone.

➤ Obtain a history of the patient's endocrine system and results of previously performed laboratory tests, surgical procedures, and other diagnostic procedures. For related tests, refer to the Endocrine System table.

➤ Note any recent procedures that can interfere with test results.

➤ Obtain a list of the medications the patient is taking, especially drugs that enhance steroid metabolism and include herbs, nutritional supplements, and nutraceuticals. The requesting health care practitioner and laboratory should be advised if the patient regularly uses these products so that their effects can be taken into consideration when reviewing results.

➤ Review the procedure with the patient. When ACTH hypersecretion is suspected, a second sample may be requested between 6 and 8 p.m. to determine if changes are the result of diurnal variation in ACTH levels. Inform the patient that more than one sample may be necessary to ensure accurate results and that the samples are obtained at specific times to determine high and low levels of the hormone. Inform the patient that each specimen collection takes approximately 5 to 10 minutes. Address concerns about pain related to the procedure. Explain to the patient that there may be some discomfort during the venipuncture.

➤ There are no food, fluid, or medication restrictions unless by medical direction.

➤ Drugs that enhance steroid metabolism may be withheld by medical direction prior to metyrapone stimulation testing.

➤ Instruct the patient to refrain from strenuous exercise for 12 hours before the test and to remain in bed or at rest for 1 hour immediately before the test. Avoid smoking and ETOH use.

➤ Prepare an ice slurry in a cup or plastic bag to have on hand for immediate transport of the specimen to the laboratory.

➤ Ensure that strenuous exercise was avoided for 12 hours before the test and that 1 hour of bed rest was taken immediately before the test. Samples should be collected between 6 and 8 a.m.

➤ Have emergency equipment readily available in case of adverse reaction to metyrapone.

➤ If the patient has a history of severe allergic reaction to latex, care should be taken to avoid the use of equipment containing latex.

➤ Instruct the patient to cooperate fully and to follow directions. Direct the patient to breathe normally and to avoid unnecessary movement.

➤ Observe standard precautions, and follow the general guidelines in Appendix A. Positively identify the patient, and label the appropriate tubes with the corresponding patient demographics, date, and time of collection. Perform a venipuncture; collect the specimen in a prechilled plastic heparinized syringe or in prechilled collection containers as listed under "Specimen."

➤ Adverse reactions to metyrapone include nausea and vomiting (N/V), abdominal pain, headache, dizziness, sedation, allergic rash, decreased white blood cell count, or bone marrow depression. Signs and symptoms of overdose or acute adrenocortical insuffiency include cardiac arrhythmias, hypotension, dehydration, anxiety, confusion, weakness, impairment of consciousness, N/V, epigastric pain, diarrhea, hyponatremia, and hyperkalemia.

➤ Remove the needle, place a gauze over the puncture site and apply gentle pressure. Observe venipuncture site for bleeding or hematoma formation. Apply paper tape over gauze or replace with adhesive bandage.

➤ Promptly transport the specimen to the laboratory for processing and analysis. The tightly capped sample should be placed in an ice slurry immediately after collection. Information on the specimen label can be protected from water in the ice slurry if the specimen is first placed in a protective plastic bag.

➤ The results are recorded manually or in a computerized system for recall and postprocedure interpretation by the appropriate health care practitioner.

Post-test:

➤ Instruct the patient to resume normal activity as directed by the health care practitioner.

➤ A written report of the examination will be sent to the requesting health care practitioner, who will discuss the results with the patient.

➤ Reinforce information given by the patient's health care provider regarding further testing, treatment, or referral to another health care provider. Answer any questions or address any concerns voiced by the patient or family.

➤ Depending on the results of this procedure, additional testing may be performed to evaluate or monitor progression of the disease process and determine the need for a change in therapy. If a diagnosis of Cushing's disease is made, pituitary computed tomography (CT) or magnetic resonance imaging (MRI) may be indicated prior to surgery. If a diagnosis of ectopic corticotropin syndrome is made, abdominal CT or MRI may be indicated prior to surgery. Evaluate test results in relation to the patient's symptoms and other tests performed.

Related laboratory tests:

➤ Related laboratory tests include cortisol, follicle-stimulating hormone, growth hormone, luteinizing hormone, testosterone, thyroid-stimulating hormone, and thyroxine.

ALANINE AMINOTRANSFERASE

SYNONYMS/ACRONYMS: Serum glutamic pyruvic transaminase (SGPT), ALT.

SPECIMEN: Serum (1 mL) collected in a red- or tiger-top tube. Plasma (1 mL) collected in a green-top (heparin) tube is also acceptable.

REFERENCE VALUE: (Method: Spectrophotometry)

Age	Conventional & SI Units
Newborn–1 y	13–45 U/L
2 y–adult	
Male	10–40 U/L
Female	7–35 U/L

DESCRIPTION & RATIONALE: Alanine aminotransferase (ALT), formerly known as serum glutamic pyruvic transaminase (SGPT), is an enzyme produced by the liver. It acts as a catalyst in the reversible transfer of an amino group between alanine and α-ketoglutarate. The highest concentration of ALT is found in liver cells, moderate amounts are found in kidney cells, and smaller amounts are found in heart and skeletal muscle cells. When liver damage occurs, serum levels of ALT rise to 50 times normal, making this a useful test in evaluating liver injury. ALT is also used to screen donated blood before transfusion because the enzyme may be elevated in the absence of detectable serologic markers of hepatitis. ∎

INDICATIONS:
• Compare serially with aspartate amino-transferase (AST) levels to track the course of liver disease.

• Monitor liver damage resulting from hepatotoxic drugs.

• Monitor response to treatment of liver disease, with tissue repair indicated by gradually declining levels.

• In blood banks, use as a routine screen for hepatitis in donor blood samples. Samples are rejected if levels are greater than 1.5 times the upper limits of normal.

RESULT

Increased in:
• Acute pancreatitis
• Biliary tract obstruction
• Burns (severe)
• Chronic alcohol abuse
• Cirrhosis
• Fatty liver
• Hepatic carcinoma
• Hepatitis
• Infectious mononucleosis
• Muscle injury from intramuscular injections, trauma, infection, and seizures (recent)
• Muscular dystrophy
• Myocardial infarction
• Myositis
• Pre-eclampsia
• Shock (severe)

Decreased in:
• Pyridoxal phosphate deficiency

CRITICAL VALUES: N/A

Interfering Factors
• Drugs that may increase ALT levels by causing cholestasis include amitriptyline, anabolic steroids, androgens, benzodiazepines, chlorothiazide, chlorpropamide, dapsone, erythromycin, estrogens, ethionamide, gold salts, imipramine, mercaptopurine, nitrofurans, oral contraceptives, penicillins, phenothiazines, progesterone, propoxy-

phene, sulfonamides, tamoxifen, and tolbutamide.

- Drugs that may increase ALT levels by causing hepatocellular damage include acetaminophen (toxic), acetylsalicylic acid, allopurinol, amiodarone, anabolic steroids, anticonvulsants, asparaginase, azithromycin, bromocriptine, captopril, cephalosporins, chloramphenicol, clindamycin, clofibrate, danazol, enflurane, ethambutol, ethionamide, fenofibrate, fluconazole, fluoroquinolones, foscarnet, gentamicin, indomethacin, interferon, interleukin-2, levamisole, levodopa, lincomycin, low-molecular-weight heparin, methyldopa, monoamine oxidase inhibitors, naproxen, nifedipine, nitrofurans, oral contraceptives, probenecid, procainamide, quinine, ranitidine, retinol, ritodrine, sulfonylureas, tetracyclines, tobramycin, and verapamil.

- Drugs that may decrease ALT levels include cyclosporine and interferon.

Nursing Implications and Procedure • • • • • • • • • • •

Pretest:

➤ Inform the patient that the test is used to assess liver function.

➤ Obtain a history of the patient's complaints, including a list of known allergens (especially allergies or sensitivities to latex), and inform the appropriate health care practitioner accordingly.

➤ Obtain a history of the patient's hepatobiliary system and results of previously performed laboratory tests, surgical procedures, and other diagnostic procedures. For related laboratory tests, refer to the Hepatobiliary System table.

➤ Obtain a list of the medications the patient is taking, including herbs, nutritional supplements, and nutraceuticals. The requesting health care practitioner and laboratory should be advised if the patient regularly uses

these products so that their effects can be taken into consideration when reviewing results.

➤ Review the procedure with the patient. Inform the patient that specimen collection takes approximately 5 to 10 minutes. Address concerns about pain related to the procedure. Explain to the patient that there may be some discomfort during the venipuncture.

➤ There are no food, fluid, or medication restrictions unless by medical direction.

Intratest:

➤ If the patient has a history of severe allergic reaction to latex, care should be taken to avoid the use of equipment containing latex.

➤ Instruct the patient to cooperate fully and to follow directions. Direct the patient to breathe normally and to avoid unnecessary movement.

➤ Observe standard precautions, and follow the general guidelines in Appendix A. Positively identify the patient, and label the appropriate tubes with the corresponding patient demographics, date, and time of collection. Perform a venipuncture; collect the specimen in a 5-mL red- or tiger-top tube.

➤ Remove the needle, place a gauze over the puncture site and apply gentle pressure to stop bleeding. Observe venipuncture site for bleeding and hematoma formation. Apply paper tape over gauze or replace with adhesive bandage.

➤ Promptly transport the specimen to the laboratory for processing and analysis.

➤ The results are recorded manually or in a computerized system for recall and postprocedure interpretation by the appropriate health care practitioner.

Post-test:

➤ Instruct the patient to resume usual diet, fluids, medications, or activity, as directed by the health care practitioner.

➤ *Nutritional considerations:* Increased ALT levels may be associated with liver disease. Dietary recommendations may be indicated and vary depending on the severity of the condition. A low-protein diet may be in order if the patient's liver has lost the ability to process the end products of protein metabolism. A diet of soft foods may be required if esophageal varices have developed. Ammonia levels may be used to determine whether protein should be added to or reduced from the diet. Patients should be encouraged to eat simple carbohydrates and emulsified fats (as in homogenized milk or eggs), as opposed to complex carbohydrates (e.g., starch, fiber, and glycogen [animal carbohydrates]) and complex fats, which would require additional bile to emulsify them so that they can be used. The cirrhotic patient should be carefully observed for the development of ascites, in which case fluid and electrolyte balance requires strict attention.

➤ A written report of the examination will be sent to the requesting health care practitioner, who will discuss the results with the patient.

➤ Reinforce information given by the patient's health care provider regarding further testing, treatment, or referral to another health care provider. Answer any questions or address any concerns voiced by the patient or family.

➤ Depending on the results of this procedure, additional testing may be performed to evaluate or monitor progression of the disease process and determine the need for a change in therapy. Evaluate test results in relation to the patient's symptoms and other tests performed.

Related laboratory tests:

➤ Related laboratory tests include acetaminophen, ammonia, AST, bilirubin, electrolytes, γ-glutamyl transpeptidase, hepatitis antigens and antibodies, lactate dehydrogenase, and liver biopsy.

ALBUMIN AND ALBUMIN/ GLOBULIN RATIO

SYNONYM/ACRONYM: Alb, A/G ratio.

SPECIMEN: Serum (1 mL) collected in a red- or tiger-top tube. Plasma (1 mL) collected in a green-top (heparin) tube is also acceptable.

REFERENCE VALUE: (Method: Spectrophotometry) Normally the albumin/globulin (A/G) ratio is greater than 1.

Age	Conventional Units	SI Units (Conventional Units × 10)
Newborn–4 d	2.8–4.4 g/dL	28–44 g/L
5 d–14 y	3.8–5.4 g/dL	38–54 g/L
15–18 y	3.2–4.5 g/dL	32–45 g/L
19–60 y	3.4–4.8 g/dL	34–48 g/L
61–90 y	3.2–4.6 g/dL	32–46 g/L
Greater than 90 y	2.9–4.5 g/dL	29–45 g/L

DESCRIPTION & RATIONALE: Most of the body's total protein is a combination of albumin and globulins. Albumin, the protein present in the highest concentrations, is the main transport protein in the body. Albumin also maintains plasma oncotic pressure. Serum albumin values are affected by the process of synthesis, distribution, and degradation. Low levels may be the result of either inadequate production or excessive loss. Albumin levels are more useful as an indicator of chronic deficiency than of short-term deficiency.

Albumin levels are affected by posture. Results from specimens collected in an upright posture are higher than results from specimens collected in a supine position.

The A/G ratio is useful in the evaluation of liver and kidney disease. The ratio is calculated using the following formula:

albumin/(total protein – albumin)

where globulin is the difference between the total protein value and the albumin value. For example, with a total protein of 7 g/dL and albumin of 4 g/dL, the A/G ratio is calculated as $4/(7 - 4)$ or $4/3 = 1.33$. A reversal in the ratio, where globulin exceeds albumin (i.e., ratio less than 1.0), is clinically significant. ■

INDICATIONS:

- Assess nutritional status of hospitalized patients, especially geriatric patients
- Evaluate chronic illness
- Evaluate liver disease

RESULT

Increased in:

- Any condition that results in a decrease of plasma water (e.g., dehydration); look for increase in hemoglobin and hematocrit
- Hyperinfusion of albumin

Decreased in:

- Insufficient intake:
  Malabsorption
  Malnutrition

- Decreased synthesis by the liver:
  Acute and chronic liver disease (e.g., alcoholism, cirrhosis, hepatitis)
  Genetic analbuminemia

- Inflammation and chronic diseases:
  Amyloidosis
  Bacterial infections
  Monoclonal gammopathies (e.g., multiple myeloma, Waldenström's macroglobulinemia)
  Neoplasm
  Parasitic infestations

Peptic ulcer
Prolonged immobilization
Rheumatic diseases
Severe skin disease

- Increased loss over body surface:
Burns
Enteropathies related to sensitivity
to ingested substances (e.g.,
gluten sensitivity, Crohn's
disease, ulcerative colitis)
Fistula (gastrointestinal or
lymphatic)
Hemorrhage
Kidney disease
Rapid hydration or overhydration
Repeated thoracentesis or
paracentesis
Trauma and crush injuries

- Increased catabolism:
Fever
Cushing's disease
Pre-eclampsia
Thyroid dysfunction

- Increased blood volume (hypervolemia):
Congestive heart failure
Monoclonal gammopathies
(Waldenström's disease,
myeloma)
Pregnancy

CRITICAL VALUES: N/A

INTERFERING FACTORS:

- Drugs that may increase albumin levels include enalapril.

- Drugs that may decrease albumin levels include acetaminophen (poisoning), dapsone, dextran, estrogens, ibuprofen, nitrofurantoin, oral contraceptives, phenytoin, prednisone (high doses), trazodone, and valproic acid.

- Availability of administered drugs is affected by variations in albumin levels.

Nursing Implications and Procedure

Pretest:

➤ Inform the patient that the test is used as a general indicator of nutritional status, hydration, and chronic disease.

➤ Obtain a history of the patient's complaints, including a list of known allergens (especially allergies or sensitivities to latex), and inform the appropriate health care practitioner accordingly.

➤ Obtain a history of the patient's gastrointestinal, genitourinary, and hepatobiliary systems and results of previously performed laboratory tests, surgical procedures, and other diagnostic procedures. For related tests, refer to the Gastrointestinal, Genitourinary, and Hepatobiliary System and Therapeutic/Toxicology tables.

➤ Obtain a list of the medications the patient is taking, including herbs, nutritional supplements, and nutraceuticals. The requesting health care practitioner and laboratory should be advised if the patient regularly uses these products so that their effects can be taken into consideration when reviewing results.

➤ Review the procedure with the patient..Inform the patient that specimen collection takes approximately 5 to 10 minutes. Address concerns about pain related to the procedure. Explain to the patient that there may be some discomfort during the venipuncture.

➤ There are no food, fluid, or medication restrictions unless by medical direction.

Intratest:

➤ If the patient has a history of severe allergic reaction to latex, care should be taken to avoid the use of equipment containing latex.

➤ Instruct the patient to cooperate fully and to follow directions.Direct the patient to breathe normally and to avoid unnecessary movement.

➤ Observe standard precautions, and follow the general guidelines in Appendix A. Positively identify the patient, and label the appropriate tubes with the corresponding patient demographics, date, and time of collection. Perform a venipuncture; collect the specimen in a 5-mL red- or tiger-top tube.

➤ Remove the needle, place a gauze over the puncture site and apply gentle pressure to stop bleeding. Observe venipuncture site for bleeding or hematoma formation. Apply paper tape over gauze or replace with adhesive bandage.

➤ Promptly transport the specimen to the laboratory for processing and analysis.

➤ The results are recorded manually or in a computerized system for recall and postprocedure interpretation by the appropriate health care practitioner.

Post-test:

➤ *Nutritional considerations:* Dietary recommendations may be indicated and vary depending on the severity of the condition. Ammonia levels may be used to determine whether protein should be added to or reduced from the diet.

➤ A written report of the examination will be sent to the requesting health care practitioner, who will discuss the results with the patient.

➤ Reinforce information given by the patient's health care provider regarding further testing, treatment, or referral to another health care provider. Answer any questions or address any concerns voiced by the patient or family.

➤ Depending on the results of this procedure, additional testing may be performed to evaluate or monitor progression of the disease process and determine the need for a change in therapy. Evaluate test results in relation to the patient's symptoms and other tests performed.

Related laboratory tests:

➤ Related laboratory tests include alanine aminotransferase, alkaline phosphatase, ammonia, anti-aspartate aminotransferase, bilirubin, electrolytes, γ-glutamyl transpeptidase, hematocrit, hemoglobin, hepatitis antibodies and antigens, liver biopsy, osmolality, prealbumin, protein, protein electrophoresis, and smooth muscle antibody.

ALDOLASE

· ·

Synonym/Acronym: ALD.

Specimen: Serum (1 mL) collected in a red- or tiger-top tube.

Reference value: (Method: Spectrophotometry)

Age	Conventional & SI Units
Newborn–2 y	3.4–11.8 U/L
25 m–16 y	1.2–8.8 U/L
Adult	Less than 7.4 U/L

DESCRIPTION & RATIONALE:

Aldolase (ALD), an enzyme found throughout the body, catalyzes the breakdown of glucose to lactate. Highest concentrations of this enzyme are found in skeletal and cardiac muscle, liver, and pancreas. When trauma or disease causes cellular breakdown of these muscles or organs, large amounts of ALD are released into the blood. Measuring serum levels helps to determine the presence, and in some cases the progress, of disease. This test is not commonly requested because the assay of other liver enzymes and creatine kinase is generally sufficient to provide the necessary information. ■

INDICATIONS:

- Assist in the diagnosis of Duchenne's muscular dystrophy
- Differentiate neuromuscular disorders from neurologic disorders, such as multiple sclerosis or myasthenia gravis

RESULT

Increased in:

- Carcinoma (lung, breast, and genitourinary tract, and metastasis to liver)
- Central nervous system tumors
- Delirium tremens
- Dermatomyositis
- Duchenne's muscular dystrophy
- Gangrene
- Hemolytic anemias
- Hepatitis (acute viral or toxic)
- Infectious mononucleosis
- Leukemia (granulocytic and megaloblastic)
- Limb girdle muscular dystrophy
- Myocardial infarction
- Pancreatitis (acute)
- Polymyositis
- Psychoses and schizophrenia (acute)
- Severe crush injuries
- Tetanus
- Trichinosis

Decreased in:

- Hereditary fructose intolerance

CRITICAL VALUES: N/A

INTERFERING FACTORS:

- Drugs that may increase aldolase levels include aminocaproic acid, carbenoxolone, chlorinated and organophosphorus insecticides, clofibrate, labetalol, and thiabendazole.
- Drugs that may decrease aldolase levels include phenothiazines (in schizophrenic patients with high initial values) and probucol.
- Intramuscular injections may increase aldolase levels as a result of muscle trauma.
- Red blood cells contain aldolase; hemolysis may cause a false elevation in values.

Nursing Implications and Procedure . . . .

Pretest:

➤ Inform the patient that the test is used to assess general liver, pancreatic, and musculoskeletal function.

Obtain a history of the patient's complaints, including a list of known allergens (especially allergies or sensitivities to latex), and inform the appropriate health care practitioner accordingly.

Obtain a history of neuromuscular disorders, related treatments, and complaints of muscle fatigue or loss of strength.

Obtain a history of the patient's hepatobiliary and musculoskeletal system and results of previously performed laboratory tests, surgical procedures, and other diagnostic procedures. For related laboratory tests, refer to the Hepatobiliary and Musculoskeletal System tables.

Obtain a list of the medications the patient is taking, including herbs, nutritional supplements, and nutraceuticals. The requesting health care practitioner and laboratory should be advised if the patient regularly uses these products so that their effects can be taken into consideration when reviewing results.

Review the procedure with the patient. Inform the patient that specimen collection takes approximately 5 to 10 minutes. Address concerns about pain related to the procedure. Explain to the patient that there may be some discomfort during the venipuncture.

There are no food, fluid, or medication restrictions unless by medical direction.

Intratest:

If the patient has a history of severe allergic reaction to latex, care should be taken to avoid the use of equipment containing latex.

Instruct the patient to cooperate fully and to follow directions. Direct the patient to breathe normally and to avoid unnecessary movement.

Observe standard precautions, and follow the general guidelines in Appendix A. Positively identify the patient, and label the appropriate tubes with the corresponding patient demographics, date, and time of collection. Perform a venipuncture; collect the specimen in a 5-mL red- or tiger-top tube.

Remove the needle, place a gauze over the puncture site and apply gentle pressure to stop bleeding. Observe venipuncture site for bleeding or hematoma formation. Apply paper tape over gauze or replace with adhesive bandage.

Promptly transport the specimen to the laboratory for processing and analysis.

The results are recorded manually or in a computerized system for recall and postprocedure interpretation by the appropriate health care practitioner.

Post-test:

A written report of the examination will be sent to the requesting health care practitioner, who will discuss the results with the patient.

Reinforce information given by the patient's health care provider regarding further testing, treatment, or referral to another health care provider. Answer any questions or address any concerns voiced by the patient or family.

Depending on the results of this procedure, additional testing may be performed to evaluate or monitor progression of the disease process and determine the need for a change in therapy. Evaluate test results in relation to the patient's symptoms and other tests performed.

Related laboratory tests:

Related laboratory tests include alkaline phosphatase, antimitochondrial antibody, aspartate aminotransferase, creatine kinase and isoenzymes, Jo-1 antibody, lactate dehydrogenase and isoenzymes, liver biopsy, muscle biopsy, and myoglobin.

ALDOSTERONE

SYNONYM/ACRONYM: N/A.

SPECIMEN: Serum (1 mL) collected in a red- or tiger-top tube. Plasma (1 mL) collected in green-top (heparin) or lavender-top (EDTA) tube is also acceptable.

REFERENCE VALUE: (Method: Radioimmunoassay)

Age	Conventional Units	SI Units (Conventional Units × 0.0277)
Cord blood	40–200 ng/dL	1.11–5.54 nmol/L
3 d–1 wk	7–184 ng/dL	0.19–5.10 nmol/L
1 mo–1 y	5–90 ng/dL	0.14–2.49 nmol/L
13–23 mo	7–54 ng/dL	0.19–1.50 nmol/L
2–10 y		
Supine	3–35 ng/dL	0.08–0.97 nmol/L
Upright	5–80 ng/dL	0.14–2.22 nmol/L
11–15 y		
Supine	2–22 ng/dL	0.06–0.61 nmol/L
Upright	4–48 ng/dL	0.11–1.33 nmol/L
Adult		
Supine	3–16 ng/dL	0.08–0.44 nmol/L
Upright	7–30 ng/dL	0.19–0.83 nmol/L

These values reflect a normal-sodium diet. Values for a low-sodium diet are three to five times higher.

DESCRIPTION & RATIONALE: Aldosterone is a mineralocorticoid secreted by the zona glomerulosa of the adrenal cortex in response to decreased serum sodium, decreased blood volume, and increased serum potassium. Aldosterone increases sodium reabsorption in the renal tubules, resulting in potassium excretion and increased water retention, blood volume, and blood pressure. A variety of factors influence serum aldosterone levels, including sodium intake, certain medications, and activity. This test is of little diagnostic value unless plasma renin activity is measured simultaneously (see monograph titled "Renin"). Patients with serum potassium less than 3.6 mEq/L and 24-hour urine potassium greater than 40 mEq/L fit the general criteria to test for aldosteronism. Renin is low in primary aldosteronism and high in secondary aldosteronism. A ratio of plasma aldosterone to plasma renin activity greater than 50 is significant. ∎

INDICATIONS:

- Evaluate hypertension of unknown cause, especially with hypokalemia not induced by diuretics
- Investigate suspected hyperaldosteronism, as indicated by elevated levels
- Investigate suspected hypoaldosteronism, as indicated by decreased levels

RESULT

Increased with Decreased Renin Levels

Primary hyperaldosteronism:
- Adenomas (Conn's syndrome)
- Bilateral hyperplasia of the aldosterone-secreting zona glomerulosa cells

Increased with Increased Renin Levels

Secondary hyperaldosteronism:
- Bartter's syndrome
- Cardiac failure
- Chronic obstructive pulmonary disease
- Cirrhosis with ascites formation
- Diuretic abuse
- Hypovolemia secondary to hemorrhage and transudation
- Laxative abuse
- Nephrotic syndrome
- Starvation (after 10 days)
- Thermal stress
- Toxemia of pregnancy

Decreased

Without hypertension:
- Addison's disease

- Hypoaldosteronism secondary to renin deficiency
- Isolated aldosterone deficiency

With hypertension:
- Acute alcohol intoxication
- Diabetes
- Excess secretion of deoxycorticosterone
- Turner's syndrome (25% of cases)

CRITICAL VALUES: N/A

INTERFERING FACTORS:

- Drugs that may increase aldosterone levels include amiloride, ammonium chloride, angiotensin, angiotensin II, dobutamine, dopamine, endralazine, fenoldopam, hydralazine, hydrochlorothiazide, laxatives (abuse), metoclopramide, nifedipine, opiates, potassium, spironolactone, and zacopride.

- Drugs that may decrease aldosterone levels include atenolol, captopril, carvedilol, cilazapril, enalapril, fadrozole, glycyrrhiza, ibopamine, indomethacin, lisinopril, nicardipine, nonsteroidal anti-inflammatory drugs, perindopril, ranitidine, saline, sinorphan, and verapamil. Prolonged heparin therapy also decreases aldosterone levels.

- Upright body posture, stress, strenuous exercise, and late pregnancy can lead to increased levels.

- Recent radioactive scans or radiation within 1 week before the test can interfere with test results when radioimmunoassay is the test method.

- Diet can significantly affect results. A low-sodium diet can increase serum aldosterone, whereas a high-sodium diet can decrease levels. Decreased serum sodium and elevated serum potassium increase aldosterone secretion. Elevated serum sodium and decreased serum potassium suppress aldosterone secretion.

Nursing Implications and Procedure • • • • • • • • • • •

Pretest:

▶ Inform the patient that the test is used to evaluate hypertension and possible hyperaldosteronism.

▶ Obtain a history of the patient's complaints, including a list of known allergens (especially allergies or sensitivities to latex), and inform the appropriate health care practitioner accordingly.

▶ Obtain a history of known or suspected fluid or electrolyte imbalance, hypertension, renal function, or stage of pregnancy. Note the amount of sodium ingested in the diet over the past 2 weeks.

▶ Obtain a history of the patient's endocrine and genitourinary systems and results of previously performed laboratory tests, surgical procedures, and other diagnostic procedures. For related laboratory tests, refer to the Endocrine and Genitourinary System tables.

▶ Note any recent procedures that can interfere with test results.

▶ Obtain a list of the medications the patient is taking, including herbs, nutritional supplements, and nutraceuticals. The requesting health care practitioner and laboratory should be advised if the patient is regularly using these products so that their effects can be taken into consideration when reviewing results.

▶ Review the procedure with the patient. Inform the patient that specimen collection takes approximately 5 to 10 minutes. Inform the patient that multiple specimens may be required. Address concerns about pain related to the procedure. Explain to the patient that there may be some discomfort during the venipuncture.

▶ Inform the patient that the required position, supine/lying down or upright/sitting up, must be maintained for 2 hours before specimen collection.

▶ The patient should be on a normal-sodium diet (1 to 2 g of sodium per day) for 2 to 4 weeks before the test.

▶ Under medical direction, the patient should avoid diuretics, antihypertensive drugs and herbals, and cyclic progestogens and estrogens for 2 to 4 weeks before the test.

Intratest:

▶ Ensure that the patient has complied with dietary, medication, and pretesting preparations regarding activity.

▶ If the patient has a history of severe allergic reaction to latex, care should be taken to avoid the use of equipment containing latex.

▶ Instruct the patient to cooperate fully and to follow directions. Direct the patient to breathe normally and to avoid unnecessary movement.

▶ Observe standard precautions, and follow the general guidelines in Appendix A. Positively identify the patient, and label the appropriate tubes with the corresponding patient demographics, date, time of collection, patient position (upright or supine), and exact source of specimen (peripheral versus arterial). Perform a venipuncture after the patient has been in the upright (sitting or standing) position for 2 hours. If a supine specimen is requested on an inpatient, the specimen should be collected early in the morning before rising. Collect the specimen in a 5-mL red- or tiger-top tube.

▶ Remove the needle, place gauze over the puncture site and apply gentle pressure to stop bleeding. Observe venipuncture site for bleeding or hematoma formation. Apply paper tape over gauze or replace with adhesive bandage.

▶ Promptly transport the specimen on ice to the laboratory for processing and analysis.

▶ The results are recorded manually or in a computerized system for recall

and postprocedure interpretation by the appropriate health care practitioner.

Post-test:

> Instruct the patient to resume usual diet, medication, and activity as directed by the health care practitioner.

> A written report of the examination will be sent to the requesting health care practitioner, who will discuss the results with the patient.

> Instruct the patient to notify the health care practitioner of any signs and symptoms of dehydration or fluid overload related to elevated aldosterone levels or compromised sodium regulatory mechanisms.

> *Nutritional considerations:* Aldosterone levels are involved in the regulation of body fluid volume. Educate patients about the importance of proper water balance. Although there is no recommended dietary allowance (RDA) for water, adults need 1 mL/kcal per day. Infants need more water because their basal metabolic heat production is much higher than in adults. Tap water may also contain other nutrients. Water-softening systems replace minerals (e.g., calcium, magnesium, iron) with sodium, so caution should be used if a low-sodium diet is prescribed.

> *Nutritional considerations:* Because aldosterone levels have an effect on sodium levels, some consideration may be given to dietary adjustment if sodium allowances need to be regulated. Educate patients with low sodium levels that the major source of dietary sodium is table salt. Many foods, such as milk and other dairy products, are also good sources of dietary sodium. Most other dietary sodium is available through consumption of processed foods. Patients who need to follow low-sodium diets should avoid beverages such as colas, ginger ale, Gatorade, lemon-lime sodas, and root beer. Many over-the-counter medications, including antacids, laxatives, analgesics, sedatives, and antitussives, contain significant amounts of sodium. The best advice is to emphasize the importance of reading all food, beverage, and medicine labels. In 1989, the Subcommittee on the 10th Edition of the RDAs established 500 mg as the recommended minimum limit for dietary intake of sodium. There are no RDAs established for potassium, but the estimated minimum intake for adults is 200 mEq/d. Potassium is present in all plant and animal cells, making dietary replacement simple. A health care practitioner or nutritionist should be consulted before considering the use of salt substitutes.

> Reinforce information given by the patient's health care provider regarding further testing, treatment, or referral to another health care provider. Answer any questions or address any concerns voiced by the patient or family.

> Depending on the results of this procedure, additional testing may be performed to evaluate or monitor progression of the disease process and determine the need for a change in therapy. Evaluate test results in relation to the patient's symptoms and other tests performed.

Related laboratory tests:

> Related laboratory tests include catecholamines (blood and urine), cortisol, creatinine (blood and urine), glucose, kidney biopsy, magnesium (blood and urine), osmolality (blood and urine), potassium (blood and urine), renin, sodium (blood and urine), urea nitrogen, urinalysis, and urine protein.

ALKALINE PHOSPHATASE AND ISOENZYMES

SYNONYMS/ACRONYM: Alk Phos, ALP and fractionation, heat-stabile ALP.

SPECIMEN: Serum (1 mL) collected in a red- or tiger-top tube. Plasma (1 mL) collected in a green-top (heparin) tube is also acceptable.

REFERENCE VALUE: (Method: Spectrophotometry for total alkaline phosphatase, inhibition/electrophoresis for fractionation)

Total ALP	Conventional & SI Units	Bone Fraction	Liver Fraction
1–5 y			
Male	56–350 U/L	39–308 U/L	Less than 8–101 U/L
Female	73–378 U/L	56–300 U/L	Less than 8–53 U/L
6–7 y			
Male	70–364 U/L	50–319 U/L	Less than 8–76 U/L
Female	73–378 U/L	56–300 U/L	Less than 8–53 U/L
8 y			
Male	70–364 U/L	50–258 U/L	Less than 8–62 U/L
Female	98–448 U/L	78–353 U/L	Less than 8–62 U/L
9–12 y			
Male	112–476 U/L	78–339 U/L	Less than 8–81 U/L
Female	98–448 U/L	78–353 U/L	Less than 8–62 U/L
13 y			
Male	112–476 U/L	78–389 U/L	Less than 8–48 U/L
Female	56–350 U/L	28–252 U/L	Less than 8–50 U/L
14 y			
Male	112–476 U/L	78–389 U/L	Less than 8–48 U/L
Female	56–266 U/L	31–190 U/L	Less than 8–48 U/L
15 y			
Male	70–378 U/L	48–311 U/L	Less than 8–39 U/L
Female	42–168 U/L	20–115 U/L	Less than 8–53 U/L
16 y			
Male	70–378 U/L	48–311 U/L	Less than 8–39 U/L
Female	28–126 U/L	14–87 U/L	Less than 8–50 U/L
17 y			
Male	56–238 U/L	34–190 U/L	Less than 8–39 U/L
Female	28–126 U/L	17–84 U/L	Less than 8–53 U/L

Total ALP	Conventional & SI Units	Bone Fraction	Liver Fraction
18 y			
Male	56–182 U/L	34–146 U/L	Less than 8–39 U/L
Female	28–126 U/L	17–84 U/L	Less than 8–53 U/L
19 y			
Male	42–154 U/L	25–123 U/L	Less than 8–39 U/L
Female	28–126 U/L	17–84 U/L	Less than 8–53 U/L
20 y			
Male	45–138 U/L	25–73 U/L	Less than 8–48 U/L
Female	33–118 U/L	17–56 U/L	Less than 8–50 U/L
Adult			
Male	35–142 U/L	11–73 U/L	0–93 U/L
Female	25–125 U/L	11–73 U/L	0–93 U/L

DESCRIPTION & RATIONALE: ALP is an enzyme found in the liver, in Kupffer cells lining the biliary tract, and in bones, intestines, and placenta. Additional sources of ALP include the proximal tubules of the kidneys, pulmonary alveolar cells, germ cells, vascular bed, lactating mammary glands, and granulocytes of circulating blood. ALP is referred to as alkaline because it functions optimally at a pH of 9.0. This test is most useful for determining the presence of liver or bone disease.

Isoelectric focusing methods can identify 12 isoenzymes of ALP. Certain cancers produce small amounts of distinctive Regan and Nagao ALP isoenzymes. Four main ALP isoenzymes, however, are of clinical significance: ALP_1 of liver origin, ALP_2 of bone origin, ALP_3 of intestinal origin (occasionally present in individuals with blood type O and B), and ALP_4 of placental origin (third trimester). ALP levels vary by age and gender. Values in children are higher than in adults because of the level of bone growth and development. An immunoassay method is available for measuring bone specific ALP as an indicator of increased bone turnover and estrogen deficiency in post-menopausal women. ∎

INDICATIONS:

- Evaluate signs and symptoms of various disorders associated with elevated ALP levels, such as biliary obstruction, hepatobiliary disease, and bone disease, including malignant processes

- Differentiate obstructive hepatobiliary tract disorders from hepatocellular disease; greater elevations of ALP are seen in the former

- Determine effects of renal disease on bone metabolism

- Determine bone growth or destruction in children with abnormal growth patterns

RESULT

Increased in:
- Liver disease:
  Biliary atresia
  Biliary obstruction (acute cholecystitis, cholelithisis, intrahepatic cholestasis of pregnancy, primary biliary cirrhosis)
  Cancer
  Chronic active hepatitis
  Cirrhosis
  Diabetes (diabetic hepatic lipidosis)
  Extrahepatic duct obstruction
  Granulomatous or infiltrative liver diseases
  Infectious mononucleosis
  Intrahepatic biliary hypoplasia
  Toxic hepatitis
  Viral hepatitis

- Bone disease:
  Healing fractures
  Metabolic bone diseases (rickets, osteomalacia)
  Metastatic tumors in bone
  Osteogenic sarcoma
  Osteoporosis
  Paget's disease (osteitis deformans)
  Parasitic infections (histoplasmosis, leptospirosis, malaria, schistosomiasis)

- Other conditions:
  Adrenal cortical hyperfunction
  Advanced pregnancy
  Amyloidosis
  Atherosclerosis
  Cancer of the breast, colon, gallbladder, lung, or pancreas
  Cancer of the lung or pancreas
  Chronic renal failure
  Congestive heart failure
  Familial hyperphosphatemia
  Galactosemia
  Hodgkin's disease
  Hyperparathyroidism (primary or secondary to chronic renal disease)
  Perforated bowel
  Pneumonia
  Pulmonary and myocardial infarctions
  Pulmonary embolism
  Sarcoidosis
  Ulcerative colitis

Decreased in:
- Anemia (severe)
- Celiac disease
- Cretinism
- Folic acid deficiency
- HIV-1 infection
- Hypervitaminosis D
- Hypophosphatasia (congenital, rare)
- Hypothyroidism (characteristic in infantile and juvenile cases)
- Milk alkali syndrome
- Kwashiorkor
- Nutritional deficiency of zinc or magnesium
- Pernicious anemia
- Scurvy
- Vitamin C deficiency
- Whipple's disease (indication of vitamin D and calcium malabsorption)
- Zollinger-Ellison syndrome (indication of vitamin D and calcium malabsorption)

CRITICAL VALUES: N/A

INTERFERING FACTORS:
- Drugs that may increase ALP levels by causing cholestasis include amitripty-

line, anabolic steroids, androgens, benzodiazepines, chlorothiazide, chlorpropamide, dapsone, erythromycin, estrogens, ethionamide, gold salts, imipramine, mercaptopurine, nitrofurans, oral contraceptives, penicillins, phenothiazines, progesterone, propoxyphene, sulfonamides, tamoxifen, and tolbutamide.

• Drugs that may increase ALP levels by causing hepatocellular damage include acetaminophen (toxic), acetylsalicylic acid, allopurinol, amiodarone, anabolic steroids, anticonvulsants, asparaginase, azithromycin, bromocriptine, captopril, cephalosporins, chloramphenicol, clindamycin, clofibrate, danazol, enflurane, ethambutol, ethionamide, fenofibrate, fluconazole, fluoroquinolones, foscarnet, gentamicin, indomethacin, interferon, interleukin-2, levamisole, levodopa, lincomycin, low-molecular-weight heparin, methyldopa, monoamine oxidase inhibitors, naproxen, nifedipine, nitrofurans, oral contraceptives, probenecid, procainamide, quinine, ranitidine, retinol, ritodrine, sulfonylureas, tetracyclines, tobramycin, and verapamil.

• Drugs that may cause an overall decrease in ALP levels include alendrolate, clofibrate, and theophylline.

• Hemolyzed specimens may cause falsely elevated results.

• Elevations of ALP may occur if the patient is nonfasting, usually 2 to 4 h after a fatty meal, and especially if the patient is a Lewis-positive secretor of blood group B or O.

Nursing Implications and Procedure • • • • • • • • • • • •

Pretest: ▮

➤ Inform the patient that the test is used to assess liver function.

➤ Obtain a history of the patient's com-

plaints, including a list of known allergens (especially allergies or sensitivities to latex), and inform the appropriate health care practitioner accordingly.

➤ Obtain a history of the patient's hepatobiliary and musculoskeletal systems and results of previously performed laboratory tests, surgical procedures, and other diagnostic procedures. For related tests, refer to the Hepatobiliary and Musculoskeletal System tables.

➤ Obtain a list of the medications the patient is taking, including herbs, nutritional supplements, and nutraceuticals. The requesting health care practitioner and laboratory should be advised if the patient is regularly using these products so that their effects can be taken into consideration when reviewing results.

➤ Review the procedure with the patient. Inform the patient that specimen collection takes approximately 5 to 10 minutes. Address concerns about pain related to the procedure. Explain to the patient that there may be some discomfort during the venipuncture.

➤ There are no food, fluid, or medication restrictions unless by medical direction.

Intratest: ▮

➤ If the patient has a history of severe allergic reaction to latex, care should be taken to avoid the use of equipment containing latex.

➤ Instruct the patient to cooperate fully and to follow directions. Direct the patient to breathe normally and to avoid unnecessary movement.

➤ Observe standard precautions, and follow the general guidelines in Appendix A. Positively identify the patient, and label the appropriate tubes with the corresponding patient demographics, date, and time of collection. Perform a venipuncture; collect the specimen in a 5-mL red- or tiger-top tube.

➤ Remove the needle, place a gauze over the puncture site and apply gentle pressure to stop bleeding. Observe venipuncture site for bleeding and hematoma formation. Apply paper tape over gauze or replace with adhesive bandage.

➤ Promptly transport the specimen to the laboratory for processing and analysis.

➤ The results are recorded manually or in a computerized system for recall and postprocedure interpretation by the appropriate health care practitioner.

Post-test:

➤ *Nutritional considerations:* Increased ALP levels may be associated with liver disease. Dietary recommendations may be indicated and vary depending on the severity of the condition. A low-protein diet may be in order if the patient's liver has lost the ability to process the end products of protein metabolism. A diet of soft foods may be required if esophageal varices have developed. Ammonia levels may be used to determine whether protein should be added to or reduced from the diet. Patients should be encouraged to eat simple carbohydrates and emulsified fats (as in homogenized milk or eggs), as opposed to complex carbohydrates (e.g., starch, fiber, and glycogen [animal carbohydrates]) and complex fats, which would require additional bile to emulsify them so that they can be used. The cirrhotic patient should be carefully observed for the development of ascites, in which case fluid and electrolyte balance requires strict attention.

➤ A written report of the examination will be sent to the requesting health care practitioner, who will discuss the results with the patient.

➤ Reinforce information given by the patient's health care provider regarding further testing, treatment, or referral to another health care provider. Answer any questions or address any concerns voiced by the patient or family.

➤ Depending on the results of this procedure, additional testing may be performed to evaluate or monitor progression of the disease process and determine the need for a change in therapy. Evaluate test results in relation to the patient's symptoms and other tests performed.

Related laboratory tests:

➤ Related laboratory tests include acetaminophen, alanine aminotransferase, albumin, ammonia, anti-DNA antibodies, antimitochondrial antibodies, antinuclear antibodies, anti–smooth muscle antibodies, α_1-antitrypsin, α_1-antitrypsin phenotyping, aspartate aminotransferase, bilirubin (total, direct, and indirect), bone biopsy, calcium, ceruloplasmin, C3 complement, C4 complement, copper, electrolytes, γ-glutamyl transpeptidase, hepatitis antigens and antibodies, liver biopsy, magnesium, parathyroid hormone, phosphorus, protein, protein electrophoresis, prothrombin time, salicylate, vitamin D, and zinc.

ALLERGEN-SPECIFIC IMMUNOGLOBULIN E
· ·

SYNONYMS/ACRONYM: Allergen profile, radioallergosorbent test (RAST).

SPECIMEN: Serum (2 mL per group of six allergens, 0.5 mL for each additional individual allergen) collected in a red- or tiger-top tube.

REFERENCE VALUE: (Method: Radioimmunoassay)

RAST Scoring Method		Alternate Scoring Method (ASM): Increasing Levels of Allergy Sensitivity	
Specific IgE Antibody Level	kIU/L	ASM Class	ASM % Reference
Absent or undetectable	Less than 0.35	0	Less than 70
Low	0.35–0.70	1	70–109
Moderate	0.71–3.50	2	110–219
High	3.51–17.50	3	220–599
Very high	Greater than 17.50	4	600–1999
		5	2000–5999
		6	Greater than 5999

DESCRIPTION & RATIONALE: Allergen-specific immunoglobulin E (IgE) or a radioallergosorbent test (RAST) is generally requested for groups of allergens commonly known to incite an allergic response in the affected individual. The test is based on the use of a radiolabeled anti-IgE reagent to detect IgE in the patient's serum, produced in response to specific allergens. The panels include allergens such as animal dander, antibiotics, dust, foods, grasses, insects, trees, mites, molds, venom, and weeds. Allergen testing is useful for evaluating the cause of hay fever, extrinsic asthma, atopic eczema, respiratory allergies, and potentially fatal reactions to insect venom, penicillin, and other drugs or chemicals. RAST has largely replaced skin tests and provocation procedures, which were inconvenient, painful, and potentially hazardous to patients. ■

INDICATIONS:

- Evaluate patients who refuse to submit to skin testing or who have generalized dermatitis or other dermatopathic conditions
- Monitor response to desensitization procedures
- Test for allergens when skin testing is inappropriate, such as in infants
- Test for allergens when there is a known history of severe allergic reaction to skin testing
- Test for specific allergic sensitivity before initiating immunotherapy or desensitization shots
- Test for specific allergic sensitivity when skin testing is unreliable

RESULT: Different scoring systems are used in the interpretation of RAST results.

Increased in:

- Allergic rhinitis
- Anaphylaxis
- Asthma (exogenous)
- Atopic dermatitis
- *Echinococcus* infection
- Eczema
- Hay fever
- Hookworm infection
- Schistosomiasis
- Visceral larva migrans

Decreased in:

- Asthma (endogenous)
- Pregnancy
- Radiation therapy

CRITICAL VALUES: N/A

INTERFERING FACTORS: Recent radioactive scans or radiation within 1 week of the test can interfere with test results when radioimmunoassay is the test method.

Nursing Implications and Procedure • • • • • • • • • • • •

Pretest:

➤ Inform the patient that the test is used to identify types of allergens that may be responsible for causing an allergic response.

➤ Obtain a history of the patient's complaints, including a list of known allergens (especially allergies or sensitivities to latex), and inform the appropriate health care practitioner accordingly.

➤ Obtain a history of the patient's immune and respiratory system and results of previously performed laboratory tests, surgical procedures, and other diagnostic procedures. For related tests, refer to the Immune and Respiratory System tables.

➤ Note any recent procedures that can interfere with test results.

➤ Obtain a list of the medications the patient is taking, including herbs, nutritional supplements, and nutraceuticals. The requesting health care practitioner and laboratory should be advised if the patient regularly uses these products so that their effects can be taken into consideration when reviewing results.

➤ Review the procedure with the patient. Inform the patient that specimen collection takes approximately 5 to 10 minutes. Address concerns about pain related to the procedure. Explain to the patient that there may be some discomfort during the venipuncture.

➤ There are no food, fluid, or medication restrictions unless by medical direction.

Intratest:

➤ If the patient has a history of severe allergic reaction to latex, care should be taken to avoid the use of equipment containing latex.

➤ Instruct the patient to cooperate fully and to follow directions. Direct the patient to breathe normally and to avoid unnecessary movement.

- Observe standard precautions, and follow the general guidelines in Appendix A. Positively identify the patient, and label the appropriate tubes with the corresponding patient demographics, date, and time of collection. Indicate the specific allergen group to be tested on the specimen requisition. Perform a venipuncture; collect the specimen in a 5-mL red- or tiger-top tube.

- Remove the needle, place a gauze over the puncture site and apply gentle pressure to stop bleeding. Observe venipuncture site for bleeding and hematoma formation. Apply paper tape over gauze or replace with adhesive bandage.

- Promptly transport the specimen to the laboratory for processing and analysis.

- The results are recorded manually or in a computerized system for recall and postprocedure interpretation by the appropriate health care practitioner.

Post-test:

- *Nutritional considerations* should be given to diet if food allergies are present. Lifestyle adjustments may be necessary depending on the specific allergens identified.

- A written report of the examination will be sent to the requesting health care practitioner, who will discuss the results with the patient.

- Reinforce information given by the patient's health care provider regarding further testing, treatment, or referral to another health care provider. Answer any questions or address any concerns voiced by the patient or family.

- Depending on the results of this procedure, additional testing may be performed to evaluate or monitor progression of the disease process and determine the need for a change in therapy. Evaluate test results in relation to the patient's symptoms and other tests performed.

Related laboratory tests:

- Related laboratory tests include arterial/alveolar oxygen ratio, blood gases, complete blood count, eosinophil count, hypersensitivity pneumonitis, IgE, ova and parasites, and theophylline.

ALVEOLAR/ARTERIAL GRADIENT AND ARTERIAL/ALVEOLAR OXYGEN RATIO

· ·

SYNONYM/ACRONYMS: Alveolar-arterial difference, A/a gradient, a/A ratio.

SPECIMEN: Arterial blood (1 mL) collected in a heparinized syringe. Specimen should be transported tightly capped and in an ice slurry.

REFERENCE VALUE: (Method: Selective electrodes that measure pO_2 and pCO_2)

Alveolar/arterial gradient	Less than 10 mm Hg at rest (room air)
	20–30 mm Hg at maximum exercise activity (room air)
Arterial/alveolar oxygen ratio	Greater than 0.75 (75%)

DESCRIPTION & RATIONALE: A test of the ability of oxygen to diffuse from the alveoli into the lungs is of use when assessing a patient's level of oxygenation. This test can help identify the cause of hypoxemia (low oxygen levels in the blood) and intrapulmonary shunting that might result from one of the following three situations: ventilated alveoli without perfusion, unventilated alveoli with perfusion, or collapse of alveoli and associated blood vessels. Information regarding the alveolar/arterial (A/a) gradient can be estimated indirectly using the partial pressure of oxygen (pO_2) (obtained from blood gas analysis) in a simple mathematical formula:

A/a gradient = pO_2 in alveolar air (estimated) – pO_2 in arterial blood (measured)

An estimate of alveolar pO_2 is accomplished by subtracting the water vapor pressure from the barometric pressure, multiplying the resulting pressure by the fraction of inspired oxygen (FIO_2; percentage of oxygen the patient is breathing), and subtracting this from 1.25 times the arterial partial pressure of carbon dioxide (pCO_2). The gradient is obtained by subtracting the patient's arterial pO_2 from the calculated alveolar pO_2:

Alveolar pO_2 = [(barometric pressure – water vapor pressure) $\times$ FIO_2] – [1.25 $\times$ pCO_2]

A/a gradient = arterial pO_2 (measured) – alveolar pO_2 (estimated)

The arterial/alveolar (a/A) ratio reflects the percentage of alveolar pO_2 that is contained in arterial pO_2. It is calculated by dividing the arterial pO_2 by the alveolar pO_2

a/A = paO_2/ pAO_2

The A/a gradient increases as the concentration of oxygen the patient inspires increases. If the gradient is abnormally high, either there is a problem with the ability of oxygen to pass across the alveolar membrane or oxygenated blood is being mixed with nonoxygenated blood. The a/A ratio is not dependent on FIO_2; it does not increase with a corresponding increase in inhaled oxygen. For patients on a mechanical ventilator with a changing FIO_2, the a/A ratio can be used to determine if oxygen diffusion is improving. ■

INDICATIONS:
- Assess intrapulmonary or coronary artery shunting
- Assist in identifying the cause of hypoxemia

RESULT

Increased in:
- Acute respiratory distress syndrome
- Atelectasis
- Atrial-venous shunts
- Bronchospasm
- Chronic obstructive pulmonary disease
- Congenital cardiac septal defects
- Underventilated alveoli (mucus plugs)
- Pneumothorax
- Pulmonary edema
- Pulmonary embolus
- Pulmonary fibrosis

CRITICAL VALUES: N/A

INTERFERING FACTORS:
- Specimens should be collected before administration of oxygen therapy.

- The temperature of the patient should be noted and reported to the laboratory if significantly elevated or depressed so that measured values can be corrected to actual body temperature.

- Exposure of sample to room air affects test results.

- Values normally increase with increasing age (see monograph titled "Blood Gases").

- ⚠ Samples for A/a gradient evaluation are obtained by arterial puncture, which carries a risk of bleeding, especially in patients with bleeding disorders or who are taking medications for a bleeding disorder.

- Prompt and proper specimen processing, storage, and analysis are important to achieve accurate results. Specimens should always be transported to the laboratory as quickly as possible after collection. Delay in transport of the sample or transportation without ice may affect test results.

Nursing Implications and Procedure • • • • • • • • • • •

Pretest:

▶ Inform the patient that the test is used to assess effective delivery of oxygen by comparing the difference between oxygen levels in the arteries and the alveoli of the lungs.

▶ Obtain a history of the patient's complaints, including a list of known allergens (especially allergies or sensitivities to latex or anesthetics), and inform the appropriate health care practitioner accordingly.

▶ Obtain a history of the patient's respiratory system and any bleeding disorders as well as results of previously performed laboratory tests, surgical procedures, and other diagnostic procedures, especially bleeding time, coagulation time, complete blood count, platelets, partial thromboplastin time, and prothrombin

time. For related laboratory tests, refer to the Cardiovascular, Genitourinary, and Respiratory System tables.

▶ Note any recent procedures that can interfere with test results.

▶ Obtain a list of medications the patient is taking, especially medications known to affect bleeding, including anticoagulants, aspirin and other salicylates, herbals, and nutraceuticals (see Appendix F: Effects of Natural Products on Laboratory Tests). It is recommended that use of such products be discontinued 14 days before dental or surgical procedures. The requesting health care practitioner and laboratory should be advised if the patient regularly uses these products so that their effects can be taken into consideration when reviewing results.

▶ Indicate the type of oxygen, mode of oxygen delivery, and delivery rate as part of the test requisition process. Wait 30 minutes after a change in type or mode of oxygen delivery or rate for specimen collection.

▶ Review the procedure with the patient, and advise rest for 30 minutes before specimen collection. Address concerns about pain related to the procedure. Be sure to explain to the patient that an arterial puncture may be painful. The site may be anesthetized with 1% to 2% lidocaine before puncture. Inform patient that specimen collection usually takes 10 to 15 minutes.

▶ ⚠ If the sample is to be collected by radial artery puncture, perform an Allen test before puncture to ensure that the patient has adequate collateral circulation to the hand. The modified Allen test is performed as follows: extend the patient's wrist over a rolled towel. Ask the patient to make a fist with the hand extended over the towel. Use the second and third fingers to locate the pulses of the ulnar and radial arteries on the palmar surface of the wrist. (The thumb should not be used to locate these arteries because it has a pulse.) Compress both arteries, and ask the patient to open and close the fist several times until the palm turns pale. Release pressure on the ulnar artery only. Color should return to the palm within 5 seconds if the ulnar artery is functioning. This is a positive Allen test, and blood gases may be drawn from the radial artery site. The Allen test should then be performed on the opposite hand. The hand to which color is restored fastest has better circulation and should be selected for specimen collection.

➤ There are no food, fluid, or medication restrictions unless by medical direction.

➤ Prepare an ice slurry in a cup or plastic bag to have ready for immediate transport of the specimen to the laboratory.

Intratest:

➤ If the patient has a history of severe allergic reaction to latex, care should be taken to avoid the use of equipment containing latex.

➤ Instruct the patient to cooperate fully and to follow directions. Direct the patient to breathe normally and to avoid unnecessary movement.

➤ Observe standard precautions, and follow the general guidelines in Appendix A. Positively identify the patient, and label the appropriate tubes with the corresponding patient demographics, date, and time of collection.

➤ Perform an arterial puncture, and collect the specimen in an air-free heparinized syringe. There is no demonstrable difference in results between samples collected in plastic syringes and samples collected in glass syringes. It is very important that no room air be introduced into the collection container, because the gases in the room and in the sample will begin equilibrating immediately. The end of the syringe must be stoppered immediately after the needle is withdrawn and removed from the puncture site. Apply a pressure dressing over the puncture site. Samples should be mixed by gentle rolling of the syringe to ensure proper mixing of the heparin with the sample, which will prevent the formation of small clots leading to rejection of the sample. The tightly capped sample should be placed in an ice slurry immediately after collection. Information on the specimen label can be protected from water in the ice slurry by first placing the specimen in a protective plastic bag. Promptly transport the specimen to the laboratory for processing and analysis.

➤ The results are recorded manually or in a computerized system for recall and postprocedure interpretation by the appropriate health care practitioner.

Post-test:

➤ Pressure should be applied to the puncture site for at least 5 minutes in the unanticoagulated patient and for at least 15 minutes in the case of a patient receiving anticoagulant therapy. Observe puncture site for bleeding or hematoma formation. Apply pressure bandage.

➤ Teach the patient breathing exercises to assist with the appropriate exchange of oxygen and carbon dioxide.

➤ Administer oxygen, if appropriate.

➤ Teach the patient how to properly use incentive spirometry or nebulizer, if ordered.

➤ Intervene appropriately for hypoxia and ventilatory disturbances.

➤ A written report of the examination will be sent to the requesting health care practitioner, who will discuss the results with the patient.

➤ Reinforce information given by the patient's health care provider regarding further testing, treatment, or referral to another health care provider. Answer any questions or address any concerns voiced by the patient or family.

> Depending on the results of this procedure, additional testing may be performed to evaluate or monitor progression of the disease process and determine the need for a change in therapy. Evaluate test results in relation to the patient's symptoms and other tests performed.

Related laboratory tests:

> Related laboratory tests include allergen-specific immunoglobulin E (IgE), α_1-antitrypsin, α_1-antitrypsin phenotyping, blood gases, D-dimer, electrolytes, eosinophil count, fibrinogen, hypersensitivity pneumonitis, IgE, and theophylline.

ALZHEIMER'S DISEASE MARKERS
· ·

SYNONYMS/ACRONYMS: CSF tau protein and β-amyloid-42, AD.

SPECIMEN: Cerebrospinal fluid (CSF) (1 to 2 mL) collected in a plain plastic conical tube.

REFERENCE VALUE: (Method: Enzyme-linked immunosorbent assay) Simultaneous tau protein and β-amyloid-42 measurements in CSF are used in conjunction as biochemical markers of Alzheimer's disease (AD). Scientific studies indicate that a combination of elevated tau protein and decreased β-amyloid-42 protein levels are consistent with the presence of AD. Values are highly dependent on the reagents and standards used in the assay. Ranges vary among laboratories; the testing laboratory should be consulted for interpretation of results.

DESCRIPTION & RATIONALE: AD is the most common cause of dementia in the elderly population. AD is a disorder of the central nervous system that results in progressive and profound memory loss followed by loss of cognitive abilities and death. It may follow years of progressive formation of amyloid plaques and brain tangles, or it may appear as an early-onset form of the disease. Two recognized pathologic features of AD are neurofibrillary tangles and amyloid plaques found in the brain. Abnormal forms of the microtubule-associated tau protein are the main component of the classic neurofibrillary tangles found in patients with AD. Tau protein concentration is believed to reflect the number of neurofibrillary tangles and may be an indication of the severity of the disease. β-Amyloid-42 is a free-floating protein normally present in CSF. It is believed to accumulate in the central nervous system of patients with AD, causing the formation of amyloid plaques on brain tissue. The result is that these patients have lower CSF values compared to age-matched non-AD control subjects. ∎

INDICATIONS:
• Assist in establishing a diagnosis of AD

RESULT

Increased in:
• Acquired immunodeficiency syndrome

• AD

• Cerebrovascular disease

• Creutzfeldt-Jakob disease

• Meningoencephalitis

• Pick's disease

CRITICAL VALUES: N/A

INTERFERING FACTORS:
• Some patients with AD may have normal levels of tau protein because of an insufficient number of neurofibrillary tangles.

Nursing Implications and Procedure • • • • • • • • • • •

Pretest:

➤ Inform the patient that the test is used to assist in predictive testing for or confirmation of Alzheimer's disease, and to monitor progression of and therapy for the disease.

➤ Obtain a history of the patient's complaints, including a list of known allergens (especially allergies or sensitivities to latex or anesthetics), and inform the appropriate health care practitioner accordingly.

➤ Obtain a history of the patient's neurologic system and results of previously performed laboratory tests, surgical procedures, and other diagnostic procedures.

➤ Obtain a list of the medications the patient is taking, including herbs, nutritional supplements, and nutraceuticals. The requesting health care practitioner and laboratory should be advised if the patient regularly uses these products so that their effects can be taken into consideration when reviewing results.

➤ Review the procedure with the patient. Inform the patient that the procedure will be performed by a health care practitioner and takes approximately 20 minutes. Address concerns about pain related to the procedure. Explain to the patient that there may be some discomfort during the lumbar puncture. Inform the patient that a stinging sensation may be felt as the local anesthetic is injected. Tell the patient to report any pain or other sensations that may require repositioning of the spinal needle.

➤ Inform the patient that the position required for the lumbar puncture may be awkward but that someone will assist. Stress the importance of remaining still and breathing normally throughout the procedure.

➤ *Sensitivity to social and cultural issues,* as well as concern for modesty, is important in providing psychological support before, during, and after the procedure.

➤ There are no food, fluid, or medication restrictions unless by medical direction.

➤ *Make sure a written and informed consent has been signed prior to the procedure and before administering any medications.*

Intratest:

➤ If the patient has a history of severe allergic reaction to latex, care should be taken to avoid the use of equipment containing latex.

➤ Instruct the patient to cooperate fully and to follow directions. Direct the patient to breathe normally and to avoid unnecessary movement.

➤ Observe standard precautions, and follow the general guidelines in Appendix A. Positively identify the patient, and label the appropriate tubes with the corresponding patient demographics, date, and time of collection.

➤ Record baseline vital signs, and

assess neurologic status. Protocols may vary from facility to facility.

▸ To perform a lumbar puncture, position the patient in the knee-chest position at the side of the bed. Provide pillows to support the spine or for the patient to grasp. The sitting position is an alternative. In this position, the patient must bend the neck and chest to the knees.

▸ Prepare the site (usually between L3 and L4 or L4 and L5) with povidone-iodine, and drape the area.

▸ A local anesthetic is injected. Using sterile technique, the health care practitioner inserts the spinal needle through the spinous processes of the vertebrae and into the subarachnoid space. The stylet is removed. CSF drips from the needle if it is properly placed.

▸ Attach the stopcock and manometer, and measure initial CSF pressure. Normal pressure for an adult in the lateral recumbent position is 90 to 180 mm H_2O. These values depend on the body position and are different in a horizontal or sitting position.

▸ If the initial pressure is elevated, the health care practitioner may perform Queckenstedt's test. To perform this test, apply pressure to the jugular vein for about 10 seconds. CSF pressure usually rises in response to the occlusion, then rapidly returns to normal within 10 seconds after the pressure is released. Sluggish response may indicate CSF obstruction.

▸ Obtain CSF, and place in specimen tubes. Take a final pressure reading, and remove the needle. Clean the puncture site with an antiseptic solution, and apply a small bandage.

▸ Promptly transport the specimen to the laboratory for processing and analysis.

▸ The results are recorded manually or in a computerized system for recall and postprocedure interpretation by the appropriate health care practitioner.

Post-test:

▸ After lumbar puncture, monitor vital signs and neurologic status every 15 minutes for 1 hour, then every 2 hours for 4 hours, and as ordered. Take the temperature every 4 hours for 24 hours. Compare with baseline values. Protocols may vary from facility to facility.

▸ Administer fluids, if permitted, to replace lost CSF and help prevent or relieve headache, which is a side effect of lumbar puncture.

▸ Check the puncture site for leakage, and frequently monitor body signs, such as temperature and blood pressure.

▸ Position the patient flat, either on the back or abdomen, although some health care practitioners allow 30 degrees of elevation. Maintain this position for 8 hours. Changing position is acceptable as long as the body remains horizontal.

▸ Observe the patient for neurologic changes, such as altered level of consciousness, change in pupils, reports of tingling or numbness, and irritability.

▸ Recognize anxiety related to test results, and be supportive of perceived loss of independence and fear of shortened life expectancy. Discuss the implications of abnormal test results on the patient's lifestyle. Provide teaching and information regarding the clinical implications of the test results, as appropriate. Educate the patient and family members regarding access to counseling and other supportive services.

▸ Reinforce information given by the patient's health care provider regarding further testing, treatment, or referral to another health care provider. Answer any questions or address any concerns voiced by the patient or family.

▸ Depending on the results of this procedure, additional testing may be performed to evaluate or monitor progression of the disease process and determine the need for a change in therapy. Evaluate test results in relation to the patient's symptoms and other tests performed.

AMINO ACID SCREEN, BLOOD

SYNONYM/ACRONYM: N/A.

SPECIMEN: Serum (1 mL) collected in a red- or tiger-top tube. Plasma (1 mL) collected in a green-top (heparin) tube is also acceptable.

REFERENCE VALUE: (Method: Chromatography) There are numerous amino acids. The following table includes those most frequently screened. All units are nanomoles per milliliter (nmol/mL).

Age	Alanine	β-Alanine	Anserine	α-Amino adipic Acid	α-Amino-N-butyric Acid
Premature	212–504	0	—	0	14–52
Newborn–1 mo	131–710	0–10	0	0	8–24
2 mo–2 y	143–439	0–7	0	0	3–26
2–18 y	152–547	0–7	0	0	4–31
Adult	177–583	0–12	0	0–6	5–41

Age	γ-Amino-butyric Acid	β-Aminoiso-butyric Acid	Arginine	Asparagine	Aspartic Acid
Premature	0	0	34–96	90–295	24–50
Newborn–1 mo	0–2	0	6–140	29–132	20–129
2 mo–2 y	0	0	12–133	21–95	0–23
2–18 y	0	0	10–140	23–112	1–24
Adult	0	0	15–128	35–74	1–25

Age	Carnosine	Citrulline	Cysta-thionine	Cystine	Ethanol-amine
Premature	—	20–87	5–10	15–70	—
Newborn–1 mo	0–19	10–45	0–3	17–98	0–115
2 mo-2 y	0	3–35	0–5	16–84	0–4
2–18 y	0	1–46	0–3	5–45	0–7
Adult	0	12–55	0–3	5–82	0–153

Age	Glutamic Acid	Glutamine	Glycine	Histidine	Homo-cystine
Premature	107–276	248–850	298–602	72–134	3–20
Newborn–1 mo	62–620	376–709	232–740	30–138	0
2 mo–2 y	10–133	246–1182	81–436	41–101	0
2–18 y	5–150	254–823	127–341	41–125	0–5
Adult	10–131	205–756	151–490	72–124	0

Age	Hydroxy-lysine	Hydroxy-proline	Isoleucine	Leucine	Lysine
Premature	0	0–80	23–85	151–220	128–255
Newborn–1 mo	0–7	0–91	26–91	48–160	92–325
2 mo–2 y	0–7	0–63	31–86	47–155	52–196
2–18 y	0–2	3–45	22–107	49–216	48–284
Adult	0	0–53	30–108	72–201	116–296

Age	Methionine	1-Methyl-histidine	3-Methyl-histidine	Ornithine	Phenyl-alanine
Premature	37–91	4–28	5–33	77–212	98–213
Newborn–1 mo	10–60	0–43	0–5	48–211	38–137
2 mo–2 y	9–42	0–44	0–5	22–103	31–75
2–18 y	7–47	0–42	0–5	10–163	26–91
Adult	10–42	0–39	0–8	48–195	35–85

Age	Phospho-ethanolamine	Phospho-serine	Proline	Sarcosine	Serine
Premature	5–35	10–45	92–310	0	127–248
Newborn–1 mo	3–27	7–47	110–417	0–625	99–395
2 mo–2 y	0–6	1–20	52–298	0	71–186
2–18 y	0–69	1–30	59–369	0–9	69–187
Adult	0–40	2–14	97–329	0	58–181

Age	Taurine	Threonine	Tryptophan	Tyrosine	Valine
Premature	151–411	150–330	28–136	147–420	99–220
Newborn–1 mo	46–492	90–329	0–60	55–147	86–190
2 mo–2 y	15–143	24–174	23–71	22–108	64–294
2–18 y	10–170	35–226	0–79	24–115	74–321
Adult	54–210	60–225	10–140	34–112	119–336

DESCRIPTION & RATIONALE: Screening for inborn errors of amino acid metabolism is generally performed on infants after an initial blood test with abnormal results. Certain congenital enzyme deficiencies interfere with normal amino acid metabolism and cause excessive accumulation of or deficiencies in amino acid levels. Reduced growth rates, mental retardation, or various unexplained symptoms can result unless the abnormality is identified and corrected early in life. ∎

INDICATIONS:
- Assist in the detection of noninherited disorders evidenced by elevated amino acid levels
- Detect inborn errors of amino acid metabolism

RESULT

Increased (total amino acids) in:
- Aminoacidopathies (usually inherited; specific amino acids are implicated)
- Brain damage (severe)
- Burns
- Diabetes
- Eclampsia
- Fructose intolerance (hereditary)
- Malabsorption
- Renal failure (acute or chronic)
- Reye's syndrome
- Severe liver damage
- Shock

Decreased (total amino acids) in:
- Adrenocortical hyperfunction
- Carcinoid syndrome
- Fever

- Glomerulonephritis
- Hartnup disease
- Huntington's chorea
- Malnutrition
- Nephrotic syndrome
- Pancreatitis (acute)
- Polycystic kidney disease
- Rheumatoid arthritis

CRITICAL VALUES: N/A

Interfering factors:
- Drugs that may increase plasma amino acid levels include bismuth salts, glucocorticoids, levarterenol, 11-oxysteroids, and testosterone (elderly).

- Drugs that may decrease plasma amino acid levels include cerulein, epinephrine, estrogens (males), glucose, oral contraceptives, progesterone (males), and secretin.

- Amino acids exhibit a strong circadian rhythm; values are highest in the afternoon and lowest in the morning. Protein intake does not influence diurnal variation but significantly affects absolute concentrations.

- Failure to follow dietary restrictions before the procedure may cause the procedure to be canceled or repeated.

Nursing Implications and Procedure • • • • • • • • • • • •

Pretest:

▶ Inform the patient (and/or caregiver) that the test is used to screen for congenital errors of protein metabolism and transport.

▶ Obtain a history of the patient's complaints, including a list of known allergens (especially allergies or sensitivities to latex), and inform the appropriate health care practitioner accordingly.

➤ Obtain a history of the patient's or parents' reproductive system as it relates to genetic disease, as well as results of previously performed laboratory tests, surgical procedures, and other diagnostic procedures. For related laboratory tests, refer to the Reproductive System table.

➤ Obtain a list of the medications the patient is taking, including herbs, nutritional supplements, and nutraceuticals. The requesting health care practitioner and laboratory should be advised if the patient regularly uses these products so that their effects can be taken into consideration when reviewing results.

➤ Review the procedure with the patient (and/or caregiver). Inform the patient (and/or caregiver) that specimen collection takes approximately 5 to 10 minutes. Address concerns about pain related to the procedure. Explain to the patient (and/or caregiver) that there may be some discomfort during the venipuncture.

➤ *Sensitivity to social and cultural issues* is important in providing psychological support before, during, and after the procedure.

➤ There are no food, fluid or medication restrictions unless by medical direction.

Intratest:

➤ Ensure that the patient has complied with dietary and other pretesting preparations; assure that food has been restricted for at least 12 hours prior to the procedure.

➤ If the patient has a history of severe allergic reaction to latex, care should be taken to avoid the use of equipment containing latex.

➤ Instruct the patient (and/or caregiver) to cooperate fully and to follow directions. Direct the patient to breathe

normally and to avoid unnecessary movement. The caregiver may assist in preventing unnecessary movement.

➤ Observe standard precautions, and follow the general guidelines in Appendix A. Positively identify the patient, and label the appropriate tubes with the corresponding patient demographics, date, and time of collection. Perform a venipuncture; collect the specimen in a 5-mL red-top tube.

➤ Remove the needle, place a gauze over the puncture site and apply gentle pressure to stop bleeding. Observe venipuncture site for bleeding or hematoma formation. Apply paper tape over gauze or replace adhesive plastic bandage.

➤ Promptly transport the specimen to the laboratory for processing and analysis.

➤ The results are recorded manually or in a computerized system for recall and postprocedure interpretation by the appropriate health care practitioner.

Post-test:

➤ Instruct the patient to resume usual diet as directed by the health care practitioner.

➤ *Nutritional considerations:* Instruct the patient (and/or caregiver) in special dietary modifications, as appropriate to treat deficiency, or refer caregiver to a qualified nutritionist. Amino acids are classified as essential (i.e., must be present simultaneously in sufficient quantities); conditionally or acquired essential (i.e., under certain stressful conditions, they become essential); and nonessential (i.e., can be produced by the body, when needed, if diet does not provide them). Essential amino acids include lysine, threonine, histidine, isoleucine, methionine, phenylalanine, tryptophan, and valine. Conditionally essential amino acids include cysteine, tyrosine, arginine, citrulline, taurine, and carnitine.

Nonessential amino acids include alanine, glutamic acid, aspartic acid, glycine, serine, proline, glutamine, and asparagine. A high intake of specific amino acids can cause other amino acids to become essential.

➤ A written report of the examination will be sent to the requesting health care practitioner, who will discuss the results with the patient (and/or caregiver).

➤ Recognize anxiety related to test results, and be supportive of perceived loss of independence and fear of shortened life expectancy. Discuss the implications of abnormal test results on the patient's lifestyle. Provide teaching and information regarding the clinical implications of the test results, as appropriate. Educate the patient (and/or care-giver) regarding access to genetic or other counseling services.

➤ Reinforce information given by the patient's health care provider regarding further testing, treatment, or referral to another health care provider. Answer any questions or address any concerns voiced by the patient or family.

➤ Depending on the results of this procedure, additional testing may be performed to evaluate or monitor progression of the disease process and determine the need for a change in therapy. Evaluate test results in relation to the patient's symptoms and other tests performed.

Related laboratory tests:

➤ Related laboratory tests include ammonia and urine amino acid screen.

AMINO ACID SCREEN, URINE

SYNONYM/ACRONYM: N/A.

SPECIMEN: Urine (10 mL) from a random or timed specimen collected in a clean plastic collection container with hydrochloric acid as a preservative.

REFERENCE VALUE: (Method: Chromatography) There are numerous amino acids. The following table includes those most frequently screened. All units are nanomoles per milligram (nmol/mg) creatinine.

Age	Alanine	β-Alanine	Anserine	a-Amino-adipic Acid	a-Amino-N-butyric Acid
Premature	1320–4040	1020–3500	—	70–460	50–710
Newborn–1 mo	982–3055	25–288	0–3	0–180	8–65
2 mo–2 y	767–6090	0–297	0–5	45–268	30–136
2–18 y	231–915	0–65	0	2–88	0–77
Adult	240–670	0–130	0	40–110	0–90

Age	γ-Amino-butyric Acid	β-Aminoiso-butyric Acid	Arginine	Asparagine	Aspartic Acid
Premature	20–260	50–470	190–820	1350–5250	580–1520
Newborn–1 mo	0–15	421–3133	35–214	185–1550	336–810
2 mo–2 y	0–105	802–4160	38–165	252–1280	230–685
2–18 y	15–30	291–1482	31–109	72–332	0–120
Adult	15–30	10–510	10–90	99–470	60–240

Age	Carnosine	Citrulline	Cystath-ionine	Cystine	Ethano amine
Premature	260–370	240–1320	260–1160	480–1690	—
Newborn–1 mo	97–665	27–181	16–147	212–668	840–3400
2 mo–2 y	203–635	22–180	33–470	68–710	0–2230
2–18 y	72–402	10–99	0–26	25–125	0–530
Adult	10–90	8–50	20–50	43–210	0–520

Age	Glutamic Acid	Glutamine	Glycine	Histidine	Homo-cystine
Premature	380–3760	520–1700	7840–23,600	1240–7240	580–2230
Newborn–1 mo	70–1058	393–1042	5749–16,423	908–2528	0–88
2 mo–2 y	54–590	670–1562	3023–11,148	815–7090	6–67
2–18 y	0–176	369–1014	897–4500	644–2430	0–32
Adult	39–330	190–510	730–4160	460–1430	0–32

Age	Hydroxy-lysine	Hydroxy-proline	Isoleucine	Leucine	Lysine
Premature	—	560–5640	250–640	190–790	1860–15,460
Newborn–1 mo	10–125	40–440	125–390	78–195	270–1850
2 mo–2 y	0–97	0–4010	38–342	70–570	189–850
2–18 y	40–102	0–3300	10–126	30–500	153–634
Adult	40–90	0–26	16–180	30–150	145–634

(Continued on the following page)

Age	Methionine	1-Methyl-histidine	3-Methyl-histidine	Ornithine	Phenyl-alanine
Premature	500–1230	170–880	420–1340	260–3350	920–2280
Newborn–1 mo	342–880	96–499	189–680	118–554	91–457
2 mo–2 y	174–1090	106–1275	147–391	55–364	175–1340
2–18 y	16–114	170–1688	182–365	31–91	61–314
Adult	38–210	170–1680	160–520	20–80	51–250

Age	Phospho-ethanolamine	Phospho-serine	Proline	Sarcosine	Serine
Premature	80–340	500–1690	1350–10,460	0	1680–6000
Newborn–1 mo	0–155	150–339	370–2323	0–56	1444–3661
2 mo–2 y	108–533	112–304	254–2195	30–358	845–3190
2–18 y	18–150	70–138	0	0–26	362–1100
Adult	20–100	40–510	0	0–80	240–670

Age	Taurine	Threonine	Tryptophan	Tyrosine	Valine
Premature	5190–23,620	840–5700	0	1090–6780	180–890
Newborn–1 mo	1650–6220	445–1122	0	220–1650	113–369
2 mo–2 y	545–3790	252–1528	0–93	333–1550	99–316
2–18 y	639–1866	121–389	0–108	122–517	58–143
Adult	380–1850	130–370	0–70	90–290	27–260

DESCRIPTION & RATIONALE: Urine amino acid testing is used in the initial screening for congenital defects and disorders of amino acid metabolism. The major genetic disorders include phenylketonuria, tyrosinuria, and alcaptonuria, a defect in the phenylalanine-tyrosine conversion pathway. Renal aminoaciduria is also associated with conditions marked by defective tubular reabsorption from congenital disorders, such as hereditary fructose intolerance, cystinuria, and Hartnup disease. Early diagnosis and treatment of certain aminoacidurias can prevent mental retardation, reduced growth rates, and various unexplained symptoms. Values are age dependent. A positive screen on a random sample should be followed up with a timed collection. Amino acid concentrations demonstrate a significant circadian rhythm with values being lowest in the morning and highest in midafternoon. ∎

INDICATIONS:
- Assist in the detection of noninherited disorders evidenced by elevated amino acid levels
- Screen for inborn errors of amino acid metabolism

RESULT

Increased (total amino acids) in:

* Primary causes (inherited):
  Aminoaciduria (specific)
  Cystinosis (may be masked
    because of decreased glomerular
    filtration rate, so values may be
    in normal range)
  Fanconi's syndrome
  Fructose intolerance
  Galactosemia
  Hartnup disease
  Lactose intolerance
  Lowe's syndrome
  Maple syrup urine disease
  Tyrosinemia type I
  Tyrosinosis
  Wilson's disease

* Secondary causes (noninherited):
  Acute leukemia
  Chronic renal failure (reduced GFR)
  Chronic renal failure
  Diabetic ketosis
  Epilepsy (transient increase due to
    disturbed renal function during
    grand mal seizure)
  Folic acid deficiency
  Hyperparathyroidism
  Liver necrosis and cirrhosis
  Multiple myeloma
  Muscular dystrophy (progressive)
  Osteomalacia (secondary to
    parathyroid hormone excess)
  Pernicious anemia
  Thalassemia major
  Vitamin deficiency (B, C, and D;
    vitamin D–deficiency rickets,
    vitamin D–resistant rickets)
  Viral hepatitis (reflects the degree
    of hepatic involvement)

Decreased in: N/A

CRITICAL VALUES: N/A

INTERFERING FACTORS:

* Drugs that may increase urine amino acid levels include acetaminophen, acetosalicylic acid, amikacin, aminocaproic acid, amphetamine, bismuth, cephalosporins, colistin, corticotropin, dopamine, ephedrine, epinephrine, erythromycin, ethylenediamine, gentamicin, hydrocortisone, hydroxyaminobutyric acid, insulin, kanamycin, levarterenol, levodopa, mafenide, metanephrine, methamphetamine, methyldopa, neomycin, normetanephrine, penicillins, phenacetin, phenobarbital, phenylephrine, phenylpropanolamine, polymixin, polythiazide, primidone, proSobee, pseudoephedrine, streptozocin, tetracycline, triamcinolone, valproic acid, and vigabatrin.

* Drugs that may decrease urine amino acid levels include antihistamines.

* Amino acids exhibit a strong circadian rhythm; values are highest in the afternoon and lowest in the morning. Protein intake does not influence diurnal variation but significantly affects absolute concentrations.

* Dilute urine (specific gravity less than 1.010) should be rejected for analysis.

* Failure to follow dietary restrictions before the procedure may cause the procedure to be canceled or repeated.

Nursing Implications and Procedure • • • • • • • • • • •

Pretest:

➤ Inform the patient (and/or caregiver) that the test is used to screen for congenital errors of protein metabolism and transport.

➤ Obtain a history of the patient's complaints, including a list of known allergens (especially allergies or sensitivities to latex), and inform the appropriate health care practitioner accordingly.

➤ Obtain a history of the patient's and parents' reproductive system as it relates to genetic disease, as well as results of previously performed laboratory tests, surgical procedures, and other diagnostic procedures. For related laboratory tests, refer to the Reproductive System table.

➤ Obtain a list of the medications the patient is taking, including herbs, nutritional supplements, and nutraceuticals. The requesting health care practitioner and laboratory should be advised if the patient regularly uses these products so that their effects can be taken into consideration when reviewing results.

➤ Review the procedure with the patient (and/or caregiver). Inform the patient and caregiver that random urine specimen collection takes approximately 5 minutes. Address concerns about pain related to the procedure. Explain to the patient (and/or caregiver) that no pain will be experienced during the test.

➤ *Sensitivity to social and cultural issues* is important in providing psychological support before, during, and after the procedure.

➤ There are no fluid or medication restrictions unless by medical direction.

➤ The patient should avoid excessive exercise and stress during the 24-hour collection of urine.

➤ Review the procedure with the patient (and/or caregiver). Provide a nonmetallic urinal, bedpan, or toilet-mounted collection device.

➤ If a timed collection is requested, inform the patient that all urine collected over a 24-hour period must be saved; if a preservative has been added to the container, instruct the patient not to discard the preservative. Instruct the patient not to void directly into the laboratory collection container. Instruct the patient to avoid defecating in the collection device and to keep toilet tissue out of the collection device to prevent contamination of the specimen. Place a sign in the bathroom to remind the patient to save all urine.

➤ Instruct the patient to void all urine into the collection device and pour the urine into the laboratory collection container. Alternatively, the specimen can be left in the collection device for a health care staff member to add to the laboratory collection container.

Intratest:

➤ Ensure that the patient has complied with dietary and other pretesting preparations; assure that food has been restricted for at least 12 hours prior to the procedure.

➤ Observe standard precautions, and follow the general guidelines in Appendix A. Positively identify the patient, and label the appropriate specimen container with the corresponding patient demographics, date, and time of collection. Include on the timed specimen label the amount of urine and test start and stop times.

➤ Promptly transport the specimen to the laboratory for processing and analysis.

➤ The results are recorded manually or in a computerized system for recall and postprocedure interpretation by the appropriate health care practitioner.

Random specimen (collect in early morning):

➤ *Infant:* Clean and dry the genital area, attach the collection device securely to prevent leakage, and observe for voiding. Remove collection device carefully from the skin to prevent irritation. Transfer the urine into a specimen container. For dipstick method, place dipstick or reagent pad into the urine specimen or on the diaper saturated with urine. Remove, compare with color chart, and record results.

➤ *Adult:* Instruct the patient to obtain a clean-catch specimen as described in Appendix A. If an indwelling catheter is in place, it may be necessary to clamp off the catheter for 15 to 30 minutes before specimen collection. Cleanse specimen port with antiseptic swab, and then aspirate 5 mL of urine with a 21- to 25-gauge needle and syringe. Transfer urine to a properly labeled plastic container.

Timed specimen:

> Obtain a clean 3-L urine specimen container, toilet-mounted collection device, and plastic bag (for transport of the specimen container). The specimen must be refrigerated or kept on ice throughout the entire collection period. If an indwelling urinary catheter is in place, the drainage bag must be kept on ice.

> Begin the test between 6 and 8 a.m., if possible. Collect first voiding and discard. Record the time the specimen was discarded as the beginning of the timed collection period. The next morning, ask the patient to void at the same time the collection was started, and add this last voiding to the container.

> If an indwelling catheter is in place, replace the tubing and container system at the start of the collection time. Keep the container system on ice during the collection period, or empty the urine into a larger container periodically during the collection period; monitor to ensure continued drainage, and conclude the test the next morning at the same hour the collection started.

> At the conclusion of the test, compare the quantity of urine with the urinary output record for the collection. If the specimen contains less than what was recorded as output, some urine may have been discarded, invalidating the test.

Post-test:

> Instruct the patient to resume usual diet as directed by the health care practitioner.

> *Nutritional considerations:* Instruct the patient (and/or caregiver) in special dietary modifications, as appropriate to treat deficiency, or refer caregiver to a qualified nutritionist.

Amino acids are classified as essential (i.e., must be present simultaneously in sufficient quantities); conditionally or acquired essential (i.e., under certain stressful conditions, they become essential); and nonessential (i.e., can be produced by the body, when needed, if diet does not provide them). Essential amino acids include lysine, threonine, histidine, isoleucine, methionine, phenylalanine, tryptophan, and valine. Conditionally essential amino acids include cysteine, tyrosine, arginine, citrulline, taurine, and carnitine. Nonessential amino acids include alanine, glutamic acid, aspartic acid, glycine, serine, proline, glutamine, and asparagine. A high intake of specific amino acids can cause other amino acids to become essential.

> A written report of the examination will be sent to the requesting health care practitioner, who will discuss the results with the patient (and/or caregiver).

> Recognize anxiety related to test results, and be supportive of perceived loss of independence and fear of shortened life expectancy. Discuss the implications of abnormal test results on the patient's lifestyle. Provide teaching and information regarding the clinical implications of the test results, as appropriate. Educate the patient regarding access to genetic or other counseling services.

> Reinforce information given by the patient's health care provider regarding further testing, treatment, or referral to another health care provider. Answer any questions or address any concerns voiced by the patient or family.

> Depending on the results of this procedure, additional testing may be performed to evaluate or monitor progression of the disease process and determine the need for a change in therapy. Evaluate test results in relation to the patient's symptoms and other tests performed.

Related laboratory tests:

> Related laboratory tests include ammonia and blood amino acid screen.

δ-AMINOLEVULINIC ACID

SYNONYM/ACRONYM: δ-ALA.

SPECIMEN: Urine (25 mL) from a timed specimen collected in a dark plastic container with hydrochloric acid as a preservative.

REFERENCE VALUE: (Method: Spectrophotometry)

Conventional Units	SI Units (Conventional Units × 7.626)
1.5–7.5 mg/24 h	11.4–57.2 μmol/24 h

DESCRIPTION & RATIONALE: δ-Aminolevulinic acid (δ-ALA) is involved in the formation of porphyrins. Disturbances in porphyrin metabolism can cause an increase in δ-ALA excretion in urine. Although lead poisoning can cause increased urinary excretion, the measurement of δ-ALA is not useful to indicate lead toxicity because it is not detectable in the urine until the blood lead level approaches and exceeds 40 μg/dL. ∎

INDICATIONS:
• Assist in the diagnosis of porphyrias

RESULT

Increased in:
• Acute porphyrias
• Aminolevulinic acid dehydrase deficiency
• Hereditary tyrosinemia
• Lead poisoning

Decreased in:
• Liver disease (alcoholic)

CRITICAL VALUES: N/A

INTERFERING FACTORS:
• Drugs that may increase δ-ALA levels include ammonia, glucosamine, and penicillins.

• Cisplatin may decrease δ-ALA levels.

• Numerous drugs are suspected as potential initiators of attacks of acute porphyria, but those classified as unsafe for high-risk individuals include aminoglutethimide, aminopyrine, antipyrine, barbiturates, carbamazepine, carbromal, chlorpropamide, danazol, dapsone, diclofenac, diphenylhydantoin, ergot preparations, ethchlorvynol, ethinamate, glutethimide, griseofulvin, mephenytoin, meprobamate, methyprylone, N-isopropyl meprobamate, novobiocin, phenylbutazone, primidone, pyrazolone preparations, succinimides, sulfomethane, sulfonamides, sulfonethylmethane, synthetic estrogens and progestins, tolazamide, tolbutamide, trimethadione, and valproic acid.

Nursing Implications and Procedure • • • • • • • • • •

▷ Inform the patient that the test is primarily used to diagnose porphyrias.

▷ Obtain a history of the patient's complaints, including a list of known allergens (especially allergies or sensitivities to latex), and inform the appropriate health care practitioner accordingly.

▷ Obtain a history of the patient's hematopoietic system and results of previously performed laboratory tests, surgical procedures, and other diagnostic procedures. For related laboratory tests, refer to the Hematopoietic System table.

▷ Obtain a list of the medications the patient is taking, including herbs, nutritional supplements, and nutraceuticals. The requesting health care practitioner and laboratory should be advised if the patient regularly uses these products so that their effects can be taken into consideration when reviewing results.

▷ Review the procedure with the patient. Provide a nonmetallic urinal, bedpan, or toilet-mounted collection device. Address concerns about pain related to the procedure. Explain to the patient that there should be no discomfort during the procedure.

▷ Usually a 24-hour time frame for urine collection is ordered. Inform the patient that all urine must be saved during that 24-hour period. Instruct the patient not to void directly into the laboratory collection container. Instruct the patient to avoid defacating in the collection device and to keep toilet tissue out of the collection device to prevent contamination of the specimen. Place a sign in the bathroom to remind the patient to save all urine.

▷ Instruct the patient to void all urine into the collection device and then to pour the urine into the laboratory col-

lection container. Alternatively, the specimen can be left in the collection device for a health care staff member to add to the laboratory collection container.

▷ *Sensitivity to social and cultural issues,* as well as concern for modesty, is important in providing psychological support before, during, and after the procedure.

▷ There are no food, fluid, or medication restrictions unless by medical direction.

▷ If the patient has a history of severe allergic reaction to latex, care should be taken to avoid the use of equipment containing latex.

▷ Instruct the patient to cooperate fully and to follow directions.

▷ Observe standard precautions, and follow the general guidelines in Appendix A. Positively identify the patient, and label the appropriate collection container with the corresponding patient demographics, date, and time of collection.

▷ Obtain a clean 3-L urine specimen container, toilet-mounted collection device, and plastic bag (for transport of the specimen container). The specimen must be refrigerated or kept on ice throughout the entire collection period. If an indwelling urinary catheter is in place, the drainage bag must be kept on ice.

▷ Begin the test between 6 and 8 a.m., if possible. Collect first voiding and discard. Record the time the specimen was discarded as the beginning of the timed collection period. The next morning, ask the patient to void at the same time the collection was started, and add this last voiding to the container.

▷ If an indwelling catheter is in place, replace the tubing and container system at the start of the collection time. Keep the container system on ice during the collection period, or empty the urine into a larger container periodically during the collection period. Monitor to ensure continued drainage, and conclude the test the next morning at the same hour the collection was begun.

➤ At the conclusion of the test, compare the quantity of urine with the urinary output record for the collection. If the specimen contains less than what was recorded as output, some urine may have been discarded, invalidating the test.

➤ Include on the specimen collection container's label the amount of urine as well as test start and stop times. Note the ingestion of any medications that may affect test results.

➤ Promptly transport the specimen to the laboratory for processing and analysis.

➤ The results are recorded manually or in a computerized system for recall and postprocedure interpretation by the appropriate health care practitioner.

care practitioner, who will discuss the results with the patient.

➤ Recognize anxiety related to test results. Discuss the implications of abnormal test results on the patient's lifestyle. Provide teaching and information regarding the clinical implications of the test results, as appropriate.

➤ Reinforce information given by the patient's health care provider regarding further testing, treatment, or referral to another health care provider. Answer any questions or address any concerns voiced by the patient or family.

➤ Depending on the results of this procedure, additional testing may be performed to evaluate or monitor progression of the disease process and determine the need for a change in therapy. Evaluate test results in relation to the patient's symptoms and other tests performed.

Post-test:

➤ A written report of the examination will be sent to the requesting health

Related laboratory tests:

➤ Related laboratory tests include lead and urine porphyrins.

AMMONIA

· ·

SYNONYM/ACRONYM: NH_3.

SPECIMEN: Plasma (1 mL) collected in completely filled green-top (heparin) tube. Specimen should be transported tightly capped and in an ice slurry.

REFERENCE VALUE: (Method: Spectrophotometry)

Age	Conventional Units	SI Units (Conventional Units × 0.714)
Newborn	90–150 μg/dL	64–107 μmol/L
Adult Male	27–102 μg/dL	19–73 μmol/L
Adult Female	19–87 μg/dL	14–62 μmol/L

DESCRIPTION & RATIONALE: Blood ammonia (NH_3) comes from two sources: deamination of amino acids during protein metabolism and degradation of proteins by colon bacteria. The liver converts ammonia in the portal blood to urea, which is excreted by the kidneys. When liver function is severely compromised, especially in situations in which decreased hepatocellular function is combined with impaired portal blood flow, ammonia levels rise. Ammonia is potentially toxic to the central nervous system. ▪

INDICATIONS:

- Evaluate advanced liver disease or other disorders associated with altered serum ammonia levels
- Identify impending hepatic encephalopathy with known liver disease
- Monitor the effectiveness of treatment for hepatic encephalopathy, indicated by declining levels
- Monitor patients receiving hyperalimentation therapy

RESULT

Increased in:

- Gastrointestinal hemorrhage
- Genitourinary tract infection with distention and stasis
- Hepatic coma
- Inborn enzyme deficiency
- Liver failure, late cirrhosis
- Reye's syndrome
- Total parenteral nutrition

Decreased in: N/A

CRITICAL VALUES: N/A

INTERFERING FACTORS:

- Drugs that may increase ammonia levels include ammonium salts, asparagi-

nase, barbiturates, diuretics, ethanol, fibrin hydrolysate, fluorides, furosemide, thiazides, and valproic acid.

- Drugs/organisms that may decrease ammonia levels include diphenhydramine, kanamycin, neomycin, tetracycline, and *Lactobacillus acidophilus.*
- Hemolysis falsely increases ammonia levels.
- Prompt and proper specimen processing, storage, and analysis are important to achieve accurate results. The specimen should be collected on ice; the collection tube should be filled completely, and then kept tightly stoppered. Ammonia increases rapidly in the collected specimen, so analysis should be performed within 20 minutes of collection.

Nursing Implications and Procedure • • • • • • • • • • •

Pretest: ▪

➤ Inform the patient that the test is used to assess liver function, particularly in the diagnosis of urea cycle deficiencies in neonates and the identification of Reye's syndrome.

➤ Obtain a history of the patient's complaints, including a list of known allergens (especially allergies or sensitivities to latex), and inform the appropriate health care practitioner accordingly.

➤ Obtain a history of the patient's gastrointestinal, genitourinary, and hepatobiliary systems, as well as results of previously performed laboratory tests, surgical procedures, and other diagnostic procedures. For related laboratory tests, refer to the Gastrointestinal, Genitourinary, and Hepatobiliary System tables.

➤ Obtain a list of the medications the patient is taking, including herbs, nutritional supplements, and nutraceuticals. The requesting health care practitioner and laboratory should be advised if the patient regularly uses these products so that their effects can be taken into consideration when reviewing results.

► Review the procedure with the patient. Inform the patient that specimen collection takes approximately 5 to 10 minutes. Address concerns about pain related to the procedure. Explain to the patient that there may be some discomfort during the venipuncture.

► There are no food, fluid, or medication restrictions unless by medical direction.

Intratest:

► If the patient has a history of severe allergic reaction to latex, care should be taken to avoid the use of equipment containing latex.

► Instruct the patient to cooperate fully and to follow directions. Direct the patient to breathe normally and to avoid unnecessary movement.

► Observe standard precautions, and follow the general guidelines in Appendix A. Positively identify the patient, and label the appropriate tubes with the corresponding patient demographics, date, and time of collection. Perform a venipuncture; collect the specimen in a 5-mL green-top tube.

► Remove the needle, place a gauze over the puncture site and apply gentle pressure to stop bleeding. Observe the venipuncture site for bleeding or hematoma formation. Apply paper tape over gauze or replace with adhesive bandage.

► Promptly transport the specimen to the laboratory for processing and analysis. The tightly capped sample should be placed in an ice slurry immediately after collection. Information on the specimen label can be protected from water in the ice slurry by first placing the specimen in a protective plastic bag.

► The results are recorded manually or in a computerized system for recall and postprocedure interpretation by the appropriate health care practitioner.

Post-test:

► *Nutritional considerations:* Increased ammonia levels may be associated with liver disease. Dietary recommendations may be indicated, depending on the severity of the condition. A low-protein diet may be in order if the patient's liver has lost the ability to process the end products of protein metabolism. A diet of soft foods may be required if esophageal varices have developed. Ammonia levels may be used to determine whether protein should be added to or reduced from the diet. Patients should be encouraged to eat simple carbohydrates and emulsified fats (as in homogenized milk or eggs), as opposed to complex carbohydrates (e.g., starch, fiber, and glycogen [animal carbohydrates]) and complex fats, which would require additional bile to emulsify them so that they could be used. The cirrhotic patient should be carefully observed for the development of ascites, in which case fluid and electrolyte balance requires strict attention.

► A written report of the examination will be sent to the requesting health care practitioner, who will discuss the results with the patient.

► Reinforce information given by the patient's health care provider regarding further testing, treatment, or referral to another health care provider. Answer any questions or address any concerns voiced by the patient or family.

► Depending on the results of this procedure, additional testing may be performed to evaluate or monitor progression of the disease process and determine the need for a change in therapy. Evaluate test results in relation to the patient's symptoms and other tests performed.

Related laboratory tests:

> Related laboratory tests include acetaminophen, alanine aminotransferase, albumin, anion gap, aspartate aminotransferase, bilirubin, blood gases, blood calcium, complete blood count, electrolytes, glucose, ketones, lactic acid, osmolality, protein, prothrombin time, urea nitrogen, and uric acid.

AMNIOTIC FLUID ANALYSIS

SYNONYM/ACRONYM: N/A.

SPECIMEN: Amniotic fluid (10 to 20 mL) collected in a clean amber glass or plastic container.

REFERENCE VALUE: (Method: Macroscopic observation of fluid for color and appearance, immunochemiluminometric assay [ZCMA] for α_1-fetoprotein, electrophoresis for acetylcholinesterase, spectrophotometry for creatinine and bilirubin, chromatography for lecithin/sphingomyelin [L/S] ratio and phosphatidylglycerol, tissue culture for chromosome analysis, dipstick for leukocyte esterase, and automated cell counter for white blood cell count and lamellar bodies)

Test	Reference Value
Color	Colorless to pale yellow
Appearance	Clear
α_1-Fetoprotein	Less than 2.0 MoM
Acetylcholinesterase	Absent
Creatinine	1.8–4.0 mg/dL at term
Bilirubin	Less than 0.075 mg/dL in early pregnancy
	Less than 0.025 mg/dL at term
L/S ratio	Greater than 2:1 at term
Phosphatidylglycerol	Present at term
Chromosome analysis	Normal karyotype
White blood cell count	None seen
Leukocyte esterase	Negative
Lamellar bodies	30,000–50,000 platelet equivalents

MoM = multiples of the median.

DESCRIPTION & RATIONALE: Amniotic fluid is formed in the membranous sac that surrounds the fetus. The total volume of fluid at term is 500 to 2500 mL. In amniocentesis, fluid is obtained by ultrasound-guided needle aspiration from the amniotic sac. This procedure is generally performed between 14 and 16 weeks' gestation, but it also can be done between 26 and 35 weeks' gestation if fetal distress is suspected. Amniotic fluid is tested to identify genetic and neural tube defects, hemolytic diseases of the newborn, fetal infection, fetal renal malfunction, or maturity of the fetal lungs (see monograph titled "Lecithin/Sphingomyelin Ratio"). ■

INDICATIONS:
- Assist in the diagnosis of (in utero) metabolic disorders, such as cystic fibrosis; or errors of lipid, carbohydrate, or amino acid metabolism.
- Detect infection secondary to ruptured membranes.
- Detect fetal ventral wall defects.
- Determine fetal maturity when preterm delivery is being considered. Fetal maturity is indicated by an L/S ratio of 2:1 or greater (see monograph titled "Lecithin/Sphingomyelin Ratio").
- Determine fetal sex when the mother is a known carrier of a sex-linked abnormal gene that could be transmitted to male offspring, such as hemophilia or Duchenne's muscular dystrophy.
- Determine the presence of fetal distress in late-stage pregnancy.
- Evaluate fetus in families with a history of genetic disorders, such as Down syndrome, Tay-Sachs disease, chromosome or enzyme anomalies, or inherited hemoglobinopathies.
- Evaluate fetus in mothers of advanced maternal age (some of the aforementioned tests are routinely requested in mothers age 35 years and older).
- Evaluate fetus in mothers with a history of miscarriage or stillbirth.
- Evaluate known or suspected hemolytic disease involving the fetus in an Rh-sensitized pregnancy, indicated by rising bilirubin levels, especially after the 30th week of gestation.
- Evaluate suspected neural tube defects, such as spina bifida or myelomeningocele, as indicated by elevated α_1-fetoprotein (see monograph titled "α_1-Fetoprotein" for information related to triple-marker testing).

RESULT:
- Yellow, green, red, or brown fluid indicates the presence of bilirubin, blood (fetal or maternal), or meconium, which indicate fetal distress or death, hemolytic disease, or growth retardation.
- Elevated bilirubin levels indicate fetal hemolytic disease or intestinal obstruction. Measurement of bilirubin is not usually performed before 20 to 24 weeks' gestation because no action can be taken before then. The severity of hemolytic disease is graded by optical density (OD) zones: A value of 0.28 to 0.46 OD at 28 to 31 weeks' gestation indicates mild hemolytic disease, which probably will not affect the fetus; 0.47 to 0.90 OD indicates a moderate effect on the fetus; and 0.91 to 1.0 OD indicates a significant effect on the fetus. A trend of increasing values with serial measurements may indicate the need for intrauterine transfusion or early delivery, depending on the fetal age. After 32 to 33 weeks' gestation, early delivery is preferred over intrauterine transfusion, because early delivery is more effective in providing the required care to the neonate.
- Creatinine concentration greater than

2.0 mg/dL indicates fetal maturity (at 36 to 37 weeks) if maternal creatinine is also within the expected range. This value should be interpreted in conjunction with other parameters evaluated in amniotic fluid and especially with the L/S ratio, because normal lung development depends on normal kidney development.

- An L/S ratio less than 2:1 and absence of phosphatidylglycerol at term indicate fetal lung immaturity and possible respiratory distress syndrome. The expected L/S ratio for the fetus of an insulin-dependent diabetic mother is higher (3.5:1). (See monograph titled "Lecithin/Sphingomyelin Ratio.")

- Lamellar bodies are specialized alveolar cells in which lung surfactant is stored. They are approximately the size of platelets. Their presence in sufficient quantities is an indicator of fetal lung maturity.

- Elevated α_1-fetoprotein levels and presence of acetylcholinesterase indicate a neural tube defect (see monograph titled "α_1-Fetoprotein").

- Abnormal karyotype indicates genetic abnormality (e.g., Tay-Sachs disease, mental retardation, chromosome or enzyme anomalies, and inherited hemoglobinopathies). (See monograph titled "Chromosome Analysis, Blood.")

- Elevated white blood cell count and positive leukocyte esterase are indicators of infection.

CRITICAL VALUES: N/A

INTERFERING FACTORS:
- Bilirubin may be falsely elevated if maternal hemoglobin or meconium is present in the sample; fetal acidosis may also lead to falsely elevated bilirubin levels.

- Bilirubin may be falsely decreased if the sample is exposed to light or if amniotic fluid volume is excessive.

- Maternal serum creatinine should be measured simultaneously for comparison with amniotic fluid creatinine for proper interpretation. Even in circumstances in which the maternal serum value is normal, the results of the amniotic fluid creatinine may be misleading. A high fluid creatinine value in the fetus of a diabetic mother may reflect the increased muscle mass of a larger fetus. If the fetus is big, the creatinine may be high, and the fetus may still have immature kidneys.

- Contamination of the sample with blood or meconium or complications in pregnancy may yield inaccurate L/S ratios.

- α_1-Fetoprotein and acetylcholinesterase may be falsely elevated if the sample is contaminated with fetal blood.

- Karyotyping cannot be performed under the following conditions: (1) failure to promptly deliver samples for chromosomal analysis to the laboratory performing the test, or (2) improper incubation of the sample, which causes cell death.

- Amniocentesis is contraindicated in women with a history of premature labor or incompetent cervix. It is also contraindicated in the presence of placenta previa or abruptio placentae.

Nursing Implications and Procedure

Pretest:

> Inform the patient that the test is used to evaluate fetal well-being.

> Obtain a history of the patient's complaints, including a list of known allergens (especially allergies or sensitivities to latex or anesthetics), and inform the appropriate health care practitioner accordingly.

➤ Obtain a history of the patient's reproductive system, previous pregnancies, and results of previously performed laboratory tests, surgical procedures, and other diagnostic procedures. Include any family history of genetic disorders such as cystic fibrosis, Duchenne's muscular dystrophy, hemophilia, sickle cell disease, Tay-Sachs disease, thalassemia, and trisomy 21. Obtain maternal Rh type. If Rh-negative, check for prior sensitization. A standard RhoGAM dose is indicated after amniocentesis; repeat doses should be considered if repeated amniocentesis is performed. For related laboratory tests, refer to the Reproductive System table.

➤ Note any recent procedures that can interfere with test results.

➤ Record the date of the last menstrual period and determine the pregnancy weeks' gestation and expected delivery date.

➤ Obtain a list of the medications the patient is taking. Include herbs, nutritional supplements, and nutraceuticals. The requesting health care practitioner and laboratory should be advised if the patient regularly uses these products so that their effects can be taken into consideration when reviewing results.

➤ Review the procedure with the patient. Warn the patient that normal results do not guarantee a normal fetus. Assure the patient that precautions to avoid injury to the fetus will be taken by localizing the fetus with ultrasound. Address concerns about pain related to the procedure. Explain that, during the transabdominal procedure, any discomfort associated with a needle biopsy will be minimized with local anesthetics. If the patient is less than 20 weeks' gestation, instruct her to drink extra fluids 1 hour before the test and to refrain from urination. The full bladder assists in raising the uterus up and out of the way to provide better visualization during the ultrasound procedure. Patients who are at 20 weeks' gestation or beyond do not need to drink extra fluids and should void before the test, because an empty bladder is less likely to be accidentally punctured during specimen collection. Encourage relaxation and controlled breathing during the procedure to aid in reducing any mild discomfort. Inform the patient that specimen collection is performed by a health care provider specializing in this procedure and usually takes approximately 20 to 30 minutes to complete.

➤ *Sensitivity to social and cultural issues*, as well as concern for modesty, is important in providing psychological support before, during, and after the procedure.

➤ There are no food, fluid, or medication restrictions unless by medical direction.

➤ *Make sure a written and informed consent has been signed prior to the procedure and before administering any medications.*

Intratest:

➤ Ensure that the patient has a full bladder before the procedure if gestation is 20 weeks or less; have patient void before the procedure if gestation is 21 weeks or more.

➤ Positively identify the patient, and label the appropriate collection containers with the corresponding patient demographics, date, time of collection, and site location.

➤ Have patient remove clothes below the waist. Assist the patient to a supine position on the exam table with the abdomen exposed. Drape the patient's legs, leaving the abdomen exposed. Raise her head or legs slightly to promote comfort and to relax the abdominal muscles. If the uterus is large, place a pillow or rolled blanket under the patient's right side to prevent hypertension caused by great-vessel compression. Instruct the patient to cooperate fully and to follow directions. Direct the patient to breathe normally and to avoid unnecessary movement during the local anesthetic and the procedure.

➤ Record maternal and fetal baseline vital signs, and continue to monitor throughout the procedure. Monitor for uterine contractions. Monitor fetal vital signs using ultrasound. Protocols may vary from facility to facility.

➤ After the administration of local anesthesia, shave and cleanse the site with an antiseptic solution, and drape the area with sterile towels.

➤ Have emergency equipment readily available.

➤ Observe standard precautions, and follow the general guidelines in Appendix A.

➤ Assess the position of the amniotic fluid, fetus, and placenta using ultrasound.

➤ Assemble the necessary equipment, including an amniocentesis tray with solution for skin preparation, local anesthetic, 10- or 20-mL syringe, needles of various sizes (including a 22-gauge, 5-inch spinal needle), sterile drapes, sterile gloves, and foil-covered or amber-colored specimen collection containers.

➤ Cleanse suprapubic area with an antiseptic solution, and protect with sterile drapes. A local anesthetic is injected. Explain that this may cause a stinging sensation.

➤ A 22-gauge, 5-inch spinal needle is inserted through the abdominal and uterine walls. Explain that a sensation of pressure may be experienced when the needle is inserted. Explain to the patient how to use focused and controlled breathing for relaxation during the procedure.

➤ After the fluid is collected and the needle is withdrawn, apply slight pressure to the site. If there is no evidence of bleeding or other drainage, apply a sterile adhesive bandage to the site.

➤ Monitor the patient for complications related to the procedure (e.g., premature labor, allergic reaction, anaphylaxis).

➤ Place samples in properly labeled specimen container, and promptly transport the specimen to the laboratory for processing and analysis.

➤ The results are recorded manually or in a computerized system for recall and postprocedure interpretation by the appropriate health care practitioner.

Post-test:

➤ ⚠ After the procedure, fetal heart rate and maternal life signs (i.e., heart rate, blood pressure, pulse, and respiration) should be compared with baseline values and closely monitored every 15 minutes for 30 to 60 minutes after the amniocentesis procedure. Protocols may vary from facility to facility.

➤ Observe for delayed allergic reactions, such as rash, urticaria, tachycardia, hyperpnea, hypertension, palpitations, nausea, or vomiting.

➤ Observe the amniocentesis site for bleeding, inflammation, or hematoma formation.

➤ Instruct the patient in the care and assessment of the amniocentesis site. Instruct the patient to report any redness, edema, bleeding, or pain at the biopsy site. Instruct the patient to keep the site clean and change the dressing as needed.

➤ Instruct the patient to expect mild cramping, leakage of small amount of amniotic fluid, and vaginal spotting for up to 2 days following the procedure. Instruct the patient to report moderate to severe abdominal pain or cramps, change in fetal activity, increased or prolonged leaking of amniotic fluid from abdominal needle site, vaginal bleeding that is heavier than spotting, and either chills or fever.

➤ Instruct the patient to rest until all symptoms have disappeared before resuming normal levels of activity.

➤ Administer standard RhoGAM dose to maternal Rh-negative patients to prevent maternal Rh sensitization should the fetus be Rh-positive.

➤ A written report of the examination will be completed by a health care practitioner specializing in this branch of medicine. A written report of the examination will be sent to the requesting health care practitioner, who will discuss the results with the patient.

➤ Recognize anxiety related to test results. Discuss the implications of abnormal test results on the patient's lifestyle. Provide teaching and information regarding the clinical implications of the test results, as appropriate. Encourage the family to seek appropriate counseling if concerned with pregnancy termination, and to seek genetic counseling if a chromosomal abnormality is determined. Decisions regarding elective abortion should take place in the presence of both parents. Provide a nonjudgmental, nonthreatening atmosphere for discussing the risks and difficulties of delivering and raising a developmentally challenged infant, as well as exploring other options (termination of pregnancy or adoption). It is also important to discuss problems the mother and father may experience (guilt, depression, anger) if fetal abnormalities are detected.

➤ Reinforce information given by the patient's health care provider regarding further testing, treatment, or referral to another health care provider. Inform the patient that it may be 2 to 4 weeks before all results are available. Answer any questions or address any concerns voiced by the patient or family.

➤ Instruct the patient in the use of any ordered medications. Explain the importance of adhering to the therapy regimen. As appropriate, instruct the patient in significant side effects and systemic reactions associated with the prescribed medication. Encourage her to review corresponding literature provided by a pharmacist.

➤ Depending on the results of this procedure, additional testing may be performed to evaluate or monitor progression of the disease process and determine the need for a change in therapy. Evaluate test results in relation to the patient's symptoms and other tests performed.

Related laboratory tests:

➤ Related laboratory tests include α_1-fetoprotein, blood groups and antibodies, chromosome analysis, and L/S ratio.

AMYLASE

SYNONYM/ACRONYM: N/A.

SPECIMEN: Serum (1 mL) collected in a red- or tiger-top tube. Plasma (1 mL) collected in a green-top (heparin) tube is also acceptable.

REFERENCE VALUE: (Method: Spectrophotometry)

Conventional & SI Units
30–110 U/L

DESCRIPTION & RATIONALE: Amylase, a digestive enzyme, splits starch into disaccharides. Although many cells have amylase activity (e.g., liver, small intestine, ovaries, skeletal muscles), circulating amylase is derived from the parotid glands and the pancreas. Amylase is a sensitive indicator of pancreatic acinar cell damage and pancreatic obstruction. Newborns and children up to 2 years old have little measurable serum amylase. In the early years of life, most of this enzyme is produced by the salivary glands. ■

INDICATIONS:
- Assist in the diagnosis of early acute pancreatitis; serum amylase begins to rise within 6 to 24 hours after onset and returns to normal in 2 to 7 days
- Assist in the diagnosis of macroamylasemia, a disorder seen in alcoholism, malabsorption syndrome, and other digestive problems
- Assist in the diagnosis of pancreatic duct obstruction, which causes serum amylase levels to remain elevated
- Detect blunt trauma or inadvertent surgical trauma to the pancreas
- Differentiate between acute pancreatitis and other causes of abdominal pain that require surgery

RESULT

Increased in:
- Abdominal trauma
- Alcoholism

- Carcinoma of the head of the pancreas (advanced)
- Common bile duct obstruction
- Diabetic ketoacidosis
- Duodenal obstruction
- Ectopic pregnancy
- Gastric resection
- Macroamylasemia
- Mumps
- Pancreatic cyst and pseudocyst
- Pancreatitis
- Parotitis
- Perforated peptic ulcer involving the pancreas
- Peritonitis
- Postoperative period
- Some tumors of the lung and ovaries
- Viral infections

Decreased in:
- Cystic fibrosis (advanced)
- Hepatic disease (severe)
- Pancreatectomy
- Pancreatic insufficiency

CRITICAL VALUES: N/A

INTERFERING FACTORS:
- Drugs and substances that may increase amylase levels include asparaginase, captopril, cimetidine, clofibrate, corticosteroids, estrogens, ethacrynic acid, furosemide, ibuprofen, methyldopa, nitrofurantoin, oral contraceptives, pentamidine, sulfonamides, tetracycline, thiazide diuretics, valproic acid, zalcitabine, and alcohol.
- Drugs that may decrease amylase levels include anabolic steroids, citrates, and fluorides.

Nursing Implications and Procedure • • • • • • • • • • •

Pretest:

➤ Inform the patient that the test is primarily used to assess pancreatic function.

➤ Obtain a history of the patient's complaints, including a list of known allergens (especially allergies or sensitivities to latex), and inform the appropriate health care practitioner accordingly.

➤ Obtain a history of the patient's endocrine, gastrointestinal, and hepatobiliary systems, as well as results of previously performed laboratory tests, surgical procedures, and other diagnostic procedures. For related laboratory tests, refer to the Endocrine, Gastrointestinal, and Hepatobiliary System tables.

➤ Obtain a list of the medications the patient is taking, including herbs, nutritional supplements, and nutraceuticals. The requesting health care practitioner and laboratory should be advised if the patient regularly uses these products so that their effects can be taken into consideration when reviewing results.

➤ Review the procedure with the patient. Inform the patient that specimen collection takes approximately 5 to 10 minutes. Address concerns about pain related to the procedure. Explain to the patient that there may be some discomfort during the venipuncture.

➤ There are no food, fluid, or medication restrictions unless by medical direction.

Intratest:

➤ If the patient has a history of severe allergic reaction to latex, care should be taken to avoid the use of equipment containing latex.

➤ Instruct the patient to cooperate fully and to follow directions. Direct the patient to breathe normally and to avoid unnecessary movement.

➤ Observe standard precautions, and follow the general guidelines in Appendix A. Positively identify the patient, and label the appropriate tubes with the corresponding patient demographics, date, and time of collection. Perform a venipuncture; collect the specimen in a 5-mL red- or tiger-top tube.

➤ Remove the needle, place a gauze over the puncture site and apply gentle pressure to stop bleeding. Observe venipuncture site for bleeding or hematoma formation. Apply paper tape over gauze or replace with adhesive bandage.

➤ Promptly transport the specimen to the laboratory for processing and analysis.

➤ The results are recorded manually or in a computerized system for recall and postprocedure interpretation by the appropriate health care practitioner.

Post-test:

➤ *Nutritional considerations:* Increased amylase levels may be associated with gastrointestinal disease or alcoholism. Small, frequent meals work best for patients with gastrointestinal disorders. Consideration should be given to dietary alterations in the case of gastrointestinal disorders. Usually after acute symptoms subside and bowel sounds return, patients are given a clear liquid diet, progressing to a low-fat, high-carbohydrate diet. Vitamin B_{12} may be ordered for parenteral administration to patients with decreased levels, especially if their disease prevents adequate absorption of the vitamin. The alcoholic patient should be encouraged to avoid alcohol and to seek appropriate counseling for substance abuse.

➤ A written report of the examination will be sent to the requesting health care practitioner, who will discuss the results with the patient.

➤ Reinforce information given by the

patient's health care provider regarding further testing, treatment, or referral to another health care provider. Answer any questions or address any concerns voiced by the patient or family.

➤ Depending on the results of this procedure, additional testing may be performed to evaluate or monitor progression of the disease process and determine the need for a change in therapy. Evaluate test results in relation to the patient's symptoms and other tests performed.

➤ Related laboratory tests include alanine aminotransferase, alkaline phosphatase, amylase (fluid), aspartate aminotransferase, bilirubin, CA 19–9, calcium, fecal fat, γ-glutamyl transpeptidase, lipase, magnesium, mumps serology, triglycerides, and white blood cell count.

ANALGESIC AND ANTIPYRETIC DRUGS: ACETAMINOPHEN, ACETYLSALICYLIC ACID

$\bullet$

SYNONYMS/ACRONYM: *Acetaminophen* (Acephen, Apacet, Aspirin Free Anacin, Banesin, Dapa, Datril, Dorcol, Gebapap, Halenol, Liquiprin, Meda Cap, Panadol, Redutemp, Tempra, Tylenol, Ty-Pap, Uni-Ace); *Acetylsalicylic acid* (salicylate, aspirin, Anacin, Aspergum, Bufferin, Ecotrin, Empirin, Measurin, Synalgos, ZORprin, ASA).

SPECIMEN: Serum (1 mL) collected in a red-top tube.

REFERENCE VALUE: (Method: Immunoassay)

Drug	Therapeutic Dose*	SI Units	Half-Life	Volume of Distribution	Protein Binding	Excretion
		(SI = Conventional Units × 6.62)				
Acetamino-phen	10–30 μg/mL	66–199 μmol/L	1–3 h	0.95 L/kg	20–50%	85–95% hepatic, metabo-lites, renal
		(SI = Conventional Units × 0.073)				
Salicylate	15–20 mg/dL	1.1–1.4 mmol/L	2–3 h	0.1–0.3 L/kg	90–95%	1° hepatic, metabo-lites, renal

* Conventional units.

DESCRIPTION & RATIONALE: Acetaminophen is used for headache, fever, and pain relief, especially for individuals unable to take salicylate products or who have bleeding conditions. It is the analgesic of choice for children less than 13 years of age; salicylates are avoided in this age group because of the association between aspirin and Reye's syndrome. Acetaminophen is rapidly absorbed from the gastrointestinal tract and reaches peak concentration within 30 to 60 minutes after administration of a therapeutic dose. It can be a silent killer because, by the time symptoms of intoxication appear 24 to 48 hours after ingestion, the antidote is ineffective. Acetylsalicylic acid (ASA) is also used for headache, fever, and pain relief. Some patients with cardiovascular disease take small prophylactic doses. The main site of toxicity for both drugs is the liver, particularly in the presence of liver disease or decreased drug metabolism and excretion.

Many factors must be considered in interpreting drug levels, including patient age, patient weight, interacting medications, electrolyte balance, protein levels, water balance, conditions that affect absorption and excretion, and foods, herbals, vitamins, and minerals that can potentiate or inhibit the intended target concentration. ▪

INDICATIONS:
- Suspected overdose
- Suspected toxicity
- Therapeutic monitoring

RESULT

Increased in:
- Acetaminophen
  Alcoholic cirrhosis

Liver disease
Toxicity

- ASA
  Toxicity

Decreased in:
- Noncompliance with therapeutic regimen

CRITICAL VALUES: ⚠ *Note:* The adverse effects of subtherapeutic levels are also important. Care should be taken to investigate signs and symptoms of too little and too much medication. Note and immediately report to the health care practitioner any critically increased values and related symptoms.

Acetaminophen: Greater Than 150 μg/mL (4 Hours Postingestion); Greater Than 50 μg/mL (12 Hours Postingestion)

Signs and symptoms of acetaminophen intoxication occur in stages over a period of time. In stage I (0 to 24 hours after ingestion), symptoms may include gastrointestinal irritation, pallor, lethargy, diaphoresis, metabolic acidosis, and possibly coma. In stage II (24 to 48 hours after ingestion), signs and symptoms may include right upper quadrant abdominal pain; elevated liver enzymes, aspartate aminotransferase (AST), and alanine aminotransferase (ALT); and possible decreased renal function. In stage III (72 to 96 hours after ingestion), signs and symptoms may include nausea, vomiting, jaundice, confusion, coagulation disorders, continued elevation of AST and ALT, decreased renal function, and coma. Intervention may include gastrointestinal decontamination (stomach pumping) if the patient presents within 6 hours of ingestion or administration of *N*-acetylcysteine (Mucomyst) in the case of an acute intoxication in which the patient presents more than 6 hours after ingestion.

ASA: Greater Than 50 mg/dL

Signs and symptoms of salicylate intoxication include ketosis, convulsions, dizziness, nausea, vomiting, hyperactivity, hyperglycemia, hyperpnea, hyperthermia, respiratory arrest, and tinnitus. Possible interventions include administration of activated charcoal as vomiting ceases, alkalinization of the urine with bicarbonate, and a single dose of vitamin K (for rare instances of hypoprothrombinemia).

Pediatric Serum Salicylate Level and Severity of Intoxication Single Dose Acute Ingestion Nomogram

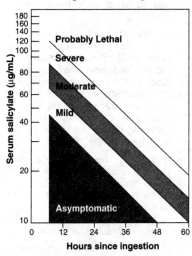

Nomogram relating serum salicylate concentration and expected severity of intoxication at varying intervals following the ingestion of a single dose of salicylate.
From Done AK, "Aspirin Overdosage: Incidence, Diagnosis, and Management," *Pediatrics*,1978, 62:890-7 with permission.

Acetaminophen Toxicity Nomogram

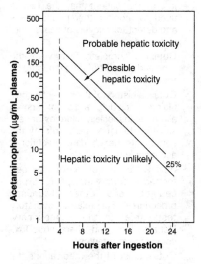

The Rumack-Matthew nomogram, relating expected severity of liver toxicity to serum acetaminophen concentrations.

From Smilkstein MJ, Bronstein AC, Linden C, et al, "Acetaminophen Overdose: A 48-Hour Intravenous N-Acetylcysteine Treatment Protocol," *Ann Emerg Med*, 1991,20(10):1058, with permission.

INTERFERING FACTORS:

- Blood drawn in serum separator tubes (gel tubes).

- Contraindicated in patients with liver disease, and caution advised in patients with renal impairment.

- Drugs that may increase acetaminophen levels include diflunisal, metoclopramide, and probenecid.

- Drugs that may decrease acetaminophen levels include cholestyramine, iron, oral contraceptives, and propantheline.

- Drugs that increase ASA levels include sulfinpyrazone.

- Drugs and substances that decrease ASA levels include activated charcoal, antacids (aluminum hydroxide), and iron.

Nursing Implications and Procedure • • • • • • • • • • •

Pretest:

➤ Inform the patient that the test is used to monitor therapeutic levels and detect toxic levels of acetaminophen and salicylate.

➤ Obtain a complete history of the time and amount of drug ingested by the patient.

➤ Obtain a history of the patient's complaints, including a list of known allergens (especially allergies or sensitivities to latex), and inform the appropriate health care practitioner accordingly.

➤ Review results of previously performed laboratory tests, surgical procedures, and other diagnostic procedures. For related laboratory tests, refer to the Genitourinary, Hepatobiliary, and Therapeutic/Toxicology System tables.

➤ Obtain a list of the medications the patient is taking, including herbs, nutritional supplements, and nutraceuticals. The requesting health care practitioner and laboratory should be advised if the patient is regularly using these products so that their effects can be taken into consideration when reviewing results.

➤ Review the procedure with the patient. Inform the patient that specimen collection takes approximately 5 to 10 minutes. Address concerns about pain related to the procedure. Explain to the patient that there may be some discomfort during the venipuncture.

➤ *Sensitivity to cultural and social issues,* as well as concern for modesty, is important in providing psychological support before, during, and after the procedure.

➤ There are no food, fluid, or medication restrictions unless by medical direction.

Intratest:

➤ If the patient has a history of severe allergic reaction to latex, care should be taken to avoid the use of equipment containing latex.

➤ Instruct the patient to cooperate fully and to follow directions. Direct the patient to breathe normally and to avoid unnecessary movement.

➤ Observe standard precautions, and follow the general guidelines in Appendix A. Positively identify the patient, and label the appropriate tubes with the corresponding patient demographics, date, and time of collection, noting the last dose of medication taken. Perform a venipuncture; collect the specimen in a 5-mL red-top tube.

➤ Remove the needle, place a gauze over the puncture site and apply gentle pressure to stop the bleeding. Observe the venipuncture site for bleeding and hematoma formation. Apply paper tape over gauze or replace with adhesive bandage.

➤ Promptly transport the specimen to the laboratory for processing and analysis.

➤ The results are recorded manually or in a computerized system for recall and postprocedure interpretation by the appropriate health care practitioner.

Post-test:

➤ *Nutritional considerations* include the avoidance of alcohol consumption.

➤ A written report of the examination will be sent to the requesting health care practitioner, who will discuss the results with the patient.

➤ Reinforce information given by the patient's health care provider regarding further testing, treatment, or referral to another health care provider. Explain to the patient the importance of following the medication regimen and instructions regarding food and drug interactions. Answer any questions or address any concerns voiced by the patient or family.

➤ Instruct the patient to be prepared to provide the pharmacist with a list of other medications he or she is already taking in the event that the requesting health care practitioner prescribes a medication.

➤ Depending on the results of this procedure, additional testing may be performed to evaluate or monitor progression of the disease process and determine the need for a change in therapy. Evaluate test results in relation to the patient's symptoms and other tests performed.

Related laboratory tests:

➤ Related laboratory tests include activated partial thromboplastin time, ALT, AST, bilirubin, blood urea nitrogen, complete blood count, creatinine, electrolytes, glucose, lactic acid, liver biopsy, and prothrombin time.

ANGIOGRAPHY, ABDOMEN

· ·

SYNONYMS/ACRONYM: Abdominal angiogram, abdominal arteriography.

AREA OF APPLICATION: Abdomen.

CONTRAST: Intravenous iodine based.

DESCRIPTION & RATIONALE: Angiography allows x-ray visualization of the large and small arteries, veins, and associated branches of the abdominal vasculature and organ parenchyma after contrast-medium injection. This visualization is accomplished by the injection of contrast medium through a catheter, which most commonly has been inserted into the femoral artery or vein and advanced through the iliac artery and aorta into the organ-specific artery or vein. Images of the organ under study and associated vessels are displayed on a monitor and recorded on film or stored electronically for future viewing and evaluation. Patterns of circulation, organ function, and changes in vessel wall appearance can be viewed to help diagnose the presence of vascular abnormalities, aneurysm, tumor, trauma, or lesions. The catheter used to administer the contrast medium to confirm the diagnosis of organ lesions may be used to deliver chemotherapeutic drugs or different types of media to stop bleeding. Catheters with attached inflatable balloons and wire mesh stents are used to widen areas of stenosis and to keep the vessels open, frequently replacing surgery. Angiography is one of the definitive tests for organ disease and may be used to evaluate chronic disease, evaluate organ failure, treat arterial stenosis, differentiate a vascular cyst from hypervascular cancers, and evaluate the effectiveness of medical or surgical treatment. ■

INDICATIONS:

- Aid in angioplasty, atherectomy, or stent placement
- Allow infusion of thrombolytic drugs into an occluded artery
- Detect arterial occlusion, which may be evidenced by a transection of the artery caused by trauma or penetrating injury
- Detect artery stenosis, evidenced by vessel dilation, collateral vessels, or increased vascular pressure
- Detect nonmalignant tumors before surgical resection
- Detect thrombosis, arteriovenous fistula, aneurysms, or emboli in abdominal vessels
- Detect tumors and arterial supply, extent of venous invasion, and tumor vascularity
- Differentiate between tumors and cysts
- Evaluate organ transplantation for function or organ rejection
- Evaluate placement of a shunt or stent
- Evaluate tumor vascularity before surgery or embolization
- Evaluate the vascular system of prospective organ donors before surgery

RESULT

Normal Findings:
- Normal structure, function, and patency of abdominal organ vessels
- Contrast medium normally circulates throughout abdomen symmetrically and without interruption
- No evidence of obstruction, variations in number and size of vessels and organs, malformations, cysts, or tumors

Abnormal Findings:
- Abscess or inflammation
- Arterial aneurysm
- Arterial stenosis, dysplasia, or organ infarction
- Arteriovenous fistula or other abnormalities
- Congenital anomalies
- Cysts or tumors
- Organ hematoma
- Trauma causing tears or other disruption

INTERFERING FACTORS

This procedure is contraindicated for:

- ⚠ Patients with allergies to shellfish or iodinated dye. The contrast medium used may cause a life-threatening allergic reaction. Patients with a known hypersensitivity to contrast medium may benefit from premedication with corticosteroids or the use of nonionic contrast medium.
- Patients with bleeding disorders.
- Patients who are pregnant or suspected of being pregnant, unless the potential benefits of the procedure far outweigh the risks to the fetus and mother.
- ⚠ Elderly and other patients who are chronically dehydrated before

the test, because of their risk of contrast-induced renal failure.

- Patients who are in renal failure.

***Factors that may impair
clear imaging:***

- Gas or feces in the gastrointestinal tract resulting from inadequate cleansing or failure to restrict food intake before the study
- Retained barium from a previous radiologic procedure
- Metallic objects within the examination field (e.g., jewelry, body rings), which may inhibit organ visualization and can produce unclear images
- Improper adjustment of the radiographic equipment to accommodate obese or thin patients, which can cause overexposure or underexposure and a poor-quality study
- Patients who are very obese, who may exceed the weight limit for the equipment
- Incorrect positioning of the patient, which may produce poor visualization of the area to be examined
- Inability of the patient to cooperate or remain still during the procedure because of age, significant pain, or mental status

Other considerations:

- Consultation with a health care practitioner should occur before the procedure for radiation safety concerns regarding younger patients or patients who are lactating.
- Risks associated with radiographic overexposure can result from frequent x-ray procedures. Personnel in the room with the patient should wear a protective lead apron, stand behind a shield, or leave the area while the examination is being done. Personnel working in the area where the examination is being done should wear badges that reveal their level of exposure to radiation.
- Failure to follow dietary restrictions and other pretesting preparations may cause the procedure to be canceled or repeated.

Nursing Implications and Procedure

Pretest: ■

➤ Inform the patient that the procedure assesses cardiovascular function.

➤ Obtain a history of the patient's complaints, including a list of known allergens (especially allergies or sensitivities to latex, iodine, seafood, contrast medium, anesthetics, or dyes), and inform the appropriate health care practitioner accordingly.

➤ Obtain a history of results of previously performed diagnostic procedures, surgical procedures, and laboratory tests. Ensure that the results of blood tests are obtained and recorded before the procedure, especially coagulation tests, blood urea nitrogen, and creatinine, if contrast medium is to be used. For related diagnostic tests, refer to the Cardiovascular System table.

➤ Note any recent procedures that can interfere with test results, including examinations using iodine-based contrast medium or barium.

➤ Record the date of the last menstrual period and determine the possibility of pregnancy in perimenopausal women.

➤ Obtain a list of the medications the patient is taking, especially medications known to affect bleeding, including anticoagulant therapy, aspirin and other salicylates. Include herbs, nutritional supplements, and nutraceuticals (see Appendix F: Effects of Natural Products on Laboratory Values). It is recommended that use of such products be discontinued 14 days before surgical procedures. The requesting health care practitioner and laboratory should be advised if the patient regularly uses these products so that their effects can be taken into consideration when reviewing results.

➤ Patients receiving metformin (glucophage) for non–insulin-dependent (type 2) diabetes should discontinue the drug on the day of the test and continue to withhold it for 48 hours after the test. Failure to do so may result in lactic acidosis.

➤ Review the procedure with the patient. Address concerns about pain related to the procedure. Explain to the patient that some pain may be experienced during the test, or there may be moments of discomfort. Inform the patient that the procedure is performed in a special department, usually in a radiology or vascular suite, by a health care practitioner and support staff and takes approximately 30 to 60 minutes.

➤ *Sensitivity to social and cultural issues,* as well as concern for modesty, is important in providing psychological support before, during, and after the procedure.

➤ Explain that an intravenous (IV) line may be inserted to allow infusion of IV fluids, contrast medium, dye, or sedatives. Usually normal saline is infused.

➤ Inform the patient that a burning and flushing sensation may be felt throughout the body during injection of the contrast medium. After injection of the contrast medium, the patient may experience an urge to cough, flushing, nausea, or a salty or metallic taste.

➤ The patient should fast and restrict fluids for 8 hours prior to the procedure. Instruct the patient to avoid taking anticoagulant medication or to reduce dosage as ordered prior to the procedure.

➤ Instruct the patient to remove dentures, jewelry (including watches), hairpins, credit cards, and other metallic objects in the area to be examined.

➤ *Make sure a written and informed consent has been signed prior to the procedure and before administering any medications.*

➤ This procedure may be terminated if chest pain, severe cardiac arrhythmias, or signs of a cerebrovascular accident occur.

Intratest:

➤ Ensure that the patient has complied with dietary and medication restrictions and pretesting preparations; assure that food and medications have been restricted for at least 8 hours prior to the procedure. Ensure that the patient has removed jewelry, dentures, all external metallic objects, and the like prior to the procedure.

➤ Have emergency equipment readily available.

➤ If the patient has a history of severe allergic reactions to any substance or drug, administer ordered prophylactic steroids or antihistamines before the procedure. Use nonionic contrast medium for the procedure.

➤ Patients are given a gown, robe, and foot coverings to wear and instructed to void prior to the procedure.

➤ Observe standard precautions, and follow the general guidelines in Appendix A.

➤ Record baseline vital signs, and assess neurologic status. Protocols may vary from facility to facility.

➤ Instruct the patient to cooperate fully and to follow directions. Instruct the patient to remain still throughout the procedure because movement produces unreliable results.

➤ Establish an IV fluid line for the injection of emergency drugs and of sedatives.

➤ Administer an antianxiety agent, as ordered, if the patient has claustrophobia. Administer a sedative to a child or to an uncooperative adult, as ordered.

➤ Place electrocardiographic electrodes on the patient for cardiac monitoring. Establish a baseline rhythm; determine if the patient has ventricular arrhythmias.

➤ Using a pen, mark the site of the patient's peripheral pulses before angiography; this allows for quicker and more consistent assessment of the pulses after the procedure.

➤ Place the patient in the supine position on an exam table. Cleanse the selected area, and cover with a sterile drape.

➤ A local anesthetic is injected at the site, and a small incision is made or a needle inserted under fluoroscopy.

➤ The contrast medium is injected, and a rapid series of images is taken during and after the filling of the vessels to be examined. Delayed images may be taken to examine the vessels after a time and to monitor the venous phase of the procedure.

➤ Instruct the patient to inhale deeply and hold his or her breath while the x-ray images are taken, and then to exhale after the images are taken.

➤ Instruct the patient to take slow, deep breaths if nausea occurs during the procedure.

➤ Monitor the patient for complications related to the procedure (e.g., allergic reaction, anaphylaxis, bronchospasm).

➤ The needle or catheter is removed, and a pressure dressing is applied over the puncture site.

➤ The results are recorded on x-ray film or electronically in a computerized system for recall and postprocedure interpretation by the appropriate health care practitioner.

Post-test:

➤ Instruct the patient to resume usual diet, fluids, medications, or activity, as directed by the health care practitioner. Renal function should be assessed before metformin is resumed.

➤ Monitor vital signs and neurologic status every 15 minutes for 1 hour, then every 2 hours for 4 hours, and as ordered. Take the temperature every 4 hours for 24 hours. Compare with baseline values. Protocols may vary from facility to facility.

➤ Observe for delayed allergic reactions, such as rash, urticaria, tachycardia, hyperpnea, hypertension, palpitations, nausea, or vomiting.

➤ Instruct the patient to immediately report symptoms such as fast heart rate, difficulty breathing, skin rash, itching, or decreased urinary output.

➤ Assess extremities for signs of ischemia or absence of distal pulse caused by a catheter-induced thrombus.

➤ Observe the needle/catheter insertion site for bleeding, inflammation, or hematoma formation.

➤ Instruct the patient to apply cold compresses to the puncture site, as needed, to reduce discomfort or edema.

➤ Instruct the patient to maintain bed rest for 4 to 6 hours after the procedure or as ordered.

➤ Instruct the patient in the care and assessment of the site and to observe for bleeding, hematoma formation, bile leakage, and inflammation. Note any pleuritic pain, persistent right shoulder pain, or abdominal pain.

➤ *Nutritional considerations:* A low-fat, low-cholesterol, and low-sodium diet should be consumed to reduce current disease processes and/or decrease risk of hypertension and coronary artery disease.

➤ No other radionuclide tests should be scheduled for 24 to 48 hours after this procedure.

➤ A written report of the examination will be completed by a health care practitioner specializing in this branch of medicine. The report will be sent to the requesting health care practitioner, who will discuss the results with the patient.

➤ Recognize anxiety related to test results, and be supportive of perceived loss of independent function. Discuss the implications of abnormal test results on the patient's lifestyle.

Provide teaching and information regarding the clinical implications of the test results, as appropriate.

➤ Reinforce information given by the patient's health care provider regarding further testing, treatment, or referral to another health care provider. Answer any questions or address any concerns voiced by the patient or family.

➤ Instruct the patient in the use of any ordered medications. Explain the importance of adhering to the therapy regimen. As appropriate, instruct the patient in significant side effects and systemic reactions associated with the prescribed medication. Encourage him or her to review cor-

responding literature provided by a pharmacist.

➤ Depending on the results of this procedure, additional testing may be performed to evaluate or monitor progression of the disease process and determine the need for a change in therapy. Evaluate test results in relation to the patient's symptoms and other tests performed.

Related diagnostic tests:

➤ Related diagnostic tests include computed tomography of the abdomen; kidney, ureter, and bladder study; magnetic resonance imaging of the abdomen, and magnetic resonance angiography.

ANGIOGRAPHY, ADRENAL

SYNONYMS/ACRONYM: Adrenal angiogram, adrenal arteriography.

AREA OF APPLICATION: Adrenal gland.

CONTRAST: Intravenous iodine based.

DESCRIPTION & RATIONALE: Adrenal angiography evaluates adrenal dysfunction by allowing x-ray visualization of the large and small arteries of the adrenal gland vasculature and parenchyma. This visualization is accomplished by the injection of contrast medium through a catheter that has been inserted into the femoral artery for viewing the artery (arteriography) or into the femoral vein for viewing the veins (venography). After the catheter is in place, a blood sample

may be taken from the vein of each gland to assess cortisol levels in determining a diagnosis of Cushing's syndrome or the presence of pheochromocytoma. After injection of the contrast medium through the catheter, images of the adrenal glands and associated vessels surrounding the adrenal tissue are displayed on a monitor and are recorded on film or electronically. Patterns of circulation, adrenal function, and changes in vessel wall appearance can be viewed to help diagnose the presence of vascular abnormalities, trauma, or lesions. This definitive test for adrenal disease may be used to evaluate chronic adrenal disease, evaluate arterial or venous stenosis, differentiate an adrenal cyst from adrenal tumors, and evaluate medical therapy or surgery of the adrenal glands. ■

INDICATIONS:

- Assist in the infusion of thrombolytic drugs into an occluded artery
- Assist with the collection of blood samples from the vein for laboratory analysis
- Detect adrenal hyperplasia
- Detect and determine the location of adrenal tumors evidenced by arterial supply, extent of venous invasion, and tumor vascularity
- Detect arterial occlusion, evidenced by a transection of the artery caused by trauma or a penetrating injury
- Detect arterial stenosis, evidenced by vessel dilation, collateral vessels, or increased vascular pressure
- Detect nonmalignant tumors before surgical resection
- Detect thrombosis, arteriovenous fistula, aneurysms, or emboli in vessels
- Differentiate between adrenal tumors and adrenal cysts
- Evaluate tumor vascularity before surgery or embolization
- Perform angioplasty, perform atherectomy, or place a stent

RESULT

Normal Findings:

- Normal structure, function, and patency of adrenal vessels
- Contrast medium circulating throughout the adrenal gland symmetrically and without interruption

- No evidence of obstruction, variations in number and size of vessels and organs, malformations, cysts, or tumors

Abnormal Findings:

- Adrenal adenoma
- Adrenal carcinoma
- Bilateral adrenal hyperplasia
- Pheochromocytoma

INTERFERING FACTORS

This procedure is contraindicated for:

- ⚠ Patients with allergies to shellfish or iodinated dye. The contrast medium used may cause a life-threatening allergic reaction. Patients with a known hypersensitivity to contrast medium may benefit from premedication with corticosteroids or the use of nonionic contrast medium.
- Patients with bleeding disorders.
- Patients who are pregnant or suspected of being pregnant, unless the potential benefits of the procedure far outweigh the risks to the fetus and mother.
- ⚠ Elderly and other patients who are chronically dehydrated before the test, because of their risk of contrast-induced renal failure.
- ⚠ Patients who are in renal failure.

Factors that may impair clear imaging:

- Gas or feces in the gastrointestinal tract resulting from inadequate cleansing or failure to restrict food intake before the study
- Retained barium from a previous radiologic procedure
- Metallic objects within the examination field (e.g., jewelry, body rings, dental amalgams), which may inhibit organ visualization and can produce unclear images

- Improper adjustment of the radiographic equipment to accommodate obese or thin patients, which can cause overexposure or underexposure and a poor-quality study

- Patients who are very obese, who may exceed the weight limit for the equipment

- Incorrect positioning of the patient, which may produce poor visualization of the area to be examined

- Inability of the patient to cooperate or remain still during the procedure because of age, significant pain, or mental status

Other considerations:

- Consultation with a health care practitioner should occur before the procedure for radiation safety concerns regarding younger patients or patients who are lactating.

- Risks associated with radiographic overexposure can result from frequent x-ray procedures. Personnel in the room with the patient should wear a protective lead apron, stand behind a shield, or leave the area while the examination is being done. Personnel working in the area where the examination is being done should wear badges that reveal their level of exposure to radiation.

- Failure to follow dietary restrictions and other pretesting preparations may cause the procedure to be canceled or repeated.

Nursing Implications and Procedure • • • • • • • • • • •

Pretest:

➤ Inform the patient that the procedure assesses cardiovascular function.

➤ Obtain a history of the patient's complaints, including a list of known allergens (especially allergies or sensitivities to latex, iodine, seafood, contrast medium, anesthetics, or dyes), and inform the appropriate health care practitioner accordingly.

➤ Obtain a history of results of previously performed diagnostic procedures, surgical procedures, and laboratory tests. Ensure that the results of blood tests are obtained and recorded before the procedure, especially coagulation tests, blood urea nitrogen, and creatinine, if contrast medium is to be used. For related diagnostic tests, refer to the Cardiovascular and Endocrine System tables.

➤ Note any recent procedures that can interfere with test results, including examinations using iodine-based contrast medium.

➤ Record the date of the last menstrual period and determine the possibility of pregnancy in perimenopausal women.

➤ Obtain a list of the medications the patient is taking, especially medications known to affect bleeding, including anticoagulant therapy, aspirin and other salicylates, herbs, nutritional supplements, and nutraceuticals (see Appendix F: Effects of Natural Products on Laboratory Values). It is recommended that use of such products be discontinued 14 days before surgical procedures. The requesting health care practitioner and laboratory should be advised if the patient regularly uses these products so that their effects can be taken into consideration when reviewing results.

➤ Patients receiving metformin (glucophage) for non–insulin-dependent (type 2) diabetes should discontinue the drug on the day of the test and continue to withhold it for 48 hours after the test. Failure to do so may result in lactic acidosis.

➤ Review the procedure with the patient. Address concerns about pain related to the procedure. Explain to the patient that some pain may be experienced during the test, or there may be moments of discomfort. Inform the patient that the procedure is performed in a special department, usually in a radiology or vascular suite, by a health care practitioner and support staff and takes approximately 30 to 60 minutes.

➤ *Sensitivity to social and cultural issues,* as well as concern for modesty, is important in providing psychological support before, during, and after the procedure.

➤ Explain that an intravenous (IV) line may be inserted to allow infusion of IV fluids, contrast medium, dye, or sedatives. Usually normal saline is infused.

➤ Inform the patient that a burning and flushing sensation may be felt throughout the body during injection of the contrast medium. After injection of the contrast medium, the patient may experience an urge to cough, flushing, nausea, or a salty or metallic taste.

➤ The patient should fast and restrict fluids for 8 hours prior to the procedure. Instruct the patient to avoid taking anticoagulant medication or to reduce dosage as ordered prior to the procedure.

➤ Instruct the patient to remove dentures, jewelry (including watches), hairpins, credit cards, and other metallic objects in the area to be examined.

➤ *Make sure a written and informed consent has been signed prior to the procedure and before administering any medications.*

➤ This procedure may be terminated if chest pain, severe cardiac arrhythmias, or signs of a cerebrovascular accident occur.

Intratest:

➤ Ensure that the patient has complied with dietary and medication restrictions and pretesting preparations; assure that food and medications have been restricted for at least 8 hours prior to the procedure. Ensure that the patient has removed jew-elry, dentures, all external metallic objects, and the like prior to the procedure.

➤ Have emergency equipment readily available.

➤ If the patient has a history of severe allergic reactions to any substance or drug, administer ordered prophylactic steroids or antihistamines before the procedure. Use nonionic contrast medium for the procedure.

➤ Patients are given a gown, robe, and foot coverings to wear and instructed to void prior to the procedure.

➤ Observe standard precautions, and follow the general guidelines in Appendix A.

➤ Record baseline vital signs, and assess neurologic status. Protocols may vary from facility to facility.

➤ Instruct the patient to cooperate fully and to follow directions. Instruct the patient to remain still throughout the procedure because movement produces unreliable results.

➤ Establish an IV fluid line for the injection of emergency drugs and of sedatives.

➤ Administer an antianxiety agent, as ordered, if the patient has claustrophobia. Administer a sedative to a child or to an uncooperative adult, as ordered.

➤ Place electrocardiographic electrodes on the patient for cardiac monitoring. Establish a baseline rhythm; determine if the patient has ventricular arrhythmias.

➤ Using a pen, mark the site of the patient's peripheral pulses before angiography; this allows for quicker and more consistent assessment of the pulses after the procedure.

➤ Place the patient in the supine position on an exam table. Cleanse the selected area, and cover with a sterile drape.

➤ A local anesthetic is injected at the site, and a small incision is made or a needle inserted under fluoroscopy.

➤ The contrast medium is injected, and a rapid series of images is taken during and after the filling of the vessels to be examined. Delayed images may be taken to examine the vessels after a time and to monitor the venous phase of the procedure.

➤ Ask the patient to inhale deeply and hold his or her breath while the x-ray images are taken, and then to exhale after the images are taken.

➤ Instruct the patient to take slow, deep breaths if nausea occurs during the procedure.

➤ Monitor the patient for complications related to the procedure (e.g., allergic reaction, anaphylaxis, bronchospasm).

➤ The needle or catheter is removed, and a pressure dressing is applied over the puncture site.

➤ The results are recorded on x-ray film or electronically in a computerized system for recall and postprocedure interpretation by the appropriate health care practitioner.

Post-test:

➤ Instruct the patient to resume usual diet, fluids, medications, or activity, as directed by the health care practitioner. Renal function should be assessed before metformin is resumed.

➤ Monitor vital signs and neurologic status every 15 minutes for 1 hour, then every 2 hours for 4 hours, and as ordered. Take the temperature every 4 hours for 24 hours. Compare with baseline values. Protocols may vary from facility to facility.

➤ Observe for delayed allergic reactions, such as rash, urticaria, tachycardia, hyperpnea, hypertension, palpitations, nausea, or vomiting.

➤ Advise the patient to immediately report symptoms such as fast heart rate, difficulty breathing, skin rash, itching, or decreased urinary output.

➤ Assess extremities for signs of ischemia or absence of distal pulse caused by a catheter-induced thrombus.

➤ Observe the needle/catheter insertion site for bleeding, inflammation, or hematoma formation.

➤ Instruct the patient to apply cold compresses to the puncture site, as needed, to reduce discomfort or edema.

➤ Instruct the patient to maintain bed rest for 4 to 6 hours after the procedure or as ordered.

➤ Instruct the patient in the care and assessment of the site and to observe for bleeding, hematoma formation, bile leakage, and inflammation. Note any pleuritic pain, persistent right shoulder pain, or abdominal pain.

➤ *Nutritional considerations:* A low-fat, low-cholesterol, and low-sodium diet should be consumed to reduce current disease processes and/or decrease risk of hypertension and coronary artery disease.

➤ No other radionuclide tests should be scheduled for 24 to 48 hours after this procedure.

➤ A written report of the examination will be completed by a health care practitioner specializing in this branch of medicine. The report will be sent to the requesting health care practitioner, who will discuss the results with the patient.

➤ Recognize anxiety related to test results, and be supportive of perceived loss of independent function. Discuss the implications of abnormal test results on the patient's lifestyle. Provide teaching and information regarding the clinical implications of the test results, as appropriate.

➤ Reinforce information given by the patient's health care provider regarding further testing, treatment, or referral to another health care provider. Answer any questions or address any concerns voiced by the patient or family.

➤ Instruct the patient in the use of any ordered medications. Explain the importance of adhering to the therapy regimen. As appropriate, instruct the patient in significant side effects and systemic reactions associated with the prescribed medication. Encourage him or her to review corresponding literature provided by a pharmacist.

➤ Depending on the results of this procedure, additional testing may be performed to evaluate or monitor progression of the disease process and determine the need for a change in therapy. Evaluate test results in relation to the patient's symptoms and other tests performed.

Related diagnostic tests:

➤ Related diagnostic tests include adrenal gland scan; computed tomography of the abdomen; kidney, ureter, and bladder study; and magnetic resonance imaging of the abdomen.

ANGIOGRAPHY, CAROTID

SYNONYMS/ACRONYM: Carotid angiogram, carotid arteriography.

AREA OF APPLICATION: Neck/cervical spine area.

CONTRAST: Intravenous iodine based.

DESCRIPTION & RATIONALE: The test evaluates blood vessels in the neck carrying arterial blood. This visualization is accomplished by the injection of contrast material through a catheter that has been inserted into the femoral artery for viewing the artery (arteriography). The angiographic catheter is a long tube about the size of a strand of spaghetti. After the injection of contrast media through the catheter, x-ray images of the carotid artery and associated vessels in surrounding tissue are displayed on a monitor and are recorded on film or electronically. The x-ray equipment is mounted on a C-shaped bed with the x-ray device beneath the table on which the patient lies. Over the patient is an image intensifier that receives the x-rays after they pass through the patient. Patterns of circulation or changes in vessel wall appearance can be viewed to help diagnose the presence of vascular abnormalities, disease, narrowing, enlargement, blockage, trauma, or lesions. This definitive test for arterial disease may be used to evaluate chronic vascular disease, arterial or venous stenosis, and medical therapy or surgery of the vasculature. Catheter angiography still is used in patients who may undergo surgery, angioplasty, or stent placement. ■

INDICATIONS:

- Aid in angioplasty, atherectomy, or stent placement
- Allow infusion of thrombolytic drugs into an occluded artery
- Detect arterial occlusion, which may be evidenced by a transection of the artery caused by trauma or penetrating injury
- Detect artery stenosis, evidenced by vessel dilation, collateral vessels, or increased vascular pressure
- Detect nonmalignant tumors before surgical resection
- Detect tumors and arterial supply, extent of venous invasion, and tumor vascularity
- Detect thrombosis, arteriovenous fistula, aneurysms, or emboli in vessels
- Differentiate between tumors and cysts
- Evaluate placement of a stent
- Evaluate tumor vascularity before surgery or embolization
- Evaluate the vascular system of prospective organ donors before surgery

RESULT

Normal Findings:

- Normal structure, function, and patency of carotid vessels
- Contrast medium normally circulates throughout neck symmetrically and without interruption
- No evidence of obstruction, variations in number and size of vessels, malformations, cysts, or tumors

Abnormal Findings:

- Abscess or inflammation
- Arterial aneurysm
- Arterial stenosis or dysplasia
- Arteriovenous fistula or other abnormalities
- Congenital anomalies
- Cysts or tumors
- Trauma causing tears or other disruption
- Vascular blockage or other disruption

INTERFERING FACTORS

This procedure is contraindicated for:

- ⚠️ Patients with allergies to shellfish or iodinated dye. The contrast medium used may cause a life-threatening allergic reaction. Patients with a known hypersensitivity to contrast medium may benefit from premedication with corticosteroids or the use of nonionic contrast medium.
- Patients with bleeding disorders.
- Patients who are pregnant or suspected of being pregnant, unless the potential benefits of the procedure far outweigh the risks to the fetus and mother.
- ⚠️ Elderly and other patients who are chronically dehydrated before the test, because of their risk of contrast-induced renal failure.
- ⚠️ Patients who are in renal failure.

Factors that may impair clear imaging:

- Gas or feces in the gastrointestinal tract resulting from inadequate cleansing or failure to restrict food intake before the study
- Retained barium from a previous radiologic procedure
- Metallic objects within the examination field (e.g., jewelry, body rings, dental amalgams), which may inhibit organ visualization and can produce unclear images
- Improper adjustment of the radiographic equipment to accommodate obese or thin patients, which can cause overexposure or underexposure and a poor-quality study

- Patients who are very obese, who may exceed the weight limit for the equipment

- Incorrect positioning of the patient, which may produce poor visualization of the area to be examined

- Inability of the patient to cooperate or remain still during the procedure because of age, significant pain, or mental status

Other considerations:
- Consultation with a health care practitioner should occur before the procedure for radiation safety concerns regarding younger patients or patients who are lactating.

- Risks associated with radiographic overexposure can result from frequent x-ray procedures. Personnel in the room with the patient should wear a protective lead apron, stand behind a shield, or leave the area while the examination is being done. Personnel working in the area where the examination is being done should wear badges that reveal their level of exposure to radiation.

- Failure to follow dietary restrictions and other pretesting preparations may cause the procedure to be canceled or repeated.

Nursing Implications and Procedure • • • • • • • • • •

Pretest:

➤ Inform the patient that the procedure assesses cardiovascular function.

➤ Obtain a history of the patient's complaints, including a list of known allergens (especially allergies or sensitivities to latex, iodine, seafood, contrast medium, anesthetics, or dyes), and inform the appropriate health care practitioner accordingly.

➤ Obtain a history of results of previously performed diagnostic procedures, surgical procedures, and laboratory tests. Ensure that the results of blood tests are obtained and recorded before the procedure, especially coagulation tests, blood urea nitrogen, and creatinine, if contrast medium is to be used. For related diagnostic tests, refer to the Cardiovascular System table.

➤ Note any recent procedures that can interfere with test results, including examinations using iodine-based contrast medium.

➤ Record the date of the last menstrual period and determine the possibility of pregnancy in perimenopausal women.

➤ Obtain a list of the medications the patient is taking, especially medications known to affect bleeding, including anticoagulant therapy, aspirin and other salicylates, herbs, nutritional supplements, and nutraceuticals (see Appendix F: Effects of Natural Products on Laboratory Values). It is recommended that use of such products be discontinued 14 days before surgical procedures. The requesting health care practitioner and laboratory should be advised if the patient regularly uses these products so that their effects can be taken into consideration when reviewing results.

➤ Patients receiving metformin (glucophage) for non–insulin-dependent (type 2) diabetes should discontinue the drug on the day of the test and continue to withhold it for 48 hours after the test. Failure to do so may result in lactic acidosis.

➤ Review the procedure with the patient. Address concerns about pain related to the procedure. Explain to the patient that some pain may be experienced during the test, or there may be moments of discomfort. Inform the patient that the procedure is performed in a special department, usually in a radiology or vascular suite, by a health care practitioner and support staff and takes approximately 30 to 60 minutes.

▶ *Sensitivity to social and cultural issues,* as well as concern for modesty, is important in providing psychological support before, during, and after the procedure.

▶ Explain that an intravenous (IV) line may be inserted to allow infusion of IV fluids, contrast medium, dye, or sedatives. Usually normal saline is infused.

▶ Inform the patient that a burning and flushing sensation may be felt throughout the body during injection of the contrast medium. After injection of the contrast medium, the patient may experience an urge to cough, flushing, nausea, or a salty or metallic taste.

▶ The patient should fast and restrict fluids for 8 hours prior to the procedure. Instruct the patient to avoid taking anticoagulant medication or to reduce dosage as ordered prior to the procedure.

▶ Instruct the patient to remove dentures, jewelry (including watches), hairpins, credit cards, and other metallic objects in the area to be examined.

▶ *Make sure a written and informed consent has been signed prior to the procedure and before administering any medications.*

▶ This procedure may be terminated if chest pain, severe cardiac arrhythmias, or signs of a cerebrovascular accident occur.

Intratest:

▶ Ensure that the patient has complied with dietary, medication, or activity restrictions and pretesting preparations; assure that food and medications have been restricted for at least 8 hours prior to the procedure. Ensure that the patient has removed jewelry, dentures, all external metallic objects, and the like prior to the procedure.

▶ Have emergency equipment readily available.

▶ If the patient has a history of severe allergic reactions to any substance or drug, administer ordered prophylactic steroids or antihistamines before the procedure. Use nonionic contrast medium for the procedure.

▶ Patients are given a gown, robe, and foot coverings to wear and instructed to void prior to the procedure.

▶ Observe standard precautions, and follow the general guidelines in Appendix A.

▶ Record baseline vital signs, and assess neurologic status. Protocols may vary from facility to facility.

▶ Instruct the patient to cooperate fully and to follow directions. Instruct the patient to remain still throughout the procedure because movement produces unreliable results.

▶ Establish an IV fluid line for the injection of emergency drugs and of sedatives.

▶ Administer an antianxiety agent, as ordered, if the patient has claustrophobia. Administer a sedative to a child or to an uncooperative adult, as ordered.

▶ Place electrocardiographic electrodes on the patient for cardiac monitoring. Establish a baseline rhythm; determine if the patient has ventricular arrhythmias.

▶ Using a pen, mark the site of the patient's peripheral pulses before angiography; this allows for quicker and more consistent assessment of the pulses after the procedure.

▶ Place the patient in the supine position on an exam table. Cleanse the selected area, and cover with a sterile drape.

▶ A local anesthetic is injected at the site, and a small incision is made or a needle inserted under fluoroscopy.

▶ The contrast medium is injected, and a rapid series of images is taken during and after the filling of the vessels to be examined. Delayed images may be taken to examine the vessels after a time and to monitor the venous phase of the procedure.

▶ Ask the patient to inhale deeply and hold his or her breath while the x-ray images are taken, and then to exhale after the images are taken.

➤ Instruct the patient to take slow, deep breaths if nausea occurs during the procedure.

➤ Monitor the patient for complications related to the procedure (e.g., allergic reaction, anaphylaxis, bronchospasm).

➤ The needle or catheter is removed, and a pressure dressing is applied over the puncture site.

➤ The results are recorded on x-ray film or electronically in a computerized system for recall and postprocedure interpretation by the appropriate health care practitioner.

Post-test:

➤ Instruct the patient to resume usual diet, fluids, medications, or activity, as directed by the health care practitioner. Renal function should be assessed before metformin is resumed.

➤ Monitor vital signs and neurologic status every 15 minutes for 1 hour, then every 2 hours for 4 hours, and as ordered. Take the temperature every 4 hours for 24 hours. Compare with baseline values. Protocols may vary from facility to facility.

➤ Observe for delayed allergic reactions, such as rash, urticaria, tachycardia, hyperpnea, hypertension, palpitations, nausea, or vomiting.

➤ Instruct the patient to immediately report symptoms such as fast heart rate, difficulty breathing, skin rash, itching, or decreased urinary output.

➤ Assess extremities for signs of ischemia or absence of distal pulse caused by a catheter-induced thrombus.

➤ Observe the needle/catheter insertion site for bleeding, inflammation, or hematoma formation.

➤ Instruct the patient to apply cold compresses to the puncture site, as needed, to reduce discomfort or edema.

➤ Instruct the patient to maintain bed rest for 4 to 6 hours after the procedure or as ordered.

➤ Instruct the patient in the care and assessment of the site and to observe for bleeding, hematoma formation, bile leakage, and inflammation. Note any pleuritic pain, persistent right shoulder pain, or abdominal pain.

➤ *Nutritional considerations:* A low-fat, low-cholesterol, and low-sodium diet should be consumed to reduce current disease processes and/or decrease risk of hypertension and coronary artery disease.

➤ No other radionuclide tests should be scheduled for 24 to 48 hours after this procedure.

➤ A written report of the examination will be completed by a health care practitioner specializing in this branch of medicine. The report will be sent to the requesting health care practitioner, who will discuss the results with the patient.

➤ Recognize anxiety related to test results, and be supportive of perceived loss of independent function. Discuss the implications of abnormal test results on the patient's lifestyle. Provide teaching and information regarding the clinical implications of the test results, as appropriate.

➤ Reinforce information given by the patient's health care provider regarding further testing, treatment, or referral to another health care provider. Answer any questions or address any concerns voiced by the patient or family.

➤ Instruct the patient in the use of any ordered medications. Explain the importance of adhering to the therapy regimen. As appropriate, instruct the patient in significant side effects and systemic reactions associated with the prescribed medication. Encourage him or her to review corresponding literature provided by a pharmacist.

➤ Depending on the results of this pro-

cedure, additional testing may be performed to evaluate or monitor progression of the disease process and determine the need for a change in therapy. Evaluate test results in relation to the patient's symptoms and other tests performed.

Related diagnostic tests:

➤ Related diagnostic tests include computed tomography angiography, magnetic resonance angiography, and ultrasound, arterial Doppler carotid studies.

ANGIOGRAPHY, CORONARY

SYNONYMS/ACRONYM: Angiocardiography, cardiac angiography, cardiac catheterization, cineangiocardiography, coronary arteriography.

AREA OF APPLICATION: Heart.

CONTRAST: Intravenous iodine based.

DESCRIPTION & RATIONALE: Angiography allows x-ray visualization of the heart, aorta, inferior vena cava, pulmonary artery and vein, and coronary arteries after injection of contrast medium. Contrast medium is injected through a catheter, which has been inserted into a peripheral vein for a right heart catheterization or an artery for a left heart catheterization; through the same catheter, cardiac pressures are recorded. Images of the heart and associated vessels are displayed on a monitor and are recorded on film or electronically. Patterns of circulation, cardiac output, cardiac functions, and changes in vessel wall appearance can be viewed to help diagnose the presence of vascular abnormalities or lesions. Pulmonary artery abnormalities are seen with right heart views, and coronary artery and thoracic aorta

abnormalities are seen with left heart views. Coronary angiography is a definitive test for coronary artery disease, and it is useful for evaluating other types of cardiac abnormalities. ■

INDICATIONS:
• Allow infusion of thrombolytic drugs into an occluded coronary artery
• Detect narrowing of coronary vessels or abnormalities of the great vessels in patients with angina, syncope, abnormal electrocardiogram, hypercholesteremia with chest pain, and persistent chest pain after revascularization
• Evaluate cardiac muscle function
• Evaluate cardiac valvular and septal defects
• Evaluate disease associated with the aortic arch
• Evaluate previous cardiac surgery or other interventional procedures

- Evaluate ventricular aneurysms
- Monitor pulmonary pressures and cardiac output
- Perform angioplasty, perform atherectomy, or place a stent
- Quantify the severity of atherosclerotic, occlusive coronary artery disease

RESULT

Normal Findings:
- Normal great vessels and coronary arteries

Abnormal Findings:
- Aortic atherosclerosis
- Aortic dissection
- Aortitis
- Aneurysms
- Cardiomyopathy
- Congenital anomalies
- Coronary artery atherosclerosis and degree of obstruction
- Graft occlusion
- Pulmonary artery abnormalities
- Septal defects
- Trauma causing tears or other disruption
- Tumors
- Valvular disease

INTERFERING FACTORS

This procedure is contraindicated for:
- Patients with allergies to shellfish or iodinated dye. The contrast medium used may cause a life-threatening allergic reaction. Patients with a known hypersensitivity to contrast medium may benefit from premedication with corticosteroids or the use of nonionic contrast medium.
- Patients with bleeding disorders.

- Patients who are pregnant or suspected of being pregnant, unless the potential benefits of the procedure far outweigh the risk of radiation exposure to the fetus.
- Elderly and compromised patients who are chronically dehydrated before the test, because of their risk of contrast-induced renal failure.
- Patients who are in renal failure.

Factors that may impair clear imaging:
- Gas or feces in the gastrointestinal tract resulting from inadequate cleansing or failure to restrict food intake before the study
- Retained barium from a previous radiologic procedure
- Metallic objects within the examination field (e.g., jewelry, body rings), which may inhibit organ visualization and can produce unclear images
- Improper adjustment of the radiographic equipment to accommodate obese or thin patients, which can cause overexposure or underexposure and a poor-quality study
- Patients who are very obese, who may exceed the weight limit for the equipment
- Incorrect positioning of the patient, which may produce poor visualization of the area to be examined
- Inability of the patient to cooperate or remain still during the procedure because of age, significant pain, or mental status

Other considerations:
- Consultation with a physician should occur before the procedure for radiation safety concerns regarding younger patients or patients who are lactating.
- Risks associated with radiographic overexposure can result from frequent x-ray procedures. Personnel in the room with the patient should wear a protective

lead apron, stand behind a shield, or leave the area while the examination is being done. Personnel working in the area where the examination is being done should wear badges that reveal their level of exposure to radiation.

• Failure to follow dietary restrictions and other pretesting preparations may cause the procedure to be canceled or repeated.

Nursing Implications and Procedure • • • • • • • • • • •

➤ Inform the patient that the procedure assesses cardiovascular function.

➤ Obtain a history of the patient's complaints, including a list of known allergens (especially allergies or sensitivities to latex, iodine, seafood, contrast medium, anesthetics, or dyes), and inform the appropriate health care practitioner accordingly.

➤ Obtain a history of results of previously performed diagnostic procedures, surgical procedures, and laboratory tests. Ensure that the results of blood tests are obtained and recorded before the procedure, especially coagulation tests, blood urea nitrogen, and creatinine, if contrast medium is to be used. For related diagnostic tests, refer to the Cardiovascular and Respiratory System tables.

➤ Note any recent procedures that can interfere with test results, including examinations using iodine-based contrast medium.

➤ Record the date of the last menstrual period and determine the possibility of pregnancy in perimenopausal women.

➤ Obtain a list of the medications the patient is taking, especially medications known to affect bleeding, including anticoagulant therapy, aspirin and other salicylates, herbs, nutritional supplements, and nutraceuticals (see Appendix F: Effects of Natural Products on Laboratory Values). It is recommended that use of such products be discontinued 14 days before surgical procedures. The requesting health care practitioner and laboratory should be advised if the patient regularly uses these products so that their effects can be taken into consideration when reviewing results.

➤ Patients receiving metformin (glucophage) for non–insulin-dependent (type 2) diabetes should discontinue the drug on the day of the test and continue to withhold it for 48 hours after the test. Failure to do so may result in lactic acidosis.

➤ Review the procedure with the patient. Address concerns about pain related to the procedure. Explain to the patient that some pain may be experienced during the test, or there may be moments of discomfort. Inform the patient that the procedure is performed in a special department, usually in a radiology or vascular suite, by a physician and support staff and takes approximately 30 to 60 minutes.

➤ *Sensitivity to cultural and social issues,* as well as concern for modesty, is important in providing psychological support before, during, and after the procedure.

➤ Explain that an intravenous (IV) line may be inserted to allow infusion of IV fluids, contrast medium, dye, or sedatives. Usually normal saline is infused.

➤ Inform the patient that a burning and flushing sensation may be felt throughout the body during injection of the contrast medium. After injection of the contrast medium, the patient may experience an urge to cough, flushing, nausea, or a salty or metallic taste.

➤ The patient should fast and restrict fluids for 8 hours prior to the procedure. Instruct the patient to avoid taking anticoagulant medication or to reduce dosage as ordered prior to the procedure.

➤ Instruct the patient to remove dentures, jewelry (including watches), hairpins, credit cards, and other metallic objects in the area to be examined.

➤ *Make sure a written and informed consent has been signed prior to the procedure and before administering any medications.*

➤ This procedure may be terminated if chest pain, severe cardiac arrhythmias, or signs of a cerebrovascular accident occur.

Intratest:

➤ Ensure that the patient has complied with dietary and medication restrictions and pretesting preparations; assure that food and medications have been restricted for at least 8 hours prior to the procedure. Ensure that the patient has removed jewelry, dentures, all external metallic objects, and the like prior to the procedure.

➤ Have emergency equipment readily available.

➤ If the patient has a history of severe allergic reactions to any substance or drug, administer ordered prophylactic steroids or antihistamines before the procedure. Use nonionic contrast medium for the procedure.

➤ Patients are given a gown, robe, and foot coverings to wear and instructed to void prior to the procedure.

➤ Observe standard precautions, and follow the general guidelines in Appendix A.

➤ Record baseline vital signs, and assess neurologic status. Protocols may vary from facility to facility.

➤ Instruct the patient to cooperate fully and to follow directions. Instruct the patient to remain still throughout the procedure because movement produces unreliable results.

➤ Establish an IV fluid line for the injection of emergency drugs and of sedatives.

➤ Administer an antianxiety agent, as ordered, if the patient has claustrophobia. Administer a sedative to a child or to an uncooperative adult, as ordered.

➤ Place electrocardiographic electrodes on the patient for cardiac monitoring. Establish a baseline rhythm; determine if the patient has ventricular arrhythmias.

➤ Using a pen, mark the site of the patient's peripheral pulses before angiography; this allows for quicker and more consistent assessment of the pulses after the procedure.

➤ Place the patient in the supine position on an exam table. Cleanse the selected area, and cover with a sterile drape.

➤ A local anesthetic is injected at the site, and a small incision is made or a needle inserted under fluoroscopy.

➤ The contrast medium is injected, and a rapid series of images is taken during and after the filling of the vessels to be examined. Delayed images may be taken to examine the vessels after a time and to monitor the venous phase of the procedure.

➤ Ask the patient to inhale deeply and hold his or her breath while the x-ray images are taken, and then to exhale after the images are taken.

➤ Instruct the patient to take slow, deep breaths if nausea occurs during the procedure.

➤ Monitor the patient for complications related to the procedure (e.g., allergic reaction, anaphylaxis, bronchospasm).

➤ The needle or catheter is removed, and a pressure dressing is applied over the puncture site.

➤ The results are recorded on x-ray film or electronically in a computerized system for recall and postprocedure interpretation by the appropriate health care practitioner.

Post-test:

➤ Instruct the patient to resume usual diet, fluids, medications, or activity, as directed by the health care practitioner. Renal function should be assessed before metformin is resumed.

➤ Monitor vital signs and neurologic status every 15 minutes for 1 hour, then every 2 hours for 4 hours, and as ordered. Take the temperature every 4 hours for 24 hours. Compare with baseline values. Protocols may vary from facility to facility.

➤ Observe for delayed allergic reactions, such as rash, urticaria, tachycardia, hyperpnea, hypertension, palpitations, nausea, or vomiting.

➤ Advise the patient to immediately report symptoms such as fast heart rate, difficulty breathing, skin rash, itching, or decreased urinary output.

➤ Assess extremities for signs of ischemia or absence of distal pulse caused by a catheter-induced thrombus.

➤ Observe the needle/catheter insertion site for bleeding, inflammation, or hematoma formation.

➤ Instruct the patient to apply cold compresses to the puncture site, as needed, to reduce discomfort or edema.

➤ Instruct the patient to maintain bed rest for 4 to 6 hours after the procedure or as ordered.

➤ Instruct the patient in the care and assessment of the site and to observe for bleeding, hematoma formation, bile leakage, and inflammation. Note any pleuritic pain, persistent right shoulder pain, or abdominal pain.

➤ A written report of the examination will be completed by a health care practitioner specializing in this branch of medicine. The report will be sent to the requesting health care practitioner, who will discuss the results with the patient.

➤ Recognize anxiety related to test results, and be supportive of perceived loss of independent function.

Discuss the implications of abnormal test results on the patient's lifestyle. Provide teaching and information regarding the clinical implications of the test results, as appropriate.

➤ Reinforce information given by the patient's health care provider regarding further testing, treatment, or referral to another health care provider. Answer any questions or address any concerns voiced by the patient or family.

➤ Instruct the patient in the use of any ordered medications. Explain the importance of adhering to the therapy regimen. As appropriate, instruct the patient in significant side effects and systemic reactions associated with the prescribed medication. Encourage him or her to review corresponding literature provided by a pharmacist.

➤ Depending on the results of this procedure, additional testing may be performed to evaluate or monitor progression of the disease process and determine the need for a change in therapy. Evaluate test results in relation to the patient's symptoms and other tests performed.

Related diagnostic tests:

➤ Related diagnostic tests include chest x-ray, computed tomography angiography, computed tomography cardiac scoring, electrocardiogram, magnetic resonance angiography, and myocardial perfusion heart scan.

ANGIOGRAPHY, PULMONARY

SYNONYMS/ACRONYM: Pulmonary angiography, pulmonary arteriography.

AREA OF APPLICATION: Pulmonary vasculature.

CONTRAST: Intravenous iodine based.

DESCRIPTION & RATIONALE: Pulmonary angiography allows x-ray visualization of the pulmonary vasculature after injection of an iodinated contrast medium into the pulmonary artery or a branch of this great vessel. Contrast medium is injected through a catheter that has been inserted into the vascular system, usually through the femoral vein. It is one of the definitive tests for pulmonary embolism, but it is also useful for evaluating other types of pulmonary vascular abnormalities. It is definitive for peripheral pulmonary artery stenosis, anomalous pulmonary venous drainage, and pulmonary fistulae. Hemodynamic measurements during pulmonary angiography can assist in the diagnosis of pulmonary hypertension and cor pulmonale. ∎

INDICATIONS:
- Detect acute pulmonary embolism
- Detect arteriovenous malformations or aneurysms
- Detect tumors; aneurysms; congenital defects; vascular changes associated with emphysema, blebs, and bullae; and heart abnormalities
- Determine the cause of recurrent or severe hemoptysis
- Evaluate pulmonary circulation

RESULT

Normal Findings:
- Normal pulmonary vasculature; radiopaque iodine contrast medium should circulate symmetrically and without interruption through the pulmonary circulatory system.

Abnormal Findings:
- Aneurysms
- Arterial hypoplasia or stenosis
- Arteriovenous malformations

- Bleeding caused by tuberculosis, bronchiectasis, sarcoidosis, or aspergilloma
- Inflammatory diseases
- Pulmonary embolism (acute or chronic)
- Pulmonary sequestration
- Tumors

CRITICAL VALUES: N/A

INTERFERING FACTORS:

This procedure is contraindicated for:

- ⚠ Patients with allergies to shellfish or iodinated dye. The contrast medium used may cause a life-threatening allergic reaction. Patients with a known hypersensitivity to contrast medium may benefit from premedication with corticosteroids or the use of nonionic contrast medium.
- Patients with bleeding disorders.
- Patients who are pregnant or suspected of being pregnant, unless the potential benefits of the procedure far outweigh the risks to the fetus and mother.
- ⚠ Elderly and other patients who are chronically dehydrated before the test, because of their risk of contrast-induced renal failure.
- ⚠ Patients who are in renal failure.

Factors that may impair clear imaging:
- Retained barium from a previous radiologic procedure
- Metallic objects within the examination field (e.g., jewelry, body rings), which may inhibit organ visualization and can produce unclear images
- Improper adjustment of the radiographic equipment to accommodate obese or thin patients, which can cause overexposure or underexposure and a poor-quality study
- Patients who are very obese, who may exceed the weight limit for the equipment

- Incorrect positioning of the patient, which may produce poor visualization of the area to be examined

- Inability of the patient to cooperate or remain still during the procedure because of age, significant pain, or mental status

Other considerations:

- Consultation with a physician should occur before the procedure for radiation safety concerns regarding younger patients or patients who are lactating.

- Risks associated with radiographic overexposure can result from frequent x-ray procedures. Personnel in the room with the patient should wear a protective lead apron, stand behind a shield, or leave the area while the examination is being done. Personnel working in the area where the examination is being done should wear badges that reveal their level of exposure to radiation.

- Failure to follow dietary restrictions and other pretesting preparations may cause the procedure to be canceled or repeated.

Nursing Implications and Procedure • • • • • • • • • • •

Pretest:

➤ Inform the patient that the procedure assesses cardiovascular function.

➤ Obtain a history of the patient's complaints, including a list of known allergens (especially allergies or sensitivities to latex, iodine, seafood, contrast medium, anesthetics, or dyes), and inform the appropriate health care practitioner accordingly.

➤ Obtain a history of results of previously performed diagnostic procedures, surgical procedures, and laboratory tests. Ensure that the results of blood tests are obtained and recorded before the procedure, especially coagulation tests, blood urea nitrogen, and creatinine, if con-

trast medium is to be used. For related diagnostic tests, refer to the Cardiovascular and Respiratory System tables.

➤ Note any recent procedures that can interfere with test results, including examinations using iodine-based contrast medium.

➤ Record the date of the last menstrual period and determine the possibility of pregnancy in perimenopausal women.

➤ Obtain a list of the medications the patient is taking, especially medications known to affect bleeding, including anticoagulant therapy, aspirin and other salicylates, herbs, nutritional supplements, and nutraceuticals (see Appendix F: Effects of Natural Products on Laboratory Values). It is recommended that use of such products be discontinued 14 days before surgical procedures. The requesting health care practitioner and laboratory should be advised if the patient regularly uses these products so that their effects can be taken into consideration when reviewing results.

➤ Patients receiving metformin (glucophage) for non–insulin-dependent (type 2) diabetes should discontinue the drug on the day of the test and continue to withhold it for 48 hours after the test. Failure to do so may result in lactic acidosis.

➤ Review the procedure with the patient. Address concerns about pain related to the procedure. Explain to the patient that some pain may be experienced during the test, or there may be moments of discomfort. Inform the patient that the procedure is performed in a special department, usually in a radiology or vascular suite, by a physician and support staff and takes approximately 30 to 60 minutes.

➤ *Sensitivity to cultural and social issues,* as well as concern for modesty, is important in providing psychological support before, during, and after the procedure.

➤ Explain that an intravenous (IV) line may be inserted to allow infusion of IV fluids, contrast medium, dye, or sedatives. Usually normal saline is infused.

➤ Inform the patient that a burning and flushing sensation may be felt throughout the body during injection of the contrast medium. After injection of the contrast medium, the patient may experience an urge to cough, flushing, nausea, or a salty or metallic taste.

➤ The patient should fast and restrict fluids for 8 hours prior to the procedure. Instruct the patient to avoid taking anticoagulant medication or to reduce dosage as ordered prior to the procedure.

➤ Instruct the patient to remove dentures, jewelry (including watches), hairpins, credit cards, and other metallic objects in the area to be examined.

➤ *Make sure a written and informed consent has been signed prior to the procedure and before administering any medications.*

➤ This procedure may be terminated if chest pain, severe cardiac arrhythmias, or signs of a cerebrovascular accident occur.

Intratest:

➤ Ensure that the patient has complied with dietary and medication restrictions and pretesting preparations; assure that food and medications have been restricted for at least 8 hours prior to the procedure. Ensure that the patient has removed jewelry, dentures, all external metallic objects, and the like prior to the procedure.

➤ Have emergency equipment readily available.

➤ If the patient has a history of severe allergic reactions to any substance or drug, administer ordered prophylactic steroids or antihistamines before the procedure. Use nonionic contrast medium for the procedure.

➤ Patients are given a gown, robe, and foot coverings to wear and instructed to void prior to the procedure.

➤ Observe standard precautions, and follow the general guidelines in Appendix A.

➤ Record baseline vital signs, and assess neurologic status. Protocols may vary from facility to facility.

➤ Instruct the patient to cooperate fully and to follow directions. Instruct the patient to remain still throughout the procedure because movement produces unreliable results.

➤ Establish an IV fluid line for the injection of emergency drugs and of sedatives.

➤ Administer an antianxiety agent, as ordered, if the patient has claustrophobia. Administer a sedative to a child or to an uncooperative adult, as ordered.

➤ Place electrocardiographic electrodes on the patient for cardiac monitoring. Establish a baseline rhythm; determine if the patient has ventricular arrhythmias.

➤ Using a pen, mark the site of the patient's peripheral pulses before angiography; this allows for quicker and more consistent assessment of the pulses after the procedure.

➤ Place the patient in the supine position on an exam table. Cleanse the selected area, and cover with a sterile drape.

➤ A local anesthetic is injected at the site, and a small incision is made or a needle inserted under fluoroscopy.

➤ The contrast medium is injected, and a rapid series of images is taken during and after the filling of the vessels to be examined. Delayed images may be taken to examine the vessels after a time and to monitor the venous phase of the procedure.

➤ Ask the patient to inhale deeply and hold his or her breath while the x-ray images are taken, and then to exhale after the images are taken.

➤ Instruct the patient to take slow, deep breaths if nausea occurs during the procedure.

> Monitor the patient for complications related to the procedure (e.g., allergic reaction, anaphylaxis, bronchospasm).

> The needle or catheter is removed, and a pressure dressing is applied over the puncture site.

> The results are recorded on x-ray film or electronically in a computerized system for recall and postprocedure interpretation by the appropriate health care practitioner.

Post-test:

> Instruct the patient to resume usual diet, fluids, medications, or activity, as directed by the health care practitioner. Renal function should be assessed before metformin is resumed.

> Monitor vital signs and neurologic status every 15 minutes for 1 hour, then every 2 hours for 4 hours, and as ordered. Take the temperature every 4 hours for 24 hours. Compare with baseline values. Protocols may vary from facility to facility.

> Observe for delayed allergic reactions, such as rash, urticaria, tachycardia, hyperpnea, hypertension, palpitations, nausea, or vomiting.

> Advise the patient to immediately report symptoms such as fast heart rate, difficulty breathing, skin rash, itching, or decreased urinary output.

> Assess extremities for signs of ischemia or absence of distal pulse caused by a catheter-induced thrombus.

> Observe the needle/catheter insertion site for bleeding, inflammation, or hematoma formation.

> Instruct the patient to apply cold compresses to the puncture site, as needed, to reduce discomfort or edema.

> Instruct the patient to maintain bed rest for 4 to 6 hours after the procedure or as ordered.

> Instruct the patient in the care and assessment of the site and to observe for bleeding, hematoma formation, bile leakage, and inflammation. Note any pleuritic pain, persistent right shoulder pain, or abdominal pain.

> A written report of the examination will be completed by a health care practitioner specializing in this branch of medicine. The report will be sent to the requesting health care practitioner, who will discuss the results with the patient.

> Recognize anxiety related to test results, and be supportive of perceived loss of independent function. Discuss the implications of abnormal test results on the patient's lifestyle. Provide teaching and information regarding the clinical implications of the test results, as appropriate.

> Reinforce information given by the patient's health care provider regarding further testing, treatment, or referral to another health care provider. Answer any questions or address any concerns voiced by the patient or family.

> Instruct the patient in the use of any ordered medications. Explain the importance of adhering to the therapy regimen. As appropriate, instruct the patient in significant side effects and systemic reactions associated with the prescribed medication. Encourage him or her to review corresponding literature provided by a pharmacist.

> Depending on the results of this procedure, additional testing may be performed to evaluate or monitor progression of the disease process and determine the need for a change in therapy. Evaluate test results in relation to the patient's symptoms and other tests performed.

Related diagnostic tests

> Related diagnostic tests include chest x-ray, computed tomography angiography, electrocardiogram, lung perfusion and lung ventilation scans, magnetic resonance angiography, magnetic resonance imaging of the chest, and thoracic computed tomography.

ANGIOGRAPHY, RENAL

SYNONYMS/ACRONYM: Renal angiogram, renal arteriography.

AREA OF APPLICATION: Kidney.

CONTRAST: Intravenous iodine based.

DESCRIPTION & RATIONALE: Renal angiography allows x-ray visualization of the large and small arteries of the renal vasculature and parenchyma or the renal veins and their branches. Contrast medium is injected through a catheter that has been inserted into the femoral artery or vein and advanced through the iliac artery and aorta into the renal artery or the inferior vena cava into the renal vein. Images of the kidneys and associated vessels are displayed on a monitor and recorded on film or electronically. Patterns of circulation, renal function, or changes in vessel wall appearance can be viewed to help diagnose the presence of vascular abnormalities, trauma, or lesions. This definitive test for renal disease may be used to evaluate chronic renal disease, renal failure, and renal artery stenosis; differentiate a vascular renal cyst from hypervascular renal cancers; and evaluate renal transplant donors, recipients, and the kidney after transplantation. ■

INDICATIONS:
- Allow infusion of thrombolytic drugs into an occluded artery
- Assist with the collection of blood samples from renal vein for renin analysis
- Detect arterial occlusion as evidenced by a transection of the renal artery caused by trauma or a penetrating injury
- Detect nonmalignant tumors before surgical resection
- Detect renal artery stenosis as evidenced by vessel dilation, collateral vessels, or increased renovascular pressure
- Detect renal tumors as evidenced by arterial supply, extent of venous invasion, and tumor vascularity
- Detect small kidney or absence of a kidney
- Detect thrombosis, arteriovenous fistulae, aneurysms, or emboli in renal vessels
- Differentiate between renal tumors and renal cysts
- Evaluate postoperative renal transplantation for function or organ rejection
- Evaluate renal function in chronic renal failure or end-stage renal disease or hydronephrosis
- Evaluate the renal vascular system of prospective kidney donors before surgery
- Evaluate tumor vascularity before surgery or embolization
- Perform angioplasty, perform atherectomy, or place a stent

RESULT

Normal Findings:
- Normal structure, function, and patency of renal vessels

- Contrast medium circulating throughout the kidneys symmetrically and without interruption
- No evidence of obstruction, variations in number and size of vessels and organs, malformations, cysts, or tumors

Abnormal Findings:
- Abscess or inflammation
- Arterial stenosis, dysplasia, or infarction
- Arteriovenous fistula or other abnormalities
- Congenital anomalies
- Intrarenal hematoma
- Renal artery aneurysm
- Renal cysts or tumors
- Trauma causing tears or other disruption

CRITICAL VALUES: N/A

INTERFERING FACTORS

This procedure is contraindicated for:

- ⚠ Patients with allergies to shellfish or iodinated dye. The contrast medium used may cause a life-threatening allergic reaction. Patients with a known hypersensitivity to contrast medium may benefit from premedication with corticosteroids or the use of nonionic contrast medium.
- Patients with bleeding disorders.
- Patients who are pregnant or suspected of being pregnant, unless the potential benefits of the procedure far outweigh the risks to the fetus and mother.
- ⚠ Elderly and other patients who are chronically dehydrated before the test, because of their risk of contrast-induced renal failure.
- ⚠ Patients who are in renal failure.

Factors that may impair clear imaging:
- Gas or feces in the gastrointestinal tract resulting from inadequate cleansing or failure to restrict food intake before the study

- Retained barium from a previous radiologic procedure
- Metallic objects within the examination field (e.g., jewelry, body rings, dental amalgams), which may inhibit organ visualization and can produce unclear images
- Improper adjustment of the radiographic equipment to accommodate obese or thin patients, which can cause overexposure or underexposure and a poor-quality study
- Patients who are very obese, who may exceed the weight limit for the equipment
- Incorrect positioning of the patient, which may produce poor visualization of the area to be examined
- Inability of the patient to cooperate or remain still during the procedure because of age, significant pain, or mental status

Other considerations:
- Consultation with a physician should occur before the procedure for radiation safety concerns regarding younger patients or patients who are lactating.
- Risks associated with radiographic overexposure can result from frequent x-ray procedures. Personnel in the room with the patient should wear a protective lead apron, stand behind a shield, or leave the area while the examination is being done. Personnel working in the area where the examination is being done should wear badges that reveal their level of exposure to radiation.
- Failure to follow dietary restrictions and other pretesting preparations may cause the procedure to be canceled or repeated.

Nursing Implications and Procedure ・・・・・・・・・・・

Pretest:

▶ Inform the patient that the procedure assesses cardiovascular function.

- Obtain a history of the patient's complaints, including a list of known allergens (especially allergies or sensitivities to latex, iodine, seafood, contrast medium, anesthetics, or dyes), and inform the appropriate health care practitioner accordingly.
- Obtain a history of results of previously performed diagnostic procedures, surgical procedures, and laboratory tests. Ensure that the results of blood tests are obtained and recorded before the procedure, especially coagulation tests, blood urea nitrogen, and creatinine, if contrast medium is to be used. For related diagnostic tests, refer to the Cardiovascular and Genitourinary System tables.
- Note any recent procedures that can interfere with test results, including examinations using iodine-based contrast medium.
- Record the date of the last menstrual period and determine the possibility of pregnancy in perimenopausal women.
- Obtain a list of the medications the patient is taking, especially medications known to affect bleeding, including anticoagulant therapy, aspirin and other salicylates, herbs, nutritional supplements, and nutraceuticals (see Appendix F: Effects of Natural Products on Laboratory Values). It is recommended that use of such products be discontinued 14 days before surgical procedures. The requesting health care practitioner and laboratory should be advised if the patient regularly uses these products so that their effects can be taken into consideration when reviewing results.
- Patients receiving metformin (glucophage) for non–insulin-dependent (type 2) diabetes should discontinue the drug on the day of the test and continue to withhold it for 48 hours after the test. Failure to do so may result in lactic acidosis.
- Review the procedure with the patient. Address concerns about pain related to the procedure. Explain to the patient that some pain may be experienced during the test, or there may be moments of discomfort. Inform the patient that the procedure is performed in a special department, usually in a radiology or vascular suite, by a physician and support staff and takes approximately 30 to 60 minutes.
- *Sensitivity to cultural and social issues,* as well as concern for modesty, is important in providing psychological support before, during, and after the procedure.
- Explain that an intravenous (IV) line may be inserted to allow infusion of IV fluids, contrast medium, dye, or sedatives. Usually normal saline is infused.
- Inform the patient that a burning and flushing sensation may be felt throughout the body during injection of the contrast medium. After injection of the contrast medium, the patient may experience an urge to cough, flushing, nausea, or a salty or metallic taste.
- The patient should fast and restrict fluids for 8 hours prior to the procedure. Instruct the patient to avoid taking anticoagulant medication or to reduce dosage as ordered prior to the procedure.
- Instruct the patient to remove dentures, jewelry (including watches), hairpins, credit cards, and other metallic objects in the area to be examined.
- *Make sure a written and informed consent has been signed prior to the procedure and before administering any medications.*
- This procedure may be terminated if chest pain, severe cardiac arrhythmias, or signs of a cerebrovascular accident occur.

- Ensure that the patient has complied with dietary and medication restrictions and pretesting preparations; assure that food and medications have been restricted for at least 8 hours prior to the procedure. Ensure that the patient has removed jewelry, dentures, all external metallic objects, and the like prior to the procedure.
- Have emergency equipment readily available.

➤ If the patient has a history of severe allergic reactions to any substance or drug, administer ordered prophylactic steroids or antihistamines before the procedure. Use nonionic contrast medium for the procedure.

➤ Patients are given a gown, robe, and foot coverings to wear and instructed to void prior to the procedure.

➤ Observe standard precautions, and follow the general guidelines in Appendix A.

➤ Record baseline vital signs, and assess neurologic status. Protocols may vary from facility to facility.

➤ Instruct the patient to cooperate fully and to follow directions. Instruct the patient to remain still throughout the procedure because movement produces unreliable results.

➤ Establish an IV fluid line for the injection of emergency drugs and of sedatives.

➤ Administer an antianxiety agent, as ordered, if the patient has claustrophobia. Administer a sedative to a child or to an uncooperative adult, as ordered.

➤ Place electrocardiographic electrodes on the patient for cardiac monitoring. Establish a baseline rhythm; determine if the patient has ventricular arrhythmias.

➤ Using a pen, mark the site of the patient's peripheral pulses before angiography; this allows for quicker and more consistent assessment of the pulses after the procedure.

➤ Place the patient in the supine position on an exam table. Cleanse the selected area, and cover with a sterile drape.

➤ A local anesthetic is injected at the site, and a small incision is made or a needle inserted under fluoroscopy.

➤ The contrast medium is injected, and a rapid series of images is taken during and after the filling of the vessels to be examined. Delayed images may be taken to examine the vessels after a time and to monitor the venous phase of the procedure.

➤ Ask the patient to inhale deeply and hold his or her breath while the x-ray images are taken, and then to exhale after the images are taken.

➤ Instruct the patient to take slow, deep breaths if nausea occurs during the procedure.

➤ Monitor the patient for complications related to the procedure (e.g., allergic reaction, anaphylaxis, bronchospasm).

➤ The needle or catheter is removed, and a pressure dressing is applied over the puncture site.

➤ The results are recorded on x-ray film or electronically in a computerized system for recall and postprocedure interpretation by the appropriate health care practitioner.

Post-test:

➤ Instruct the patient to resume usual diet, fluids, medications, or activity, as directed by the health care practitioner. Renal function should be assessed before metformin is resumed.

➤ Monitor vital signs and neurologic status every 15 minutes for 1 hour, then every 2 hours for 4 hours, and as ordered. Take the temperature every 4 hours for 24 hours. Compare with baseline values. Protocols may vary from facility to facility.

➤ Observe for delayed allergic reactions, such as rash, urticaria, tachycardia, hyperpnea, hypertension, palpitations, nausea, or vomiting.

➤ Advise the patient to immediately report symptoms such as fast heart rate, difficulty breathing, skin rash, itching, or decreased urinary output.

➤ Assess extremities for signs of ischemia or absence of distal pulse caused by a catheter-induced thrombus.

➤ Observe the needle/catheter insertion site for bleeding, inflammation, or hematoma formation.

➤ Instruct the patient to apply cold compresses to the puncture site, as needed, to reduce discomfort or edema.

➤ Instruct the patient to maintain bed rest for 4 to 6 hours after the procedure or as ordered.

➤ Instruct the patient in the care and

assessment of the site and to observe for bleeding, hematoma formation, bile leakage, and inflammation. Note any pleuritic pain, persistent right shoulder pain, or abdominal pain.

➤ A written report of the examination will be completed by a health care practitioner specializing in this branch of medicine. The report will be sent to the requesting health care practitioner, who will discuss the results with the patient.

➤ Recognize anxiety related to test results, and be supportive of perceived loss of independent function. Discuss the implications of abnormal test results on the patient's lifestyle. Provide teaching and information regarding the clinical implications of the test results, as appropriate.

➤ Reinforce information given by the patient's health care provider regarding further testing, treatment, or referral to another health care provider. Answer any questions or address any concerns voiced by the patient or family.

➤ Instruct the patient in the use of any ordered medications. Explain the importance of adhering to the therapy regimen. As appropriate, instruct the patient in significant side effects and systemic reactions associated with the prescribed medication. Encourage him or her to review corresponding literature provided by a pharmacist.

➤ Depending on the results of this procedure, additional testing may be performed to evaluate or monitor progression of the disease process and determine the need for a change in therapy. Evaluate test results in relation to the patient's symptoms and other tests performed.

Related diagnostic tests

➤ Related diagnostic tests include computed tomography of the abdomen; computed tomography angiography; kidney, ureter, and bladder study; magnetic resonance angiography and magnetic resonance imaging of the abdomen.

ANGIOTENSIN-CONVERTING ENZYME

· ·

SYNONYM/ACRONYM: Angiotensin I–converting enzyme (ACE).

SPECIMEN: Serum (1 mL) collected in a red- or tiger-top tube.

REFERENCE VALUE: (Method: Spectrophotometry)

Age	Conventional Units	SI Units (Conventional Units × 0.017)
0–2 y	5–83 U/L	0.09–1.41 μKat/L
3–7 y	8–76 U/L	0.14–1.29 μKat/L
8–14 y	6–89 U/L	0.10–1.51 μKat/L
Greater than 14 y	8–52 U/L	0.14–0.88 μKat/L

DESCRIPTION & RATIONALE:

Angiotensin-converting enzyme (ACE) production occurs mainly in the epithelial cells of the pulmonary bed. Smaller amounts are found in blood vessels and renal tissue, where ACE converts angiotensin I to angiotensin II; this conversion helps regulate arterial blood pressure. Angiotensin II stimulates the adrenal cortex to produce aldosterone. Aldosterone is a hormone that helps the kidneys maintain water balance by retaining sodium and promoting the excretion of potassium.

ACE levels are used primarily in the evaluation of hypertension and active sarcoidosis, a granulomatous disease that can affect many organs, including the lungs. Serial levels are useful in correlating the therapeutic response to corticosteroid treatment. Increasing ACE levels with positive gallium scans in sarcoidosis patients receiving steroids indicate a poor response to therapy. Monitoring ACE levels may also have some utility in assessing the risk of pulmonary damage in affected patients receiving antineoplastic agents. Thyroid hormones may play a role in regulating ACE levels: Decreased levels have been noted in patients with clinical hypothyroidism and anorexia nervosa, whereas increased levels have been noted in patients with hyperthyroidism. Elevations of serum ACE have been reported in 20% to 30% of patients with abnormal α_1-antitrypsin variants. ACE levels are sometimes ordered on cerebrospinal fluid to evaluate patients with neurosarcoidosis. Results must be interpreted with care because of the nonspecificity of increased and decreased ACE levels. ACE is normally elevated in pediatric patients and therefore is not a useful marker in the evaluation of disease for patients less than 20 years of age. ■

INDICATIONS:

• Assist in establishing a diagnosis of sarcoidosis
• Assist in the evaluation of Gaucher's disease
• Assist in the treatment of sarcoidosis
• Evaluate hypertension
• Evaluate the severity and activity of sarcoidosis

RESULT

Increased in:

• Bronchitis (acute and chronic)
• Connective tissue disease
• Gaucher's disease
• Hansen's disease (leprosy)
• Histoplasmosis and other fungal diseases
• Hyperthyroidism (untreated)
• Pulmonary fibrosis
• Rheumatoid arthritis
• Sarcoidosis

Decreased in:

• Advanced pulmonary carcinoma
• The period following corticosteroid therapy for sarcoidosis

CRITICAL VALUES: N/A

INTERFERING FACTORS:

• Drugs that may increase serum ACE levels include triiodothyronine.
• Drugs that may decrease serum ACE levels include captopril, cilazapril, enalapril, fosinopril, lisinopril, nicardipine, pentopril, perindopril, propranolol, quinapril, ramipril, and trandolapril.
• Prompt and proper specimen processing, storage, and analysis are important to achieve accurate results. Failure to freeze sample if not tested immediately

may cause falsely decreased values because ACE degrades rapidly.

Nursing Implications and Procedure ● ● ● ● ● ● ● ● ● ● ●

Pretest:

➤ Inform the patient that the test is primarily used to diagnose and monitor treatment of sarcoidosis.

➤ Obtain a history of the patient's complaints, including a list of known allergens (especially allergies or sensitivities to latex), and inform the appropriate health care practitioner accordingly.

➤ Obtain a history of the patient's endocrine, immune, musculoskeletal, and respiratory systems, as well as results of previously performed laboratory tests, surgical procedures, and other diagnostic procedures. For related laboratory tests, refer to the Endocrine, Immune, Musculoskeletal, and Respiratory System tables.

➤ Obtain a list of the medications the patient is taking, including herbs, nutritional supplements, and nutraceuticals. The requesting health care practitioner and laboratory should be advised if the patient regularly uses these products so that their effects can be taken into consideration when reviewing results.

➤ Review the procedure with the patient. Note the patient's age. This test is rarely ordered on patients less than 20 years old. Inform the patient that specimen collection takes approximately 5 to 10 minutes. Address concerns about pain related to the procedure. Explain to the patient that there may be some discomfort during the venipuncture.

➤ There are no food, fluid, or medication restrictions unless by medical direction.

Intratest:

➤ If the patient has a history of severe allergic reaction to latex, care should be taken to avoid the use of equipment containing latex.

➤ Instruct the patient to cooperate fully and to follow directions. Direct the patient to breathe normally and to avoid unnecessary movement.

➤ Observe standard precautions, and follow the general guidelines in Appendix A. Positively identify the patient, and label the appropriate tubes with the corresponding patient demographics, date, and time of collection. Perform a venipuncture; collect the specimen in a 5-mL red- or tiger-top tube.

➤ Remove the needle, place a gauze over the puncture site and apply gentle pressure to stop bleeding. Observe venipuncture site for bleeding or hematoma formation. Apply paper tape over gauze or replace with adhesive bandage.

➤ Promptly transport the specimen to the laboratory for processing and analysis.

➤ The results are recorded manually or in a computerized system for recall and postprocedure interpretation by the appropriate health care practitioner.

Post-test:

➤ *Nutritional considerations:* ACE levels affect the regulation of fluid balance and electrolytes. Dietary adjustment may be considered if sodium allowances need to be regulated. Educate patients with low sodium levels that the major source of dietary sodium is found in table salt. Many foods such as milk and other dairy products are also good sources of dietary sodium. Most other dietary sodium is available through consumption of processed foods. Patients who need to follow low-sodium diets should be advised to avoid beverages such as colas, ginger ale, Gatorade, lemon-lime sodas, and root beer. Many over-the-counter medications, including antacids, laxatives, analgesics, sedatives, and antitussives, contain significant amounts of sodium. The best advice is to emphasize the importance of reading all food, beverage, and medicine labels. In 1989, the Sub-committee on the 10th Edition of the Recommended Dietary Allowances (RDAs) established 500 mg as the recommended minimum limit for dietary intake of sodium. There are no RDAs established for potassium, but the estimated minimum intake for adults is 200 mEq/d. Potassium is present in all plant and animal cells, making dietary replacement fairly simple. A health care practitioner or nutritionist should be consulted before considering the use of salt substitutes.

➤ A written report of the examination will be sent to the requesting health care practitioner, who will discuss the results with the patient.

➤ Reinforce information given by the patient's health care provider regarding further testing, treatment, or referral to another health care provider. Answer any questions or address any concerns voiced by the patient or family.

➤ Depending on the results of this procedure, additional testing may be performed to evaluate or monitor progression of the disease process and determine the need for a change in therapy. Evaluate test results in relation to the patient's symptoms and other tests performed.

Related laboratory tests:

➤ Related laboratory tests include aldosterone, alkaline phosphatase, anion gap, α_1-antitrypsin, α_1-antitrypsin phenotyping, arterial/alveolar oxygen ratio, blood gases, serum and urine calcium, electrolytes, erythrocyte sedimentation rate, liver biopsy, lymph node biopsy, phosphorus, potassium, protein electrophoresis, renin, rheumatoid factor, skin biopsy, sodium, thyroid hormone levels, and urine protein.

ANION GAP

SYNONYM/ACRONYM: Agap.

SPECIMEN: Serum (1 mL) for electrolytes collected in a red- or tiger-top tube. Plasma (1 mL) collected in a green-top (heparin) tube is also acceptable.

REFERENCE VALUE: (Method: Anion gap is derived mathematically from the direct measurement of sodium, chloride, and total carbon dioxide.) There are differences between serum and plasma values for some electrolytes. The reference ranges listed are based on serum values.

Age	Conventional Units	SI Units (Conventional Units × 1)
Child	8–16 mEq/L	8–16 mmol/L
Adult	8–16 mEq/L	8–16 mmol/L

DESCRIPTION & RATIONALE: The anion gap is used most frequently as a clinical indicator of metabolic acidosis. It does not include measurement of important cations, such as calcium, potassium (usually), and magnesium; or anions, such as proteins, forms of phosphorus, sulfur, and organic acids. The anion gap is calculated as follows:

(sodium – [chloride + HCO_3^-])

Because bicarbonate (HCO_3^-) is not directly measured on most chemistry analyzers, it is estimated by substitution of the total carbon dioxide (TCO_2) value in the calculation. Some laboratories may include potassium in the calculation of the anion gap. Calculations including potassium can be invalidated because minor amounts of hemolysis can contribute significant levels of potassium leaked into the serum as a result of cell rupture. The anion gap is also widely used as a laboratory quality control measure because low gaps usually indicate a reagent, calibration, or instrument error. ∎

INDICATIONS:
- Evaluate metabolic acidosis
- Indicate the need for laboratory instrument recalibration or review of electrolyte reagent preparation and stability
- Indicate the presence of a disturbance in electrolyte balance

RESULT

Increased in:
- Dehydration (severe)
- Excessive exercise
- Ketoacidosis caused by starvation, high-protein/low-carbohydrate diet, diabetes, and alcoholism
- Lactic acidosis
- Poisoning (salicylate, methanol, ethylene glycol, or paraldehyde)
- Renal failure
- Uremia

Decreased in:
- Hyperchloremia
- Hypergammaglobulinemia (multiple myeloma)
- Hypoalbuminemia
- Hyponatremia (hyperviscosity syndromes)

TCO_2 is commonly substituted for HCO_3^- in anion gap calculations. It is important to note the clinical significance of excessive HCO_3^-, which occurs in renal alkalosis, gastrointestinal alkalosis, and excessive ingestion of exogenous sources of alkali, the effects of which may not be accurately reflected by the calculated anion gap.

CRITICAL VALUES: N/A

INTERFERING FACTORS:
- Drugs that can increase or decrease the anion gap include those listed in the individual electrolyte (i.e., sodium, chloride, calcium, magnesium, and total carbon dioxide), total protein, lactic acid, and phosphorus monographs.
- Specimens should never be collected above an intravenous line because of the potential for dilution when the specimen and the intravenous solution combine in the collection container, falsely decreasing the result. There is also the potential of contaminating the sample with the substance of interest, if it is present in the intravenous solution, falsely increasing the result.

Nursing Implications and Procedure • • • • • • • • • • •

Pretest:

> Inform the patient that the test is used to assist in the evaluation of electrolyte balance.

> Obtain a history of the patient's complaints, including a list of known allergens (especially allergies or sensitivities to latex), and inform the appropriate health care practitioner accordingly.

> Obtain a history of the patient's cardiovascular, endocrine, gastrointestinal, genitourinary, hematopoietic, immune, and respiratory systems, as well as results of previously performed laboratory tests, surgical procedures, and other diagnostic procedures. For related laboratory tests, refer to the Cardiovascular, Endocrine, Gastrointestinal, Genitourinary, Hematopoietic, Immune, and Respiratory System tables.

> Obtain a list of the medications the patient is taking, including herbs, nutritional supplements, and nutraceuticals. The requesting health care practitioner and laboratory should be advised if the patient regularly uses these products so that their effects can be taken into consideration when reviewing results.

> Review the procedure with the patient. Inform the patient that specimen collection takes approximately 5 to 10 minutes. Address concerns about pain related to the procedure. Explain to the patient that there may be some discomfort during the venipuncture.

> There are no food, fluid, or medication restrictions unless by medical direction.

Intratest:

> If the patient has a history of severe allergic reaction to latex, care should be taken to avoid the use of equipment containing latex.

> Instruct the patient to cooperate fully and to follow directions. Direct the patient to breathe normally and to avoid unnecessary movement.

> Observe standard precautions, and follow the general guidelines in Appendix A. Positively identify the patient, and label the appropriate tubes with the corresponding patient demographics, date, and time of collection. Perform a venipuncture; collect the specimen in a 5-mL red- or tiger-top tube.

> Remove the needle, place a gauze over the puncture site and apply gentle pressure to stop bleeding. Observe venipuncture site for bleeding and hematoma formation. Apply paper tape over gauze or replace with adhesive bandage.

> Promptly transport the specimen to the laboratory for processing and analysis.

> The results are recorded manually or in a computerized system for recall and postprocedure interpretation by the appropriate health care practitioner.

Post-test:

> *Nutritional considerations:* Specific dietary considerations are listed in the monographs on individual electrolytes (i.e., sodium, chloride, calcium, and magnesium), total protein, and phosphorus.

> *Nutritional considerations:* The anion gap can be used to indicate the presence of dehydration. Evaluate the patient for signs and symptoms of dehydration. Dehydration is a significant and common finding in geriatric patients and patients with decreased renal function.

> A written report of the examination will be sent to the requesting health care practitioner, who will discuss the results with the patient.

> Reinforce information given by the patient's health care provider regarding further testing, treatment, or re-

ferral to another health care provider. Answer any questions or address any concerns voiced by the patient or family.

➤ Depending on the results of this procedure, additional testing may be performed to evaluate or monitor progression of the disease process and determine the need for a change in therapy. Evaluate test results in relation to the patient's symptoms and other tests performed.

Related laboratory tests:

➤ Related laboratory tests include albumin, blood gases, blood urea nitrogen, creatinine, electrolytes, ethanol, glucose, ketones, lactic acid, osmolality, protein, protein electrophoresis, salicylate, and urinalysis.

ANTIARRHYTHMIC DRUGS: DIGOXIN, DISOPYRAMIDE, FLECAINIDE, LIDOCAINE, PROCAINAMIDE, QUINIDINE

SYNONYMS/ACRONYMS: *Digoxin* (Digitek, Lanoxicaps, Lanoxin); *disopyramide* (Norpace, Norpace CR); *flecainide* (flecainide acetate, Tambocor); *lidocaine* (Xylocaine); *procainamide* (Procanbid, Pronestyl, Pronestyl SR); *quinidine* (Quinidex Extentabs, quinidine sulface SR, quinidine gluconate SR).

SPECIMEN: Serum (1 mL) collected in a red-top tube.

Drug	Route of Administration	Recommended Collection Time
Digoxin	Oral	Trough: 12–24 h after dose Never draw peak samples
Disopyramide	Oral	Trough: immediately before next dose Peak: 2–5 h after dose
Flecainide	Oral	Trough: immediately before next dose Peak: 3 h after dose
Lidocaine	IV	15 min, 1 h, then every 24 h
Procainamide	IV	15 min; 2, 6, 12 hours; then every 24 h
Procainamide	Oral	Trough: immediately before next dose Peak: 75 min after dose
Quinidine sulfate	Oral	Trough: immediately before next dose Peak: 1 h after dose
Quinidine gluconate	Oral	Trough: immediately before next dose Peak: 5 h after dose
Quinidine polygalac-turonate	Oral	Trough: immediately before next dose Peak: 2 h after dose

IV = intravenous.

Drug (Indication)	Therapeutic Dose*	SI Units	Half-Life (h)	Volume of Distribution (L/kg)	Protein Binding (%)	Excretion
Digoxin	0.5–2.0 ng/mL	*(SI = Conventional Units × 1.28)* 0.6–2.6 nmol/L	20–60	7	20–30	1° renal
Disopyramide (atrial arrhythmias)	2.8–3.2 μg/mL	*(SI = Conventional Units × 2.95)* 8.3–9.4 μmol/L	4–10	0.7–0.9	20–60	1° renal
Disopyramide (ventricular arrhythmias)	3.3–5.0 μg/mL	9.7–15.0 μmol/L				1° renal
Flecainide	0.2–1.0 μg/mL	*(SI = Conventional Units × 2.41)* 0.5–2.4 μmol/L	7–19	5–13	40–50	1° renal
Lidocaine	1.5–5.0 μg/mL	*(SI = Conventional Units × 4.27)* 6.4–21.4 μmol/L	1.5–2	1–1.5	60–80	1° hepatic
Procainamide	4–10 μg/mL	*(SI = Conventional Units × 4.23)* 17–42 μmol/L	2–6	2–4	10–20	1° renal
Procainamide + N-acetyl procainamide	10–30 μg/mL	*(SI = Conventional Units × 3.61)* 36–108 μmol/L	8			1° renal
Quinidine	2–5 μg/mL	*(SI = Conventional Units × 3.08)* 6–15 μmol/L	6–8	2–3	70–90	Renal and hepatic

* Conventional units.
CHF = congestive heart failure.

DESCRIPTION & RATIONALE: Cardiac glycosides are used in the prophylactic management and treatment of heart failure and ventricular and atrial arrhythmias. Because these drugs have narrow therapeutic windows, they must be monitored closely. The signs and symptoms of toxicity are often difficult to distinguish from those of cardiac disease. Patients with toxic levels may show gastrointestinal, ocular, and central nervous system effects and disturbances in potassium balance.

Many factors must be considered in effective dosing and monitoring of therapeutic drugs, including patient age, patient weight, interacting medications, electrolyte balance, protein levels, water balance, conditions that affect absorption and excretion, and the ingestion of substances (e.g., foods, herbals, vitamins, and minerals) that can either potentiate or inhibit the intended target concentra-tion. Peak and trough collection times should be documented carefully in relation to the time of medication administration. ▪

IMPORTANT NOTE: This information must be communicated clearly and accurately to avoid misunderstanding of the dose time in relation to the collection time. Miscommunication between the individual administering the medication and the individual collecting the specimen is the most frequent cause of subtherapeutic levels, toxic levels, and misleading information used in the calculation of future doses.

INDICATIONS:
- Assist in the diagnosis and prevention of toxicity
- Monitor compliance with therapeutic regimen
- Monitor patients who have a pacemaker, who have impaired renal or hepatic function, or who are taking interacting drugs

RESULT

Level	Result
Normal levels	Therapeutic effect
Subtherapeutic levels	Adjust dose as indicated
Toxic levels	Adjust dose as indicated
Digoxin	Renal impairment, CHF, elderly patients
Disopyramide	Renal impairment
Flecainide	Renal impairment, CHF
Lidocaine	Hepatic impairment, CHF
Procainamide	Renal impairment
Quinidine	Renal and hepatic impairment, CHF, elderly patients

CHF = congestive heart failure.

CRITICAL VALUES: ⚠ Adverse effects of subtherapeutic levels are important. Care should be taken to investigate the signs and symptoms of too little and too much medication. Note and immediately report to the health care practitioner any critically increased values and related symptoms.

Digoxin: Greater Than 2.5 ng/mL

Signs and symptoms of digoxin toxicity include arrhythmias, anorexia, hyperkalemia, nausea, vomiting, diarrhea, changes in mental status, and visual disturbances (objects appear yellow or have halos around them). Possible interventions include discontinuing the medication, continuous electrocardiographic (ECG) monitoring (prolonged P-R interval, widening QRS interval, lengthening Q-Tc interval, and atrioventricular block), transcutaneous pacing, administration of activated charcoal (if the patient has a gag reflex and central nervous system function), support and treatment of electrolyte disturbance, and administration of Digibind (digoxin immune Fab). The amount of Digibind given depends on the level of digoxin to be neutralized. Digoxin levels must be measured before the administration of Digibind. Digoxin levels should not be measured for several days after administration of Digibind in patients with normal renal function (1 week or longer in patients with decreased renal function). Digibind cross-reacts in the digoxin assay and may provide misleading elevations or decreases in values depending on the particular assay in use by the laboratory.

Disopyramide: Greater Than 7 μg/mL

Signs and symptoms of disopyramide toxicity include prolonged Q-T interval, ventricular tachycardia, hypotension, and heart failure. Possible interventions include discontinuing the medication, airway support, and ECG and blood pressure monitoring.

Flecainide: Greater Than 1 μg/mL

Signs and symptoms of flecainide toxicity include exaggerated pharmacologic effects resulting in arrhythmia. Possible interventions include discontinuing the medication as well as continuous ECG, respiratory, and blood pressure monitoring.

Lidocaine: Greater Than 6 μg/mL

Signs and symptoms of lidocaine toxicity include slurred speech, central nervous system depression, cardiovascular depression, convulsions, muscle twitches, and possible coma. Possible interventions include continuous ECG monitoring, airway support, seizure precautions, and hourly monitoring of temperature for hyperthermia.

Procainamide: Greater Than 12 μg/mL; Procainamide + N-acetyl Procainamide: Greater Than 30 μg/mL

The active metabolite of procainamide is N-acetyl procainamide (NAPA). Signs and symptoms of procainamide toxicity include torsades de pointes (ventricular tachycardia), nausea, vomiting, agranulocytosis, and hepatic disturbances. Possible interventions include airway protection, emesis, gastric lavage, and administration of sodium lactate.

Quinidine: Greater Than 8 μg/mL

Signs and symptoms of quinidine toxicity include ataxia, nausea, vomiting, diarrhea, respiratory system depression, hypotension, syncope, anuria, arrhythmias (heart block, widening of QRS and Q-T intervals), asystole, hallucinations, paresthesia, and irritability. Possible interventions include airway support, emesis, gastric lavage, administration of activated charcoal, administration of sodium lactate, and temporary transcutaneous or transvenous pacemaker.

INTERFERING FACTORS:

- Blood drawn in serum separator tubes (gel tubes).

- Contraindicated in patients with liver disease, and caution advised in patients with renal impairment.

- Drugs that may increase digoxin levels or increase risk of toxicity include amiodarone, amphotericin B, diclofenac, diltiazem, erythromycin, propantheline, quinidine, spironolactone, tetracycline, and verapamil.

- Drugs that may decrease digoxin levels include aluminum hydroxide (antacids), cholestyramine, colestipol, kaolin-pectin, metoclopramide, neomycin, phenytoin, and sulfasalazine.

- Drugs that may increase disopyramide levels or increase risk of toxicity include amiodarone and troleandomycin.

- Drugs that may decrease disopyramide levels include rifampin.

- Drugs that may increase flecainide levels or increase risk of toxicity include amiodarone and cimetidine.

- Drugs that may increase lidocaine levels or increase risk of toxicity include anticonvulsants, β-blockers, cimetidine, metoprolol, nadolol, and propranolol.

- Drugs that may increase procainamide levels or increase risk of toxicity include amiodarone, cimetidine, other antiarrhythmics, ranitidine, and trimethoprim.

- Drugs that may increase quinidine levels or increase risk of toxicity include amiodarone, cimetidine, thiazide diuretics, and verapamil.

- Drugs that may decrease quinidine levels include disopyramide, nifedipine, phenobarbital, phenytoin, and rifampin.

- Digitoxin cross-reacts with digoxin; results are falsely elevated if digoxin is measured when the patient is taking digitoxin.

- Digitalis-like immunoreactive substances are found in the serum of some patients who are not taking digoxin, causing false-positive results. Patients whose serum contain digitalis-like immunoreactive substances usually have a condition related to salt and fluid retention, such as renal failure, hepatic failure, low-renin hypertension, and pregnancy.

- Unexpectedly low digoxin levels may be found in patients with thyroid disease.

- Disopyramide may cause a decrease in glucose levels. It may also potentiate the anticoagulating effects of warfarin.

- Long-term administration of procainamide can cause false-positive antinuclear antibody results and development of a lupus-like syndrome in some patients.

- Quinidine may potentiate the effects of neuromuscular blocking medications and warfarin anticoagulants.

- Concomitant administration of quinidine and digoxin can rapidly raise digoxin to toxic levels. If both drugs are to be given together, the digoxin level should be measured before the first dose of quinidine and again in 4 to 6 days.

Nursing Implications and Procedure • • • • • • • • • • •

Pretest:

▶ Inform the patient that the test is used to monitor for therapeutic and toxic drug levels.

▶ Obtain a history of the patient's complaints, including a list of known allergens (especially allergies or sensitivities to latex), and inform the appropriate health care practitioner accordingly.

▶ Obtain a history of the patient's genitourinary and hepatobiliary systems as well as results of previously performed laboratory tests, surgical procedures, and other diagnostic procedures. For related laboratory tests, refer to the Genitourinary and Hepatobiliary Systems and Therapeutic/Toxicology tables.

Obtain a list of the medications the patient is taking, including herbs, nutritional supplements, and nutraceuticals. Note the last time and dose of medication taken. The requesting health care practitioner and laboratory should be advised if the patient regularly uses these products so that their effects can be taken into consideration when reviewing results.

Review the procedure with the patient. Inform the patient that specimen collection takes approximately 5 to 10 minutes. Address concerns about pain related to the procedure. Explain to the patient that there may be some discomfort during the venipuncture.

Sensitivity to cultural and social issues, as well as concern for modesty, is important in providing psychological support before, during, and after the procedure.

There are no food, fluid, or medication restrictions unless by medical direction.

Intratest:

If the patient has a history of severe allergic reaction to latex, care should be taken to avoid the use of equipment containing latex.

Instruct the patient to cooperate fully and to follow directions. Direct the patient to breathe normally and to avoid unnecessary movement.

Observe standard precautions, and follow the general guidelines in Appendix A. Consider recommended collection time in relation to the dosing schedule. Positively identify the patient, and label the appropriate tubes with the corresponding patient demographics, date, and time of collection, noting the last dose of medication taken. Perform a venipuncture; collect the specimen in a 5-mL red top tube.

Remove the needle, place a gauze over the puncture site and apply gentle pressure to stop bleeding. Observe venipuncture site for bleed-ing or hematoma formation. Apply paper tape over gauze or replace with adhesive bandage.

Promptly transport the specimen to the laboratory for processing and analysis.

The results are recorded manually or in a computerized system for recall and postprocedure interpretation by the appropriate health care practitioner.

Post-test:

Nutritional considerations include the avoidance of alcohol consumption.

A written report of the examination will be sent to the requesting health care practitioner, who will discuss the results with the patient.

Reinforce information given by the patient's health care provider regarding further testing, treatment, or referral to another health care provider. Explain to the patient the importance of following the medication regimen and instructions regarding drug interactions. Instruct the patient to immediately report any unusual sensations (e.g., dizziness, changes in vision, loss of appetite, nausea, vomiting, diarrhea, weakness, or irregular heartbeat) to his or her health care practitioner. Instruct the patient not to take medicine within 1 hour of food high in fiber. Answer any questions or address any concerns voiced by the patient or family.

Instruct the patient to be prepared to provide the pharmacist with a list of other medications he or she is already taking in the event that the requesting health care practitioner prescribes a medication.

Depending on the results of this procedure, additional testing may be performed to evaluate or monitor progression of the disease process and determine the need for a change in therapy. Evaluate test results in relation to the patient's symptoms and other tests performed.

> Related laboratory tests include alanine aminotransferase, albumin, alkaline phosphatase, apolipoprotein A, apolipoprotein B, aspartate aminotransferase, atrial natriuretic peptide, B-type natriuretic peptide, blood gases, C-reactive protein, calcium, cholesterol (total, HDL, and LDL), creatine kinase and isoenzymes, creatinine, glucose, glycated hemoglobin, homocysteine, ionized calcium, ketones, lactate dehydrogenase and isoenzymes, magnesium, myoglobin, platelet count, potassium, triglycerides, troponin, and urea nitrogen.

ANTIBIOTIC DRUGS— AMINOGLYCOSIDES: AMIKACIN, GENTAMICIN, TOBRAMYCIN; TRICYCLIC GLYCOPEPTIDE: VANCOMYCIN

SYNONYMS: *Amikacin* (Amikin); *gentamicin* (Garamycin, Genoptic, Gentacidin, Gentafair, Gentak, Gentamar, Gentrasul, G-myticin, Oco-Mycin, Spectro-Genta); *tobramycin* (Nebcin, Tobrex); *vancomycin* (Lyphocin, Vancocin, Vancoled).

SPECIMEN: Serum (1 mL) collected in a red-top tube.

Antibiotic Type	Route of Administration	Recommended Collection Time*
Aminoglycosides		
Amikacin	IV, IM	Trough: immediately before next dose Peak: 30 min after the end of a 30-min IV infusion
Gentamicin	IV, IM	Trough: immediately before next dose Peak: 30 min after the end of a 30-min IV infusion
Tobramycin	IV, IM	Trough: immediately before next dose Peak: 30 min after the end of a 30-min IV infusion
Tricyclic glycopeptide		
Vancomycin	IV, PO	Trough: immediately before next dose Peak: 30-60 min after the end of a 60-min IV infusion

* Usually after fifth dose if given every 8 hours or third dose if given every 12 hours.
IV = intravenous; IM = intramuscular; PO = by mouth.

Drug	Therapeutic Dose*	SI Units	Half-Life (h)	Distribution (L/kg)	Volume of Binding (%)	Protein Excretion
Amikacin		*(SI = Conventional Units × 1.71)*				
Peak	20–30 µg/mL	34–51 µmol/L	4–8	0.4–1.3	50	1° renal
Trough	1–8 µg/mL	2–14 µmol/L				
Gentamicin (Standard Dosing)		*(SI = Conventional Units × 2.09)*				
Peak	6–10 µg/mL	12–21 µmol/L	4–8	0.4–1.3	50	1° renal
Trough	0.5–1.5 µg/mL	1–3 µmol/L				
Tobramycin		*(SI = Conventional Units × 2.14)*				
Peak	6–10 µg/mL	13–21 µmol/L	4–8	0.4–1.3	50	1° renal
Trough	0.5–1.5 µg/mL	1–3 µmol/L				
Vancomycin		*(SI = Conventional Units × 0.69)*				
Peak	30–40 µg/mL	21–28 µmol/L	4–8	0.4–1.3	50	1° renal
Trough	5–10 µg/mL	3–7 µmol/L				

* Conventional units.

DESCRIPTION & RATIONALE: The aminoglycoside antibiotics amikacin, gentamicin, and tobramycin are used against many gram-negative *(Acinetobacter, Citrobacter, Enterobacter, Escherichia coli, Klebsiella, Proteus, Providencia, Pseudomonas, Salmonella, Serratia,* and *Shigella)* and some gram-positive *(Staphylococcus aureus)* pathogenic microorganisms. Aminoglycosides are poorly absorbed through the gastrointestinal tract and are most frequently administered intravenously.

Vancomycin is a tricyclic glycopeptide antibiotic used against many gram-positive microorganisms, such as staphylococci, *Streptococcus pneumoniae,* group A β-hemolytic streptococci, enterococci, *Corynebacterium,* and *Clostridium.* Vancomycin has also been used in an oral form for the treatment of pseudomembranous colitis resulting from *Clostridium difficile* infection. This approach is less frequently used because of the emergence of vancomycin-resistant enterococci (VRE).

Many factors must be considered in effective dosing and monitoring of therapeutic drugs, including patient age, patient weight, interacting medications, electrolyte balance, protein levels, water balance, conditions that affect absorption and excretion, and ingestion of substances (e.g., foods, herbals, vitamins, and minerals) that can either potentiate or inhibit the intended target concentration. The most serious side effects of the aminoglycosides and vancomycin are nephrotoxicity and irreversible ototoxicity (uncommon). Peak and trough collection times should be documented carefully in relation to the time of medication administration. Creatinine levels should be monitored every 2 to 3 days to detect renal impairment due to toxic drug levels. ■

IMPORTANT NOTE: This information must be clearly and accurately communicated to avoid misunderstanding of the dose time in relation to the collection time. Miscommunication between the individual administering the medication and the individual collecting the specimen is the most frequent cause of subtherapeutic levels, toxic levels, and misleading information used in the calculation of future doses. Some pharmacies use a computerized pharmacokinetics approach to dosing that eliminates the need to be concerned about peak and trough collections; random specimens are adequate.

INDICATIONS:
• Assist in the diagnosis and prevention of toxicity
• Monitor renal dialysis patients or patients with rapidly changing renal function
• Monitor therapeutic regimen

RESULT

Level	Result
Normal levels	Therapeutic effect
Subtherapeutic levels	Adjust dose as indicated
Toxic levels	Adjust dose as indicated
Amikacin	Renal, hearing impairment
Gentamicin	Renal, hearing impairment
Tobramycin	Renal, hearing impairment
Vancomycin	Renal, hearing impairment

CRITICAL VALUES: The adverse effects of subtherapeutic levels are important. Care should be taken to investigate signs and symptoms of too little and too much medication. Note and immediately report to the health care practitioner any critically increased or subtherapeutic values and related symptoms.

Signs and symptoms of toxic levels of these antibiotics are similar and include loss of hearing and decreased renal function. The most important intervention is accurate therapeutic drug monitoring so the medication can be discontinued before irreversible damage is done.

Drug Name	Toxic Levels
Amikacin	Peak greater than 30 μg/mL, trough greater than 8 μg/mL
Gentamicin	Peak greater than 12 μg/mL, trough greater than 2 μg/mL
Tobramycin	Peak greater than 12 μg/mL, trough greater than 2 μg/mL
Vancomycin	Peak greater than 80 μg/mL, trough greater than 20 μg/mL

INTERFERING FACTORS:

- Blood drawn in serum separator tubes (gel tubes).

- Contraindicated in patients with liver disease, and caution advised in patients with renal impairment.

- Drugs that may decrease aminoglycoside efficacy include bleomycin, daunorubicin, doxorubicin, and penicillins (e.g., carbenicillin, piperacillin).

- Obtain a culture before and after the first dose of aminoglycosides.

- The risks of ototoxicity and nephrotoxicity are increased by the concomitant administration of aminoglycosides.

Nursing Implications and Procedure . . . .

Pretest:

➤ Inform the patient that the test is used to monitor for therapeutic and toxic drug levels.

➤ Obtain a history of the patient's complaints, including a list of known allergens (especially allergies or sensitivities to latex), and inform the appropriate health care practitioner accordingly.

➤ Obtain a history of the patient's genitourinary system as well as results of previously performed laboratory tests, surgical procedures, and other diagnostic procedures. For related laboratory tests, refer to the Genitourinary System and Therapeutic/Toxicology tables.

➤ Obtain a list of the medications the patient is taking, including herbs, nutritional supplements, and nutraceuticals. Note the last time and dose of medication taken. The requesting health care practitioner and laboratory should be advised if the patient regularly uses such products so that their effects can be taken into consideration when reviewing results.

➤ Review the procedure with the patient. Inform the patient that specimen collection takes approximately 5 to 10 minutes. Address concerns about pain related to the procedure. Explain to the patient that there may be some discomfort during the venipuncture.

➤ *Sensitivity to cultural and social issues,* as well as concern for modesty, is important in providing psychological support before, during, and after the procedure.

➤ There are no food, fluid, or medication restrictions unless by medical direction.

Intratest:

➤ If the patient has a history of severe allergic reaction to latex, care should

be taken to avoid the use of equipment containing latex.

➤ Instruct the patient to cooperate fully and to follow directions. Direct the patient to breathe normally and to avoid unnecessary movement.

➤ Observe standard precautions, and follow the general guidelines in Appendix A. Consider recommended collection time in relation to the dosing schedule. Positively identify the patient and label the appropriate tubes with the corresponding patient demographics, date, and time of collection, noting the last dose of medication taken. Perform a venipuncture; collect the specimen in a 5-mL red- or tiger-top tube.

➤ Remove the needle, place a gauze over the puncture site and apply gentle pressure to stop bleeding. Observe venipuncture site for bleeding or hematoma formation. Apply paper tape over gauze or replace with adhesive bandage.

➤ Promptly transport the specimen to the laboratory for processing and analysis.

➤ The results are recorded manually or in a computerized system for recall and postprocedure interpretation by the appropriate health care practitioner.

Post-test:

➤ Instruct the patient receiving aminoglycosides to immediately report any unusual symptoms (e.g., hearing loss, decreased urinary output) to his or her health care practitioner.

➤ *Nutritional considerations* include the avoidance of alcohol consumption.

➤ Administer antibiotic therapy if ordered. Remind the patient of the importance of completing the entire course of antibiotic therapy, even if signs and symptoms disappear before completion of therapy.

➤ A written report of the examination will be sent to the requesting health care practitioner, who will discuss the results with the patient.

➤ Reinforce information given by the patient's health care provider regarding further testing, treatment, or referral to another health care provider. Explain to the patient the importance of following the medication regimen and instructions regarding food and drug interactions. Answer any questions or address any concerns voiced by the patient or family.

➤ Instruct the patient to be prepared to provide the pharmacist with a list of other medications he or she is already taking in the event that the requesting health care practitioner prescribes a medication.

➤ Depending on the results of this procedure, additional testing may be performed to evaluate or monitor progression of the disease process and determine the need for a change in therapy. Evaluate test results in relation to the patient's symptoms and other tests performed.

Related laboratory tests:

➤ Related laboratory tests include albumin, blood urea nitrogen, creatinine, creatinine clearance, potassium, and urinalysis.

ANTIBODIES, ANTICYTOPLASMIC NEUTROPHILIC

SYNONYMS/ACRONYMS: Cytoplasmic antineutrophil cytoplasmic antibody (c-ANCA), perinuclear antineutrophil cytoplasmic antibody (p-ANCA).

SPECIMEN: Serum (1 mL) collected in a red-top tube.

REFERENCE VALUE: (Method: Indirect immunofluorescence) Negative.

DESCRIPTION & RATIONALE: There are two types of cytoplasmic neutrophil antibodies (ANCA), identified by their cellular staining characteristics. c-ANCA (cytoplasmic) is specific for proteinase 3 in neutrophils and monocytes and is found in the sera of patients with Wegener's granulomatosis. Wegener's syndrome includes granulomatous inflammation of the upper and lower respiratory tract and vasculitis. p-ANCA (perinuclear) is specific for myeloperoxidase, elastase, and lactoferrin, as well as other enzymes in neutrophils. p-ANCA is present in the sera of patients with pauci-immune necrotizing glomerulonephritis. ■

INDICATIONS:
- Assist in the diagnosis of Wegener's granulomatosis and its variants
- Differential diagnosis of ulcerative colitis
- Distinguish between biliary cirrhosis and sclerosing cholangitis
- Distinguish between vasculitic disease and the effects of therapy

RESULT

Increased in:
- c-ANCA
  Wegener's granulomatosis and its variants
- p-ANCA
  Alveolar hemorrhage
  Angiitis and polyangiitis
  Autoimmune liver disease
  Capillaritis
  Churg-Strauss syndrome
  Felty's syndrome
  Inflammatory bowel disease
  Leukocytoclastic skin vasculitis
  Necrotizing-crescentic glomerulonephritis
  Rheumatoid arthritis
  Vasculitis

Decreased in: N/A

CRITICAL VALUES: N/A

INTERFERING FACTORS: N/A

Nursing Implications and Procedure • • • • • • • • • • •

Pretest:

➤ Inform the patient that the test is used to assist in the diagnosis and monitoring of inflammatory activity in primary systemic small vessel vasculitides.

➤ Obtain a history of the patient's complaints, including a list of known allergens (especially allergies or sensitivities to latex), and inform the appropriate health care practitioner accordingly.

➤ Obtain a history of the patient's gastrointestinal, genitourinary, hepatobiliary, immune, and musculoskeletal systems and results of previously performed laboratory tests, surgical procedures, and other diagnostic procedures. For related laboratory tests, refer to the Gastrointestinal, Genitourinary, Hepatobiliary, Immune, and Musculoskeletal System tables.

➤ Obtain a list of the medications the patient is taking, including herbs, nutritional supplements, and nutraceuticals. The requesting health care practitioner and laboratory should be advised if the patient regularly uses these products so that their effects can be taken into consideration when reviewing results.

➤ Review the procedure with the patient. Inform the patient that specimen collection takes approximately 5 to 10 minutes. Address concerns about pain related to the procedure. Explain to the patient that there may be some discomfort during the venipuncture.

➤ There are no food, fluid, or medication restrictions unless by medical direction.

Intratest:

➤ If the patient has a history of severe allergic reaction to latex, care should be taken to avoid the use of equipment containing latex.

➤ Instruct the patient to cooperate fully and to follow directions. Direct the patient to breathe normally and to avoid unnecessary movement.

➤ Observe standard precautions, and follow the general guidelines in Appendix A. Positively identify the patient, and label the appropriate tubes with the corresponding patient demographics, date, and time of collection. Perform a venipuncture; collect the specimen in a 5-mL red-top tube.

➤ Remove the needle, place a gauze over the puncture site and apply gentle pressure to stop bleeding. Observe venipuncture site for bleeding or hematoma formation. Apply paper tape over gauze or replace with adhesive bandage.

➤ Promptly transport the specimen to the laboratory for processing and analysis.

➤ The results are recorded manually or in a computerized system for recall and postprocedure interpretation by the appropriate health care practitioner.

Post-test:

➤ A written report of the examination will be sent to the requesting health care practitioner, who will discuss the results with the patient.

➤ Recognize anxiety related to test results, and be supportive of perceived loss of independence and fear of shortened life expectancy. Discuss the implications of abnormal test results on the patient's lifestyle. Provide teaching and information regarding the clinical implications of the test results, as appropriate. Educate the patient regarding access to counseling services.

➤ Reinforce information given by the patient's health care provider regarding further testing, treatment, or referral to another health care provider.

Answer any questions or address any concerns voiced by the patient or family.

➤ Depending on the results of this procedure, additional testing may be performed to evaluate or monitor progression of the disease process and determine the need for a change in therapy. Evaluate test results in relation to the patient's symptoms and other tests performed.

Related laboratory tests:

➤ Related laboratory tests include anti–glomerular basement membrane antibody, antimitochondrial antibody, eosinophil count, kidney biopsy, rheumatoid factor, and urinalysis.

ANTIBODIES, ANTI–GLOMERULAR BASEMENT MEMBRANE

SYNONYMS/ACRONYM: Goodpasture's antibody, anti-GBM.

SPECIMEN: Serum (1 mL) collected in a red- or tiger-top tube. Lung or kidney tissue also may be submitted for testing. Refer to related biopsy monographs for specimen collection instructions.

REFERENCE VALUE: (Method: Direct or indirect immunofluorescence) Negative.

DESCRIPTION & RATIONALE: Goodpasture syndrome is a rare hypersensitivity condition characterized by the presence of circulating anti–glomerular basement membrane antibodies in the blood and the deposition of immunoglobulin and complement in renal basement membrane tissue. Severe and progressive glomerulonephritis can result from the presence of antibodies to renal glomerular basement membrane (GBM). Autoantibodies may also be directed to act against lung tissue in Goodpasture's syndrome. ■

INDICATIONS:

• Differentiate glomerulonephritis caused by anti-GBM from glomerulonephritis from other causes

RESULT

Increased in:
• Glomerulonephritis

• Goodpasture's syndrome

• Idiopathic pulmonary hemosiderosis

Decreased in: N/A

CRITICAL VALUES: N/A

INTERFERING FACTORS: N/A

Nursing Implications and Procedure • • • • • • • • • • •

Pretest:

➤ Inform the patient that the test is used to assist in detection and monitoring of glomerular basement membrane antibodies present in Goodpasture's syndrome.

➤ Obtain a history of the patient's complaints, including a list of known allergens (especially allergies or sensitivities to latex), and inform the appropriate health care practitioner accordingly.

➤ Obtain a history of the patient's genitourinary, immune, and respiratory systems and results of previously performed laboratory tests, surgical procedures, and other diagnostic procedures. For related laboratory tests, refer to the Genitourinary, Immune, and Respiratory System tables.

➤ Obtain a list of the medications the patient is taking, including herbs, nutritional supplements, and nutraceuticals. The requesting health care practitioner and laboratory should be advised if the patient regularly uses such products so that their effects can be taken into consideration when reviewing results.

➤ Review the procedure with the patient. Inform the patient that specimen collection takes approximately 5 to 10 minutes. Address concerns about pain related to the procedure. Explain to the patient that there may be some discomfort during the venipuncture.

➤ There are no food, fluid, or medication restrictions unless by medical direction.

Intratest:

➤ If the patient has a history of severe allergic reaction to latex, care should be taken to avoid the use of equipment containing latex.

➤ Instruct the patient to cooperate fully and to follow directions. Direct the patient to breathe normally and to avoid unnecessary movement.

➤ Observe standard precautions, and follow the general guidelines in Appendix A. Positively identify the patient, and label the appropriate tubes with the corresponding patient demographics, date, and time of collection. Perform a venipuncture; collect the specimen in a 5-mL red-top tube.

➤ Remove the needle, place a gauze over the puncture site and apply gentle pressure to stop bleeding. Observe venipuncture site for bleeding or hematoma formation. Apply paper tape over gauze or replace with adhesive bandage.

➤ Promptly transport the specimen to the laboratory for processing and analysis.

➤ The results are recorded manually or in a computerized system for recall and postprocedure interpretation by the appropriate health care practitioner.

Post-test:

➤ A written report of the examination will be sent to the requesting health care practitioner, who will discuss the results with the patient.

➤ Recognize anxiety related to test results, and be supportive of perceived loss of independence and fear of shortened life expectancy. Discuss the implications of abnormal test results on the patient's lifestyle. Provide teaching and information regarding the clinical implications of the test results, as appropriate. Educate the patient regarding access to counseling services.

➤ Reinforce information given by the patient's health care provider regarding further testing, treatment, or referral to another health care provider. Answer any questions or address any concerns voiced by the patient or family.

▶ Depending on the results of this procedure, additional testing may be performed to evaluate or monitor progression of the disease process and determine the need for a change in therapy. Evaluate test results in relation to the patient's symptoms and other tests performed.

Related laboratory tests:

▶ Related laboratory tests include antineutrophilic anti-cytoplasmic antibody, kidney biopsy, lung biopsy, and urinalysis.

ANTIBODIES, ANTINUCLEAR, ANTI-DNA, AND ANTICENTROMERE

SYNONYMS/ACRONYMS: Antinuclear antibodies (ANA), anti-DNA (anti-ds DNA).

SPECIMEN: Serum (2 mL) collected in a red-top tube.

REFERENCE VALUE: (Method: Indirect fluorescent antibody for ANA and anticentromere; enzyme-linked immunosorbent assay [ELISA] for anti-DNA)
ANA and anticentromere: titer of 1:40 or less

ANTI-DNA:

Negative	Less than 24 IU
Borderline	25–30 IU
Positive	31–200 IU
Strong positive	Greater than 200 IU

DESCRIPTION & RATIONALE: Antinuclear antibodies (ANA) are autoantibodies mainly located in the nucleus of affected cells. The presence of ANA indicates systemic lupus erythematosus (SLE), related collagen vascular diseases, and immune complex diseases. Antibodies against cellular DNA are strongly associated with SLE. Anticentromere antibodies are a subset of ANA. Their presence is strongly associated with CREST syndrome (*c*alcinosis, *R*aynaud's phenomenon, *e*sophageal dysfunction, *s*clerodactyly, and *t*elangiectasia). ANA and anticentromere antibodies are detected using Hep-2 cells (human epithelial cultured cells). Anti-DNA antibodies can be detected using a *Crithidia luciliae* substrate. Women are much more likely than men to be diagnosed with SLE. ■

INDICATIONS:

• Assist in the diagnosis and evaluation of SLE

• Evaluate suspected immune disorders, such as rheumatoid arthritis, systemic sclerosis, polymyositis, Sjögren's syndrome, and mixed connective tissue disease

RESULT

ANA Pattern*	Associated Antibody
Rim and/or homogeneous	Double-stranded DNA
	Single- or double-stranded DNA
Homogeneous	Histones
Speckled	Sm (Smith) antibody
	RNP
	SS-B/La, SS-A/Ro
Diffuse speckled with positive mitotic figures	Centromere
Nucleolar	Nucleolar, RNP

*ANA patterns are helpful in that certain conditions are frequently associated with specific patterns, but the patterns are not diagnostic for a particular disease. RNP = ribonucleoprotein.

Increased in:

• Drug-induced lupus erythematosus

• Lupoid hepatitis

• Mixed connective tissue disease

• Polymyositis

• Progressive systemic sclerosis

• Rheumatoid arthritis

• Sjögren's syndrome

• SLE

Decreased in: N/A

CRITICAL VALUES: N/A

INTERFERING FACTORS:

• Drugs that may cause positive results include carbamazepine, chlorpromazine, ethosuximide, hydralazine, isoniazid, mephenytoin, methyldopa, penicillins, phenytoin, primidone, procainamide, and quinidine.

• A patient can have lupus and test ANA negative.

• Inability of the patient to cooperate or remain still during the procedure because of age, significant pain, or mental status may interfere with the test results.

Nursing Implications and Procedure

Pretest:

➤ Inform the patient that the test is used to detect the presence of antinuclear antibodies associated with a variety of musculoskeletal and connective tissue diseases.

➤ Obtain a history of the patient's complaints, including a list of known allergens (especially allergies or sensitivities to latex), and inform the appropriate health care practitioner accordingly.

➤ Obtain a history of the patient's immune and musculoskeletal systems and results of previously performed laboratory tests, surgical procedures, and other diagnostic procedures. For related laboratory tests, refer to the Immune and Musculoskeletal System tables.

➤ Obtain a list of the medications the patient is taking, including herbs, nutritional supplements, and nutraceuticals. The requesting health care practitioner and laboratory should be advised if the patient regularly uses these products so that their effects can be taken into consideration when reviewing results.

➤ Review the procedure with the patient. Inform the patient that specimen collection takes approximately 5 to 10 minutes. Address concerns about pain related to the procedure. Explain to the patient that there may be some discomfort during the venipuncture.

➤ There are no food, fluid, or medication restrictions unless by medical direction.

Intratest:

➤ If the patient has a history of severe allergic reaction to latex, care should be taken to avoid the use of equipment containing latex.

➤ Instruct the patient to cooperate fully and to follow directions. Direct the patient to breathe normally and to avoid unnecessary movement.

➤ Observe standard precautions, and follow the general guidelines in Appendix A. Positively identify the patient, and label the appropriate tubes with the corresponding patient demographics, date, and time of collection. Perform a venipuncture; collect the specimen in a 5-mL red-top tube.

➤ Remove the needle, place a gauze over the puncture site and apply gentle pressure to stop bleeding. Observe venipuncture site for bleeding or hematoma formation. Apply paper tape over gauze or replace with adhesive bandage.

➤ Promptly transport the specimen to the laboratory for processing and analysis.

➤ The results are recorded manually or in a computerized system for recall and postprocedure interpretation by the appropriate health care practitioner.

Post-test:

➤ A written report of the examination will be sent to the requesting health care practitioner, who will discuss the results with the patient.

➤ Recognize anxiety related to test results, and be supportive of perceived loss of independence and fear of shortened life expectancy. Collagen and connective tissue diseases are chronic and, as such, they must be addressed on a continuous basis. Discuss the implications of abnormal test results on the patient's lifestyle. Provide teaching and information regarding the clinical implications of the test results, as appropriate. Educate the patient regarding access to counseling services.

➤ Educate the patient, as appropriate, regarding the importance of preventing infection, which is a significant cause of death in immunosuppressed individuals.

➤ Reinforce information given by the patient's health care provider regarding further testing, treatment, or referral to another health care provider. Answer any questions or address any concerns voiced by the patient or family.

➤ Depending on the results of this procedure, additional testing may be performed to evaluate or monitor progression of the disease process and determine the need for a change in therapy. Evaluate test results in relation to the patient's symptoms and other tests performed.

Related laboratory tests:

➤ Related laboratory tests include anticardiolipin antibody, antisclerodermal antibodies, C3, C4, erythrocyte sedimentation rate, extractable nuclear antibodies, Jo-1 antibody, kidney biopsy, procainamide, rheumatoid factor, skin biopsy, and total complement.

ANTIBODIES, ANTISCLERODERMA

SYNONYMS/ACRONYM: Progressive systemic sclerosis antibody, Scl-70 antibody.

SPECIMEN: Serum (1 mL) collected in a red-top tube.

REFERENCE VALUE: (Method: Indirect fluorescent antibody) Negative.

DESCRIPTION & RATIONALE: Antiscleroderma antibodies are associated with progressive systemic sclerosis, a condition that affects multiple systems, including the skin, gastrointestinal tract, lungs, blood vessels, heart, and kidneys. These antibodies are present in the sera of patients with CREST syndrome (*c*alcinosis, *R*aynaud's phenomenon, *e*sophageal dysfunction, *s*clerodactyly, and *t*elangiectasia). ▪

INDICATIONS:

• Assist in the diagnosis of scleroderma

RESULT

Increased in:
• CREST syndrome

• Progressive diffuse scleroderma

Decreased in: N/A

CRITICAL VALUES: N/A

INTERFERING FACTORS: N/A

Nursing Implications and Procedure

Pretest:

➤ Inform the patient that the test is used in the differential diagnosis of scleroderma and other autoimmune diseases of the musculoskeletal system.

➤ Obtain a history of the patient's complaints, including a list of known allergens (especially allergies or sensitivities to latex), and inform the appropriate health care practitioner accordingly.

➤ Obtain a history of the patient's immune and musculoskeletal systems and results of previously performed laboratory tests, surgical procedures, and other diagnostic procedures. For related laboratory tests, refer to the Immune and Musculoskeletal System tables.

➤ Obtain a list of the medications the patient is taking, including herbs, nutritional supplements, and nutraceuticals. The requesting health care practitioner and laboratory should be advised if the patient regularly uses these products so that their effects can be taken into consideration when reviewing results.

➤ Review the procedure with the

patient. Inform the patient that specimen collection takes approximately 5 to 10 minutes. Address concerns about pain related to the procedure. Explain to the patient that there may be some discomfort during the venipuncture.

➤ There are no food, fluid, or medication restrictions unless by medical direction.

Intratest:

➤ If the patient has a history of severe allergic reaction to latex, care should be taken to avoid the use of equipment containing latex.

➤ Instruct the patient to cooperate fully and to follow directions. Direct the patient to breathe normally and to avoid unnecessary movement.

➤ Observe standard precautions, and follow the general guidelines in Appendix A. Positively identify the patient, and label the appropriate tubes with the corresponding patient demographics, date, and time of collection. Perform a venipuncture; collect the specimen in a 5-mL red-top tube.

➤ Remove the needle, place a gauze over the puncture site and apply gentle pressure to stop bleeding. Observe venipuncture site for bleeding or hematoma formation. Apply paper tape over gauze or replace with adhesive bandage.

➤ Promptly transport the specimen to the laboratory for processing and analysis.

➤ The results are recorded manually or in a computerized system for recall and postprocedure interpretation by the appropriate health care practitioner.

Post-test:

➤ A written report of the examination will be sent to the requesting health care practitioner, who will discuss the results with the patient.

➤ Recognize anxiety related to test results, and be supportive of perceived loss of independence and fear of shortened life expectancy. Collagen and connective tissue diseases are chronic and, as such, they must be addressed on a continuous basis. Discuss the implications of abnormal test results on the patient's lifestyle. Provide teaching and information regarding the clinical implications of the test results, as appropriate. Educate the patient regarding access to counseling services.

➤ Educate the patient, as appropriate, regarding the importance of preventing infection, which is a significant cause of death in immunosuppressed individuals.

➤ Reinforce information given by the patient's health care provider regarding further testing, treatment, or referral to another health care provider. Answer any questions or address any concerns voiced by the patient or family.

➤ Depending on the results of this procedure, additional testing may be performed to evaluate or monitor progression of the disease process and determine the need for a change in therapy. Evaluate test results in relation to the patient's symptoms and other tests performed.

Related laboratory tests:

➤ Related laboratory tests include anticentromere antibodies, anti-DNA antibodies, antinuclear antibodies, extractable nuclear antibodies, Jo-1 antibody, kidney biopsy, rheumatoid factor, and skin biopsy.

ANTIBODIES, ANTISPERM

SYNONYMS/ACRONYM: N/A.

SPECIMEN: Serum (1 mL) collected in a red-top tube.

REFERENCE VALUE: (Method: Immunoassay)

Result	Sperm Bound by Immunobead (%)
Negative	0–15
Weak positive	16–30
Moderate positive	31–50
Strong positive	51–100

DESCRIPTION & RATIONALE: A major cause of infertility in men is blocked efferent testicular ducts. As a result of the reabsorption of sperm from the blocked ducts, antibodies against the sperm may be produced over time and thereby may lower the patient's fertility. Semen and cervical mucus can also be tested for antisperm antibodies. ∎

INDICATIONS:

• Evaluation of infertility

RESULT

Increased in:
• Blocked testicular efferent duct
• Postvasectomy

Decreased in: N/A

CRITICAL VALUES: N/A

INTERFERING FACTORS:

• The patient should not ejaculate for 3 to 4 days before specimen collection if semen will be evaluated.

• Sperm antibodies have been detected in pregnant women and in women with primary infertility.

Nursing Implications and Procedure

Pretest:

➤ Inform the patient that the test is used in the evaluation of infertility and guidance through assisted reproductive techniques.

➤ Obtain a history of the patient's complaints, including a list of known allergens (especially allergies or sensitivities to latex), and inform the appropriate health care practitioner accordingly.

➤ Obtain a history of the patient's immune and reproductive systems and results of previously performed laboratory tests, surgical procedures, and other diagnostic procedures. For related laboratory tests, refer to the Immune and Reproductive System tables.

➤ Obtain a list of the medications the

patient is taking, including herbs, nutritional supplements, and nutraceuticals. The requesting health care practitioner and laboratory should be advised if the patient regularly uses these products so that their effects can be taken into consideration when reviewing results.

➤ Review the procedure with the patient. Inform the patient that specimen collection takes approximately 5 to 10 minutes and that additional specimens may be required. Address concerns about pain related to the procedure. Explain to the patient that there may be some discomfort during the venipuncture.

➤ *Sensitivity to social and cultural issues,* as well as concern for modesty, is important in providing psychological support before, during, and after the procedure.

➤ There are no food, fluid, or medication restrictions unless by medical direction.

Intratest:

➤ If the patient has a history of severe allergic reaction to latex, care should be taken to avoid the use of equipment containing latex.

➤ Instruct the patient to cooperate fully and to follow directions. Direct the patient to breathe normally and to avoid unnecessary movement.

➤ Observe standard precautions, and follow the general guidelines in Appendix A. Positively identify the patient, and label the appropriate tubes with the corresponding patient demographics, date, and time of collection. Perform a venipuncture; collect the specimen in a 5-mL red-top tube.

➤ Remove the needle, place a gauze over the puncture site and apply gentle pressure to stop bleeding. Observe venipuncture site for bleeding or hematoma formation. Apply paper tape over gauze or replace with adhesive bandage.

➤ Promptly transport the specimen to the laboratory for processing and analysis.

➤ The results are recorded manually or in a computerized system for recall and postprocedure interpretation by the appropriate health care practitioner.

Post-test:

➤ A written report of the examination will be sent to the requesting health care practitioner, who will discuss the results with the patient.

➤ Recognize anxiety related to test results. Discuss the implications of abnormal test results on the patient's lifestyle. Educate the patient regarding access to counseling services. Provide a supportive, nonjudgmental environment when assisting a patient through the process of fertility testing. Educate the patient regarding access to counseling services, as appropriate.

➤ Reinforce information given by the patient's health care provider regarding further testing, treatment, or referral to another health care provider. Answer any questions or address any concerns voiced by the patient or family.

➤ Depending on the results of this procedure, additional testing may be performed to evaluate or monitor progression of the disease process and determine the need for a change in therapy. Evaluate test results in relation to the patient's symptoms and other tests performed.

Related laboratory tests:

➤ Related laboratory tests include human chorionic gonadotropin, luteinizing hormone, progesterone, semen analysis, and testosterone.

ANTIBODIES, ANTISTREPTOLYSIN *O*

SYNONYM/ACRONYM: Streptozyme, ASO.

SPECIMEN: Serum (1 mL) collected in a red-top tube.

REFERENCE VALUE: (Method: Nephelometry) Less than 200 IU/mL.

DESCRIPTION & RATIONALE: Group A β-hemolytic streptococci secrete the enzyme streptolysin *O*, which can destroy red blood cells. The enzyme acts as an antigen and stimulates the immune system to develop streptolysin *O* antibodies. These antistreptolysin *O* (ASO) antibodies occur within 1 month after the onset of a streptococcal infection. Detection of the antibody over several weeks strongly suggests exposure to group A β-hemolytic streptococci. ■

INDICATIONS:
- Assist in establishing a diagnosis of streptococcal infection
- Evaluate patients with streptococcal infections for the development of acute rheumatic fever or nephritis
- Monitor response to therapy in streptococcal illnesses

RESULT

Increased in:
- Endocarditis
- Glomerulonephritis
- Rheumatic fever
- Scarlet fever

Decreased in: N/A

CRITICAL VALUES: N/A

INTERFERING FACTORS:
- Drugs that may decrease ASO titers include antibiotics and corticosteroids, because therapy suppresses antibody response.

Nursing Implications and Procedure

Pretest:

➤ Inform the patient that the test is used to document exposure to group A streptococci bacteria.

➤ Obtain a history of the patient's complaints, including a list of known allergens (especially allergies or sensitivities to latex), and inform the appropriate health care practitioner accordingly.

➤ Obtain a history of the patient's immune system and results of previously performed laboratory tests, surgical procedures, and other diagnostic procedures. For related laboratory tests, refer to the Immune System table.

➤ Obtain a list of the medications the patient is taking, including herbs, nutritional supplements, and nutraceuticals. The requesting health care practitioner and laboratory should be advised if the patient regularly uses these products so that their effects can be taken into consideration when reviewing results.

➤ Review the procedure with the patient. Inform the patient that specimen collection takes approximately 5 to 10 minutes. Address concerns about pain related to the procedure. Explain to the patient that there may be some discomfort during the venipuncture.

➤ There are no food, fluid, or medication restrictions unless by medical direction.

Intratest:

➤ If the patient has a history of severe allergic reaction to latex, care should be taken to avoid the use of equipment containing latex.

➤ Instruct the patient to cooperate fully and to follow directions. Direct the patient to breathe normally and to avoid unnecessary movement.

➤ Observe standard precautions, and follow the general guidelines in Appendix A. Positively identify the patient, and label the appropriate tubes with the corresponding patient demographics, date, and time of collection. Perform a venipuncture; collect the specimen in a 5-mL red-top tube.

➤ Remove the needle, place a gauze over the puncture site and apply gentle pressure to stop bleeding. Observe venipuncture site for bleeding or hematoma formation. Apply paper tape over gauze or replace with adhesive bandage.

➤ Promptly transport the specimen to the laboratory for processing and analysis.

➤ The results are recorded manually or in a computerized system for recall and postprocedure interpretation by the appropriate health care practitioner.

Post-test:

➤ Administer antibiotics as ordered. Remind the patient of the importance of completing the entire course of antibiotic therapy even if signs and symptoms disappear before completion of therapy.

➤ A written report of the examination will be sent to the requesting health care practitioner, who will discuss the results with the patient.

➤ Reinforce information given by the patient's health care provider regarding further testing, treatment, or referral to another health care provider. Answer any questions or address any concerns voiced by the patient or family.

➤ Depending on the results of this procedure, additional testing may be performed to evaluate or monitor progression of the disease process and determine the need for a change in therapy. Evaluate test results in relation to the patient's symptoms and other tests performed.

Related laboratory tests:

➤ Related laboratory tests include group A streptococcal screen, streptococcal anti-DNAse B, and throat culture.

ANTIBODIES, ANTITHYROGLOBULIN AND ANTITHYROID PEROXIDASE

SYNONYMS/ACRONYM: Thyroid antibodies, antithyroid peroxidase antibodies (thyroid peroxidase [TPO] antibodies were previously called thyroid antimicrosomal antibodies).

SPECIMEN: Serum (1 mL) collected in a red-top tube.

REFERENCE VALUE: (Method: Radioimmunoassay)

Antibody	Conventional Units	SI Units (Conversion Factor × 1)
Antithyroglobulin antibody	Less than 0.3 U/mL	Less than 0.3 kU/L
Antiperoxidase antibody	Less than 0.3 U/mL	Less than 0.3 kU/L

DESCRIPTION & RATIONALE: Thyroid antibodies are mainly immunoglobulin G–type antibodies. Antithyroid peroxidase antibodies bind with microsomal antigens on cells lining the microsomal membrane. They are thought to destroy thyroid tissue as a result of stimulation by lymphocytic killer cells. These antibodies are present in hypothyroid and hyperthyroid conditions. Antithyroglobulin antibodies are autoantibodies directed against thyroglobulin. The function of these antibodies is unclear. Both tests are normally requested together. ▪

INDICATIONS:
• Assist in confirming suspected inflammation of thyroid gland
• Assist in the diagnosis of suspected hypothyroidism caused by thyroid tissue destruction
• Assist in the diagnosis of suspected thyroid autoimmunity in patients with other autoimmune disorders

RESULT

Increased in:
• Autoimmune disorders
• Graves' disease
• Goiter
• Hashimoto's thyroiditis
• Idiopathic myxedema
• Pernicious anemia
• Thyroid carcinoma

Decreased in: N/A

CRITICAL VALUES: N/A

INTERFERING FACTORS:
- Lithium may increase thyroid antibody levels.

- Recent radioactive scans or radiation within 1 week before the test can interfere with test results when radioimmunoassay is the test method.

Nursing Implications and Procedure . . . .

Pretest:

➤ Inform the patient that the test is used to assess thyroid gland function.

➤ Obtain a history of the patient's complaints, including a list of known allergens (especially allergies or sensitivities to latex), and inform the appropriate health care practitioner accordingly.

➤ Obtain a history of the patient's endocrine and immune system and results of previously performed laboratory tests, surgical procedures, and other diagnostic procedures. For related laboratory tests, refer to the Endocrine and Immune System tables.

➤ Obtain a list of the medications the patient is taking, including herbs, nutritional supplements, and nutraceuticals. The requesting health care practitioner and laboratory should be advised if the patient regularly uses these products so that their effects can be taken into consideration when reviewing results.

➤ Note any recent procedures that can interfere with test results.

➤ Review the procedure with the patient. Inform the patient that specimen collection takes approximately 5 to 10 minutes. Address concerns about pain related to the procedure.

Explain to the patient that there may be some discomfort during the venipuncture.

➤ There are no food, fluid, or medication restrictions unless by medical direction.

Intratest:

➤ If the patient has a history of severe allergic reaction to latex, care should be taken to avoid the use of equipment containing latex.

➤ Instruct the patient to cooperate fully and to follow directions. Direct the patient to breathe normally and to avoid unnecessary movement.

➤ Observe standard precautions, and follow the general guidelines in Appendix A. Positively identify the patient, and label the appropriate tubes with the corresponding patient demographics, date, and time of collection. Perform a venipuncture; collect the specimen in a 5-mL red-top tube.

➤ Remove the needle, place a gauze over the puncture site and apply gentle pressure to stop bleeding. Observe venipuncture site for bleeding or hematoma formation. Apply paper tape over gauze or replace with adhesive bandage.

➤ Promptly transport the specimen to the laboratory for processing and analysis.

➤ The results are recorded manually or in a computerized system for recall and postprocedure interpretation by the appropriate health care practitioner.

Post-test:

➤ A written report of the examination will be sent to the requesting health care practitioner, who will discuss the results with the patient.

➤ Reinforce information given by the patient's health care provider regarding further testing, treatment, or referral to another health care provider.

Answer any questions or address any concerns voiced by the patient or family.

➤ Depending on the results of this procedure, additional testing may be performed to evaluate or monitor progression of the disease process and determine the need for a change in therapy. Evaluate test results in relation to the patient's symptoms and other tests performed.

Related laboratory tests:

➤ Related laboratory tests include complete blood count, thyroid biopsy, thyroid-stimulating hormone, free thyroxine, thyroxine, and triiodothyronine.

ANTIBODIES, CARDIOLIPIN, IMMUNOGLOBULIN G, AND IMMUNOGLOBULIN M

SYNONYMS/ACRONYMS: Antiphospholipid antibody, lupus anticoagulant, LA, ACA.

SPECIMEN: Serum (1 mL) collected in a red-top tube.

REFERENCE VALUE: (Method: Immunoassay, enzyme-linked immunosorbent assay [ELISA]) Negative.

DESCRIPTION & RATIONALE: Cardiolipin antibody is one of several identified antiphospholipid antibodies. These antibodies react with proteins in the blood that are bound to phospholipid and interfere with normal blood vessel function. The two primary types of problems they cause are narrowing and irregularity of the blood vessels and blood clots in the blood vessels. Cardiolipin antibodies are found in individuals with lupus erythematosus, lupus-related conditions, infectious diseases, drug reactions, and sometimes fetal loss.

Cardiolipin antibodies are often found in association with lupus anticoagulant. Increased antiphospholipid antibody levels have been found in pregnant women with lupus who have had miscarriages. The combination of noninflammatory thrombosis of blood vessels, low platelet count, and history of miscarriage is termed *antiphospholipid antibody syndrome*. ■

INDICATIONS:

• Assist in the diagnosis of antiphospholipid antibody syndrome

RESULT

Increased in:

- Antiphospholipid antibody syndrome
- Chorea
- Drug reactions
- Epilepsy
- Infectious diseases
- Mitral valve endocarditis
- Patients with lupus-like symptoms (often antinuclear antibody negative)
- Placental infarction
- Recurrent fetal loss (strong association with two or more occurrences)
- Recurrent venous and arterial thromboses

Decreased in: N/A

CRITICAL VALUES: N/A

INTERFERING FACTORS: Cardiolipin antibody is partially cross-reactive with syphilis reagin antibody and lupus anticoagulant. False-positive rapid plasma reagin results may occur.

Nursing Implications and Procedure • • • • • • • • • • •

Pretest:

➤ Inform the patient that the test is used to detect the presence of antiphospholipid antibodies, which can lead to the development of blood vessel problems, complications of which include stroke, heart attack, and miscarriage.

➤ Obtain a history of the patient's complaints, including a list of known allergens (especially allergies or sensitivities to latex), and inform the appropriate health care practitioner accordingly.

➤ Obtain a history of the patient's hematopoietic, immune, and reproductive systems and results of previously performed laboratory tests, surgical procedures, and other diagnostic procedures. For related laboratory tests, refer to the Hematopoietic, Immune, and Reproductive System tables.

➤ Obtain a list of the medications the patient is taking, including herbs, nutritional supplements, and nutraceuticals. The requesting health care practitioner and laboratory should be advised if the patient regularly uses these products so that their effects can be taken into consideration when reviewing results.

➤ Review the procedure with the patient. Inform the patient that specimen collection takes approximately 5 to 10 minutes. Address concerns about pain related to the procedure. Explain to the patient that there may be some discomfort during the venipuncture.

➤ There are no food, fluid, or medication restrictions unless by medical direction.

Intratest:

➤ If the patient has a history of severe allergic reaction to latex, care should be taken to avoid the use of equipment containing latex.

➤ Instruct the patient to cooperate fully and to follow directions. Direct the patient to breathe normally and to avoid unnecessary movement.

➤ Observe standard precautions, and follow the general guidelines in Appendix A. Positively identify the patient, and label the appropriate tubes with the corresponding patient demographics, date, and time of collection. Perform a venipuncture; collect the specimen in a 5-mL red-top tube.

➤ Remove the needle, place a gauze over the puncture site and apply gentle pressure to stop bleeding.

Observe venipuncture site for bleeding or hematoma formation. Apply paper tape over gauze or replace with adhesive bandage.

➤ Promptly transport the specimen to the laboratory for processing and analysis.

➤ The results are recorded manually or in a computerized system for recall and postprocedure interpretation by the appropriate health care practitioner.

Post-test:

➤ A written report of the examination will be sent to the requesting health care practitioner, who will discuss the results with the patient.

➤ Recognize anxiety related to test results, and be supportive of fear of shortened life expectancy. Discuss the implications of abnormal test results on the patient's lifestyle. Provide teaching and information regarding the clinical implications of the test results, as appropriate.

Educate the patient regarding access to counseling services. Provide contact information, if desired, for the Lupus Foundation of America (*http://www.lupus.org*).

➤ Reinforce information given by the patient's health care provider regarding further testing, treatment, or referral to another health care provider. Answer any questions or address any concerns voiced by the patient or family.

➤ Depending on the results of this procedure, additional testing may be performed to evaluate or monitor progression of the disease process and determine the need for a change in therapy. Evaluate test results in relation to the patient's symptoms and other tests performed.

Related laboratory tests:

➤ Related laboratory tests include antinuclear antibodies, complete blood count, fibrinogen, lupus anticoagulant antibodies, platelet count, protein C, protein S, and syphilis serology.

ANTIBODIES, GLIADIN (IMMUNOGLOBULIN G AND IMMUNOGLOBULIN A)

SYNONYMS/ACRONYMS: Endomysial antibodies, gliadin (IgG and IgA) antibodies, EMA.

SPECIMEN: Serum (1 mL) collected in a red-top tube.

REFERENCE VALUE: (Method: Immunoassay)

Gliadin Antibody	Conventional Units
IgA	Less than 5 U
IgG	Less than 57 U

DESCRIPTION & RATIONALE: Gliadin is a water-soluble protein found in the gluten of wheat, rye, oats, and barley. The intestinal mucosa of certain individuals does not digest gluten, allowing a toxic buildup of gliadin. Antibodies to gliadin form and result in damage to the intestinal mucosa. In severe cases, intestinal mucosa can be lost. Immunoglobulin G (IgG) and immunoglobulin A (IgA) gliadin antibodies are detectable in the serum of patients with gluten-sensitive enteropathy. ■

INDICATIONS:
- Assist in the diagnosis of asymptomatic gluten-sensitive enteropathy in some patients with dermatitis herpetiformis
- Assist in the diagnosis of gluten-sensitive enteropathies
- Assist in the diagnosis of nontropical sprue
- Monitor dietary compliance of patients with gluten-sensitive enteropathies

RESULT

Increased in:
- Asymptomatic gluten-sensitive enteropathy
- Celiac disease
- Dermatitis herpetiformis
- Nontropical sprue

Decreased in: N/A

CRITICAL VALUES: N/A

INTERFERING FACTORS:
- Conditions other than gluten-sensitive enteropathy can result in elevated antibody levels without corresponding histologic evidence. These conditions include Crohn's disease, postinfection malabsorption, and food protein intolerance.
- A negative IgA gliadin result, especially with a positive IgG gliadin result in an untreated patient, does not rule out active gluten-sensitive enteropathy.

Nursing Implications and Procedure

Pretest:

➤ Inform the patient that the test is used to assist in the diagnosis and monitoring of gluten-sensitive enteropathies.

➤ Obtain a history of the patient's complaints, including a list of known allergens (especially allergies or sensitivities to latex), and inform the appropriate health care practitioner accordingly.

➤ Obtain a history of the patient's gastrointestinal and immune systems as well as results of previously performed laboratory tests, surgical procedures, and other diagnostic procedures. For related laboratory tests, refer to the Gastrointestinal and Immune System tables.

➤ Obtain a list of foods and medications the patient is taking, including herbs, nutritional supplements, and nutraceuticals. The requesting health care practitioner and laboratory should be advised if the patient regularly uses these products so that their effects can be taken into consideration when reviewing results.

➤ Review the procedure with the patient. Inform the patient that specimen collection takes approximately 5 to 10 minutes. Address concerns about pain related to the procedure. Explain to the patient that there may be some discomfort during the venipuncture.

➤ There are no food, fluid, or medication restrictions unless by medical direction.

Intratest:

➤ If the patient has a history of severe allergic reaction to latex, care should be taken to avoid the use of equipment containing latex.

➤ Instruct the patient to cooperate fully and to follow directions. Direct the patient to breathe normally and to avoid unnecessary movement.

➤ Observe standard precautions, and follow the general guidelines in Appendix A. Positively identify the patient, and label the appropriate tubes with the corresponding patient demographics, date, and time of collection. Perform a venipuncture; collect the specimen in a 5-mL red-top tube.

➤ Remove the needle, place a gauze over the puncture site and apply gentle pressure to stop bleeding. Observe venipuncture site for bleeding or hematoma formation. Apply paper tape over gauze or replace with adhesive bandage.

➤ Promptly transport the specimen to the laboratory for processing and analysis.

➤ The results are recorded manually or in a computerized system for recall and postprocedure interpretation by the appropriate health care practitioner.

Post-test:

➤ *Nutritional considerations:* Encourage the patient with abnormal findings to consult with a qualified nutritionist to plan a gluten-free diet. This dietary planning is complex because patients are often malnourished and have other related nutritional problems.

➤ A written report of the examination will be sent to the requesting health care practitioner, who will discuss the results with the patient.

➤ Recognize anxiety related to test results, and offer support. Discuss the implications of abnormal test results on the patient's lifestyle. Provide teaching and information regarding the clinical implications of the test results, as appropriate. Educate the patient regarding access to appropriate counseling services.

➤ Reinforce information given by the patient's health care provider regarding further testing, treatment, or referral to another health care provider. Answer any questions or address any concerns voiced by the patient or family.

➤ Depending on the results of this procedure, additional testing may be performed to evaluate or monitor progression of the disease process and determine the need for a change in therapy. Evaluate test results in relation to the patient's symptoms and other tests performed.

Related laboratory tests:

➤ Related laboratory tests include albumin, calcium, D-xylose tolerance test, electrolytes, fecal analysis, fecal fat, folic acid, iron, lactose tolerance test, and skin biopsy.

ANTIBODY, ANTIMITOCHONDRIAL

SYNONYM/ACRONYM: AMA.

SPECIMEN: Serum (1 mL) collected in a red-top tube.

REFERENCE VALUE: (Method: Indirect fluorescent antibody) Negative or titer less than 1:20.

DESCRIPTION & RATIONALE: Antimitochondrial antibodies are found in 90% of patients with primary biliary cirrhosis (PBC). PBC is identified most frequently in women ages 35 to 60 years. Testing is useful in the differential diagnosis of chronic liver disease as antimitochondrial antibodies are rarely detected in extrahepatic biliary obstruction, various forms of hepatitis, and cirrhosis. ■

INDICATIONS:
• Assist in the diagnosis of PBC
• Assist in the differential diagnosis of chronic liver disease

RESULT

Increased in:
• Hepatitis (alcoholic, viral)
• PBC
• Rheumatoid arthritis (occasionally)
• Systemic lupus erythematosus (occasionally)
• Thyroid disease (occasionally)

Decreased in: N/A

CRITICAL VALUES: N/A

INTERFERING FACTORS: N/A

Nursing Implications and Procedure ● ● ● ● ● ● ● ● ● ● ●

Pretest:

➤ Inform the patient that the test is used in the differential diagnosis of chronic liver disease.

➤ Obtain a history of the patient's complaints, including a list of known allergens (especially allergies or sensitivities to latex), and inform the appropriate health care practitioner accordingly.

➤ Obtain a history of the patient's hepatobiliary and immune systems, as well as results of previously performed laboratory tests, surgical procedures, and other diagnostic procedures. For related laboratory tests, refer to the Hepatobiliary and Immune System tables.

➤ Obtain a list of the medications the patient is taking, including herbs, nutritional supplements, and nutraceuticals. The requesting health care practitioner and laboratory should be advised if the patient regularly uses these products so that their effects can be taken into consideration when reviewing results.

➤ Review the procedure with the patient. Inform the patient that specimen collection takes approximately 5 to 10 minutes. Address concerns about pain related to the procedure. Explain to the patient that there may be some discomfort during the venipuncture.

➤ There are no food, fluid, or medication restrictions unless by medical direction.

Intratest:

➤ If the patient has a history of severe allergic reaction to latex, care should be taken to avoid the use of equipment containing latex.

➤ Instruct the patient to cooperate fully and to follow directions. Direct the patient to breathe normally and to avoid unnecessary movement.

➤ Observe standard precautions, and follow the general guidelines in Appendix A. Positively identify the patient, and label the appropriate tubes with the corresponding patient demographics, date, and time of collection. Perform a venipuncture; collect the specimen in a 5-mL red-top tube.

➤ Remove the needle, place a gauze over the puncture site and apply gentle pressure to stop bleeding. Observe venipuncture site for bleeding or hematoma formation. Apply paper tape over gauze or replace with adhesive bandage.

➤ Promptly transport the specimen to the laboratory for processing and analysis.

➤ The results are recorded manually or in a computerized system for recall and postprocedure interpretation by the appropriate health care practitioner.

Post-test:

➤ *Nutritional considerations:* The presence of antimitochondrial antibodies may be associated with liver disease. Dietary recommendations may be indicated and vary depending on the severity of the condition. A low-protein diet may be in order if the liver cannot process the end products of protein metabolism. A diet of soft foods may be required if esophageal varices have developed. Ammonia levels may be used to determine whether protein should be added to or reduced from the diet. Patients should be encouraged to eat simple carbohydrates and emulsified fats (as in homogenized milk or eggs), as opposed to complex carbohydrates (e.g., starch, fiber, and glycogen [animal carbohydrates]) and complex fats, which would require additional bile to emulsify them so that they could be used. Observe the cirrhotic patient carefully for the development of ascites; if ascites develops, pay strict attention to fluid and electrolyte balance.

➤ A written report of the examination will be sent to the requesting health care practitioner, who will discuss the results with the patient.

➤ Reinforce information given by the patient's health care provider regarding further testing, treatment, or referral to another health care provider. Answer any questions or address any concerns voiced by the patient or family.

➤ Depending on the results of this procedure, additional testing may be performed to evaluate or monitor progression of the disease process and determine the need for a change in therapy. Evaluate test results in relation to the patient's symptoms and other tests performed.

Related laboratory tests:

➤ Related laboratory tests include albumin, alkaline phosphatase, ammonia, anticytoplasmic neutrophilic antibodies, antinuclear antibodies, anti–smooth muscle antibodies, bilirubin, electrolytes, γ-glutamyl transpeptidase, and liver biopsy.

ANTIBODY, ANTI–SMOOTH MUSCLE

SYNONYM/ACRONYM: ASMA.

SPECIMEN: Serum (1 mL) collected in a red-top tube.

REFERENCE VALUE: (Method: Indirect fluorescent antibody) Negative.

DESCRIPTION & RATIONALE: Anti–smooth muscle antibodies are autoantibodies found in high titers in the sera of patients with autoimmune diseases of the liver and bile duct. Simultaneous testing for antimitochondrial antibodies can be useful in the differential diagnosis of chronic liver diesease. ∎

INDICATIONS:
• Differential diagnosis of liver disease

RESULT

Increased in:
• Autoimmune hepatitis
• Chronic active viral hepatitis
• Infectious mononucleosis

Decreased in: N/A

CRITICAL VALUES: N/A

INTERFERING FACTORS: N/A

Nursing Implications and Procedure • • • • • • • • • • •

Pretest:

> Inform the patient that the test is used in the differential diagnosis of chronic liver disease.

> Obtain a history of the patient's complaints, including a list of known allergens (especially allergies or sensitivities to latex), and inform the appropriate health care practitioner accordingly.

> Obtain a history of the patient's hepatobiliary and immune systems, as well as results of previously performed laboratory tests, surgical procedures, and other diagnostic procedures. For related laboratory tests, refer to the Hepatobiliary and Immune System tables.

> Obtain a list of the medications the patient is taking, including herbs, nutritional supplements, and nutraceuticals. The requesting health care practitioner and laboratory should be advised if the patient regularly uses these products so that their effects can be taken into consideration when reviewing results.

> Review the procedure with the patient. Inform the patient that specimen collection takes approximately 5 to 10 minutes. Address concerns about pain related to the procedure. Explain to the patient that there may be some discomfort during the venipuncture.

> There are no food, fluid, or medication restrictions unless by medical direction.

Intratest:

> If the patient has a history of severe allergic reaction to latex, care should be taken to avoid the use of equipment containing latex.

> Instruct the patient to cooperate fully and to follow directions. Direct the patient to breathe normally and to avoid unnecessary movement.

> Observe standard precautions, and follow the general guidelines in Appendix A. Positively identify the patient, and label the appropriate tubes with the corresponding patient demographics, date, and time of collection. Perform a venipuncture; collect the specimen in a 5-mL red-top tube.

> Remove the needle, place a gauze over the puncture site and apply gentle pressure to stop bleeding. Observe venipuncture site for bleeding or hematoma formation. Apply paper tape over gauze or replace with adhesive bandage.

> Promptly transport the specimen to the laboratory for processing and analysis.

> The results are recorded manually or in a computerized system for recall and postprocedure interpretation by the appropriate health care practitioner.

➤ *Nutritional considerations:* The presence of anti–smooth muscle antibodies may be associated with liver disease. Dietary recommendations may be indicated and vary depending on the severity of the condition. A low-protein diet may be in order if the liver cannot process the end products of protein metabolism. A diet of soft foods may be required if esophageal varices have developed. Ammonia levels may be used to determine whether protein should be added to or reduced from the diet. Patients should be encouraged to eat simple carbohydrates and emulsified fats (as in homogenized milk or eggs), as opposed to complex carbohydrates (e.g., starch, fiber, and glycogen [animal carbohydrates]) and complex fats, which would require additional bile to emulsify them so that they could be used. Observe the cirrhotic patient carefully for the development of ascites; if ascites develops, pay strict attention to fluid and electrolyte balance.

➤ A written report of the examination will be sent to the requesting health care practitioner, who will discuss the results with the patient.

➤ Reinforce information given by the patient's health care provider regarding further testing, treatment, or referral to another health care provider. Answer any questions or address any concerns voiced by the patient or family.

➤ Depending on the results of this procedure, additional testing may be performed to evaluate or monitor progression of the disease process and determine the need for a change in therapy. Evaluate test results in relation to the patient's symptoms and other tests performed.

Related laboratory tests:

➤ Related laboratory tests include alkaline phosphatase, ammonia, antimitochondrial antibody, antinuclear antibody, aspartate aminotransferase, bilirubin, hepatitis serology, liver biopsy, prothrombin time, and serum protein electrophoresis.

ANTIBODY, Jo-1

SYNONYM/ACRONYM: Antihistidyl transfer RNA (tRNA) synthase.

SPECIMEN: Serum (1 mL) collected in a red-top tube.

REFERENCE VALUE: (Method: Immunoassay) Negative.

DESCRIPTION & RATIONALE: Jo-1 is an autoantibody found in the serum of some antinuclear antibody–positive patients. Compared to the presence of other autoantibodies, the presence of Jo-1 suggests a more aggressive disease course and a higher risk of mortality. The clinical effects of this autoantibody include acute onset, fever, dry and cracked skin on the hands, Raynaud's phenomenon, and arthritis.

INDICATIONS:

- Test for idiopathic inflammatory myopathies

RESULT

Increased in:

- Dermatomyositis

- Polymyositis

Decreased in: N/A

CRITICAL VALUES: N/A

INTERFERING FACTORS: N/A

Nursing Implications and Procedure • • • • • • • • • • •

Pretest:

▷ Inform the patient that the test is used to identify and monitor idiopathic myopathies.

▷ Obtain a history of the patient's complaints, including a list of known allergens (especially allergies or sensitivities to latex), and inform the appropriate health care practitioner accordingly.

▷ Obtain a history of the patient's immune and musculoskeletal systems, as well as results of previously performed laboratory tests, surgical procedures, and other diagnostic procedures. For related laboratory tests, refer to the Immune and Musculoskeletal System tables.

▷ Obtain a list of the medications the patient is taking, including herbs, nutritional supplements, and nutraceuticals. The requesting health care practitioner and laboratory should be advised if the patient regularly uses these products so that their effects can be taken into consideration when reviewing results.

▷ Review the procedure with the patient. Inform the patient that specimen collection takes approximately 5 to 10 minutes. Address concerns about pain related to the procedure. Explain to the patient that there may be some discomfort during the venipuncture.

▷ There are no food, fluid, or medication restrictions unless by medical direction.

Intratest:

▷ If the patient has a history of severe allergic reaction to latex, care should be taken to avoid the use of equipment containing latex.

▷ Instruct the patient to cooperate fully and to follow directions. Direct the patient to breathe normally and to avoid unnecessary movement.

▷ Observe standard precautions, and follow the general guidelines in Appendix A. Positively identify the patient, and label the appropriate tubes with the corresponding patient demographics, date, and time of collection. Perform a venipuncture; collect the specimen in a 5-mL red-top tube.

▷ Remove the needle, place a gauze over the puncture site and apply gentle pressure to stop bleeding. Observe venipuncture site for bleeding or hematoma formation. Apply paper tape over gauze or replace with adhesive bandage..

▷ Promptly transport the specimen to the laboratory for processing and analysis.

▷ The results are recorded manually or in a computerized system for recall and postprocedure interpretation by the appropriate health care practitioner.

Post-test:

▷ A written report of the examination will be sent to the requesting health care practitioner, who will discuss the results with the patient.

▷ Reinforce information given by the patient's health care provider regard-

ing further testing, treatment, or referral to another health care provider. Answer any questions or address any concerns voiced by the patient or family.

➤ Depending on the results of this procedure, additional testing may be performed to evaluate or monitor progression of the disease process and determine the need for a change in therapy. Evaluate test results in relation to the patient's symptoms and other tests performed.

Related laboratory tests:

➤ Related laboratory tests include alanine aminotransferase, aldolase, antinuclear antibody, aspartate aminotransferase, creatine kinase, erythrocyte sedimentation rate, extractable nuclear antibodies, lactate dehydrogenase and isoenzymes, muscle biopsy, myoglobin, rheumatoid factor, anti-scleroderma antibody, skin biopsy, and urine creatinine.

ANTICONVULSANT DRUGS: CARBAMAZEPINE, ETHOSUXIMIDE, PHENOBARBITAL, PHENYTOIN, PRIMIDONE, VALPROIC ACID

SYNONYMS/ACRONYM: *Carbamazepine* (Carbatrol, Tegretol, Tegretol XR); *Ethosuximide* (Zarontin); *Phenobarbital* (Luminal, Phenobarb); *Phenytoin* (Cerebyx, Dilantin, Fenytoin, Phenytek); *Primidone* (Mysoline); *Valproic acid* (Depacon, Depakene, Depakote).

SPECIMEN: Serum (1 mL) collected in a red-top tube.

Drug	Route of Administration
Carbamazepine*	Oral
Ethosuximide*	Oral
Phenobarbital*	Oral
Phenytoin*	Oral
Primidone*	Oral
Valproic Acid*	Oral

* Recommended collection time = trough: immediately before next dose (at steady state) or at a consistent sampling time.

Drug	Therapeutic Dose*	SI Units	Half-Life (h)	Volume of Distribution (L/kg)	Protein Binding (%)	Excretion
Carbamazepine	4–12 µg/mL	*(SI = Conventional Units × 4.23)* 17–51 µmol/L	15–40	0.8–1.8	60–80	Hepatic
Ethosuximide	40–100 µg/mL	*(SI = Conventional Units × 7.08)* 283–708 µmol/L	25–70	0.7	0–5	Renal
Phenobarbital	*Adult:* 15–40 µg/mL *Child:* 15–30 µg/mL	*(SI = Conventional Units × 4.31)* *Adult:* 65–172 µmol/L *Child:* 65–129 µmol/L	*Adult:* 50–140 *Child:* 40–70	0.5–1.0 L/kg	40–50	80% Hepatic 20% Renal
Phenytoin	10–20 µg/mL *Neonatal:* 6–14 µg/mL	*(SI = Conventional Units × 3.96)* 40–79 µmol/L *Neonatal:* 24–55 µmol/L	*Adult:* 20–40 *Child:* 10	0.6–0.7	85–95	Hepatic
Primidone	*Adult:* 5–12 µg/mL *Child:* 7–10 µg/mL	*(SI = Conventional Units × 4.58)* *Adult:* 23–55 µmol/L *Child:* 32–46 µmol/L	4–12	0.5–1.0	0–20	Hepatic
Valproic Acid	50–120 µg/mL	*(SI = Conventional Units × 6.93)* 347–832 µmol/L	12–16	0.1–0.5	85–95	Hepatic

* Conventional units.

DESCRIPTION & RATIONALE: Anticonvulsants are used to reduce the frequency and severity of seizures for patients with epilepsy. Carbamazepine is also used for controlling neurogenic pain in trigeminal neuralgia and diabetic neuropathy and for treating for bipolar disease and other neurologic and psychiatric conditions. Valproic acid is also used for some psychiatric conditions like bipolar disease and for prevention of migrane headache.

Many factors must be considered in effective dosing and monitoring of therapeutic drugs, including patient age, patient weight, interacting medications, electrolyte balance, protein levels, water balance, conditions that affect absorption and excretion, and foods, herbals, vitamins, and minerals that can either potentiate or inhibit the intended target concentration.

Peak and trough collection times should be documented carefully in relation to the time of medication administration. ■

IMPORTANT NOTE: This information must be clearly and accurately communicated to avoid misunderstanding of the dose time in relation to the collection time. Miscommunication between the individual administering the medication and the individual collecting the specimen is the most frequent cause of subtherapeutic levels, toxic levels, and misleading information used in calculation of future doses.

INDICATIONS:
- Assist in the diagnosis of and prevention of toxicity
- Evaluate overdose, especially in combination with ethanol
- Monitor compliance with therapeutic regimen

RESULT

Level	Response
Normal levels	Therapeutic effect
Subtherapeutic levels	Adjust dose as indicated
Toxic levels	Adjust dose as indicated
Carbamazepine	Hepatic impairment
Ethosuximide	Hepatic impairment
Phenobarbital	Hepatic impairment
Phenytoin	Hepatic impairment
Primidone	Hepatic impairment
Valproic acid	Hepatic impairment

CRITICAL VALUES: ⚠ It is important to note the adverse effects of toxic and subtherapeutic levels. Care must be taken to investigate the signs and symptoms of too little and too much medication. Note and immediately report to the health care practitioner any critically increased values and related symptoms.

Carbamazepine: Greater Than 12 μg/mL

Signs and symptoms of carbamazepine toxicity include respiratory depression, seizures, leukopenia, hyponatremia, hypotension, stupor, and possible coma. Possible interventions include gastric lavage (contraindicated if ileus is present); airway protection; administration of fluids and vasopressors for hypotension; treatment of seizures with diazepam, phenobarbital, or phenytoin; cardiac monitoring; monitoring of vital signs; and discontinuing the medication. Emetics are contraindicated.

Ethosuximide: Greater Than 100 μg/mL

Signs and symptoms of ethosuximide toxicity include nausea, vomiting, and lethargy. Possible interventions include administration of activated charcoal, administration of saline cathartic and gastric lavage (contraindicated if ileus is present), airway protection, hourly assessment of neurologic function, and discontinuing the medication.

Phenobarbital: Greater Than 40 μg/mL

Signs and symptoms of phenobarbital toxicity include cold, clammy skin; ataxia; central nervous system depression; hypothermia; hypotension; cyanosis; Cheyne-Stokes respiration; tachycardia; possible coma; and possible renal impairment. Possible interventions include gastric lavage, administration of activated charcoal with cathartic, airway protection, possible intubation and mechanical ventilation (especially during gastric lavage if there is no gag reflex), monitoring for hypotension, and discontinuing the medication.

Phenytoin: Adults: Greater Than 20 μg/mL; Neonatal: Greater Than 14 μg/mL

Signs and symptoms of phenytoin toxicity include double vision, nystagmus, lethargy, central nervous system depression, and possible coma. Possible interventions include airway support, electrocardiographic monitoring, administration of activated charcoal, gastric lavage with warm saline or tap water,

administration of saline or sorbitol cathartic, and discontinuing the medication.

Primidone: Greater Than 12 μg/mL

Signs and symptoms of primidone toxicity include ataxia, anemia, and central nervous system depression. Possible interventions include airway protection, treatment of anemia with vitamin B_{12} and folate, and discontinuing the medication.

Valproic Acid: Greater Than 120 μg/mL

Signs and symptoms of valproic acid toxicity include numbness, tingling, weakness, loss of appetite, and mental changes. Possible interventions include administration of activated charcoal and naloxone and discontinuing the medication.

INTERFERING FACTORS:

- Blood drawn in serum separator tubes (gel tubes).
- Contraindicated in patients with liver disease, and caution advised in patients with renal impairment.
- Drugs that may increase carbamazepine levels or increase risk of toxicity include cimetidine, clozapine, danazol, diazepam, diltiazem, erythromycin, haloperidol, isoniazid, propoxyphene, risperidone, triacetyloleandomycin, tricyclic antidepressants, valproic acid, and verapamil.
- Drugs that may decrease carbamazepine levels include phenobarbital, phenytoin, and primidone.
- Drugs that may increase ethosuximide levels include isoniazid, ritonavir, and valproic acid.
- Drugs that may decrease ethosuximide levels include phenobarbital, phenytoin, and primidone.
- Drugs that may increase phenobarbital levels or increase risk of toxicity include barbital drugs, furosemide, primidone, salicylates, and valproic acid.

• Phenobarbital may affect the metabolism of other drugs, increasing their effectiveness, such as β-blockers, chloramphenicol, corticosteroids, doxycycline, griseofulvin, haloperidol, methylphenidate, phenothiazines, phenylbutazone, propoxyphene, quinidine, theophylline, tricyclic antidepressants, and valproic acid.

• Phenobarbital may affect the metabolism of other drugs, decreasing their effectiveness, such as chloramphenicol, cyclosporine, ethosuximide, oral anticoagulants, oral contraceptives, phenytoin, and theophylline.

• Phenobarbital is an active metabolite of primidone, and both drug levels should be monitored while the patient is receiving primidone to avoid either toxic or subtherapeutic levels of both medications.

• Drugs that may increase phenytoin levels or increase the risk of phenytoin toxicity include amiodarone, azapropazone, carbamazepine, chloramphenicol, cimetidine, disulfiram, ethanol, fluconazole, halothane, ibuprofen, imipramine, levodopa, metronidazole, miconazole, nifedipine, phenylbutazone, sulfonamides, trazodone, tricyclic antidepressants, and trimethoprim. Small changes in formulation (i.e., changes in brand) also may increase phenytoin levels or increase the risk of phenytoin toxicity.

• Drugs that may decrease phenytoin levels include bleomycin, carbamazepine, cisplatin, disulfiram, folic acid, intravenous fluids containing glucose, nitrofurantoin, oxacillin, rifampin, salicylates, and vinblastine.

• Primidone decreases the effectiveness of carbamazepine, ethosuximide, felbamate, lamotrigine, oral anticoagulants, oxcarbazepine, topiramate, and valproate.

• Drugs that may increase valproic acid levels or increase risk of toxicity include dicumarol, phenylbutazone, and high doses of salicylate.

• Drugs that may decrease valproic acid levels include carbamazepine, phenobarbital, phenytoin, and primidone.

Nursing Implications and Procedure

Pretest:

➤ Inform the patient that the test is used to monitor for therapeutic and toxic drug levels.

➤ Obtain a history of the patient's complaints, including a list of known allergens (especially allergies or sensitivities to latex), and inform the appropriate health care practitioner accordingly.

➤ Obtain a history of the patient's genitourinary and hepatobiliary systems as well as results of previously performed laboratory tests, surgical procedures, and other diagnostic procedures. For related laboratory tests, refer to the Genitourinary and Hepatobiliary Systems and Therapeutic/Toxicology tables.

➤ Obtain a list of medications the patient is taking, including herbs, nutritional supplements, and nutraceuticals. Note the last time and dose of medication taken. The requesting health care practitioner and laboratory should be advised if the patient regularly uses these products so that their effects can be taken into consideration when reviewing results.

➤ Review the procedure with the patient. Inform the patient that specimen collection takes approximately 5 to 10 minutes. Address concerns about pain related to the procedure. Explain to the patient that there may be some discomfort during the venipuncture.

Sensitivity to cultural and social issues, as well as concern for modesty, is important in providing psychological support before, during, and after the procedure.

There are no food, fluid, or medication restrictions unless by medical direction.

Intratest:

➤ If the patient has a history of severe allergic reaction to latex, care should be taken to avoid the use of equipment containing latex.

➤ Direct the patient to breathe normally and to avoid unnecessary movement.

➤ Observe standard precautions, and follow the general guidelines in Appendix A. Consider recommended collection time in relation to dosing schedule. Positively identify the patient, and label the appropriate tubes with the corresponding patient demographics, date, and time of collection, noting the last dose of medication taken. Perform a venipuncture; collect the specimen in a 5-mL red-top tube.

➤ Remove the needle, place a gauze over the puncture site and apply gentle pressure to stop bleeding. Observe venipuncture site for bleeding or hematoma formation. Apply paper tape over gauze or replace with adhesive bandage.

➤ Promptly transport the specimen to the laboratory for processing and analysis.

➤ The results are recorded manually or in a computerized system for recall and postprocedure interpretation by the appropriate health care practitioner

Post-test:

➤ A written report of the examination will be sent to the requesting health care practitioner, who will discuss the results with the patient.

➤ Reinforce information given by the patient's health care provider regarding further testing, treatment, or referral to another health care provider. Explain to the patient the importance of following the medication regimen and instructions regarding drug interactions. Instruct the patient to immediately report any unusual sensations (e.g., ataxia, dizziness, dyspnea, lethargy, rash, tremors, mental changes, weakness, or visual disturbances) to his or her health care practitioner. Answer any questions or address any concerns voiced by the patient or family.

➤ Instruct the patient to be prepared to provide the pharmacist with a list of other medications he or she is already taking in the event that the requesting health care practitioner prescribes a medication.

➤ Depending on the results of this procedure, additional testing may be performed to evaluate or monitor progression of the disease process and determine the need for a change in therapy. Evaluate test results in relation to the patient's symptoms and other tests performed.

Related laboratory tests:

➤ Related laboratory tests include albumin, blood urea nitrogen, creatinine, complete blood count, electrolytes, liver function tests, and total protein.

ANTIDEOXYRIBONUCLEASE-B, STREPTOCOCCAL

· ·

SYNONYMS/ACRONYM: ADNase-B, AntiDNase-B titer, antistreptococcal DNase-B titer, streptodornase.

SPECIMEN: Serum (1 mL) collected in a red-top tube.

REFERENCE VALUE: (Method: Spectrophotometry)

Age	Normal Results
Preschoolers	Less than 61 U
School-age children	Less than 171 U
Adults	Less than 86 U

DESCRIPTION & RATIONALE: The presence of streptococcal deoxyribonuclease (DNase) antibodies is an indicator of recent infection, especially if a rise in antibody titer can be shown. This test is more sensitive than the antistreptolysin *O* test. A rise in titer of two or more dilution increments between acute and convalescent specimens is clinically significant. ■

INDICATIONS:
• Investigate the presence of streptococcal antibodies as a source of recent infection

RESULT

Increased in:
• Streptococcal infections (systemic)

Decreased in: N/A

CRITICAL VALUES: N/A

INTERFERING FACTORS: N/A

Nursing Implications and Procedure · · · · · · · · · · · ·

Pretest:

➤ Inform the patient that the test is used to document recent streptococcal infection.

➤ Obtain a history of the patient's complaints, including a list of known allergens (especially allergies or sensitivities to latex), and inform the appropriate health care practitioner accordingly.

➤ Obtain a history of the patient's immune system and results of previously performed laboratory tests, surgical procedures, and other diagnostic procedures. For related laboratory tests, refer to the Immune System table.

➤ Obtain a list of the medications the patient is taking, including herbs, nutritional supplements, and nutraceuticals. The requesting health care practitioner and laboratory should be advised if the patient regularly uses these products so that their effects can be taken into consideration when reviewing results.

- Review the procedure with the patient. Inform the patient that specimen collection takes approximately 5 to 10 minutes. Address concerns about pain related to the procedure. Explain to the patient that there may be some discomfort during the venipuncture.
- There are no food, fluid, or medication restrictions unless by medical direction.

Intratest:

- If the patient has a history of severe allergic reaction to latex, care should be taken to avoid the use of equipment containing latex.
- Instruct the patient to cooperate fully and to follow directions. Direct the patient to breathe normally and to avoid unnecessary movement.
- Observe standard precautions, and follow the general guidelines in Appendix A. Positively identify the patient, and label the appropriate tubes with the corresponding patient demographics, date, and time of collection. Perform a venipuncture; collect the specimen in a 5-mL red-top tube.
- Remove the needle, place a gauze over the puncture site and apply gentle pressure to stop bleeding. Observe venipuncture site for bleeding or hematoma formation. Apply paper tape over gauze or replace with adhesive bandage.
- Promptly transport the specimen to the laboratory for processing and analysis.

- The results are recorded manually or in a computerized system for recall and postprocedure interpretation by the appropriate health care practitioner.

Post-test:

- Administer analgesics and antibiotics if ordered. Remind the patient of the importance of completing the entire course of antibiotic therapy, even if signs and symptoms disappear before completion of therapy.
- A written report of the examination will be sent to the requesting health care practitioner, who will discuss the results with the patient.
- Reinforce information given by the patient's health care provider regarding further testing, treatment, or referral to another health care provider. Inform the patient that a convalescent specimen may be requested in 7 to 10 days. Answer any questions or address any concerns voiced by the patient or family.
- Depending on the results of this procedure, additional testing may be performed to evaluate or monitor progression of the disease process and determine the need for a change in therapy. Evaluate test results in relation to the patient's symptoms and other tests performed.

Related laboratory tests:

- Related laboratory tests include antistreptolysin *O* antibody, group A streptococcal screen, and throat culture.

ANTIDEPRESSANT DRUGS (Cyclic): AMITRIPTYLINE, NORTRIPTYLINE, DOXEPIN, IMIPRAMINE, DESIPRAMINE

SYNONYMS/ACRONYM: *Cyclic antidepressants: amitriptyline* (Elavil, Endep, Etrafon, Limbitrol DS, Triavil); *nortriptyline* (Aventyl HCL, Pamelor); *doxepin* (Adapin, Sinequan); *imipramine* (Anafranil, Clomipramine, Imavate, Presamine, Surmontil, Tofranil PM, Trimipramine); *desipramine* (Norpramin, pertofrane).

SPECIMEN: Serum (1 mL) collected in a red-top tube.

Drug	Route of Administration	Recommended Collection Time
Amitriptyline	Oral	Trough: immediately before next dose (at steady state)
Nortriptyline	Oral	Trough: immediately before next dose (at steady state)
Doxepin	Oral	Trough: immediately before next dose (at steady state)
Imipramine	Oral	Trough: immediately before next dose (at steady state)
Desipramine	Oral	Trough: immediately before next dose (at steady state)

REFERENCE VALUE: (Method: Chromatography for amitriptyline, nortriptyline, and doxepin; immunoassay for imipramine and desipramine)

Drug	Therapeutic Dose*	SI Units	Half-Life (h)	Volume of Distribution (L/kg)	Protein Binding (%)	Excretion
		(SI = Conventional Units × 3.61)				
Amitriptyline, alone	80–200 ng/mL	289–722 nmol/L	17–40	10–36	85–95	Hepatic
		(SI = Conventional Units × 3.8)				
Nortriptyline, alone	50–150 ng/mL	190–570 nmol/L	20–90	15–23	90–95	Hepatic
		(SI = Conventional Units × 3.58)				
Combined doxepin and desmethyldoxepin	150–250 ng/mL	540–900 nmol/L	10–25	10–30	75–85	Hepatic
		(SI = Conventional Units × 3.57)				
Imipramine	150–250 ng/mL	536–892 nmol/L	6–28	9–23	60–95	Hepatic
		(Conventional Units × 3.75)				
Desipramine	150–250 ng/mL	562–938 nmol/L	6–28	9–23	60–95	Hepatic

* Conventional units.

DESCRIPTION & RATIONALE: Cyclic antidepressants are used in the treatment of major depression. They have also been used effectively to treat bipolar disorder, panic disorder, attention-deficit hyperactivity disorder (ADHD), obsessive-compulsive disorder (OCD), enuresis, eating disorders (bulimia nervosa in particular), nicotine dependence (tobacco), and cocaine dependence. Numerous drug interactions occur with the cyclic antidepressants.

Many factors must be considered in effective dosing and monitoring of therapeutic drugs, including patient age, patient weight, interacting medications, electrolyte balance, protein levels, water balance, conditions that affect absorption and excretion, and foods, herbals, vitamins, and minerals that can either potentiate or inhibit the intended target concentration.

Trough collection times should be documented carefully in relation to the time of medication administration. ■

IMPORTANT NOTE: This information must be clearly and accurately communicated to avoid misunderstanding of the dose time in relation to the collection time. Miscommunication between the individual administering the medication and the individual collecting the specimen is the most frequent cause of subtherapeutic levels, toxic levels, and misleading information used in calculation of future doses.

INDICATIONS:
• Assist in the diagnosis and prevention of toxicity

• Evaluate overdose, especially in combination with ethanol (*Note:* Doxepin abuse is unusual)

• Monitor compliance with therapeutic regimen

RESULT

Level	Response
Normal levels	Therapeutic effect
Subtherapeutic levels	Adjust dose as indicated
Toxic levels	Adjust dose as indicated
Amitriptyline	Hepatic impairment
Nortriptyline	Hepatic impairment
Doxepin	Hepatic impairment
Imipramine	Hepatic impairment
Desipramine	Hepatic impairment

CRITICAL VALUES: ⚠ It is important to note the adverse effects of toxic and subtherapeutic levels of antidepressants. Care must be taken to investigate signs and symptoms of too little and too much medication. Note and immediately report to the health care practitioner any critically increased values and related symptoms.

Cyclic Antidepressants:
• Amitriptyline: Greater than 300 ng/mL

• Combined amitriptyline and nortriptyline: Greater than 250 ng/mL

• Combined doxepin and desmethyldoxepin: Greater than 150 ng/mL

• Desipramine: Greater than 300 ng/mL

• Imipramine: Greater than 250 ng/mL

Signs and symptoms of cyclic antidepressant toxicity include agitation, hallucinations, confusion, seizures, arrhythmias, hyperthermia, flushing, dilation of the pupils, and possible coma. Possible interventions include administration of activated charcoal; emesis; gastric lavage with saline; administration of physostigmine to counteract seizures, hypertension, or respiratory depression; administration of bicarbonate, propranolol, lidocaine, or phenytoin to counteract arrhythmias; and electrocardiographic monitoring.

INTERFERING FACTORS:
• Blood drawn in serum separator tubes (gel tubes).

• Contraindicated in patients with liver disease, and caution advised in patients with renal impairment.

• Cyclic antidepressants may potentiate the effects of oral anticoagulants.

Nursing Implications and Procedure • • • • • • • • • •

Pretest:

➤ Inform the patient that the test is used to monitor for therapeutic and toxic drug levels.

➤ Obtain a history of the patient's complaints, including a list of known allergens (especially allergies or sensitivities to latex), and inform the appropriate health care practitioner accordingly.

➤ Obtain a history of the patient's genitourinary and hepatobiliary systems as well as results of previously performed laboratory tests, surgical procedures, and other diagnostic procedures. For related laboratory tests, refer to the Genitourinary and Hepatobiliary Systems and Therapeutic/Toxicology tables.

➤ Obtain a list of the medications the patient is taking, including herbs, nutritional supplements, and nutraceuticals. Note the last time and dose of medication taken. The requesting health care practitioner and laboratory should be advised if the patient regularly uses these products so that their effects can be taken into consideration when reviewing results.

➤ Review the procedure with the patient. Inform the patient that specimen collection takes approximately 5 to 10 minutes. Address concerns about pain related to the procedure. Explain to the patient that there may be some discomfort during the venipuncture.

➤ *Sensitivity to cultural and social issues,* as well as concern for modesty, is important in providing psychological support before, during, and after the procedure.

➤ There are no food, fluid, or medication restrictions unless by medical direction.

Intratest:

➤ If the patient has a history of severe allergic reaction to latex, care should be taken to avoid the use of equipment containing latex.

➤ Instruct the patient to cooperate fully and to follow directions. Direct the patient to breathe normally and to avoid unnecessary movement.

➤ Observe standard precautions, and follow the general guidelines in Appendix A. Consider recommended collection time in relation to dosing schedule. Positively identify the patient, and label the appropriate tubes with the corresponding patient demographics, date, and time of collection, noting the last dose of medication taken. Perform a venipuncture; collect the specimen in a 5-mL red-top tube.

➤ Remove the needle, place a gauze over the puncture site and apply gentle pressure to stop bleeding. Observe venipuncture site for bleeding or hematoma formation. Apply paper tape over gauze or replace with adhesive bandage.

➤ Promptly transport the specimen to the laboratory for processing and analysis.

➤ The results are recorded manually or in a computerized system for recall and postprocedure interpretation by the appropriate health care practitioner

Post-test:

➤ *Nutritional considerations* include the avoidance of alcohol consumption.

➤ A written report of the examination will be sent to the requesting health care practitioner, who will discuss the results with the patient.

➤ Reinforce information given by the patient's health care provider regarding further testing, treatment, or referral to another health care provider. Explain to the patient the importance of following the medication regimen and instructions regarding drug interactions. Instruct the patient to immediately report any unusual sensations (e.g., severe headache, vomiting, sweating, diaphoresis, visual disturbances) to his or her health care practitioner. Blood pressure should be monitored regularly. Answer any questions or address any concerns voiced by the patient or family.

➤ Instruct the patient to be prepared to provide the pharmacist with a list of other medications he or she is already taking in the event that the requesting health care practitioner prescribes a medication.

➤ Depending on the results of this procedure, additional testing may be performed to evaluate or monitor progression of the disease process and determine the need for a change in therapy. Evaluate test results in relation to the patient's symptoms and other tests performed.

Related laboratory tests:

➤ Related laboratory tests include albumin, blood urea nitrogen, creatinine, complete blood count, electrolytes, liver function tests, and total protein.

ANTIDIURETIC HORMONE

SYNONYMS/ACRONYM: Vasopressin, arginine vasopressin hormone, ADH.

SPECIMEN: Plasma (1 mL) collected in lavender-top (ethylenediaminetetraacetic acid [EDTA]) tube.

REFERENCE VALUE: (Method: Radioimmunoassay)

RECOMMENDATION: This test should be ordered and interpreted with results of a serum osmolality.

Serum Osmolality*	Antidiuretic Hormone*	SI Units (Conversion Factor × 0.926)
270–280 mOsm/kg	Less than 1.5 pg/mL	Less than 1.4 pmol/L
280–285 mOsm/kg	Less than 2.5 pg/mL	Less than 2.3 pmol/L
285–290 mOsm/kg	1–5 pg/mL	0.9–4.6 pmol/L
290–295 mOsm/kg	2–7 pg/mL	1.9–6.5 pmol/L
295–300 mOsm/kg	4–12 pg/mL	3.7–11.1 pmol/L

* Conventional units.

DESCRIPTION & RATIONALE: Antidiuretic hormone (ADH) is formed by the hypothalamus and stored in the posterior pituitary gland. ADH is released in response to increased serum osmolality or decreased blood volume. When the hormone is active, small amounts of concentrated urine are produced; in its absence, large amounts of dilute urine are produced. Although a 1% change in serum osmolality stimulates ADH secretion, blood volume must decrease by approximately 10% for ADH secretion to be induced. Psychogenic stimuli, such as stress, pain, and anxiety, may also stimulate ADH release, but the mechanism is unclear. ■

INDICATIONS:
- Assist in the diagnosis of known or suspected malignancy associated with syndrome of inappropriate ADH secretion (SIADH), such as oat cell lung cancer, thymoma, lymphoma, leukemia, pancreatic carcinoma, prostate gland carcinoma, and intestinal carcinoma; elevated ADH levels indicate the presence of this syndrome.
- Assist in the diagnosis of known or suspected pulmonary conditions associated with SIADH, such as tuberculosis, pneumonia, and positive-pressure mechanical ventilation.
- Detect central nervous system trauma, surgery, or disease that may lead to impaired ADH secretion.
- Differentiate neurogenic (central) diabetes insipidus from nephrogenic diabetes insipidus by decreased ADH levels in neurogenic diabetes insipidus or elevated levels in nephrogenic diabetes insipidus if normal feedback mechanisms are intact.
- Evaluate polyuria or altered serum osmolality to identify possible alterations in ADH secretion as the cause.

RESULT

Increased in:
- Acute intermittent porphyria
- Brain tumor
- Disorders involving the central nervous system, thyroid gland, and adrenal gland
- Ectopic production (systemic neoplasm)
- Guillain-Barré syndrome
- Nephrogenic diabetes insipidus
- Pain, stress, or exercise
- Pneumonia
- Pulmonary tuberculosis
- SIADH
- Tuberculous meningitis

Decreased in:
- Nephrotic syndrome
- Pituitary (central) diabetes insipidus
- Psychogenic polydipsia

CRITICAL VALUES: Effective treatment of SIADH depends on identifying and resolving the cause of increased ADH production. Signs and symptoms of SIADH are the same as those for hyponatremia, including irritability, tremors, muscle spasms, convulsions, and neurologic changes. The patient has enough sodium, but it is diluted in excess retained water.

INTERFERING FACTORS:
• Drugs that may increase ADH levels include barbiturates, carbamazepine, chlorpropamide, chlorthalidone, cisplatin, clofibrate, ether, furosemide, haloperidol, hydrochlorothiazide, lithium, methyclothiazide, narcotic analgesics, phenothiazides, polythiazide, tolbutamide, tricyclic antidepressants, vidarabine, vinblastine, and vincristine.
• Drugs that may decrease ADH levels include clonidine, demeclocycline, ethanol, lithium carbonate, and phenytoin.
• Recent radioactive scans or radiation within 1 week before the test can interfere with test results when radioimmunoassay is the test method.
• ADH exhibits diurnal variation, with highest levels of secretion occurring at night; first morning collection is recommended.
• ADH secretion is also affected by posture, with higher levels measured while upright.

Nursing Implications and Procedure ....

Pretest:

➤ Inform the patient that the test is used to assist in the diagnosis of disorders affecting urine concentration.
➤ Obtain a history of the patient's complaints, including a list of known allergens (especially allergies or sensitivities to latex), and inform the appropriate health care practitioner accordingly.

➤ Obtain a history of the patient's endocrine and genitourinary systems, as well as results of previously performed laboratory tests, surgical procedures, and other diagnostic procedures. For related laboratory tests, refer to the Endocrine and Genitourinary System tables.
➤ Note any recent procedures that can interfere with test results.
➤ Obtain a list of the medications the patient is taking, including herbs, nutritional supplements, and nutraceuticals. The requesting health care practitioner and laboratory should be advised if the patient regularly uses these products so that their effects can be taken into consideration when reviewing results.
➤ Review the procedure with the patient. Inform the patient that specimen collection takes approximately 5 to 10 minutes. Address concerns about pain related to the procedure. Explain to the patient that there may be some discomfort during the venipuncture.
➤ There are no food, fluid, or medication restrictions unless by medical direction.
➤ Prepare an ice slurry in a cup or plastic bag to have ready for immediate transport of the specimen to the laboratory. Prechill the lavender-top tube in the ice slurry.

Intratest:

➤ If the patient has a history of severe allergic reaction to latex, care should be taken to avoid the use of equipment containing latex.
➤ Instruct the patient to cooperate fully and to follow directions. The patient should be encouraged to be calm and in a sitting position for specimen collection. Direct the patient to breathe normally and to avoid unnecessary movement.
➤ Observe standard precautions, and follow the general guidelines in Appendix A. Positively identify the patient, and label the appropriate tubes with the corresponding patient demographics, date, and time of col-

lection. Perform a venipuncture; collect the specimen in a prechilled 5-mL lavender-top tube.

➤ Remove the needle, place a gauze over the puncture site and apply gentle pressure to stop bleeding. Observe venipuncture site for bleeding or hematoma formation. Apply paper tape over gauze or replace with adhesive bandage.

➤ The sample should be placed in an ice slurry immediately after collection. Information on the specimen label can be protected from water in the ice slurry by first placing the specimen in a protective plastic bag. Promptly transport the specimen to the laboratory for processing and analysis.

➤ The results are recorded manually or in a computerized system for recall and postprocedure interpretation by the appropriate health care practitioner.

Post-test:

➤ A written report of the examination will be sent to the requesting health care practitioner, who will discuss the results with the patient.

➤ Reinforce information given by the patient's health care provider regarding further testing, treatment, or referral to another health care provider. Inform the patient, as appropriate, that treatment may include diuretic therapy and fluid restriction to successfully eliminate the excess water. Answer any questions or address any concerns voiced by the patient or family.

➤ Depending on the results of this procedure, additional testing may be performed to evaluate or monitor progression of the disease process and determine the need for a change in therapy. Evaluate test results in relation to the patient's symptoms and other tests performed.

Related laboratory tests:

➤ Related laboratory tests include serum and urine electrolytes, serum and urine osmolality, serum and urine sodium, thyroid-stimulating hormone, blood urea nitrogen, uric acid, and urinalysis.

ANTIGENS/ANTIBODIES, ANTI–EXTRACTABLE NUCLEAR

SYNONYMS/ACRONYMS: La antibodies, Ro antibodies, SS-A antibodies, SS-B antibodies, ENA.

SPECIMEN: Serum (1 mL) collected in a red-top tube.

REFERENCE VALUE: (Method: Immunoassay) Negative.

DESCRIPTION & RATIONALE: The extractable nuclear antigens (ENAs) include ribonucleoprotein (RNP), Smith (Sm), SS-A/Ro, and SS-B/La antigens. ENAs and antibodies to them are found in various combinations in individuals with combinations of overlapping rheumatologic symptoms. ∎

INDICATIONS:
• Assist in the diagnosis of mixed connective tissue disease
• Assist in the diagnosis of Sjögren's syndrome
• Assist in the diagnosis of systemic lupus erythematosus (SLE)

RESULT

Increased in:
• Anti-RNP is associated with mixed connective tissue disease.

• Anti-SS-A and anti-SS-B are helpful in antinuclear antibody (ANA)–negative cases of SLE.

• Anti-SS-A/ANA–positive, anti-SS-B–negative patients are likely to have nephritis.

• Anti-SS-A/anti-SS-B–positive sera are found in patients with neonatal lupus.

• Anti-SS-A–positive patients may also have antibodies associated with antiphospholipid syndrome.

• Anti-SS-A/La is associated with primary Sjögren's syndrome.

• Anti-SS-A/Ro is a predictor of congenital heart block in neonates born to mothers with SLE.

• Anti-SS-A/Ro–positive patients have photosensitivity.

Decreased in: N/A

CRITICAL VALUES: N/A

INTERFERING FACTORS: N/A

Nursing Implications and Procedure ∙∙∙∙∙∙∙∙∙∙∙∙

Pretest:

➤ Inform the patient that the test is used to detect the presence of antibodies associated with autoimmune disorders such as systemic lupus erythematosus and mixed connective tissue disease.

➤ Obtain a history of the patient's complaints, including a list of known allergens (especially allergies or sensitivities to latex), and inform the appropriate health care practitioner accordingly.

➤ Obtain a history of the patient's immune and musculoskeletal systems, as well as results of previously performed laboratory tests, surgical procedures, and other diagnostic procedures. For related laboratory tests, refer to the Immune and Musculoskeletal System tables.

➤ Obtain a list of medications the patient is taking, including herbs, nutritional supplements, and nutraceuticals. The requesting health care practitioner and laboratory should be advised if the patient regularly uses these products so that their effects can be taken into consideration when reviewing results.

➤ Review the procedure with the patient. Inform the patient that specimen collection takes approximately 5 to 10 minutes. Address concerns about pain related to the procedure. Explain to the patient that there may be some discomfort during the venipuncture.

➤ There are no food, fluid, or medication restrictions unless by medical direction.

Intratest:

➤ If the patient has a history of severe allergic reaction to latex, care should be taken to avoid the use of equipment containing latex.

➤ Instruct the patient to cooperate fully and to follow directions. Direct the patient to breathe normally and to avoid unnecessary movement.

➤ Observe standard precautions, and follow the general guidelines in Appendix A. Positively identify the patient, and label the appropriate tubes with the corresponding patient demographics, date, and time of collection. Perform a venipuncture; collect the specimen in a 5-mL red-top tube.

➤ Remove the needle, place a gauze over the puncture site and apply gentle pressure to stop bleeding. Observe venipuncture site for bleeding or hematoma formation. Apply paper tape over gauze or replace with adhesive bandage.

➤ Promptly transport the specimen to the laboratory for processing and analysis.

➤ The results are recorded manually or in a computerized system for recall and postprocedure interpretation by the appropriate health care practitioner.

Post-test:

➤ A written report of the examination will be sent to the requesting health care practitioner, who will discuss the results with the patient.

➤ Recognize anxiety related to test results, and be supportive of impaired activity, perceived loss of independence, and fear of shortened life expectancy. Collagen and connective tissue diseases are chronic. As such, they must be addressed on a continuous basis and may require significant changes in lifestyle. Discuss the implications of abnormal test results on the patient's lifestyle. Provide teaching and information regarding the clinical implications of the test results, as appropriate. Educate the patient in the importance of preventing infection, which is a significant cause of death in immunosuppressed individuals. Educate the patient regarding access to counseling services.

➤ Reinforce information given by the patient's health care provider regarding further testing, treatment, or referral to another health care provider. Answer any questions or address any concerns voiced by the patient or family.

➤ Depending on the results of this procedure, additional testing may be performed to evaluate or monitor progression of the disease process and determine the need for a change in therapy. Evaluate test results in relation to the patient's symptoms and other tests performed.

Related laboratory tests:

➤ Related laboratory tests include ANA, anticardiolipin antibodies, anti-DNA antibodies, and anti-scleroderma antibody.

ANTIPSYCHOTIC DRUGS AND ANTIMANIC DRUGS: HALOPERIDOL, LITHIUM

SYNONYMS/ACRONYM: *Antipsychotic drugs: haloperidol* (Haldol, Haldol Decanoate, Haldol Lactate); *antimanic drugs: lithium* (Eskalith, Eskalith-CR, Lithobid).

SPECIMEN: Serum (1 mL) collected in a red-top tube.

Drug	Route of Administration	Recommended Collection Time
Haloperidol	Oral	Peak: 3–6 h
Lithium	Oral	Trough: at least 12 h after last dose

REFERENCE VALUE: (Method: Chromatography for haloperidol; ion-selective electrode for lithium)

Drug	Therapeutic Dose*	SI Units	Half-Life (h)	Volume of Distribution (L/kg)	Protein Binding (%)	Excretion
		(SI = Conventional Units × 2.66)				
Haloperidol	4–26 ng/mL	11–69 nmo/L	15–40	18–30	90	Hepatic
		(SI = Conventional Units × 1)				
Lithium	0.6–1.4 mEq/L	0.6–1.4 mmol/L	18–24	0.7–1.0	0	Renal

* Conventional units.

DESCRIPTION & RATIONALE: Haloperidol is an antipsychotic tranquilizer used for the following indications: acute and chronic psychotic disorders, Tourette's syndrome, and hyperactive children with severe behavioral problems. Lithium is used in the treatment of manic depression.

Many factors must be considered in effective dosing and monitoring of therapeutic drugs, including patient age, patient weight, interacting medications, electrolyte balance, protein levels, water balance, conditions that affect absorption and excretion, and foods, herbals, vitamins, and minerals that can either potentiate or inhibit the intended target concentration. Peak collection times should be documented carefully in relation to the time of medication administration. ▪

IMPORTANT NOTE: This information must be clearly and accurately communicated to avoid misunderstanding of the dose time in relation to the collection time. Miscommunication between the individual administering the medication and the individual collecting the specimen is the most frequent cause of subtherapeutic levels, toxic levels, and misleading information used in calculation of future doses.

INDICATIONS:
- Assist in the diagnosis and prevention of toxicity

- Monitor compliance with therapeutic regimen

RESULT

Level	Response
Normal levels	Therapeutic effect
Subtherapeutic levels	Adjust dose as indicated
Toxic levels	Adjust dose as indicated
Haloperidol	Hepatic impairment
Lithium	Renal impairment

CRITICAL VALUES: ⚠ It is important to note the adverse effects of toxic and subtherapeutic levels. Care must be taken to investigate signs and symptoms of not enough medication and too much medication. Note and immediately report to the health care practitioner any critically increased values and related symptoms.

Haloperidol: Greater Than 50 ng/mL

Signs and symptoms of haloperidol toxicity include hypotension, respiratory depression, and extrapyramidal neuromuscular reactions. Possible interventions include emesis (contraindicated in the absence of gag reflex or central nervous system depression or excitation), and gastric lavage followed by administration of activated charcoal.

Lithium: Greater Than 1.5 mEq/L

Signs and symptoms of lithium toxicity include ataxia, coarse tremors, muscle weakness, vomiting, diarrhea, confusion, convulsions, stupor, T-wave flattening, loss of consciousness, and possible coma. Possible interventions include administration of activated charcoal, gastric lavage, and administration of intravenous fluids with diuresis.

INTERFERING FACTORS:
- Blood drawn in serum separator tubes (gel tubes).

- Contraindicated in patients with liver disease, and caution advised in patients with renal impairment.

- Haloperidol may increase levels of tricyclic antidepressants and increase the risk of lithium toxicity.

- Drugs that may increase lithium levels include angiotensin-converting enzyme inhibitors, some nonsteroidal anti-inflammatory drugs, and thiazide diuretics.

- Drugs and substances that may decrease lithium levels include acetazolamide, osmotic diuretics, theophylline, and caffeine.

Nursing Implications and Procedure • • • • • • • • • • • •

Pretest:

➤ Inform the patient that the test is used to monitor for therapeutic and toxic drug levels.

➤ Obtain a history of the patient's complaints, including a list of known allergens (especially allergies or sensitivities to latex), and inform the appropriate health care practitioner accordingly.

➤ Obtain a history of the patient's genitourinary and hepatobiliary systems as well as results of previously performed laboratory tests, surgical procedures, and other diagnostic procedures. For related laboratory tests, refer to the Genitourinary and Hepatobiliary System and Therapeutic/Toxicology tables.

➤ Obtain a list of medications the patient is taking, including herbs, nutritional supplements, and nutraceuticals. Note the last time and dose of medication taken. The requesting health care practitioner and laboratory should be advised if the patient regularly uses these products so that their effects can be taken into consideration when reviewing results.

➤ Review the procedure with the patient. Inform the patient that specimen collection takes approximately 5 to 10 minutes. Address concerns about pain related to the procedure. Explain to the patient that there may be some discomfort during the venipuncture.

➤ *Sensitivity to cultural and social issues,* as well as concern for modesty, is important in providing psychological support before, during, and after the procedure.

➤ There are no food, fluid, or medication restrictions unless by medical direction.

Intratest:

➤ If the patient has a history of severe allergic reaction to latex, care should be taken to avoid the use of equipment containing latex.

➤ Instruct the patient to cooperate fully and to follow directions. Direct the patient to breathe normally and to avoid unnecessary movement.

➤ Observe standard precautions, and follow the general guidelines in Appendix A. Consider recommended collection time in relation to dosing schedule. Positively identify the patient, and label the appropriate tubes with the corresponding patient demographics, date, and time of collection, noting the last dose of medication taken. Perform a venipuncture; collect the specimen in a 5-mL red-top tube.

➤ Remove the needle, place a gauze over the puncture site and apply gentle pressure to stop bleeding. Observe venipuncture site for bleeding or hematoma formation. Apply paper tape over gauze or replace with adhesive bandage.

➤ Promptly transport the specimen to the laboratory for processing and analysis.

➤ The results are recorded manually or in a computerized system for recall and postprocedure interpretation by the appropriate health care practitioner.

Post-test:

➤ *Nutritional considerations* include the avoidance of alcohol consumption.

➤ A written report of the examination will be sent to the requesting health

care practitioner, who will discuss the results with the patient.

➤ Reinforce information given by the patient's health care provider regarding further testing, treatment, or referral to another health care provider. Explain to the patient the importance of following the medication regimen and instructions regarding drug interactions.

➤ Instruct the patient receiving haloperidol to immediately report any unusual symptoms (e.g., arrhythmias, blurred vision, dry eyes, repetitive uncontrolled movements) to his or her health care practitioner. Instruct the patient receiving lithium to immediately report any unusual symptoms (e.g., anorexia, nausea, vomiting, diarrhea, dizziness, drowsiness, dysarthria, tremor, muscle twitching, visual disturbances) to his or her health care practitioner. Answer any questions or address any concerns voiced by the patient or family.

➤ Instruct the patient to be prepared to provide the pharmacist with a list of other medications he or she is already taking in the event that the requesting health care practitioner prescribes a medication.

➤ Depending on the results of this procedure, additional testing may be performed to evaluate or monitor progression of the disease process and determine the need for a change in therapy. Evaluate test results in relation to the patient's symptoms and other tests performed.

Related laboratory tests:

➤ Related laboratory tests include albumin, blood urea nitrogen, calcium, creatinine, glucose, magnesium, potassium, and sodium.

ANTITHROMBIN III

· ·

Sʏɴoɴʏᴍ/Aᴄʀoɴʏᴍ: Heparin cofactor assay, AT-III.

Sᴘᴇᴄɪᴍᴇɴ: Plasma (1 mL) collected in a blue-top (sodium citrate) tube.

Rᴇꜰᴇʀᴇɴᴄᴇ Vᴀʟᴜᴇ: (Method: Radioimmunodiffusion)

	Conventional Units	SI Units (Conventional Units × 10)
Immunologic assay	21–30 mg/dL	210–300 mg/L
	Conventional Units	**SI Units (Conventional Units × 0.01)**
Functional assay	85–115% of standard	0.85–1.15

DESCRIPTION & RATIONALE: Antithrombin III (AT-III) can inhibit thrombin and factors IX, X, XI, and XII. It is a heparin cofactor, interacting with heparin and thrombin. AT-III acts to increase the rate at which thrombin is neutralized or inhibited, and it decreases the total quantity of thrombin inhibited. Patients with low levels show some level of resistance to heparin therapy. ▪

INDICATIONS:
• Investigate tendency for thrombosis

RESULT

Increased in:
• Acute hepatitis
• Inflammation
• Menstruation
• Obstructive jaundice
• Renal transplantation
• Vitamin K deficiency

Decreased in:
• Carcinoma
• Chronic liver failure
• Cirrhosis
• Congenital deficiency
• Disseminated intravascular coagulation
• Liver transplantation or partial hepatectomy
• Nephrotic syndrome
• Pulmonary embolism

CRITICAL VALUES: N/A

INTERFERING FACTORS:
• Drugs that may increase AT-III levels include anabolic steroids, gemfibrozil, and warfarin.

• Drugs that may decrease AT-III levels include asparaginase, estrogens, gestodene, heparin, and oral contraceptives.

• Placement of the tourniquet for longer than 1 minute can result in venous stasis and changes in the concentration of the plasma proteins to be measured. Platelet activation may also occur under these conditions, resulting in erroneous measurements.

Nursing Implications and Procedure

Pretest:

➤ Inform the patient that the test is used to assist in the diagnosis of coagulation disorders.

➤ Obtain a history of the patient's complaints, including a list of known allergens (especially allergies or sensitivities to latex), and inform the appropriate health care practitioner accordingly.

➤ Obtain a history of the patient's hematopoietic system and results of previously performed laboratory tests, surgical procedures, and other diagnostic procedures. For related laboratory tests, refer to the Hematopoietic System table.

➤ Obtain a list of medications the patient is taking, including herbs, nutritional supplements, and nutraceuticals. The requesting health care practitioner and laboratory should be advised if the patient regularly uses these products so that their effects can be taken into consideration when reviewing results.

➤ Review the procedure with the patient. Inform the patient that specimen collection takes approximately 5 to 10 minutes. Address concerns about pain related to the procedure. Explain to the patient that there may be some discomfort during the venipuncture.

➤ There are no food, fluid, or medication restrictions unless by medical direction.

Intratest:

➤ If the patient has a history of severe allergic reaction to latex, care should be taken to avoid the use of equipment containing latex.

➤ Instruct the patient to cooperate fully and to follow directions. Direct the patient to breathe normally and to avoid unnecessary movement.

➤ Observe standard precautions, and follow the general guidelines in Appendix A. Positively identify the patient, and label the appropriate tubes with the corresponding patient demographics, date, and time of collection. Perform a venipuncture; collect the specimen in a 5-mL blue-top tube. *Important note:* Two different concentrations of sodium citrate preservative are currently added to blue-top tubes for coagulation studies: 3.2% and 3.8%. The Clinical and Laboratory Standards Institute/CLSI (formerly the National Committee for Clinical Laboratory Standards/ NCCLS) guideline for sodium citrate is 3.2%. Laboratories establish reference ranges for coagulation testing based on numerous factors, including sodium citrate concentration, test equipment, and test reagents. It is important to ask the laboratory which concentration it recommends, because each concentration will have its own specific reference range. When multiple specimens are drawn, the blue-top tube should be collected after sterile (i.e., blood culture) and red-top tubes. When coagulation testing is the only work to be done, an extra red-top tube should be collected before the blue-top tube to avoid contaminating the specimen with tissue thromboplastin.

➤ Remove the needle, place a gauze over the puncture site and apply gentle pressure to stop bleeding. Observe venipuncture site for bleeding or hematoma formation. Apply paper tape over gauze or replace with adhesive bandage.

➤ Promptly transport the specimen to the laboratory for processing and analysis. The CLSI recommendation for processed and unprocessed samples stored in unopened tubes is that testing should be completed within 1 to 4 hours of collection.

➤ The results are recorded manually or in a computerized system for recall and postprocedure interpretation by the appropriate health care practitioner.

Post-test:

➤ A written report of the examination will be sent to the requesting health care practitioner, who will discuss the results with the patient.

➤ Reinforce information given by the patient's health care provider regarding further testing, treatment, or referral to another health care provider. Answer any questions or address any concerns voiced by the patient or family.

➤ Depending on the results of this procedure, additional testing may be performed to evaluate or monitor progression of the disease process and determine the need for a change in therapy. Evaluate test results in relation to the patient's symptoms and other tests performed.

Related laboratory tests:

➤ Related laboratory tests include activated partial thromboplastin time, protein C, protein S, and vitamin K.

α_1-ANTITRYPSIN AND α_1-ANTITRYPSIN PHENOTYPING

SYNONYMS/ACRONYMS: α_1-antitrypsin: A_1AT, α_1-AT, AAT; α_1-antitrypsin phenotyping: A_1AT phenotype, α_1-AT phenotype, AAT phenotype, Pi phenotype.

SPECIMEN: Serum (1 mL) for α_1-antitrypsin (α_1-AT) and serum (2 mL) for α_1-AT phenotyping collected in a red- or tiger-top tube.

REFERENCE VALUE: (Method: Rate nephelometry for α_1-AT, isoelectric focusing/high-resolution electrophoresis for α_1-AT phenotyping)

α_1-Antitrypsin

Age	Conventional Units	SI Units (Conventional Units × 0.01)
0–1 mo	124–348 mg/dL	1.24–3.48 g/L
2–6 mo	111–297 mg/dL	1.11–2.97 g/L
7 mo–2 y	95–251 mg/dL	0.95–2.51 g/L
3 y–19 y	110–279 mg/dL	1.10–2.79 g/L
Adult	126–226 mg/dL	1.26–2.26 g/L

α_1-Antitrypsin Phenotyping

There are three major protease inhibitor phenotypes:
MM—Normal
SS—Intermediate; heterozygous
ZZ—Markedly abnormal; homozygous
The total level of measurable α_1-AT varies with genotype. The effects of α_1-AT deficiency depend on the patient's personal habits, but are most severe in patients who smoke tobacco.

DESCRIPTION & RATIONALE: α_1-AT is the main glycoprotein produced by the liver. Its inhibitory function is directed against proteolytic enzymes, such as trypsin, elastin, and plasmin, released by alveolar macrophages and bacteria. In the absence of α_1-AT, functional tissue is destroyed by proteolytic enzymes and replaced with excessive connective tissue. Emphysema develops at an earlier age in α_1-AT–deficient emphysema patients than in other emphysema patients. α_1-AT deficiency is passed on as an autosomal recessive trait. Inherited deficiencies are associated early in life with development of lung and liver disorders. In the pediatric population, the ZZ phenotype usually presents as liver disease, cholestasis, and cirrhosis.

Greater than 80% of ZZ-deficient individuals ultimately develop chronic lung or liver disease. It is important to identify inherited deficiencies early in life. Typically, α_1-AT–deficient patients have circulating levels less than 50 mg/dL. Patients who have α_1-AT values less than 140 mg/dL should be phenotyped.

Elevated levels are found in normal individuals when an inflammatory process, such as rheumatoid arthritis, bacterial infection, neoplasm, or vasculitis, is present. Decreased levels are found in affected patients with chronic obstructive pulmonary disease (COPD) and in children with cirrhosis of the liver. Decreased α_1-AT levels also may be elevated into the normal range in heterozygous α_1-AT–deficient patients during concurrent infection, pregnancy, estrogen therapy, steroid therapy, cancer, and postoperative periods. Homozygous α_1-AT–deficient patients do not show such an elevation. ■

INDICATIONS:

- Assist in establishing a diagnosis of COPD
- Assist in establishing a diagnosis of liver disease
- Detect hereditary absence or deficiency of α_1-AT

RESULT

Increased in:

- Acute and chronic inflammatory conditions
- Carcinomas
- Estrogen therapy
- Postoperative recovery
- Pregnancy
- Steroid therapy
- Stress (extreme physical)

Decreased in:

- COPD
- Homozygous α_1-AT–deficient patients
- Liver disease (severe)
- Liver cirrhosis (child)
- Malnutrition
- Nephrotic syndrome

CRITICAL VALUES: N/A

INTERFERING FACTORS:

- α_1-AT is an acute-phase reactant protein, and any inflammatory process elevates levels. If a serum C-reactive protein is performed simultaneously and is positive, the patient should be retested for α_1-AT in 10 to 14 days.

- Rheumatoid factor causes false-positive elevations.

- Drugs that may increase serum α_1-AT levels include aminocaproic acid, estrogen therapy, oral contraceptives (high-dose preparations), oxymetholone, streptokinase, tamoxifen, and typhoid vaccine.

Nursing Implications and Procedure . . . .

Pretest:

▶ Inform the patient that the test is used to identify chronic obstructive pulmonary disease and liver disease associated with α_1-antitrypsin deficiency.

▶ Obtain a history of the patient's complaints, including a list of known allergens (especially allergies or sensitivities to latex), and inform the appropriate health care practitioner accordingly.

▶ Obtain a history of the patient's hepatobiliary and respiratory system and results of previously performed laboratory tests, surgical procedures, and other diagnostic procedures. For related laboratory tests, refer to the Hepatobiliary and Respiratory System tables.

➤ Obtain a list of the medications the patient is taking, including herbs, nutritional supplements, and nutraceuticals. Oral contraceptives should be withheld 24 hours before the specimen is collected, although this restriction should first be confirmed with the person ordering the test. The requesting health care practitioner and laboratory should be advised if the patient regularly uses these products so that their effects can be taken into consideration when reviewing results.

➤ Review the procedure with the patient. Inform the patient that specimen collection takes approximately 5 to 10 minutes. Address concerns about pain related to the procedure. Explain to the patient that there may be some discomfort during the venipuncture.

➤ There are no food, fluid, or medication restrictions unless by medical direction.

Intratest:

➤ If the patient has a history of severe allergic reaction to latex, care should be taken to avoid the use of equipment containing latex.

➤ Instruct the patient to cooperate fully and to follow directions. Direct the patient to breathe normally and to avoid unnecessary movement.

➤ Observe standard precautions, and follow the general guidelines in Appendix A. Positively identify the patient, and label the appropriate tubes with the corresponding patient demographics, date, and time of collection. Perform a venipuncture; collect the specimen in a 5-mL red- or tiger-top tube.

➤ Remove the needle, place a gauze over the puncture site and apply gentle pressure to stop bleeding. Observe venipuncture site for bleeding or hematoma formation. Apply paper tape over gauze or replace with adhesive bandage.

➤ Promptly transport the specimen to the laboratory for processing and analysis.

➤ The results are recorded manually or in a computerized system for recall and postprocedure interpretation by the appropriate health care practitioner.

Post-test:

➤ Instruct the patient to resume usual medication as directed by the health care practitioner.

➤ *Nutritional considerations:* Malnutrition is commonly seen in α_1-AT–deficient patients with severe respiratory disease for many reasons, including fatigue, lack of appetite, and gastrointestinal distress. Research has estimated that the daily caloric intake required for respiration in patients with COPD is 10 times higher than that required of normal individuals. Inadequate nutrition can result in hypophosphatemia, especially in the respirator-dependent patient. During periods of starvation, phosphorus leaves the intracellular space and moves outside the tissue, resulting in dangerously decreased phosphorus levels. Adequate intake of vitamins A and C is important to prevent pulmonary infection and to decrease the extent of lung tissue damage. The importance of following the prescribed diet should be stressed to the patient and caregiver.

➤ *Nutritional considerations:* Water balance must be closely monitored in α_1-AT–deficient patients with COPD. Fluid retention can lead to pulmonary edema.

➤ Educate the patient with abnormal findings in preventive measures for protection of the lungs (e.g., avoid contact with persons who have respiratory or other infections; avoid the use of tobacco; avoid areas having highly polluted air; and avoid work environments with hazards such as fumes, dust, and other respiratory pollutants).

➤ Instruct the affected patient in deep breathing and pursed-lip breathing to enhance breathing patterns as appropriate. Inform the patient of smoking cessation programs, as appropriate.

> A written report of the examination will be sent to the requesting health care practitioner, who will discuss the results with the patient.

> Recognize anxiety related to test results, and be supportive of fear of shortened life expectancy. Discuss the implications of abnormal test results on the patient's lifestyle. Provide teaching and information regarding the clinical implications of the test results, as appropriate. Because decreased α_1-AT can be an inherited disorder, it may be appropriate to recommend resources for genetic counseling if levels less than 140 mg/dL are reported. It may also be appropriate to inform the patient that α_1-AT phenotype testing can be performed on family members to determine the homozygous or heterozygous nature of the deficiency.

> Reinforce information given by the patient's health care provider regarding further testing, treatment, or referral to another health care provider. Inform the patient of the importance of medical follow-up, and suggest ongoing support resources to assist the patient in coping with chronic illness and possible early death. Answer any questions or address any concerns voiced by the patient or family.

> Depending on the results of this procedure, additional testing may be performed to evaluate or monitor progression of the disease process and determine the need for a change in therapy. Evaluate test results in relation to the patient's symptoms and other tests performed.

Related laboratory tests:

> Related laboratory tests include angiotensin-converting enzyme, anion gap, arterial/alveolar oxygen ratio, blood gases, electrolytes, osmolality, and phosphorus.

APOLIPOPROTEIN A

SYNONYM/ACRONYM: Apo A.

SPECIMEN: Serum (1 mL) collected in a red- or tiger-top tube.

REFERENCE VALUE: (Method: Immunonephelometry)

Sex/Age	Conventional Units	SI Units (Conventional Units × 0.01)
Male		
Newborn	41–93 mg/dL	0.41–0.93 g/L
6 mo–4 y	67–163 mg/dL	0.67–1.63 g/L
Adult	81–166 mg/dL	0.81–1.66 g/L
Female		
Newborn	38–106 mg/dL	0.38–1.06 g/L
6 mo–4 y	60–148 mg/dL	0.60–1.48 g/L
Adult	80–214 mg/dL	0.80–2.14 g/L

DESCRIPTION & RATIONALE: Apolipoprotein A (Apo A), the major component of high-density lipoprotein (HDL), is synthesized in the liver and intestines. Apolipoproteins assist in the regulation of lipid metabolism by activating and inhibiting enzymes required for this process. Apo A-I activates the enzyme lecithin-cholesterol acyltransferase (LCAT), whereas Apo A-II inhibits LCAT. The apolipoproteins also help keep lipids in solution as they circulate in the blood and direct the lipids toward the correct target organs and tissues in the body. It is believed that Apo A measurements may be more important than HDL cholesterol measurements as a predictor of coronary artery disease (CAD). There is an inverse relationship between Apo A levels and risk for developing CAD. Because of difficulties with method standardization, the above-listed reference ranges should be used as a rough guide in assessing abnormal conditions. Values for African Americans are 5 to 10 mg/dL higher than values for whites. ■

INDICATIONS:
• Evaluation for risk of CAD

RESULT

Increased in:
• Familial hyper-α-lipoproteinemia
• Weight reduction

Decreased in:
• Abetalipoproteinemia
• Cholestasis
• Chronic renal failure
• Diabetes (uncontrolled)
• Diet high in carbohydrates or polyunsaturated fats

• Familial deficiencies of related enzymes and lipoproteins
• Hepatocellular disorders
• Hypertriglyceridemia
• Nephrotic syndrome
• Premature coronary heart disease
• Smoking

CRITICAL VALUES: N/A

INTERFERING FACTORS:
• Drugs and substances that may increase Apo A levels include anticonvulsants, beclobrate, bezafibrate, ciprofibrate, estrogens, furosemide, lovastatin, pravastatin, prednisolone, simvastatin, and ethanol (abuse).

• Drugs that may decrease Apo A levels include androgens, β-blockers, diuretics, and probucol.

• Failure to follow dietary restrictions before the procedure may cause the procedure to be canceled or repeated.

Nursing Implications and Procedure • • • • • • • • • • • •

Pretest:

➤ Inform the patient that the test is used to assess and monitor risk for coronary artery disease.

➤ Obtain a history of the patient's complaints, including a list of known allergens (especially allergies or sensitivities to latex), and inform the appropriate health care practitioner accordingly.

➤ Obtain a history of the patient's cardiovascular system and results of previously performed laboratory tests, surgical procedures, and other diagnostic procedures. For related laboratory tests, refer to the Cardiovascular System table.

➤ Obtain a list of medications the patient is taking, including herbs, nutritional supplements, and nutraceuticals. The requesting health care practitioner and laboratory should be advised if the patient regularly uses these products so that their effects can be taken into consideration when reviewing results.

➤ Review the procedure with the patient. Inform the patient that specimen collection takes approximately 5 to 10 minutes. Address concerns about pain related to the procedure. Explain to the patient that there may be some discomfort during the venipuncture.

➤ The patient should abstain from food for 6 to 12 hours before specimen collection.

➤ There are no fluid or medication restrictions unless by medical direction.

Intratest:

➤ Ensure that the patient has complied with dietary, medication, or activity restrictions and pretesting preparations; assure that food has been restricted for at least 6 to 12 hours prior to the procedure.

➤ If the patient has a history of severe allergic reaction to latex, care should be taken to avoid the use of equipment containing latex.

➤ Instruct the patient to cooperate fully and to follow directions. Direct the patient to breathe normally and to avoid unnecessary movement.

➤ Observe standard precautions, and follow the general guidelines in Appendix A. Positively identify the patient, and label the appropriate tubes with the corresponding patient demographics, date, and time of collection. Perform a venipuncture; collect the specimen in a 5-mL red- or tiger-top tube.

➤ Remove the needle, place a gauze over the puncture site and apply gentle pressure to stop bleeding. Observe venipuncture site for bleeding or hematoma formation. Apply paper tape over gauze or replace with adhesive bandage.

➤ Promptly transport the specimen to the laboratory for processing and analysis.

➤ The results are recorded manually or in a computerized system for recall and postprocedure interpretation by the appropriate health care practitioner.

Post-test:

➤ Instruct the patient to resume usual diet as directed by the health care practitioner.

➤ *Nutritional considerations:* Decreased Apo A levels may be associated with CAD. Nutritional therapy is recommended for individuals identified to be at high risk for developing CAD. Overweight patients should be encouraged to achieve a normal weight. The American Heart Association Step 1 and Step 2 diets may be helpful in achieving a goal of reducing total cholesterol and triglyceride levels. The Step 1 diet emphasizes a reduction in foods high in saturated fats and cholesterol. Red meats, eggs, and dairy products are the major sources of saturated fats and cholesterol. If triglycerides are also elevated, the patient should be advised to eliminate or reduce alcohol and simple carbohydrates from the diet. The Step 2 diet recommends stricter reductions.

➤ A written report of the examination will be sent to the requesting health care practitioner, who will discuss the results with the patient.

➤ Recognize anxiety related to test results, and be supportive of fear of shortened life expectancy. Discuss the implications of abnormal test results on the patient's lifestyle. Provide teaching and information regarding the clinical implications of the test results, as appropriate. Educate the patient regarding access to counseling services. Provide contact information, if desired, for the American Heart Association (*http://www.americanheart. org*).

➤ Reinforce information given by the patient's health care provider regarding further testing, treatment, or referral to another health care provider. Answer any questions or address any concerns voiced by the patient or family.

➤ Depending on the results of this procedure, additional testing may be performed to evaluate or monitor progression of the disease process and determine the need for a change in therapy. Evaluate test results in relation to the patient's symptoms and other tests performed.

Related laboratory tests:

➤ Related laboratory tests include antiarrhythmic drugs, apolipoprotein B, aspartate aminotransferase, atrial natriuretic peptide, B-type natriuretic peptide, blood gases, C-reactive protein, calcium and ionized calcium, cholesterol (total, HDL, and LDL), creatine kinase and isoenzymes, glucose, glycated hemoglobin, homocysteine, ketones, lactate dehydrogenase and isoenzymes, lipoprotein electrophoresis, magnesium, myoglobin, potassium, triglycerides, and troponin.

APOLIPOPROTEIN B

SYNONYM/ACRONYM: Apo B.

SPECIMEN: Serum (1 mL) collected in a red- or tiger-top tube.

REFERENCE VALUE: (Method: Immunonephelometry)

Age	Conventional Units	SI Units (Conventional Units × 0.01)
Newborn–5 y	11–31 mg/dL	0.11–0.31 g/L
5–17 y		
Male	47–139 mg/dL	0.47–1.39 g/L
Female	41–96 mg/dL	0.41–0.96 g/L
Adult		
Male	46–174 mg/dL	0.46–1.74 g/L
Female	46–142 mg/dL	0.46–1.42 g/L

DESCRIPTION & RATIONALE: Apolipoprotein B (Apo B), the major component of the low-density lipoproteins (chylomicrons, LDL, and very-low-density lipoprotein), is synthesized in the liver and intestines. Apolipoproteins assist in the regulation of lipid metabolism by activating and inhibiting enzymes required for this process. The apolipoproteins also help keep lipids in solution as they circulate in the blood and direct the lipids toward the correct target organs and tissues in the body. ■

INDICATIONS:
• Evaluation for risk of coronary artery disease (CAD)

RESULT

Increased in:
• Anorexia nervosa
• Cushing's syndrome
• Diabetes
• Dysglobulinemia
• Emotional stress
• Hepatic disease
• Hepatic obstruction
• Hyperlipoproteinemias
• Hypothyroidism
• Infantile hypercalcemia
• Nephrotic syndrome
• Porphyria
• Pregnancy
• Premature CAD
• Renal failure
• Werner's syndrome

Decreased in:
• Acute stress (burns, illness)
• Chronic anemias
• Chronic pulmonary disease
• Familial deficiencies of related enzymes and lipoproteins
• Hyperthyroidism
• Inflammatory joint disease
• Intestinal malabsorption
• α-Lipoprotein deficiency (Tangier disease)
• Malnutrition
• Myeloma
• Reye's syndrome
• Weight reduction

CRITICAL VALUES: N/A

INTERFERING FACTORS:
• Drugs that may increase Apo B levels include amiodarone, androgens, β-blockers, catecholamines, cyclosporine, diuretics, ethanol (abuse), etretinate, glucogenic corticosteroids, oral contraceptives, and phenobarbital.

• Drugs that may decrease Apo B levels include beclobrate, captopril, cholestyramine, fibrates, ketanserin, lovastatin, niacin, nifedipine, pravastatin, prazosin, probucol, and simvastatin.

• Failure to follow dietary restrictions before the procedure may cause the procedure to be canceled or repeated.

Nursing Implications and Procedure . . . .

Pretest:

➤ Inform the patient that the test is used to assess and monitor risk for coronary artery disease.

➤ Obtain a history of the patient's complaints, including a list of known allergens (especially allergies or sensitivities to latex), and inform the appropriate health care practitioner accordingly.

➤ Obtain a history of the patient's cardiovascular system and results of previously performed laboratory tests, surgical procedures, and other diagnostic procedures. For related laboratory tests, refer to the Cardiovascular System table.

➤ Obtain a list of medications the patient is taking, including herbs, nutritional supplements, and nutraceuticals. The requesting health care practitioner and laboratory should be advised if the patient regularly uses these products so that their effects can be taken into consideration when reviewing results.

➤ Review the procedure with the patient. Inform the patient that specimen collection takes approximately

5 to 10 minutes. Address concerns about pain related to the procedure. Explain to the patient that there may be some discomfort during the venipuncture.

➤ The patient should abstain from food for 6 to 12 hours before specimen collection.

➤ There are no fluid or medication restrictions unless by medical direction.

Intratest:

➤ Ensure that the patient has complied with dietary, medication, or activity restrictions and pretesting preparations; assure that food has been restricted for at least 6 to 12 hours prior to the procedure.

➤ If the patient has a history of severe allergic reaction to latex, care should be taken to avoid the use of equipment containing latex.

➤ Instruct the patient to cooperate fully and to follow directions. Direct the patient to breathe normally and to avoid unnecessary movement.

➤ Observe standard precautions, and follow the general guidelines in Appendix A. Positively identify the patient, and label the appropriate tubes with the corresponding patient demographics, date, and time of collection. Perform a venipuncture; collect the specimen in a 5-mL red- or tiger-top tube.

➤ Remove the needle, place a gauze over the puncture site and apply gentle pressure to stop bleeding. Observe venipuncture site for bleeding or hematoma formation. Apply paper tape over gauze or replace with adhesive bandage.

➤ Promptly transport the specimen to the laboratory for processing and analysis.

➤ The results are recorded manually or in a computerized system for recall and postprocedure interpretation by the appropriate health care practitioner.

Post-test:

➤ Instruct the patient to resume usual diet as directed by the health care practitioner.

➤ *Nutritional considerations:* Increased Apo B levels may be associated with CAD. Nutritional therapy is recommended for individuals identified to be at high risk for developing CAD. Overweight patients should be encouraged to achieve a normal weight. The American Heart Association Step 1 and Step 2 diets may be helpful in achieving a goal of reducing total cholesterol and triglyceride levels. The Step 1 diet emphasizes a reduction in foods high in saturated fats and cholesterol. Red meats, eggs, and dairy products are the major sources of saturated fats and cholesterol. If triglycerides are also elevated, the patient should be advised to eliminate or reduce alcohol and simple carbohydrates from the diet. The Step 2 diet recommends stricter reductions.

➤ A written report of the examination will be sent to the requesting health care practitioner, who will discuss the results with the patient.

➤ Recognize anxiety related to test results, and be supportive of fear of shortened life expectancy. Discuss the implications of abnormal test results on the patient's lifestyle. Provide teaching and information regarding the clinical implications of the test results, as appropriate. Educate the patient regarding access to counseling services. Provide contact information, if desired, for the American Heart Association *(http://www.americanheart.org)*.

➤ Reinforce information given by the patient's health care provider regarding further testing, treatment, or referral to another health care provider. Answer any questions or address any concerns voiced by the patient or family.

➤ Depending on the results of this procedure, additional testing may be performed to evaluate or monitor

progression of the disease process and determine the need for a change in therapy. Evaluate test results in relation to the patient's symptoms and other tests performed.

Related laboratory tests:

Related laboratory tests include antiarrhythmic drugs, apolipoprotein A, aspartate aminotransferase, atrial natriuretic peptide, B-type natriuretic peptide, blood gases, C-reactive protein, calcium and ionized calcium, cholesterol (total, HDL, and LDL), creatine kinase and isoenzymes, glucose, glycated hemoglobin, homocysteine, ketones, lactate dehydrogenase and isoenzymes, lipoprotein electrophoresis, magnesium, myoglobin, potassium, triglycerides, and troponin.

ARTHROGRAM

Sʏɴᴏɴʏᴍ/Aᴄʀᴏɴʏᴍ: Joint study.

Aʀᴇᴀ ᴏꜰ Aᴘᴘʟɪᴄᴀᴛɪᴏɴ: Shoulder, elbow, wrist, hip, knee, ankle, temporomandibular joint.

Cᴏɴᴛʀᴀsᴛ: Iodinated or gadolinium.

Dᴇsᴄʀɪᴘᴛɪᴏɴ & Rᴀᴛɪᴏɴᴀʟᴇ: An arthrogram evaluates the cartilage, ligaments, and bony structures that compose a joint. After local anesthesia is administered to the area of interest, a fluoroscopically guided small-gauge needle is inserted into the joint space. Fluid in the joint space is aspirated and sent to the laboratory for analysis. Contrast medium is inserted into the joint space to outline the soft tissue structures and the contour of the joint. After brief exercise of the joint, radiographs or magnetic resonance images (MRIs) are obtained. Arthrograms are used primarily for assessment of persistent, unexplained joint discomfort. ∎

INDICATIONS:

* Evaluate pain, swelling, or dysfunction of a joint

* Monitor disease progression

RESULT

Normal Findings:

* Normal bursae, menisci, ligaments, and articular cartilage of the joint (*note:* the cartilaginous surfaces and menisci should be smooth, without evidence of erosion, tears, or disintegration)

Abnormal Findings:

* Arthritis

* Cysts

* Diseases of the cartilage (chondromalacia)

- Injury to the ligaments
- Joint derangement
- Meniscal tears or laceration
- Muscle tears
- Osteochondral fractures
- Osteochondritis dissecans
- Synovial tumor
- Synovitis

INTERFERING FACTORS

This procedure is contraindicated for:

- Patients who are pregnant or suspected of being pregnant, unless the potential benefits of the procedure far outweigh the risks to the fetus and mother.

- Patients with bleeding disorders, active arthritis, or joint infections.

- ⚠ Patients with allergies to shellfish or iodinated dye. The contrast medium used may cause a life-threatening allergic reaction. Patients with a known hypersensitivity to the medium may benefit from premedication with corticosteroids or the use of a nonionic contrast medium.

Factors that may impair clear imaging:

- Inability of the patient to cooperate or remain still during the procedure because of age, significant pain, or mental status

- Metallic objects within the examination field (e.g., jewelry, earrings, dental amalgams), which may inhibit organ visualization and can produce unclear images

- Improper adjustment of the radiographic equipment to accommodate obese or thin patients, which can cause overexposure or underexposure and a poor-quality study

- Patients who are very obese, who may exceed the weight limit for the equipment

- Incorrect positioning of the patient, which may produce poor visualization of the area to be examined

Other considerations:

- Consultation with a physician should occur before the procedure for radiation safety concerns regarding younger patients or patients who are lactating.

- Risks associated with radiographic overexposure can result from frequent x-ray procedures. Personnel in the room with the patient should wear a protective lead apron, stand behind a shield, or leave the area while the examination is being done. Personnel working in the area where the examination is being done should wear badges that reveal their level of exposure to radiation.

Nursing Implications and Procedure • • • • • • • • • • •

Pretest:

➤ Inform the patient that the procedure assesses the joint being examined.

➤ Obtain a history of the patient's complaints or symptoms, including a list of known allergens, especially allergies or sensitivities to latex, iodine, seafood, contrast medium, and dyes.

➤ Obtain a history of results of previously performed diagnostic procedures, surgical procedures, and laboratory tests. For related diagnostic tests, refer to the Musculoskeletal System table.

➤ Record the date of the last menstrual period and determine the possibility of pregnancy in perimenopausal women.

➤ Obtain a list of the medications the patient is taking.

➤ Explain to the patient that some pain may be experienced during the test, and there may be moments of discomfort. Explain the purpose of the test and how the procedure is performed. Inform the patient that the procedure is performed in the radiology department, usually by a physician and support staff, and takes approximately 30 to 60 minutes.

> *Sensitivity to cultural and social issues,* as well as concern for modesty, is important in providing psychological support before, during, and after the procedure.

> There are no food, fluid, or medication restrictions.

> *Make sure a written and informed consent has been signed prior to the procedure and before administering any medications.*

Intratest:

> Observe standard precautions and follow the general guidelines in Appendix A.

> Instruct the patient to cooperate fully and to follow directions. Instruct the patient to remain still throughout the procedure because movement produces unreliable results.

> Have the patient void before the procedure begins.

> Patients are given a gown and robe to wear. Clothing and metallic objects are removed from the joint to be examined.

> When x-rays are used, lead protection is placed over the gonads to prevent their irradiation.

> Place the patient on the table in a supine position.

> The skin surrounding the joint is aseptically cleaned and anesthetized.

> A small-gauge needle is inserted into the joint space.

> Any fluid in the space is aspirated and sent to the laboratory for analysis.

> Contrast medium is inserted into the joint space with fluoroscopic guidance.

> The needle is removed, and the joint is exercised to help distribute the contrast medium.

> X-rays or MRIs are taken of the joint.

> The patient is instructed to inhale deeply and hold his or her breath while the x-ray film is taken, and then to exhale after the film is taken.

Post-test:

> Inform the patient that further examinations may be needed to evaluate disease progression and to determine the need for a change in therapy.

> Answer any questions or concerns voiced by the patient or family.

> Assess the joint for swelling after the test. Apply ice as needed.

> Instruct the patient to use a mild analgesic (aspirin, acetaminophen), as ordered, if there is discomfort.

> Advise the patient to avoid strenuous activity until approved by the physician.

> Instruct the patient to notify the health care provider if he or she experiences fever or increased pain, drainage, warmth, edema, or swelling of the joint.

> Inform the patient that noises from the joint after the procedure are common and should disappear 24 to 48 hours after the procedure.

> A written report of the examination will be completed by a health care practitioner specializing in this branch of medicine. The report will be sent to the requesting health care practitioner, who will discuss the results with the patient.

> Depending on the results of this procedure, additional testing may be needed to evaluate or monitor progression of the disease process and determine the need for a change in therapy. Evaluate test results in relation to the patient's symptoms and other tests performed.

Related diagnostic tests:

> Related diagnostic tests include bone scan and radiography of the bone.

ARTHROSCOPY

SYNONYM/ACRONYM: N/A.

AREA OF APPLICATION: Joints.

CONTRAST: None.

DESCRIPTION & RATIONALE: Arthroscopy provides direct visualization of a joint through the use of a fiberoptic endoscope. The arthroscope has a light, fiberoptics, and lenses; it connects to a monitor, and the images are recorded for future study and comparison. This procedure is used for inspection of joint structures, performance of a biopsy, and surgical repairs to the joint. Meniscus removal, spur removal, and ligamentous repair are some of the surgical procedures that may be performed. This procedure is most commonly performed to diagnose athletic injuries and acute or chronic joint disorders. Because arthroscopy allows direct visualization, degenerative processes can be accurately differentiated from injuries. A local anesthetic allows the arthroscope to be inserted through the skin with minimal discomfort. This procedure may also be done under a spinal or general anesthetic, especially if surgery is anticipated. ∎

INDICATIONS:
• Detect torn ligament or tendon
• Evaluate joint pain and damaged cartilage
• Evaluate meniscal, patellar, condylar, extrasynovial, and synovial injuries or diseases of the knee
• Evaluate the extent of arthritis
• Evaluate the presence of gout
• Monitor effectiveness of therapy
• Remove loose objects

RESULT

Normal Findings:
• Normal muscle, ligament, cartilage, synovial, and tendon structures of the joint

Abnormal Findings:
• Arthritis
• Chondromalacia
• Cysts
• Degenerative joint changes
• Ganglion or Baker's cyst
• Gout or pseudogout
• Joint tumors
• Loose bodies
• Meniscal disease
• Osteoarthritis
• Osteochondritis

- Rheumatoid arthritis
- Subluxation, fracture, or dislocation
- Synovitis
- Torn cartilage
- Torn ligament
- Torn rotator cuff
- Trapped synovium

INTERFERING FACTORS

This procedure is contraindicated for:
- Patients with bleeding disorders, active arthritis, or cardiac conditions
- Patients with joint infection or skin infection near proposed arthroscopic site
- Patients who have had an arthrogram within the last 14 days

Factors that may impair clear imaging:
- Inability of the patient to cooperate or remain still during the procedure because of age, significant pain, or mental status
- Improper adjustment of the radiographic equipment to accommodate obese or thin patients, which can cause overexposure or underexposure and a poor-quality study
- Patients who are very obese, who may exceed the weight limit for the equipment
- Incorrect positioning of the patient, which may produce poor visualization of the area to be examined
- Fibrous ankylosis of the joint preventing effective use of the arthroscope
- Joints with flexion of less than 50°

Other considerations:
- Failure to follow dietary restrictions before the procedure may cause the procedure to be canceled or repeated.

Nursing Implications and Procedure • • • • • • • • • •

Pretest:

- ► Inform the patient that the procedure assesses the joint to be examined.
- ► Obtain a history of the patient's complaints or symptoms, including a list of known allergens, especially allergies or sensitivities to latex.
- ► Obtain a history of results of previously performed diagnostic procedures, surgical procedures, and laboratory tests. For related diagnostic tests, refer to the Musculoskeletal System table.
- ► Record the date of the last menstrual period and determine the possibility of pregnancy in perimenopausal women.
- ► Obtain a list of the medications the patient is taking,
- ► Explain to the patient that some pain may be experienced during the test, and there may be moments of discomfort. Explain the purpose of the test and how the procedure is performed. Inform the patient that the procedure is performed in the radiology department, usually by a physician and support staff, and takes approximately 30 to 60 minutes.
- ► *Sensitivity to cultural and social issues,* as well as concern for modesty, is important in providing psychological support before, during, and after the procedure.
- ► Instruct the patient to refrain from food and fluids for 6 to 8 hours before the test.
- ► *Make sure a written and informed consent has been signed prior to the procedure and before administering any medications.*
- ► Determine previous abnormalities in laboratory test results, particularly hematologic or coagulation tests.
- ► Crutch walking should be taught before the procedure if it is anticipated postoperatively.
- ► The joint area and areas 5 to 6 inches

above and below the joint are shaved and prepared for the procedure.

➤ The patient is given a preprocedure sedative, as ordered.

Intratest:

➤ Resuscitation equipment and patient monitoring equipment must be available.

➤ Have the patient remove dentures, contact lenses, eyeglasses, and jewelry. Notify the physician if the patient has crownwork that could affect the examination. Have the patient remove clothing and change into a gown for the procedure.

➤ The extremity is scrubbed, elevated, and wrapped with an elastic bandage from the distal portion of the extremity to the proximal portion to drain as much blood from the limb as possible.

➤ A pneumatic tourniquet placed around the proximal portion of the limb is inflated, and the elastic bandage is removed.

➤ As an alternative to a tourniquet, a mixture of lidocaine with epinephrine and sterile normal saline may be instilled into the joint to help reduce bleeding.

➤ The joint is placed in a 45° angle, and a local anesthetic is administered.

➤ A small incision is made in the skin in the lateral or medial aspect of the joint.

➤ The arthroscope is inserted into the joint spaces. The joint is manipulated as it is visualized. Added puncture sites may be needed to provide a full view of the joint.

➤ Biopsy or treatment can be performed at this time, and photographs should be taken for future reference.

➤ After inspection, specimens may be obtained for cytologic and microbiologic study. All specimens are placed in appropriate containers, labeled with the corresponding patient demographics, date and time of collection, site location, and promptly sent to the laboratory.

➤ The joint is irrigated, and the arthroscope is removed. Manual pressure is applied to the joint to remove remaining irrigation solution.

➤ The incision sites are sutured, and a pressure dressing is applied.

➤ Gloves and gowns are worn throughout the procedure.

Post-test:

➤ Advise the patient to avoid strenuous activity involving the joint until approved by the health care practitioner.

➤ Instruct the patient to resume normal diet and medications, as directed by the health care practitioner.

➤ Instruct the patient to take an analgesic for joint discomfort after the procedure; ice bags may be used to reduce postprocedure swelling.

➤ Monitor the patient's circulation and sensations in the joint area.

➤ Emphasize that any fever as well as excessive bleeding, difficulty breathing, incision site redness, swelling, and tenderness must be reported to the health care practitioner.

➤ To reduce swelling, instruct the patient to elevate the joint when sitting and to avoid overbending of the joint.

➤ Inform the patient to shower after 48 hours but to avoid a tub bath until after his or her appointment with the health care practitioner.

➤ A written report of the examination will be completed by a health care practitioner specializing in this branch of medicine. The report will be sent to the requesting health care practitioner, who will discuss the results with the patient.

➤ Depending on the results of this procedure, additional testing may be needed to evaluate or monitor progression of the disease process and determine the need for a change in therapy. Evaluate test results in relation to the patient's symptoms and other tests performed.

Related diagnostic tests:

➤ Related diagnostic tests include bone scan and radiography of the bone.

ASPARTATE AMINOTRANSFERASE

SYNONYM/ACRONYMS: Serum glutamic-oxaloacetic transaminase, AST, SGOT.

SPECIMEN: Serum (1 mL) collected in a red- or tiger-top tube.

REFERENCE VALUE: (Method: Spectrophotometry, enzymatic at 37°C)

Age	Conventional & SI Units
Newborn	47–150 U/L
10 d–23 m	9–80 U/L
2–59 y	
Male	15–40 U/L
Female	13–35 U/L
60–90 y	
Male	19–48 U/L
Female	9–36 U/L

DESCRIPTION & RATIONALE: Aspartate aminotransferase (AST) is an enzyme that catalyzes the reversible transfer of an amino group between aspartate and α-ketoglutaric acid. It was formerly known as serum glutamic-oxaloacetic transaminase (SGOT). AST exists in large amounts in liver and myocardial cells and in smaller but significant amounts in skeletal muscle, kidneys, pancreas, and the brain. Serum AST rises when there is cellular damage to the tissues where the enzyme is found. AST values greater than 500 U/L are usually associated with hepatitis and other hepatocellular diseases in an acute phase. AST levels are very elevated at birth and decrease with age. *Note:*

Measurement of AST in evaluation of myocardial infarction has been replaced by more sensitive tests, such as creatine kinase–MB fraction (CK-MB) and troponin. ∎

INDICATIONS:
- Assist in the diagnosis of disorders or injuries involving the tissues where AST is normally found
- Assist (formerly) in the diagnosis of myocardial infarction (*Note:* AST rises within 6 to 8 hours, peaks at 24 to 48 hours, and declines to normal within 72 to 96 hours of a myocardial infarction)
- Compare serially with alanine aminotransferase levels to track the course of hepatitis
- Monitor response to therapy with potentially hepatotoxic or nephrotoxic drugs
- Monitor response to treatment for various disorders in which AST may be elevated, with tissue repair indicated by declining levels

RESULT

Significantly increased in (greater than five times normal levels):
- Acute hepatitis
- Acute hepatocellular disease

- Acute pancreatitis
- Shock

Moderately increased in (three to five times normal levels):
- Biliary tract obstruction
- Cardiac arrhythmias
- Chronic hepatitis
- Congestive heart failure
- Dermatomyositis
- Liver tumors
- Muscular dystrophy

Slightly increased in (two to three times normal):
- Cerebrovascular accident
- Cirrhosis, fatty liver
- Delirium tremens
- Hemolytic anemia
- Pericarditis
- Pulmonary infarction

CRITICAL VALUES: N/A

INTERFERING FACTORS
- Drugs that may increase AST levels by causing cholestasis include amitriptyline, anabolic steroids, androgens, benzodiazepines, chlorothiazide, chlorpropamide, dapsone, erythromycin, estrogens, ethionamide, gold salts, imipramine, mercaptopurine, nitrofurans, oral contraceptives, penicillins, phenothiazines, progesterone, propoxyphene, sulfonamides, tamoxifen, and tolbutamide.

- Drugs that may increase AST levels by causing hepatocellular damage include acetaminophen (toxic), acetylsalicylic acid, allopurinol, amiodarone, anabolic steroids, anticonvulsants, asparaginase, azithromycin, bromocriptine, captopril, cephalosporins, chloramphenicol, clindamycin, clofibrate, danazol, enflurane, ethambutol, ethionamide, fenofibrate, fluconazole, fluoroquinolones, foscarnet, gentamicin, indomethacin, interferon, interleukin-2, levamisole, levodopa, lincomycin, low-molecular-weight heparin, methyldopa, monoamine oxidase inhibitors, naproxen, nifedipine, nitrofurans, oral contraceptives, probenecid, procainamide, quinine, ranitidine, retinol, ritodrine, sulfonylureas, tetracyclines, tobramycin, and verapamil.

- Hemolysis falsely increases AST values.

Nursing Implications and Procedure ⚫⚫⚫⚫⚫⚫⚫⚫⚫⚫⚫

Pretest: ▪

➤ Inform the patient that the test is primarily used to assess liver function.

➤ Obtain a history of the patient's complaints, including a list of known allergens (especially allergies or sensitivities to latex), and inform the appropriate health care practitioner accordingly.

➤ Obtain a history of the patient's cardiovascular and hepatobiliary systems, as well as results of previously performed laboratory tests, surgical procedures, and other diagnostic procedures. For related laboratory tests, refer to the Cardiovascular and Hepatobiliary System tables.

➤ Obtain a list of medications the patient is taking, including herbs, nutritional supplements, and nutraceuticals. The requesting health care practitioner and laboratory should be advised if the patient regularly uses these products so that their effects can be taken into consideration when reviewing results.

➤ Review the procedure with the patient. Inform the patient that specimen collection takes approximately 5 to 10 minutes. Address concerns about pain related to the procedure. Explain to the patient that there may be some discomfort during the venipuncture.

➤ There are no food, fluid, or medication restrictions unless by medical direction.

> If the patient has a history of severe allergic reaction to latex, care should be taken to avoid the use of equipment containing latex.

> Instruct the patient to cooperate fully and to follow directions. Direct the patient to breathe normally and to avoid unnecessary movement.

> Observe standard precautions, and follow the general guidelines in Appendix A. Positively identify the patient, and label the appropriate tubes with the corresponding patient demographics, date, and time of collection. Perform a venipuncture; collect the specimen in a 5-mL red- or tiger-top tube.

> Remove the needle, place a gauze over the puncture site and apply gentle pressure to stop bleeding. Observe venipuncture site for bleeding or hematoma formation. Apply paper tape over gauze or replace with adhesive bandage.

> Promptly transport the specimen to the laboratory for processing and analysis.

> The results are recorded manually or in a computerized system for recall and postprocedure interpretation by the appropriate health care practitioner.

Post-test:

> *Nutritional considerations:* Increased AST levels may be associated with liver disease. Dietary recommendations may be indicated and vary depending on the condition and its severity. Currently, there are no specific medications that can be given to cure hepatitis, but elimination of alcohol ingestion and a diet optimized for convalescence are commonly included in the treatment plan. A high-calorie, high-protein, moderate-fat diet with a high fluid intake is often recommended for patients with hepatitis. Treatment of cirrhosis is different; a low-protein diet may be in order if the patient's liver can no longer process the end products of protein metabolism. A diet of soft foods may be required if esophageal varices have developed. Ammonia levels may be used to determine whether protein should be added to or reduced from the diet. Patients should be encouraged to eat simple carbohydrates and emulsified fats (as in homogenized milk or eggs), as opposed to complex carbohydrates (e.g., starch, fiber, and glycogen [animal carbohydrates]) and complex fats, which would require additional bile to emulsify them so that they can be used. The cirrhotic patient should be observed carefully for the development of ascites, in which case fluid and electrolyte balance requires strict attention.

> *Nutrional considerations:* Increased AST levels may be associated with coronary artery disease (CAD). Nutritional therapy is recommended for individuals identified to be at high risk for CAD. Overweight patients should be encouraged to achieve a normal weight. The American Heart Association Step 1 and Step 2 diets may be helpful in achieving a goal of reducing total cholesterol and triglyceride levels. The Step 1 diet emphasizes a reduction in foods high in saturated fats and cholesterol. Red meats, eggs, and dairy products are the major sources of saturated fats and cholesterol. If triglycerides are also elevated, the patient should be advised to eliminate or reduce alcohol and simple carbohydrates from the diet. The Step 2 diet recommends stricter reductions.

> Instruct the patient to immediately report chest pain and changes in breathing pattern to the health care practitioner.

> A written report of the examination will be sent to the requesting health care practitioner, who will discuss the results with the patient.

> Reinforce information given by the patient's health care provider regard-

ing further testing, treatment, or referral to another health care provider. Answer any questions or address any concerns voiced by the patient or family.

➤ Depending on the results of this procedure, additional testing may be performed to evaluate or monitor progression of the disease process and determine the need for a change in therapy. Evaluate test results in relation to the patient's symptoms and other tests performed.

Related laboratory tests:

➤ Related laboratory tests include acetaminophen, alanine aminotransferase, albumin, alkaline phosphatase, ammonia, antimitochondrial antibody, α_1-antitrypsin/phenotyping, bilirubin, ethanol, ferritin, γ-glutamyltransferase, hepatitis antigens and antibodies, iron/total iron-binding capacity, liver biopsy, protein, and prothrombin time if liver disease is suspected; and antiarrhythmic drugs, apolipoprotein A, apolipoprotein B, atrial natriuretic peptide, B-type natriuretic peptide, blood gases, C-reactive protein, calcium/ionized calcium, cholesterol (total, HDL, & LDL), creatine kinase, homocysteine, lactate dehydrogenase, myoglobin, potassium, triglycerides, and troponin if myocardial infarction is suspected.

ATRIAL NATRIURETIC PEPTIDE

• •

SYNONYMS/ACRONYMS: Atrial natriuretic hormone, atrial natriuretic factor, ANF, ANH.

SPECIMEN: Plasma (1 mL) collected in a chilled, lavender-top tube. Specimen should be transported tightly capped and in an ice slurry.

REFERENCE VALUE: (Method: Radioimmunoassay)

Conventional Units	SI Units (Conventional Units × 1)
20–77 pg/mL	20–77 ng/L

DESCRIPTION & RATIONALE: Atrial natriuretic peptide or atrial natriuretic factor (ANF) is a hormone secreted from cells in the right atrium of the heart when right atrial pressure

increases. The release of this cardiac peptide is stimulated by increases in the stretch of the atrial wall caused by an increase in blood pressure or blood volume. ANF receptors are also stimulated by elevated sodium levels. This extremely potent hormone enhances salt and water excretions by blocking aldosterone and renin secretion. ANF inhibits angiotensin II and vasopressin, resulting in vasodilation and a decrease in blood volume and blood pressure. ■

INDICATIONS:
• Assist in the confirmation of congestive heart failure (CHF), as indicated by increased level
• Identify asymptomatic cardiac volume overload, as indicated by increased level

RESULT

Increased in:
• Asymptomatic cardiac volume overload
• CHF
• Elevated cardiac filling pressure
• Paroxysmal atrial tachycardia

Decreased in: N/A

CRITICAL VALUES: N/A

INTERFERING FACTORS:
• Drugs that may increase ANF levels include atenolol, candoxatril, captopril, carteolol, dopamine, morphine, oral contraceptives, vasopressin, and verapamil.
• Drugs that may decrease ANF levels include clonidine, prazosin, and urapidil.
• Recent radioactive scans or radiation within 1 week before the test can interfere with test results when radioimmunoassay is the test method.
• Failure to follow dietary and medication restrictions before the procedure may cause the procedure to be canceled or repeated.

Nursing Implications and Procedure • • • • • • • • • • •

Pretest:

▶ Inform the patient that the test is used to assess cardiac function.

▶ Obtain a history of the patient's complaints, including a list of known allergens, (especially allergies or sensitivities to latex), and inform the appropriate health care practitioner accordingly. Be alert to signs and symptoms of altered cardiopulmonary tissue perfusion related to ventilation-perfusion imbalance, decreased cardiac output related to altered muscle contractility, and fluid-volume excess related to glomerular filtration rate.

▶ Obtain a history of the patient's cardiovascular system and results of previously performed laboratory tests, surgical procedures, and other diagnostic procedures. For related laboratory tests, refer to the Cardio-vascular System table.

▶ Obtain a list of medications the patient is taking, including herbs, nutritional supplements, and nutraceuticals. The requesting health care practitioner and laboratory should be advised if the patient regularly uses these products so that their effects can be taken into consideration when reviewing results.

▶ Note any recent procedures that may interfere with test results.

▶ Review the procedure with the patient. Inform the patient that specimen collection takes approximately 5 to 10 minutes. Address concerns about pain related to the procedure. Explain to the patient that there may be some discomfort during the venipuncture.

▶ Instruct the patient to fast for 6 to 12 hours before the test and to avoid taking medications that interfere with test results, as directed by the health care practitioner. *Note:* Drugs such as β-blocking agents, calcium antagonists, cardiac glycosides, and vasodilators can affect results.

➤ Prepare an ice slurry in a cup or plastic bag to have ready for immediate transport of the specimen to the laboratory. Prechill the lavender-top tube in the ice slurry.

Intratest:

➤ Ensure that the patient has complied with dietary, medication, or activity restrictions and pretesting preparations; assure that food has been restricted for at least 6 to 12 hours prior to the procedure.

➤ If the patient has a history of severe allergic reaction to latex, care should be taken to avoid the use of equipment containing latex.

➤ Instruct the patient to cooperate fully and to follow directions. Direct the patient to breathe normally and to avoid unnecessary movement.

➤ Observe standard precautions, and follow the general guidelines in Appendix A. Positively identify the patient, and label the appropriate tubes with the corresponding patient demographics, date, and time of collection. Perform a venipuncture; collect the specimen in a prechilled 5-mL lavender-top tube.

➤ Remove the needle, place a gauze over the puncture site and apply gentle pressure to stop bleeding. Observe venipuncture site for bleeding or hematoma formation. Apply paper tape over gauze or replace with adhesive bandage.

➤ The sample should be placed in an ice slurry immediately after collection. Information on the specimen label can be protected from water in the ice slurry by first placing the specimen in a protective plastic bag. Promptly transport the specimen to the laboratory for processing and analysis.

➤ The results are recorded manually or in a computerized system for recall and postprocedure interpretation by the appropriate health care practitioner.

Post-test:

➤ Instruct the patient to resume usual diet and medication, as directed by the health care practitioner.

➤ *Nutritional considerations:* Increased ANF may be associated with coronary artery disease (CAD). Nutritional therapy is recommended for the patient identified to be at high risk for developing CAD. If overweight, the patient should be encouraged to achieve a normal weight. The American Heart Association Step 1 and Step 2 diets may be helpful in achieving a goal of lowering total cholesterol and triglyceride levels. The Step 1 diet emphasizes a reduction in foods high in saturated fats and cholesterol. Red meats, eggs, and dairy products are the major sources of saturated fats and cholesterol. If triglycerides also are elevated, the patient should be advised to eliminate or reduce alcohol and simple carbohydrates from the diet. The Step 2 diet recommends stricter reductions.

➤ *Nutritional considerations:* Overweight patients with high blood pressure should be encouraged to achieve a normal weight. Other changeable risk factors warranting patient education include strategies to safely decrease sodium intake, increase physical activity, decrease alcohol consumption, eliminate tobacco use, and decrease cholesterol levels.

➤ A written report of the examination will be sent to the requesting health care practitioner, who will discuss the results with the patient.

➤ Recognize anxiety related to test results, and be supportive of fear of shortened life expectancy. Discuss the implications of abnormal test results on the patient's lifestyle. Provide teaching and information regarding the clinical implications of the test results, as appropriate. Educate the patient regarding access to counseling services. Provide contact information, if desired, for the

American Heart Association (*www. americanheart.org*).

➤ Reinforce information given by the patient's health care provider regarding further testing, treatment, or referral to another health care provider. Answer any questions or address any concerns voiced by the patient or family.

➤ Depending on the results of this procedure, additional testing may be performed to evaluate or monitor progression of the disease process and determine the need for a change in therapy. Evaluate test results in relation to the patient's symptoms and other tests performed.

Related laboratory tests: ■

➤ Related laboratory tests include aldosterone, antiarrhythmic drugs, antidiuretic hormone, apolipoprotein A, apolipoprotein B, aspartate aminotranspeptidase, B-type natriuretic peptide, blood gases, C-reactive protein, calcium/ionized calcium, cholesterol (total, HDL, & LDL), creatine kinase and isoenzymes, glucose, glycated hemoglobin, homocysteine, ketones, lactate dehydrogenase and isoenzymes, lipoprotein electrophoresis, magnesium, myoglobin, potassium, renin, triglycerides, and troponin.

AUDIOMETRY, HEARING LOSS

SYNONYMS/ACRONYMS: N/A.

AREA OF APPLICATION: Ears.

CONTRAST: N/A.

DESCRIPTION & RATIONALE: Hearing loss audiometry involves the quantitative testing for a hearing deficit using an electronic instrument called an audiometer that measures and records thresholds of hearing by air conduction and bone conduction tests. These results determine if hearing loss is conductive, sensorineural, or a combination of both. An elevated air-conduction threshold with a normal bone-conduction threshold indicates a conductive hearing loss. An equally elevated threshold for both air and bone conduction indicates a sensorineural hearing loss. An elevated threshold of air conduction that is more than an elevated threshold of bone conduction indicates a composite of both types of hearing loss. A conductive hearing loss is caused by an abnormality in the external auditory canal or middle ear, and a sensorineural hearing loss by an abnormality in the inner ear or of the VIII (auditory) nerve. Sensorineural hearing loss can be further differentiated clinically by sensory (cochlear) or neural (VIII nerve) lesions. Additional information for comparing and differentiating between conductive and sensorineural hearing loss can be obtained by performing hearing loss tuning fork tests. ■

INDICATIONS:

• Determine the need for a type of hearing aid and evaluate its effectiveness.

• Determine the type and extent of hearing loss (conductive, as evidenced by a reduced air threshold and unchanged bone threshold, or sensorineural, as evidenced by a reduced air and bone threshold, or mixed, as evidenced by abnormal air and bone thresholds) and if further radiologic, audiologic, or vestibular procedures are needed to identify the cause.

• Evaluate communication disabilities and plan for rehabilitation interventions.

• Evaluate degree and extent of preoperative and postoperative hearing loss following stapedectomy in patients with otosclerosis.

• Screen for hearing loss in infants and children and determine the need for a referral to an audiologist.

RESULT

ANSI 1996 scale	Elevated Pure Tone Averages
Slight Loss	16–25 dB
Mild Loss	26–40 dB
Moderate Loss	41–55 dB
Moderately Severe Loss	56–70 dB
Severe Loss	71–90 dB
Profound Loss	Greater than 91 dB

Normal Findings:
• Normal pure tone average of −10 to 15 dB.

Abnormal Findings:
• Causes of conductive hearing loss
  Obstruction of external ear canal
  Otitis externa
  Otitis media
  Otosclerosis
• Causes of sensorineural hearing loss
  Congenital damage or
    malformations of the inner ear
  Ototoxic drugs
  Serious infections
  Trauma to the inner ear
  Tumor
  Vascular disorders

CRITICAL VALUES: N/A

INTERFERING FACTORS:

Factors that may impair the results of the examination:

• Inability of the patient to cooperate or remain still during the procedure because of age, significant pain, or mental status may interfere with the test results.

• Obstructions of the ear canal by cerumen or other material or object will affect decibel (dB) perception.

• Noisy environment or extraneous movements can affect results.

• Tinnitus or other sensations can cause abnormal responses.

• Improper earphone fit or audiometer calibration can affect results.

- Failure to follow pretesting preparations before the procedure may cause the procedure to be canceled or repeated.

Nursing Implications and Procedure • • • • • • • • • • •

 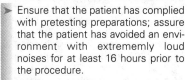

➤ Inform the patient that the procedure detects hearing loss.

➤ Obtain a history of the patient's complaints, including a list of known allergens.

➤ Obtain a history of the patient's known or suspected hearing loss, including type and cause; ear conditions with treatment regimens; ear surgery; and other tests and procedures to assess and diagnose auditory deficit.

➤ Obtain a history of results of previously performed laboratory tests, surgical procedures, and other diagnostic procedures.

➤ Obtain a list of the medications the patient is taking, including herbs, nutritional supplements, and nutraceuticals. The requesting health care practitioner should be advised if the patient regularly uses these products so that their effects can be taken into consideration when reviewing results.

➤ Review the procedure with the patient. Instruct the patient to avoid an environment with extremely loud noises for at least 16 hours prior to the procedure. Address concerns about pain related to the procedure. Explain to the patient that no discomfort will be experienced during the test. Inform the patient that an audiologist, physician, or nurse performs the test, in a quiet, darkened room, and that the test can take up 20 minutes to evaluate both ears.

➤ There are no food, fluid, or medication restrictions unless by medical direction.

➤ Ensure that the external auditory canal is clear of impacted cerumen.

➤ Ensure that the patient has complied with pretesting preparations; assure that the patient has avoided an environment with extrememly loud noises for at least 16 hours prior to the procedure.

➤ Instruct the patient to cooperate fully and to follow directions. Instruct the patient to remain still during the procedure because movement produces unreliable results.

➤ Perform otoscopy examination to ensure that the external ear canal is free from any obstruction (see monograph titled "Otoscopy").

➤ Test for closure of the canal by the pressure of the earphones by compressing the tragus. Tendency for the canal to close (often the case in children and elderly patients) can be corrected by the careful insertion of a small stiff plastic tube into the anterior canal.

➤ Place the patient in a sitting position in comfortable proximity to the audiometer in a soundproof room. The ear not being tested is masked to prevent crossover of test tones, and the earphones are positioned on the head and over the ear canals.

➤ Start the test by providing a trial tone of 30 dB (ASHA 1978 Guidelines) to the ear for 1 to 2 seconds to familiarize the patient with the sounds. Instruct the patient to press the button each time a tone is heard, no matter how loudly or faintly it is perceived. If no response is indicated, the level is increased to 50 dB and then raised in 10-dB increments until a response is obtained or until the audiometer's limit is reached for the test frequency. The test results are plotted on a graph called an audiogram using symbols that indicate the ear tested and responses using earphones (air conduction) or oscillator (bone conduction).

Air Conduction:

➤ Air conduction is tested first by starting at 1000 Hz and gradually decreasing the intensity 10 dB at a time until the patient no longer presses the button, indicating that the tone is no longer heard. The intensity is then increased 5 dB at a time until the tone is heard again. This is repeated until the same response is achieved at a 50% response rate at the same hertz (Hz) level. The threshold is derived from the lowest decibel level at which the patient correctly identifies three out of six responses to a tone at that hertz level. The test is continued for each ear, testing the better ear first, with tones delivered at 1000 Hz, 2000 Hz, 4000 Hz, and 8000 Hz, and then again at 1000 Hz, 500 Hz, and 250 Hz to determine a second threshold. Results are recorded on a graph called an audiogram. Averaging the air conduction thresholds at the 500-Hz, 1000-Hz, and 2000-Hz levels reveals the degree of hearing loss and is called the pure tone average (PTA).

Bone Conduction:

➤ Bone conduction is then tested using an oscillator placed on the mastoid process behind the ear(s) after removal of the earphones. The raised and lowered tones are delivered as in air conduction using 250 Hz, 500 Hz, 1000 Hz, 2000 Hz, and 4000 Hz to determine the thresholds. An analysis of thresholds for air and bone conduction tones is done to determine the type of hearing loss (conductive, sensorineural, or mixed).

➤ In children between 6 months and 2 years of age, minimal response levels can be determined by behavioral responses to test tone. In the child 2 years of age and older, play audiometry that requires the child to perform a task or raise a hand in response to a specific tone is performed. In children 12 years of age and older, the child is asked to follow directions in identifying objects; response to speech of specific intensities can be used to evaluate hearing loss that is affected by speech frequencies.

➤ The results are recorded manually or on a paper strip from the automated equipment for recall and postprocedure interpretation by the appropriate health care practitioner.

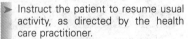
Post-test:

➤ Instruct the patient to resume usual activity, as directed by the health care practitioner.

➤ A written report of the examination will be completed by a health care practitioner specializing in this branch of medicine. The report will be sent to the requesting health care practitioner, who will discuss the results with the patient.

➤ Recognize anxiety related to test results, and be supportive of impaired activity related to hearing loss or perceived loss of independence. Discuss the implications of abnormal test results on the patient's lifestyle. Provide teaching and information regarding the clinical implications of the test results, as appropriate.

➤ Reinforce information given by the patient's health care provider regarding further testing, treatment, or referral to another health care provider. As appropriate, instruct the patient in the use, cleaning, and storing of a hearing aid. Answer any questions or address any concerns voiced by the patient or family.

➤ Depending on the results of this procedure, additional testing may be performed to evaluate or monitor progression of the disease process and determine the need for a change in therapy. Evaluate test results in relation to the patient's symptoms and other tests performed.

Related diagnostic tests:

➤ Related diagnostic tests include evoked brain potential studies for hearing loss, otoscopy, spondee speech reception threshold, and tuning fork tests (Webber, Rinne).

BARIUM ENEMA

. . . .

SYNONYMS/ACRONYMS: Air-contrast barium enema, double-contrast barium enema, lower GI series, BE.

AREA OF APPLICATION: Colon.

CONTRAST: Barium sulfate, air, iodine mixture.

DESCRIPTION & RATIONALE: This radiologic examination of the colon, distal small bowel, and occasionally the appendix follows instillation of barium using a rectal tube inserted into the rectum or an existing ostomy. The patient must retain the barium while a series of radiographs are obtained. Visualization can be improved by using air or barium as the contrast medium (double-contrast study). A combination of x-ray and fluoroscopy techniques is used to complete the study. This test is especially useful in the evaluation of patients experiencing lower abdominal pain, changes in bowel habits, or the passage of stools containing blood or mucus, and for visualizing polyps, diverticula, and tumors. A barium enema may be therapeutic; it may reduce an obstruction caused by intussusception, or telescoping of the intestine. Barium enema should be performed before an upper gastrointestinal study or barium swallow. ∎

INDICATIONS:
- Determine the cause of rectal bleeding, blood, pus, or mucus in feces
- Evaluate suspected inflammatory process, congenital anomaly, motility disorder, or structural change
- Evaluate unexplained weight loss, anemia, or a change in bowel pattern
- Identify and locate benign or malignant polyps or tumors

RESULT

Normal Findings:
- Normal size, filling, shape, position, and motility of the colon
- Normal filling of the appendix and terminal ileum

Abnormal Findings:
- Appendicitis
- Colorectal cancer
- Congenital anomalies
- Crohn's disease
- Diverticular disease
- Fistulas
- Gastroenteritis
- Granulomatous colitis
- Hirschsprung's disease
- Intussusception
- Perforation of the colon

- Polyps
- Sarcoma
- Sigmoid torsion
- Sigmoid volvulus
- Stenosis
- Tumors
- Ulcerative colitis

INTERFERING FACTORS:

This procedure is contraindicated for:

- ⚠ Patients with allergies to shellfish or iodinated dye, when iodinated contrast medium is used. The contrast medium, when used, may cause a life-threatening allergic reaction. Patients with a known hypersensitivity to contrast medium may benefit from premedication with corticosteroids or the use of nonionic contrast medium.

- Patients who are pregnant or suspected of being pregnant, unless the potential benefits of the procedure far outweigh the risks to the fetus and mother.

- Patients with intestinal obstruction, acute ulcerative colitis, acute diverticulitis, megacolon, or suspected rupture of the colon.

Factors that may impair clear imaging:

- Gas or feces in the gastrointestinal tract resulting from inadequate cleansing or failure to restrict food intake before the study

- Retained barium from a previous radiologic procedure

- Metallic objects within the examination field (e.g., jewelry, body rings), which may inhibit organ visualization and can produce unclear images

- Improper adjustment of the radiographic equipment to accommodate obese or thin patients, which can cause

overexposure or underexposure and a poor-quality study

- Patients who are very obese, who may exceed the weight limit for the equipment

- Incorrect positioning of the patient, which may produce poor visualization of the area to be examined

- Inability of the patient to cooperate or remain still during the procedure because of age, significant pain, or mental status

- Spasm of the colon, which can mimic the radiographic signs of cancer (*Note:* the use of intravenous glucagon minimizes spasm)

- Inability of the patient to tolerate introduction of or retention of barium, air, or both in the bowel

Other considerations:

- Complications of the procedure may include hemorrhage and cardiac arrhythmias.

- The procedure may be terminated if chest pain or severe cardiac arrhythmias occur.

- Failure to follow dietary restrictions and other pretesting preparations may cause the procedure to be canceled or repeated.

- Consultation with a physician should occur before the procedure for radiation safety concerns regarding younger patients or patients who are lactating.

- Risks associated with radiographic overexposure can result from frequent x-ray procedures. Personnel in the room with the patient should wear a protective lead apron, stand behind a shield, or leave the area while the examination is being done. Personnel working in the area where the examination is being done should wear badges that reveal their level of exposure to radiation.

Nursing Implications and Procedure • • • • • • • • • •

➤ Inform the patient that the procedure assesses the colon.

➤ Obtain a history of the patient's complaints or symptoms, including a list of known allergens, especially allergies or sensitivities to latex, iodine, seafood, contrast medium, and dyes.

➤ Obtain a history of results of previously performed diagnostic procedures, surgical procedures, and laboratory tests. For related diagnostic tests, refer to the Gastrointestinal System table.

➤ Ensure that this procedure is performed before an upper gastrointestinal study or barium swallow.

➤ Record the date of the last menstrual period and determine the possibility of pregnancy in perimenopausal women.

➤ Obtain a list of the medications the patient is taking.

➤ Explain to the patient that some pain may be experienced during the test, and there may be moments of discomfort. Explain the purpose of the test and how the procedure is performed. Inform the patient that the procedure is performed in a radiology department, usually by a physician and support staff, and takes approximately 30 to 60 minutes.

➤ *Sensitivity to cultural and social issues,* as well as concern for modesty, is important in providing psychological support before, during, and after the procedure.

➤ Instruct the patient to eat a low-residue diet for several days before the procedure and to consume only clear liquids the evening before the test. The patient should fast and restrict fluids for 8 hours prior to the procedure.

➤ Instruct patients with a colostomy to follow the same dietary preparation, take laxatives the evening before, and perform colostomy irrigation before the study.

➤ Inform the patient that a laxative and cleansing enema may be needed the day before the procedure, with cleansing enemas on the morning of the procedure, depending on the institution's policy.

➤ Instruct the patient to remove jewelry (including watches), credit cards, and other metallic objects.

➤ Ensure that the patient has complied with dietary, and medication restrictions and pretesting preparations for at least 6 hours prior to the procedure. Ensure that the patient has removed all external metallic objects prior to the procedure.

➤ Assess for completion of bowel preparation according to the institution's procedure.

➤ Have emergency equipment readily available.

➤ Patients are given a gown, robe, and foot coverings to wear and instructed to void prior to the procedure.

➤ Observe standard precautions, and follow the general guidelines in Appendix A.

➤ Instruct the patient to cooperate fully and to follow directions. Instruct the patient to remain still throughout the procedure because movement produces unreliable results.

➤ Place the patient in the supine position on an exam table.

➤ An initial image is taken. The patient is helped to a side-lying position (Sims' position). A rectal tube is inserted into the anus while an attached balloon is inflated after it is situated against the anal sphincter.

➤ Barium is instilled into the colon, and then its movement through the colon is observed by fluoroscopy.

➤ Images are taken at different angles and positions to aid in the evaluation of the patient's problem.

➤ For patients with a colostomy, an indwelling urinary catheter is inserted into the stoma and barium is administered.

➤ The patient is returned to a position of comfort, and is placed on a bedpan or helped to the bathroom to expel the barium.

➤ After the expulsion of the barium, an additional film is taken of the intestine.

➤ If a double-contrast barium enema has been ordered, air is then instilled in the intestine and additional films are taken.

➤ The results are recorded manually, on film, or by automated equipment in a computerized system for recall and postprocedure interpretation by the appropriate health care practitioner.

Post-test:

➤ Instruct the patient to resume usual diet, fluids, medications, or activity, as directed by the health care practitioner.

➤ If iodine is used, monitor for reaction to iodinated contrast medium, including rash, urticaria, tachycardia, hyperpnea, hypertension, palpitations, nausea, or vomiting.

➤ Carefully monitor the patient for fatigue and fluid and electrolyte imbalance.

➤ Instruct the patient to take a mild laxative and increase fluid intake (four 8-ounce glasses) to aid in elimination of barium, unless contraindicated.

➤ Instruct the patient that stools will be white or light in color for 2 to 3 days. If the patient is unable to eliminate the barium, or if stools do not return to normal color, the patient should notify the physician.

➤ Advise patients with a colostomy to administer tap water colostomy irrigation to aid in barium removal.

➤ A written report of the examination will be completed by a health care practitioner specializing in this branch of medicine. The report will be sent to the requesting health care practitioner, who will discuss the results with the patient.

➤ Depending on the results of this procedure, additional testing may be needed to evaluate or monitor progression of the disease process and determine the need for a change in therapy. Evaluate test results in relation to the patient's symptoms and other tests performed.

Related diagnostic tests:

➤ Related diagnostic tests include colonoscopy, computed tomography abdomen and magnetic resonance imaging abdomen.

BARIUM SWALLOW

· ·

SYNONYMS/ACRONYM: Esophagram, video swallow, esophagus x-ray, swallowing function, esophagography.

AREA OF APPLICATION: Esophagus.

CONTRAST: Barium sulfate, water-soluble iodinated contrast.

DESCRIPTION & RATIONALE: This radiologic examination of the esophagus evaluates motion and anatomic structures of the esophageal lumen by recording images of the lumen while the patient swallows a barium solution of milkshake consistency and chalky taste. The procedure uses fluoroscopic and cineradiographic techniques. The barium swallow is often performed as part of an upper gastrointestinal series or cardiac series and is indicated for patients with a history of dysphagia and regurgitation. In patients with esophageal reflux, the radiologist may identify reflux of the barium from the stomach back into the esophagus. Muscular abnormalities such as achalasia, as well as diffuse esophageal spasm, can be easily detected with this procedure. ■

INDICATIONS:
- Confirm the integrity of esophageal anastomoses in the postoperative patient
- Detect esophageal reflux, tracheoesophageal fistulas, and varices
- Determine the cause of dysphagia, heartburn, or regurgitation
- Determine the type and location of foreign bodies within the pharynx and esophagus
- Evaluate suspected esophageal motility disorders
- Evaluate suspected polyps, strictures, Zenker's diverticula, tumor, or inflammation

RESULT

Normal Findings:
- Normal peristalsis through the esophagus into the stomach with normal size, filling, patency, and shape of the esophagus

Abnormal Findings:
- Achalasia
- Acute or chronic esophagitis
- Benign or malignant tumors
- Chalasia
- Diverticula
- Esophageal ulcers
- Esophageal varices
- Hiatal hernia
- Perforation of the esophagus
- Strictures or polyps

INTERFERING FACTORS:

This procedure is contraindicated for:
- Patients who are pregnant or suspected of being pregnant, unless the potential benefits of the procedure far outweigh the risks to the fetus and mother
- Patients with intestinal obstruction or suspected esophageal rupture, unless water-soluble iodinated contrast medium is used
- Patients with suspected tracheoesophageal fistula, unless barium is used

Factors that may impair clear imaging:
- Gas or feces in the gastrointestinal tract resulting from inadequate cleansing or failure to restrict food intake before the study
- Retained barium from a previous radiologic procedure
- Metallic objects within the examination field (e.g., jewelry, body rings), which may inhibit organ visualization and can produce unclear images
- Improper adjustment of the radiographic equipment to accommodate obese or thin patients, which can cause overexposure or underexposure and a poor-quality study

- Patients who are very obese, who may exceed the weight limit for the equipment
- Incorrect positioning of the patient, which may produce poor visualization of the area to be examined
- Inability of the patient to cooperate or remain still during the procedure because of age, significant pain, or mental status

Other considerations:

- The procedure may be terminated if chest pain, or severe cardiac arrhythmias occur.

- Failure to follow dietary restrictions and other pretesting preparations may cause the procedure to be canceled or repeated.

- A potential complication of a barium swallow is barium-induced fecal impaction.

- Ensure that the procedure is done after cholangiography and barium enema.

- Consultation with a physician should occur before the procedure for radiation safety concerns regarding younger patients or patients who are lactating.

- Risks associated with radiographic overexposure can result from frequent x-ray procedures. Personnel in the room with the patient should wear a protective lead apron, stand behind a shield, or leave the area while the examination is being done. Personnel working in the area where the examination is being done should wear badges that reveal their level of exposure to radiation.

Nursing Implications and Procedure • • • • • • • • • • •

Pretest:

➤ Inform the patient that the procedure assesses the esophagus.

➤ Obtain a history of the patient's complaints or symptoms, including a list of known allergens, especially allergies or sensitivities to latex, iodine, seafood, contrast medium, and dyes.

➤ Obtain a history of results of previously performed diagnostic procedures, surgical procedures, and laboratory tests. For related diagnostic tests, refer to the Gastrointestinal System table.

➤ Ensure that this procedure is performed before an upper gastrointestinal study or video swallow.

➤ Record the date of the last menstrual period and determine the possibility of pregnancy in perimenopausal women.

➤ Obtain a list of the medications the patient is taking.

➤ Explain to the patient that some pain may be experienced during the test, and there may be moments of discomfort. Explain the purpose of the test, how the procedure is performed, and the need to swallow contrast medium. Inform the patient that the procedure is performed in a radiology department, usually by a physician and support staff, and takes approximately 15 to 30 minutes.

➤ *Sensitivity to cultural and social issues,* as well as concern for modesty, is important in providing psychological support before, during, and after the procedure.

➤ Instruct the patient to fast and restrict fluids for 8 hours prior to the procedure.

➤ Instruct the patient to remove jewelry or other metallic objects.

Intratest:

➤ Ensure that the patient has complied with dietary and medication restrictions and pretesting preparations for at least 6 hours prior to the procedure. Ensure that the patient has removed all external metallic objects prior to the procedure.

➤ Have emergency equipment readily available.

➤ Patients are given a gown, robe, and foot coverings to wear and instructed to void prior to the procedure.

➤ Observe standard precautions, and follow the general guidelines in Appendix A.

➤ Instruct the patient to cooperate fully and to follow directions. Instruct the patient to remain still throughout the procedure because movement produces unreliable results.

➤ Place the patient in the supine position on an exam table, or have the patient stand in front of an x-ray fluoroscopy screen.

➤ An initial image is taken, and the patient is asked to swallow a barium solution with or without a straw.

➤ Images are taken at different angles and positions to aid in the evaluation of patient's problem.

➤ The patient may be asked to drink additional barium to complete the study. Swallowing the additional barium evaluates the passage of barium from the esophagus into the stomach.

➤ Return the patient to a comfortable position; help the patient from the x-ray table to a chair or stretcher.

➤ The results are recorded manually, on film, or by automated equipment in a computerized system for recall and postprocedure interpretation by the appropriate health care practitioner.

Post-test:

➤ Instruct the patient to resume usual diet, fluids, medications, or activity, as directed by the health care practitioner.

➤ If iodine is used, monitor for reaction to iodinated contrast medium, including rash, urticaria, tachycardia, hyperpnea, hypertension, palpitations, nausea, or vomiting.

➤ Carefully monitor the patient for fatigue and fluid and electrolyte imbalance.

➤ Instruct the patient to take a mild laxative and increase fluid intake (four 8-ounce glasses) to aid in elimination of barium, unless contraindicated.

➤ Instruct the patient that stools will be white or light in color for 2 to 3 days. If the patient is unable to eliminate the barium, or if stools do not return to normal color, the patient should notify the physician.

➤ A written report of the examination will be completed by a health care practitioner specializing in this branch of medicine. The report will be sent to the requesting health care practitioner, who will discuss the results with the patient.

➤ Depending on the results of this procedure, additional testing may be needed to evaluate or monitor progression of the disease process and determine the need for a change in therapy. Evaluate test results in relation to the patient's symptoms and other tests performed.

Related diagnostic tests:

➤ Related diagnostic tests include chest x-ray, computed tomography thoracic, endoscopy, magnetic resonance imaging chest, and thyroid scan.

BILIRUBIN AND BILIRUBIN FRACTIONS

SYNONYMS/ACRONYM: Conjugated/direct bilirubin, unconjugated/indirect bilirubin, delta bilirubin, TBil.

SPECIMEN: Serum (1 mL) collected in a red- or tiger-top tube. Plasma (1 mL) collected in green-top (heparin) tube or in a heparinized microtainer is also acceptable.

REFERENCE VALUE: (Method: Spectrophotometry) Total bilirubin levels in infants should decrease to adult levels by day 10 as the development of the hepatic circulatory system matures. Values in breast-fed infants may take longer to reach normal adult levels. Values in premature infants may initially be higher than in full-term infants and also take longer to decrease to normal levels.

Bilirubin	Conventional Units	SI Units (Conventional Units × 17.1)
Total bilirubin		
Newborn–1 d	1.4–8.7 mg/dL	24–149 μmol/L
1–2 d	3.4–11.5 mg/dL	58–97 μmol/L
3–5 d	1.5–12.0 mg/dL	26–205 μmol/L
1 mo–adult	0.3–1.2 mg/dL	5–21 μmol/L
Unconjugated bilirubin	Less than 1.1 mg/dL	Less than 19 μmol/L
Conjugated bilirubin	Less than 0.3 mg/dL	Less than 5 μmol/L
Delta bilirubin	Less than 0.2 mg/dL	Less than 3 μmol/L

DESCRIPTION & RATIONALE: Bilirubin is a byproduct of heme catabolism from aged red blood cells. Bilirubin is primarily produced in the liver, spleen, and bone marrow. Total bilirubin is the sum of unconjugated bilirubin, monoglucuronide and diglucuronide, conjugated bilirubin, and albumin-bound delta bilirubin. Unconjugated bilirubin is carried to the liver by albumin, where it becomes conjugated. In the small intestine, conjugated bilirubin converts to urobilinogen and then to urobilin. Urobilin is then excreted in the feces. Increases in bilirubin levels can result from prehepatic and/or posthepatic conditions, making fractionation useful in determining the cause of the increase in total bilirubin levels. Delta bilirubin has a longer half-life than the other bilirubin fractions and therefore remains elevated during convalescence after the other fractions have decreased to normal levels. When bilirubin concentration increases, the yellowish pigment deposits in skin and sclera. This increase in yellow pigmentation is termed *jaundice* or *icterus*. ∎

INDICATIONS:
- Assist in the differential diagnosis of obstructive jaundice
- Assist in the evaluation of liver and biliary disease
- Monitor the effects of drug reactions on liver function
- Monitor the effects of phototherapy on jaundiced newborns
- Monitor jaundice in newborn patients

RESULT

Increased in:
- Prehepatic (hemolytic) jaundice
  Erythroblastosis fetalis
  Hematoma
  Hemolytic anemias
  Pernicious anemia
  Physiologic jaundice of the newborn
  The post–blood transfusion period, when a number of units are rapidly infused or in the case of a delayed transfusion reaction
  Red blood cell enzyme abnormalities (i.e., glucose-6-phosphate dehydrogenase, pyruvate kinase, spherocytosis)
- Hepatic jaundice—bilirubin conjugation failure
  Crigler-Najjar syndrome
- Hepatic jaundice—disturbance in bilirubin transport
  Dubin-Johnson syndrome (preconjugation transport failure)
  Gilbert's syndrome (postconjugation transport failure)
- Hepatic jaundice—liver damage or necrosis
  Alcoholism
  Cholangitis
  Cholecystitis

  Cholestatic drug reactions
  Cirrhosis
  Hepatitis
  Hepatocellular damage
  Infectious mononucleosis
- Posthepatic jaundice
  Advanced tumors of the liver
  Biliary obstruction
- Other conditions
  Anorexia or starvation
  Premature or breastfed infants
  Hypothyroidism

Decreased in: N/A

CRITICAL VALUES: ⚠ Greater than 15 mg/dL

Note and immediately report to the health care practitioner any critically increased values and related symptoms.

Sustained hyperbilirubinemia can result in brain damage. *Kernicterus* refers to the deposition of bilirubin in the basal ganglia and brainstem nuclei. There is no exact level of bilirubin that puts infants at risk for developing kernicterus. Symptoms of kernicterus in infants include lethargy, poor feeding, upward deviation of the eyes, and seizures. Intervention for infants may include early frequent feedings to stimulate gastrointestinal motility, phototherapy, and exchange transfusion.

INTERFERING FACTORS:
- Drugs that may increase bilirubin levels by causing cholestasis include amitriptyline, anabolic steroids, androgens, benzodiazepines, chlorothiazide, chlorpropamide, dapsone, erythromycin, estrogens, ethionamide, gold salts, imipramine, mercaptopurine, nitrofurans, oral contraceptives, penicillins, phenothiazines, progesterone, propoxyphene, sulfonamides, tamoxifen, and tolbutamide.
- Drugs that may increase bilirubin levels by causing hepatocellular damage include acetaminophen (toxic), acetyl-

salicylic acid, allopurinol, amiodarone, anabolic steroids, anticonvulsants, asparaginase, azithromycin, bromocriptine, captopril, cephalosporins, chloramphenicol, clindamycin, clofibrate, danazol, enflurane, ethambutol, ethionamide, fenofibrate, fluconazole, fluoroquinolones, foscarnet, gentamicin, indomethacin, interferon, interleukin-2, levamisole, levodopa, lincomycin, low-molecular-weight heparin, methyldopa, monoamine oxidase inhibitors, naproxen, nifedipine, nitrofurans, oral contraceptives, probenecid, procainamide, quinine, ranitidine, retinol, ritodrine, sulfonylureas, tetracyclines, tobramycin, and verapamil.

- Drugs that may increase bilirubin levels by causing hemolysis include amphotericin B, carbamazepine, carbutamide, cephaloridine, cephalothin, chlorpromazine, chlorpropamide, dinitrophenol, ibuprofen, insulin, isoniazid, levodopa, mefenamic acid, melphalan, methotrexate, methyldopa, penicillins, phenacetin, procainamide, quinidine, quinine, rifampin, stibophen, sulfonamides, and tolbutamide.

- Bilirubin is light sensitive. Therefore, the collection container should be suitably covered to protect the specimen from light between the time of collection and analysis.

Nursing Implications and Procedure • • • • • • • • • • • •

Pretest:

➤ Inform the patient that the test is used to assess liver function.

➤ Obtain a history of the patient's complaints, including a list of known allergens (especially allergies or sensitivities to latex), and inform the appropriate health care practitioner accordingly.

➤ Obtain a history of the patient's hepatobiliary system, as well as results of previously performed laboratory tests, surgical procedures, and other diagnostic procedures. For related laboratory tests, refer to the Hepatobiliary System table.

➤ Obtain a list of the medications the patient is taking, including herbs, nutritional supplements, and nutraceuticals. The requesting health care practitioner and laboratory should be advised if the patient regularly uses these products so their effects can be taken into consideration when reviewing results.

➤ Review the procedure with the patient. Inform the patient that specimen collection takes approximately 5 to 10 minutes. Address concerns about pain related to the procedure. Explain to the patient that there may be some discomfort during the venipuncture.

➤ *Sensitivity to cultural and social issues,* as well as concern for modesty, is important in providing psychological support before, during, and after the procedure.

➤ There are no food, fluid, or medication restrictions unless by medical direction.

Intratest:

➤ If the patient has a history of severe allergic reaction to latex, care should be taken to avoid the use of equipment containing latex.

➤ Instruct the patient to cooperate fully and to follow directions. Direct the patient to breathe normally and to avoid unnecessary movement.

➤ Observe standard precautions, and follow the general guidelines in Appendix A. Positively identify the patient, and label the appropriate tubes with the corresponding patient demographics, date, and time of collection. Perform a venipuncture; collect the specimen in a 5-mL red- or tiger-top tube.

➤ Remove the needle and place a gauze over the puncture site and apply gentle pressure to stop bleeding. Observe venipuncture site for bleeding or hematoma formation. Apply paper tape over gauze or replace with adhesive bandage.

➤ Protect the specimen from light and promptly transport the specimen to the laboratory for processing and analysis.

➤ The results are recorded manually or in a computerized system for re-call and postprocedure interpretation by the appropriate health care practitioner.

Post-test:

➤ *Nutritional considerations:* Increased bilirubin levels may be associated with liver disease. Dietary recommendations may be indicated depending on the condition and severity of the condition. Currently, for example, there are no specific medications that can be given to cure hepatitis, but elimination of alcohol ingestion and a diet optimized for convalescence are commonly included in the treatment plan. A high-calorie, high-protein, moderate-fat diet with a high fluid intake is often recommended for the patient with hepatitis. Treatment of cirrhosis is different because a low-protein diet may be in order if the patient's liver has lost the ability to process the end products of protein metabolism. A diet of soft foods may also be required if esophageal varices have developed. Ammonia levels may be used to determine whether protein should be added to or reduced from the diet. Patients should be encouraged to eat simple carbohydrates and emulsified fats (as in homogenized milk or eggs), as opposed to complex carbohydrates (e.g., starch, fiber, and glycogen [animal carbohydrates]) and complex fats, which would require additional bile to emulsify them so that they can be used.

The cirrhotic patient should be carefully observed for the development of ascites, in which case, fluid and electrolyte balance requires strict attention. The alcoholic patient should be encouraged to avoid alcohol and also to seek appropriate counseling for substance abuse.

➤ Intervention for hyperbilirubinemia in the neonatal patient may include early frequent feedings (to stimulate gastrointestinal motility), phototherapy, and exchange transfusion.

➤ A written report of the examination will be sent to the requesting health care practitioner, who will discuss the results with the patient.

➤ Reinforce information given by the patient's health care provider regarding further testing, treatment, or referral to another health care provider. Answer any questions or address any concerns voiced by the patient or family.

➤ Depending on the results of this procedure, additional testing may be performed to evaluate or monitor progression of the disease process and determine the need for a change in therapy. Evaluate test results in relation to the patient's symptoms and other tests performed.

Related laboratory tests:

➤ Related laboratory tests include alanine aminotransferase, albumin, alkaline phosphatase, ammonia, amylase, antimitochondrial antibody, anti–smooth muscle antibody, α_1-antitrypsin/phenotyping, aspartate aminotransferase, cholesterol, coagulation factor assays, complete blood count, copper, γ-glutamyltransferase, hepatitis serologies, infectious mononucleosis screen, lipase, liver biopsy, protein, prothrombin time, and urinalysis.

BIOPSY, BLADDER

SYNONYM/ACRONYM: N/A.

SPECIMEN: Bladder tissue or cells.

REFERENCE VALUE: (Method: Macroscopic and microscopic examination of tissue) No abnormal tissue or cells.

DESCRIPTION & RATIONALE: A urologist performs a biopsy of the bladder during cystoscopic examination. The procedure is usually carried out under general anesthesia. After the bladder is filled with saline for irrigation, the bladder and urethra are examined by direct and lighted visualization using a cystoscope. A sample of suspicious bladder tissue is then excised and examined macroscopically and microscopically to determine the presence of cell morphology and tissue abnormalities. ■

INDICATIONS:
• Assist in confirmation of malignant lesions of the bladder or ureter, especially if tumor is seen by radiological examination

• Assist in the evaluation of cases in which symptoms such as hematuria persist after previous treatment (e.g., removal of polyps or kidney stones)

• Monitor existing recurrent benign lesions for malignant changes

RESULT: Positive findings in neoplasm of the bladder or ureter.

CRITICAL VALUES: N/A

INTERFERING FACTORS:
• This test is contraindicated in patients with an acute infection of the bladder, urethra, or prostate.

• ⚠ This procedure is contraindicated in patients with bleeding disorders.

• Failure to follow dietary restrictions before the procedure may cause the procedure to be canceled or repeated.

Nursing Implications and Procedure

Pretest:

➤ Inform the patient that the test is used to establish a histologic diagnosis of bladder disease.

➤ Obtain a history of the patient's complaints, including a list of known allergens (especially allergies or sensitivities to latex or anesthetics), and inform the appropriate health care practitioner accordingly.

➤ Obtain a history of the patient's genitourinary and immune systems, any bleeding disorders, and results of previously performed laboratory tests (especially bleeding time, complete blood count, partial thromboplastin time, platelets, and prothrombin time), surgical procedures, and other diagnostic procedures. For related tests, refer to the Genitourinary and Immune System tables.

> Record the date of the last menstrual period and determine the possibility of pregnancy in perimenopausal women.

> Note any recent procedures that can interfere with test results.

> Obtain a list of the medications the patient is taking, including anticoagulant therapy, acetylsalicylic acid, herbs, nutritional supplements, and nutraceuticals, especially those known to affect coagulation. It is recommended that use be discontinued 14 days before dental or surgical procedures. The requesting health care practitioner and laboratory should be advised if the patient regularly uses these products so that their effects can be taken into consideration when reviewing results.

> Review the procedure with the patient. Inform patients that they may experience back pain and burning or pressure in the genital area after the procedure. Prophylactic antibiotics may be administered before the procedure in certain cases. Address concerns about pain related to the procedure. Explain to the patient that a general anesthesia will be administered prior to the biopsy. Explain to the patient that no pain will be experienced during the biopsy. Inform the patient that the biopsy is performed under sterile conditions by a health care practitioner specializing in this procedure. The procedure usually takes about 30 to 45 minutes to complete.

> *Sensitivity to cultural and social issues,* as well as concern for modesty, is important in providing psychological support before, during, and after the procedure.

> Explain that an intravenous (IV) line will be inserted to allow infusion of IV fluids, antibiotics, anesthetics, and analgesics.

> Instruct the patient that nothing should be taken by mouth for 6 to 8 hours prior to a general anesthetic.

> *Make sure a written and informed consent has been signed prior to the procedure and before administering any medications.*

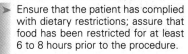
Intratest:

> Ensure that the patient has complied with dietary restrictions; assure that food has been restricted for at least 6 to 8 hours prior to the procedure.

> Ensure that anticoagulant therapy has been withheld for the appropriate amount of days prior to the procedure. Amount of days to withhold medication is dependent on the type of anticoagulant. Notify the health care practitioner if patient anticoagulant therapy has not been withheld.

> Have emergency equipment readily available.

> Have the patient void before the procedure.

> Observe standard precautions, and follow the general guidelines in Appendix A. Positively identify the patient, and label the appropriate collection containers with the corresponding patient demographics, date and time of collection, and site location.

> Assist the patient to a comfortable position, and direct the patient to breathe normally during the beginning of the general anesthetic.

> Record baseline vital signs, and continue to monitor throughout the procedure. Protocols may vary from facility to facility.

Cystoscopy:

> After administration of general anesthesia, place the patient in a lithotomy position on the examination table (with the feet up in stirrups). Drape the patient's legs. Clean the external genitalia with a suitable antiseptic solution and drape the area with sterile towels.

> Once the cystoscope is inserted, the bladder is irrigated with saline. A tissue sample is removed using a cytology brush or biopsy forceps. Catheters may be used to obtain samples from the ureter.

Open biopsy:

➤ After administration of general anesthesia and surgical prep are completed, an incision is made, suspicious areas are located, and tissue samples are collected.

General:

➤ Monitor the patient for complications related to the procedure (e.g., allergic reaction, anaphylaxis).

➤ Place tissue samples in properly labeled specimen container containing formalin solution, and promptly transport the specimen to the laboratory for processing and analysis.

➤ The results are recorded manually or in a computerized system for recall and postprocedure interpretation by the appropriate health care practitioner.

Post-test:

➤ Instruct the patient to resume preoperative diet, as directed by the health care practitioner. Assess the patient's ability to swallow before allowing the patient to attempt liquids or solid foods.

➤ Monitor vital signs and neurologic status every 15 minutes for 1 hour, then every 2 hours for 4 hours, and then as ordered by the health care practitioner. Monitor temperature every 4 hours for 24 hours. Compare with baseline values. Notify the health care practitioner if temperature is elevated. Protocols may vary from facility to facility.

➤ Monitor fluid intake and output for 24 hours. Instruct the patient on intake and output recording and provide appropriate measuring containers.

➤ Encourage fluid intake of 3000 mL in 24 hours, unless contraindicated.

➤ Observe for delayed allergic reactions, such as rash, urticaria, tachycardia, hyperpnea, hypertension, palpitations, nausea, or vomiting.

➤ Instruct the patient to immediately report pain, chills, or fever. Assess for infection, hemorrhage, or perforation of the bladder.

➤ Inform the patient that blood may be seen in the urine after the first or second postprocedural voiding.

➤ Instruct the patient to report any further changes in urinary pattern, volume, or appearance.

Open biopsy:

➤ Observe the biopsy site for bleeding, inflammation, or hematoma formation.

➤ Instruct the patient in the care and assessment of the site. Instruct the patient to report any redness, edema, bleeding, or pain at the biopsy site. Instruct the patient to keep the site clean and change the dressing as needed.

General:

➤ Assess for nausea, pain, and bladder spasms. Administer antiemetic, analgesic, and antispasmodic medications as needed and as directed by the health care practitioner.

➤ Administer antibiotic therapy if ordered. Remind the patient of the importance of completing the entire course of antibiotic therapy, even if signs and symptoms disappear before completion of therapy.

➤ A written report of the examination will be completed by a health care practitioner specializing in this branch of medicine. The report will be sent to the requesting health care practitioner, who will discuss the results with the patient.

➤ Recognize anxiety related to test results. Discuss the implications of abnormal test results on the patient's lifestyle. Provide teaching and information regarding the clinical implications of the test results, as appropriate. Educate the patient regarding access to counseling services.

➤ Reinforce information given by the patient's health care provider regarding further testing, treatment, or referral to another health care provider. Answer any questions or address any concerns voiced by the patient or family.

Instruct the patient in the use of any ordered medications. Explain the importance of adhering to the therapy regimen. As appropriate, instruct the patient in significant side effects and systemic reactions associated with the prescribed medication. Encourage him or her to review corresponding literature provided by a pharmacist.

Depending on the results of this procedure, additional testing may be performed to evaluate or monitor progression of the disease process and determine the need for a change in therapy. Evaluate test results in relation to the patient's symptoms and other tests performed.

Related laboratory tests:

Related laboratory tests include routine urinalysis and urine bladder cancer test.

BIOPSY, BONE

SYNONYM/ACRONYM: N/A.

SPECIMEN: Bone tissue.

REFERENCE VALUE: (Method: Microscopic study of bone samples) No abnormal tissue or cells.

DESCRIPTION & RATIONALE: Biopsy is the excision of a sample of tissue that can be analyzed microscopically to determine cell morphology and the presence of tissue abnormalities. This test is used to assist in confirming the diagnosis of cancer when clinical symptoms or x-rays are suspicious. After surgical incision to reveal the affected area, bone biopsy is obtained. An alternative collection method is needle biopsy, in which a plug of bone is removed using a special serrated needle. ∎

INDICATIONS:
- Differentiation of a benign from a malignant bone lesion
- Radiographic evidence of a bone lesion

RESULT

Abnormal findings in:
- Ewing's sarcoma
- Multiple myeloma
- Osteoma
- Osteosarcoma

CRITICAL VALUES: N/A

INTERFERING FACTORS:
- ⚠ This procedure is contraindicated in patients with bleeding disorders.
- Failure to follow dietary restrictions before the procedure may cause the procedure to be canceled or repeated.

Nursing Implications and Procedure • • • • • • • • • •

➤ Inform the patient that the test is used to establish a histologic diagnosis of bone disease.

➤ Obtain a history of the patient's complaints, including a list of known allergens (especially allergies or sensitivities to latex or anesthetics), and inform the appropriate health care practitioner accordingly.

➤ Obtain a history of the patient's immune and musculoskeletal systems, any bleeding disorders, and results of previously performed laboratory tests (especially complete bleeding time, complete blood count, partial thromboplastin time, platelets, and prothrombin time), surgical procedures, and other diagnostic procedures. For related laboratory tests, refer to the Immune and Musculoskeletal System tables.

➤ Record the date of the last menstrual period and determine the possibility of pregnancy in perimenopausal women.

➤ Note any recent procedures that can interfere with test results.

➤ Obtain a list of the medications the patient is taking, including anticoagulant therapy, acetylsalicylic acid, herbs, nutritional supplements, and nutraceuticals, especially those known to affect coagulation. It is recommended that use be discontinued 14 days before dental or surgical procedures. The requesting health care practitioner and laboratory should be advised if the patient regularly uses these products so that their effects can be taken into consideration when reviewing results.

➤ Review the procedure with the patient. Inform the patient that it may be necessary to shave the site before the procedure. Address concerns about pain related to the procedure. Explain that a sedative and/or analgesia will be administered to promote relaxation and reduce discomfort prior to the percutaneous biopsy; a general anesthesia will be administered prior to the open biopsy. Explain to the patient that no pain will be experienced during the test when general anesthesia is used, but that any discomfort with a needle biopsy will be minimized with local anesthetics and systemic analgesics. Inform the patient that the biopsy is performed under sterile conditions by a health care practitioner specializing in this procedure. The surgical procedure usually takes about 30 minutes to complete, and sutures may be necessary to close the site. A needle biopsy usually takes about 20 minutes to complete.

➤ *Sensitivity to cultural and social issues,* as well as concern for modesty, is important in providing psychological support before, during, and after the procedure.

➤ Explain that an intravenous (IV) line will be inserted to allow infusion of IV fluids, anesthetics, analgesics, or IV sedation.

Open biopsy:

➤ Instruct the patient that nothing should be taken by mouth for 6 to 8 hours prior to a general anesthetic.

Needle biopsy:

➤ Instruct the patient that nothing should be taken by mouth for at least 4 hours prior to the procedure to reduce the risk of nausea and vomiting.

General:

➤ *Make sure a written and informed consent has been signed prior to the procedure and before administering any medications.*

➤ Ensure that the patient has complied with dietary restrictions; assure that food has been restricted for at least 4 to 8 hours depending on the anesthetic chosen for the procedure.

Ensure that anticoagulant therapy has been withheld for the appropriate amount of days prior to the procedure. Amount of days to withhold medication is dependent on the type of anticoagulant. Notify the health care practitioner if patient anticoagulant therapy has not been withheld.

Have emergency equipment readily available.

Have the patient void before the procedure.

Observe standard precautions, and follow the general guidelines in Appendix A. Positively identify the patient, and label the appropriate collection containers with the corresponding patient demographics, date and time of collection, and site location.

Assist the patient to the desired position depending on the test site to be used, and direct the patient to breathe normally during the beginning of the general anesthetic. Instruct the patient to cooperate fully and to follow directions. Direct the patient to breathe normally and to avoid unnecessary movement during the local anesthetic and the procedure.

Record baseline vital signs, and continue to monitor throughout the procedure. Protocols may vary from facility to facility.

After the administration of general or local anesthesia, shave and cleanse the site with an antiseptic solution, and drape the area with sterile towels.

Open biopsy:

After administration of general anesthesia and surgical prep are completed, an incision is made, suspicious area(s) are located, and tissue samples are collected.

Needle biopsy:

Instruct the patient to take slow deep breaths when the local anesthetic is injected. Protect the site with sterile drapes. A small incision is made and the biopsy needle is inserted to remove the specimen. Pressure is applied to the site for 3 to 5 minutes, then a sterile pressure dressing is applied.

General:

Monitor the patient for complications related to the procedure (e.g., allergic reaction, anaphylaxis).

Place tissue samples in properly labeled specimen container containing formalin solution, and promptly transport the specimen to the laboratory for processing and analysis.

The results are recorded manually or in a computerized system for recall and postprocedure interpretation by the appropriate health care practitioner.

Post-test:

Instruct the patient to resume preoperative diet, as directed by the health care practitioner. Assess the patient's ability to swallow before allowing the patient to attempt liquids or solid foods.

Monitor vital signs and neurologic status every 15 minutes for 1 hour, then every 2 hours for 4 hours, and then as ordered by the health care practitioner. Monitor temperature every 4 hours for 24 hours. Compare with baseline values. Notify the health care practitioner if temperature is elevated. Protocols may vary from facility to facility.

Observe for delayed allergic reactions, such as rash, urticaria, tachycardia, hyperpnea, hypertension, palpitations, nausea, or vomiting.

Observe the biopsy site for bleeding, inflammation, or hematoma formation.

Instruct the patient in the care and assessment of the site. Instruct the patient to report any redness, edema, bleeding, or pain at the biopsy site. Instruct the patient to immediately report chills or fever. Instruct the patient to keep the site clean and change the dressing as needed.

➤ Assess for nausea and pain. Administer antiemetic and analgesic medications as needed and as directed by the health care practitioner.

➤ Administer antibiotic therapy if ordered. Remind the patient of the importance of completing the entire course of antibiotic therapy, even if signs and symptoms disappear before completion of therapy.

➤ A written report of the examination will be completed by a health care practitioner specializing in this branch of medicine. The report will be sent to the requesting health care practitioner, who will discuss the results with the patient.

➤ Recognize anxiety related to test results. Discuss the implications of abnormal test results on the patient's lifestyle. Provide teaching and information regarding the clinical implications of the test results, as appropriate. Educate the patient regarding access to counseling services.

➤ Reinforce information given by the patient's health care provider regarding further testing, treatment, or referral to another health care provider. Inform the patient of a follow-up appointment for removal of sutures, if indicated. Answer any questions or address any concerns voiced by the patient or family.

➤ Instruct the patient in the use of any ordered medications. Explain the importance of adhering to the therapy regimen. As appropriate, instruct the patient in significant side effects and systemic reactions associated with the prescribed medication. Encourage him or her to review corresponding literature provided by a pharmacist.

➤ Depending on the results of this procedure, additional testing may be performed to evaluate or monitor progression of the disease process and determine the need for a change in therapy. Evaluate test results in relation to the patient's symptoms and other tests performed.

Related laboratory tests:

➤ Related laboratory tests include alkaline phosphatase; bone marrow biopsy; calcium and urine calcium; complete blood count; cortisol; immunofixation electrophoresis; immunoglobulins A, G, and M; β_2-microglobulin; parathyroid hormone; phosphorus; urine and serum protein electrophoresis; urine and serum total protein; urinalysis; and vitamin D.

BIOPSY, BONE MARROW

SYNONYM/ACRONYM: N/A.

SPECIMEN: Bone marrow aspirate, bone core biopsy, marrow and peripheral smears.

REFERENCE VALUE: (Method: Microscopic study of bone and bone marrow samples, flow cytometry) Reference ranges are subject to many variables, and therefore the laboratory should be consulted for their specific interpretation. Some generalities may be commented on regarding findings as follows:

- Ratio of marrow fat to cellular elements is related to age, with the amount of fat increasing with increasing age.

- Normal cellularity, cellular distribution, presence of megakaryocytes, and absence of fibrosis or tumor cells.

- The myeloid-to-erythrocyte ratio (M:E) is 2:1 to 4:1 in adults. It may be slightly higher in children.

Differential Parameter	Conventional Units
Erythrocyte precursors	18–32%
Myeloblasts	0–2%
Promyelocytes	2–6%
Myelocytes	9–17%
Metamyelocytes	7–25%
Bands	10–16%
Neutrophils	18–28%
Eosinophils and precursors	1–5%
Basophils and precursors	0–1%
Monocytes and precursors	1–5%
Lymphocytes	9–19%
Plasma cells	0–1%

DESCRIPTION & RATIONALE: This test involves the removal of a small sample of bone marrow by aspiration, needle biopsy, or open surgical biopsy for a complete hematologic analysis. The marrow is a suspension of blood, fat, and developing blood cells, which is evaluated for morphology and examined for all stages of maturation; iron stores; and M:E. Sudan black B and periodic acid–Schiff (PAS) stains can be performed for microscopic examination to differentiate the types of leukemia, although flow cytometry and cytogenetics have become more commonly used techniques for this purpose. ∎

INDICATIONS:
- Determine marrow differential (proportion of the various types of cells present in the marrow) and M:E

- Evaluate abnormal results of complete blood count or white blood cell count with differential showing increased numbers of leukocyte precursors

- Evaluate hepatomegaly or splenomegaly

- Identify bone marrow hyperplasia or hypoplasia

- Monitor effects of exposure to bone marrow depressants

- Monitor bone marrow response to chemotherapy or radiation therapy

RESULT

Increased reticulocytes:
- Compensated red blood cell (RBC) loss
- Response to vitamin B_{12} therapy

Decreased reticulocytes:
- Aplastic crisis of sickle cell anemia or hereditary spherocytosis

Increased neutrophils (total):
- Acute myeloblastic leukemia
- Myeloid (chronic) leukemias

Decreased neutrophils (total):

• Aplastic anemia
• Leukemias (monocytic and lymphoblastic)

Increased lymphocytes:

• Aplastic anemia
• Lymphatic leukemia
• Lymphomas
• Lymphosarcoma
• Mononucleosis
• Viral infections

Increased plasma cells:

• Cancer
• Cirrhosis of the liver
• Connective tissue disorders
• Hypersensitivity reactions
• Infections
• Macroglobulinemia
• Ulcerative colitis

Increased megakaryocytes:

• Hemorrhage
• Increasing age
• Infections
• Megakaryocytic myelosis
• Myeloid leukemia
• Pneumonia
• Polycythemia vera
• Thrombocytopenia

Decreased megakaryocytes:

• Agranulocytosis
• Cirrhosis of the liver
• Pernicious aplastic anemia
• Radiation therapy
• Thrombocytopenic purpura

Increased M:E:

• Bone marrow failure
• Infections
• Leukemoid reactions
• Myeloid leukemia

Decreased M:E:

• Anemias
• Hepatic disease
• Polycythemia vera
• Posthemorrhagic hematopoiesis

Increased normoblasts:

• Anemias
• Chronic blood loss
• Polycythemia vera

Decreased normoblasts:

• Aplastic anemia
• Folic acid or vitamin B_{12} deficiency
• Hemolytic anemia

Increased eosinophils:

• Bone marrow cancer
• Lymphadenoma
• Myeloid leukemia

CRITICAL VALUES: N/A

INTERFERING FACTORS:
• Recent blood transfusions, iron therapy, or administration of cytotoxic agents may alter test results.

• ⚠ This procedure is contraindicated in patients with known bleeding disorders.

• Failure to follow dietary restrictions before the procedure may cause the procedure to be canceled or repeated.

Nursing Implications and Procedure • • • • • • • • • • •

➤ Inform the patient that the test is used to establish a histologic diagnosis of bone marrow and immune system disease.

➤ Obtain a history of the patient's complaints, including a list of known allergens (especially allergies or sensitivities to latex or anesthetics), and inform the appropriate health care practitioner accordingly.

➤ Obtain a history of the patient's hematopoietic and immune systems, any bleeding disorders, and results of previously performed laboratory tests (especially bleeding time, complete blood count, partial thromboplastin time, platelets, and prothrombin time), surgical procedures, and other diagnostic procedures. For related laboratory tests, refer to the Hematopoietic and Immune System tables.

➤ Record the date of the last menstrual period and determine the possibility of pregnancy in perimenopausal women.

➤ Note any recent procedures that can interfere with test results.

➤ Obtain a list of the medications the patient is taking, including anticoagulant therapy, acetylsalicylic acid, herbs, nutritional supplements, and nutraceuticals, especially those known to affect coagulation. It is recommended that use be discontinued 14 days before dental or surgical procedures. The requesting health care practitioner and laboratory should be advised if the patient regularly uses these products so that their effects can be taken into consideration when reviewing results.

➤ Review the procedure with the patient. Inform the patient that it may be necessary to shave the site before the procedure. Address concerns about pain related to the pro-

cedure. Explain that a sedative and/or analgesia will be administered to promote relaxation and reduce discomfort prior to the percutaneous biopsy; a general anesthesia will be administered prior to the open biopsy. Explain to the patient that no pain will be experienced during the test when general anesthesia is used, but that any discomfort with a needle biopsy will be minimized with local anesthetics and systemic analgesics. Inform the patient that the biopsy is performed under sterile conditions by a health care practitioner specializing in this procedure. The surgical procedure usually takes about 30 minutes to complete, and sutures may be necessary to close the site. A needle biopsy usually takes about 20 minutes to complete.

➤ *Sensitivity to cultural and social issues,* as well as concern for modesty, is important in providing psychological support before, during, and after the procedure.

➤ Explain that an intravenous (IV) line may be inserted to allow infusion of IV fluids, anesthetics, or sedatives.

➤ Instruct the patient that nothing should be taken by mouth for at least 4 hours prior to the procedure to reduce the risk of nausea and vomiting.

➤ *Make sure a written and informed consent has been signed prior to the procedure and before administering any medications.*

➤ Ensure that the patient has complied with dietary restrictions; assure that food has been restricted for at least 4 to 8 hours depending on the anesthetic chosen for the procedure.

➤ Ensure that anticoagulant therapy has been withheld for the appropriate amount of days prior to the procedure. Amount of days to withhold medication is dependent on the type of anticoagulant. Notify the health care practitioner if patient anticoagulant therapy has not been withheld.

➤ Have emergency equipment readily available.

➤ Have the patient void before the procedure.

➤ Observe standard precautions, and follow the general guidelines in Appendix A.

➤ Positively identify the patient, and label the appropriate collection containers with the corresponding patient demographics, date and time of collection, and site location.

➤ Assist the patient to the desired position depending on the test site to be used. In young children, the most frequently chosen site is the proximal tibia. Vertebral bodies T10 through L4 are preferred in older children. In adults, the sternum or iliac crests are the preferred sites. Place the patient in the prone, sitting, or side-lying position for the vertebral bodies; the side-lying position for iliac crest or tibial sites; or the supine position for the sternum. Instruct the patient to cooperate fully and to follow directions. Direct the patient to breathe normally and to avoid unnecessary movement during the local anesthetic and the procedure.

➤ Record baseline vital signs, and continue to monitor throughout the procedure. Protocols may vary from facility to facility.

➤ After the administration of general or local anesthesia, shave and cleanse the site with an antiseptic solution, and drape the area with sterile towels.

Needle aspiration:

➤ The health care practitioner will anesthetize the site with procaine or lidocaine, and then insert a needle with stylet into the marrow. The stylet is removed, a syringe attached, and a 0.5-mL aliquot of marrow withdrawn. The needle is removed, and pressure is applied to the site. The aspirate is applied to slides, and, when dry, a fixative is applied.

Needle biopsy:

➤ Instruct the patient to take slow deep breaths when the local anesthetic is injected. Protect the site with sterile drapes.

➤ Local anesthetic is introduced deeply enough to include periosteum. A cutting biopsy needle is introduced through a small skin incision and bored into the marrow cavity. A core needle is introduced through the cutting needle, and a plug of marrow is removed. The needles are withdrawn, and the specimen is placed in a preservative solution. Pressure is applied to the site for 3 to 5 minutes, and then a pressure dressing is applied.

General:

➤ Monitor the patient for complications related to the procedure (e.g., allergic reaction, anaphylaxis).

➤ Place tissue samples in properly labeled specimen container containing formalin solution, and promptly transport the specimen to the laboratory for processing and analysis.

➤ The results are recorded manually or in a computerized system for recall and postprocedure interpretation by the appropriate health care practitioner

Post-test:

➤ Instruct the patient to resume preoperative diet, as directed by the health care practitioner.

➤ Monitor vital signs and neurologic status every 15 minutes for 1 hour, then every 2 hours for 4 hours, and then as ordered by the health care practitioner. Monitor temperature every 4 hours for 24 hours. Compare with baseline values. Notify the health care practitioner if temperature is elevated. Protocols may vary from facility to facility.

➤ Observe for delayed allergic reactions, such as rash, urticaria, tachycardia, hyperpnea, hypertension, palpitations, nausea, or vomiting.

➤ Observe the biopsy site for bleeding, inflammation, or hematoma formation.

➤ Instruct the patient in the care and assessment of the site. Instruct the patient to report any redness, edema, bleeding, or pain at the biopsy site. Instruct the patient to immediately report chills or fever. Instruct the patient to keep the site clean and change the dressing as needed.

➤ Assess for nausea and pain. Administer antiemetic and analgesic medications as needed and as directed by the health care practitioner.

➤ Administer antibiotic therapy if ordered. Remind the patient of the importance of completing the entire course of antibiotic therapy, even if signs and symptoms disappear before completion of therapy.

➤ A written report of the examination will be completed by a health care practitioner specializing in this branch of medicine. The report will be sent to the requesting health care practitioner, who will discuss the results with the patient.

➤ Recognize anxiety related to test results. Discuss the implications of abnormal test results on the patient's lifestyle. Provide teaching and information regarding the clinical implications of the test results, as appropriate. Educate the patient regarding access to counseling services.

➤ Reinforce information given by the patient's health care provider regarding further testing, treatment, or referral to another health care provider. Inform the patient of a follow-up appointment for removal of sutures, if indicated. Answer any questions or address any concerns voiced by the patient or family.

➤ Instruct the patient in the use of any ordered medications. Explain the importance of adhering to the therapy regimen. As appropriate, instruct the patient in significant side effects and systemic reactions associated with the prescribed medication. Encourage him or her to review corresponding literature provided by a pharmacist.

➤ Depending on the results of this procedure, additional testing may be performed to evaluate or monitor progression of the disease process and determine the need for a change in therapy. Evaluate test results in relation to the patient's symptoms and other tests performed.

Related laboratory tests:

➤ Related laboratory tests include complete blood count, leukocyte alkaline phosphatase, lymph node biopsy, serum immunofixation electrophoresis, urine immunofixation electrophoresis, and vitamin B_{12}.

BIOSY, BREAST

SYNONYM/ACRONYM: N/A.

SPECIMEN: Breast tissue or cells.

REFERENCE VALUE: (Method: Macroscopic and microscopic examination of tissue) No abnormal cells or tissue.

DESCRIPTION & RATIONALE: Biopsy is the excision of a sample of tissue that can be analyzed microscopically to determine cell morphology and the presence of tissue abnormalities. Fine needle and open biopsies of the breast have become more commonly ordered in recent years as increasing emphasis on early detection of breast cancer has become stronger. Breast biopsies are used to assist in the identification and prognosis of breast cancer. ■

INDICATIONS:

• Evidence of breast lesion by palpation, mammography, or ultrasound

• Observable breast changes such as "peau d'orange" skin, scaly skin of the areola, drainage from the nipple, or ulceration of the skin

RESULT: Positive findings in carcinoma of the breast.

CRITICAL VALUES: N/A

INTERFERING FACTORS:

• ⚠ This procedure is contraindicated in patients with bleeding disorders.

• Failure to follow dietary restrictions before the procedure may cause the procedure to be canceled or repeated.

Nursing Implications and Procedure • • • • • • • • • • • •

Pretest:

➤ Inform the patient that the test is used to establish a histologic diagnosis of breast disease.

➤ Obtain a history of the patient's complaints, including a list of known allergens (especially allergies or sensitivities to latex or anesthetics), and inform the appropriate health care practitioner accordingly.

➤ Obtain a history of the patient's immune and reproductive systems,

any bleeding disorders, and results of previously performed laboratory tests (especially bleeding time, complete blood count, partial thromboplastin time, platelets, and prothrombin time), surgical procedures, and other diagnostic procedures. For related laboratory tests, refer to the Immune and Reproductive System tables.

➤ Record the date of the last menstrual period and determine the possibility of pregnancy in perimenopausal women.

➤ Note any recent procedures that can interfere with test results.

➤ Obtain a list of the medications the patient is taking, including anticoagulant therapy, acetylsalicylic acid, herbs, nutritional supplements, and nutraceuticals, especially those known to affect coagulation. It is recommended that use be discontinued 14 days before dental or surgical procedures. The requesting health care practitioner and laboratory should be advised if the patient regularly uses these products so that their effects can be taken into consideration when reviewing results.

➤ Review the procedure with the patient. Inform the patient that it may be necessary to shave the site before the procedure. Instruct that prophylactic antibiotics may be administered prior to the procedure. Address concerns about pain related to the procedure. Explain that a sedative and/or analgesia will be administered to promote relaxation and reduce discomfort prior to the percutaneous biopsy; a general anesthesia will be administered prior to the open biopsy. Explain to the patient that no pain will be experienced during the test when general anesthesia is used, but that any discomfort with a needle biopsy will be minimized with local anesthetics and systemic analgesics. Inform the patient that the biopsy is performed under sterile conditions by a health care practitioner specializing in this procedure. The surgical procedure usually takes about 20 to 30 minutes to complete, and sutures may be necessary to close the site. A needle biopsy usually takes about 15 minutes to complete.

▶ *Sensitivity to cultural and social issues,* as well as concern for modesty, is important in providing psychological support before, during, and after the procedure.

▶ Explain that an intravenous (IV) line may be inserted to allow infusion of IV fluids, anesthetics, analgesics, or IV sedation.

Open biopsy:

▶ Instruct the patient that nothing should be taken by mouth for 6 to 8 hours prior to a general anesthetic.

Needle biopsy:

▶ Instruct the patient that nothing should be taken by mouth for at least 4 hours prior to the procedure to reduce the risk of nausea and vomiting.

General:

▶ *Make sure a written and informed consent has been signed prior to the procedure and before administering any medications.*

Intratest:

▶ Ensure that the patient has complied with dietary restrictions; assure that food has been restricted for at least 4 to 8 hours depending on the anesthetic chosen for the procedure.

▶ Ensure that anticoagulant therapy has been withheld for the appropriate amount of days prior to the procedure. Amount of days to withhold medication is dependent on the type of anticoagulant. Notify the health care practitioner if patient anticoagulant therapy has not been withheld.

▶ Have emergency equipment readily available.

▶ Have the patient void before the procedure.

▶ Observe standard precautions, and follow the general guidelines in Appendix A. Positively identify the patient and label the appropriate collection containers with the corresponding patient demographics, date and time of collection, and site location, especially left or right breast.

▶ Assist the patient to the desired position depending on the test site to be used, and direct the patient to breathe normally during the beginning of the general anesthesic. Instruct the patient to cooperate fully and to follow directions. Direct the patient to breathe normally and to avoid unnecessary movement during the local anesthetic and the procedure.

▶ Record baseline vital signs, and continue to monitor throughout the procedure. Protocols may vary from facility to facility.

▶ After the administration of general or local anesthesia, shave and cleanse the site with an antiseptic solution, and drape the area with sterile towels.

Open biopsy:

▶ After administration of general anesthesia and surgical prep are completed, an incision is made, suspicious area(s) are located, and tissue samples are collected.

Needle biopsy:

▶ Direct the patient to take slow deep breaths when the local anesthetic is injected. Protect the site with sterile drapes. Instruct the patient to take a deep breath, exhale forcefully, and hold the breath while the biopsy needle is inserted and rotated to obtain a core of breast tissue. Once the needle is removed, the patient may breathe. Pressure is applied to the site for 3 to 5 minutes, then a sterile pressure dressing is applied.

General:

▶ Monitor the patient for complications related to the procedure (e.g., allergic reaction, anaphylaxis).

▶ Place tissue samples in formalin solution. Label the specimen, indicating site location, and promptly transport the specimen to the laboratory for processing and analysis.

➤ The results are recorded manually or in a computerized system for recall and postprocedure interpretation by the appropriate health care practitioner

Post-test:

➤ Instruct the patient to resume preoperative diet, as directed by the health care practitioner. Assess the patient's ability to swallow before allowing the patient to attempt liquids or solid foods.

➤ Monitor vital signs and neurologic status every 15 minutes for 1 hour, then every 2 hours for 4 hours, and then as ordered by the health care practitioner. Monitor temperature every 4 hours for 24 hours. Compare with baseline values. Notify the health care practitioner if temperature is elevated. Protocols may vary from facility to facility.

➤ Observe for delayed allergic reactions, such as rash, urticaria, tachycardia, hyperpnea, hypertension, palpitations, nausea, or vomiting.

➤ Observe the biopsy site for bleeding, inflammation, or hematoma formation.

➤ Instruct the patient in the care and assessment of the site. Instruct the patient to report any redness, edema, bleeding, or pain at the biopsy site. Instruct the patient to immediately report chills or fever. Instruct the patient to keep the site clean and change the dressing as needed.

➤ Assess for nausea and pain. Administer antiemetic and analgesic medications as needed and as directed by the health care practitioner.

➤ Administer antibiotic therapy if ordered. Remind the patient of the importance of completing the entire course of antibiotic therapy, even if signs and symptoms disappear before completion of therapy.

➤ A written report of the examination will be completed by a health care practitioner specializing in this branch of medicine. The report will be sent to the requesting health care practitioner, who will discuss the results with the patient.

➤ Recognize anxiety related to test results. Discuss the implications of abnormal test results on the patient's lifestyle. Provide teaching and information regarding the clinical implications of the test results, as appropriate. Educate the patient regarding access to counseling services.

➤ Reinforce information given by the patient's health care provider regarding further testing, treatment, or referral to another health care provider. Inform the patient of a follow-up appointment for removal of sutures, if indicated. Instruct and educate the patient how to perform monthly breast self-examination and emphasize, as appropriate, the importance of having a mammogram performed annually. Answer any questions or address any concerns voiced by the patient or family.

➤ Instruct the patient in the use of any ordered medications. Explain the importance of adhering to the therapy regimen. As appropriate, instruct the patient in significant side effects and systemic reactions associated with the prescribed medication. Encourage the patient to review corresponding literature provided by a pharmacist.

➤ Depending on the results of this procedure, additional testing may be performed to evaluate or monitor progression of the disease process and determine the need for a change in therapy. Evaluate test results in relation to the patient's symptoms and other tests performed.

Related laboratory tests:

➤ Related laboratory tests include cancer antigen 15-3, carcinoembryonic antigen, estrogen receptors, HER-2/neu oncoprotein, and progesterone receptors.

BIOPSY, CERVICAL

SYNONYM/ACRONYM: Cone Biopsy, LEEP.

SPECIMEN: Cervical tissue.

REFERENCE VALUE: (Method: Microscopic examination of tissue cells) No abnormal cells or tissue.

DESCRIPTION & RATIONALE: Biopsy is the excision of a sample of tissue that can be analyzed microscopically to determine cell morphology and the presence of tissue abnormalities. The cervical biopsy is used to assist in confirmation of cancer when screening tests are positive. Cervical biopsy is obtained using an instrument that punches into the tissue and retrieves a tissue sample. Schiller's test entails applying an iodine solution to the cervix. Normal cells pick up the iodine and stain brown. Abnormal cells do not pick up any color. Punch biopsy results may indicate the need for a cone biopsy of the cervix. Cone biopsy is where a wedge shape of tissue is removed from the cervix by using a loop electrosurgical excision procedure (LEEP). The LEEP procedure can be performed by placing the patient under a general anesthetic; by a regional anesthesia, such as a spinal or epidural; or by a cervical block, where a local anesthetic is injected into the cervix. The patient is given oral or intravenous (IV) pain medicine in conjunction with the local anesthetic when this method is used. ■

INDICATIONS:
• Follow-up to abnormal Papanicolaou (Pap) smear, Schiller's test, or colposcopy

• Suspected cervical malignancy

RESULT

Positive findings in:
• Carcinoma in situ

• Cervical dysplasia

• Cervical polyps

CRITICAL VALUES: N/A

INTERFERING FACTORS:
• ⚠ The test is contraindicated in cases of acute pelvic inflammatory disease or bleeding disorders.

• This test should not be performed while the patient is menstruating.

• Failure to follow dietary restrictions before the procedure may cause the procedure to be canceled or repeated.

Nursing Implications and Procedure • • • • • • • • • •

➤ Inform the patient that the test is used to establish a histologic diagnosis of cervical disease.

➤ Obtain a history of the patient's complaints, including a list of known allergens (especially allergies or sensitivities to latex or anesthetics), and inform the appropriate health care practitioner accordingly.

➤ Obtain a history of the patient's immune and reproductive systems, any bleeding disorders, and results of previously performed laboratory tests (especially bleeding time, complete blood count, partial thromboplastin time, platelets, and prothrombin time), surgical procedures, and other diagnostic procedures. For related laboratory tests, refer to the Immune and Reproductive System tables.

➤ Record the date of the last menstrual period and determine the possibility of pregnancy in perimenopausal women.

➤ Obtain a list of the medications the patient is taking, including anticoagulant therapy, acetylsalicylic acid, herbs, nutritional supplements, and nutraceuticals, especially those known to affect coagulation. It is recommended that use be discontinued 14 days before dental or surgical procedures. The requesting health care practitioner and laboratory should be advised if the patient regularly uses these products so that their effects can be taken into consideration when reviewing results.

➤ Review the procedure with the patient. Inform the patient that it may be necessary to shave the site before the procedure. Instruct that prophylactic antibiotics may be administered prior to the procedure. Address concerns about pain related to the procedure. Explain that a sedative and/or analgesia will be administered to promote relaxation and reduce discomfort prior to the percutaneous biopsy; a general anesthesia will be administered prior to the open biopsy. Explain to the patient that no pain will be experienced during the test when general anesthesia is used, but that any discomfort with a needle biopsy will be minimized with local anesthetics and systemic analgesics. Inform the patient that the biopsy is performed under sterile conditions by a health care practitioner specializing in this procedure. The surgical procedure usually takes about 20 to 30 minutes to complete, and sutures may be necessary to close the site.

➤ *Sensitivity to cultural and social issues, as well as concern for modesty, is important in providing psychological support before, during, and after the procedure.*

➤ Explain that an IV line may be inserted to allow infusion of IV fluids, anesthetics, analgesics, or IV sedation.

LEEP as an outpatient procedure:

➤ Instruct the patient that nothing should be taken by mouth for at least 6 to 8 hours prior to a general anesthetic.

LEEP in health care practitioner's office:

➤ Instruct the patient that nothing should be taken by mouth for at least 4 hours prior to the procedure to reduce the risk of nausea and vomiting.

General:

➤ *Make sure a written and informed consent has been signed prior to the procedure and before administering any medications.*

➤ Ensure that the patient has complied with dietary restrictions; assure that food has been restricted for at least

4 to 8 hours depending on the anesthetic chosen for the procedure.

➤ Ensure that anticoagulant therapy has been withheld for the appropriate amount of days prior to the procedure. Amount of days to withhold medication is dependent on the type of anticoagulant. Notify health care practitioner if patient anticoagulant therapy has not been withheld.

➤ Have emergency equipment readily available.

➤ Have the patient void before the procedure.

➤ Observe standard precautions, and follow the general guidelines in Appendix A. Positively identify the patient and label the appropriate collection containers with the corresponding patient demographics, date and time of collection, and site location.

➤ Have the patient remove clothes below the waist. Assist the patient into a lithotomy position on a gynecologic exam table (with feet in stirrups). Drape the patient's legs. Instruct the patient to cooperate fully and to follow directions. Direct the patient to breathe normally and to avoid unnecessary movement during the local or general anesthetic and the procedure.

➤ Punch biopsy: A small round punch is rotated into the skin to the desired depth. The cylinder of skin is pulled upward with forceps and separated at its base with a scalpel or scissors. If needed, sutures are applied. A sterile dressing is applied over the site.

➤ Record baseline vital signs, and continue to monitor throughout the procedure. Protocols may vary from facility to facility.

➤ After the administration of general or local anesthesia, shave and cleanse the site with an antiseptic solution, and drape the area with sterile towels.

LEEP in the health care practitioner's office:

➤ A speculum is inserted into the vagina and is opened to gently spread apart the vagina for inspection of the cervix.

➤ The diseased tissue is removed along with a small amount of healthy tissue along the margins of the biopsy to ensure that no diseased tissue is left in the cervix after the procedure.

LEEP as an outpatient procedure:

➤ After administration of general anesthesia and surgical prep are completed, the procedure is carried out as noted above.

General:

➤ Monitor the patient for complications related to the procedure (e.g., allergic reaction, anaphylaxis).

➤ Place tissue samples in properly labeled specimen container containing formalin solution, and promptly transport the specimen to the laboratory for processing and analysis.

➤ The results are recorded manually or in a computerized system for recall and postprocedure interpretation by the appropriate health care practitioner.

Post-test:

➤ Instruct the patient to resume preoperative diet, as directed by the health care practitioner. Assess the patient's ability to swallow before allowing the patient to attempt liquids or solid foods.

➤ Monitor vital signs and neurologic status every 15 minutes for 1 hour, then every 2 hours for 4 hours, and then as ordered by the health care practitioner. Monitor temperature every 4 hours for 24 hours. Compare with baseline values. Notify the health care practitioner if temperature is elevated. Protocols may vary from facility to facility.

➤ Observe for delayed allergic reactions, such as rash, urticaria, tachycardia, hyperpnea, hypertension, palpitations, nausea, or vomiting.

➤ Instruct the patient to expect a gray-green vaginal discharge for several days, some vaginal bleeding may occur for up to 1 week but should not be heavier than a normal menses, some pelvic pain may occur. Instruct the patient to avoid strenuous activity for 8 to 24 hours, to avoid douching or intercourse for 2 weeks or as instructed by the health care practitioner, and to report excessive bleeding, chills, fever or any other unusual findings to the health care practitioner.

➤ Assess for nausea and pain. Administer antiemetic and analgesic medications as needed and as directed by the health care practitioner.

➤ Administer antibiotic therapy if ordered. Remind the patient of the importance of completing the entire course of antibiotic therapy, even if signs and symptoms disappear before completion of therapy.

➤ A written report of the examination will be completed by a health care practitioner specializing in this branch of medicine. The report will be sent to the requesting health care practitioner, who will discuss the results with the patient.

➤ Recognize anxiety related to test results and offer support. Discuss the implications of abnormal test results on the patient's lifestyle.

➤ Provide teaching and information regarding the clinical implications of the test results, as appropriate. Educate the patient regarding access to counseling services.

➤ Reinforce information given by the patient's health care provider regarding further testing, treatment, or referral to another health care provider. Answer any questions or address any concerns voiced by the patient or family.

➤ Instruct the patient in the use of any ordered medications. Explain the importance of adhering to the therapy regimen. As appropriate, instruct the patient in significant side effects and systemic reactions associated with the prescribed medication. Encourage her to review corresponding literature provided by a pharmacist.

➤ Depending on the results of this procedure, additional testing may be performed to evaluate or monitor progression of the disease process and determine the need for a change in therapy. Evaluate test results in relation to the patient's symptoms and other tests performed.

Related laboratory tests:

➤ A related laboratory test is the Pap smear.

BIOPSY, CHORIONIC VILLUS

SYNONYM/ACRONYM: N/A.

SPECIMEN: Chorionic villus tissue.

REFERENCE VALUE: (Method: Tissue culture) Normal karyotype.

DESCRIPTION & RATIONALE: This test is used to detect fetal abnormalities caused by numerous genetic disorders. The advantage over amniocentesis is that it can be performed as early as the 8th week of pregnancy, permitting earlier decisions regarding termination of pregnancy. However, unlike amniocentesis, this test will not detect neural tube defects. ■

INDICATIONS:

• Assist in the diagnosis of in utero metabolic disorders such as cystic fibrosis or other errors of lipid, carbohydrate, or amino acid metabolism

• Detect abnormalities in the fetus of women of advanced maternal age

• Determine fetal gender when the mother is a known carrier of a sex-linked abnormal gene that could be transmitted to male offspring, such as hemophilia or Duchenne's muscular dystrophy

• Evaluate fetus in families with a history of genetic disorders, such as Down syndrome, Tay-Sachs disease, chromosome or enzyme anomalies, or inherited hemoglobinopathies

RESULT

ABNORMAL KARYOTYPE: Numerous genetic disorders. Generally, the laboratory provides detailed interpretive information regarding the specific chromosome abnormality detected.

CRITICAL VALUES: N/A

INTERFERING FACTORS:

• ⚠ The test is contraindicated in the patient with a history of or in the presence of incompetent cervix.

• Failure to follow dietary restrictions before the procedure may cause the procedure to be canceled or repeated.

Nursing Implications and Procedure • • • • • • • • • • •

Pretest:

➤ Inform the patient that the test is used to establish a histologic diagnosis of in-utero genetic disorders.

➤ Obtain a history of the patient's complaints, including a list of known allergens (especially allergies or sensitivities to latex or anesthetics), and inform the appropriate health care practitioner accordingly.

➤ Obtain a history of the patient's reproductive system, as well as results of previously performed laboratory tests, surgical procedures, and other diagnostic procedures. Include any family history of genetic disorders such as cystic fibrosis, Duchenne's muscular dystrophy, hemophilia, sickle cell anemia, Tay-Sachs disease, thalassemia, and trisomy 21. Obtain maternal Rh type. If Rh-negative, check for prior sensitization. For related laboratory tests, refer to the Reproductive System table.

➤ Record the date of the last menstrual period and determine that the pregnancy is in the first trimester between the 10th and 12th weeks.

➤ Obtain a history of intravenous drug use, high-risk sexual activity, or occupational exposure.

➤ Obtain a list of the medications the patient is taking, including herbs, nutritional supplements, and nutraceuticals. The requesting health care practitioner and laboratory should be advised if the patient regularly uses these products so that their effects can be taken into consideration when reviewing results.

➤ Review the procedure with the patient. Warn the patient that normal results do not guarantee a normal fetus. Assure the patient that precautions to avoid injury to the fetus will be taken by localizing the fetus with ultrasound. Address concerns about pain related to the procedure. Explain that, during the transabdominal procedure, any discomfort with a needle biopsy will be minimized with local anesthetics. Explain that, during the transvaginal procedure, some cramping may be experienced as the catheter is guided through the cervix. Encourage relaxation and controlled breathing during the procedure to aid in reducing any mild discomfort. Inform the patient that specimen collection is performed by health care provider specializing in this procedure and usually takes approximately 10 to 15 minutes to complete.

➤ *Sensitivity to cultural and social issues*, as well as concern for modesty, is important in providing psychological support before, during, and after the procedure.

➤ There are no food, fluid, or medication restrictions unless by medical direction.

➤ Have the patient drink a glass of water about 30 minutes prior to testing so that the bladder is full. This elevates the uterus higher in the pelvis. The patient should not void before the procedure.

➤ *Make sure a written and informed consent has been signed prior to the procedure and before administering any medications.*

Intratest:

➤ Ensure that the patient has a full bladder before the procedure.

➤ Have emergency equipment readily available.

➤ Observe standard precautions, and follow the general guidelines in Appendix A. Positively identify the patient, and label the appropriate collection containers with the corresponding patient demographics, date and time of collection, and site location.

➤ Have the patient remove clothes below the waist. *Transabdominal:* Assist the patient into a supine position on the exam table with abdomen exposed. Drape the patient's legs, leaving abdomen exposed. *Transvaginal:* Assist the patient into a lithotomy

position on a gynecologic examination table (with feet in stirrups). Drape the patient's legs. Instruct the patient to cooperate fully and to follow directions. Direct the patient to breathe normally and to avoid unnecessary movement during the local anesthetic and the procedure.

➤ Record maternal and fetal baseline vital signs, and continue to monitor throughout the procedure. Monitor for uterine contractions. Monitor fetal vital signs using ultrasound. Protocols may vary from facility to facility.

➤ After the administration of local anesthesia, shave and cleanse the site with an antiseptic solution, and drape the area with sterile towels.

Transabdominal biopsy:

➤ Assess the position of the amniotic fluid, fetus, and placenta using ultrasound.

➤ A needle is inserted through the abdomen into the uterus, avoiding contact with the fetus. A syringe is connected to the needle and the specimen of chorionic villus cells is withdrawn from the uteroplacental area. Pressure is applied to the site for 3 to 5 minutes, then a sterile pressure dressing is applied.

Transvaginal biopsy:

➤ Assess the position of the fetus and placenta using ultrasound.

➤ A speculum is inserted into the vagina and is opened to gently spread apart the vagina for inspection of the cervix. The cervix is cleansed with a swab of antiseptic solution.

➤ A catheter is inserted through the cervix into the uterus, avoiding contact with the fetus. A syringe is connected to the catheter and the specimen of chorionic villus cells is withdrawn from the uteroplacental area.

General:

➤ Monitor the patient for complications related to the procedure (e.g., premature labor, allergic reaction, ana-phylaxis).

➤ Place tissue samples in formalin solution. Label the specimen, indicating site location, and promptly transport the specimen to the laboratory for processing and analysis.

➤ The results are recorded manually or in a computerized system for recall and postprocedure interpretation by the appropriate health care practitioner.

Post-test:

➤ After the procedure, the patient is placed in the left side-lying position, and both maternal and fetal vital signs are monitored for at least 30 minutes. Protocols may vary from facility to facility.

➤ Observe for delayed allergic reactions, such as rash, urticaria, tachycardia, hyperpnea, hypertension, palpitations, nausea, or vomiting.

➤ Observe the biopsy site for bleeding, inflammation, or hematoma formation.

➤ Instruct the patient in the care and assessment of the site. Instruct the patient to report any redness, edema, bleeding, or pain at the biopsy site. Instruct the patient to keep the site clean and change the dressing as needed.

➤ Instruct the patient to expect mild cramping, leakage of small amount of amniotic fluid, and vaginal spotting for up to 2 days following the procedure. Instruct the patient to report moderate to severe abdominal pain or cramps, increased or prolonged leaking of amniotic fluid from vagina or abdominal needle site, vaginal bleeding that is heavier than spotting, and either chills or fever.

➤ Administer RhoGAM to maternal Rh-negative patients to prevent maternal Rh sensitization should the fetus be Rh-positive.

➤ Administer mild analgesic and antibiotic therapy as ordered. Remind the patient of the importance of completing the entire course of antibiotic therapy, even if signs and symptoms disappear before completion of therapy.

➤ A written report of the examination will be completed by a health care practitioner specializing in this branch of medicine. The report will be sent to the requesting health care practitioner, who will discuss the results with the patient.

➤ Recognize anxiety related to test results. Discuss the implications of abnormal test results on the patient's lifestyle. Provide teaching and information regarding the clinical implications of the test results, as appropriate. Encourage family to seek counseling if concerned with pregnancy termination or to seek genetic counseling if chromosomal abnormality is determined. Decisions regarding elective abortion should take place in the presence of both parents. Provide a nonjudgmental, nonthreatening atmosphere for a discussion during which risks of delivering a developmentally challenged infant are discussed with options (termination of pregnancy or adoption). It is also important to discuss problems the mother and father may experience (guilt, depression, anger) if fetal abnormalities are detected.

➤ Reinforce information given by the patient's health care provider regarding further testing, treatment, or referral to another health care provider. Answer any questions or address any concerns voiced by the patient or family.

➤ Instruct the patient in the use of any ordered medications. Explain the importance of adhering to the therapy regimen. As appropriate, instruct the patient in significant side effects and systemic reactions associated with the prescribed medication. Encourage her to review corresponding literature provided by a pharmacist.

➤ Depending on the results of this pro-

cedure, additional testing may be performed to evaluate or monitor progression of the disease process and determine the need for a change in therapy. Evaluate test results in relation to the patient's symptoms and other tests performed.

Related laboratory tests:

➤ Related laboratory tests include amniotic fluid analysis, chromosome analysis, α-fetoprotein, hexosaminidase A and B, and lecithin/sphingomyelin ratio.

BIOPSY, INTESTINAL

SYNONYM/ACRONYM: N/A.

SPECIMEN: Intestinal tissue or cells.

REFERENCE VALUE: (Method: Macroscopic and microscopic examination of tissue) No abnormal tissue or cells.

DESCRIPTION & RATIONALE: Intestinal biopsy is the excision of a tissue sample from the small intestine for microscopic analysis to determine cell morphology and the presence of tissue abnormalities. This test assists in confirming the diagnosis of cancer or intestinal disorders. Biopsy specimen is usually obtained during endoscopic examination. ▪

INDICATIONS:
• Assist in the diagnosis of various intestinal disorders, such as lactose and other enzyme deficiencies, celiac disease, and parasitic infections
• Confirm suspected intestinal malignancy
• Confirm suspicious findings during endoscopic visualization of the intestinal wall

RESULT

Abnormal findings in:
• Cancer
• Celiac disease
• Lactose deficiency
• Parasitic infestation
• Tropical sprue

CRITICAL VALUES: N/A

INTERFERING FACTORS:
• Barium swallow within 48 hours of small intestine biopsy affects results.
• ⚠ This procedure is contraindicated in patients with bleeding disorders and aortic arch aneurysm.
• Failure to follow dietary restrictions before the procedure may cause the procedure to be canceled or repeated.

Nursing Implications and Procedure • • • • • • • • • • •

➤ Inform the patient that the test is used to establish a histologic diagnosis of intestinal disease.

➤ Obtain a history of the patient's complaints, including a list of known allergens (especially allergies or sensitivities to latex or anesthetics), and inform the appropriate health care practitioner accordingly.

➤ Obtain a history of the patient's gastrointestinal and immune systems, any bleeding disorders, and results of previously performed laboratory tests (especially bleeding time, complete blood count, partial thromboplastin time, platelets, and prothrombin time), surgical procedures, and other diagnostic procedures. For related laboratory tests, refer to the Gastrointestinal and Immune System tables.

➤ Record the date of the last menstrual period and determine the possibility of pregnancy in perimenopausal women.

➤ Note any recent procedures that can interfere with test results.

➤ Obtain a list of the medications the patient is taking, including anticoagulant therapy, acetylsalicylic acid, herbs, nutritional supplements, and nutraceuticals, especially those known to affect coagulation. It is recommended that use be discontinued 14 days before dental or surgical procedures. The requesting health care practitioner and laboratory should be advised if the patient regularly uses these products so that their effects can be taken into consideration when reviewing results.

➤ Review the procedure with the patient. Address concerns about pain related to the procedure. Explain that a sedative may be administered to promote relaxation during the procedure. Inform the patient that the procedure is performed by a health care practitioner specializing in this procedure and usually takes about 60 minutes to complete.

➤ *Sensitivity to cultural and social issues, as well as concern for modesty, is important in providing psychological support before, during, and after the procedure.*

➤ Explain that an intravenous (IV) line will be inserted to allow infusion of IV fluids, anesthetics, and analgesics.

➤ Explain that a clear liquid diet is to be consumed 1 day prior to the procedure. Then food and fluids are restricted for 6 to 8 hours before the test.

➤ Patients are given a gown, robe, and foot coverings to wear and instructed to void prior to the procedure.

➤ Instruct the patient to remove dentures, jewelry (including watches), hairpins, credit cards, and other metallic objects. Inform the health care practitioner if the patient has any crowns or caps on the teeth.

➤ *Make sure a written and informed consent has been signed prior to the procedure and before administering any medications.*

➤ Ensure that the patient has complied with dietary restrictions; assure that food has been restricted for at least 6 to 8 hours prior to the procedure if general anesthesia will be used.

➤ Ensure that anticoagulant therapy has been withheld for the appropriate amount of days prior to the procedure. Amount of days to withhold medication is dependent on the type of anticoagulant. Notify the health care practitioner if patient anticoagulant therapy has not been withheld.

➤ Have emergency equipment readily available.

➤ Observe standard precautions and follow the general guidelines in Appendix A. Positively identify the patient, and label the appropriate collection containers with the corresponding patient demographics, date and time of collection, and site location.

➤ Assist the patient into a semireclining position. Instruct the patient to cooperate fully and to follow directions. Direct the patient to breathe normally and to avoid unnecessary movement.

➤ Record baseline vital signs, and continue to monitor throughout the procedure. Protocols may vary from facility to facility.

Esophagogastroduodeno-scopy (EGD) biopsy:

➤ A local anesthetic is sprayed into the throat. A protective tooth guard and a bite block may be placed in the mouth.

➤ The flexible endoscope is passed into and through the mouth, and the patient is asked to swallow. Once the endoscope passes into the esophagus, assist the patient into the left lateral position. A suction device is used to drain saliva.

➤ The esophagus, stomach, and duodenum are visually examined as the endoscope passes through each section. A biopsy specimen can be taken from any suspicious sites.

➤ Tissue samples are obtained by inserting a cytology brush or biopsy forceps through the endoscope.

➤ When the examination and tissue removal are complete, the endoscope and suction device are withdrawn and the tooth guard and bite block are removed.

➤ Monitor the patient for complications related to the procedure (e.g., allergic reaction, anaphylaxis).

➤ Place tissue samples in formalin solution. Label the specimen, indicating site location, and promptly transport the specimen to the laboratory for processing and analysis.

➤ The results are recorded manually or in a computerized system for recall and postprocedure interpretation by the appropriate health care practitioner.

Post-test:

➤ Instruct the patient to resume usual diet, as directed by the health care practitioner. Assess the patient's ability to swallow before allowing the patient to attempt liquids or solid foods.

➤ Monitor vital signs and neurologic status every 15 minutes for 1 hour, then every 2 hours for 4 hours, and then as ordered by the health care practitioner. Monitor temperature every 4 hours for 24 hours. Compare with baseline values. Notify the health care practitioner if temperature is elevated. Protocols may vary from facility to facility.

➤ Instruct the patient to report any chest pain, upper abdominal pain, pain on swallowing, difficulty breathing, or expectoration of blood. Report these to the health care practitioner immediately.

➤ Observe for delayed allergic reactions, such as rash, urticaria, tachycardia, hyperpnea, hypertension, palpitations, nausea, or vomiting.

➤ Administer mild analgesic and antibiotic therapy as ordered. Remind the patient of the importance of completing the entire course of antibiotic therapy, even if signs and symptoms disappear before completion of therapy.

➤ A written report of the examination will be completed by a health care practitioner specializing in this branch of medicine. The report will be sent to the requesting health care practitioner, who will discuss the results with the patient.

➤ Recognize anxiety related to test results. Discuss the implications of abnormal test results on the patient's lifestyle. Provide teaching and information regarding the clinical implications of the test results, as appropriate. Educate the patient regarding access to counseling services.

➤ Reinforce information given by the patient's health care provider regarding further testing, treatment, or referral to another health care provider. Answer any questions or address any concerns voiced by the patient or family.

➤ Instruct the patient in the use of any

ordered medications. Explain the importance of adhering to the therapy regimen. As appropriate, instruct the patient in significant side effects and systemic reactions associated with the prescribed medication. Encourage him or her to review corresponding literature provided by a pharmacist.

➤ Depending on the results of this procedure, additional testing may be performed to evaluate or monitor progression of the disease process and determine the need for a change in therapy. Evaluate test results in relation to the patient's symptoms and other tests performed.

Related laboratory tests:

➤ Related laboratory tests include albumin, calcium, D-xylose tolerance, fecal analysis (occult blood), fecal fat, folic acid, gliadin antibodies, iron/total iron-binding capacity, lactose tolerance, ova and parasites, potassium, prothrombin time, sodium, vitamin B_{12}, and vitamin D.

BIOPSY, KIDNEY

SYNONYM/ACRONYM: Renal biopsy.

SPECIMEN: Kidney tissue or cells.

REFERENCE VALUE: (Method: Macroscopic and microscopic examination of tissue) No abnormal cells or tissue.

DESCRIPTION & RATIONALE: Kidney or renal biopsy is the excision of a tissue sample from the kidney for microscopic analysis to determine cell morphology and the presence of tissue abnormalities. This test assists in confirming a diagnosis of cancer found on x-ray or ultrasound or to diagnose certain inflammatory or immunologic conditions. Biopsy specimen is usually obtained either percutaneously or after surgical incision. ∎

INDICATIONS:

• Assist in confirming suspected renal malignancy

• Assist in the diagnosis of the cause of renal disease

• Determine extent of involvement in systemic lupus erythematosus or other immunologic disorders

• Monitor progression of nephrotic syndrome

• Monitor renal function after transplantation

RESULT

Positive findings in:

• Acute and chronic poststreptococcal glomerulonephritis

• Amyloidosis infiltration

- Cancer

- Disseminated lupus erythematosus

- Goodpasture's syndrome

- Immunologic rejection of transplanted kidney

- Nephrotic syndrome

- Pyelonephritis

- Renal venous thrombosis

CRITICAL VALUES: N/A

INTERFERING FACTORS:

- ⚠ This procedure is contraindicated in bleeding disorders, advanced renal disease, uncontrolled hypertension, or solitary kidney (except transplanted kidney).

- Obesity and severe spinal deformity can make percutaneous biopsy impossible.

- Failure to follow dietary restrictions before the procedure may cause the procedure to be canceled or repeated.

Nursing Implications and Procedure • • • • • • • • • • •

Pretest:

▸ Inform the patient that the test is used to establish a histologic diagnosis of kidney disease.

▸ Obtain a history of the patient's complaints, including a list of known allergens (especially allergies or sensitivities to latex or anesthetics), and inform the appropriate health care practitioner accordingly.

▸ Obtain a history of the patient's genitourinary and immune system, any bleeding disorders, and results of previously performed laboratory tests (especially bleeding time, complete blood count, partial thromboplastin time, platelets, prothrombin time, blood urea nitrogen, and creatinine), surgical procedures, and other

diagnostic procedures. For related laboratory tests, refer to the Genitourinary and Immune System tables.

▸ Record the date of the last menstrual period and determine the possibility of pregnancy in perimenopausal women.

▸ Note any recent procedures that can interfere with test results.

▸ Obtain a list of the medications the patient is taking, including anticoagulant therapy, acetylsalicylic acid, herbs, nutritional supplements, and nutraceuticals, especially those known to affect coagulation. It is recommended that use be discontinued 14 days before dental or surgical procedures. The requesting health care practitioner and laboratory should be advised if the patient regularly uses these products so that their effects can be taken into consideration when reviewing results.

▸ Review the procedure with the patient. Inform the patient that it may be necessary to shave the site before the procedure. Instruct that prophylactic antibiotics may be administered prior to the procedure. Address concerns about pain related to the procedure. Explain that a sedative and/or analgesia will be administered to promote relaxation and reduce discomfort prior to the percutaneous biopsy; a general anesthesia will be administered prior to the open biopsy. Explain to the patient that no pain will be experienced during the test when general anesthesia is used, but that any discomfort with a needle biopsy will be minimized with local anesthetics and systemic analgesics. Inform the patient that the biopsy is performed under sterile conditions by a health care practitioner specializing in this procedure. The surgical procedure usually takes about 60 minutes to complete, and sutures may be necessary to close the site. A needle biopsy usually takes about 40 minutes to complete.

▸ *Sensitivity to cultural and social issues*, as well as concern for mod-

esty, is important in providing psychological support before, during, and after the procedure.

➤ Explain that an intravenous (IV) line will be inserted to allow infusion of IV fluids, anesthetics, analgesics, or IV sedation.

Open biopsy:

➤ Instruct the patient that nothing should be taken by mouth for 6 to 8 hours prior to a general anesthetic.

Needle biopsy:

➤ Instruct the patient that nothing should be taken by mouth for at least 4 hours prior to the procedure to reduce the risk of nausea and vomiting.

General:

➤ *Make sure a written and informed consent has been signed prior to the procedure and before administering any medications.*

Intratest:

➤ Ensure that the patient has complied with dietary restrictions; assure that food has been restricted for at least 4 to 8 hours depending on the anesthetic chosen for the procedure.

➤ Ensure that anticoagulant therapy has been withheld for the appropriate amount of days prior to the procedure. Amount of days to withhold medication is dependent on the type of anticoagulant. Notify the health care practitioner if patient anticoagulant therapy has not been withheld.

➤ Have emergency equipment readily available.

➤ Have the patient void before the procedure.

➤ Observe standard precautions, and follow the general guidelines in Appendix A. Positively identify the patient, and label the appropriate collection containers with the corresponding patient demographics, date and time of collection, and site location, especially left or right kidney.

➤ Assist the patient to the desired position depending on the test site to be used, and direct the patient to breathe normally during the beginning of the general anesthesic. Instruct the patient to cooperate fully and to follow directions. Direct the patient to breathe normally and to avoid unnecessary movement.

➤ Record baseline vital signs, and continue to monitor throughout the procedure. Protocols may vary from facility to facility.

➤ After the administration of general or local anesthesia, shave and cleanse the site with an antiseptic solution, and drape the area with sterile towels.

Open biopsy:

➤ After administration of general anesthesia and surgical prep are completed, an incision is made, suspicious area(s) are located, and tissue samples are collected.

Needle biopsy:

➤ A sandbag may be placed under the abdomen to aid in moving the kidneys to the desired position. Direct the patient to take slow deep breaths when the local anesthetic is injected. Protect the site with sterile drapes. Instruct the patient to take a deep breath, exhale forcefully, and hold the breath while the biopsy needle is inserted and rotated to obtain a core of renal tissue. Once the needle is removed, the patient may breathe. Pressure is applied to the site for 5 to 20 minutes, then a sterile pressure dressing is applied.

General:

➤ Monitor the patient for complications related to the procedure (e.g., allergic reaction, anaphylaxis).

➤ Place tissue samples in formalin solution. Label the specimen, indicating site location, and promptly transport the specimen to the laboratory for processing and analysis.

➤ The results are recorded manually or in a computerized system for recall

and postprocedure interpretation by the appropriate health care practitioner.

Post-test:

▶ Instruct the patient to resume preoperative diet, as directed by the health care practitioner. Assess the patient's ability to swallow before allowing the patient to attempt liquids or solid foods.

▶ Monitor vital signs and neurologic status every 15 minutes for 1 hour, then every 2 hours for 4 hours, and then as ordered by the health care practitioner. Monitor temperature every 4 hours for 24 hours. Compare with baseline values. Notify the health care practitioner if temperature is elevated. Protocols may vary from facility to facility.

▶ Observe for delayed allergic reactions, such as rash, urticaria, tachycardia, hyperpnea, hypertension, palpitations, nausea, or vomiting.

▶ Observe the biopsy site for bleeding, inflammation, or hematoma formation.

▶ Instruct the patient in the care and assessment of the site. Instruct the patient to report any redness, edema, bleeding, or pain at the biopsy site. Instruct the patient to immediately report chills or fever. Instruct the patient to keep the site clean and change the dressing as needed. Instruct the patient to immediately report symptoms such as backache, flank pain, shoulder pain, light-headedness, burning on urination, hematuria, chills, or fever, which may indicate the presence of infection, hemorrhage, or inadvertent puncture of other internal organs. Observe the patient for other signs of distress, including hypotension and tachycardia.

▶ Inform the patient that blood may be seen in the urine after the first or second postprocedural voiding.

▶ Monitor fluid intake and output for 24 hours. Instruct the patient on intake and output recording and provide appropriate measuring containers.

▶ Instruct the patient to report any changes in urinary pattern or volume or any unusual appearance of the urine. If urinary volume is less than 200 mL in the first 8 hours, encourage the patient to increase fluid intake unless contraindicated by another medical condition.

▶ Assess for nausea and pain. Administer antiemetic and analgesic medications as needed and as directed by the health care practitioner.

▶ Administer antibiotic therapy if ordered. Remind the patient of the importance of completing the entire course of antibiotic therapy, even if signs and symptoms disappear before completion of therapy.

▶ A written report of the examination will be completed by a health care practitioner specializing in this branch of medicine. The report will be sent to the requesting health care practitioner, who will discuss the results with the patient.

▶ Recognize anxiety related to test results. Discuss the implications of abnormal test results on the patient's lifestyle. Provide teaching and information regarding the clinical implications of the test results, as appropriate. Educate the patient regarding access to counseling services.

▶ Reinforce information given by the patient's health care provider regarding further testing, treatment, or referral to another health care provider. Inform the patient of a follow-up appointment for removal of sutures, if indicated. Answer any questions or address any concerns voiced by the patient or family.

▶ Instruct the patient in the use of any ordered medications. Explain the importance of adhering to the therapy regimen. As appropriate, instruct the patient in significant side effects and systemic reactions associated with the prescribed medication. Encourage him or her to review corresponding literature provided by a pharmacist.

➤ Depending on the results of this procedure, additional testing may be performed to evaluate or monitor progression of the disease process and determine the need for a change in therapy. Evaluate test results in relation to the patient's symptoms and other tests performed.

➤ Related laboratory tests include albumin, aldosterone, anti–glomerular basement membrane antibody, β_2-microglobulin, creatinine, creatinine clearance, osmolality (blood and urine), potassium (blood and urine), protein (blood and urine), renin, sodium (blood and urine), urea nitrogen, urinalysis, and urine cytology.

BIOPSY, LIVER

SYNONYM/ACRONYM: N/A.

SPECIMEN: Liver tissue or cells.

REFERENCE VALUE: (Method: Macroscopic and microscopic examination of tissue) No abnormal cells or tissue.

DESCRIPTION & RATIONALE: Liver biopsy is the excision of a tissue sample from the liver for microscopic analysis to determine cell morphology and the presence of tissue abnormalities. This test is used to assist in confirming a diagnosis of cancer or certain disorders of the hepatic parenchyma. Biopsy specimen is usually obtained either percutaneously or after surgical incision. ∎

INDICATIONS:
- Assist in confirming suspected hepatic malignancy

- Assist in confirming suspected hepatic parenchymal disease

- Assist in diagnosing the cause of persistently elevated liver enzymes, hepatomegaly, or jaundice

RESULT

Positive findings in:
- Benign tumor

- Cancer

- Cholesterol ester storage disease

- Cirrhosis

- Galactosemia

- Hemochromatosis

- Hepatic involvement with systemic lupus erythematosus, sarcoidosis, or amyloidosis

- Hepatitis

- Parasitic infestations (e.g., amebiasis, malaria, visceral larva migrans)

- Reye's syndrome

- Wilson's disease

CRITICAL VALUES: N/A

INTERFERING FACTORS:

- ⚠️ This procedure is contraindicated in patients with bleeding disorders, suspected vascular tumor of the liver, ascites that may obscure proper insertion site for needle biopsy, subdiaphragmatic or right hemothoracic infection, or biliary tract infection.

- Failure to follow dietary restrictions before the procedure may cause the procedure to be canceled or repeated.

Nursing Implications and Procedure • • • • • • • • • • •

Pretest:

➤ Inform the patient that the test is used to establish a histologic diagnosis of liver disease.

➤ Obtain a history of the patient's complaints, especially fatigue and pain related to inflammation and swelling of the liver. Include a list of known allergens, especially allergies or sensitivities to latex or anesthetics, and inform the appropriate health care practitioner accordingly.

➤ Obtain a history of the patient's hepatobiliary and immune system, any bleeding disorders, and results of previously performed laboratory tests (especially bleeding time, complete blood count, partial thromboplastin time, platelets, prothrombin time, and liver function tests), surgical procedures, and other diagnostic procedures. For related laboratory tests, refer to the Hepatobiliary and Immune System tables.

➤ Record the date of the last menstrual period and determine the possibility of pregnancy in perimenopausal women.

➤ Note any recent procedures that can interfere with test results.

➤ Obtain a list of the medications the patient is taking, including anticoagulant therapy, acetylsalicylic acid, herbs, nutritional supplements, and nutraceuticals, especially those known to affect coagulation. It is recommended that use be discontinued 14 days before dental or surgical procedures. The requesting health care practitioner and laboratory should be advised if the patient regularly uses these products so that their effects can be taken into consideration when reviewing results.

➤ Review the procedure with the patient. Inform the patient that it may be necessary to shave the site before the procedure. Instruct that prophylactic antibiotics may be administered prior to the procedure. Address concerns about pain related to the procedure. Explain that a sedative and/or analgesia will be administered to promote relaxation and reduce discomfort prior to the percutaneous biopsy; a general anesthesia will be administered prior to the open biopsy. Explain to the patient that no pain will be experienced during the test when general anesthesia is used, but that any discomfort with a needle biopsy will be minimized with local anesthetics and systemic analgesics. Inform the patient that the biopsy is performed under sterile conditions by a health care practitioner specializing in this procedure. The surgical procedure usually takes about 90 minutes to complete, and sutures may be necessary to close the site. A needle biopsy usually takes about 15 minutes to complete.

➤ *Sensitivity to cultural and social issues*, as well as concern for modesty, is important in providing psychological support before, during, and after the procedure.

➤ Explain that an intravenous (IV) line will be inserted to allow infusion of IV fluids, anesthetics, analgesics, or IV sedation.

Open biopsy:

➤ Instruct the patient that nothing should be taken by mouth for 6 to 8 hours prior to a general anesthetic.

Needle biopsy:

➤ Instruct the patient that nothing should be taken by mouth for at least 4 hours prior to the procedure to reduce the risk of nausea and vomiting.

General:

➤ *Make sure a written and informed consent has been signed prior to the procedure and before administering any medications.*

Intratest:

➤ Ensure that the patient has complied with dietary restrictions; assure that food has been restricted for at least 4 to 8 hours depending on the anesthetic chosen for the procedure.

➤ Ensure that anticoagulant therapy has been withheld for the appropriate amount of days prior to the procedure. Amount of days to withhold medication is dependent on the type of anticoagulant. Notify the health care practitioner if patient anticoagulant therapy has not been withheld.

➤ Have emergency equipment readily available.

➤ Have the patient void before the procedure.

➤ Observe standard precautions, and follow the general guidelines in Appendix A. Positively identify the patient, and label the appropriate collection containers with the corresponding patient demographics, date and time of collection, and site location.

➤ Assist the patient to the desired position depending on the test site to be used and direct the patient to breathe normally during the beginning of the general anesthesic. Instruct the patient to cooperate fully and to follow directions. Direct the patient to breathe normally and to avoid unnecessary movement during the local anesthetic and the procedure. Instruct the patient to avoid

coughing or straining, as this may increase intra-abdominal pressure.

➤ Record baseline vital signs, and continue to monitor throughout the procedure. Protocols may vary from facility to facility.

➤ After the administration of general or local anesthesia, shave and cleanse the site with an antiseptic solution, and drape the area with sterile towels.

Open biopsy:

➤ After administration of general anesthesia and surgical prep are completed, an incision is made, suspicious area(s) are located, and tissue samples are collected.

Needle biopsy:

➤ Direct the patient to take slow deep breaths when the local anesthetic is injected. Protect the site with sterile drapes. Instruct the patient to take a deep breath, exhale forcefully, and hold the breath while the biopsy needle is inserted and rotated to obtain a core of liver tissue. Once the needle is removed, the patient may breathe. Pressure is applied to the site for 3 to 5 minutes, then a sterile pressure dressing is applied.

General:

➤ Monitor the patient for complications related to the procedure (e.g., allergic reaction, anaphylaxis).

➤ Place tissue samples in formalin solution. Label the specimen, indicating site location, and promptly transport the specimen to the laboratory for processing and analysis.

➤ The results are recorded manually or in a computerized system for recall and postprocedure interpretation by the appropriate health care practitioner.

Post-test:

➤ Instruct the patient to resume preoperative diet, as directed by the health care practitioner. Assess the patient's ability to swallow before allowing the patient to attempt liquids or solid foods.

➤ Monitor vital signs and neurologic status every 15 minutes for 1 hour, then every 2 hours for 4 hours, and then as ordered by the health care practitioner. Monitor temperature every 4 hours for 24 hours. Compare with baseline values. Notify the health care practitioner if temperature is elevated. Protocols may vary from facility to facility.

➤ Observe for delayed allergic reactions, such as rash, urticaria, tachycardia, hyperpnea, hypertension, palpitations, nausea, or vomiting.

➤ Observe the biopsy site for bleeding, inflammation, or hematoma formation.

➤ Instruct the patient in the care and assessment of the site. Instruct the patient to report any redness, edema, bleeding, or pain at the biopsy site. Instruct the patient to immediately report chills or fever. Instruct the patient to keep the site clean and change the dressing as needed. Instruct the patient to immediately report any pleuritic pain, persistent right shoulder pain, or abdominal pain.

➤ Assess for nausea and pain. Administer antiemetic and analgesic medications as needed and as directed by the health care practitioner.

➤ Administer antibiotic therapy if ordered. Remind the patient of the importance of completing the entire course of antibiotic therapy, even if signs and symptoms disappear before completion of therapy.

➤ A written report of the examination will be completed by a health care practitioner specializing in this branch of medicine. The report of the examination will be sent to the requesting health care practitioner, who will discuss the results with the patient.

➤ Recognize anxiety related to test results. Discuss the implications of abnormal test results on the patient's lifestyle. Provide teaching and information regarding the clinical implications of the test results, as appropriate. Educate the patient regarding access to counseling services.

➤ Reinforce information given by the patient's health care provider regarding further testing, treatment, or referral to another health care provider. Inform the patient of a follow-up appointment for removal of sutures, if indicated. Answer any questions or address any concerns voiced by the patient or family.

➤ Instruct the patient in the use of any ordered medications. Explain the importance of adhering to the therapy regimen. As appropriate, instruct the patient in significant side effects and systemic reactions associated with the prescribed medication. Encourage him or her to review corresponding literature provided by a pharmacist.

➤ Depending on the results of this procedure, additional testing may be performed to evaluate or monitor progression of the disease process and determine the need for a change in therapy. Evaluate test results in relation to the patient's symptoms and other tests performed.

Related laboratory tests:

➤ Related laboratory tests include alanine aminotransferase, albumin, alkaline phosphatase, ammonia, amylase, antimitochondrial antibody, anti–smooth muscle antibody, α_1-antitrypsin/phenotyping, aspartate aminotransferase, bilirubin, bilirubin fractions, cholesterol, coagulation factor assays, complete blood count, copper, γ-glutamyltransferase, infectious mononucleosis screen, lipase, prothrombin time, and urinalysis.

BIOPSY, LUNG

SYNONYM/ACRONYM: Transbronchial lung biopsy, open lung biopsy.

SPECIMEN: Lung tissue or cells.

REFERENCE VALUE: (Method: Macroscopic and microscopic examination of tissue) No abnormal tissue or cells; no growth in culture.

DESCRIPTION & RATIONALE: A biopsy of the lung is performed to obtain lung tissue for examination of pathologic features. The specimen can be obtained transbronchially or by open lung biopsy. In a transbronchial biopsy, forceps pass through the bronchoscope to obtain the specimen. In a transbronchial needle aspiration biopsy, a needle passes through a bronchoscope to obtain the specimen. In a transcatheter bronchial brushing, a brush is inserted through the bronchoscope. In an open lung biopsy, the chest is opened and a small thoracic incision is made to remove tissue from the chest wall. Lung biopsies are used to differentiate between infection and other sources of disease indicated by initial radiology studies, computed tomography scans, or sputum analysis. Specimens are cultured to detect pathogenic organisms or directly examined for the presence of malignant cells. ■

INDICATIONS:
- Assist in the diagnosis of lung cancer
- Assist in the diagnosis of fibrosis and degenerative or inflammatory diseases of the lung
- Assist in the diagnosis of sarcoidosis

RESULT

Abnormal findings in:
- Amyloidosis
- Cancer
- Granulomas
- Infections caused by *Blastomyces, Histoplasma, Legionella* spp., and *Pneumocystis jiroveci* (formerly *carinii*)
- Sarcoidosis
- Systemic lupus erythematosus
- Tuberculosis

CRITICAL VALUES:
- Shortness of breath, cyanosis, or rapid pulse during the procedure must be reported immediately.
- Any postprocedural decrease in breath sounds noted at the biopsy site should be reported immediately.

INTERFERING FACTORS:
- ⚠ Conditions such as vascular anomalies of the lung, bleeding abnormalities, or pulmonary hypertension may increase the risk of bleeding.
- ⚠ Conditions such as bullae or cysts and respiratory insufficiency increase the risk of pneumothorax.

• Failure to follow dietary restrictions before the procedure may cause the procedure to be canceled or repeated.

Nursing Implications and Procedure • • • • • • • • • • •

Pretest:

➤ Inform the patient that the test is used to establish a histologic diagnosis of lung disease.

➤ Obtain a history of the patient's complaints, including a list of known allergens (especially allergies or sensitivities to latex or anesthetics), and inform the appropriate health care practitioner accordingly.

➤ Obtain a history of the patient's immune and respiratory systems, any bleeding disorders, and results of previously performed laboratory tests, (especially bleeding time, complete blood count, partial thromboplastin time, platelets, and prothrombin time), surgical procedures, and other diagnostic procedures. For related laboratory tests, refer to the Immune and Respiratory System tables.

➤ Note any recent procedures that can interfere with test results.

➤ Record the date of the last menstrual period and determine the possibility of pregnancy in perimenopausal women.

➤ Obtain a list of the medications the patient is taking, including anticoagulant therapy, acetylsalicylic acid, herbs, nutritional supplements, and nutraceuticals, especially those known to affect coagulation. It is recommended that use be discontinued 14 days before dental or surgical procedures. The requesting health care practitioner and laboratory should be advised if the patient regularly uses these products so that their effects can be taken into consideration when reviewing results.

➤ Review the procedure with the patient. Inform the patient that it may be necessary to shave the site before the procedure. Instruct that prophylactic antibiotics may be administered prior to the procedure. Address concerns about pain related to the procedure. Explain that a sedative and/or analgesia will be administered to promote relaxation and reduce discomfort prior to the transbronchial needle aspiration biopsy; a general anesthesia will be administered prior to the open biopsy. Explain to the patient that no pain will be experienced during the test when general anesthesia is used, but that any discomfort with a needle biopsy will be minimized with local anesthetics and systemic analgesics. Atropine is usually given before bronchoscopy examinations to reduce bronchial secretions and prevent vagally induced bradycardia. Meperidine (Demerol) or morphine may be given as a sedative. Lidocaine is sprayed in the patient's throat to reduce discomfort caused by the presence of the tube. Inform the patient that the biopsy is performed under sterile conditions by a health care practitioner specializing in this procedure. The surgical procedure usually takes about 30 minutes to complete, and sutures may be necessary to close the site. A needle biopsy usually takes about 15 to 30 minutes to complete.

➤ *Sensitivity to cultural and social issues,* as well as concern for modesty, is important in providing psychological support before, during, and after the procedure.

➤ Explain that an intravenous (IV) line will be inserted to allow infusion of IV fluids, antibiotics, anesthetics, and analgesics.

➤ Instruct the patient that nothing should be taken by mouth for 6 to 8 hours prior to a general anesthetic.

➤ Have the patient void before the procedure.

➤ *Make sure a written and informed consent has been signed prior to the procedure and before administering any medications.*

Intratest: ▨

▶ Ensure that the patient has complied with dietary restrictions; assure that food has been restricted for at least 6 to 8 hours prior to the procedure.

▶ Ensure that anticoagulant therapy has been withheld for the appropriate amount of days prior to the procedure. Amount of days to withhold medication is dependent on the type of anticoagulant. Notify the health care practitioner if patient anticoagulant therapy has not been withheld.

▶ Have emergency equipment readily available. Keep resuscitation equipment on hand in the case of respiratory impairment or laryngospasm after the procedure.

▶ Avoid using morphine sulfate in those with asthma or other pulmonary disease. This drug can further exacerbate bronchospasms and respiratory impairment.

▶ Observe standard precautions, and follow the general guidelines in Appendix A. Positively identify the patient, and label the appropriate collection containers with the corresponding patient demographics, date and time of collection, and site location, especially left or right lung.

▶ Have patient remove dentures, contact lenses, eyeglasses, and jewelry. Notify the physician if the patient has permanent crowns on teeth. Have the patient remove clothing and change into a gown for the procedure.

▶ Assist the patient to a comfortable position, and direct the patient to breath normally during the beginning of the general anesthesia. Instruct the patient to cooperate fully and to follow directions. Direct the patient to breathe normally and to avoid unnecessary movement during the local anesthetic and the procedure.

▶ Record baseline vital signs and continue to monitor throughout the procedure. Protocols may vary from facility to facility.

▶ After the administration of general or local anesthesia, shave and cleanse the site with an antiseptic solution, and drape the area with sterile towels.

Open biopsy:

▶ The patient is prepared for thoracotomy under general anesthesia in the operating room. Tissue specimens are collected from suspicious sites. Place specimen from needle aspiration or brushing on clean glass microscope slides. Place tissue or aspirate specimens in appropriate sterile container for culture or appropriate fixative container for histologic studies.

▶ Carefully observe the patient for any signs of respiratory distress during the procedure.

▶ A chest tube is inserted after the procedure.

Needle biopsy:

▶ Instruct the patient to take slow deep breaths when the local anesthetic is injected. Protect the site with sterile drapes. Assist patient to a sitting position with arms on a pillow over a bed table. Instruct patient to avoid coughing during the procedure. The needle is inserted through the posterior chest wall and into the intercostal space. The needle is rotated to obtain the sample and then withdrawn. Pressure is applied to the site with a Vaseline gauze, and a pressure dressing is applied over the Vaseline gauze.

Bronchoscopy:

▶ Provide mouth care to reduce oral bacterial flora.

▶ After administration of general anesthesia, position the patient in a supine position with the neck hyperextended. If local anesthesia is used, the patient is seated while the tongue and oropharynx are sprayed and swabbed with anesthetic. Provide an emesis basin for the increased saliva and encourage the patient to spit out the saliva because the gag reflex may be impaired. When loss of sensation is adequate, the patient is placed in a supine or side-lying position. The fiberoptic scope can be introduced through the nose, the mouth, an endotracheal tube, a tracheostomy tube, or a rigid bronchoscope. Most common insertion is through the nose. Patients with copious secretions or massive hemoptysis, or in whom airway complications are more likely, may be intubated before the bronchoscopy. Additional local anesthetic is applied through the scope as it approaches the vocal cords and the carina, eliminating reflexes in these sensitive areas. The fiberoptic approach allows visualization of airway segments without having to move the patient's head through various positions.

➤ After visual inspection of the lungs, tissue samples are collected from suspicious sites by bronchial brush or biopsy forceps to be used for cytologic and microbiologic studies.

➤ After the procedure, the bronchoscope is removed. Patients who had local anesthesia are placed in a semi-Fowler's position to recover.

General:

➤ Monitor the patient for complications related to the procedure (e.g., allergic reaction, anaphylaxis).

➤ Place tissue samples in properly labeled specimen containers containing formalin solution, and promptly transport the specimen to the laboratory for processing and analysis.

➤ The results are recorded manually or in a computerized system for recall and postprocedure interpretation by the appropriate health care practitioner.

Post-test:

➤ Instruct the patient to resume preoperative diet, as directed by the health care practitioner. Assess the patient's ability to swallow before allowing the patient to attempt liquids or solid foods.

➤ Inform the patient that he or she may experience some throat soreness and hoarseness. Instruct patient to treat throat discomfort with lozenges and warm gargles when the gag reflex returns.

➤ Monitor vital signs and neurologic status every 15 minutes for 1 hour, then every 2 hours for 4 hours, and then as ordered by the health care practitioner. Monitor temperature every 4 hours for 24 hours. Compare with baseline values. Notify the health care practitioner if temperature is elevated. Protocols may vary from facility to facility.

➤ Emergency resuscitation equipment should be readily available if the vocal cords become spastic after intubation.

➤ Observe for delayed allergic reactions, such as rash, urticaria, tachycardia, hyperpnea, hypertension, palpitations, nausea, or vomiting.

➤ Observe the biopsy site for bleeding, inflammation, or hematoma formation.

➤ Observe the patient for hemoptysis, difficulty breathing, cough, air hunger, excessive coughing, pain, or absent breath sounds over the affected area. Report to health care provider. Monitor chest tube patency and drainage after a thoracotomy.

➤ Evaluate the patient for symptoms indicating the development of pneumothorax, such as dyspnea, tachypnea, anxiety, decreased breathing sounds, or restlessness. A chest x-ray may be ordered to check for the presence of this complication.

➤ Evaluate the patient for symptoms of empyema, such as fever, tachycardia, malaise, or elevated white blood cell count.

➤ Observe the patient's sputum for blood if a biopsy was taken, because large amounts of blood may indicate the development of a problem; a small amount of streaking is expected. Evaluate the patient for signs of bleeding, such as tachycardia, hypotension, or restlessness.

➤ Instruct the patient in the care and assessment of the biopsy site. Instruct the patient to report any redness, edema, bleeding, or pain at the biopsy site. Instruct the patient to keep the site clean and change the dressing as needed.

➤ Instruct the patient to remain in a semi-Fowler's position after bronchoscopy or fine needle aspiration to maximize ventilation. Semi-Fowler's position is a semisitting position with the knees flexed and supported by pillows on the bed or examination table. Instruct the patient to stay in bed lying on the affected side for at least 2 hours with a pillow or rolled towel under the site to prevent bleeding. The patient will also need to remain on bed rest for 24 hours.

➤ Assess for nausea and pain. Administer antiemetic and analgesic medications as needed and as directed by the health care practitioner.

➤ Administer antibiotic therapy if ordered. Remind the patient of the importance of completing the entire course of antibiotic therapy, even if signs and symptoms disappear before completion of therapy.

➤ A written report of the examination will be completed by a health care practitioner specializing in this branch of medicine. The report will be sent to the requesting health care practitioner, who will discuss the results with the patient.

➤ Recognize anxiety related to test results. Discuss the implications of abnormal test results on the patient's lifestyle. Provide teaching and information regarding the clinical implications of the test results, as appropriate. Educate the patient regarding access to counseling services.

➤ Reinforce information given by the patient's health care provider regarding further testing, treatment, or referral to another health care provider. Instruct the patient to use lozenges or gargle for throat discomfort. Inform the patient of smoking cessation programs as appropriate. Malnutrition is commonly seen in patients with severe respiratory disease for numerous reasons, including fatigue, lack of appetite, and gastrointestinal distress. Adequate intake of vitamins A and C are also important to prevent pulmonary infection and to decrease the extent of lung tissue damage. The importance of following the prescribed diet should be stressed to the patient/caregiver. Educate the patient regarding access to counseling services, as appropriate. Answer any questions or address any concerns voiced by the patient or family.

➤ Instruct the patient in the use of any ordered medications. Explain the importance of adhering to the therapy regimen. As appropriate, instruct the patient in significant side effects and systemic reactions associated with the prescribed medication. Encourage him or her to review corresponding literature provided by a pharmacist.

➤ Depending on the results of this procedure, additional testing may be performed to evaluate or monitor progression of the disease process and determine the need for a change in therapy. Evaluate test results in relation to the patient's symptoms and other tests performed.

Related laboratory tests:

➤ Related laboratory tests include arterial/alveolar oxygen ratio, anti–glomerular basement membrane antibody, blood gases, chest x-ray, complete blood count, computed tomography of the thorax, magnetic resonance imaging of the chest, lung perfusion scan, culture, Gram/acid-fast stain, cytology, and sputum findings.

BIOPSY, LYMPH NODE

SYNONYM/ACRONYM: N/A.

SPECIMEN: Lymph node tissue or cells.

REFERENCE VALUE: (Method: Macroscopic and microscopic examination of tissue) No abnormal tissue or cells.

DESCRIPTION & RATIONALE: Lymph node biopsy is the excision of a tissue sample from one or more lymph nodes for microscopic analysis to determine cell morphology and the presence of tissue abnormalities. This test assists in confirming a diagnosis of cancer, diagnosing disorders causing systemic illness, or determining the stage of metastatic cancer. A biopsy specimen is usually obtained either by needle biopsy or after surgical incision. Biopsies are most commonly performed on the following types of lymph nodes: cervical nodes, which drain the face and scalp; axillary nodes, which drain the arms, breasts, and upper chest; and inguinal nodes, which drain the legs, external genitalia, and lower abdominal wall. ■

INDICATIONS:
• Assist in confirming suspected fungal or parasitic infections of the lymphatics
• Assist in confirming suspected malignant involvement of the lymphatics
• Determine the stage of metastatic cancer
• Differentiate between benign and malignant disorders that may cause lymph node enlargement

• Evaluate persistent enlargement of one or more lymph nodes for unknown reasons

RESULT

Abnormal findings in:
• Chancroid
• Fungal infection (e.g., cat scratch disease)
• Immunodeficiency
• Infectious mononucleosis
• Lymph involvement of systemic diseases (e.g., systemic lupus erythematosus, sarcoidosis)
• Lymphangitis
• Lymphogranuloma venereum
• Malignancy (e.g., lymphomas, leukemias)
• Metastatic disease
• Parasitic infestation (e.g., pneumoconiosis)

CRITICAL VALUES: N/A

INTERFERING FACTORS:
• ⚠ This procedure is contraindicated in patients with bleeding disorders.
• Failure to follow dietary restrictions before the procedure may cause

the procedure to be canceled or repeated.

Nursing Implications and Procedure • • • • • • • • • • •

➤ Inform the patient that the test is used to establish a histologic diagnosis of lymph node disease.

➤ Obtain a history of the patient's complaints, including a list of known allergens (especially allergies or sensitivities to latex or anesthetics), and inform the appropriate health care practitioner accordingly.

➤ Obtain a history of the patient's immune and musculoskeletal systems, any bleeding disorders, and results of previously performed laboratory tests (especially bleeding time, complete blood count, partial thromboplastin time, platelets, and prothrombin time), surgical procedures, and other diagnostic procedures. For related laboratory tests, refer to the Immune and Musculoskeletal System tables.

➤ Record the date of the last menstrual period and determine the possibility of pregnancy in perimenopausal women.

➤ Note any recent procedures that can interfere with test results.

➤ Obtain a list of the medications the patient is taking, including anticoagulant therapy, acetylsalicylic acid, herbs, nutritional supplements, and nutraceuticals, especially those known to affect coagulation. It is recommended that use be discontinued 14 days before dental or surgical procedures. The requesting health care practitioner and laboratory should be advised if the patient regularly uses these products so that their effects can be taken into consideration when reviewing results.

➤ Review the procedure with the patient. Inform the patient that it may be necessary to shave the site before the procedure. Instruct that prophylactic antibiotics may be administered prior to the procedure. Address concerns about pain related to the procedure. Explain that a sedative and/or analgesia will be administered to promote relaxation and reduce discomfort prior to the percutaneous biopsy; a general anesthesia will be administered prior to the open biopsy. Explain to the patient that no pain will be experienced during the test when general anesthesia is used, but that any discomfort with a needle biopsy will be minimized with local anesthetics and systemic analgesics. Inform the patient that the biopsy is performed under sterile conditions by a health care practitioner specializing in this procedure. The surgical procedure usually takes about 30 minutes to complete, and sutures may be necessary to close the site. A needle biopsy usually takes about 15 minutes to complete.

➤ *Sensitivity to cultural and social issues*, as well as concern for modesty, is important in providing psychological support before, during, and after the procedure.

➤ Explain that an intravenous (IV) line will be inserted to allow infusion of IV fluids, anesthetics, analgesics, or IV sedation.

Open biopsy:

➤ Instruct the patient that nothing should be taken by mouth for 6 to 8 hours prior to a general anesthetic.

Needle biopsy:

➤ Instruct the patient that nothing should be taken by mouth for at least 4 hours prior to the procedure to reduce the risk of nausea and vomiting.

General:

➤ *Make sure a written and informed consent has been signed prior to the procedure and before administering any medications.*

Intratest:

➤ Ensure that the patient has complied with dietary restrictions; assure that food has been restricted for at least 4 to 8 hours depending on the anesthetic chosen for the procedure.

➤ Ensure that anticoagulant therapy has been withheld for the appropriate amount of days prior to the procedure. Amount of days to withhold medication is dependent on the type of anticoagulant. Notify the health care practitioner if patient anticoagulant therapy has not been withheld.

➤ Have emergency equipment readily available.

➤ Have the patient void before the procedure.

➤ Observe standard precautions, and follow the general guidelines in Appendix A. Positively identify the patient, and label the appropriate collection containers with the corresponding patient demographics, date and time of collection, and site location.

➤ Assist the patient to the desired position depending on the test site to be used and direct the patient to breathe normally during the beginning of the general anesthesic. Instruct the patient to cooperate fully and to follow directions. Direct the patient to breathe normally and to avoid unnecessary movement during the local anesthetic and the procedure.

➤ Record baseline vital signs, and continue to monitor throughout the procedure. Protocols may vary from facility to facility.

➤ After the administration of general or local anesthesia, shave and cleanse the site with an antiseptic solution, and drape the area with sterile towels.

Open biopsy:

➤ After administration of general anesthesia and surgical prep are completed, an incision is made, suspicious area(s) are located.and tissue samples are collected.

Needle biopsy:

➤ Instruct the patient to take slow deep breaths when the local anesthetic is injected. Protect the site with sterile drapes. The node is grasped with sterile gloved fingers, and a needle (with attached syringe) is inserted directly into the node. The node is aspirated to collect the specimen. Pressure is applied to the site for 3 to 5 minutes, then a sterile dressing is applied.

General:

➤ Monitor the patient for complications related to the procedure (e.g., allergic reaction, anaphylaxis).

➤ Place tissue samples in formalin solution. Label the specimen, indicating site location, and promptly transport the specimen to the laboratory for processing and analysis.

➤ The results are recorded manually or in a computerized system for recall and postprocedure interpretation by the appropriate health care practitioner.

Post-test:

➤ Instruct the patient to resume preoperative diet, as directed by the health care practitioner. Assess the patient's ability to swallow before allowing the patient to attempt liquids or solid foods.

➤ Monitor vital signs and neurologic status every 15 minutes for 1 hour, then every 2 hours for 4 hours, and then as ordered by the health care practitioner. Monitor temperature every 4 hours for 24 hours. Compare with baseline values. Notify the health care practitioner if temperature is elevated. Protocols may vary from facility to facility.

➤ Observe for delayed allergic reactions, such as rash, urticaria, tachycardia, hyperpnea, hypertension, palpitations, nausea, or vomiting.

➤ Observe the biopsy site for bleeding, inflammation, or hematoma formation.

Instruct the patient in the care and assessment of the site. Instruct the patient to report any redness, edema, bleeding, or pain at the biopsy site. Instruct the patient to immediately report chills or fever. Instruct the patient to keep the site clean and change the dressing as needed.

Assess for nausea and pain. Administer antiemetic and analgesic medications as needed and as directed by the health care practitioner.

Administer antibiotic therapy if ordered. Remind the patient of the importance of completing the entire course of antibiotic therapy, even if signs and symptoms disappear before completion of therapy.

A written report of the examination will be completed by a health care practitioner specializing in this branch of medicine. The report will be sent to the requesting health care practitioner, who will discuss the results with the patient.

Recognize anxiety related to test results. Discuss the implications of abnormal test results on the patient's lifestyle. Provide teaching and information regarding the clinical implications of the test results, as appropriate. Educate the patient regarding access to counseling services.

Reinforce information given by the patient's health care provider regarding further testing, treatment, or referral to another health care provider. Inform the patient of a follow-up appointment for removal of sutures, if indicated. Answer any questions or address any concerns voiced by the patient or family.

Instruct the patient in the use of any ordered medications. Explain the importance of adhering to the therapy regimen. As appropriate, instruct the patient in significant side effects and systemic reactions associated with the prescribed medication. Encourage him or her to review corresponding literature provided by a pharmacist.

Depending on the results of this procedure, additional testing may be performed to evaluate or monitor progression of the disease process and determine the need for a change in therapy. Evaluate test results in relation to the patient's symptoms and other tests performed.

Related laboratory tests:

Related laboratory tests include CD4/CD8 enumeration; cerebrospinal fluid analysis; *Chlamydia* serology; complete blood count; culture for bacteria/fungus; cytomegalovirus serology; Gram stain; HIV-1/HIV-2 serology; immunofixation electrophoresis; immunoglobulins A, G, and M; infectious mononucleosis screen; rheumatoid factor; total protein; total protein electrophoresis; and toxoplasmosis serology.

BIOPSY, MUSCLE

SYNONYM/ACRONYM: N/A.

SPECIMEN: Muscle tissue or cells.

REFERENCE VALUE: (Method: Macroscopic and microscopic examination of tissue) No abnormal tissue or cells.

DESCRIPTION & RATIONALE: Muscle biopsy is the excision of a muscle tissue sample for microscopic analysis to determine cell morphology and the presence of tissue abnormalities. This test is used to confirm a diagnosis of neuropathy or myopathy and to diagnose parasitic infestation. A biopsy specimen is usually obtained from the deltoid or gastrocnemius muscle after a surgical incision. ■

INDICATIONS:

• Assist in confirming suspected fungal infection or parasitic infestation of the muscle

• Assist in diagnosing the cause of neuropathy or myopathy

• Assist in the diagnosis of Duchenne's muscular dystrophy

RESULT

Abnormal findings in:

• Alcoholic myopathy

• Amyotrophic lateral sclerosis

• Duchenne's muscular dystrophy

• Fungal infection

• Myasthenia gravis

• Myotonia congenita

• Parasitic infestation

• Polymyalgia rheumatica

• Polymyositis

CRITICAL VALUES: N/A

INTERFERING FACTORS:

• If electromyography is performed before muscle biopsy, residual inflammation may lead to false-positive biopsy results.

• ⚠ This procedure is contraindicated in patients with bleeding disorders.

• Failure to follow dietary restrictions before the procedure may cause the procedure to be canceled or repeated.

Nursing Implications and Procedure • • • • • • • • • • •

Pretest:

➤ Inform the patient that the test is used to establish a histologic diagnosis of musculoskeletal disease.

➤ Obtain a history of the patient's complaints, including a list of known allergens (especially allergies or sensitivities to latex or anesthetics), and inform the appropriate health care practitioner accordingly.

➤ Obtain a history of the patient's immune and musculoskeletal systems, any bleeding disorders, and results of previously performed laboratory tests, (especially bleeding time, complete blood count, partial thromboplastin time, platelets, and prothrombin time), surgical procedures, and other diagnostic procedures. For related laboratory tests, refer to the Immune and Musculoskeletal System tables.

➤ Record the date of the last menstrual period and determine the possibility of pregnancy in perimenopausal women.

➤ Note any recent procedures that can interfere with test results.

➤ Obtain a list of the medications the

patient is taking, including anticoagulant therapy, acetylsalicylic acid, herbs, nutritional supplements, and nutraceuticals, especially those known to affect coagulation. It is recommended that use be discontinued 14 days before dental or surgical procedures. The requesting health care practitioner and laboratory should be advised if the patient regularly uses these products so that their effects can be taken into consideration when reviewing results.

➤ Review the procedure with the patient. Inform the patient that it may be necessary to shave the site before the procedure. Instruct that prophylactic antibiotics may be administered prior to the procedure. Address concerns about pain related to the procedure. Explain that a sedative and/or analgesia will be administered to promote relaxation and reduce discomfort prior to the percutaneous biopsy; a general anesthesia will be administered prior to the open biopsy. Explain to the patient that no pain will be experienced during the test when general anesthesia is used, but that any discomfort with a needle biopsy will be minimized with local anesthetics and systemic analgesics. Inform the patient that the biopsy is performed under sterile conditions by a health care practitioner specializing in this procedure. The surgical procedure usually takes about 20 minutes to complete, and sutures may be necessary to close the site. A needle biopsy usually takes about 15 minutes to complete.

➤ *Sensitivity to cultural and social issues,* as well as concern for modesty, is important in providing psychological support before, during, and after the procedure.

➤ Explain that an intravenous (IV) line may be inserted to allow infusion of IV fluids, anesthetics, or sedatives.

➤ Instruct the patient that nothing should be taken by mouth for at least 4 hours prior to the procedure to reduce the risk of nausea and vomiting.

➤ *Make sure a written and informed consent has been signed prior to the procedure and before administering any medications.*

Intratest:

➤ Ensure that the patient has complied with dietary restrictions; assure that food has been restricted for at least 4 hours prior to the procedure.

➤ Ensure that anticoagulant therapy has been withheld for the appropriate amount of days prior to the procedure. Amount of days to withhold medication is dependent on the type of anticoagulant. Notify the health care practitioner if patient anticoagulant therapy has not been withheld.

➤ Have emergency equipment readily available.

➤ Have the patient void before the procedure.

➤ Observe standard precautions, and follow the general guidelines in Appendix A. Positively identify the patient, and label the appropriate collection containers with the corresponding patient demographics, date and time of collection, and site location.

➤ Assist the patient to a comfortable position: a supine position (for deltoid biopsy) or prone position (for gastrocnemius biopsy). Instruct the patient to cooperate fully and to follow directions. Direct the patient to breathe normally and to avoid unnecessary movement during the local anesthetic and the procedure.

➤ Record baseline vital signs, and continue to monitor throughout the procedure. Protocols may vary from facility to facility.

➤ After the administration of general or local anesthesia, shave and cleanse the site with an antiseptic solution, and drape the area with sterile towels.

Open biopsy:

➤ Assess baseline neurologic status. Instruct the patient to take slow deep breaths when the local anesthetic is injected. Protect the site with sterile drapes.

➤ After infiltration of the site with local anesthetic, a small incision is made through the dermis, exposing the muscle. A small area of muscle is excised and removed with forceps. The area is then closed with sutures or similar material, and a sterile dressing is applied.

Needle biopsy:

➤ Instruct the patient to take slow deep breaths when the local anesthetic is injected. Protect the site with sterile drapes.

➤ After infiltration of the site with local anesthetic, a cutting biopsy needle is introduced through a small skin incision and bored into the muscle. A core needle is introduced through the cutting needle, and a plug of muscle is removed. The needles are withdrawn, and the specimen is placed in a preservative solution. Pressure is applied to the site for 3 to 5 minutes, and then a pressure dressing is applied.

General:

➤ Monitor the patient for complications related to the procedure (e.g., allergic reaction, anaphylaxis).

➤ Place tissue samples in properly labeled specimen container containing formalin solution, and promptly transport the specimen to the laboratory for processing and analysis.

➤ The results are recorded manually or in a computerized systemfor recall and postprocedure interpretation by the appropriate health care practitioner.

Post-test:

➤ Instruct the patient to resume preoperative diet, as directed by the health care practitioner.

➤ Monitor vital signs and neurologic status every 15 minutes for 1 hour, then every 2 hours for 4 hours, and then as ordered by the health care practitioner. Monitor temperature every 4 hours for 24 hours. Compare with baseline values. Notify the health care practitioner if temperature is elevated. Protocols may vary from facility to facility.

➤ Observe for delayed allergic reactions, such as rash, urticaria, tachycardia, hyperpnea, hypertension, palpitations, nausea, or vomiting.

➤ Observe the biopsy site for bleeding, inflammation, or hematoma formation.

➤ Instruct the patient in the care and assessment of the site. Instruct the patient to report any redness, edema, bleeding, or pain at the biopsy site. Instruct the patient to immediately report chills or fever. Instruct the patient to keep the site clean and change the dressing as needed.

➤ Assess for nausea and pain. Administer antiemetic and analgesic medications as needed and as directed by the health care practitioner.

➤ Administer antibiotic therapy if ordered. Remind the patient of the importance of completing the entire course of antibiotic therapy, even if signs and symptoms disappear before completion of therapy.

➤ A written report of the examination will be completed by a health care practitioner specializing in this branch of medicine. The report will be sent to the requesting health care practitioner, who will discuss the results with the patient. .

➤ Recognize anxiety related to test results. Discuss the implications of abnormal test results on the patient's lifestyle. Provide teaching and information regarding the clinical implications of the test results, as appropriate. Educate the patient regarding access to counseling services.

➤ Reinforce information given by the patient's health care provider regarding further testing, treatment, or referral to another health care provider. Inform the patient of a follow-up appointment for removal of sutures, if indicated. Answer any questions or address any concerns voiced by the patient or family.

➤ Instruct the patient in the use of any ordered medications. Explain the importance of adhering to the therapy regimen. As appropriate, instruct the patient in significant side effects and systemic reactions associated with the prescribed medication. Encourage him or her to review corresponding literature provided by a pharmacist.

➤ Depending on the results of this procedure, additional testing may be performed to evaluate or monitor progression of the disease process and determine the need for a change in therapy. Evaluate test results in relation to the patient's symptoms and other tests performed.

Related laboratory tests:

➤ Related laboratory tests include acetylcholine receptor antibody, aldolase, antinuclear antibodies, antithyroglobulin antibodies, creatine kinase and isoenzymes, Jo-1 antibody, myoglobin, and rheumatoid factor.

BIOPSY, PROSTATE

SYNONYM/ACRONYM: N/A.

SPECIMEN: Prostate tissue.

REFERENCE VALUE: (Method: Microscopic examination of tissue cells) No abnormal cells or tissue.

DESCRIPTION & RATIONALE: Biopsy of the prostate gland is performed to identify cancerous cells, especially if serum prostate-specific antigen is increased. ∎

INDICATIONS:
• Evaluate prostatic hypertrophy of unknown etiology
• Investigate suspected cancer of the prostate

RESULT: Positive findings in prostate cancer.

CRITICAL VALUES: N/A

INTERFERING FACTORS:
• ⚠ This procedure is contraindicated in patients with bleeding disorders.

• Failure to follow dietary restrictions before the procedure may cause the procedure to be canceled or repeated.

• ⚠ The various sampling approaches have individual drawbacks that should be considered: transurethral sampling does not always ensure that malignant cells will be included in the specimen, whereas transrectal sampling carries the risk of perforating the rectum and creating a channel through which malignant cells can seed normal tissue.

Nursing Implications and Procedure • • • • • • • • • • • •

➤ Inform the patient that the test is used to establish a histologic diagnosis of prostate disease.

➤ Obtain a history of the patient's complaints, including a list of known allergens (especially allergies or sensitivities to latex or anesthetics), and inform the appropriate health care practitioner accordingly.

➤ Obtain a history of the patient's genitourinary and immune systems, any bleeding disorders, and results of previously performed laboratory tests (especially bleeding time, complete blood count, partial thromboplastin time, platelets, and prothrombin time), surgical procedures, and other diagnostic procedures. For related laboratory tests, refer to the Genitourinary and Immune System tables.

➤ Note any recent procedures that can interfere with test results.

➤ Obtain a list of the medications the patient is taking, including anticoagulant therapy, acetylsalicylic acid, herbs, nutritional supplements, and nutraceuticals, especially those known to affect coagulation. It is recommended that use be discontinued 14 days before dental or surgical procedures. The requesting health care practitioner and laboratory should be advised if the patient regularly uses these products so that their effects can be taken into consideration when reviewing results.

➤ Review the procedure with the patient. Inform the patient that it may be necessary to shave the site before the procedure. Instruct that prophylactic antibiotics may be administered prior to the procedure. Address concerns about pain related to the procedure. Explain that a sedative and/or analgesia will be administered to promote relaxation and reduce discomfort prior to the percutaneous biopsy; a general anesthesia will be administered prior to the open biopsy. Explain to the patient that no pain will be experienced during the test when general anesthesia is used, but that any discomfort with a needle biopsy will be minimized with local anesthetics and systemic analgesics. Inform the patient that the biopsy is performed under sterile conditions by a health care practitioner specializing in this procedure. The surgical procedure usually takes about 30 minutes to complete, and sutures may be necessary to close the site. A needle biopsy usually takes about 20 minutes to complete.

➤ *Sensitivity to cultural and social issues,* as well as concern for modesty, is important in providing psychological support before, during, and after the procedure.

➤ Explain that an intravenous (IV) line will be inserted to allow infusion of IV fluids, antibiotics, anesthetics, and analgesics.

➤ Ensure that anticoagulant therapy has been withheld for the appropriate amount of days prior to the procedure. Amount of days to withhold medication is dependent on the type of anticoagulant. Notify the health care practitioner if patient anticoagulant therapy has not been withheld.

➤ Instruct the patient that nothing should be taken by mouth for 6 to 8 hours prior to a general anesthetic.

➤ *Make sure a written and informed consent has been signed prior to the procedure and before administering any medications.*

➤ Ensure that the patient has complied with dietary restrictions; assure that food has been restricted for at least 6 to 8 hours prior to the procedure.

➤ Have emergency equipment readily available.

➤ Have the patient void before the procedure. Administer enemas if ordered.

➤ Observe standard precautions, and

follow the general guidelines in Appendix A. Positively identify the patient, and label the appropriate collection containers with the corresponding patient demographics, date and time of collection, and site location.

➤ Assist the patient to a comfortable position, and direct the patient to breath normally during the beginning of the general anesthesia..

➤ Cleanse the biopsy site with an antiseptic solution, and drape the area with sterile towels.

➤ Record baseline vital signs, and continue to monitor throughout the procedure. Protocols may vary from facility to facility.

Transurethral approach:

➤ After administration of general anesthesia, position the patient on a urologic exam table with the feet in stirrups. The endoscope is inserted into the urethra. The tissue is excised with a cutting loop and is placed in formalin solution.

Transrectal approach:

➤ After administration of general anesthesia, position the patient in the Sims' position. A rectal examination is performed to locate suspicious nodules. A biopsy needle guide is placed at the biopsy site, and the biopsy needle is inserted through the needle guide. The cells are aspirated, the needle is withdrawn, and the sample is placed in formalin solution.

Perineal approach:

➤ After administration of general anesthesia, position the patient in the lithotomy position. Clean the perineum with an antiseptic solution, and protect the biopsy site with sterile drapes. A small incision is made and the sample is removed by needle biopsy or biopsy punch and placed in formalin solution.

General:

➤ Monitor the patient for complications related to the procedure (e.g., allergic reaction, anaphylaxis).

➤ Apply digital pressure to the biopsy site. If there is no bleeding after the perineal approach, place a sterile dressing on the biopsy site.

➤ Place tissue samples in properly labeled specimen containers containing formalin solution, and promptly transport the specimen to the laboratory for processing and analysis.

➤ The results are recorded manually or in a computerized system for recall and postprocedure interpretation by the appropriate health care practitioner.

Post-test:

➤ Instruct the patient to resume preoperative diet, as directed by the health care practitioner. Assess the patient's ability to swallow before allowing the patient to attempt liquids or solid foods.

➤ Monitor vital signs and neurologic status every 15 minutes for 1 hour, then every 2 hours for 4 hours, and then as ordered by the health care practitioner. Monitor temperature every 4 hours for 24 hours. Compare with baseline values. Notify the health care practitioner if temperature is elevated. Protocols may vary from facility to facility.

➤ Monitor fluid intake and output for 24 hours. Instruct the patient on intake and output recording and provide appropriate measuring containers.

➤ Encourage fluid intake of 3000 mL, unless contraindicated.

➤ Observe for delayed allergic reactions, such as rash, urticaria, tachycardia, hyperpnea, hypertension, palpitations, nausea, or vomiting.

➤ Observe the perineal approach biopsy site for bleeding, inflammation, or hematoma formation. Instruct the patient to keep the site clean and change the dressing as needed.

➤ Instruct the patient to immediately report pain, chills, of fever. Assess for infection, hemorrhage, or perforation of the urethra or rectum.

➤ Inform the patient that blood may be

seen in the urine after the first or second post procedural voiding.

➤ Instruct the patient to report any further changes in urinary pattern, volume, or appearance.

➤ Assess for nausea, pain, and bladder spasms. Administer antiemetic, analgesic, and antispasmodic medications as needed and as directed by the health care practitioner.

➤ Administer antibiotic therapy if ordered. Remind the patient of the importance of completing the entire course of antibiotic therapy, even if signs and symptoms disappear before completion of therapy.

➤ A written report of the examination will be completed by a health care practitioner specializing in this branch of medicine. The report will be sent to the requesting health care practitioner, who will discuss the results with the patient.

➤ Recognize anxiety related to test results. Discuss the implications of abnormal test results on the patient's lifestyle. Provide teaching and information regarding the clinical implications of the test results, as appropriate. Educate the patient regarding access to counseling services.

➤ Reinforce information given by the patient's health care provider regarding further testing, treatment, or referral to another health care provider. Counsel the patient, as appropriate, that sexual dysfunction related to altered body function, drugs, or radiation may occur. Educate the patient regarding access to counseling services, as appropriate. Answer any questions or address any concerns voiced by the patient or family.

➤ Instruct the patient in the use of any ordered medications. Explain the importance of adhering to the therapy regimen. As appropriate, instruct the patient in significant side effects and systemic reactions associated with the prescribed medication. Encourage him to review corresponding literature provided by a pharmacist.

➤ Depending on the results of this procedure, additional testing may be performed to evaluate or monitor progression of the disease process and determine the need for a change in therapy. Evaluate test results in relation to the patient's symptoms and other tests performed.

Related laboratory tests:

➤ Related laboratory tests include prostate-specific antigen and prostatic acid phosphatase.

BIOPSY, SKIN

. . . .

SYNONYM/ACRONYM: N/A.

SPECIMEN: Skin tissue or cells.

REFERENCE VALUE: (Method: Macroscopic and microscopic examination of tissue) No abnormal tissue or cells.

DESCRIPTION & RATIONALE: Skin biopsy is the excision of a tissue sample from suspicious skin lesions. The microscopic analysis can determine cell morphology and the presence of tissue abnormalities. This test assists in confirming the diagnosis of malignant or benign skin lesions. A skin biopsy can be obtained by any of these four ways: curettage, shaving, excision, or punch. ▪

INDICATIONS:
• Assist in the diagnosis of keratoses, warts, moles, keloids, fibromas, cysts, or inflamed lesions

• Assist in the diagnosis of skin cancer

• Evaluate suspicious skin lesions

RESULT

Abnormal findings in:
• Basal cell carcinoma

• Cysts

• Dermatitis

• Dermatofibroma

• Keloids

• Malignant melanoma

• Neurofibroma

• Pemphigus

• Pigmented nevi

• Seborrheic keratosis

• Skin involvement in systemic lupus erythematosus, discoid lupus erythematosus, and scleroderma

• Squamous cell carcinoma

• Warts

CRITICAL VALUES: N/A

INTERFERING FACTORS:
• ⚠ This procedure is contraindicated in patients with bleeding disorders.

• Failure to follow dietary restrictions before the procedure may cause the procedure to be canceled or repeated.

Nursing Implications and Procedure • • • • • • • • • • •

Pretest:

➤ Inform the patient that the test is used to establish a histologic diagnosis of skin disease.

➤ Obtain a history of the patient's complaints, including a list of known allergens (especially allergies or sensitivities to latex or anesthetics), and inform the appropriate health care practitioner accordingly.

➤ Obtain a history of the patient's immune and musculoskeletal systems, any bleeding disorders, and results of previously performed laboratory tests (especially bleeding time, complete blood count, partial thromboplastin time, platelets, and prothrombin time), surgical procedures, and other diagnostic procedures. For related laboratory tests, refer to the Immune and Musculoskeletal System tables.

➤ Record the date of the last menstrual period and determine the possibility of pregnancy in perimenopausal women.

➤ Note any recent procedures that can interfere with test results.

➤ Obtain a list of the medications the patient is taking, including anticoagulant therapy, acetylsalicylic acid, herbs, nutritional supplements, and nutraceuticals, especially those known to affect coagulation. It is recommended that use be discontinued 14 days before dental or surgical procedures. The requesting health care practitioner and laboratory should be advised if the patient regularly uses these products so that their effects can be taken into consideration when reviewing results.

➤ Review the procedure with the patient. Inform the patient that it may be necessary to shave the site before the procedure. Instruct that prophylactic antibiotics may be administered prior to the procedure. Address concerns about pain related to the procedure. Explain that a sedative and/or analgesia will be administered to promote relaxation and reduce discomfort prior to the punch biopsy; a general anesthesia will be administered prior to the open biopsy. Explain to the patient that no pain will be experienced during the test when general anesthesia is used, but that any discomfort with a punch biopsy will be minimized with local anesthetics and systemic analgesics. Inform the patient that the biopsy is performed under sterile conditions by a health care practitioner specializing in this procedure. The surgical procedure usually takes about 30 minutes to complete, and sutures may be necessary to close the site. A punch biopsy usually takes about 20 minutes to complete.

➤ *Sensitivity to cultural and social issues,* as well as concern for modesty, is important in providing psychological support before, during, and after the procedure.

➤ Explain that an intravenous (IV) line may be inserted to allow infusion of IV fluids, anesthetics, or sedatives, depending on the type of biopsy.

➤ There are no food, fluid, or medication restrictions unless by medical direction.

➤ *Make sure a written and informed consent has been signed prior to the procedure and before administering any medications.*

Intratest:

➤ Ensure that the patient has complied with dietary restrictions, if ordered by the health care practitioner.

➤ Ensure that anticoagulant therapy has been withheld for the appropriate amount of days prior to the procedure. Amount of days to withhold medication is dependent on the type of anticoagulant. Notify the health care practitioner if patient anticoagulant therapy has not been withheld.

➤ Have emergency equipment readily available.

➤ Have the patient void before the procedure.

➤ Observe standard precautions, and follow the general guidelines in Appendix A. Positively identify the patient, and label the appropriate collection containers with the corresponding patient demographics, date and time of collection, and site location.

➤ Assist the patient to the desired position depending on the test site to be used, and direct the patient to breathe normally during the local anesthetic and the procedure. Instruct the patient to cooperate fully and to follow directions and to avoid unnecessary movement.

➤ Record baseline vital signs, and continue to monitor throughout the procedure. Protocols may vary from facility to facility.

➤ After the administration of general or local anesthesia, shave and cleanse the site with an antiseptic solution, and drape the area with sterile towels.

➤ *Curettage:* The skin is scraped with a curette to obtain specimen.

➤ *Shaving or excision:* A scalpel is used to remove a portion of the lesion that protrudes above the epidermis. If the lesion is to be excised, the incision is made as wide and as deep as needed to ensure that the entire lesion is removed. Bleeding is controlled with external pressure to the site. Large wounds are closed with sutures. An adhesive bandage is applied when excision is complete.

➤ *Punch biopsy:* A small, round punch about 4 to 6 mm in diameter is rotated into the skin to the desired depth. The cylinder of skin is pulled upward with forceps and separated at its base with a scalpel or scissors. If needed, sutures are applied. A sterile dressing is applied over the site.

➤ Monitor the patient for complications related to the procedure (e.g., allergic reaction, anaphylaxis).

➤ Place tissue samples in properly labeled specimen container containing formalin solution, and promptly transport the specimen to the laboratory for processing and analysis.

➤ The results are recorded manually or in a computerized system for recall and postprocedure interpretation by the appropriate health care practitioner.

Post-test:

➤ Instruct the patient to resume preoperative diet, as directed by the health care practitioner. Assess the patient's ability to swallow before allowing the patient to attempt liquids or solid foods.

➤ Monitor vital signs and neurologic status every 15 minutes for 1 hour, then every 2 hours for 4 hours, and then as ordered by the health care practitioner. Monitor temperature every 4 hours for 24 hours. Compare with baseline values. Notify the health care practitioner if temperature is elevated. Protocols may vary from facility to facility.

➤ Observe for delayed allergic reactions, such as rash, urticaria, tachycardia, hyperpnea, hypertension, palpitations, nausea, or vomiting.

➤ Observe the biopsy site for bleeding, inflammation, or hematoma formation.

➤ Instruct the patient in the care and assessment of the site. Instruct the patient to report any redness, edema, bleeding, or pain at the biopsy site. Instruct the patient to immediately report chills or fever. Instruct the patient to keep the site clean and change the dressing as needed.

➤ Assess for nausea and pain. Administer antiemetic and analgesic medications as needed and as directed by the health care practitioner.

➤ Administer antibiotic therapy if ordered. Remind the patient of the importance of completing the entire course of antibiotic therapy, even if signs and symptoms disappear before completion of therapy.

➤ A written report of the examination will be completed by a health care practitioner specializing in this branch of medicine. The report will be sent to the requesting health care practitioner, who will discuss the results with the patient.

➤ Recognize anxiety related to test results. Discuss the implications of abnormal test results on the patient's lifestyle. Provide teaching and information regarding the clinical implications of the test results, as appropriate. Educate the patient regarding access to counseling services.

➤ Reinforce information given by the patient's health care provider regarding further testing, treatment, or referral to another health care provider. Inform the patient of a follow-up appointment for the removal of sutures, if indicated. Answer any questions or address any concerns voiced by the patient or family.

➤ Instruct the patient in the use of any ordered medications. Explain the importance of adhering to the therapy regimen. As appropriate, instruct the patient in significant side effects and systemic reactions associated with the prescribed medication. Encourage him or her to review corresponding literature provided by a pharmacist.

➤ Depending on the results of this procedure, additional testing may be performed to evaluate or monitor progression of the disease process and determine the need for a change in therapy. Evaluate test results in relation to the patient's symptoms and other tests performed.

Related laboratory tests:

➤ Related laboratory tests include allergen-specific immunoglobulin E (IgE), antinuclear antibody, eosinophil count, erythrocyte sedimentation rate, IgE, and skin culture.

BIOPSY, THYROID

SYNONYM/ACRONYM: N/A.

SPECIMEN: Thyroid gland tissue or cells.

REFERENCE VALUE: (Method: Macroscopic and microscopic examination of tissue) No abnormal cells or tissue.

DESCRIPTION & RATIONALE: Thyroid biopsy is the excision of a tissue sample for microscopic analysis to determine cell morphology and the presence of tissue abnormalities. This test assists in confirming a diagnosis of cancer or determining the cause of persistent thyroid symptoms. A biopsy specimen can be obtained by needle aspiration or by surgical excision. ■

INDICATIONS:
- Assist in the diagnosis of thyroid cancer or benign cysts or tumors
- Determine the cause of inflammatory thyroid disease
- Determine the cause of hyperthyroidism
- Evaluate enlargement of the thyroid gland

RESULT

Positive findings in:
- Benign thyroid cyst
- Granulomatous thyroiditis
- Hashimoto's thyroiditis
- Nontoxic nodular goiter
- Thyroid cancer

CRITICAL VALUES: N/A

INTERFERING FACTORS:
- ⚠ This procedure is contraindicated in patients with bleeding disorders.
- Failure to follow dietary restrictions before the procedure may cause the procedure to be canceled or repeated.

Nursing Implications and Procedure ....

Pretest:

➤ Inform the patient that the test is used to establish a histologic diagnosis of thyroid disease.

➤ Obtain a history of the patient's complaints, including a list of known allergens, especially allergies or sensitivities to latex or anesthetics and inform the appropriate health care practitioner accordingly.

➤ Obtain a history of the patient's endocrine and immune systems, any bleeding disorders, and results of previously performed laboratory tests (especially bleeding time, complete blood count, partial thromboplastin time, platelets, and prothrombin time), surgical procedures, and other diagnostic procedures. For related laboratory tests, refer to the

Endocrine and Immune system tables.

➤ Record the date of the last menstrual period and determine possibility of pregnancy in perimenopausal women.

➤ Note any recent procedures that can interfere with test results.

➤ Obtain a list of the medications the patient is taking. Include herbs, nutritional supplements, and nutraceuticals, including anticoagulant therapy, acetylsalicylic acid, herbs, and nutraceuticals known to affect coagulation. It is recommended that use be discontinued 14 days before dental or surgical procedures. The requesting health care practitioner and laboratory should be advised if the patient regularly uses these products so that their effects can be taken nto consideration when reviewing results.

➤ Review the procedure with the patient. Inform the patient that it may be necessary to shave the site before the procedure. Instruct that prophylactic antibiotics may be administered prior to the procedure. Address concerns about pain related to the procedure. Explain that a sedative and/or analgesia will be administered to promote relaxation and reduce discomfort prior to the percutaneous biopsy; a general anesthesia will be administered prior to the open biopsy. Explain to the patient that no pain will be experienced during the test when general anesthesia is used, but that any discomfort with a needle biopsy will be minimized with local anesthetics and systemic analgesics. Inform the patient that the biopsy is performed under sterile conditions by a health care practitioner specializing in this procedure., The surgical procedure usually takes about 30 minutes to complete, and that sutures may be necessary to close the site. A needle biopsy usually takes about 15 minutes to complete.

➤ *Sensitivity to cultural and social issues*, as well as concern for modesty, is important in providing psy-chological support before, during and after the procedure.

➤ Explain that an IV line may be inserted to allow infusion of IV fluids, anesthetics, analgesics, or IV sedation.

Open biopsy:

➤ Instruct the patient that nothing should be taken by mouth for 6 to 8 hours prior to a general anesthetic.

Needle biopsy:

➤ Instruct the patient that nothing should be taken by mouth for at least 4 hours prior to the procedure to reduce the risk of nausea and vomiting.

➤ Have the patient void before the procedure.

General:

➤ *Make sure a written and informed consent has been signed prior to the procedure and before administering any medications.*

Intratest:

➤ Ensure that the patient has complied with dietary restrictions; assure food has been restricted for at least 4 to 8 hours depending on the anesthetic chosen for the procedure.

➤ Ensure that anticoagulant therapy has been withheld for the appropriate amount of days prior to the procedure. Amount of days to withhold medication is dependant on the type of anticoagulant. Notify health care practitioner if patient anticoagulant therapy has not been withheld.

➤ Have emergency equipment readily available.

➤ Observe standard precautions, and follow the general guidelines in Appendix A. Positively identify the patient and label the appropriate collection containers with the corresponding patient demographics, date and time of collection, and site location.

➤ Assist the patient to the desired position depending on the test site to be used and direct the patient to breathe normally during the beginning of the general anesthesic.

Instruct the patient to cooperate fully and to follow directions. Direct the patient to breathe normally and to avoid unnecessary movement during the local anesthetic and the procedure..

➤ Record baseline vital signs and continue to monitor throughout the procedure. Protocols may vary from facility to facility.

➤ After the administration of general or local anesthesia, shave and cleanse the site with an antiseptic solution, and drape the area with sterile towels.

Open biopsy:

➤ After administration of general anesthesia and surgical prep is completed, an incision is made, suspicious area(s) are located, and tissue samples are collected.

Needle biopsy:

➤ Direct the patient to take slow deep breaths when the local anesthetic is injected. Protect the site with sterile drapes. Instruct the patient to take a deep breath, exhale forcefully, and hold the breath while the biopsy needle is inserted and rotated to obtain a core of breast tissue. Once the needle is removed, the patient may breathe. Pressure is applied to the site for 3 to 5 minutes, then a sterile pressure dressing is applied.

General:

➤ Monitor the patient for complications related to the procedure (e.g., allergic reaction, anaphylaxis).

➤ Place tissue samples in properly labelled specimen container containing formalin solution, and promptly transport the specimen to the laboratory for processing and analysis.

➤ The results are recorded manually or in a computerized system for recall and postprocedure interpretation by the appropriate healthcare practitioner.

Post-test:

➤ Instruct the patient to resume pre-op diet, as directed by the health care practitioner. Assess the patient's ability to swallow before allowing the patient to attempt liquids or solid foods.

➤ Monitor vital signs and neurologic status every 15 minutes for 1 hour, then every 2 hours for 4 hours, and then as ordered by the health care practitioner. Monitor temperature every 4 hours for 24 hours. Notify the health care practitioner if elevated tempterature. Protocols may vary from facility to facility.

➤ Observe for delayed allergic reactions, such as rash, urticaria, tachycardia, hyperpnea, hypertension, palpitations, nausea, or vomiting.

➤ Observe the biopsy site for bleeding, inflammation, or hematoma formation.

➤ Instruct the patient in the care and assessment of the site. Instruct the patient to report any redness, edema, bleeding, or pain at the biopsy site. Instruct the patient to immediately report chills or fever. Instruct the patient to keep the site clean and change the dressing as needed.

➤ Assess for nausea and pain. Administer antiemetic and analgesic medications as needed and as directed by the health care practitioner.

➤ Administer antibiotic therapy if ordered. Remind the patient of the importance of completing the entire course of antibiotic therapy, even if signs and symptoms disappear before completion of therapy.

➤ A written report of the examination will be completed by a health care practitioner specializing in this branch of medicine. The report will be sent to the requesting health care practitioner who will discuss the results with the patient.

➤ Recognize anxiety related to test. Discuss the implications of the abnormal test results on the patient's lifestyle. Provide teaching and information regarding the clinical impli-cations of the test results, as appro-priate. Educate the patient regarding access to counseling services.

➤ Reinforce information given by the patient's health care provider regard-ing further testing, treatment or referral to another health care provider. Inform the patient of a follow-up appointment for removal of sutures, if indicated. Answer any questions or address any concerns voiced by the patient or family.

➤ Instruct the patient in the use of any ordered medications. Explain the importance of adhering to the ther-apy regimen. As appropriate, instruct the patient in significant side effects and systemic reactions associated

with the prescribed medication. Encourage them to review corre-sponding literature provided by a pharmacist.

➤ Depending on the results of this procedure, additional testing may be performed to evaluate or monitor progression of the disease process and determine the need for a change in therapy. Evaluate test results in relation to the patient's symptoms and other tests performed.

Related laboratory tests

➤ Related laboratory tests include antithyroglobulin antibodies, thyroid-stimulating hormone, and free thy-roxine.

BLADDER CANCER MARKERS, URINE

. . . .

SYNONYMS/ACRONYMS: NMP22, Bard BTA.

SPECIMEN: Urine (5 mL), unpreserved random specimen collected in a clean plastic collection container.

REFERENCE VALUE: (Method: Enzyme immunoassay for NMP22, immunochromatographic for Bard BTA)

NMP22: Less than 10 units/mL
Bard BTA: Negative

DESCRIPTION & RATIONALE: Cys-toscopy is still considered the gold standard for detection of bladder can-cer, but other noninvasive tests are being developed, including several urine assays approved by the Food and

Drug Administration. Compared to cytologic studies, these assays are believed to be more sensitive but less specific for detecting transitional cell carcinoma.

NMP22: Nuclear matrix proteins (NMPs) are involved in the regulation and expression of various genes. The NMP identified as NuMA is abundant in bladder tumor cells. The dying tumor cells release the soluble NMP into the urine. This assay is quantitative.

Bladder tumor antigen (BTA): A human complement factor H–related protein (hCFHrp) is thought to be produced by bladder tumor cells as protection from the body's natural immune response. The bladder tumor antigen is released from tumor cells into the urine. This assay is qualitative. ▪

INDICATIONS:
• Detection of bladder carcinoma

• Management of recurrent bladder cancer

RESULT: Increased in bladder carcinoma.

CRITICAL VALUES: N/A

INTERFERING FACTORS:
• *NMP22:* Any condition that results in inflammation of the bladder or urinary tract may cause falsely elevated values.

• *Bard BTA:* Recent surgery, biopsy, or other trauma to the bladder or urinary tract may cause falsely elevated values. Active urinary tract infection, renal or bladder calculi, gross hemolysis, and positive leukocyte dipstick may also cause false-positive results.

Nursing Implications and Procedure • • • • • • • • • • •

Pretest:

➤ Inform the patient that the test is used to diagnose bladder cancer.

➤ Obtain a history of the patient's complaints, including a list of known allergens, and inform the appropriate health care practitioner accordingly.

➤ Obtain a history of the patient's gen-

itourinary and immune systems and results of previously performed laboratory tests, surgical procedures, and other diagnostic procedures. For related laboratory tests, refer to the Genitourinary and Immune System tables.

➤ Note any recent procedures that can interfere with test results.

➤ Obtain a list of the medications the patient is taking, including herbs, nutritional supplements, and nutraceuticals. The requesting health care practitioner and laboratory should be advised if the patient regularly uses these products so their effects can be taken into consideration when reviewing results.

➤ Review the procedure with the patient. Address concerns about pain related to the procedure. Explain to the patient that there should be no discomfort during the procedure. Inform the patient that specimen collection takes approximately 5 minutes, depending on the cooperation and ability of the patient.

➤ *Sensitivity to social and cultural issues*, as well as concern for modesty, is important in providing psychological support before, during, and after the procedure.

➤ There are no food, fluid, or medication restrictions unless by medical direction.

Intratest:

➤ Instruct the patient to cooperate fully and to follow directions.

➤ Observe standard precautions, and follow the general guidelines in Appendix A. Positively identify the patient, and label the appropriate collection container with the corresponding patient demographics, date, and time of collection.

➤ Obtain urine specimen in a clean plastic collection container. Promptly transport the specimen to the laboratory for processing and analysis.

➤ The results are recorded manually

or in a computerized system for recall and postprocedure interpretation by the appropriate health care practitioner.

Post-test:

➤ A written report of the examination will be sent to the requesting health care practitioner, who will discuss the results with the patient.

➤ Recognize anxiety related to test results, and be supportive of fear of shortened life expectancy. Discuss the implications of abnormal test results on the patient's lifestyle. Provide teaching and information regarding the clinical implications of the test results, as appropriate. Educate the patient regarding access to counseling services.

➤ Reinforce information given by the patient's health care provider regarding further testing, treatment, or referral to another health care provider. Answer any questions or address any concerns voiced by the patient or family.

➤ Depending on the results of this procedure, additional testing may be performed to evaluate or monitor progression of the disease process and determine the need for a change in therapy. Evaluate test results in relation to the patient's symptoms and other tests performed.

Related laboratory tests:

➤ Related laboratory tests include bladder biopsy and urine cytology.

BLEEDING TIME

SYNONYM/ACRONYM: Mielke bleeding time, Simplate bleeding time, Template bleeding time, Surgicutt, Ivy bleeding time.

SPECIMEN: Whole blood.

REFERENCE VALUE: (Method: Timed observation of incision)

Template: 2.5 to 10 minutes
Ivy: 2 to 7 minutes
There are slight differences in the disposable devices used to make the incision. Although the Mielke or Template bleeding time is believed to offer greater standardization to a fairly subjective procedure, both methods are thought to be of equal sensitivity and reproducibility.

DESCRIPTION & RATIONALE: Bleeding time assesses platelet and capillary function. ■

INDICATIONS:

Many laboratories have discounted the use of bleeding time testing in favor of PT, aPTT, platelet count or platelet function testing as appropriate. This change in laboratory practice is based on the results of studies that do not support its clinical value in either surgical or nonsurgical applications.

RESULT

This test does not predict excessive bleeding during a surgical procedure.

Prolonged in:

- Bernard-Soulier syndrome
- Fibrinogen disorders
- Glanzmann's thrombasthenia
- Hereditary telangiectasia
- Liver disease
- Macroglobulinemia
- Some myeloproliferative disorders
- Renal disease
- Thrombocytopenia
- von Willebrand's disease

Decreased in: N/A

CRITICAL VALUES:

Greater than 14 minutes

Note and immediately report to the health care practitioner any critically increased values and related symptoms.

INTERFERING FACTORS:

- Drugs that may prolong bleeding time include acetylsalicylic acid, aminocaproic acid, ampicillin, asparaginase, carbenicillin, cefoperazone, cilostazol, dextran, diltiazem, ethanol, flurbiprofen, fluroxene, halothane, heparin, ketorolac, mezlocillin, moxalactam, nafcillin, naproxen, nifedipine, nonsteroidal anti-inflammatory drugs, penicillin, piroxicam, plicamycin, propranolol, streptokinase, sulindac, ticarcillin, tolmetin, urokinase, valproic acid, and warfarin.
- Drugs that may decrease bleeding time include desmopressin and erythropoietin.
- ⚠ The test should not be performed

on patients who must be restrained, have excessively cold or edematous arms, have a platelet count less than 50,000/mm^3, have an infectious skin disease, or cannot have a blood pressure cuff placed on the arm.

Nursing Implications and Procedure • • • • • • • • • • •

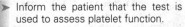

Pretest:

➤ Inform the patient that the test is used to assess platelet function.

➤ Obtain a history of the patient's complaints, including a list of known allergens (especially allergies or sensitivities to latex), and inform the appropriate health care practitioner accordingly.

➤ Obtain a history of the patient's hematopoietic system, as well as results of previously performed laboratory tests, surgical procedures, and other diagnostic procedures. For related laboratory tests, refer to the Hematopoietic System table.

➤ The test should not be performed until a minimum of 10 days after the last dose of any medication containing acetylsalicylic acid.

➤ Obtain a list of the medications the patient is taking, including herbs, nutritional supplements, and nutraceuticals. The requesting health care practitioner and laboratory should be advised if the patient regularly uses these products so their effects can be taken into consideration when reviewing results.

➤ Review the procedure with the patient. Inform the patient that specimen collection takes approximately 2 to 15 minutes. Address concerns about pain related to the procedure. Explain to the patient that there may be some discomfort during the procedure. Inform the patient that scarring, keloid formation, or infection may occur.

➤ There are no food or fluid restrictions unless by medical direction.

Intratest:

➤ Instruct the patient to cooperate fully and to follow directions. Direct the patient to breathe normally and to avoid unnecessary movement.

➤ Observe standard precautions, and follow the general guidelines in Appendix A. Positively identify the patient. Place a blood pressure cuff on the arm above the elbow and inflate to 40 mm Hg. Cleanse the site with alcohol and wait until it is air-dry. Hold skin taut. Avoid superficial veins and use bleeding time device to make a parallel incision about 3 mm deep into the muscular outside area of the forearm distal to the antecubital fossa (in the direction of wrist to elbow). Start stopwatch immediately. At 30-second intervals, blot the incision site, in a clockwise fashion, on the edge of a piece of filter paper. The test concludes when the bleeding stops or if bleeding continues longer than 15 minutes. Bleeding time is determined by adding the total number of blots on the filter paper (30 seconds or 0.5 minutes).

➤ The results are recorded manually or in a computerized system for recall and postprocedure interpretation by the appropriate health care practitioner.

Post-test:

➤ Observe the incision site for bleeding. It may be necessary to place a dressing or butterfly bandage on the site after the test.

➤ Inform the patient with a bleeding disorder of the importance of taking precautions against bruising and bleeding. These precautions may include the use of soft-bristle toothbrush, use of an electric razor, avoidance of constipation, avoidance of acetylsalicylic acid and similar products, and avoidance of intramuscular injections.

➤ A written report of the examination will be sent to the requesting health care practitioner, who will discuss the results with the patient.

➤ Reinforce information given by the patient's health care provider regarding further testing, treatment, or referral to another health care provider. Answer any questions or address any concerns voiced by the patient or family.

➤ Depending on the results of this procedure, additional testing may be performed to evaluate or monitor progression of the disease process and determine the need for a change in therapy. Evaluate test results in relation to the patient's symptoms and other tests performed.

Related laboratory tests:

➤ Related laboratory tests include clot retraction and platelet count.

BLOOD GASES

SYNONYMS/ACRONYM: Arterial blood gases (ABGs), venous blood gases, capillary blood gases, cord blood gases.

SPECIMEN: Whole blood. Specimen volume and collection container may vary with collection method. See Intratest section for specific collection instructions. Specimen should be tightly capped and transported in an ice slurry.

REFERENCE VALUE: (Method: Selective electrodes for pH, pCO_2 and pO_2)

Blood Gas Value (pH)	Birth, Cord, Full Term	Adult/Child
Arterial	7.11–7.36	7.35–7.45
Venous	7.25–7.45	7.32–7.43
Capillary	7.32–7.49	7.35–7.45
Scalp	7.25–7.40	N/A

SI units (conversion factor × 1).

pCO_2	Arterial	SI Units (Conventional Units ×0.133)	Venous	SI Units (Conventional Units ×0.133)	Capillary	SI Units (Conventional Units ×0.133)
Birth, cord, full term	32–66 mm Hg	4.3–8.8 kPa	27–49 mm Hg	3.6–6.5 kPa	—	—
Adult/child	35–45 mm Hg	4.66–5.98 kPa	41–51 mm Hg	5.4–6.8 kPa	26–41 mm Hg	3.5–5.4 kPa

pO_2	Arterial	SI Units (Conventional Units ×0.133)	Venous	SI Units (Conventional Units ×0.133)	Capillary	SI Units (Conversion Units ×0.133)
Birth, cord, full term	8–24 mm Hg	1.1–3.2 kPa	17–41 mm Hg	2.3–5.4 kPa	—	—
Adult/child	80–95 mm Hg	10.6–12.6 kPa	20–49 mm Hg	2.6–6.5 kPa	80–95 mm Hg	10.6–12.6 kPa

HCO₃⁻	Arterial SI Units mmol/L (Conventional Units ×1)	Venous SI Units mmol/L (Conventional Units ×1)	Capillary SI Units mmol/L (Conventional Units ×1)
Birth, cord, full term	17–24 mEq/L	17–24 mEq/L	N/A
Adult/child	18–23 mEq/L	24–28 mEq/L	18–23 mEq/L

O₂ Sat	Arterial	Venous	Capillary
Birth, cord, full term	40–90%	40–70%	—
Adult/child	95–99%	70–75%	95–98%

tCO₂	Arterial SI Units mmol/L (Conventional Units ×1)	Venous SI Units mmol/L (Conventional Units ×1)
Birth, cord, full term	13–22 mEq/L	14–22 mEq/L
Adult/child	22–29 mEq/L	25–30 mEq/L

BE Arterial	SI Units mmol/L (Conventional Units ×1)
Birth, cord, full term	(−10)–(−2) mEq/L
Adult/child	(−2)–(+3) mEq/L

DESCRIPTION & RATIONALE: Blood gas analysis is used to evaluate respiratory function and provide a measure for determining acid-base balance. Respiratory, renal, and cardiovascular system functions are integrated in order to maintain normal acid-base balance. Therefore, respiratory or metabolic disorders may cause abnormal blood gas findings. The blood gas measurements commonly reported are pH, partial pressure of carbon dioxide in the blood (pCO_2), partial pressure of oxygen in the blood (pO_2), bicarbonate (HCO_3^-), O_2 saturation, and base excess (BE) or base deficit (BD).

pH reflects the number of free hydrogen ions (H^+) in the body. A pH less than 7.35 indicates acidosis. A pH greater than 7.45 indicates alkalosis. Changes in the ratio of free hydrogen ions to bicarbonate will result in a compensatory response from the lungs or kidneys to restore proper acid-base balance.

pCO_2 is an important indicator of ventilation. The level of pCO_2 is controlled primarily by the lungs and is referred to as the respiratory component of acid-base balance. The main buffer system in the body is the bicarbonate–carbonic acid system.

Bicarbonate is an important alkaline ion that participates along with other anions such as hemoglobin, proteins, and phosphates to neutralize acids. For the body to maintain proper balance, there must be a ratio of 20 parts bicarbonate to one part carbonic acid (20:1). Carbonic acid level is indirectly measured by pCO_2. Bicarbonate level is indirectly measured by the total carbon dioxide content (tCO_2). The carbonic acid level is not measured directly, but can be estimated because it is 3% of the pCO_2. Bicarbonate can also be calculated from these numbers once the carbonic acid value has been obtained because of the 20:1 ratio. For example, if the pCO_2 was 40, the carbonic acid would be 1.2 (3% $\times$ 40) and the HCO_3^- would be 24 (20 $\times$ 1.2). The main acid in the acid-base system is carbonic acid. It is the metabolic or nonrespiratory component of the acid-base system and is controlled by the kidney. Bicarbonate levels can either be measured directly or estimated from the tCO_2 in the blood. BE/BD reflects the amount of anions available in the blood to help buffer changes in pH. A BD (negative BE) indicates metabolic acidosis, whereas positive BE indicates metabolic alkalosis.

Extremes in acidosis are generally more life threatening than alkalosis. Acidosis can develop either very quickly (e.g., cardiac arrest) or over a longer period of time (e.g., renal failure). Infants can develop acidosis very quickly if they are not kept warm and given enough calories. Children with diabetes tend to go into acidosis more quickly than do adults who have been dealing with the disease over a longer period of time. In many cases a venous or capillary specimen is satisfactory to obtain the necessary information regarding acid-base balance without subjecting the patient to an arterial puncture with its associated risks.

As seen in the table of reference ranges, pO_2 is lower in infants than in children and adults owing to the respective level of maturation of the lungs at birth. pO_2 tends to trail off after age 30 years, decreasing by approximately 3 to 5 mm Hg per decade as the organs age and begin to lose elasticity. There is a formula that can be used to approximate the relationship between age and pO_2:

$$pO_2 = 104 - (age \times 0.27)$$

Like carbon dioxide, oxygen is carried in the body in a dissolved and combined (oxyhemoglobin) form. Oxygen content is the sum of the dissolved and combined oxygen. The oxygen-carrying capacity of the blood indicates how much oxygen could be carried if all the hemoglobin were saturated with oxygen. Percent oxygen saturation is [oxyhemoglobin concentration divided by (oxyhemoglobin concentration+deoxyhemoglobin concentration)] times 100.

Testing on specimens other than arterial blood is often ordered when oxygen measurements are not needed or when the information regarding oxygen can be obtained by noninvasive techniques such as pulse oximetry. Capillary blood is satisfactory for most purposes for pH and pCO_2; the use of capillary pO_2 is limited to the exclusion of hypoxia. Measurements involving oxygen are usually not useful when performed on venous samples; arterial blood is required to accurately measure pO_2 and oxygen saturation. There is considerable evidence that prolonged exposure to high levels of oxygen can result in injury, such as retinopathy of prematurity in infants or the drying of airways in any patient. Monitoring pO_2 from blood gases is especially appropriate under such circumstances. ■

INDICATIONS: This group of tests is used to assess conditions such as asthma, chronic obstructive pulmonary disease (COPD), embolism (e.g., fatty or other embolism) during coronary arterial bypass surgery, and hypoxia. It is also used to assist in the diagnosis of respiratory failure, which is defined as a pO_2 less than 50 mm Hg and pCO_2 greater than 50 mm Hg. Blood gases can be valuable in the management of patients on ventilators or being weaned from ventilators. Blood gas values are used to determine acid-base status, the type of imbalance, and the degree of compensation as summarized in the following section. Restoration of pH to near-normal values is referred to as fully compensated balance. When pH values are moving in the same direction (i.e., increasing or decreasing) as the pCO_2 or HCO_3^-, the imbalance is metabolic. When the pH values are moving in the opposite direction from the pCO_2 or HCO_3^-, the imbalance is caused by respiratory disturbances. To remember this concept, the following mnemonic can be useful: MeTRO = **Metabolic Together, Respiratory Opposite.**

Acid-Base Disturbance	pH	pCO_2	pO_2	HCO_3^-
Respiratory Acidosis				
Uncompensated	Decreased	Increased	Normal	Normal
Compensated	Normal	Increased	Increased	Increased
Respiratory Alkalosis				
Uncompensated	Increased	Decreased	Normal	Normal
Compensated	Normal	Decreased	Decreased	Decreased
Metabolic (Nonrespiratory) Acidosis				
Uncompensated	Decreased	Normal	Decreased	Decreased
Compensated	Normal	Decreased	Decreased	Decreased
Metabolic (Nonrespiratory) Alkalosis				
Uncompensated	Increased	Normal	Increased	Increased
Compensated	Normal	Increased	Increased	Increased

RESULT:
• Acid-base imbalance is determined by evaluating pH, pCO_2, and HCO_3^- values. pH less than 7.35 reflects an acidic state, whereas pH greater than 7.45 reflects alkalosis. pCO_2 and HCO_3^- determine whether the imbalance is respiratory or nonrespiratory. Because a patient may have more than one imbalance and may also be in the process of compensating, the interpretation of blood gas values may not always seem straightforward.

• Respiratory conditions that interfere with normal breathing will cause CO_2 to be retained in the blood. This results in an increase of circulating carbonic acid and a corresponding decrease in pH (respiratory acidosis). Acute respiratory acidosis can occur in acute pulmonary edema, severe respiratory infections, bronchial obstruction, pneumothorax, hemothorax, open chest wounds, opiate poisoning, respiratory depressant drug therapy, and inhalation of air with a high CO_2 content. Chronic respiratory acidosis can be seen in patients with asthma, pulmonary fibrosis, emphysema, bronchiectasis, and respiratory depressant drug therapy. Alternately, respiratory conditions that increase the breathing rate will cause CO_2 to be removed from the alveoli more rapidly than it is being produced. This will result in an alkaline pH. Acute respiratory alkalosis may be seen in anxiety, hysteria, hyperventilation, and pulmonary embolus and with an increase in artificial ventilation. Chronic respiratory alkalosis may be seen in high fever, administration of drugs (e.g., salicylate and sulfa) that stimulate the respiratory system, hepatic coma, hypoxia of high altitude, and central nervous system (CNS) lesions or injury that result in stimulation of the respiratory center.

- Metabolic (nonrespiratory) conditions that cause the excessive formation or decreased excretion of organic or inorganic acids result in metabolic acidosis. Some of these conditions include ingestion of salicylates, ethylene glycol, and methanol, as well as uncontrolled diabetes, starvation, shock, renal disease, and biliary or pancreatic fistula. Metabolic alkalosis results from conditions that increase pH, as can be seen in excessive intake of antacids to treat gastritis or peptic ulcer, excessive administration of HCO_3^-, loss of stomach acid caused by protracted vomiting, cystic fibrosis, or potassium and chloride deficiencies.

Respiratory Acidosis

- Decreased pH:

- Decreased O_2 saturation:

- Increased pCO_2:
  Acute intermittent porphyria

Anemia (severe)
Anorexia
Anoxia
Asthma
Atelectasis
Bronchitis
Bronchoconstriction
Carbon monoxide poisoning
Cardiac disorders
Congenital heart defects
Congestive heart failure
COPD
Cystic fibrosis
Depression of respiratory center
Drugs depressing the respiratory system
Electrolyte disturbances (severe)
Emphysema
Fever
Head injury
Hypercapnia
Hypothyroidism (severe)
Near drowning
Pleural effusion
Pneumonia
Pneumothorax
Poisoning
Poliomyelitis
Pulmonary edema
Pulmonary embolism
Pulmonary tuberculosis
Respiratory distress syndrome (adult and neonatal)
Respiratory failure
Sarcoidosis
Smoking
Tumor

- A decreased pO_2 that increases pCO_2:
  Decreased alveolar gas exchange: cancer, compression or resection of lung, respiratory distress syndrome (newborns), sarcoidosis
  Decreased ventilation or perfusion: asthma, bronchiectasis,

bronchitis, cancer, croup, cystic fibrosis (mucoviscidosis), emphysema, granulomata, pneumonia, pulmonary infarction, shock

Hypoxemia: anesthesia, carbon monoxide exposure, cardiac disorders, high altitudes, near drowning, presence of abnormal hemoglobins

Hypoventilation: cerebrovascular incident, drugs depressing the respiratory system, head injury

Right-to-left shunt: congenital heart disease, intrapulmonary venoarterial shunting

Compensation

- Increased pO_2:
  Hyperbaric oxygenation
  Hyperventilation

- Increased base excess:
  Increased HCO_3^- to bring pH to (near) normal

Respiratory Alkalosis

- Increased pH:

- Decreased pCO_2:
  Anxiety
  CNS lesions or injuries that cause stimulation of the respiratory center
  Excessive artificial ventilation
  Fever
  Head injury
  Hyperthermia
  Hyperventilation
  Hysteria
  Salicylate intoxication

Compensation

- Decreased pO_2:
  Rebreather mask

- Decreased base excess:
  Decreased HCO_3^- to bring pH to (near) normal

Metabolic Acidosis

- Decreased pH:

- Decreased HCO_3^-:

- Decrease base excess:

- Decreased tCO_2:
  Decreased excretion of H^+: acquired (e.g., drugs, hypercalcemia), Addison's disease, diabetic ketoacidosis, Fanconi's syndrome, inherited (e.g., cystinosis, Wilson's disease), renal failure, renal tubular acidosis
  Increased acid intake
  Increased formation of acids: diabetic ketoacidosis, high-fat/low-carbohydrate diets
  Increased loss of alkaline body fluids: diarrhea, excess potassium, fistula
  Renal disease

Compensation

- Decreased pCO_2:
  Hyperventilation

Metabolic Alkalosis

- Increased pH:

- Increased HCO_3^-:

- Increased base excess:

- Increased tCO_2:
  Alkali ingestion (excessive)
  Anoxia
  Gastric suctioning
  Hypochloremic states
  Hypokalemic states
  Potassium depletion: Cushing's disease, diarrhea, diuresis, excessive vomiting, excessive ingestion of licorice, inadequate potassium intake, potassium-losing nephropathy, steroid administration
  Salicylate intoxication
  Shock
  Vomiting

Compensation

- Increased tCO_2:
  Hypoventilation

CRITICAL VALUES: ⚠ Note and immediately report to the health care practitioner any critically increased or decreased values and related symptoms.

Arterial Blood Gas Parameter	Less Than	Greater Than
pH	7.20	7.60
HCO_3^-	10 mmol/L	40 mmol/L
pCO_2	20 mm Hg	67 mm Hg
pO_2	45 mm Hg	

INTERFERING FACTORS:

- Drugs that may cause an increase in HCO_3^- include acetylsalicylic acid (initially), antacids, carbenicillin, carbenoxolone, ethacrynic acid, glycyrrhiza (licorice), laxatives, mafenide, and sodium bicarbonate.

- Drugs that may cause a decrease in HCO_3^- include acetazolamide, acetylsalicylic acid (long term or high doses), citrates, dimethadione, ether, ethylene glycol, fluorides, mercury compounds (laxatives), methylenedioxyamphetamine, paraldehyde, and xylitol.

- Drugs that may cause an increase in pCO_2 include acetylsalicylic acid, aldosterone bicarbonate, carbenicillin, carbenoxolone, corticosteroids, dexamethasone, ethacrynic acid, laxatives (chronic abuse), and x-ray contrast agents.

- Drugs that may cause a decrease in pCO_2 include acetazolamide, acetylsalicylic acid, ethamivan, neuromuscular relaxants (secondary to postoperative hyperventilation), NSD 3004 (arterial long-acting carbonic anhydrase inhibitor), theophylline, tromethamine, and xylitol.

- Drugs that may cause an increase in pO_2 include theophylline and urokinase.

- Drugs that may cause a decrease in pO_2 include althesin, barbiturates, granulocyte-macrophage colony-stimulating factor, isoproterenol, and meperidine.

- Samples for blood gases are obtained by arterial puncture, which carries a risk of bleeding, especially in patients who have bleeding disorders or are taking medications for a bleeding disorder.

- Recent blood transfusion may produce misleading values.

- Specimens with extremely elevated white blood cell counts will undergo misleading decreases in pH resulting from cellular metabolism, if transport to the laboratory is delayed.

- Specimens collected soon after a change in inspired oxygen has occurred will not accurately reflect the patient's oxygenation status.

- Specimens collected within 20 to 30 minutes of respiratory passage suctioning or other respiratory therapy will not be accurate.

- Excessive differences in actual body temperature relative to normal body temperature will not be reflected in the results. Temperature affects the amount of gas in solution. Blood gas analyzers measure samples at 37°C (98.6°F); therefore, if the patient is hyperthermic or hypothermic, it is important to notify the laboratory of the patient's actual body temperature at the time the specimen was collected. Fever will increase actual pO_2 and pCO_2 values; therefore the uncorrected values measured at 37°C will be falsely decreased. Hypothermia decreases actual pO_2 and pCO_2 values; therefore the uncorrected values measured at 37°C will be falsely increased.

- A falsely increased O_2 saturation may occur because of elevated levels of carbon monoxide in the blood.

- O_2 saturation is a calculated parameter based on an assumption of 100% hemoglobin A. Values may be misleading when hemoglobin variants with different oxygen dissociation curves are present. Hemoglobin S will cause a shift to the right, indicating decreased oxygen binding. Fetal hemoglobin and methemoglobin will cause a shift to the left, indicating increased oxygen binding.

- Excessive amounts of heparin in the sample may falsely decrease pH, pCO_2, and pO_2.

- Citrates should never be used as an anticoagulant in evacuated collection tubes for venous blood gas determinations because citrates will cause a marked analytic decrease in pH.

- Air bubbles or blood clots in the specimen are cause for rejection. Air bubbles in the specimen can falsely elevate or decrease the results depending on the patient's blood gas status. If an evacuated tube is used for venous blood gas specimen collection, the tube must be removed from the needle before the needle is withdrawn from the arm or else the sample will be contaminated with room air.

- Specimens should be placed in ice slurry immediately after collection because blood cells continue to carry out metabolic processes in the specimen after it has been removed from the patient. These natural life processes can affect pH, pO_2, pCO_2, and the other calculated values in a short period of time. The cold temperature provided by the ice slurry will slow down but not completely stop metabolic changes occurring in the sample over time. Iced specimens not analyzed within 60 minutes of collection should be rejected for analysis.

Nursing Implications and Procedure

Pretest:

▶ Inform the patient that the test is used to assess acid-base balance and oxygenation level of the blood.

▶ Obtain a history of the patient's complaints, including a list of known allergens (especially allergies or sensitivities to latex and anesthetics), and inform the appropriate health care practitioner accordingly.

▶ Obtain a history of the patient's respiratory system and any bleeding disorders as well as results of previously performed laboratory tests, surgical procedures, and other diagnostic procedures, especially bleeding time, clotting time, complete blood count, partial thromboplastin time, platelets, and prothrombin time. For other related laboratory tests, refer to the Cardiovascular, Genitourinary, and Respiratory System tables.

▶ Note any recent procedures that can interfere with test results.

▶ Obtain a list of the medications the patient is taking, including anticoagulant therapy, acetylsalicylic acid, herbs, and nutraceuticals known to affect coagulation. It is recommended that use of these products be discontinued 14 days before dental or surgical procedures. The requesting health care practitioner and laboratory should be advised if the patient is regularly using these products so their effects can be taken into consideration when reviewing results.

▶ Record the patient's temperature.

➤ Indicate the type of oxygen, mode of oxygen delivery, and delivery rate as part of the test requisition process. Wait 30 minutes after a change in type or mode of oxygen delivery or rate for specimen collection.

➤ ⚠ If the sample is to be collected by radial artery puncture, perform an Allen test before puncture to ensure that the patient has adequate collateral circulation to the hand if thrombosis of the radial artery occurs after arterial puncture. The modified Allen test is performed as follows: extend the patient's wrist over a rolled towel. Ask the patient to make a fist with the hand extended over the towel. Use the second and third fingers to locate the pulses of the ulnar and radial arteries on the palmar surface of the wrist. (The thumb should not be used to locate these arteries because it has a pulse.) Compress both arteries and ask the patient to open and close the fist several times until the palm turns pale. Release pressure on the ulnar artery only. Color should return to the palm within 5 seconds if the ulnar artery is functioning. This is a positive Allen test, and blood gases may be drawn from the radial artery site. The Allen test should then be performed on the opposite hand. The hand to which color is restored fastest has better circulation and should be selected for specimen collection.

➤ Review the procedure with the patient and advise rest for 30 minutes before specimen collection. Be sure to explain to the patient that an arterial puncture may be painful. The site may be anesthetized with 1% to 2% lidocaine before puncture. Assess if the patient has an allergy to local anesthetics, and inform the health care practitioner accordingly.

➤ Inform the patient that specimen collection usually takes 10 to 15 minutes. The person collecting the specimen should be notified beforehand if the patient is receiving anticoagulant therapy, or taking aspirin or other natural products that may prolong bleeding from the puncture site.

➤ There are no food, fluid, or medication restrictions unless by medical direction.

➤ Prepare an ice slurry in a cup or plastic bag to have ready for immediate transport of the specimen to the laboratory.

Intratest:

➤ If the patient has a history of severe allergic reaction to latex, care should be taken to avoid the use of equipment containing latex.

➤ Instruct the patient to cooperate fully and to follow directions. Direct the patient to breathe normally and to avoid unnecessary movement.

➤ Observe standard precautions and follow the general guidelines in Appendix A. Positively identify the patient and label the appropriate tubes with the corresponding patient demographics, date, and time of collection.

➤ The results are recorded manually or in a computerized system for recall and post-procedure interpretation by the appropriate health care practitioner.

Arterial

➤ Perform an arterial puncture and collect the specimen in an air-free heparinized syringe. There is no demonstrable difference in results between samples collected in plastic syringes and samples collected in glass syringes. It is very important that no room air be introduced into the collection container because the gases in the room and in the sample will begin equilibrating immediately. The end of the syringe must be stoppered immediately after the needle is withdrawn and removed. Apply a pressure dressing over the puncture site. Samples should be mixed by gentle rolling of the syringe to ensure proper mixing of the heparin with the sample, which will prevent the formation of small clots leading to rejection of the sample. The tightly capped sample should be placed in an ice slurry immediately after collection. Information on the specimen label can be protected from water in the ice slurry by first placing the specimen in a protective plastic bag. Promptly transport the specimen to the laboratory for processing and analysis.

Venous

➤ Central venous blood is collected in a heparinized syringe.

➤ Venous blood collected percutaneously by venipuncture in a 5-mL green-top (heparin) tube (for adult patients) or a heparinized microtainer (for pediatric patients). The vacuum collection tube must be removed from the needle before the needle is removed from the patient's arm. Apply a pressure dressing over the puncture site. Samples should be mixed by gentle rolling of the syringe to ensure proper mixing of the heparin with the sample, which will prevent the formation of small clots leading to rejection of the sample. The tightly capped sample should be placed in an ice slurry immediately after collection. Information on the specimen label can be protected from water in the ice slurry by first placing the specimen in a protective plastic bag. Promptly transport the specimen to the laboratory for processing and analysis.

Capillary

➤ Perform a capillary puncture and collect the specimen in two 250-µL heparinized capillaries (scalp or heel for neonatal patients) or a heparinized microtainer (for pediatric patients). Observe standard precautions and follow the general guidelines in Appendix A. The capillary tubes should be filled as much as possible and capped on both ends. Some hospitals recommend that metal "fleas" be added to the capillary tube before the ends are capped. During transport, a magnet can be moved up and down the outside of the capillary tube to facilitate mixing and prevent the formation of clots, which would cause rejection of the sample. It is important to inform

the laboratory or respiratory therapy staff of the number of fleas used so the fleas can be accounted for and removed before the sample is introduced into the blood gas analyzers. Fleas left in the sample may damage the blood gas equipment if allowed to enter the analyzer. Microtainer samples should be mixed by gentle rolling of the capillary tube to ensure proper mixing of the heparin with the sample, which will prevent the formation of small clots leading to rejection of the sample. Promptly transport the specimen to the laboratory for processing and analysis.

Cord blood

➤ The sample may be collected directly from the cord, using a syringe. The tightly capped sample should be placed in an ice slurry immediately after collection. Information on the specimen label can be protected from water in the ice slurry by first placing the specimen in a protective plastic bag. Promptly transport the specimen to the laboratory for processing and analysis.

Scalp sample

➤ Samples for scalp pH may be collected anaerobically before delivery in special, scalp-sample collection capillaries and transported immediately to the laboratory for analysis. Some hospitals recommend that fleas be added to the scalp tube before the ends are capped. See preceding section on capillary collection for discussion of fleas.

Post-test:

➤ Pressure should be applied to the puncture site for at least 5 minutes in the unanticoagulated patient and for at least 15 minutes in the case of a patient receiving anticoagulant therapy. Observe puncture site for bleeding or hematoma formation. Apply pressure bandage.

➤ Observe the patient for signs or symptoms of respiratory acidosis, such as dyspnea, headache, tachycardia, pallor, diaphoresis,

➤ apprehension, drowsiness, coma, hypertension, or disorientation.

➤ Teach the patient breathing exercises to assist with the appropriate exchange of oxygen and carbon dioxide.

➤ Administer oxygen, if appropriate.

➤ Teach the patient how to properly use the incentive spirometer device or mininebulizer, if ordered.

➤ Observe the patient for signs or symptoms of respiratory alkalosis, such as tachypnea, restlessness, agitation, tetany, numbness, seizures, muscle cramps, dizziness, or tingling fingertips.

➤ Instruct the patient to breathe deeply and slowly; performing this type of breathing exercise into a paper bag decreases hyperventilation and quickly helps the patient's breathing return to normal.

➤ Observe the patient for signs or symptoms of metabolic acidosis, such as rapid breathing, flushed skin, nausea, vomiting, dysrhythmias, coma, hypotension, hyperventilation, and restlessness.

➤ Observe the patient for signs or symptoms of metabolic alkalosis, such as shallow breathing, weakness, dysrhythmias, tetany, hypokalemia, hyperactive reflexes, and excessive vomiting.

➤ *Nutritional considerations:* Abnormal blood gas values may be associated with diseases of the respiratory system. Malnutrition is commonly seen in patients with severe respiratory disease for reasons including fatigue, lack of appetite, and gastrointestinal distress. Research has estimated that the daily caloric intake required for respiration of patients with COPD is 10 times higher than that of normal individuals. Inadequate nutrition can result in hypophosphatemia, especially in the respirator-dependent patient. During periods of starvation, phosphorus leaves the intracellular space and moves outside the tissue, resulting in dangerously decreased phosphorus levels. Adequate intake of vitamins A and C is also important to prevent pulmonary infection and to decrease the extent of lung tissue damage. The importance of following the prescribed diet should be stressed to the patient and/or caregiver.

➤ Water balance needs to be closely monitored in COPD patients. Fluid retention can lead to pulmonary edema.

➤ A written report of the examination will be sent to the requesting health care practitioner, who will discuss the results with the patient.

➤ Reinforce information given by the patient's health care provider regarding further testing, treatment, or referral to another health care provider. Answer any questions or address any concerns voiced by the patient or family.

➤ Depending on the results of this procedure, additional testing may be performed to evaluate or monitor progression of the disease process and determine the need for a change in therapy. Evaluate test results in relation to the patient's symptoms and other tests performed.

Related laboratory tests:

➤ Related laboratory tests include anion gap, arterial/alveolar oxygen ratio, chloride sweat, culture and smear for mycobacteria, electrolytes, Gram stain, osmolality, phosphorus, pleural fluid analysis, lactic acid, lung biopsy, sputum bacterial culture, sputum cytology, tuberculin skin tests, and white blood cell count and cell differential.

BLOOD GROUPS AND ANTIBODIES

SYNONYMS/ACRONYM: ABO group and Rh typing, blood group antibodies, type and screen, type and crossmatch.

SPECIMEN: Serum (2 mL) collected in a red-top tube or whole blood (2 mL) collected in a lavender-top (EDTA) tube.

REFERENCE VALUE: (Method: FDA-licensed reagents with glass slides, glass tubes, or automated systems) Compatibility (no clumping or hemolysis).

Blood Type	Rh Type (with any ABO)	Other Antibodies That React at 37°C or with Antiglobulin	Other Antibodies That React at Room Temperature or Below
A	Positive	Kell	Lewis
B	Negative	Duffy	P
AB		Kidd	MN
O		S	Cold agglutinins
		s	
		U	

DESCRIPTION & RATIONALE: Blood typing is a series of tests that include the ABO and Rh blood-group system performed to detect surface antigens on red blood cells by an agglutination test and compatibility tests to determine antibodies against these antigens. The major antigens in the ABO system are A and B, although AB and O are also common phenotypes. The patient with A antigens has type A blood; the patient with B antigens has type B blood. The patient with both A and B antigens has type AB blood (universal recipient); the patient with neither A nor B antigens has type O blood (universal donor). Blood type is genetically determined. After 6 months of age, individuals develop serum antibodies that react with A or B antigen absent from their own red blood cells. These are called *anti-A* and *anti-B antibodies.*

In ABO blood typing, the patient's red blood cells mix with anti-A and anti-B sera, a process known as *forward grouping.* The process then reverses, and the patient's serum mixes with type A and B cells in *reverse grouping.*

Generally, only blood with the same ABO and Rh group as the recip-

ient is transfused because the anti-A and anti-B antibodies are strong agglutinins that cause a rapid, complement-mediated destruction of incompatible cells. ABO and Rh testing is also performed as a prenatal screen in pregnant women to identify the risk of hemolytic disease of the newborn. Although most of the anti-A and anti-B activity resides in the immunoglobulin M (IgM) class of immunoglobulins, some activity rests with immunoglobulin G (IgG). Anti-A and anti-B antibodies of the IgG class coat the red blood cells without immediately affecting their viability and can readily cross the placenta, resulting in hemolytic disease of the newborn. Individuals with type O blood frequently have more IgG anti-A and anti-B; thus, ABO hemolytic disease of the newborn will affect infants of type O mothers almost exclusively (unless the newborn is also type O).

Major antigens of the Rh system are D (or Rh$_o$), C, E, c, and e. Individuals whose red blood cells possess D antigen are called Rh-positive; those who lack D antigen are called Rh-negative, no matter what other Rh antigens are present. Individuals who are Rh-negative produce anti-D antibodies when exposed to Rh-positive cells by either transfusions or pregnancy. These anti-D antibodies cross the placenta to the fetus and can cause hemolytic disease of the newborn or transfusion reactions if Rh-positive blood is administered. ∎

INDICATIONS:
- Determine ABO and Rh compatibility of donor and recipient before transfusion (Type and Screen or Crossmatch)
- Determine anti-D antibody titer of Rh-negative mothers after sensitization by pregnancy with an Rh-positive fetus
- Determine the need for a microdose of immunosuppressive therapy (e.g., with RhoGAM) during the first 12 weeks of gestation or a standard dose after 12 weeks' gestation for complications such as abortion, miscarriage, vaginal hemorrhage, ectopic pregnancy, or abdominal trauma
- Determine Rh blood type and perform antibody screen of prenatal patients on initial visit to determine maternal Rh type and to indicate whether maternal red blood cells have been sensitized by any antibodies known to cause hemolytic disease of the newborn, especially anti-D antibody. Rh blood type, antibody screen, and antibody titration (if an antibody has been indentified) will be rechecked at 28 weeks' gestation and prior to injection of prophylactic standard RhoGAM dose for Rh-negative mothers. These tests will also be repeated after delivery of an Rh-positive fetus to an Rh-negative mother and prior to injection of prophylactic standard RhoGAM dose (if maternal Rh-negative blood has not been previously sensitized with Rh-positive cells resulting in a positive anti-D antibody titer). A postpartum blood sample must be evaluated for fetal-maternal bleed on all Rh-negative mothers to determine the need for additional doses of Rh immune globulin. One in 300 cases will demonstrate hemorrhage greater than 15 mL of blood and require additional RhoGAM.
- Identify donor ABO and Rh blood type for stored blood
- Identify maternal and infant ABO and Rh blood types to predict risk of hemolytic disease of the newborn
- Identify the patient's ABO and Rh blood type, especially before a procedure in which blood loss is a threat or blood replacement may be needed

RESULT:
- ABO system: A, B, AB, or O specific to person
- Rh system: positive or negative specific to person
- Cross-matching: compatibility between donor and recipient
- Incompatibility indicated by clumping (agglutination) of red blood cells

Group and Type	Incidence (%)	Alternative Transfusion Group and Type of PACKED CELL UNITS in Order of Preference If Patient's Own Group and Type Not Available
O Positive	37.4	O Negative
O Negative	6.6	O Positive*
A Positive	35.7	A Negative, O Positive, O Negative
A Negative	6.3	O Negative, A Positive,* O Positive*
B Positive	8.5	B Negative, O Positive, O Negative
B Negative	1.5	O Negative, B Positive,* O Positive*
AB Positive	3.4	AB Negative, A Positive, B Positive, A Negative, B Negative, O Positive, O Negative
AB Negative	0.6	A Negative, B Negative, O Negative, AB Positive,* A Positive,* B Positive,* O Positive*
Rh Type		
Rh Positive	85–90	
Rh Negative	10–15	

*If blood units of exact match to the patient's group and type are not available, a switch in ABO blood group is preferable to a change in Rh type. However, in extreme circumstances, Rh-positive blood can be issued to an Rh-negative recipient. It is very likely that the recipient will develop antibodies as the result of receiving Rh-positive red blood cells. Rh antibodies are highly immunogenic, and, once developed, the recipient can only receive Rh-negative blood for subsequent red blood cell transfusion.

CRITICAL VALUES: Note and immediately report to the health care practitioner any signs and symptoms associated with a blood transfusion reaction.

Signs and symptoms of blood transfusion reaction range from mildly febrile to anaphylactic and may include chills, dyspnea, fever, headache, nausea, vomiting, palpitations and tachycardia, chest or back pain, apprehension, flushing, hives, angioedema, diarrhea, hypotension, oliguria, hemoglobinuria, renal failure, sepsis, shock, and jaundice. Complications from disseminated intravascular coagulation (DIC) may also occur.

Possible interventions in mildly febrile reactions would include slowing the rate of infusion, then verifying and comparing patient identification, transfusion requisition, and blood bag label. The patient should be monitored closely for further development of signs and symptoms. Administration of epinephrine may be ordered.

Possible interventions in a more severe transfusion reaction may include immediate cessation of infusion, notification of the health care practitioner, keeping the intravenous (IV) line open with saline or lactated Ringer's solution, collection of

red- and lavender-top tubes for post-transfusion workup, collection of urine, monitoring vital signs every 5 minutes, ordering additional testing if DIC is suspected, maintaining patent airway and blood pressure, and administering mannitol. See Appendix D for a more detailed description of transfusion reactions and potential nursing inteventions.

INTERFERING FACTORS:

- Drugs including levodopa, methyldopa, methyldopate hydrochloride, and cephalexin may cause a false-positive result in Rh typing and in antibody screens.

- Recent administration of blood, blood products, dextran, or IV contrast medium causes cellular aggregation resembling agglutination in ABO typing.

- Contrast material such as iodine, barium, and gadolinium may interfere with testing.

- Abnormal proteins, cold agglutinins, and bacteremia may interfere with testing.

- Testing does not detect every antibody and may miss the presence of a weak antibody.

- History of bone marrow transplant, cancer, or leukemia (may cause discrepancy in ABO typing).

Nursing Implications and Procedure • • • • • • • • • • • •

Pretest:

➤ Inform the patient that the test is used to determine ABO blood group and Rh type.

➤ Obtain a history of the patient's complaints, including a list of known allergens (especially allergies or sensitivities to latex), and inform the appropriate health care practitioner accordingly.

➤ Obtain a history of the patient's immune and hematopoietic systems, as well as results of previously performed laboratory tests, surgical procedures, and other diagnostic procedures. For related laboratory tests, refer to the Immune and Hematopoietic System tables.

➤ Note any recent procedures that could interfere with test results.

➤ Obtain a list of the medications the patient is taking, including herbs, nutritional supplements, and nutraceuticals. The requesting health care practitioner and laboratory should be advised if the patient regularly uses these products so their effects can be taken into consideration when reviewing results.

➤ Review the procedure with the patient. Inform the patient that specimen collection takes approximately 5 to 10 minutes. Address concerns about pain related to the procedure. Explain to the patient that there may be some discomfort during the venipuncture.

➤ *Sensitivity to social and cultural issues,* as well as concern for modesty, is important in providing psychological support before, during, and after the procedure.

➤ There are no food, fluid, or medication restrictions unless by medical direction.

➤ *Make sure a written and informed consent has been signed prior to any transfusion of ABO- and Rh-compatible blood products.*

Intratest:

➤ If the patient has a history of severe allergic reaction to latex, care should be taken to avoid the use of equipment containing latex.

➤ Instruct the patient to cooperate fully and to follow directions. Direct the patient to breathe normally and to avoid unnecessary movement.

➤ Observe standard precautions, and follow the general guidelines in Appendix A. Positively identify the patient, and label the appropriate tubes with the corresponding patient demographics, date, and time of collection. Perform a venipuncture; collect the specimen in 5-mL red- and lavender-top tubes.

➤ Although correct patient identification is important for test specimens, it is crucial when blood is collected for type and crossmatch. Therefore, additional requirements are necessary, including the verification of two unique identifiers that could include any two unique patient demographics such as name, social security number, hospital number, date, or blood bank number on requisition and specimen labels; completing and applying a wristband on the arm with the same information; and placing labels with the same information and blood bank number on blood sample tubes.

➤ Remove the needle, and apply a pressure dressing over the puncture site.

➤ Promptly transport the specimen to the laboratory for processing and analysis.

➤ The results are recorded manually or in a computerized system for recall and postprocedure interpretation by the appropriate health care practitioner.

➤ Inform patient of ABO blood and Rh type, and advise the patient to record the information on a card or other document normally carried.

➤ Inform women who are Rh-negative to inform the health care practitioner of their Rh-negative status if they become pregnant or need a transfusion.

➤ A written report of the examination will be sent to the requesting health care practitioner, who will discuss the results with the patient.

➤ Reinforce information given by the patient's health care provider regarding further testing, treatment, or referral to another health care provider. Answer any questions or address any concerns voiced by the patient or family.

➤ Depending on the results of this procedure, additional testing may be performed to evaluate or monitor progression of the disease process and determine the need for a change in therapy. Evaluate test results in relation to the patient's symptoms and other tests performed.

Post-test:

➤ Observe venipuncture site for bleeding or hematoma formation. Apply paper tape or other adhesive to hold pressure bandage in place, or replace with a plastic bandage.

Related laboratory tests:

➤ Related laboratory tests include direct and indirect antiglobulin, bilirubin, cold agglutinin, gram stain, haptoglobin, immunoglobulin A, Kleihauer-Betke, and urinalysis.

BLOOD POOL IMAGING

SYNONYMS/ACRONYM: Cardiac blood pool scan, ejection fraction study, gated cardiac scan, radionuclide ventriculogram, wall motion study, MUGA.

AREA OF APPLICATION: Heart.

CONTRAST: Intravenous radioactive material.

DESCRIPTION & RATIONALE: Multigated blood pool imaging (MUGA; also known as *cardiac blood pool scan*) is used to diagnose cardiac abnormalities involving the left ventricle and myocardial wall abnormalities by imaging the blood within the cardiac chamber rather than the myocardium. The ventricular blood pool can be imaged during the initial transit of a peripherally injected, intravenous bolus of radionuclide (first-pass technique) or when the radionuclide has reached equilibrium concentration. The patient's electrocardiogram (ECG) is synchronized to the gamma camera imager and computer and thereby termed "gated." For multigated studies, technetium-99m (Tc-99m) pertechnetate is injected after an injection of pyrophosphate, allowing the labeling of circulating red blood cells; Tc-99m sulfur colloid is used for first-pass studies. Studies detect abnormalities in heart wall motion at rest or with exercise, ejection fraction, ventricular dilation, stroke volume, and cardiac output. The MUGA procedure, performed with the heart in motion, is used to obtain multiple images of the heart in contraction and relaxation during an R-to-R cardiac cycle. The resulting images can be displayed in a cinematic mode to visualize cardiac function. Repetitive data acquisitions are possible during graded levels of exercise, usually a bicycle ergometer or handgrip, to assess ventricular functional response to exercise.

After the administration of sublingual nitroglycerin, the MUGA scan can evaluate the effectiveness of the drug on ventricular function. Heart shunt imaging is done in conjunction with a resting MUGA scan to obtain ejection fraction and assess regional wall motion.

First-pass cardiac flow study is done to study heart chamber disorders, including left-to-right and right-to-left shunts, determine both right and left ventricular ejection fractions, and assess blood flow through the great vessels. The study uses a jugular or antecubital vein injection of the radionuclide. ∎

INDICATIONS:

- Aid in the diagnosis of myocardial infarction

- Aid in the diagnosis of true or false ventricular aneurysms

- Aid in the diagnosis of valvular heart disease and determine the optimal time for valve replacement surgery

- Detect left-to-right shunts and determine pulmonary-to-systemic blood flow ratios, especially in children

- Determine cardiomyopathy

- Determine drug cardiotoxicity to stop therapy before development of congestive heart failure

- Determine ischemic coronary artery disease

- Differentiate between chronic obstructive pulmonary disease and left ventricular failure

- Evaluate ventricular size, function, and wall motion after an acute episode or in chronic heart disease

- Quantitate cardiac output by calculating global or regional ejection fraction

RESULT

Normal Findings:

- Normal wall motion, ejection fraction (55% to 65%), coronary blood flow, ventricular size and function, and symmetry in contractions of the left ventricle

Abnormal Findings:
- Abnormal wall motion (akinesia or dyskinesia)
- Cardiac hypertrophy
- Cardiac ischemia
- Enlarged left ventricle
- Infarcted areas are akinetic
- Ischemic areas are hypokinetic
- Myocardial infarction

INTERFERING FACTORS:

This procedure is contraindicated for:
- Testing is contraindicated in patients with hypersensitivity to the radionuclide and in pregnancy and lactation unless the benefits of performing the test greatly outweigh the risks.
- Dipyridamole testing is not performed in patients with anginal pain at rest or in patients with severe atherosclerotic coronary vessels.
- Chemical stress with vasodilators should not be done to patients having asthma; bronchospasm can occur.

Factors that may impair clear imaging:
- Inability of the patient to cooperate or remain still during the procedure because of age, significant pain, or mental status
- Metallic objects within the examination field (e.g., jewelry, body rings), which may inhibit organ visualization and can produce unclear images
- Improper adjustment of the radiographic equipment to accommodate obese or thin patients, which can cause overexposure or underexposure and poor-quality study
- Patients who are very obese, who

may exceed the weight limit for the equipment
- Incorrect positioning of the patient, which may produce poor visualization of the area to be examined

Other considerations:
- Conditions such as chest wall trauma, cardiac trauma, angina that is difficult to control, significant cardiac arrhythmias, or a recent cardioversion procedure may affect test results.
- Atrial fibrillation and extrasystoles invalidate the procedure.
- Suboptimal cardiac stress or patient exhaustion, preventing maximum heart rate testing, will affect results when the procedure is done in conjunction with exercise testing.
- Consultation with a physician should occur before the procedure for radiation safety concerns regarding younger patients or patients who are lactating.
- Risks associated with radiographic overexposure can result from frequent x-ray procedures. Personnel in the room with the patient should wear a protective lead apron, stand behind a shield, or leave the area while the examination is being done. Badges that reveal the level of exposure to radiation should be worn by persons working in the area where the examination is being done.

Nursing Implications and Procedure • • • • • • • • • • •

Pretest:

➤ Inform the patient that the test permits assessment of the pumping action of the heart.

➤ Obtain a history of the patient's complaints and symptoms, including a list of known allergens.

➤ Obtain a history of results of previously performed diagnostic procedures, surgical procedures, and laboratory tests. For related tests, refer to the Cardiovascular System table.

➤ Obtain a list of the patient's current medications.

➤ Explain to the patient that some pain may be experienced during the test, and there may be moments of discomfort. Explain the purpose of the test and how the procedure is performed. Inform the patient that the procedure is performed in a nuclear medicine department, usually by a technologist and support staff, and takes approximately 30 to 60 minutes.

➤ *Sensitivity to cultural and social issues,* as well as concern for modesty, is important in providing psychological support before, during, and after the procedure.

➤ Record the date of the last menstrual period and determine the possibility of pregnancy in perimenopausal women.

➤ Reassure the patient that radioactive material poses no radioactive hazard and rarely produces side effects.

➤ Tell the patient to wear walking shoes for the treadmill or bicycle exercise. Emphasize to the patient the importance of reporting fatigue, pain, or shortness of breath.

➤ Ask the patient to lie very still during the procedure, as movement will produce unclear images.

➤ Restrict food for 4 hours, and medications for 24 hours before the test as ordered by the physician.

Intratest:

➤ Ensure that the patient has complied with dietary preparations and other pretesting restrictions.

➤ Ensure that emergency equipment is readily available during the procedure.

➤ Have the patient remove all jewelry or other metallic objects, put on a hospital gown, and then void.

➤ The patient is placed at rest in the supine position on the scanning table.

➤ Observe standard precautions, and follow the general guidelines in Appendix A.

➤ Expose the chest and attach the ECG leads. Record baseline readings.

➤ The radionuclide is administered intravenously, and, after 1 minute, scanning is done to obtain views of the heart in the anterior, oblique, and lateral views. Between 12 and 64 images are obtained reflecting the motion of heart over the entire cardiac cycle.

➤ When the scan is done under exercise conditions, the patient is assisted onto the treadmill or bicycle ergometer and is exercised to a calculated 80% to 85% of the maximum heart rate as determined by the protocol selected. Images are done at each exercise level and begun immediately after injection of the radionuclide.

➤ If nitroglycerin is given, a cardiologist assessing the baseline MUGA scan injects the medication and records another scan, and then repeats this procedure until blood pressure reaches the desired level.

➤ Patients who cannot exercise are given dipyridamole before the radionuclide is injected.

➤ Patient movement during the procedure will affect the results and make interpretation difficult.

➤ The results are recorded manually on film or in a computerized system for recall and postprocedure interpretation by the appropriate health care practitioner.

Post-test:

➤ Monitor ECG tracings and compare with baseline readings until stable.

➤ Observe the injection site for redness, swelling, or hematoma.

➤ Observe the patient for up to 60 minutes after the procedure for possible reaction to the radionuclide or complications from the procedure.

➤ Advise the patient to drink fluids to eliminate the radionuclide from the body, unless otherwise contraindicated.

➤ If a woman who is breast-feeding must have a nuclear scan, she should not breast-feed the infant until the radionuclide has been eliminated. This could take as long as 3 days. She should be instructed to express the milk and discard it during the 3-day period to prevent cessation of milk production.

➤ Instruct the patient to wash hands with soap and water after each voiding for 24 hours.

➤ Instruct the patient to resume normal activity and diet, unless otherwise indicated.

➤ A written report of the examination will be completed by a health care practitioner who specializes in this branch of medicine. The report will be sent to the requesting health care practitioner, who will discuss the results with the patient.

➤ Inform the patient that abnormalities of the heart scan can indicate the need for further studies, including cardiac catheterization and echocardiography.

➤ If possible, pregnant health care workers should avoid caring for a patient who has had a nuclear medicine procedure for the first 24 hours.

➤ Depending on the results of this procedure, additional testing may be needed to evaluate and determine the need for a change in therapy or progression of the disease process. Evaluate test results in relation to the patient's symptoms and other tests performed.

Related diagnostic tests:

➤ Related diagnostic tests include echocardiogram and myocardial perfusion scan.

BONE MINERAL DENSITOMETRY

SYNONYM/ACRONYMS: Ultrasound densitometry, DEXA, DXA, SXA, QCT, RA.

Dual-energy x-ray absorptiometry (DEXA, DXA): Two x-rays of different energy levels measure bone mineral density and predict risk of fracture.

Single-energy x-ray absorptiometry (SXA): A single-energy x-ray measures bone density at peripheral sites.

Quantitative computed tomography (QCT): QCT is used to examine the lumbar vertebrae. It measures trabecular and cortical bone density. Results are compared to a known standard. This test is the most expensive and involves the highest radiation dose of all techniques.

Radiographic absorptiometry (RA): A standard x-ray of the hand. Results are compared to a known standard.

Ultrasound densitometry: Studies bone mineral content in peripheral densitometry sites such as the heel or wrist. It is not as precise as x-ray techniques, but less expensive than other techniques.

AREA OF APPLICATION: Lumbar spine, heel, hip, wrist, whole body.

CONTRAST: None.

DESCRIPTION & RATIONALE: Bone mineral density (BMD) can be measured at any of several body sites, including the spine, hip, wrist, and heel. Machines to measure BMD include computed tomography (CT), radiographic absorptiometry, ultrasound, single-energy x-ray absorptiometry (SXA), and most commonly, dual-energy x-ray absorptiometry (DEXA). The radiation exposure from SXA and DEXA machines is approximately one-tenth that of a standard chest x-ray.

The BMD values measured by the various techniques cannot be directly compared. Therefore, they are stated in terms of standard deviation (SD) units. The patient's *T-score* is the number of SD units above or below the average BMD in young adults. A *Z-score* is the number of SD units above or below the average value for a person of the same age as the measured patient. For most BMD readings, 1 SD is equivalent to 10% to 12% of the average young-normal BMD value. A T-score of –2.5 is therefore equivalent to a bone mineral loss of 30% when compared to a young adult. ■

INDICATIONS:
Osteoporosis is a condition characterized by low BMD, which results in increased risk of fracture. The National Osteoporosis Foundation estimates that 4 to 6 million postmenopausal women in the United States have osteoporosis, and an additional 13 to 17 million (30% to 50%) have low bone density at the hip. It is estimated that one of every two women will experience a fracture as a result of low bone mineral content in her lifetime. The measurement of BMD gives the best indication of risk for a fracture. The lower the BMD, the greater the risk of fracture. The most common fractures are those of the hip, vertebrae, and distal forearm. Bone mineral loss is a disease of the entire skeleton and not restricted to the areas listed. The effect of the fractures has a wide range, from complete recovery to chronic pain, disability, and possible death.

- Determine the mineral content of bone
- Determine a possible cause of amenorrhea
- Establish a diagnosis of osteoporosis
- Evaluate bone demineralization associated with chronic renal failure
- Evaluate bone demineralization associated with immobilization
- Monitor changes in BMD due to medical problems or therapeutic intervention
- Predict future fracture risk

RESULT
- T-score estimates the actual fracture risk compared to young adults.
- Normal bone mass is designated as a T-score value not less than –1.
- Osteoporosis is defined as a BMD T-score value less than –2.5.
- Low bone mass or osteopenia has T-scores from –1 to –2.5.
- Fracture risk increases as BMD declines from young-normal levels (low T-scores).
- Low Z-scores in older adults can be misleading because low BMD is very common.
- Z-scores estimate fracture risk compared to others of the same age (versus young-normal adults).

INTERFERING FACTORS (OR FACTORS ASSOCIATED WITH INCREASED RISK OF OSTEOPOROSIS):

This procedure is contraindicated for:
- Patients who are pregnant or suspected of being pregnant, unless the potential

benefits of the procedure far outweigh the risks to the fetus and mother.

Factors that may impair clear imaging:

• Inability of the patient to cooperate or remain still during the procedure because of age, significant pain, or mental status

• Metallic objects within the examination field (e.g., jewelry, earrings, and/or dental amalgams), which may inhibit organ visualization and can produce unclear images

• Improper adjustment of the radiographic equipment to accommodate obese or thin patients, which can cause overexposure or underexposure and poor-quality study

• Patients who are very obese, who may exceed the weight limit for the equipment

• Incorrect positioning of the patient, which may produce poor visualization of the area to be examined

Other considerations:

• The use of anticonvulsant drugs, cytotoxic drugs, tamoxifen, glucocorticoid, lithium, or heparin, as well as increased alcohol intake, increased aluminum levels, excessive thyroxin, renal dialysis, or smoking, may affect the test results by either increasing or decreasing the bone mineral content.

• Consultation with a physician should occur before the procedure for radiation safety concerns regarding younger patients or patients who are lactating.

• Risks associated with radiographic overexposure can result from frequent x-ray procedures. Personnel in the room with the patient should wear a protective lead apron, stand behind a shield, or leave the area while the examination is being done. Badges that reveal the level of exposure to radiation should be worn by persons working in the area where the examination is being done.

Nursing Implications and Procedure · · · · · · · · · · ·

As a result of altered BMD, not the BMD testing process:

➤ Vertebral fractures may cause complications including back pain, height loss, and kyphosis.

➤ Limited activity may result including difficulty bending and reaching.

➤ Patient may have poor self-esteem resulting from the cosmetic effects of kyphosis.

➤ Potential restricted lung function may result from fractures.

➤ Fractures may alter abdominal anatomy, resulting in constipation, pain, distention, and diminished appetite.

➤ Potential for a restricted lifestyle may result in depression and other psychological symptoms.

➤ Possible increased dependency on family for basic care may occur.

Pretest:

➤ Obtain a history of the patient's complaints and symptoms, including a list of known allergens.

➤ Obtain a list of the patient's current medications.

➤ Obtain a history of the patient's bone mineral status, as well as results of previously performed diagnostic procedures, surgical procedures, and laboratory tests. For related tests, refer to the Musculoskeletal System table.

➤ Explain the purpose of the test and how the procedure is performed. Inform the patient that the test usually takes 15 minutes.

➤ Make special note of age, previous fractures, thinness, smoking, family history, fall risk, alcohol and coffee intake, age of menopause, and calcium intake.

➤ Record the date of the last menstrual period and determine the possibility of pregnancy in perimenopausal women.

➤ *Sensitivity to cultural and social issues,* as well as concern for modesty, is important in providing psychological support before, during, and after the procedure.

➤ There are no food, fluid, or medication restrictions unless by medical direction.

Intratest:

➤ Clothing is not usually removed unless it contains metal or other items that would interfere with the test.

➤ Patients may want to wear a gown and robe, depending on the area to be examined.

➤ Remove all metal objects from the area to be examined.

➤ Observe standard precautions, and follow the general guidelines in Appendix A.

➤ Direct the patient to breathe normally and to avoid unnecessary movement.

➤ The results are recorded manually on film or in a computerized system for recall and postprocedure interpretation by the appropriate health care practitioner.

Post-test:

➤ Post-test instructions should include instructions for adequate intake of calcium and vitamin D, weight-bearing exercise, and avoidance of tobacco use and alcohol abuse.

➤ Recognize anxiety related to test results, and be supportive of perceived loss of independent function. Discuss the implications of abnormal test results on the patient's lifestyle. Provide teaching and information regarding the clinical implications of the test results, as appropriate.

➤ Reinforce information given by the patient's health care provider regarding further testing, treatment, or referral to another health care provider. Answer any questions or address any concerns voiced by the patient or family.

➤ A written report of the examination will be completed by a health care practitioner specializing in this branch of medicine. The report will be sent to the requesting health care practitioner, who will discuss the results with the patient.

➤ Depending on the results of this procedure, additional testing may be needed to evaluate or monitor progression of the disease process and determine the need for a change in therapy. Evaluate test results in relation to the patient's symptoms, previous BMD values, and other tests performed.

Related diagnostic tests:

➤ Related diagnostic tests include CT of the spine or pelvis, and magnetic resonance imaging of the pelvis.

BONE SCAN

SYNONYMS/ACRONYM: Bone imaging, radionuclide bone scan, bone scintigraphy, whole-body bone scan.

AREA OF APPLICATION: Bone/skeleton.

CONTRAST & RATIONALE: Intravenous radioactive material (diphosphonate compounds), usually combined with technetium-99m.

DESCRIPTION: This nuclear medicine scan assists in diagnosing and determining the extent of primary and metastatic bone disease and bone trauma, and monitors the progression of degenerative disorders. Abnormalities are identified by scanning 1 to 3 hours after the intravenous injection of a radionuclide such as technetium-99m methylene diphosphonate. Areas of increased uptake and activity on the bone scan represent abnormalities unless they occur in normal areas of increased activity, such as the sternum, sacroiliac, clavicle, and scapular joints in adults, and growth centers and cranial sutures in children. The radionuclide mimics calcium physiologically and therefore localizes in bone with an intensity proportional to the degree of metabolic activity. Gallium, magnetic resonance imaging (MRI), or white blood cell scanning can follow a bone scan to obtain a more sensitive study if acute inflammatory conditions such as osteomyelitis or septic arthritis are suspected. In addition, bone scan can detect fractures in patients who continue to have pain, even though x-rays have proved negative. A gamma camera detects the radiation emitted from the injected radioactive material. Whole-body or representative images of the skeletal system can be obtained. ∎

INDICATIONS:
- Aid in the diagnosis of benign tumors or cysts
- Aid in the diagnosis of metabolic bone diseases
- Aid in the diagnosis of osteomyelitis
- Aid in the diagnosis of primary malignant bone tumors (e.g., osteogenic sarcoma, chondrosarcoma, Ewing's sarcoma, metastatic malignant tumors)
- Aid in the detection of traumatic or stress fractures
- Assess degenerative joint changes or acute septic arthritis
- Assess suspected child abuse
- Confirm temporomandibular joint derangement
- Detect Legg-Calvé-Perthes disease
- Determine the cause of unexplained bone or joint pain

- Evaluate the healing process following fracture, especially if an underlying bone disease is present

- Evaluate prosthetic joints for infection, loosening, dislocation, or breakage

- Evaluate tumor response to radiation or chemotherapy

- Identify appropriate site for bone biopsy, lesion excision, or débridement

RESULT

Normal Findings:
- No abnormalities, as indicated by homogeneous and symmetric distribution of the radionuclide throughout all skeletal structures

Abnormal Findings:
- Bone necrosis
- Degenerative arthritis
- Fracture
- Legg-Calvé-Perthes disease
- Metastatic bone neoplasm
- Osteomyelitis
- Paget's disease
- Primary metastatic bone tumors
- Renal osteodystrophy
- Rheumatoid arthritis

INTERFERING FACTORS

This procedure is contraindicated for:
- Patients who are pregnant or suspected of being pregnant, unless the potential benefits of the procedure far outweigh the risks to the fetus and mother

Factors that may impair clear imaging:
- Inability of the patient to cooperate or remain still during the procedure because of age, significant pain, or mental status.

- Metallic objects within the examination field (e.g., jewelry, earrings, and/or dental amalgams), which may inhibit organ visualization and can produce unclear images.

- Improper adjustment of the radiographic equipment to accommodate obese or thin patients, which can cause overexposure or underexposure and poor-quality study.

- Patients who are very obese, who may exceed the weight limit for the equipment.

- Incorrect positioning of the patient, which may produce poor visualization of the area to be examined.

- Retained barium from a previous radiologic procedure may affect the image.

- A distended bladder may obscure pelvic detail.

- Other nuclear scans done within the previous 24 to 48 hours may alter image.

Other considerations:
- The existence of multiple myeloma or thyroid cancer can result in a false-negative scan for bone abnormalities.

- Improper injection of the radionuclide may allow the tracer to seep deep into the muscle tissue, producing erroneous hot spots.

- Consultation with a physician should occur before the procedure for radiation safety concerns regarding younger patients or patients who are lactating.

- Risks associated with radiologic overexposure can result from frequent x-ray procedures. Personnel in the room with the patient should wear a protective lead apron, stand behind a shield, or leave the area while the examination is being done. Badges that reveal the level of exposure to radiation should be worn by persons working in the area where the examination is being done.

Nursing Implications and Procedure • • • • • • • • • • •

Pretest:

➤ Inform the patient that the bone scan can detect bone disease before the disease can be detected with plain film x-rays.

➤ Obtain a history of the patient's complaints and symptoms, including a list of known allergens.

➤ Obtain a history of results of previously performed diagnostic procedures, surgical procedures, and laboratory tests. For related tests, refer to the Musculoskeletal System table.

➤ Obtain a list of the patient's current medications.

➤ Explain to the patient that some pain may be experienced during the test, and there may be moments of discomfort. Explain the purpose of the test and how the procedure is performed. Inform the patient that the procedure is performed in a nuclear medicine department, usually by a technologist and support staff, and takes approximately 30 to 60 minutes.

➤ *Sensitivity to cultural and social issues,* as well as concern for modesty, is important in providing psychological support before, during, and after the procedure.

➤ There are no food, fluid, or medication restrictions unless by medical direction.

➤ Record the date of the last menstrual period and determine the possibility of pregnancy in perimenopausal women.

➤ Inform the patient that the technologist will administer an intravenous injection of the radionuclide, and that he or she will need to return 2 to 3 hours later for the scan.

➤ After the injection, the patient should be encouraged to increase fluid intake and continue normal physical activity.

➤ Instruct the patient to lie very still during the procedure because movement will produce unclear images.

➤ Sedate children who are unable to lie still.

Intratest:

➤ Ask patient to remove jewelry, including watches, and any other metallic objects.

➤ Patients are given a gown, robe, and foot coverings to wear and instructed to void prior to the procedure.

➤ Observe standard precautions, and follow the general guidelines in Appendix A.

➤ Place the patient in a supine position on a flat table with foam wedges to help maintain position and immobilization. The radionuclide is administered intravenously, with images taken every 3 seconds for the first minute over the area to be examined. This will evaluate the blood flow to the area. A blood pool image is then obtained over the area to be examined (usually taking 2 to 3 minutes). A 2- to 3-hour delay is required between the injection and the actual bone scan to improve tumor imaging.

➤ After the delay that allows the radionuclide to be taken up by the bones, multiple images are obtained over the complete skeleton. A camera with a large field of view is used to cover the whole area. Delayed views may be taken up to 24 hours after the injection.

➤ The results are recorded manually on film or in a computerized system for recall and postprocedure interpretation by the appropriate health care practitioner.

➤ The patient may be imaged by single-photon emission computed tomography (SPECT) techniques to further clarify areas of suspicious radionuclide localization.

➤ Instruct the patient to resume usual diet, medication, and activity as directed by the health care practitioner.

➤ Unless contraindicated, advise patient to drink increased amounts of fluids for 24 to 48 hours to eliminate the radionuclide from the body. Tell the patient that radionuclide is eliminated from the body within 24 to 48 hours.

➤ If a woman who is breast-feeding must have a nuclear scan, she should not breast-feed the infant until the radionuclide has been eliminated. This could take as long as 3 days. She should be instructed to express the milk and discard it during the 3-day period to prevent cessation of milk production.

➤ No other radionuclide tests should be scheduled for 24 to 48 hours after this procedure.

➤ Inform the patient to immediately flush the toilet after each voiding after the procedure and to meticulously wash hands with soap and water after each voiding for 48 hours after the procedure.

➤ Tell all caregivers to wear gloves when discarding urine for 48 hours after the procedure. Wash gloved hands with soap and water before removing gloves. Then wash ungloved hands after the gloves are removed.

➤ Instruct the patient in the care and assessment of the injection site. Observe for bleeding, hematoma formation, and inflammation.

➤ A written report of the examination will be completed by a health care practitioner specializing in this branch of medicine. The report will be sent to the requesting health care practitioner, who will discuss the results with the patient.

➤ Depending on the results of this procedure, additional testing may be needed to evaluate or monitor progression of the disease process and determine the need for a change in therapy. Evaluate test results in relation to the patient's symptoms and other tests performed.

Related diagnostic tests:

➤ Related diagnostic tests include computed tomography of the spine or pelvis, and MRI of the pelvis.

BRONCHOSCOPY

. . . .

SYNONYM/ACRONYM: Flexible bronchoscopy.

AREA OF APPLICATION: Bronchial tree, larynx, trachea.

CONTRAST: None.

DESCRIPTION & RATIONALE: This procedure provides direct visualization of the larynx, trachea, and bronchial tree by means of either a rigid or a flexible bronchoscope. A fiberoptic bronchoscope with a light incorporated is guided into the tracheobronchial tree. A local anesthetic may be used to allow the scope to be inserted through the mouth or nose into the trachea and into the bronchi. The patient must breathe during insertion and with the scope in place. The purpose of the procedure is both diagnostic and therapeutic.

The rigid bronchoscope allows visualization of the larger airways, including the lobar, segmental, and subsegmental bronchi, while maintaining effective gas exchange. Rigid bronchoscopy is preferred when large volumes of blood or secretions need to be aspirated, when foreign bodies are to be removed, when large-sized biopsy specimens are to be obtained, and for most bronchoscopies in children.

The flexible fiberoptic bronchoscope has a smaller lumen that is designed to allow for visualization of all segments of the bronchial tree. The accessory lumen of the bronchoscope is used for tissue biopsy, bronchial washings, instillation of anesthetic agents and medications, and to obtain specimens with brushes for cytologic examination. In general, fiberoptic bronchoscopy is less traumatic to the surrounding tissues than the larger rigid bronchoscopes. Fiberoptic bronchoscopy is performed under local anesthesia; patient tolerance is better for fiberoptic bronchoscopy than for rigid bronchoscopy. ■

INDICATIONS:

- Detect end-stage bronchogenic cancer
- Detect lung infections and inflammation
- Determine etiology of persistent cough, hemoptysis, hoarseness, unexplained chest x-ray abnormalities, and/or abnormal cytologic findings in sputum
- Determine extent of smoke-inhalation or other traumatic injury
- Evaluate airway patency; aspirate deep or retained secretions
- Evaluate endotracheal tube placement or possible adverse sequelae to tube placement
- Evaluate possible airway obstruction in patients with known or suspected sleep apnea
- Evaluate respiratory distress and tachypnea in an infant to rule out tracheoesophageal fistula or other congenital anomaly
- Identify bleeding sites and remove clots within the tracheobronchial tree
- Identify hemorrhagic and inflammatory changes in Kaposi's sarcoma
- Intubate patients with cervical spine injuries or massive upper airway edema
- Remove foreign body
- Treat lung cancer through instillation of chemotherapeutic agents, implantation of radioisotopes, or laser palliative therapy

RESULT

Normal Findings:
- Normal larynx, trachea, bronchi, bronchioles, and alveoli

Abnormal Findings:
- Abscess
- Bronchial diverticulum

- Bronchial stenosis
- Bronchogenic cancer
- Coccidioidomycosis, histoplasmosis, blastomycosis, phycomycosis
- Foreign bodies
- Inflammation
- Interstitial pulmonary disease
- Opportunistic lung infections (e.g., pneumocystitis, nocardia, cytomegalovirus)
- Strictures
- Tuberculosis
- Tumors

INTERFERING FACTORS

This procedure is contraindicated for:
- Patients with bleeding disorders, especially those associated with uremia and cytotoxic chemotherapy
- Patients with pulmonary hypertension
- Patients with cardiac conditions or dysrhythmias
- Patients with disorders that limit extension of the neck
- Patients with severe obstructive tracheal conditions
- Patients with or having the potential for respiratory failure; introduction of the bronchoscope alone may cause a 10 to 20 mm Hg drop in PaO_2

Factors that may impair a complete examination:
- Inability of the patient to cooperate or remain still during the procedure because of age, significant pain, or mental status
- Metallic objects within the examination field (e.g., jewelry, earrings, and/or dental amalgams), which may inhibit

organ visualization and can produce unclear images
- Improper adjustment of the radiographic equipment to accommodate obese or thin patients, which can cause overexposure or underexposure and poor-quality study
- Patients who are very obese, who may exceed the weight limit for the equipment
- Incorrect positioning of the patient, which may produce poor visualization of the area to be examined

Other considerations:
- Hypoxemic or hypercapnic states require continuous oxygen administration.
- Failure to follow dietary restrictions before the procedure may cause the procedure to be canceled or repeated.

Nursing Implications and Procedure • • • • • • • • • • •

Pretest:

➤ Inform the patient that the procedure assesses the lungs and respiratory system.

➤ Obtain a history of the patient's complaints or symptoms, including a list of known allergens, especially allergies or sensitivities to latex and anesthetics.

➤ Obtain a history of the patient's immune and respiratory systems, any bleeding disorders, and results of previously performed laboratory tests (especially bleeding time, complete blood count, partial thromboplastin time, platelets, and prothrombin time), surgical procedures, and other diagnostic procedures. For related laboratory tests, refer to the Immune and Respiratory System tables.

➤ Note any recent procedures that can

interfere with test results. Ensure that this procedure is performed before an upper gastrointestinal study or barium swallow.

➤ Record the date of the last menstrual period and determine the possibility of pregnancy in perimenopausal women.

➤ Obtain a list of the medications the patient is taking, including anticoagulant therapy, acetylsalicylic acid, herbs, nutritional supplements, and nutraceuticals, especially those known to affect coagulation. It is recommended that use be discontinued 14 days before dental or surgical procedures. The requesting health care practitioner and laboratory should be advised if the patient regularly uses these products so that their effects can be taken into consideration when reviewing results.

➤ Review the procedure with the patient. Instruct that prophylactic antibiotics may be administered prior to the procedure. Address concerns about pain related to the procedure. Explain that a sedative and/or analgesia may be administered to promote relaxation and reduce discomfort prior to the bronchoscopy. Explain to the patient that some pain may be experienced during the test, and there may be moments of discomfort. Atropine is usually given before bronchoscopy examinations to reduce bronchial secretions and prevent vagally induced bradycardia. Meperidine (Demerol) or morphine may be given as a sedative. Lidocaine is sprayed in the patient's throat to reduce discomfort caused by the presence of the tube. Inform the patient that the procedure is performed in a GI lab or radiology department, under sterile conditions, by a health care practitioner specializing in this procedure. The procedure usually takes about 30 to 60 minutes to complete.

➤ *Sensitivity to cultural and social issues,* as well as concern for modesty, is important in providing psychological support before, during, and after the procedure.

➤ Explain that an intravenous (IV) line will be inserted to allow infusion of IV fluids, antibiotics, anesthetics, and analgesics.

➤ Instruct the patient that nothing should be taken by mouth for 6 to 8 hours prior to a general anesthetic.

➤ Have the patient void before the procedure.

➤ *Make sure a written and informed consent has been signed prior to the procedure and before administering any medications.*

Intratest:

➤ Ensure that the patient has complied with dietary restrictions; assure that food has been restricted for at least 6 to 8 hours prior to the procedure. Ensure that the patient has removed (jewelry, dentures, all external metallic objects, etc.) prior to the procedure.

➤ Ensure that anticoagulant therapy has been withheld for the appropriate amount of days prior to the procedure. Amount of days to withhold medication is dependent on the type of anticoagulant. Notify the health care practitioner if patient anticoagulant therapy has not been withheld.

➤ Have emergency equipment readily available. Keep resuscitation equipment on hand in the case of respiratory impairment or laryngospasm after the procedure.

➤ Avoid using morphine sulfate in those with asthma or other pulmonary disease. This drug can further exacerbate bronchospasms and respiratory impairment.

➤ Observe standard precautions, and follow the general guidelines in Appendix A. Positively identify the patient, and label the appropriate collection containers with the corresponding patient demographics, date and time of collection, and site location, especially left or right lung.

➤ Have patient remove dentures, contact lenses, eyeglasses, and jewelry. Notify the physician if the patient has permanent crowns on teeth.

Have the patient remove clothing and change into a gown for the procedure.

➤ Assist the patient to a comfortable position, and direct the patient to breath normally during the beginning of the general anesthesia. Instruct the patient to cooperate fully and to follow directions. Direct the patient to breathe normally and to avoid unnecessary movement during the local anesthetic and the procedure.

➤ Record baseline vital signs and continue to monitor throughout the procedure. Protocols may vary from facility to facility.

➤ After the administration of general or local anesthesia, shave and cleanse the site with an antiseptic solution, and drape the area with sterile towels.

Rigid bronchoscopy:

➤ The patient is placed in the supine position and a general anesthetic is administered. The patient's neck is hyperextended, and the lightly lubricated bronchoscope is inserted orally and passed through the glottis. The patient's head is turned or repositioned to aid visualization of various segments.

➤ After inspection, the bronchial brush, suction catheter, biopsy forceps, laser, and electrocautery devices are introduced to obtain specimens for cytologic or microbiologic study or for therapeutic procedures.

➤ If a bronchial washing is performed, small amounts of solution are instilled into the airways and removed.

➤ After the procedure, the bronchoscope is removed and the patient is placed in a side-lying position with the head slightly elevated.

Fiberoptic bronchoscopy:

➤ Provide mouth care to reduce oral bacterial flora.

➤ The patient is placed in a sitting position while the tongue and oropharynx is sprayed or swabbed with local anesthetic. Provide an emesis basin for the increased saliva and encourage the patient to spit out the saliva because the gag reflex may be impaired. When loss of sensation is adequate, the patient is placed in a supine or side-lying position. The fiberoptic scope can be introduced through the nose, the mouth, an endotracheal tube, a tracheostomy tube, or a rigid bronchoscope. Most common insertion is through the nose. Patients with copious secretions or massive hemoptysis, or in whom airway complications are more likely, may be intubated before the bronchoscopy. Additional local anesthetic is applied through the scope as it approaches the vocal cords and the carina, eliminating reflexes in these sensitive areas. The fiberoptic approach allows visualization of airway segments without having to move the patient's head through various positions.

➤ After visual inspection of the lungs, tissue samples are collected from suspicious sites by bronchial brush or biopsy forceps to be used for cytologic and microbiologic studies.

➤ After the procedure, the bronchoscope is removed. Patients who had local anesthesia are placed in a semi-Fowler's position to recover.

General:

➤ Monitor the patient for complications related to the procedure (e.g., allergic reaction, anaphylaxis).

➤ Place tissue samples in properly labeled specimen containers containing formalin solution, and promptly transport the specimen to the laboratory for processing and analysis.

➤ The results are recorded manually or in a computerized system for recall and postprocedure interpretation by the appropriate health care practitioner.

Post-test:

➤ Instruct the patient to resume preoperative diet, as directed by the health care practitioner. Assess the patient's ability to swallow before allowing the patient to attempt liquids or solid foods.

➤ Inform the patient that he or she may experience some throat soreness and hoarseness. Instruct patient to treat throat discomfort with lozenges and warm gargles when the gag reflex returns.

➤ Monitor vital signs and neurologic status every 15 minutes for 1 hour, then every 2 hours for 4 hours, and then as ordered by the health care practitioner. Monitor temperature every 4 hours for 24 hours. Compare with baseline values. Notify the health care practitioner if temperature changes. Protocols may vary from facility to facility.

➤ Emergency resuscitation equipment should be readily available if the vocal cords become spastic after intubation.

➤ Observe for delayed allergic reactions, such as rash, urticaria, tachycardia, hyperpnea, hypertension, palpitations, nausea, or vomiting.

➤ Observe the patient for hemoptysis, difficulty breathing, cough, air hunger, excessive coughing, pain, or absent breathing sounds over the affected area. Report to health care provider.

➤ Evaluate the patient for symptoms indicating the development of pneumothorax, such as dyspnea, tachypnea, anxiety, decreased breathing sounds, or restlessness. A chest x-ray may be ordered to check for the presence of this complication.

➤ Evaluate the patient for symptoms of empyema, such as fever, tachycardia, malaise, or elevated white blood cell count.

➤ Observe the patient's sputum for blood if a biopsy was taken, because large amounts of blood may indicate the development of a problem; a small amount of streaking is expected. Evaluate the patient for signs of bleeding such as tachycardia, hypotension, or restlessness.

➤ Assess for nausea and pain. Administer antiemetic and analgesic medications as needed and as directed by the health care practitioner.

➤ Administer antibiotic therapy if ordered. Remind the patient of the importance of completing the entire course of antibiotic therapy, even if signs and symptoms disappear before completion of therapy.

➤ A written report of the examination will be completed by a health care practitioner specializing in this branch of medicine. The report will be sent to the requesting health care practitioner, who will discuss the results with the patient.

➤ Recognize anxiety related to test results. Discuss the implications of abnormal test results on the patient's lifestyle. Provide teaching and information regarding the clinical implications of the test results, as appropriate. Educate the patient regarding access to counseling services.

➤ Reinforce information given by the patient's health care provider regarding further testing, treatment, or referral to another health care provider. Instruct the patient to use lozenges or gargle for throat discomfort. Inform the patient of smoking cessation programs as appropriate. Malnutrition is commonly seen in patients with severe respiratory disease for numerous reasons, including fatigue, lack of appetite, and gastrointestinal distress. Adequate intake of vitamins A and C is also important to prevent pulmonary infection and to decrease the extent of lung tissue damage. The importance of following the prescribed diet should be stressed to the patient/caregiver. Educate the patient regarding access to counseling services, as appropriate. Answer any questions or address any concerns voiced by the patient or family.

➤ Instruct the patient in the use of any ordered medications. Explain the importance of adhering to the therapy regimen. As appropriate, instruct the patient in significant side effects and systemic reactions associated with the prescribed medication. Encourage him or her to review corresponding literature provided by a pharmacist.

➤ Depending on the results of this procedure, additional testing may be needed to evaluate or monitor progression of the disease process and determine the need for a change in therapy. Evaluate test results in relation to the patient's symptoms and other tests performed.

Related laboratory tests:

➤ Related laboratory and diagnostic tests include arterial/alveolar oxygen ratio, anti–glomerular basement membrane antibody, blood gases, chest x-ray, complete blood count, computed tomography of the thorax, magnetic resonance imaging of the chest, lung scan, gram stain, culture and smear mycobacteria, culture sputum, culture from gel cytology sputum.

B-TYPE NATRIURETIC PEPTIDE AND PRO-B-TYPE NATRIURETIC PEPTIDE

· ·

SYNONYMS/ACRONYMS: BNP and Pro-BNP.

SPECIMEN: Plasma (1 mL) collected in a plastic, lavender-top (EDTA) tube.

REFERENCE VALUE: (Method: Immunochemiluminometric for BNP; immuno(electro)chemiluminescence for Pro-BNP)

	BNP	Pro-BNP (N-Terminal)
Male	Less than 100 pg/mL	Less than or equal to 60 pg/mL
Female	Less than 100 pg/mL	12–150 pg/mL

DESCRIPTION & RATIONALE: The peptides B-type natriuretic peptide (BNP) and atrial natriuretic peptide (ANP) assist in the regulation of fluid balance and blood pressure. BNP, Pro-BNP, and ANP are useful markers in the diagnosis of congestive heart failure. BNP or brain natriuretic peptide, first isolated in the brain of pigs, is a neurohormone synthesized primarily in the ventricles of the human heart in response to increases in ventricular pressure and volume. Circulating levels of BNP and Pro-BNP increase in proportion to the severity of heart failure. ■

INDICATIONS:

* Assist in determining the prognosis and therapy of patients with heart failure
* Assist in the diagnosis of heart failure
* Assist in differentiating heart failure from pulmonary disease
* Screen for left ventricular dysfunction and therefore need for echocardiography for further assessment

RESULT

Increased in:

* Cardiac inflammation (myocarditis, cardiac allograft rejection)
* Cirrhosis
* Cushing's syndrome
* Heart failure
* Kawasaki disease
* Left ventricular hypertrophy
* Myocardial infarction
* Primary hyperaldosteronism
* Primary pulmonary hypertension
* Renal failure
* Ventricular dysfunction

Decreased in: N/A

CRITICAL VALUES: N/A

Nursing Implications and Procedure • • • • • • • • • • •

Pretest:

▶ Inform the patient that the test is primarily used to identify congestive heart failure.

▶ Obtain a history of the patient's complaints, including a list of known allergens (especially allergies or sensitivities to latex), and inform the appropriate health care practitioner accordingly.

▶ Obtain a history of the patient's cardiovascular system and results of previously performed laboratory tests, surgical procedures, and other diagnostic procedures. For related laboratory tests, refer to the Cardiovascular System table.

▶ Obtain a list of the medications the patient is taking, including herbs, nutritional supplements, and nutraceuticals. The requesting health care practitioner and laboratory should be advised if the patient regularly uses these products so that their effects can be taken into consideration when reviewing results.

▶ Review the procedure with the patient. Inform the patient that specimen collection takes approximately 5 to 10 minutes. Address concerns about pain related to the procedure. Explain to the patient that there may be some discomfort during the venipuncture.

▶ *Sensitivity to social and cultural issues,* as well as concern for modesty, is important in providing psychological support before, during, and after the procedure.

▶ There are no food, fluid, or medication restrictions unless by medical direction.

Intratest:

▶ If the patient has a history of severe allergic reaction to latex, care should be taken to avoid the use of equipment containing latex.

▶ Instruct the patient to cooperate fully and to follow directions. Direct the patient to breathe normally and to avoid unnecessary movement.

▶ Observe standard precautions, and follow the general guidelines in Appendix A. Positively identify the patient, and label the appropriate tubes with the corresponding patient demographics, date, and time of collection. Perform a venipuncture; collect the specimen in a 5-mL plastic, lavender-top tube.

▶ Remove the needle, and apply a pressure dressing over the puncture site.

▶ Promptly transport the specimen to the laboratory for processing and analysis.

The results are recorded manually or in a computerized system for recall and postprocedure interpretation by the appropriate health care practitioner.

Post-test:

> Observe venipuncture site for bleeding or hematoma formation. Apply paper tape or other adhesive to hold pressure bandage in place, or replace with a plastic bandage.

> *Treatment considerations for CHF:* Ensure that the patient (if not currently taking) is placed on an angiotensin-converting enzyme inhibitor, β-blocker, and diuretic; and monitored with daily weights.

> *Nutritional considerations:* Instruct patients to consume a variety of foods within the basic food groups, eat foods high in potassium when taking diuretics, eat a diet high in fiber (25 to 35 g/d), maintain a healthy weight, be physically active, limit salt intake to 2000 mg/d, limit alcohol intake, and be a nonsmoker.

> *Nutritional considerations:* Foods high in potassium include citrus fruits such as bananas, strawberries, oranges; cantaloupe; green leafy vegetables such as spinach and broccoli; dried fruits such as dates, prunes, and raisins; legumes such as peas and pinto beans; nuts and whole grains.

> A written report of the examination will be completed by a health care practitioner specializing in this branch of medicine. The report will be sent to the requesting health care practitioner, who will discuss the results with the patient.

> Reinforce information given by the patient's health care provider regarding further testing, treatment, or referral to another health care provider. Answer any questions or address any concerns voiced by the patient or family.

> Depending on the results of this procedure, additional testing may be performed to evaluate or monitor progression of the disease process and determine the need for a change in therapy. Evaluate test results in relation to the patient's symptoms and other tests performed.

Related laboratory tests:

> Related laboratory tests include aspartate aminotransferase, atrial natriuretic factor, calcium and ionized calcium, C-reactive protein, creatine kinase and isoenzymes, glucose, homocysteine, lactate dehydrogenase and isoenzymes, magnesium, myoglobin, potassium, and tropinin.

> A Rapid BNP point-of-care immunoassay may be performed, in which a venous blood sample is collected, placed on a strip, and inserted into a device that measures BNP. Results are completed in 10 to 15 minutes.

CA 125

SYNONYMS/ACRONYM: Carbohydrate antigen 125, cancer antigen 125.

SPECIMEN: Serum (1 mL) collected in a red-top tube.

REFERENCE VALUE: (Method: Enzyme immunoassay)

Conventional Units	SI Units (Conventional Units ×1)
Less than 35 U/mL	Less than 35 kU/L

DESCRIPTION & RATIONALE: CA 125, a glycoprotein present in normal endometrial tissue, appears in the blood when natural endometrial protective barriers are destroyed, as occurs in cancer or endometriosis. Persistently rising levels indicate a poor prognosis, but absence of the tumor marker does not rule out tumor presence. Levels may also rise in pancreatic, liver, colon, breast, and lung cancers. It is not useful as a screening test when used alone. ■

INDICATIONS:
• Assist in the diagnosis of carcinoma of the cervix and endometrium

• Assist in the diagnosis of ovarian cancer

• Monitor response to treatment of ovarian cancer

RESULT

Increased in:
• Breast, colon, endometrial, liver, lung, ovarian, and pancreatic cancer

• Endometriosis

• First-trimester pregnancy

• Menses

• Ovarian abscess

• Pelvic inflammatory disease

• Peritonitis

Decreased in:

• Effective therapy or removal of the tumor

CRITICAL VALUES: N/A

INTERFERING FACTORS: N/A

Nursing Implications and Procedure • • • • • • • • • •

Pretest:

➤ Inform the patient that the test is primarily used in the serial monitoring of ovarian cancers.

➤ Obtain a history of the patient's complaints, including a list of known allergens (especially allergies or sensitivities to latex), and inform the appropriate health care practitioner accordingly.

➤ Obtain a history of the patient's immune and reproductive systems, as well as results of previously performed laboratory tests, surgical procedures, and other diagnostic procedures. For related laboratory tests, refer to the Immune and Reproductive System tables.

➤ Obtain a list of the medications the patient is taking, including herbs, nutritional supplements, and nutraceuticals. The requesting health care practitioner and laboratory should be advised if the patient regularly uses these products so that their effects can be taken into consideration when reviewing results.

➤ Review the procedure with the patient. Inform the patient that specimen collection takes approximately 5 to 10 minutes. Address concerns about pain related to the procedure. Explain to the patient that there may be some discomfort during the venipuncture.

➤ There are no food, fluid, or medication restrictions unless by medical direction.

Intratest:

➤ If the patient has a history of severe allergic reaction to latex, care should be taken to avoid the use of equipment containing latex.

➤ Instruct the patient to cooperate fully and to follow directions. Direct the patient to breathe normally and to avoid unnecessary movement.

➤ Observe standard precautions, and follow the general guidelines in Appendix A. Positively identify the patient, and label the appropriate tubes with the corresponding patient demographics, date, and time of collection. Perform a venipuncture; collect the specimen in a 5-mL red-top tube.

➤ Remove the needle, and apply a pressure dressing over the puncture site.

➤ Promptly transport the specimen to the laboratory for processing and analysis.

➤ The results are recorded manually or in a computerized system for recall and postprocedure interpretation by the appropriate health care practitioner.

Post-test:

➤ Observe venipuncture site for bleeding or hematoma formation. Apply paper tape or other adhesive to hold pressure bandage in place, or replace with a plastic bandage.

➤ A written report of the examination will be sent to the requesting health care practitioner, who will discuss the results with the patient.

➤ Recognize anxiety related to test results, and be supportive of fear of shortened life expectancy. Discuss the implications of abnormal test results on the patient's lifestyle. Provide teaching and information regarding the clinical implications of the test results, as appropriate. Educate the patient regarding access to counseling services.

➤ Reinforce information given by the patient's health care provider regarding further testing, treatment, or referral to another health care provider. Inform the patient that serial specimens may be requested at regular intervals. Answer any questions or address any concerns voiced by the patient or family.

➤ Depending on the results of this procedure, additional testing may be performed to evaluate or monitor progression of the disease process and determine the need for a change in therapy. Evaluate test results in relation to the patient's symptoms and other tests performed.

Related laboratory tests:

➤ Related laboratory tests include breast biopsy, CA 15-3, CA 19-9, and carcinoembryonic antigen (CEA).

CA 15-3

. . . .

SYNONYMS/ACRONYM: Carbohydrate antigen 15-3, cancer antigen 15-3.

SPECIMEN: Serum (1 mL) collected in a red-top tube.

REFERENCE VALUE: (Method: Microparticle immunoassay, MEIA)

Conventional Units	SI Units (Conventional Units ×1)
Less than 30 U/mL	Less than 30 kU/L

DESCRIPTION & RATIONALE: CA 15-3 monitors patients for recurrence of breast carcinoma. CA 27.29 (reference range less than 38 U/mL), a more recently approved protein marker, is replacing CA 15-3 in some reference laboratories. ∎

INDICATIONS: Monitor recurrent carcinoma of the breast

RESULT

Increased in: Recurrent carcinoma of the breast

Decreased in: Effective therapy or removal of the tumor

CRITICAL VALUES: N/A

INTERFERING FACTORS: N/A

Nursing Implications and Procedure • • • • • • • • • • •

Pretest:

➤ Inform the patient that the test is used to monitor progression of therapy for various tumors.

➤ Obtain a history of the patient's complaints, including a list of known allergens (especially allergies or sensitivities to latex), and inform the appropriate health care practitioner accordingly.

➤ Obtain a history of the patient's immune and reproductive systems, as well as results of previously performed laboratory tests, surgical procedures, and other diagnostic procedures. For related laboratory tests, refer to the Immune and Reproductive System tables.

➤ Obtain a list of the medications the patient is taking, including herbs, nutritional supplements, and nutraceuticals. Advise the requesting health care practitioner and laboratory if the patient regularly uses these products so that their effects can be taken into consideration when reviewing results.

➤ Review the procedure with the patient. Inform the patient that specimen collection takes approximately 5 to 10 minutes. Address concerns about pain related to the procedure. Explain to the patient that there may be some discomfort during the venipuncture.

➤ There are no food, fluid, or medication restrictions unless by medical direction.

Intratest:

➤ If the patient has a history of severe allergic reaction to latex, care should be taken to avoid the use of equipment containing latex.

➤ Instruct the patient to cooperate fully and to follow directions. Direct the patient to breathe normally and to avoid unnecessary movement.

➤ Observe standard precautions, and follow the general guidelines in Appendix A. Positively identify the patient, and label the appropriate tubes with the corresponding patient demographics, date, and time of collection. Perform a venipuncture; collect the specimen in a 5-mL red-top tube.

➤ Remove the needle, and apply a pressure dressing over the puncture site.

➤ Promptly transport the specimen to the laboratory for processing and analysis.

➤ The results are recorded manually or in a computerized system for recall and postprocedure interpretation by the appropriate health care practitioner.

Post-test:

➤ Observe venipuncture site for bleeding or hematoma formation. Apply paper tape or other adhesive to hold pressure bandage in place, or replace with a plastic bandage.

➤ A written report of the examination will be sent to the requesting health care practitioner, who will discuss the results with the patient.

➤ Recognize anxiety related to test results and be supportive of perceived loss of independence and fear of shortened life expectancy. Discuss the implications of abnormal test results on the patient's lifestyle. Provide teaching and information regarding the clinical implications of the test results, as appropriate.

➤ Reinforce information given by the patient's health care provider regarding further testing, treatment, or referral to another health care provider. Inform the patient that serial specimens may be requested at regular intervals. Answer any questions or address any concerns voiced by the patient or family.

➤ Depending on the results of this procedure, additional testing may be performed to evaluate or monitor progression of the disease process and determine the need for a change in therapy. Evaluate test results in relation to the patient's symptoms and other tests performed.

Related laboratory tests:

➤ Related laboratory tests include breast biopsy, CA 125, and carcinoembryonic antigen.

CA 19-9

• •

SYNONYMS/ACRONYM: Carbohydrate antigen 19-9, cancer antigen 19-9.

SPECIMEN: Serum (1 mL) collected in a red-top tube.

REFERENCE VALUE: (Method: Immunoradiometric)

Conventional Units	SI Units (Conventional Units ×1)
Less than 37 U/mL	Less than 37 kU/L

DESCRIPTION & RATIONALE: CA 19–9 is used to monitor patients with various types of cancer. ∎

INDICATIONS:
• Monitor effectiveness of therapy
• Monitor gastrointestinal, head and neck, and gynecologic carcinomas

• Predict recurrence of cholangiocarcinoma

• Predict recurrence of stomach, pancreatic, colorectal, gallbladder, liver, and urothelial carcinomas

RESULT

Increased in:

• Gastrointestinal, head and neck, and gynecologic carcinomas

• Recurrence of stomach, pancreatic, colorectal, gallbladder, liver, and urothelial carcinomas

• Recurrence of cholangiocarcinoma

Decreased in:

• Effective therapy or removal of the tumor

CRITICAL VALUES: N/A

INTERFERING FACTORS:

• Recent radioactive scans or radiation within 1 week before the test can interfere with test results when radioimmunoassay is the test method.

Nursing Implications and Procedure • • • • • • • • • • •

Pretest:

➤ Inform the patient that the test is used to monitor progression of therapy for various tumors.

➤ Obtain a history of the patient's complaints, including a list of known allergens (especially allergies or sensitivities to latex), and inform the appropriate health care practitioner accordingly.

➤ Obtain a history of the patient's gastrointestinal and immune systems, as well as results of previously performed laboratory tests, surgical procedures, and other diagnostic procedures. For related laboratory tests, refer to the Gastrointestinal and Immune System tables.

➤ Note any recent procedures that can interfere with test results.

➤ Obtain a list of the medications the patient is taking, including herbs, nutritional supplements, and nutraceuticals. The requesting health care practitioner and laboratory should be advised if the patient regularly uses these products so that their effects can be taken into consideration when reviewing results.

➤ Review the procedure with the patient. Inform the patient that specimen collection takes approximately 5 to 10 minutes. Address concerns about pain related to the procedure. Explain to the patient that there may be some discomfort during the venipuncture.

➤ There are no food, fluid, or medication restrictions unless by medical direction.

Intratest:

➤ If the patient has a history of severe allergic reaction to latex, care should be taken to avoid the use of equipment containing latex.

➤ Instruct the patient to cooperate fully and to follow directions. Direct the patient to breathe normally and to avoid unnecessary movement.

➤ Observe standard precautions, and follow the general guidelines in Appendix A. Positively identify the patient, and label the appropriate tubes with the corresponding patient demographics, date, and time of collection. Perform a venipuncture; collect the specimen in a 5-mL red-top tube.

➤ Remove the needle, and apply a pressure dressing over the puncture site.

➤ Promptly transport the specimen to the laboratory for processing and analysis.

➤ The results are recorded manually or in a computerized system for recall and postprocedure interpretation by the appropriate health care practitioner.

Post-test:

➤ Observe venipuncture site for bleeding or hematoma formation. Apply

paper tape or other adhesive to hold pressure bandage in place, or replace with a plastic bandage.

➤ A written report of the examination will be sent to the requesting health care practitioner, who will discuss the results with the patient.

➤ Recognize anxiety related to test results and be supportive of perceived loss of independence and fear of shortened life expectancy. Discuss the implications of abnormal test results on the patient's lifestyle. Provide teaching and information regarding the clinical implications of the test results, as appropriate. Educate the patient regarding access to counseling services.

➤ Reinforce information given by the patient's health care provider regarding further testing, treatment, or referral to another health care provider. Inform the patient that serial specimens may be requested at regular intervals. Answer any questions or address any concerns voiced by the patient or family.

➤ Depending on the results of this procedure, additional testing may be performed to evaluate or monitor progression of the disease process and determine the need for a change in therapy. Evaluate test results in relation to the patient's symptoms and other tests performed.

Related laboratory tests:

➤ Related laboratory tests include biopsy of suspect tissue, CA 125, CA 15-3, and carcinoembryonic antigen.

CALCITONIN AND CALCITONIN STIMULATION TESTS

· ·

SYNONYM/ACRONYM: Thyrocalcitonin, hCT.

SPECIMEN: Serum (3 mL) collected in a red- or tiger-top tube.

REFERENCE VALUE: (Method: Radioimmunoassay)

Procedure	Medication Administered	Recommended Collection Times
Calcium and pentagastrin stimulation	Calcium, 2 mg/kg IV for 1 min, followed by pentagastrin 0.5 μg/kg	4 calcitonin levels—baseline immediately before bolus; and 1 min, 2 min, and 5 min postbolus
Pentagastrin stimulation	Pentagastrin, 0.5 μg/kg IV push	4 calcitonin levels—baseline immediately before bolus; and 1.5 min, 2 min, and 5 min postbolus

IV = intravenous.

	Conventional Units	SI Units (Conventional Units ×1)
Calcitonin		
Male	Less than 19 pg/mL	Less than 19 ng/L
Female	Less than 14 pg/mL	Less than 14 ng/L
Maximum Response		
After Calcium and Pentagastrin Stimulation		
Male	Less than 350 pg/mL	Less than 350 ng/L
Female	Less than 94 pg/mL	Less than 94 ng/L
After Pentagastrin Stimulation		
Male	Less than 110 pg/mL	Less than 110 ng/L
Female	Less than 30 pg/mL	Less than 30 ng/L

DESCRIPTION & RATIONALE: Calcitonin, also called thyrocalcitonin, is secreted by the parafollicular or C cells of the thyroid gland in response to elevated serum calcium levels. Calcitonin antagonizes the effects of parathyroid hormone and vitamin D so that calcium continues to be laid down in bone rather than reabsorbed into the blood. Calcitonin also increases renal clearance of magnesium and inhibits tubular reabsorption of phosphates. The net result is that calcitonin decreases the serum calcium level. The pentagastrin (Peptavlon) provocation test and the calcium pentagastrin provocation test are useful for diagnosing medullary thyroid cancer. ■

INDICATIONS:
- Assist in the diagnosis of hyperparathyroidism
- Assist in the diagnosis of medullary thyroid cancer
- Evaluate altered serum calcium levels
- Monitor response to therapy for medullary thyroid carcinoma
- Predict recurrence of medullary thyroid carcinoma

- Screen family members of patients with medullary thyroid carcinoma (20% have a familial pattern)

RESULT

Increased in:
- Alcoholic cirrhosis
- Cancer of the breast, lung, and pancreas
- Carcinoid syndrome
- C-cell hyperplasia
- Chronic renal failure
- Ectopic secretion (especially neuroendocrine origins)
- Hypercalcemia (any cause)
- Medullary thyroid cancer
- Pancreatitis
- Pernicious anemia
- Pregnancy (late)
- Pseudohypoparathyroidism
- Thyroiditis
- Zollinger-Ellison syndrome

Decreased in: N/A

CRITICAL VALUES: N/A

INTERFERING FACTORS:

- Drugs that may increase calcitonin levels include calcium, epinephrine, estrogens, glucagon, oral contraceptives, pentagastrin, and sincalide.

- Recent radioactive scans or radiation within 1 week before the test can interfere with test results when radioimmunoassay is the test method.

- Failure to follow dietary restrictions before the procedure may cause the procedure to be canceled or repeated.

Nursing Implications and Procedure • • • • • • • • • •

Pretest:

- Inform the patient that the test is used to detect C-cell hyperplasia of the the thyroid gland and to detect and monitor tumors of the thyroid gland.

- Obtain a history of the patient's complaints, including a list of known allergens (especially allergies or sensitivities to latex), and inform the appropriate health care practitioner accordingly.

- Obtain a history of the patient's endocrine, genitourinary, and musculoskeletal systems, as well as results of previously performed laboratory tests, surgical procedures, and other diagnostic procedures. For related laboratory tests, refer to the Endocrine, Genitourinary, and Musculoskeletal System tables.

- Note any recent procedures that can interfere with test results.

- Obtain a list of medications the patient is taking, including herbs, nutritional supplements, and nutraceuticals. The requesting health care practitioner and laboratory should be advised if the patient regularly uses these products so that their effects can be taken into consideration when reviewing results.

- Review the procedure with the patient. Inform the patient that specimen collection takes approximately 5 to 10 minutes; a few extra minutes are required to administer the stimulation tests. Address concerns about pain related to the procedure. Explain to the patient that there may be some discomfort during the venipuncture.

- The patient should fast for 10 to 12 hours before specimen collection.

- There are no fluid or medication restrictions unless by medical direction.

- Prepare an ice slurry in a cup or plastic bag to have ready for immediate transport of the specimen to the laboratory. Prechill the red-top tube in the ice slurry.

Intratest:

- Ensure that the patient has complied with dietary restrictions and pretesting preparations; assure that food has been restricted for at least 10 to 12 hours prior to the procedure.

- If the patient has a history of severe allergic reaction to latex, care should be taken to avoid the use of equipment containing latex.

- Instruct the patient to cooperate fully and to follow directions. Direct the patient to breathe normally and to avoid unnecessary movement.

- Observe standard precautions, and follow the general guidelines in Appendix A. Positively identify the patient, and label the appropriate tubes with the corresponding patient demographics, date, and time of collection. Perform a venipuncture; collect the specimen in a prechilled 5-mL red- or tiger-top tube.

- Remove the needle and apply a pressure dressing over the puncture site.

- The sample should be placed in an ice slurry immediately after collection. Information on the specimen label can be protected from water in the ice slurry by first placing the specimen in a protective plastic bag. Promptly transport the specimen to the laboratory for processing and analysis.

➤ The results are recorded manually or in a computerized system for recall and postprocedure interpretation by the appropriate health care practitioner.

Post-test:

➤ Observe venipuncture site for bleeding or hematoma formation. Apply paper tape or other adhesive to hold pressure bandage in place, or replace with a plastic bandage.

➤ Instruct the patient to resume usual diet as directed by the health care practitioner.

➤ A written report of the examination will be sent to the requesting health care practitioner, who will discuss the results with the patient.

➤ Reinforce information given by the patient's health care provider regarding further testing, treatment, or referral to another health care provider. Answer any questions or address any concerns voiced by the patient or family.

➤ Depending on the results of this procedure, additional testing may be performed to evaluate or monitor progression of the disease process and determine the need for a change in therapy. Evaluate test results in relation to the patient's symptoms and other tests performed.

Related laboratory tests:

➤ Related laboratory tests include adrenocorticotropic hormone, calcium, carcinoembrionic antigen, catecholamines, complete blood count, magnesium, metanephrines, thyroid biopsy, urine phosphorus, and vitamin D.

CALCIUM, BLOOD

SYNONYM/ACRONYM: Total calcium, Ca.

SPECIMEN: Serum (1 mL) collected in a red- or tiger-top tube. Plasma (1 mL) collected in green-top (heparin) tube is also acceptable.

REFERENCE VALUE: (Method: Spectrophotometry)

Age	Conventional Units	SI Units (Conventional Units × 0.25)
Cord	8.2–11.2 mg/dL	2.05–2.80 mmol/L
0–10 d	7.6–10.4 mg/dL	1.90–2.60 mmol/L
11 d–2 y	9.0–11.0 mg/dL	2.25–2.75 mmol/L
3–12 y	8.8–10.8 mg/dL	2.20–2.70 mmol/L
13–18 y	8.4–10.2 mg/dL	2.10–2.55 mmol/L
Adult	8.2–10.2 mg/dL	2.05–2.55 mmol/L
Adult older than 90 y	8.2–9.6 mg/dL	2.05–2.40 mmol/L

DESCRIPTION & RATIONALE: Calcium, the most abundant cation in the body, participates in almost all of the vital processes. Calcium concentration is largely regulated by the parathyroid glands and by the action of vitamin D. Of the body's calcium reserves, 98% to 99% is stored in the teeth and skeleton. Calcium values are higher in children because of growth and active bone formation. About 45% of the total amount of blood calcium circulates as free ions that participate in coagulation, neuromuscular conduction, intracellular regulation, glandular secretion, and control of skeletal and cardiac muscle contractility. The remaining calcium is bound to circulating proteins (40% bound mostly to albumin) and anions (15% bound to anions such as bicarbonate, citrate, phosphate, and lactate) and plays no physiologic role. Calcium values can be adjusted up or down by 0.8 mg/dL for every 1 g/dL that albumin is greater than or less than 4 g/dL. Calcium and phosphorus levels are inversely proportional.

Fluid and electrolyte imbalances are often seen in patients with serious illness or injury; in these clinical situations, the normal homeostatic balance of the body is altered. During surgery or in the case of a critical illness, bicarbonate, phosphate, and lactate concentrations can change dramatically. Therapeutic treatments may also cause or contribute to electrolyte imbalance. This is why total calcium values can sometimes be misleading. Abnormal calcium levels are used to indicate general malfunctions in various body systems. Ionized calcium is used in more specific conditions (see monograph titled "Calcium, Ionized").

Calcium values should be interpreted in conjunction with results of other tests. Normal calcium with an abnormal phosphorus value indicates impaired calcium absorption (possibly because of altered parathyroid hormone level or activity). Normal calcium with an elevated urea nitrogen value indicates possible hyperparathyroidism (primary or secondary). Normal calcium with decreased albumin value is an indication of hypercalcemia. The most common cause of hypocalcemia (low calcium levels) is hypoalbuminemia. The most common causes of hypercalcemia (high calcium levels) are hyperparathyroidism and cancer (with or without bone metastases). ▪

INDICATIONS:

- Detect parathyroid gland loss after thyroid or other neck surgery, as indicated by decreased levels

- Evaluate cardiac arrhythmias and coagulation disorders to determine if altered serum calcium level is contributing to the problem

- Evaluate the effects of various disorders on calcium metabolism, especially diseases involving bone

- Monitor the effectiveness of therapy being administered to correct abnormal calcium levels, especially calcium deficiencies

- Monitor the effects of renal failure and various drugs on calcium levels

RESULT

Increased in:
- Acidosis

- Acromegaly

- Addison's disease

- Cancers (bone, Burkitt's lymphoma,

Hodgkin's lymphoma, leukemia, myeloma, and metastases from other organs)
- Dehydration
- Excessive intake (milk, antacids)
- Hyperparathyroidism
- Idiopathic hypercalcemia of infancy
- Lung disease (tuberculosis, histoplasmosis, coccidioidomycosis, berylliosis)
- Malignant disease without bone involvement (squamous cell carcinoma of the lung, kidney cancer)
- Milk-alkali syndrome (Burnett's syndrome)
- Paget's disease
- Pheochromocytoma
- Polycythemia vera
- Renal transplant
- Rhabdomyolysis
- Sarcoidosis
- Thyrotoxicosis
- Vitamin D toxicity

Decreased in:
- Acute pancreatitis
- Alcoholism
- Alkalosis
- Chronic renal failure
- Cystinosis
- Hepatic cirrhosis
- Hyperphosphatemia
- Hypoalbuminemia
- Hypomagnesemia
- Hypoparathyroidism (congenital, idiopathic, surgical)
- Inadequate nutrition
- Leprosy

- Long-term anticonvulsant therapy
- Malabsorption (celiac disease, tropical sprue, pancreatic insufficiency)
- Massive blood transfusion
- Neonatal prematurity
- Osteomalacia (advanced)
- Renal tubular disease
- Vitamin D deficiency (rickets)

CRITICAL VALUES:

Less than 7 mg/dL
Greater than 12 mg/dL (some patients can tolerate higher concentrations)

Note and immediately report to the health care practitioner any critically increased or decreased values and related symptoms.

Observe the patient for symptoms of critically decreased or elevated calcium levels. Hypocalcemia is evidenced by convulsions, arrhythmias, changes in electrocardiogram (ECG) in the form of prolonged ST segment and Q-T interval, facial spasms (positive Chvostek's sign), tetany, muscle cramps, numbness in extremities, tingling, and muscle twitching (positive Trousseau's sign). Possible interventions include seizure precautions, increased frequency of ECG monitoring, and administration of calcium or magnesium.

Severe hypercalcemia is manifested by polyuria, constipation, changes in ECG (shortened ST segment), lethargy, muscle weakness, apathy, anorexia, headache, and nausea and ultimately may result in coma. Possible interventions include the administration of normal saline and diuretics to speed up excretion or administration of calcitonin or steroids to force the circulating calcium into the cells.

INTERFERING FACTORS:

- Drugs that may increase calcium levels include anabolic steroids, some antacids, calcitriol, calcium salts, danazol, diuretics (long-term), ergocalciferol, isotretinoin, lithium, oral contraceptives, parathyroid extract, parathyroid hormone, prednisone, progesterone, tamoxifen, vitamin A, and vitamin D.

• Drugs that may decrease calcium levels include albuterol, alprostadil, aminoglycosides, anticonvulsants, calcitonin, diuretics (initially), gastrin, glucagon, glucocorticoids, glucose, insulin, laxatives (excessive use), magnesium salts, methicillin, phosphates, plicamycin, sodium sulfate (given intravenously), tetracycline (in pregnancy), trazodone, and viomycin.

• Calcium exhibits diurnal variation; serial samples should be collected at the same time of day for comparison.

• Venous hemostasis caused by prolonged use of a tourniquet during venipuncture can falsely elevate calcium levels.

• Patients on ethylenediaminetetra-acetic acid (EDTA) therapy (chelation) may show falsely decreased calcium values.

• Hemolysis and icterus cause false-positive results because of interference from biologic pigments.

• Specimens should never be collected above an intravenous (IV) line because of the potential for dilution when the specimen and the IV solution combine in the collection container, falsely decreasing the result. There is also the potential of contaminating the sample with the substance of interest, if it is present in the IV solution, falsely increasing the result.

Nursing Implications and Procedure • • • • • • • • • • •

Pretest:

➤ Inform the patient that the test is used to investigate various conditions indicated by abnormally increased or decreased calcium levels.

➤ Obtain a history of the patient's complaints, including a list of known allergens (especially allergies or sensitivities to latex), and inform the appropriate health care practitioner accordingly.

➤ Obtain a history of the patient's cardiovascular, gastrointestinal, genitourinary, hematopoietic, hepatobiliary, and musculoskeletal systems, as well as results of previously performed laboratory tests, surgical procedures, and other diagnostic procedures. For related laboratory tests, refer to the Cardiovascular, Gastrointestinal, Genitourinary, Hematopoietic, Hepatobiliary, and Musculoskeletal System tables.

➤ Note any recent procedures that can interfere with test results.

➤ Obtain a list of medications the patient is taking, including herbs, nutritional supplements, and nutraceuticals. The requesting health care practitioner and laboratory should be advised if the patient regularly uses these products so that their effects can be taken into consideration when reviewing results.

➤ Review the procedure with the patient. Inform the patient that specimen collection takes approximately 5 to 10 minutes. Address concerns about pain related to the procedure. Explain to the patient that there may be some discomfort during the venipuncture.

➤ *Sensitivity to cultural and social issues,* as well as concern for modesty, is important in providing psychological support before, during, and after the procedure.

➤ There are no food, fluid, or medication restrictions unless by medical direction.

Intratest:

➤ If the patient has a history of severe allergic reaction to latex, care should be taken to avoid the use of equipment containing latex.

➤ Instruct the patient to cooperate fully and to follow directions. Direct the patient to breathe normally and to avoid unnecessary movement.

➤ Observe standard precautions, and follow the general guidelines in Appendix A. Positively identify the patient, and label the appropriate tubes with the corresponding patient demographics, date, and time of collection. Perform a venipuncture; collect the specimen in a 5-mL red- or tiger-top tube.

➤ Remove the needle, and apply a pressure dressing over the puncture site.

➤ Promptly transport the specimen to the laboratory for processing and analysis.

➤ The results are recorded manually or in a computerized system for recall and postprocedure interpretation by the appropriate health care practitioner.

Post-test:

➤ Observe venipuncture site for bleeding or hematoma formation. Apply paper tape or other adhesive to hold pressure bandage in place, or replace with a plastic bandage.

➤ *Nutritional considerations:* Patients with abnormal calcium values should be informed that daily intake of calcium is important even though body stores in the bones can be called on to supplement circulating levels. Dietary calcium can be obtained from animal or plant sources. Milk and milk products, sardines, clams, oysters, salmon, rhubarb, spinach, beet greens, broccoli, kale, tofu, legumes, and fortified orange juice are high in calcium. Milk and milk products also contain vitamin D and lactose, which assist calcium absorp-

tion. Cooked vegetables yield more absorbable calcium than raw vegetables. Patients should be informed of the substances that can inhibit calcium absorption by irreversibly binding to some of the calcium, making it unavailable for absorption, such as oxalates, which naturally occur in some vegetables and are found in tea; phytic acid, found in some cereals; phosphoric acid, found in dark cola; and insoluble dietary fiber (in excessive amounts). Excessive protein intake can also negatively affect calcium absorption, especially if it is combined with foods high in phosphorus and in the presence of a reduced dietary calcium intake.

➤ A written report of the examination will be sent to the requesting health care practitioner, who will discuss the results with the patient.

➤ Reinforce information given by the patient's health care provider regarding further testing, treatment, or referral to another health care provider. Answer any questions or address any concerns voiced by the patient or family.

➤ Depending on the results of this procedure, additional testing may be performed to evaluate or monitor progression of the disease process and determine the need for a change in therapy. Evaluate test results in relation to the patient's symptoms and other tests performed.

Related laboratory tests:

➤ Related laboratory tests include albumin, alkaline phosphatase, calcitonin, calcium (ionized and urine), electrolytes, kidney stone analysis, magnesium (blood and urine), parathyroid hormone, phosphorus (blood and urine), total protein, urinalysis, and vitamin D.

CALCIUM, IONIZED

SYNONYM/ACRONYM: free calcium, unbound calcium, Ca++, Ca^{2+}.

SPECIMEN: Serum (1 mL) collected in a red- or tiger-top tube. Specimen should be transported tightly capped and remain unopened until testing. Exposure of serum to room air changes the pH of the specimen due to the release of carbon dioxide and can cause erroneous results.

REFERENCE VALUE: (Method: Ion-selective electrode)

	Conventional Units	SI Units (Conventional Units × 0.25)
Whole blood		
Cord blood	5.20–5.84 mg/dL	1.30–1.46 mmol/L
Adult	4.60–5.08 mg/dL	1.12–1.32 mmol/L
Plasma		
Adult	4.12–4.92 mg/dL	1.03–1.23 mmol/L
Serum		
Cord blood	5.20–6.40 mg/dL	1.30–1.60 mmol/L
Adult	4.64–5.28 mg/dL	1.16–1.32 mmol/L

DESCRIPTION & RATIONALE: Calcium is the most abundant cation in the body and participates in almost all vital body processes (see other calcium monographs). Circulating calcium is found in the free or ionized form; bound to organic anions such as lactate, phosphate, or citrate; and bound to proteins such as albumin. Ionized calcium is the physiologically active form of circulating calcium. About half of the total amount of calcium circulates as free ions that participate in blood coagulation, neuromuscular conduction, intracellular regulation, glandular secretion, and control of skeletal and cardiac muscle contractility. Calcium levels are regulated largely by the parathyroid glands and by vitamin D. Compared to total calcium level, ionized calcium is a better measurement of calcium metabolism. Ionized calcium levels are not influenced by protein concentrations, as seen in patients with chronic renal failure, nephrotic syndrome, malabsorption, and multiple myeloma. Levels are also not affected in patients with metabolic acid-base balance disturbances. Elevations in ionized calcium may be seen when the total calcium is normal. Measurement of ionized calcium is useful to monitor patients undergoing cardiothoracic surgery or organ transplantation. It is also useful in the evaluation of patients in cardiac arrest. ∎

INDICATIONS:

- Detect ectopic parathyroid hormone–producing neoplasms
- Evaluate the effect of protein on calcium levels
- Identify individuals with hypocalcemia
- Identify individuals with toxic levels of vitamin D
- Investigate suspected hyperparathyroidism
- Monitor patients with renal failure or organ transplantation, in whom secondary hyperparathyroidism may be a complication
- Monitor patients with sepsis or magnesium deficiency

RESULT

Increased in:
- Hyperparathyroidism
- Parathyroid hormone–producing neoplasms
- Vitamin D toxicity

Decreased in:
- Burns
- Hypoparathyroidism (primary)
- Magnesium deficiency
- Multiple organ failure
- Pancreatitis
- The post-dialysis period, as a result of low-calcium dialysate administration
- The post-surgical period (i.e., major surgeries)
- The post-transfusion period, as a result of the use of citrated preservative (calcium chelator)
- Premature infants with hypoproteinemia and acidosis
- Pseudohypoparathyroidism
- Sepsis

- Trauma
- Vitamin D deficiency

CRITICAL VALUES:
Less than 3.2 mg/dL
Greater than 6.2 mg/dL

Note and immediately report to the health care practitioner any critically increased or decreased values and related symptoms.

Observe the patient for symptoms of critically decreased or elevated calcium levels. Hypocalcemia is evidenced by convulsions, arrhythmias, changes in electrocardiogram (ECG) in the form of prolonged ST segment and Q-T interval, facial spasms (positive Chvostek's sign), tetany, muscle cramps, numbness in extremities, tingling, and muscle twitching (positive Trousseau's sign). Possible interventions include seizure precautions, increased frequency of ECG monitoring, and administration of calcium or magnesium.

Severe hypercalcemia is manifested by polyuria, constipation, changes in ECG (shortened ST segment), lethargy, muscle weakness, apathy, anorexia, headache, and nausea, and ultimately may result in coma. Possible interventions include the administration of normal saline and diuretics to speed up excretion or administration of calcitonin or steroids to force the circulating calcium into the cells.

INTERFERING FACTORS:
- Drugs that may increase calcium levels include antacids (some), calcitriol, and lithium.
- Drugs that may decrease calcium levels include calcitonin, citrates, foscarnet, and pamidronate (initially).
- Calcium exhibits diurnal variation; serial samples should be collected at the same time of day for comparison.
- Venous hemostasis caused by prolonged use of a tourniquet during venipuncture can falsely elevate calcium levels.
- Patients on ethylenediaminetetra-acetic

acid (EDTA) therapy (chelation) may show falsely decreased calcium values.

• Specimens should never be collected above an intravenous (IV) line because of the potential for dilution when the specimen and the IV solution combine in the collection container, falsely decreasing the result. There is also the potential of contaminating the sample with the substance of interest, if it is present in the IV solution, falsely increasing the result.

Nursing Implications and Procedure • • • • • • • • • • •

Pretest:

➤ Inform the patient that the test is used to investigate various conditions indicated by abnormally increased or decreased levels of ionized calcium.

➤ Obtain a history of the patient's complaints, including a list of known allergens (especially allergies or sensitivities to latex), and inform the appropriate health care practitioner accordingly.

➤ Obtain a history of the patient's cardiovascular, gastrointestinal, genitourinary, hematopoietic, hepatobiliary, and musculoskeletal systems, as well as results of previously performed laboratory tests, surgical procedures, and other diagnostic procedures. For related laboratory tests, refer to the Cardiovascular, Gastrointestinal, Genitourinary, Hematopoietic, Hepatobiliary, and Musculoskeletal System tables.

➤ Note any recent procedures that could interfere with test results.

➤ Obtain a list of the medications the patient is taking, including herbs, nutritional supplements, and nutraceuticals. The requesting health care practitioner and laboratory should be advised if the patient regularly uses these products so that their effects can be taken into consideration when reviewing results.

➤ Review the procedure with the patient. Inform the patient that specimen collection takes approximately 5 to 10 minutes. Address concerns about pain related to the procedure. Explain to the patient that there may be some discomfort during the venipuncture.

➤ *Sensitivity to cultural and social issues,* as well as concern for modesty, is important in providing psychological support before, during, and after the procedure.

➤ There are no food, fluid, or medication restrictions unless by medical direction.

Intratest:

➤ If the patient has a history of severe allergic reaction to latex, care should be taken to avoid the use of equipment containing latex.

➤ Instruct the patient to cooperate fully and to follow directions. Direct the patient to breathe normally and to avoid unnecessary movement.

➤ Observe standard precautions, and follow the general guidelines in Appendix A. Positively identify the patient, and label the appropriate tubes with the corresponding patient demographics, date, and time of collection. Perform a venipuncture and, without using a tourniquet, collect the specimen in a 5-mL red- or tiger-top tube. The specimen must be maintained in an anaerobic environment.

➤ Remove the needle, and apply a pressure dressing over the puncture site.

➤ The specimen should be stored under anaerobic conditions after collection to prevent the diffusion of gas from the specimen. Falsely decreased values result from uncovered specimens. Promptly transport the specimen to the laboratory for processing and analysis.

➤ The results are recorded manually or in a computerized system for recall and postprocedure interpretation by the appropriate health care practitioner.

Post-test:

➤ Observe venipuncture site for bleeding or hematoma formation. Apply paper tape or other adhesive to hold pressure bandage in place, or replace with a plastic bandage.

➤ *Nutritional considerations:* Patients with abnormal calcium values should be informed that daily intake of calcium is important even though body stores in the bones can be called on to supplement circulating levels. Dietary calcium can be obtained from animal or plant sources. Milk and milk products, sardines, clams, oysters, salmon, rhubarb, spinach, beet greens, broccoli, kale, tofu, legumes, and fortified orange juice are high in calcium. Milk and milk products also contain vitamin D and lactose, which assist calcium absorption. Cooked vegetables yield more absorbable calcium than raw vegetables. Patients should be informed of the substances that can inhibit calcium absorption by irreversibly binding to some of the calcium, making it unavailable for absorption, such as oxalates, which naturally occur in some vegetables and are found in tea; phytic acid, found in some cereals; phosphoric acid, found in dark cola; and insoluble dietary fiber (in excessive amounts). Excessive protein intake can also negatively affect calcium absorption, especially if it is combined with foods high in phosphorus and in the presence of a reduced dietary calcium intake.

➤ A written report of the examination will be sent to the requesting health care practitioner, who will discuss the results with the patient.

➤ Reinforce information given by the patient's health care provider regarding further testing, treatment, or referral to another health care provider. Answer any questions or address any concerns voiced by the patient or family.

➤ Depending on the results of this procedure, additional testing may be performed to evaluate or monitor progression of the disease process and determine the need for a change in therapy. Evaluate test results in relation to the patient's symptoms and other tests performed.

Related laboratory tests:

➤ Related laboratory tests include albumin, alkaline phosphatase, calcitonin, calcium (blood and urine), electrolytes, kidney stone panel, magnesium (blood and urine), parathyroid hormone, phosphorus (blood and urine), total protein, urinalysis, and vitamin D.

CALCIUM, URINE

SYNONYM/ACRONYM: N/A.

SPECIMEN: Urine (5 mL) from an unpreserved random or timed specimen collected in a clean plastic collection container.

REFERENCE VALUE: (Method: Spectrophotometry)

Age	Conventional Units*	SI Units (Conventional Units × 0.025)*
Infant and child	Up to 6 mg/kg per 24 h	Up to 0.15 mmol/kg per 24 h
Adult on average diet	100–300 mg/24 h	2.5–7.5 mmol/24 h

*Values depend on diet. Average daily intake of calcium: 600–800 mg/24 h.

DESCRIPTION & RATIONALE: Regulating electrolyte balance is a major function of the kidneys. In normally functioning kidneys, urine levels increase when serum levels are high and decrease when serum levels are low to maintain homeostasis. Analyzing urinary electrolyte levels can provide important clues to the functioning of the kidneys and other major organs. Tests for calcium in urine usually involve timed urine collections during a 12- or 24-hour period. Measurement of random specimens may also be requested. Urinary calcium excretion may also be expressed as calcium-to-creatinine ratio: In a healthy individual with constant muscle mass, the ratio is less than 0.14. ∎

INDICATIONS:
- Assist in establishing the presence of kidney stones
- Evaluate bone disease
- Evaluate dietary intake and absorption
- Evaluate renal loss
- Monitor patients on calcium replacement

RESULT

Increased in:
- Acromegaly
- Diabetes
- Fanconi's syndrome
- Glucocorticoid excess
- Hepatolenticular degeneration
- Hyperparathyroidism
- Hyperthyroidism
- Idiopathic hypercalciuria
- Immobilization
- Kidney stones
- Leukemia and lymphoma (some instances)
- Myeloma
- Neoplasm of the breast or bladder
- Osteitis deformans
- Osteolytic bone metastases (carcinoma, sarcoma)
- Osteoporosis
- Paget's disease
- Renal tubular acidosis
- Sarcoidosis
- Schistosomiasis
- Thyrotoxicosis
- Vitamin D intoxication

Decreased in:
- Hypocalcemia (other than renal disease)
- Hypocalciuric hypercalcemia (familial, nonfamilial)
- Hypoparathyroidism
- Hypothyroidism

- Malabsorption (celiac disease, tropical sprue)
- Malignant bone neoplasm
- Nephrosis and acute nephritis
- Osteoblastic metastases
- Osteomalacia
- Pre-eclampsia
- Pseudohypoparathyroidism
- Renal osteodystrophy
- Rickets
- Vitamin D deficiency

CRITICAL VALUES: N/A

INTERFERING FACTORS:

- Drugs that can increase urine calcium levels include acetazolamide, ammonium chloride, asparaginase, calcitonin, calcitriol, corticosteroids, corticotropin, dexamethasone, diuretics (initially), ergocalciferol, ethacrynic acid, mannitol (initially), meralluride, mercaptomerin, mersalyl, nandrolone, parathyroid extract, parathyroid hormone, plicamycin, sodium sulfate, sulfates, triamterene, viomycin, and vitamin D.

- Drugs that can decrease urine calcium levels include angiotensin, bicarbonate, calcitonin, citrates, diuretics (chronic), lithium, neomycin, oral contraceptives, and spironolactone.

- Failure to collect all the urine and store the specimen properly during the 24-hour test period invalidates the results.

Nursing Implications and Procedure

Pretest:

➤ Inform the patient that the test is used to indicate sufficiency of dietary calcium intake and rate of absorption. Urine calcium levels are also used to assess bone resorption, renal stones, and renal loss of calcium.

➤ Obtain a history of the patient's complaints, including a list of known allergens (especially allergies or sensitivities to latex), and inform the appropriate health care practitioner accordingly.

➤ Obtain a history of the patient's endocrine, genitourinary, and musculoskeletal systems and results of previously performed laboratory tests, surgical procedures, and other diagnostic procedures. For related laboratory tests, refer to the Endocrine, Genitourinary, and Musculoskeletal System tables.

➤ Obtain a list of the medications the patient is taking, including herbs, nutritional supplements, and nutraceuticals. The requesting health care practitioner and laboratory should be advised if the patient regularly uses these products so that their effects can be taken into consideration when reviewing results.

➤ Review the procedure with the patient. Provide a nonmetallic urinal, bedpan, or toilet-mounted collection device. Address concerns about pain related to the procedure. Explain to the patient that there should be no discomfort during the procedure.

➤ Usually a 24-hour time frame for urine collection is ordered. Inform the patient that all urine must be saved during that 24-hour period. Instruct the patient not to void directly into the laboratory collection container. Instruct the patient to avoid defecating in the collection device and to keep toilet tissue out of the collection device to prevent contamination of the specimen. Place a sign in the bathroom to remind the patient to save all urine.

➤ Instruct the patient to void all urine into the collection device and then to pour the urine into the laboratory collection container. Alternatively, the specimen can be left in the collection device for a health care staff member to add to the laboratory collection container.

➤ *Sensitivity to social and cultural issues,* as well as concern for modesty, is important in providing psychological support before, during, and after the procedure.

➤ There are no fluid or medication restrictions unless by medical direction.

➤ Instruct the patient to follow a normal calcium diet for at least 4 days before test.

Intratest:

➤ Ensure that the patient has complied with dietary restrictions; assure that a normal calcium diet has been followed for at least 4 days prior to the procedure.

➤ If the patient has a history of severe allergic reaction to latex, care should be taken to avoid the use of equipment containing latex.

➤ Instruct the patient to cooperate fully and to follow directions.

➤ Observe standard precautions, and follow the general guidelines in Appendix A. Positively identify the patient, and label the appropriate collection container with the corresponding patient demographics, date, and time of collection.

Random specimen (collect in early morning):

➤ Obtain urine specimen in a properly labeled plastic collection container and immediately transport urine. If an indwelling catheter is in place, it may be necessary to clamp off the catheter for 15 to 30 minutes before specimen collection. Cleanse specimen port with antiseptic swab, and then aspirate 5 mL of urine with a 21- to 25-gauge needle and syringe. Transfer urine to a plastic container.

Timed specimen:

➤ Obtain a clean 3-L urine specimen container, toilet-mounted collection device, and plastic bag (for transport of the specimen container). The specimen must be refrigerated or kept on ice throughout the

collection period. If an indwelling urinary catheter is in place, the drainage bag must be kept on ice.

➤ Begin the test between 6 and 8 a.m., if possible. Collect first voiding and discard. Record the time the specimen was discarded as the beginning of the timed collection period. The next morning, ask the patient to void at the same time the collection was started, and add this last voiding to the container.

➤ If an indwelling catheter is in place, replace the tubing and container system at the start of the collection time. Keep the container system on ice during the collection period or empty the urine into a larger container periodically during the collection period; monitor to ensure continued drainage, and conclude the test the next morning at the same hour the collection began.

➤ At the conclusion of the test, compare the quantity of urine with the urinary output record for the collection; if the specimen contains less than the recorded output, some urine may have been discarded, invalidating the test.

➤ Include on the collection container's label the amount of urine collected and test start and stop times. Promptly transport the specimen to the laboratory for processing and analysis.

General:

➤ The results are recorded manually or in a computerized system for recall and postprocedure interpretation by the appropriate health care practitioner.

Post-test:

➤ Instruct the patient to resume usual diet as directed by the health care practitioner.

➤ *Nutritional considerations:* Increased urine calcium levels may be associated with kidney stones. Educate the patient, if appropriate, as to the importance of drinking a sufficient amount of water when kidney stones are suspected.

➤ A written report of the examination will be sent to the requesting health care practitioner, who will discuss the results with the patient.

➤ Recognize anxiety related to test results. Discuss the implications of abnormal test results on the patient's lifestyle. Provide teaching and information regarding the clinical implications of the test results, as appropriate.

➤ Reinforce information given by the patient's health care provider regarding further testing, treatment, or referral to another health care provider. Answer any questions or address any concerns voiced by the patient or family.

➤ Depending on the results of this procedure, additional testing may be performed to evaluate or monitor progression of the disease process and determine the need for a change in therapy. Evaluate test results in relation to the patient's symptoms and other tests performed.

Related laboratory tests:

➤ Related laboratory tests include calcium, kidney stone panel, magnesium (blood and urine), parathyroid hormone, phosphorus (blood and urine) potassium (blood and urine), uric acid (blood and urine), urinalysis, urine oxalate, and vitamin D.

CALCULUS, KIDNEY STONE PANEL

· ·

SYNONYMS/ACRONYM: Kidney stone analysis, nephrolithiasis analysis.

SPECIMEN: Kidney stones.

REFERENCE VALUE: (Method: Infrared spectrometry) None detected.

DESCRIPTION & RATIONALE: Renal calculi (kidney stones) are formed by the crystallization of calcium oxalate (most common), magnesium ammonium phosphate, calcium phosphate, uric acid, and cystine. Formation of stones may be due to reduced urine flow and excessive amounts of the previously mentioned insoluble substances. The presence of stones is confirmed by diagnostic visualization or passing of the stones in the urine.

The chemical nature of the stones is confirmed qualitatively. ■

INDICATIONS: Identify substances present in renal calculi

RESULT

Positive findings in:
Presence of renal calculi

Negative findings in: N/A

CRITICAL VALUES: N/A

INTERFERING FACTORS:

- Drugs and substances that may increase the formation of urine calculi include probenecid and vitamin D.

- Adhesive tape should not be used to attach stones to any transportation or collection container, because the adhesive interferes with infrared spectrometry.

Nursing Implications and Procedure • • • • • • • • • • •

Pretest:

▶ Inform the patient that the test is used to identify the presence of kidney stones.

▶ Obtain a history of the patient's complaints, especially hematuria, recurrent urinary tract infection, and abdominal pain. Also, obtain a list of known allergens and inform the appropriate health care practitioner accordingly.

▶ Obtain a history of the patient's genitourinary system and results of previously performed laboratory tests, surgical procedures, and other diagnostic procedures. For related laboratory tests, refer to the Genitourinary System table.

▶ Obtain a list of the medications the patient is taking, including herbs, nutritional supplements, and nutraceuticals. The requesting health care practitioner and laboratory should be advised if the patient regularly uses these products so that their effects can be taken into consideration when reviewing results.

▶ Review the procedure with the patient. Address concerns about pain related to the procedure. Explain to the patient that there may be some discomfort during the procedure.

▶ *Sensitivity to social and cultural issues,* as well as concern for modesty, is important in providing psychological support before, during, and after the procedure.

▶ There are no food, fluid, or medication restrictions unless by medical direction.

Intratest:

▶ Instruct the patient to cooperate fully and to follow directions.

▶ Observe standard precautions, and follow the general guidelines in Appendix A. Positively identify the patient, and label the appropriate collection container with the corresponding patient demographics, date, and time of collection.

▶ The patient presenting with symptoms indicating the presence of kidney stones may be provided with a device to strain the urine. The patient should be informed to transfer any particulate matter remaining in the strainer into the specimen collection container provided. Stones removed by the health care practitioner should be placed in the appropriate collection container.

▶ Promptly transport the specimen to the laboratory for processing and analysis.

▶ The results are recorded manually or in a computerized system for recall and postprocedure interpretation by the appropriate health care practitioner.

Post-test:

▶ Inform the patient with kidney stones that the likelihood of recurrence is high. Educate the patient regarding risk factors that contribute to the likelihood of kidney stone formation, including family history, osteoporosis, urinary tract infections, gout, magnesium deficiency, Crohn's disease with prior resection, age, gender (males are two to three times more likely to develop stones than females), and climate.

▶ *Dietary considerations:* Nutritional therapy is indicated for individuals identified as being at high risk for developing kidney stones. Educate the patient that diets rich in protein, salt, and oxalates increase the risk of stone formation. Adequate fluid intake should be encouraged.

➤ A written report of the examination will be sent to the requesting health care practitioner, who will discuss the results with the patient.

➤ Recognize anxiety related to test results. Discuss the implications of abnormal test results on the patient's lifestyle. Provide teaching and information regarding the clinical implications of the test results, as appropriate.

➤ Reinforce information given by the patient's health care provider regarding further testing, treatment, or referral to another health care provider. Follow-up testing of urine may be requested, but usually not

for 1 month after the stones have passed or been removed. Answer any questions or address any concerns voiced by the patient or family.

➤ Depending on the results of this procedure, additional testing may be performed to evaluate or monitor progression of the disease process and determine the need for a change in therapy. Evaluate test results in relation to the patient's symptoms and other tests performed.

Related laboratory tests:

➤ Related laboratory tests include creatinine clearance, urine calcium, urine culture, urine magnesium, urine oxalate, urine phosphorus, urine uric acid, and urinalysis.

CAPSULE ENDOSCOPY

· ·

SYNONYMS/ACRONYMS: Pill GI endoscopy .

AREA OF APPLICATION: Esophagus, stomach, upper duodenum, and small bowel.

CONTRAST: None.

DESCRIPTION & RATIONALE: This outpatient procedure involves ingesting a small (size of a large vitamin pill) capsule that is wireless and contains a small video camera that will pass naturally through the digestive system while taking pictures of the intestine. The capsule is 11 mm by 30 mm and contains a camera, light source, radio transmitter, and battery. The patient swallows the capsule, and the camera takes and transmits two images per

second. The images are transmitted to a recording device, which saves all images for review later by a health care practitioner. This device is approximately the size of a personal compact disc player. The recording device is worn on a belt around the patient's waist, and the video images are transmited to aerials taped to the body and stored on the device. After 8 hours, the device is removed and returned to the health care practitioner for processing. Thousand of images are downloaded onto a computer for viewing by a health care practitioner specialist. The capsule is disposable and will be excreted naturally in the patient's bowel movements. In the rare case that it will not be excreted naturally, it will need to be removed endoscopically or surgically. ▪

INDICATIONS:
• Assist in differentiating between benign and neoplastic tumors

• Detect gastric or duodenal ulcers

• Detect gastrointestinal tract (GI) inflammatory disease

• Determine the presence and location of GI bleeding, and vascular abnormalities

• Evaluate the extent of esophageal injury after ingestion of chemicals

• Evaluate stomach or duodenum after surgical procedures

• Evaluate suspected gastric obstruction

• Identify Crohn's disease, infectious enteritis, and celiac sprue

• Identify source of chronic diarrhea

• Investigate the cause of abdominal pain, celiac syndrome, and other malabsorption syndromes

RESULT

Normal Findings:
• Esophageal mucosa is normally yellow-pink. At about 9 inches from the incisor teeth, a pulsation indicates the location of the aortic arch. The gastric mucosa is orange-red and contains rugae. The proximal duodenum is reddish and contains a few longitudinal folds, whereas the distal duodenum has circular folds lined with villi. No abnormal structures or functions are observed in the esophagus, stomach, or duodenum.

Abnormal Findings:
• Achalasia

• Acute and chronic gastric and duodenal ulcers

• Crohn's disease, infectious enteritis, and celiac sprue

• Diverticular disease

• Duodenal cancer, diverticula, and ulcers

• Duodenitis

• Esophageal or pyloric stenosis

• Esophageal varices

• Esophagitis or strictures

• Gastric cancer, tumors, and ulcers

• Gastritis

• Hiatal hernia

• Mallory-Weiss syndrome

• Perforation of the esophagus, stomach, or small bowel

• Polyps

• Small bowel tumors

• Strictures

• Tumors (benign or malignant)

CRITICAL VALUES: N/A

INTERFERING FACTORS:

This procedure is contraindicated for:
• Patients who have had surgery involving the stomach or duodenum, which can make locating the duodenal papilla difficult

• Patients with a bleeding disorder

• Patients with unstable cardiopulmonary status, blood coagulation defects, or cholangitis, unless the patient received prophylactic antibiotic therapy before the test (otherwise the examination must be rescheduled)

- Patients with unstable cardiopulmonary status, blood coagulation defects, known aortic arch aneurysm, large esophageal Zenker's diverticulum, recent GI surgery, esophageal varices, or known esophageal perforation

Factors that may impair clear imaging:

- Gas or feces in the gastrointestinal tract resulting from inadequate cleansing or failure to restrict food intake before the study

- Retained barium from a previous radiologic procedure

Other considerations:

- The patient should not be near any electromangetic source, such as magnetic resonance imaging (MRI) or amateur (ham) radio equipment.

- Undergoing an MRI during the procedure may result in serious damage to the patient's intestestinal tract or abdomen. The patient should contact his or her health care practitioner for evaluation prior to any other procedure.

- Delayed capsule transit times may be a result of narcotic use, somatostatin use, gastroparesis, or psychiatric illness.

Nursing Implications and Procedure • • • • • • • • • • •

Pretest:

➤ Inform the patient that the procedure assesses the gastrointestinal tract.

➤ Obtain a history of the patient's complaints or symptoms.

➤ Obtain a history of results of previously performed diagnostic procedures, surgical procedures, and laboratory tests. For related diagnostic tests, refer to the Gastrointestinal System table.

➤ Ensure that this procedure is performed before an upper GI series or barium swallow.

➤ Obtain a list of the medications the patient is taking.

➤ Explain the purpose of the test and how the procedure is performed. Inform the patient that the procedure is begun in a GI lab or health care practitioner's office, usually by a health care practitioner or support staff, and that it takes approximately 30 to 60 minutes to begin the procedure.

➤ *Sensitivity to cultural and social issues,* as well as concern for modesty, is important in providing psychological support before, during, and after the procedure.

➤ Instruct the patient to start a liquid diet on the day before the procedure. From 10 p.m. the evening before the procedure, the patient should not eat or drink except for necessary medication with a sip of water.

➤ Instruct the patient not to take any medication for 2 hours prior to the procedure.

➤ Instruct the patient to abstain from smoking for 24 hours prior to the procedure.

➤ Instruct the patient to stop taking medications that have a coating effect, such as Sucralfate and Pepto-Bismol, 3 days before the procedure.

➤ Inform the patient that there is a chance of intestinal obstruction associated with the procedure.

➤ Instruct the patient to take a standard bowel prep the night before the procedure.

➤ Instruct the patient to wear loose, two-piece clothing on the day of the procedure. This assists with the placement of the sensors on the patient's abdomen.

➤ *Make sure a written and informed consent has been signed prior to the procedure.*

Intratest:

➤ Ensure that the patient has complied with dietary and medication restrictions and pretesting preparations for at least 8 hours prior to the procedure.

➤ Observe standard precautions, and follow the general guidelines in Appendix A.

➤ Obtain accurate height, weight, and abdominal girth measurements prior to beginning the examination.

➤ Instruct the patient to cooperate fully and to follow directions.

➤ Ask the patient to ingest the capsule with a full glass of water. The water may have Simethicone in it to reduce gastric and bile bubbles.

➤ After ingesting the capsule, the patient should not eat or drink for at least 2 hours. After 4 hours, the patient may have a light snack.

➤ After ingesting the capsule and until it is excreted, the patient should not be near any source of powerful electromagnetic fields, such as MRI or amateur (ham) radio equipment.

➤ The procedure lasts approximately 8 hours.

➤ Instruct the patient not to disconnect the equipment or remove the belt at any time during the test.

➤ If the data recorder stops functioning, instruct the patient to record the time and the nature of any event such as eating or drinking.

➤ Instruct the patient to keep a timed diary for the day detailing the food and liquids ingested and symptoms during the recording period.

➤ Instruct the patient to avoid any strenuous physical activity, bending, or stooping during the test.

Post-test:

➤ Instruct the patient to resume normal activity, medication, and diet after the test is ended, or as tolerated after the examination, as directed by the health care practitioner.

➤ Instruct the patient to remove the recorder and return it to the health care practitioner.

➤ Patients are asked to verify the elimination of the capsule, but not to retrieve the capsule.

➤ Inform the patient that the capsule is a single-use device that does not harbor any environmental hazards.

➤ Emphasize that any abdominal pain, fever, nausea, vomiting, or difficulty breathing must be immediately reported to the health care practitioner.

➤ A written report of the examination will be completed by a health care practitioner specializing in this branch of medicine. The report will be sent to the requesting health care practitioner, who will discuss the results with the patient.

➤ Depending on the results of this procedure, additional testing may be needed to evaluate or monitor progression of the disease process and determine the need for a change in therapy. Evaluate test results in relation to the patient's symptoms and other tests performed.

Related diagnostic tests:

➤ Related diagnostic tests include computed tomography of the abdomen; esophagogastroduodenoscopy (upper GI series); kidney, ureter, and bladder study; magnetic resonance imaging of the abdomen, and ultrasound of the abdomen.

CARBON DIOXIDE

SYNONYMS/ACRONYMS: CO_2 combining power, CO_2, tCO_2.

SPECIMEN: Serum (1 mL) collected in a red- or tiger-top tube, plasma (1 mL) collected in a green-top (lithium or sodium heparin) tube; or whole blood (1 mL) collected in a green-top (lithium or sodium heparin) tube or heparinized syringe.

REFERENCE VALUE: (Method: Colorimetry, enzyme assay, or pCO_2 electrode)

Carbon Dioxide	Conventional Units	SI Units (Conventional Units × 1)
Plasma or serum (venous)		
Infant–2 y	13–29 mmol/L	13–29 mmol/L
2 y and older	23–29 mmol/L	23–29 mmol/L
Whole blood (venous)		
Infant–2 y	18–28 mmol/L	18–28 mmol/L
2 y and older	22–26 mmol/L	22–26 mmol/L

DESCRIPTION & RATIONALE: Serum or plasma carbon dioxide (CO_2) measurement is usually done as part of an electrolyte panel. Total CO_2 (tCO_2) is an important component of the body's buffering capability, and measurements are used mainly in the evaluation of acid-base balance. It is important to understand the differences between tCO_2 (CO_2 content) and CO_2 gas (pCO_2). *Total CO_2* reflects the majority of CO_2 in the body, mainly in the form of bicarbonate (HCO_3^-); is present as a base; and is regulated by the kidneys. *CO_2 gas* contributes little to the tCO_2 level, is acidic, and is regulated by the lungs. (See monograph titled "Blood Gases" for more information.)

CO_2 provides the basis for the principal buffering system of the extracellular fluid system, which is the bicarbonate–carbonic acid buffer system. CO_2 circulates in the body either bound to protein or physically dissolved. Constituents in the blood that contribute to tCO_2 levels are bicarbonate, carbamino compounds, and carbonic acid (carbonic acid includes undissociated carbonic acid and dissolved CO_2). Bicarbonate is the second largest group of anions in the extracellular fluid (chloride being the largest group of extracellular anions). tCO_2 levels closely reflect bicarbonate (HCO_3^-) levels in the blood, because 90% to 95% of CO_2 circulates as HCO_3^-. ∎

INDICATIONS:

- Evaluate decreased venous CO_2 in the case of compensated metabolic acidosis
- Evaluate increased venous CO_2 in the case of compensated metabolic alkalosis
- Monitor decreased venous CO_2 as a result of compensated respiratory alkalosis
- Monitor increased venous CO_2 as a result of compensation for respiratory acidosis secondary to significant respiratory system infection or cancer; decreased respiratory rate

RESULT

Increased in:

- Acute intermittent porphyria
- Airway obstruction
- Asthmatic shock
- Brain tumor
- Bronchitis (chronic)
- Cardiac disorders
- Depression of respiratory center
- Electrolyte disturbance (severe)
- Emphysema
- Hypothyroidism
- Hypoventilation
- Metabolic alkalosis
- Myopathy
- Pneumonia
- Poliomyelitis
- Respiratory acidosis
- Tuberculosis (pulmonary)

Decreased in:

- Acute renal failure
- Anxiety
- Dehydration

- Diabetic ketoacidosis
- Diarrhea (severe)
- High fever
- Metabolic acidosis
- Respiratory alkalosis
- Salicylate intoxication
- Starvation

CRITICAL VALUES:

Less than 15 mmol/L
Greater than 40 mmol/L

Observe the patient for signs and symptoms of excessive or insufficient CO_2 levels, and report these findings to the health care practitioner. If the patient has been vomiting for several days and is breathing shallowly, or if the patient has had gastric suctioning and is breathing shallowly, this may indicate elevated CO_2 levels. Decreased CO_2 levels are evidenced by deep, vigorous breathing and flushed skin.

INTERFERING FACTORS:

- Drugs that may cause an increase in tCO_2 levels include acetylsalicylic acid, aldosterone, bicarbonate, carbenicillin, carbenoxolone, corticosteroids, dexamethasone, ethacrinic acid, laxatives (chronic abuse), and x-ray contrast agents.

- Drugs that may cause a decrease in tCO_2 levels include acetazolamide, acetylsalicylic acid (initially), amiloride, ammonium chloride, fluorides, metformin, methicillin, nitrofurantoin, NSD 3004 (long-acting carbonic anhydrase inhibitor), paraldehyde, tetracycline, triamterene, and xylitol.

- Prompt and proper specimen processing, storage, and analysis are important to achieve accurate results. The specimen should be stored under anaerobic conditions after collection to prevent the diffusion of CO_2 gas from the specimen. Falsely decreased values result from uncovered specimens. It is estimated that CO_2 diffuses from the sample at the rate of 6 mmol/h.

Nursing Implications and Procedure • • • • • • • • • • •

➤ Inform the patient that the test is used to assess the effect of total carbon dioxide levels on respiratory and metabolic acid-base balance.

➤ Obtain a history of the patient's complaints, including a list of known allergens (especially allergies or sensitivities to latex), and inform the appropriate health care practitioner accordingly.

➤ Obtain a history of the patient's genitourinary and respiratory systems, as well as results of previously performed laboratory tests, surgical procedures, and other diagnostic procedures. For related laboratory tests, refer to the Cardiovascular, Genitourinary, and Respiratory System tables.

➤ Note any recent procedures that can interfere with test results.

➤ Obtain a list of the medications the patient is taking, including herbs, nutritional supplements, and nutraceuticals. The requesting health care practitioner and laboratory should be advised if the patient regularly uses these products so that their effects can be taken into consideration when reviewing results.

➤ Review the procedure with the patient. Inform the patient that specimen collection takes approximately 5 to 10 minutes. Address concerns about pain related to the procedure. Explain to the patient that there may be some discomfort during the venipuncture.

➤ There are no food, fluid, or medication restrictions unless by medical direction.

➤ If the patient has a history of severe allergic reaction to latex, care should be taken to avoid the use of equipment containing latex.

➤ Instruct the patient to cooperate fully and to follow directions. Direct the patient to breathe normally and to avoid unnecessary movement.

➤ Observe standard precautions, and follow the general guidelines in Appendix A. Positively identify the patient, and label the appropriate tubes with the corresponding patient demographics, date, and time of collection. Perform a venipuncture; collect the specimen in a 5-mL red- or tiger-, or green-top tube.

➤ Remove the needle, and apply a pressure dressing over the puncture site.

➤ Promptly transport the specimen to the laboratory for processing and analysis.

➤ The results are recorded manually or in a computerized system for recall and postprocedure interpretation by the appropriate health care practitioner.

➤ Observe venipuncture site for bleeding or hematoma formation. Apply paper tape or other adhesive to hold pressure bandage in place, or replace with a plastic bandage.

➤ *Nutritional considerations:* Abnormal CO_2 values may be associated with diseases of the respiratory system. Malnutrition is commonly seen in patients with severe respiratory disease for reasons including fatigue, lack of appetite, and gastrointestinal distress. Research has estimated that the daily caloric intake required for respiration of patients with chronic obstructive pulmonary disease is 10 times higher than that of normal individuals. Adequate intake of vitamins A and C is also important to prevent pulmonary infection and to decrease the extent of lung tissue

- damage. The importance of following the prescribed diet should be stressed to the patient and/or caregiver.
- ➤ A written report of the examination will be sent to the requesting health care practitioner, who will discuss the results with the patient.
- ➤ Reinforce information given by the patient's health care provider regarding further testing, treatment, or referral to another health care provider. Answer any questions or address any concerns voiced by the patient or family.

- ➤ Depending on the results of this procedure, additional testing may be performed to evaluate or monitor progression of the disease process and determine the need for a change in therapy. Evaluate test results in relation to the patient's symptoms and other tests performed.

Related laboratory tests:

- ➤ Related laboratory tests include anion gap, arterial/alveolar oxygen ratio, blood gases, electrolytes, ketones, and salicylate.

CARBOXYHEMOGLOBIN

SYNONYMS/ACRONYMS: Carbon monoxide, CO, COHb, COH.

SPECIMEN: Whole blood (1 mL) collected in a green-top (heparin) or lavender-top (EDTA) tube, depending on laboratory requirement. Specimen should be transported tightly capped (anaerobic) and in an ice slurry if blood gases are to be performed simultaneously. Carboxyhemoglobin is stable at room temperature.

REFERENCE VALUE: (Method: Spectrophotometry, co-oximetry)

	% Saturation of Hemoglobin
Newborns	10–12%
Nonsmokers	Up to 2%
Smokers	Up to 12%

DESCRIPTION & RATIONALE: Exogenous carbon monoxide (CO) is a colorless, odorless, tasteless byproduct of incomplete combustion derived from the exhaust of automobiles, coal and gas burning, and tobacco smoke. Endogenous CO is produced as a result of red blood cell catabolism. CO levels are elevated in newborns as a result of the combined effects of high hemoglobin turnover and the inefficiency of the infant's respiratory system. CO binds tightly to hemoglobin with an affinity 250 times greater than oxygen, competitively and dramatically reducing the oxygen-carrying capacity of hemoglobin. The increased percentage of bound CO reflects the extent to which normal transport of oxygen has been negatively affected. Overexposure causes hypoxia, which results in headache, nausea, vomiting, vertigo, collapse, or convulsions. Toxic exposure causes anoxia, increased levels of lactic acid, and irreversible tissue damage, which can result in coma or death. Acute exposure may be evidenced by a cherry red color to the lips, skin, and nail beds; this observation may not be apparent in cases of chronic exposure. A direct correlation has been implicated between carboxyhemoglobin levels and symptoms of atherosclerotic disease, angina, and myocardial infarction. ■

INDICATIONS:

• Assist in the diagnosis of suspected CO poisoning

• Evaluate the effect of smoking on the patient

• Evaluate exposure to fires and smoke inhalation

RESULT

Increased in:
• CO poisoning

• Hemolytic disease

• Tobacco smoking

Decreased in: N/A

CRITICAL VALUES:

Percent of total hemoglobin	Symptoms
10%–20%	Asymptomatic
10%–30%	Disturbance of judgment, headache, dizziness
30%–40%	Dizziness, muscle weakness, vision problems, confusion, increased heart rate, increased breathing rate
50%–60%	Loss of consciousness
Greater than 60%	Seizures, coma, death

Women and children may suffer more severe symptoms of carbon monoxide poisoning at lower levels of carbon monoxide than men because women and children usually have lower red blood cell counts.

A possible intervention in moderate CO poisoning is the administration of supplemental oxygen given at atmospheric pressure. In severe CO poisoning, hyperbaric oxygen treatments may be used.

INTERFERING FACTORS: Specimen should

be collected before administration of oxygen therapy.

Nursing Implications and Procedure

Pretest:

▶ Inform the patient that the test is used to evaluate the extent of carbon monoxide poisoning and toxicity.

▶ Obtain a history of the patient's complaints, including a list of known allergens (especially allergies or sensitivities to latex), and inform the appropriate health care practitioner accordingly.

➤ Obtain a history of the patient's respiratory system and results of previously performed laboratory tests, surgical procedures, and other diagnostic procedures. For related laboratory tests, refer to the Respiratory System table.

➤ Note any recent procedures that can interfere with test results.

➤ Obtain a list of medications the patient is taking, including herbs, nutritional supplements, and nutraceuticals. The requesting health care practitioner and laboratory should be advised if the patient regularly uses these products so that their effects can be taken into consideration when reviewing results.

➤ Review the procedure with the patient. Explain to the patient or family members that the cause of the headache, vomiting, dizziness, convulsions, or coma could be related to CO exposure. Inform the patient that specimen collection takes approximately 5 to 10 minutes. Address concerns about pain related to the procedure. Explain to the patient that there may be some discomfort during the venipuncture.

➤ If carboxyhemoglobin measurement will be performed simultaneously with arterial blood gases, prepare an ice slurry in a cup or plastic bag and have it on hand for immediate transport of the specimen to the laboratory.

➤ There are no food, fluid, or medication restrictions unless by medical direction.

Intratest: ■

➤ If the patient has a history of severe allergic reaction to latex, care should be taken to avoid the use of equipment containing latex.

➤ Instruct the patient to cooperate fully and to follow directions. Direct the patient to breathe normally and to avoid unnecessary movement.

➤ Observe standard precautions, and follow the general guidelines in Appendix A. Positively identify the patient, and label the appropriate tubes with the corresponding patient demographics, date, and time of collection. Perform a venipuncture; collect the specimen in a 5-mL red- or lavender-top tube. The tightly capped sample should be placed in an ice slurry immediately after collection. Information on the specimen label can be protected from water in the ice slurry if the specimen is first placed in a protective plastic bag.

➤ Remove the needle, and apply a pressure dressing over the puncture site.

➤ Promptly transport the specimen to the laboratory for processing and analysis.

➤ The results are recorded manually or in a computerized system for recall and postprocedure interpretation by the appropriate health care practitioner.

Post-test: ■

➤ Observe venipuncture site for bleeding or hematoma formation. Apply paper tape or other adhesive to hold pressure bandage in place, or replace with a plastic bandage.

➤ A written report of the examination will be sent to the requesting health care practitioner, who will discuss the results with the patient.

➤ Recognize anxiety related to test results, and be supportive of impaired activity related to fear of shortened life expectancy. Discuss the implications of abnormal test results on the patient's lifestyle. Provide teaching and information regarding the clinical implications of the test results, as appropriate. Educate the patient regarding access to counseling services. Educate the patient regarding avoiding gas heaters and indoor cooking fires without adequate ventilation, and the need to have gas furnaces checked yearly for CO leakage. Inform the patient of smoking cessation programs, as appropriate.

➤ Reinforce information given by the patient's health care provider regarding further testing, treatment, or referral to another health care provider. Answer any questions or address any concerns voiced by the patient or family.

➤ Depending on the results of this procedure, additional testing may be performed to evaluate or monitor progression of the disease process and determine the need for a change in therapy. Evaluate test results in relation to the patient's symptoms and other tests performed.

Related laboratory tests

➤ Related laboratory tests include arterial/alveolar oxygen ratio, blood gases, and complete blood count.

CARCINOEMBRYONIC ANTIGEN

SYNONYM/ACRONYM: CEA.

SPECIMEN: Serum (1 mL) collected in a red-top tube. Plasma (1 mL) collected in lavender-top (EDTA) tube is also acceptable. Care must be taken to use the same type of collection container if serial measurements are to be taken.

REFERENCE VALUE: (Method: Enzyme immunoassay)

Smoking Status	Conventional Units	SI Units (Conventional Units × 1)
Smoker	Less than 5.0 ng/mL	Less than 5.0 µg/L
Nonsmoker	Less than 2.5 ng/mL	Less than 2.5 µg/L

DESCRIPTION & RATIONALE: Carcinoembryonic antigen (CEA) is a glycoprotein normally produced only during early fetal life and rapid multiplication of epithelial cells, especially those of the digestive system. CEA also appears in the blood of chronic smokers. Although the test is not diagnostic for any specific disease and is not useful as a screening test for cancer, it is useful for monitoring response to antineoplastic therapy in breast and gastrointestinal cancer. ■

INDICATIONS:
• Determine stage of colorectal cancer and test for recurrence
• Monitor response to treatment of breast and gastrointestinal cancers

RESULT

Increased in:

- Benign tumors, including benign breast disease

- Chronic tobacco smoking

- Colorectal, pulmonary, gastric, pancreatic, breast, head or neck, esophageal, ovarian, or prostate cancer

- Radiation therapy (transient)

Decreased in: N/A

CRITICAL VALUES: N/A

INTERFERING FACTORS: N/A

Nursing Implications and Procedure ....

Pretest:

▶ Inform the patient that the test is used to monitor the progress of various types of cancer and evaluate the response to therapy.

▶ Obtain a history of the patient's complaints, including a list of known allergens (especially allergies or sensitivities to latex), and inform the appropriate health care practitioner accordingly.

▶ Obtain a history of the patient's gastrointestinal, immune, and reproductive systems, as well as results of previously performed laboratory tests, surgical procedures, and other diagnostic procedures. For related laboratory tests, refer to the Gastrointestinal, Immune, and Reproductive System tables.

▶ Obtain a list of medications the patient is taking, including herbs, nutritional supplements, and nutraceuticals. The requesting health care practitioner and laboratory should be advised if the patient regularly uses these products so that their effects can be taken into consideration when reviewing results.

▶ Determine if the patient smokes, because smokers may have false elevations.

▶ Review the procedure with the patient. Inform the patient that specimen collection takes approximately 5 to 10 minutes. Address concerns about pain related to the procedure. Explain to the patient that there may be some discomfort during the venipuncture.

▶ There are no food, fluid, or medication restrictions unless by medical direction.

Intratest:

▶ If the patient has a history of severe allergic reaction to latex, care should be taken to avoid the use of equipment containing latex.

▶ Instruct the patient to cooperate fully and to follow directions. Direct the patient to breathe normally and to avoid unnecessary movement.

▶ Observe standard precautions, and follow the general guidelines in Appendix A. Positively identify the patient, and label the appropriate tubes with the corresponding patient demographics, date, and time of collection. Perform a venipuncture; collect the specimen in a 5-mL red- or lavender -top tube.

▶ Remove the needle, and apply a pressure dressing over the puncture site.

▶ Promptly transport the specimen to the laboratory for processing and analysis.

▶ The results are recorded manually or in a computerized system for recall and postprocedure interpretation by the appropriate health care practitioner.

Post-test:

▶ Observe venipuncture site for bleeding or hematoma formation. Apply paper tape or other adhesive to hold pressure bandage in place, or replace with a plastic bandage.

▶ A written report of the examination will be sent to the requesting health care practitioner, who will discuss the results with the patient.

▶ Recognize anxiety related to test

results, and be supportive of perceived loss of independence and fear of shortened life expectancy. Discuss the implications of abnormal test results on the patient's lifestyle. Provide teaching and information regarding the clinical implications of the test results, as appropriate. Educate the patient regarding access to counseling services.

➤ Reinforce information given by the patient's health care provider regarding further testing, treatment, or referral to another health care provider. Inform the patient that the test may be repeated periodically to monitor response to therapy. Instruct the patient in the importance of con-

tinuing scheduled therapy or follow-up visits. Answer any questions or address any concerns voiced by the patient or family.

➤ Depending on the results of this procedure, additional testing may be performed to evaluate or monitor progression of the disease process and determine the need for a change in therapy. Evaluate test results in relation to the patient's symptoms and other tests performed.

Related laboratory tests

➤ Related laboratory tests include biopsy of suspicious tissue, CA 15–3, CA 19–9, and CA 125.

CATECHOLAMINES, BLOOD

· ·

SYNONYMS/ACRONYM: Epinephrine, norepinephrine, dopamine.

SPECIMEN: Plasma (2 mL) collected in green-top (heparin) tube.

REFERENCE VALUE: (Method: High-performance liquid chromatography)

	Conventional Units	SI Units
		(Conventional Units × 5.46)
Epinephrine		
Supine, 30 min	0–110 pg/mL	0–600 pmol/L
Standing, 30 min	0–140 pg/mL	0–764 pmol/L
		(Conventional Units × 5.91)
Norepinephrine		
Supine, 30 min	70–750 pg/mL	414–4432 pmol/L
Standing, 30 min	200–1700 pg/mL	1182–10,047 pmol/L
		(Conventional Units × 6.53)
Dopamine		
Supine or standing	0–30 pg/mL	0–196 pmol/L

DESCRIPTION & RATIONALE: Cate-
cholamines are produced by the chromaffin tissue of the adrenal medulla. They are also found in sympathetic nerve endings and in the brain. The major catecholamines are epinephrine, norepinephrine, and dopamine. They prepare the body for the fight-or-flight stress response, help regulate metabolism, and are excreted from the body by the kidneys. Catecholamine levels are affected by diurnal variations, fluctuating in response to stress, postural changes, diet, smoking, drugs, and temperature changes. As a result, blood measurement is not as reliable as a 24-hour timed urine test. Results are most reliable when the specimen is collected during a hypertensive episode. Catecholamines are measured when there is high suspicion of pheochromocytoma but urine results are normal or borderline. Findings should be compared with the metabolites of epinephrine and norepinephrine, metanephrines and vanillylmandelic acid, and with the product of dopamine metabolism, homovanillic acid. Use of a clonidine suppression test with measurement of plasma catecholamines may be requested. Failure to suppress production of catecholamines after administration of clonidine supports the diagnosis of pheochromocytoma. ∎

INDICATIONS:
- Assist in the diagnosis of neuroblastoma, ganglioneuroma, or dysautonomia

- Assist in the diagnosis of paragangliomas

- Assist in the diagnosis of pheochromocytoma

- Evaluate acute hypertensive episode

- Evaluate hypertension of unknown origin

- Screen for pheochromocytoma among family members with an autosomal dominant inheritance pattern for Lindau–von Hippel disease or multiple endocrine neoplasia

RESULT

Increased in:
- Diabetic acidosis (epinephrine and norepinephrine)

- Ganglioblastoma (epinephrine, slight increase; norepinephrine, large increase)

- Ganglioneuroma (all are increased; norepinephrine, largest increase)

- Hypothyroidism (epinephrine and norepinephrine)

- Long-term manic-depressive disorders (epinephrine and norepinephrine)

- Myocardial infarction (epinephrine and norepinephrine)

- Neuroblastoma (all are increased; norepinephrine and dopamine, largest increase)

- Pheochromocytoma (epinephrine, continuous or intermittent increase; norepinephrine, slight increase)

- Shock (epinephrine and norepinephrine)

- Strenuous exercise (epinephrine and norepinephrine)

Decreased in:
- Autonomic nervous system dysfunction (norepinephrine)

- Orthostatic hypotension (norepinephrine)

- Parkinson's disease (dopamine)

CRITICAL VALUES: N/A

INTERFERING FACTORS:

- Drugs that may increase catecholamine levels include ajmaline, chlorpromazine, cyclopropane, diazoxide, ether, monoamine oxidase inhibitors, nitroglycerin, pentazocine, perphenazine, phenothiazine, promethazine, and theophylline.

- Drugs that may decrease catecholamine levels include clonidine, metyrosine, and reserpine.

- Stress, hypoglycemia, smoking, and drugs can produce elevated plasma catecholamines.

- Secretion of catecholamines exhibits diurnal variation, with the lowest levels occurring at night.

- Secretion of catecholamines varies during the menstrual cycle, with higher levels excreted during the luteal phase and lowest levels during ovulation.

- Diets high in amines (e.g., bananas, avocados, beer, aged cheese, chocolate, cocoa, coffee, fava beans, grains, tea, vanilla, walnuts, Chianti wine) can produce elevated plasma catecholamine levels, although this effect is more likely to be seen relative to certain urinary metabolites.

- Recent radioactive scans within 1 week of the test can interfere with test results.

- Failure to follow dietary restrictions before the procedure may cause the procedure to be canceled or repeated.

Nursing Implications and Procedure . . . .

Pretest:

➤ Inform the patient that the test is used to diagnose catecholamine-secreting tumors and in the investigation of hypertension.

➤ Obtain a history of the patient's complaints, including a list of known allergens (especially allergies or sensitivities to latex), and inform the appropriate health care practitioner accordingly.

➤ Obtain a history of the patient's endocrine system, as well as results of previously performed laboratory tests, surgical procedures, and other diagnostic procedures. For related laboratory tests, refer to the Endocrine System table.

➤ Record the date of the last menstrual period.

➤ Obtain a list of the medications the patient is taking, including herbs, nutritional supplements, and nutraceuticals. The requesting health care practitioner and laboratory should be advised if the patient regularly uses these products so that their effects can be taken into consideration when reviewing results.

➤ Review the procedure with the patient. Inform the patient that he or she may be asked to keep warm and to rest for 45 to 60 minutes before the test. Inform the patient that multiple specimens may be required. Inform the patient that specimen collection takes approximately 5 to 10 minutes. Address concerns about pain related to the procedure. Explain to the patient that there may be some discomfort during the venipuncture.

➤ *Sensitivity to social and cultural issues*, as well as concern for modesty, is important in providing psychological support before, during, and after the procedure.

➤ Inform the patient that a saline lock may be inserted before the test because the stress of repeated venipunctures may increase catecholamine levels.

➤ Instruct the patient to follow a normal-sodium diet for 3 days before testing, abstain from smoking tobacco for 24 hours before testing, and avoid consumption of foods high in amines for 48 hours before testing.

➤ Instruct the patient to avoid self-prescribed medications for 2 weeks before testing (especially appetite suppressants and cold and allergy medications, such as nose drops, cough suppressants, and bronchodilators).

➤ Instruct the patient to withhold prescribed medication (especially methyldopa, epinephrine, levodopa, and methenamine mandelate) if directed by the health care practitioner.

➤ Instruct the patient to fast from food and fluids for 10 to 12 hours before the test.

➤ Prepare an ice slurry in a cup or plastic bag to have ready for immediate transport of the specimen to the laboratory. Prechill the green-top tube in the ice slurry.

Intratest:

➤ Ensure that the patient has complied with dietary and medication restrictions as well as other pretesting preparations; assure that food and fluids have been restricted for at least 10 to 12 hours prior to the procedure.

➤ If the patient has a history of severe allergic reaction to latex, care should be taken to avoid the use of equipment containing latex.

➤ Instruct the patient to cooperate fully and to follow directions. Direct the patient to breathe normally and to avoid unnecessary movement.

➤ Observe standard precautions, and follow the general guidelines in Appendix A. Positively identify the patient, and label the appropriate tubes with the corresponding patient demographics, position of the patient, date, and time of collection. Perform a venipuncture between 6 and 8 a.m.; collect the specimen in a prechilled 5-mL green-top tube.

➤ Remove the needle, and apply a pressure dressing over the puncture site.

➤ Ask the patient to stand for 10 minutes, and then obtain a second sample as previously described.

➤ The sample should be placed in an ice slurry immediately after collection. Information on the specimen label can be protected from water in the ice slurry if the specimen is first placed in a protective plastic bag. Promptly transport the specimen to the laboratory for processing and analysis.

➤ The results are recorded manually or in a computerized system for recall and postprocedure interpretation by the appropriate health care practitioner.

Post-test:

➤ Observe venipuncture site for bleeding or hematoma formation. Apply paper tape or other adhesive to hold pressure bandage in place, or replace with a plastic bandage.

➤ Instruct the patient to resume usual diet, fluids, medications or activity, as directed by the health care practitioner.

➤ Assess the patient for increased pulse and blood pressure, hyperglycemia, shakiness, and palpitations associated with increased values.

➤ A written report of the examination will be sent to the requesting health care practitioner, who will discuss the results with the patient.

➤ Recognize anxiety related to test results. Discuss the implications of abnormal test results on the patient's lifestyle. Provide teaching and information regarding the clinical implications of the test results, as appropriate. Educate the patient regarding access to counseling services.

➤ Reinforce information given by the patient's health care provider regarding further testing, treatment, or referral to another health care provider. Answer any questions or address any concerns voiced by the patient or family.

➤ Depending on the results of this pro-

cedure, additional testing may be performed to evaluate or monitor progression of the disease process and determine the need for a change in therapy. Evaluate test results in relation to the patient's symptoms and other tests performed.

Related laboratory tests:

➤ Related laboratory tests include calcitonin, urine catecholamines, urine homovanillic acid, urine metanephrines, and urine vanillylmandelic acid.

CATECHOLAMINES, URINE

SYNONYMS/ACRONYM: Epinephrine, norepinephrine, dopamine.

SPECIMEN: Urine (25 mL) from a timed specimen collected in a clean plastic, amber collection container with 6N hydrochloric acid as a preservative.

REFERENCE VALUE: (Method: High-performance liquid chromatography)

	Conventional Units	SI Units
		(Conventional Units × 5.46)
Epinephrine		
1–4 y	0–6.0 μg/24 h	0–32.8 nmol/24 h
4 – 10 y	0–10.0 μg/24 h	0–54.6 nmol/24 h
10–15 y	0.5–20 μg/24 h	2.7–109 nmol/24 h
Adult	0–20 μg/24 h	0–109 nmol/24 h
		(Conventional Units × 5.91)
Norepinephrine		
1–4 y	0–29 μg/24 h	0–171 nmol/24 h
4–10 y	8–65 μg/24 h	47–384 nmol/24 h
10 y–adult	15–80 μg/24 h	89–473 nmol/24 h
		(Conventional Units × 6.53)
Dopamine		
1–4 y	10–260 μg/24 h	65–1698 nmol/24 h
4 y–adult	65–400 μg/24 h	424–2612 nmol/24 h

DESCRIPTION & RATIONALE: Catecholamines are produced by the chromaffin tissue of the adrenal medulla. They also are found in sympathetic nerve endings and in the brain. The major catecholamines are epinephrine, norepinephrine, and dopamine. They prepare the body for the fight-or-flight stress response, help regulate metabolism, and are excreted from the body by the kidneys. Levels are affected by diurnal variations, fluctuating in response to stress, postural changes, diet, smoking, drugs, and temperature changes. As a result, blood measurement is not as reliable as a 24-hour timed urine test. For test results to be valid, all of the previously mentioned environmental variables must be controlled when the test is performed. Elevated homovanillic acid levels rule out pheochromocytoma because this tumor primarily secretes epinephrine. Elevated catecholamines without hypertension suggest neuroblastoma or ganglioneuroma. Findings should be compared with metanephrines and vanillylmandelic acid, which are the metabolites of epinephrine and norepinephrine. Findings should also be compared with homovanillic acid, which is the product of dopamine metabolism. ■

INDICATIONS:
- Assist in the diagnosis of neuroblastoma, ganglioneuroma, or dysautonomia
- Assist in the diagnosis of pheochromocytoma
- Evaluate acute hypertensive episode
- Evaluate hypertension of unknown origin
- Screen for pheochromocytoma among family members with an autosomal dominant inheritance pattern for Lindau–von Hippel disease or multiple endocrine neoplasia

RESULT

Increased in:
- Diabetic acidosis (epinephrine and norepinephrine)

- Ganglioblastoma (epinephrine, slight increase; norepinephrine, large increase)
- Ganglioneuroma (all are increased; norepinephrine, largest increase)
- Hypothyroidism (epinephrine and norepinephrine)
- Long-term manic-depressive disorders (epinephrine and norepinephrine)
- Myocardial infarction (epinephrine and norepinephrine)
- Neuroblastoma (all are increased; norepinephrine and dopamine, largest increase)
- Pheochromocytoma (epinephrine, continuous or intermittent increase; norepinephrine, slight increase)
- Shock (epinephrine and norepinephrine)
- Strenuous exercise (epinephrine and norepinephrine)

Decreased in:
- Autonomic nervous system dysfunction (norepinephrine)
- Orthostatic hypotension (norepinephrine)
- Parkinson's disease (dopamine)

CRITICAL VALUES: N/A

INTERFERING FACTORS:
- Drugs that may increase urine catecholamine levels include acetaminophen, atenolol, dopamine (intravenous), isoproterenol, methyldopa, niacin, nitroglycerin, prochlorperazine, rauwolfia, reserpine, syrosingopine, and theophylline.
- Drugs that may decrease urine catecholamine levels include bretylium tosylate, clonidine, decaborane, guanethidine, guanfacine, methyldopa, ouabain, radiographic substances, and reserpine.
- Stress, hypoglycemia, smoking, and

drugs can produce elevated catecholamines.

• Secretion of catecholamines exhibits diurnal variation, with the lowest levels occurring at night.

• Secretion of catecholamines varies during the menstrual cycle, with higher levels excreted during the luteal phase and lowest levels during ovulation.

• Diets high in amines (e.g., bananas, avocados, beer, aged cheese, chocolate, cocoa, coffee, fava beans, grains, tea, vanilla, walnuts, Chianti wine) can produce elevated catecholamine levels.

• Failure to collect all urine and store 24-hour specimen properly will yield a falsely low result.

• Failure to follow dietary restrictions before the procedure may cause the procedure to be canceled or repeated.

Nursing Implications and Procedure • • • • • • • • • • •

Pretest:

➤ Inform the patient that the test is used to diagnose pheochromocytoma and in the workup of neuroblastoma.

➤ Obtain a history of the patient's complaints, including a list of known allergens (especially allergies or sensitivities to latex), and inform the appropriate health care practitioner accordingly.

➤ Obtain a history of the patient's endocrine system and results of previously performed laboratory tests, surgical procedures, and other diagnostic procedures. For related laboratory tests, refer to the Endocrine System table.

➤ Record the date of the last menstrual period.

➤ Obtain a list of medications the patient is taking, including herbs, nutritional supplements, and nutraceuticals. The requesting health care

practitioner and laboratory should be advised if the patient regularly uses these products so that their effects can be taken into consideration when reviewing results.

➤ Review the procedure with the patient. Provide a nonmetallic urinal, bedpan, or toilet-mounted collection device. Address concerns about pain related to the procedure. Explain to the patient that there should be no discomfort during the procedure.

➤ Usually a 24-hour time frame for urine collection is ordered. Inform the patient that all urine over a 24-hour period must be saved; if a preservative has been added to the container, instruct the patient not to discard the preservative. Instruct the patient not to void directly into the laboratory collection container. Instruct the patient to avoid defecating in the collection device and to keep toilet tissue out of the collection device to prevent contamination of the specimen. Place a sign in the bathroom as a reminder to save all urine.

➤ Instruct the patient to void all urine into the collection device, then pour the urine into the laboratory collection container. Alternatively, the specimen can be left in the collection device for a health care staff member to add to the laboratory collection container.

➤ *Sensitivity to social and cultural issues,* as well as concern for modesty, is important in providing psychological support before, during, and after the procedure.

Instruct the patient to:

➤ Follow a normal-sodium diet for 3 days before testing.

➤ Avoid consumption of foods high in amines for 48 hours before testing.

➤ Avoid excessive stress and exercise during the 24-hour collection period.

➤ Abstain from smoking tobacco for 24 hours before testing.

➤ Avoid self-prescribed medications for 2 weeks before testing (especially appetite suppressants and cold and allergy medications, such as nose drops, cough suppressants, and bronchodilators).

➤ Withhold prescribed medication (especially methyldopa, epinephrine, levodopa, and methenamine mandelate) if directed by the health care practitioner.

➤ Fast from food and fluids for 10 to 12 hours before the test.

Intratest:

➤ Ensure that the patient has complied with dietary, medication, and activity restrictions and with pretesting preparations: assure that food and fluids have been restricted for at least 10 to 12 hours prior to the procedure, and that excessive exercise and stress have been avoided prior to the procedure. Instruct the patient to continue to avoid excessive exercise and stress during the 24-hour collection of urine.

➤ If the patient has a history of severe allergic reaction to latex, care should be taken to avoid the use of equipment containing latex.

➤ Instruct the patient to cooperate fully and to follow directions.

➤ Observe standard precautions, and follow the general guidelines in Appendix A. Positively identify the patient, and label the appropriate collection container with the corresponding patient demographics, date, and time of collection.

Timed specimen:

➤ Obtain a clean 3-L urine specimen container, toilet-mounted collection device, and plastic bag (for transport of the specimen container). The specimen must be refrigerated or kept on ice throughout the collection period. If an indwelling urinary catheter is in place, the drainage bag must be kept on ice.

➤ Begin the test between 6 and 8 a.m., if possible. Collect first voiding and discard. Record the time the specimen was discarded as the beginning of the timed collection period. The next morning, ask the patient to void at the same time the collection was started and add this last voiding to the container.

➤ If an indwelling catheter is in place, replace the tubing and container system at the start of the collection time. Keep the container system on ice during the collection period or empty the urine into a larger container periodically during the collection period; monitor to ensure continued drainage, and conclude the test the next morning at the same hour the collection was begun.

➤ At the conclusion of the test, compare the quantity of urine with the urinary output record for the collection; if the specimen contains less than what was recorded as output, some urine may have been discarded, invalidating the test.

➤ Include on the collection container's label the amount of urine, test start and stop times, and ingestion of any foods or medications that can affect test results.

➤ Promptly transport the specimen to the laboratory for processing and analysis.

➤ The results are recorded manually or in a computerized system for recall and postprocedure interpretation by the appropriate health care practitioner.

Post-test:

➤ Instruct the patient to resume usual diet, fluids, medications, or activity, as directed by the health care practitioner.

➤ A written report of the examination will be sent to the requesting health care practitioner, who will discuss the results with the patient.

➤ Recognize anxiety related to test results. Discuss the implications of abnormal test results on the patient's lifestyle. Provide teaching and information regarding the clinical implications of the test results, as appropriate.

▶ Reinforce information given by the patient's health care provider regarding further testing, treatment, or referral to another health care provider. Answer any questions or address any concerns voiced by the patient or family.

▶ Depending on the results of this procedure, additional testing may be performed to evaluate or monitor progression of the disease process and determine the need for a change in therapy. Evaluate test results in relation to the patient's symptoms and other tests performed.

Related laboratory tests:

▶ Related laboratory tests include calcitonin, plasma catecholamines, urine homovanillic acid, urine metanephrines, and urine vanillylmandelic acid.

CD4/CD8 ENUMERATION

SYNONYM/ACRONYM: T-cell profile.

SPECIMEN: Whole blood (1 mL) collected in green-top (heparin) tube.

REFERENCE VALUE: (Method: Flow cytometry)

Total lymphocytes	1500–4000/mm^3
CD3	876–1900/mm^3
CD4	450–1400/mm^3
CD8	190–725/mm^3
CD20	64–475/mm^3
CD4/CD8 ratio	1.0–3.5

DESCRIPTION & RATIONALE: Enumeration of lymphocytes, identification of cell lineage, and identification of cellular stage of development are used to diagnose and classify malignant myeloproliferative diseases and to plan treatment. T-cell enumeration is also useful in the evaluation and management of immunodeficiency and autoimmune disease. A severely depressed CD4 count is an excellent predictor of imminent opportunistic infection. ∎

INDICATIONS:

• Assist in the diagnosis of acquired immunodeficiency syndrome (AIDS) and plan treatment

• Evaluate malignant myeloproliferative diseases and plan treatment

• Evaluate thymus-dependent or cellular immunocompetence

RESULT

Increased in:

• Malignant myeloproliferative diseases (e.g., acute and chronic lymphocytic leukemia, lymphoma)

Decreased in:

• AIDS

• Aplastic anemia

• Hodgkin's disease

CRITICAL VALUES: N/A

INTERFERING FACTORS:

• Drugs that may increase T-cell count include interferon-γ.

• Drugs that may decrease T-cell count include chlorpromazine and prednisone.

• Specimens should be stored at room temperature.

• Recent radioactive scans or radiation can decrease T-cell counts.

• Values may be abnormal in patients with severe recurrent illness or after recent surgery requiring general anesthesia.

Nursing Implications and Procedure • • • • • • • • • • •

Pretest:

➤ Inform the patient that the test is primarily used to monitor disease progression and effectiveness of retroviral therapy.

➤ Obtain a history of the patient's complaints, including a list of known allergens (especially allergies or sensitivities to latex), and inform the appropriate health care practitioner accordingly.

➤ Obtain a history of the patient's hematopoietic and immune systems and results of previously performed laboratory tests, surgical procedures, and other diagnostic procedures. For related laboratory tests, refer to the Hematopoietic and Immune System tables.

➤ Note any recent procedures that can interfere with test results.

➤ Obtain a list of medications the patient is taking, including herbs, nutritional supplements, and nutraceuticals. The requesting health care practitioner and laboratory should be advised if the patient regularly uses these products so that their effects can be taken into consideration when reviewing results.

➤ There are no food, fluid, or medication restrictions unless by medical direction.

Intratest:

➤ If the patient has a history of severe allergic reaction to latex, care should be taken to avoid the use of equipment containing latex.

➤ Instruct the patient to cooperate fully and to follow directions. Direct the patient to breathe normally and to avoid unnecessary movement.

➤ Observe standard precautions, and follow the general guidelines in Appendix A. Positively identify the patient, and label the appropriate tubes with the corresponding patient demographics, date, and time of collection. Perform a venipuncture; collect the specimen in a 5-mL green-top tube.

➤ Remove the needle, and apply a pressure dressing over the puncture site.

➤ Promptly transport the specimen to the laboratory for processing and analysis.

➤ The results are recorded manually or in a computerized system for recall and postprocedure interpretation by the appropriate health care practitioner.

➤ Observe venipuncture site for bleeding or hematoma formation. Apply paper tape or other adhesive to hold pressure bandage in place, or replace with a plastic bandage.

➤ *Nutritional considerations:* As appropriate, stress the importance of good nutrition and suggest that the patient meet with a nutritional specialist. Stress the importance of following the care plan for medications and follow-up visits. Inform the patient that subsequent requests for follow-up blood work at regular intervals should be anticipated.

➤ A written report of the examination will be sent to the requesting health care practitioner, who will discuss the results with the patient.

➤ Recognize anxiety related to test results, and be supportive of impaired activity related to perceived loss of independence and fear of shortened life expectancy. Discuss the implications of abnormal test results on the patient's lifestyle. Provide teaching and information regarding the clinical implications of the test results, as appropriate. Educate the patient as to the risk of infection related to immunosuppressed inflammatory response and fatigue related to decreased energy production. Educate the patient regarding access to counseling services.

➤ Reinforce information given by the patient's health care provider regarding further testing, treatment, or referral to another health care provider. Answer any questions or address any concerns voiced by the patient or family.

➤ Depending on the results of this procedure, additional testing may be performed to evaluate or monitor progression of the disease process and determine the need for a change in therapy. Evaluate test results in relation to the patient's symptoms and other tests performed.

Related laboratory tests:

➤ Related laboratory tests include bone marrow, complete blood count, HIV-1/HIV-2 antibodies, and β_2-microglobulin.

CEREBROSPINAL FLUID ANALYSIS

SYNONYM/ACRONYM: CSF analysis.

SPECIMEN: CSF (1 to 3 mL) collected in three or four separate plastic conical tubes. Tube 1 is used for chemistry and serology testing, tube 2 is used for microbiology, tube 3 is used for cell count, and tube 4 is used for miscellaneous testing.

REFERENCE VALUE: (Method: Macroscopic evaluation of appearance; spectrophotometry for glucose, lactic acid, and protein; radioimmunoassay for myelin basic protein; nephelometry for immunoglobulin G [IgG]; electrophoresis for oligoclonal banding; Gram stain, India ink preparation, and culture for microbiology; microscopic examination of fluid for cell count; flocculation for Venereal Disease Research Laboratory [VDRL])

Lumbar Puncture	Conventional Units	SI Units
Color and appearance	Crystal clear	
Protein	15–45 mg/dL	*(Conventional Units × 10)* 150–450 mg/L
Glucose		*(Conventional Units × 0.0555)*
Infant or child	60–80 mg/dL	3.3–4.4 mmol/L
Adult	40–70 mg/dL	2.2–3.9 mmol/L
Lactic acid		*(Conventional Units × 0.111)*
Neonate	10–60 mg/dL	1.1–6.7 mmol/L
3–10 d	10–40 mg/dL	1.1–4.4 mmol/L
Adult	Less than 25.2 mg/dL	Less than 2.8 mmol/L
Myelin basic protein	Less than 2.5 ng/mL	*(Conventional Units × 1)* Less than 2.5 µg/L
Oligoclonal bands	Absent	
IgG	Less than 3.4 mg/dL	*(Conventional Units × 10)* Less than 34 mg/L
Gram stain	Negative	
India ink	Negative	
Culture	No growth	
RBC count	0	0
WBC count		*(Conventional Units × 1)*
Less than 1 y	0–30/mL	$0–30 × 10^6$/L
1–4 y	0–20/mL	$0–20 × 10^6$/L
5–12 y	0–10/mL	$0–10 × 10^6$/L
Adult	0–5/mL	$0–5 × 10^6$/L

WBC Differential	Adult	Children	Adult	Children
Lymphocytes	40%–80%	5%–13%	0.4–0.8	0.55–0.35
Monocytes	15%–45%	50%–90%	0.15–0.45	0.50–0.90
Neutrophils	0%–6%	0%–8%	0–0.6	0–0.8
VDRL	Nonreactive			
Cytology	No abnormal cells seen			

RBC = red blood cell; VDRL = Venereal Disease Research Laboratory; WBC = white blood cell.

DESCRIPTION & RATIONALE: Cerebrospinal fluid (CSF) circulates in the subarachnoid space and has a twofold function: to protect the brain and spinal cord from injury and to transport products of cellular metabolism and neurosecretion. CSF analysis helps determine the presence and cause of bleeding and assists in diagnosing cancer, infections, and degenerative and autoimmune diseases of the brain and spinal cord. Specimens for analysis are most frequently obtained by lumbar puncture and sometimes by ventricular or cisternal puncture. Lumbar puncture can also have therapeutic uses, including injection of drugs and anesthesia. ▪

INDICATIONS:
- Assist in the diagnosis and differentiation of subarachnoid or intracranial hemorrhage
- Assist in the diagnosis and differentiation of viral or bacterial meningitis or encephalitis
- Assist in the diagnosis of diseases such as multiple sclerosis, autoimmune disorders, or degenerative brain disease
- Assist in the diagnosis of neurosyphilis and chronic central nervous system (CNS) infections
- Detect obstruction of CSF circulation due to hemorrhage, tumor, or edema
- Establish the presence of any condition decreasing the flow of oxygen to the brain
- Monitor for metastases of cancer into the CNS
- Monitor severe brain injuries

RESULT

Increases in:
- Color and appearance: bloody—hemorrhage; xanthochromic—old hemorrhage, red blood cell (RBC) breakdown, methemoglobin, bilirubin (greater than 6 mg/dL), increased protein (greater than 150 mg/dL), melanin (meningeal melanosarcoma), carotene (systemic carotenemia); hazy—meningitis; pink to dark yellow—aspiration of epidural fat; turbid—cells, microorganisms, protein, fat, or contrast medium
- Protein: meningitis, encephalitis
- Lactic acid: bacterial, tubercular, fungal meningitis

- Myelin basic protein: trauma, stroke, tumor, multiple sclerosis, subacute sclerosing panencephalitis
- IgG and oligoclonal banding: multiple sclerosis, CNS syphilis, and subacute sclerosing panencephalitis
- Gram stain: meningitis due to *Streptococcus pneumoniae, Haemophilus influenzae, Neisseria meningitidis, Cryptococcus neoformans*
- India ink preparation: meningitis due to *C. neoformans*
- Culture: encephalitis or meningitis due to herpes simplex virus, *S. pneumoniae, H. influenzae, N. meningitidis, C. neoformans*
- RBC count: hemorrhage
- White blood cell (WBC) count:
  General increase—injection of contrast media or anticancer drugs in subarachnoid space; CSF infarct; metastatic tumor in contact with CSF; reaction to repeated lumbar puncture
  Elevated WBC count with a predominance of neutrophils indicative of bacterial meningitis
  Elevated WBC count with a predominance of lymphocytes indicative of viral, tubercular, parasitic, or fungal meningitis; multiple sclerosis
  Elevated WBC count with a predominance of monocytes indicative of chronic bacterial meningitis, amebic meningitis, multiple sclerosis, toxoplasmosis
  Increased plasma cells indicative of acute viral infections, multiple sclerosis, sarcoidosis, syphilitic meningoencephalitis, subacute sclerosing panencephalitis, tubercular meningitis, parasitic infections, Guillain-Barré syndrome
  Presence of eosinophils indicative of parasitic and fungal infections, acute polyneuritis, idiopathic

hypereosinophilic syndrome, reaction to drugs or a shunt in CSF

- VDRL: syphilis

Positive findings in:

- Cytology: malignant cells

Decreases in:

- Glucose: bacterial and tubercular meningitis

CRITICAL VALUES:
- Positive Gram stain, India ink preparation, or culture

- Presence of malignant cells or blasts

- Elevated white blood cell count

- Glucose greater than 37 mg/dL

Note and immediately report to the health care practitioner any positive or critically increased results and related symptoms.

INTERFERING FACTORS:

This procedure is contraindicated for:

- ⚠ This procedure is contraindicated if infection is present at the needle insertion site.

- ⚠ It may also be contraindicated in patients with degenerative joint disease or coagulation defects and in patients who are uncooperative during the procedure.

- ⚠ Use with extreme caution in patients with increased intracranial pressure because overly rapid removal of CSF can result in herniation.

Other considerations:

- Drugs that may decrease CSF protein levels include cefotaxime and dexamethasone.

- Interferon-β may increase myelin basic protein levels.

- Drugs that may increase CSF glucose levels include cefotaxime and dexamethasone.

- RBC count may be falsely elevated with a traumatic spinal tap.

- Recent radioactive scans or radiation within 1 week before the test can interfere with test results when radioimmunoassay is the test method.

Nursing Implications and Procedure • • • • • • • • • • • •

Pretest:

➤ Inform the patient that the test is primarily used to assist in the differential diagnosis of infection or hemorrhaging in the brain. It is also used in the evaluation of other conditions with significant neuromuscular affects.

➤ Obtain a history of the patient's complaints, including a list of known allergens (especially allergies or sensitivities to latex or anesthetics), and inform the appropriate health care practitioner accordingly.

➤ Obtain a history of the patient's immune and musculoskeletal systems and results of previously performed laboratory tests, surgical procedures, and other diagnostic procedures. For related laboratory tests, refer to the Immune and Musculoskeletal System tables.

➤ Note any recent procedures that can interfere with test results.

➤ Obtain a list of the medications the patient is taking. Include herbs, nutritional supplements, and nutraceuticals. The requesting health care practitioner and laboratory should be advised if the patient regularly uses these products so that their effects can be taken into consideration when reviewing results.

➤ Review the procedure with the patient. Inform the patient that the position required may be awkward, but that someone will assist during the procedure. Stress the importance of remaining still and breathing normally throughout the procedure. Inform the patient that specimen collection takes approximately 20 minutes. Address concerns about pain related to the procedure. Inform the patient that a stinging sensation may be felt when the local anesthetic is injected. Tell the patient to report any pain or other sensations that may require repositioning the spinal needle. Explain to the patient that there may be some discomfort during the procedure. Tell the patient the procedure will be performed by a health care practitioner.

➤ *Sensitivity to cultural and social issues,* as well as concern for modesty, is important in providing psychological support before, during, and after the procedure.

➤ There are no food, fluid, or medication restrictions unless by medical direction.

➤ *Make sure a written and informed consent has been signed prior to the procedure and before administering any medications.*

Intratest:

➤ If the patient has a history of severe allergic reaction to latex, care should be taken to avoid the use of equipment containing latex.

➤ Ensure that anticoagulant therapy has been withheld for the appropriate amount of days prior to the procedure. Amount of days to withhold medication is dependant on the type of anticoagulant. Notify health care practitioner if patient anticoagulant therapy has not been withheld.

➤ Have emergency equipment readily available.

➤ Instruct the patient to cooperate fully and to follow directions. Direct the patient to breathe normally and to avoid unnecessary movement.

➤ Observe standard precautions, and follow the general guidelines in Appendix A. Positively identify the patient, and label the appropriate

tubes with the corresponding patient demographics, date, and time of collection. Collect the specimen in four plastic conical tubes.

➤ Record baseline vital signs.

➤ To perform a lumbar puncture, position the patient in the knee-chest position at the side of the bed. Provide pillows to support the spine or for the patient to grasp. The sitting position is an alternative. In this position, the patient must bend the neck and chest to the knees.

➤ Prepare the site—usually between L3 and L4, or between L4 and L5—with povidone-iodine and drape the area.

➤ A local anesthetic is injected. Using sterile technique, the health care practitioner inserts the spinal needle through the spinous processes of the vertebrae and into the subarachnoid space. The stylet is removed. If the needle is properly placed, CSF drips from the needle.

➤ Attach the stopcock and manometer, and measure initial pressure. Normal pressure for an adult in the lateral recumbent position is 90 to 180 mm H_2O; normal pressure for a child age 8 years or younger is 10 to 100 mm H_2O. These values depend on the body position and are different in a horizontal or sitting position.

➤ CSF pressure may be elevated if the patient is anxious, holding his or her breath, or tensing muscles. It may also be elevated if the patient's knees are flexed too firmly against the abdomen. CSF pressure may be significantly elevated in patients with intracranial tumors. If the initial pressure is elevated, the health care practitioner may perform Queckenstedt's test. To perform this test, pressure is applied to the jugular vein for about 10 seconds. CSF pressure usually rises rapidly in response to the occlusion, and then returns to the pretest level within 10 seconds after the pressure is released. Sluggish response may indicate CSF obstruction.

➤ Obtain four vials of spinal fluid in

separate tubes (1 to 3 mL in each), and label them numerically (1-4 or 5) in the order they were filled.

➤ A final pressure reading is taken, and the needle is removed. Clean the puncture site with an antiseptic solution, and apply a small bandage.

➤ Promptly transport the specimen to the laboratory for processing and analysis.

➤ The results are recorded manually or in a computerized system for recall and postprocedure interpretation by the appropriate health care practitioner.

Post-test:

➤ Observe puncture site for bleeding, CSF leakage, or hematoma formation. Apply paper tape or other adhesive to hold pressure bandage in place, or replace with a plastic bandage.

➤ Monitor vital signs and neurologic status and for headache every 15 minutes for 1 hour, then every 2 hours for 4 hours, and then as ordered by the health care practitioner. Monitor temperature every 4 hours for 24 hours. Compare with baseline values. Notify the health care practitioner if temperature is elevated. Protocols may vary from facility to facility.

➤ If permitted, administer fluids to replace lost CSF and help prevent or relieve headache—a side effect of lumbar puncture.

➤ Position the patient flat in the supine position with head of bed at not more than a 30° elevation, following the health care provider's instructions. Maintain position for 8 hours.

Changing position is acceptable as long as the body remains horizontal.

➤ A written report of the examination will be sent to the requesting health care practitioner, who will discuss the results with the patient.

➤ Recognize anxiety related to test results. Discuss the implications of abnormal test results on the patient's lifestyle. Provide teaching and information regarding the clinical implications of the test results, as appropriate.

➤ Reinforce information given by the patient's health care provider regarding further testing, treatment, or referral to another health care provider. Answer any questions or address any concerns voiced by the patient or family.

➤ Instruct the patient in the use of any ordered medications. Explain the importance of adhering to the therapy regimen. As appropriate, instruct the patient in significant side effects and systemic reactions associated with the prescribed medication. Encourage him or her to review corresponding literature provided by a pharmacist.

➤ Depending on the results of this procedure, additional testing may be performed to evaluate or monitor progression of the disease process and determine the need for a change in therapy. Evaluate test results in relation to the patient's symptoms and other tests performed.

Related laboratory tests:

➤ Related laboratory tests include complete blood count, culture for appropriate organisms, Gram stain, and syphilis serology.

CERULOPLASMIN

SYNONYM/ACRONYM: Copper oxidase, Cp.

SPECIMEN: Serum (1 mL) collected in a red- or tiger-top tube.

REFERENCE VALUE: (Method: Nephelometry)

Age	Conventional Units	SI Units (Conventional Units × 10)
Newborn–3 mo	5–18 mg/dL	50–180 mg/L
6–12 mo	33–43 mg/dL	330–430 mg/L
1–3 y	26–55 mg/dL	260–550 mg/L
4–5 y	27–56 mg/dL	270–560 mg/L
6–7 y	24–48 mg/dL	240–480 mg/L
Greater than 7 y	20–54 mg/dL	200–540 mg/L

DESCRIPTION & RATIONALE: Ceruloplasmin is an α_2-globulin produced by the liver that binds copper for transport in the blood after it is absorbed from the gastrointestinal system. Decreased production of this globulin causes copper to be deposited in body tissues such as the brain, liver, corneas, and kidneys. ■

INDICATIONS:
• Assist in the diagnosis of Menkes (kinky hair) disease
• Assist in the diagnosis of Wilson's disease
• Determine genetic predisposition to Wilson's disease
• Monitor patient response to total parenteral nutrition (hyperalimentation)

RESULT

Increased in:
• Acute infections
• Biliary cirrhosis
• Cancer of the bone, lung, stomach
• Copper intoxication
• Hodgkin's disease
• Leukemia
• Pregnancy (last trimester)
• Rheumatoid arthritis
• Tissue necrosis

Decreased in:
• Menkes disease
• Nutritional deficiency of copper
• Wilson's disease

CRITICAL VALUES: N/A

INTERFERING FACTORS:

- Drugs that may increase ceruloplasmin levels include anticonvulsants, norethindrone, oral contraceptives, and tamoxifen.

- Drugs that may decrease ceruloplasmin levels include asparaginase and levonorgestrel (Norplant).

- Excessive therapeutic intake of zinc may interfere with intestinal absorption of copper.

Nursing Implications and Procedure ....

Pretest:

- Inform the patient that the test is used in the evaluation of copper intoxication and liver disease, especially Wilson's disease.

- Obtain a history of the patient's complaints, including a list of known allergens (especially allergies or sensitivities to latex), and inform the appropriate health care practitioner accordingly.

- Obtain a history of the patient's hepatobiliary system and results of previously performed laboratory tests, surgical procedures, and other diagnostic procedures. For related laboratory tests, refer to the Hepatobiliary System table.

- Obtain a list of medications the patient is taking, including herbs, nutritional supplements, and nutraceuticals. The requesting health care practitioner and laboratory should be advised if the patient regularly uses these products so that their effects can be taken into consideration when reviewing results.

- There are no food, fluid, or medication restrictions unless by medical direction.

Intratest:

- If the patient has a history of severe allergic reaction to latex, care should be taken to avoid the use of equipment containing latex.

- Instruct the patient to cooperate fully and to follow directions. Direct the patient to breathe normally and to avoid unnecessary movement.

- Observe standard precautions, and follow the general guidelines in Appendix A. Positively identify the patient, and label the appropriate tubes with the corresponding patient demographics, date, and time of collection. Perform a venipuncture; collect the specimen in a 5-mL red- or tiger-top tube.

- Remove the needle, and apply a pressure dressing over the puncture site.

- Promptly transport the specimen to the laboratory for processing and analysis.

- The results are recorded manually or in a computerized system for recall and postprocedure interpretation by the appropriate health care practitioner.

Post-test:

- Observe venipuncture site for bleeding or hematoma formation. Apply paper tape or other adhesive to hold pressure bandage in place, or replace with a plastic bandage.

- *Nutritional considerations:* Instruct the patient with copper deficiency to increase intake of foods rich in copper, as appropriate. Organ meats, shellfish, nuts, and legumes are good sources of dietary copper. High intake of zinc, iron, calcium, and manganese interferes with copper absorption. Copper deficiency does not normally occur in adults; however, patients receiving long-term total parenteral nutrition should be evaluated if signs and symptoms of copper deficiency appear, such as jaundice or eye color changes. Kayser-Fleischer rings (green-gold rings) in the cornea and a liver biopsy specimen showing more than 250 μg of copper per gram confirms Wilson's disease.

- A written report of the examination

will be sent to the requesting health care practitioner, who will discuss the results with the patient.

➤ Reinforce information given by the patient's health care provider regarding further testing, treatment, or referral to another health care provider. Answer any questions or address any concerns voiced by the patient or family.

➤ Depending on the results of this pro-

cedure, additional testing may be performed to evaluate or monitor progression of the disease process and determine the need for a change in therapy. Evaluate test results in relation to the patient's symptoms and other tests performed.

Related laboratory tests:

➤ Related laboratory tests include copper, liver biopsy, and zinc.

CHEST X-RAY

· ·

SYNONYM/ACRONYM: Chest radiography, CXR.

AREA OF APPLICATION: Lungs.

CONTRAST: None.

DESCRIPTION & RATIONALE: Chest radiography, commonly called chest x-ray, is one of the most frequently performed radiologic diagnostic studies. This study yields information about the pulmonary, cardiac, and skeletal systems. X-rays penetrate air easily; areas filled with air appear dark or black on x-ray film. Bones appear near-white on the film because x-rays cannot penetrate them to reach the film. Organs and tissues appear as shades of gray because they absorb more x-ray than air but less than bone. A routine chest x-ray includes a posteroanterior view, in which x-rays are passing from the posterior to the anterior, and a lateral view. Portable x-rays, done in more acute or critical situa-

tions, can be done at the bedside and include only the anteroposterior projection. Films may be taken with the patient supine or in a lateral decubitus position, if the presence of free pleural fluid is in question. Other projections that can be obtained are the obliques, lateral decubitus, and lordotic; in general, the part being studied is placed next to the film. Films may be taken on full inspiration and on full expiration to detect a pneumothorax. Rib detail films may be taken to delineate rib pathology, useful when chest radiographs suggest fractures or metastatic lesions. Fluoroscopic studies of the chest can also be done to evaluate movement of the chest and diaphragm during breathing and coughing. In the beginning of the disease process of tuberculosis, asthma, and chronic obstructive pulmonary disease, the results of the chest x-ray may not correlate with the clinical status of the patient and may even be normal. ■

INDICATIONS:

- Aid in the diagnosis of diaphragmatic hernia, lung tumors, intravenous devices, and metastasis.

- Evaluate known or suspected pulmonary disorders, chest trauma, cardiovascular disorders, and skeletal disorders

- Evaluate placement and position of an endotracheal tube, tracheostomy tube, nasogastric feeding tube, pacemaker wires, central venous catheters, Swan-Ganz catheters, chest tubes, and intra-aortic balloon pump

- Evaluate positive PPD or Mantoux tests.

- Monitor resolution, progression, or maintenance of disease

- Monitor effectiveness of the treatment regimen

RESULT

Normal Findings:
- Normal lung fields, cardiac size, mediastinal structures, thoracic spine, ribs, and diaphragm

Abnormal Findings:
- Atelectasis
- Bronchitis
- Curvature of the spinal column (scoliosis)
- Enlarged heart
- Enlarged lymph nodes
- Flattened diaphragm

- Foreign bodies lodged in the pulmonary system
- Fractures of the sternum, ribs, and spine
- Lung pathology, including tumors
- Malposition of tubes or wires
- Mediastinal tumor and pathology
- Pericardial effusion
- Pericarditis
- Pleural effusion
- Pneumonia
- Pneumothorax
- Pulmonary bases, fibrosis, infiltrates
- Tuberculosis
- Vascular abnormalities

CRITICAL VALUES: N/A

INTERFERING FACTORS:

This procedure is contraindicated for:
- Patients who are pregnant or suspected of being pregnant, unless the potential benefits of the procedure far outweigh the risks to the fetus and mother

Factors that may impair the results of the examination:
- Metallic objects within the examination field (e.g., jewelry, body rings), which may inhibit organ visualization and can produce unclear images

- Improper adjustment of the radiographic equipment to accommodate obese or thin patients, which can cause overexposure or underexposure and a poor-quality study

- Patients who are very obese, who may exceed the weight limit for the equipment

- Incorrect positioning of the patient,

which may produce poor visualization of the area to be examined

• Inability of the patient to cooperate or remain still during the procedure because of age, significant pain, or mental status

Other considerations:
• The procedure may be terminated if chest pain or severe cardiac arrhythmias occur.

• Consultation with a physician should occur before the procedure for radiation safety concerns regarding younger patients or patients who are lactating.

• Risks associated with radiographic overexposure can result from frequent x-ray procedures. Personnel in the room with the patient should wear a protective lead apron, stand behind a shield, or leave the area while the examination is being done. Personnel working in the area where the examination is being done should wear badges that reveal their level of exposure to radiation.

Nursing Implications and Procedure • • • • • • • • • • •

Pretest:

➤ Inform the patient that the procedure assesses cardiopulmonary status.

➤ Obtain a history of the patient's symptoms and complaints, including a list of known allergens.

➤ Obtain a history of results of previously performed laboratory tests, surgical procedures, and other diagnostic procedures. For related diagnostic tests, refer to the Cardiovascular and Respiratory System table.

➤ Record the date of the last menstrual period and determine the possibility of pregnancy in perimenopausal women.

➤ Obtain a list of the medications the patient is taking.

➤ Review the procedure with the patient. Explain to the patient that no pain will be experienced during the test, but there may be moments of discomfort. Inform the patient that the procedure is performed in the radiology department or at the bedside, by a registered radiologic techologist, and takes approximately 5 to 15 minutes to complete.

➤ *Sensitivity to cultural and social issues,* as well as concern for modesty, is important in providing psychological support before, during, and after the procedure.

➤ There are no food, fluid, or medication restrictions unless by medical direction.

➤ Instruct the patient to remove dentures, jewelry (including watches), hairpins, credit cards, and other metallic objects.

Intratest:

➤ Ensure that the patient has removed jewelry, dentures, all external metallic objects, wires, and the like prior to the procedure.

➤ Patients are given a gown, robe, and foot coverings to wear and instructed to void prior to the procedure.

➤ Observe standard precautions, and follow the general guidelines in Appendix A.

➤ Instruct the patient to cooperate fully and to follow directions. Instruct the patient to remain still throughout the procedure because movement produces unreliable results.

➤ Place the patient in the standing position in front of the x-ray film or detector.

➤ Have the patient place hands on hips, extend neck, and position shoulders forward.

➤ Position the chest with the left side against the film holder for a lateral view.

➤ For portable examinations, elevate the head of the bed to the high Fowler's position.

➤ Ask the patient to inhale deeply and hold his or her breath while the x-ray images are taken, and then to exhale after the images are taken.

➤ The results are recorded on a sheet of x-ray film or electronically, in a computerized system, for recall and postprocedure interpretation by the appropriate health care practitioner.

Post-test:

➤ A written report of the examination will be completed by a health care practitioner specializing in this branch of medicine. The report will be sent to the requesting health care practitioner, who will discuss the results with the patient.

➤ Recognize anxiety related to test results and be supportive of impaired activity related to respiratory capacity and perceived loss of physical activity. Discuss the implications of abnormal test results on the patient's lifestyle. Provide teaching and information regarding the clinical implications of the test results, as appropriate.

➤ Reinforce information given by the patient's health care provider regarding further testing, treatment, or referral to another health care provider. Answer any questions or address any concerns voiced by the patient or family.

➤ Depending on the results of this procedure, additional testing may be performed to evaluate and determine the need for a change in therapy or progression of the disease process. Evaluate test results in relation to the patient's symptoms and other tests performed.

Related diagnostic tests:

➤ Related diagnostic tests include computed tomography of the thorax, electrocardiogram, lung perfusion scan, magnetic resonance imaging of the chest, and pulmonary function.

CHLAMYDIA GROUP ANTIBODY

SYNONYM/ACRONYM: N/A.

SPECIMEN: Serum (1 mL) collected in a red-top tube.

REFERENCE VALUE: (Method: Indirect fluorescent antibody, polymerase chain reaction) Negative or less than fourfold increase in titer.

DESCRIPTION & RATIONALE: Chlamydia, one of the most common sexually transmitted infections, is caused by *Chlamydia trachomatis*. These gram-negative bacteria are called *obligate cell parasites* because they require living cells for growth. There are three serotypes of *C. trachomatis:* One group causes lymphogranuloma venereum, with symptoms of the first phase of the disease appearing 2 to 6 weeks after infection; another causes a genital tract infection different from lymphogranuloma venereum, in which symptoms in men appear 7 to 28 days after intercourse (women are generally asymptomatic); and the third causes the ocular disease trachoma (incubation period, 7 to 10 days). *Chlamydia psittaci* is the cause of psittacosis in birds and humans. It is increasing in prevalence as a pathogen responsible for other significant diseases of the respiratory system. The incubation period for *C. psittaci* infections in humans is 7 to 15 days, which is followed by chills, fever, and a persistent nonproductive cough.

Chlamydia is difficult to culture and grow, so antibody testing has become the technology of choice. The antigen used in many screening kits is not species specific and can confirm only the presence of *Chlamydia* spp. Newer technology using DNA probes can identify the species. Assays that can specifically identify *C. trachomatis* require special collection and transport kits. They also have specific collection instructions, and the specimens are collected on swabs. The laboratory performing this testing should be consulted before specimen collection. ■

INDICATIONS:

- Establish *Chlamydia* as the cause of atypical pneumonia
- Establish the presence of chlamydial infection

RESULT

Positive findings in:
- Chlamydial infection
- Infantile pneumonia
- Infertility
- Lymphogranuloma venereum
- Ophthalmia neonatorum
- Pelvic inflammatory disease
- Urethritis

CRITICAL VALUES: N/A

INTERFERING FACTORS: N/A

Nursing Implications and Procedure • • • • • • • • • • • •

Pretest:

➤ Inform the patient that the test is used to assist in the diagnosis of chlamydia infection.

➤ Obtain a history of the patient's complaints, including a list of known allergens (especially allergies or sensitivities to latex), and inform the appropriate health care practitioner accordingly.

➤ Obtain a history of the patient's immune and reproductive systems, as well as results of previously performed laboratory tests, surgical procedures, and other diagnostic procedures. For related laboratory tests, refer to the Immune and Reproductive System tables.

➤ Obtain a list of medications the patient is taking, including herbs, nutritional supplements, and nutraceuticals. The requesting health care practitioner and laboratory should be advised if the patient regularly uses these products so that their effects can be taken into consideration when reviewing results.

➤ Review the procedure with the patient. Inform the patient that specimen collection takes approximately 5 to 10 minutes. Address concerns about pain related to the procedure.

Explain to the patient that there may be some discomfort during the venipuncture.

➤ Inform the patient that several tests may be necessary to confirm diagnosis. Any individual positive result should be repeated in 7 to 10 days to monitor a change in titer.

➤ There are no food, fluid, or medication restrictions unless by medical direction.

Intratest:

➤ If the patient has a history of severe allergic reaction to latex, care should be taken to avoid the use of equipment containing latex.

➤ Instruct the patient to cooperate fully and to follow directions. Direct the patient to breathe normally and to avoid unnecessary movement.

➤ Observe standard precautions, and follow the general guidelines in Appendix A. Positively identify the patient, and label the appropriate tubes with the corresponding patient demographics, date, and time of collection. Perform a venipuncture; collect the specimen in a 5-mL red-top tube.

➤ Remove the needle, and apply a pressure dressing over the puncture site.

➤ Promptly transport the specimen to the laboratory for processing and analysis.

➤ The results are recorded manually or in a computerized system for recall and postprocedure interpretation by the appropriate health care practitioner.

Post-test:

➤ Observe venipuncture site for bleeding or hematoma formation. Apply paper tape or other adhesive to hold pressure bandage in place, or replace with a plastic bandage.

➤ A written report of the examination will be sent to the requesting health care practitioner, who will discuss the results with the patient.

➤ Recognize anxiety related to test results, and be supportive. Discuss the implications of abnormal test results on the patient's lifestyle. Provide teaching and information regarding the clinical implications of the test results, as appropriate. Emphasize the need to return to have a convalescent blood sample taken in 7 to 14 days. Educate the patient regarding access to counseling services.

➤ *Social and cultural considerations:* Counsel the patient, as appropriate, as to the risk of sexual transmission and educate the patient regarding proper prophylaxis. Reinforce the importance of strict adherence to the treatment regimen.

➤ *Social and cultural considerations:* Inform the patient with positive *C. trachomatis* that findings must be reported to a local health department official, who will question the patient regarding his or her sexual partners.

➤ *Social and cultural considerations:* Offer support, as appropriate, to patients who may be the victim of rape or sexual assault. Educate the patient regarding access to counseling services. Provide a nonjudgmental, nonthreatening atmosphere for a discussion during which you explain the risks of sexually transmitted diseases. It is also important to discuss emotions the patient may experience (guilt, depression, anger) as a victim of rape or sexual assault.

➤ Provide emotional support if the patient is pregnant and if results are positive. Inform the patient that *Chlamydia* infection during pregnancy places the newborn at risk for pneumonia and conjunctivitis.

➤ Reinforce information given by the patient's health care provider regarding further testing, treatment, or referral to another health care provider. Answer any questions or address any concerns voiced by the patient or family.

➤ Depending on the results of this procedure, additional testing may be performed to evaluate or monitor

progression of the disease process and determine the need for a change in therapy. Evaluate test results in relation to the patient's symptoms and other tests performed.

CHLORIDE, BLOOD

SYNONYM/ACRONYM: Cl⁻.

SPECIMEN: Serum (1 mL) collected in a red- or tiger-top tube. Plasma (1 mL) collected in green-top (heparin) tube is also acceptable.

REFERENCE VALUE: (Method: Ion-selective electrode)

Age	Conventional Units	SI Units (Conventional Units × 1)
Premature	95–110 mEq/L	95–110 mmol/L
0–1 mo	98–113 mEq/L	98–113 mmol/L
2 mo–adult	97–107 mEq/L	97–107mmol/L

DESCRIPTION & RATIONALE: Chloride is the most abundant anion in the extracellular fluid. Its most important function is in the maintenance of acid-base balance, in which it competes with bicarbonate for sodium. Chloride levels generally increase and decrease proportional to sodium levels and inversely proportional to bicarbonate levels. Chloride also participates with sodium in the maintenance of water balance and aids in the regulation of osmotic pressure. Chloride contributes to gastric acid (hydrochloric acid) for digestion and activation of enzymes. The chloride content of venous blood is slightly higher than that of arterial blood because chloride ions enter red blood cells in response to absorption of carbon dioxide into the cell. As carbon dioxide enters the blood cell, bicarbonate leaves and chloride is absorbed in exchange to maintain electrical neutrality within the cell.

Chloride is provided by dietary intake, mostly in the form of sodium chloride. It is absorbed by the gastrointestinal system, filtered out by the glomeruli, and reabsorbed by the renal tubules. Excess chloride is excreted in the urine. Serum values normally remain fairly stable. A slight decrease may be detectable after meals because chloride is used to produce hydrochloric acid as part of the digestive process. Measurement of chloride levels is not as essential as measurement of other electrolytes such as sodium or potassium. Chloride is usually included in standard electrolyte panels to detect the presence of unmeasured anions via calculation of the anion gap. Chloride levels are usually not interpreted apart from sodium, potassium, carbon dioxide, and anion gap.

The patient's clinical picture needs to be considered in the evaluation of electrolytes. Fluid and electrolyte imbalances are often seen in patients with serious illness or injury because in these cases the clinical situation has affected the normal homeostatic balance of the body. It is also possible that therapeutic treatments being administered are causing or contributing to the electrolyte imbalance. Children and adults are at high risk for fluid and electrolyte imbalances when chloride levels are depleted. Children are considered to be at high risk during chloride imbalance because a positive serum chloride balance is important for expansion of the extracellular fluid compartment. Anemia, the result of decreased hemoglobin levels, is a frequent issue for elderly patients. Because hemoglobin participates in a major buffer system in the body, depleted hemoglobin levels affect the efficiency of chloride ion exchange for bicarbonate in red blood cells, which in turn affects acid-base balance. Elderly patients are also at high risk because their renal response to change in pH is slower, resulting in a more rapid development of electrolyte imbalance. ■

INDICATIONS:

* Assist in confirming a diagnosis of disorders associated with abnormal chloride values, as seen in acid-base and fluid imbalances

* Differentiate between types of acidosis (hyperchloremic versus anion gap)

* Monitor effectiveness of drug therapy to increase or decrease serum chloride levels

RESULT

Increased in:

* Acute renal failure

* Cushing's disease

* Dehydration

* Diabetes insipidus

* Excessive infusion of normal saline

* Head trauma with hypothalamic stimulation or damage

* Hyperparathyroidism (primary)

* Metabolic acidosis (associated with prolonged diarrhea)

* Renal tubular acidosis

* Respiratory alkalosis (e.g., hyperventilation)

* Salicylate intoxication

Decreased in:

* Addison's disease

* Burns

* Congestive heart failure

* Cushing's syndrome

* Diabetic ketoacidosis

* Excessive sweating

- Gastrointestinal loss from vomiting (severe), diarrhea, nasogastric suction, or fistula

- Metabolic alkalosis

- Overhydration

- Respiratory acidosis (chronic)

- Salt-losing nephritis

- Syndrome of inappropriate antidiuretic hormone secretion

- Water intoxication

CRITICAL VALUES:

Less than 80 mEq/L

Greater than 115 mEq/L

Note and immediately report to the health care practitioner any critically increased or decreased values and related symptoms. Observe the patient for symptoms of critically decreased or elevated chloride levels. Proper interpretation of chloride values must be made within the context of other electrolyte values and requires clinical knowledge of the patient.

The following may be seen in hypochloremia: twitching or tremors, which may indicate excitability of the nervous system; slow and shallow breathing; and decreased blood pressure as a result of fluid loss. Possible interventions relate to treatment of the underlying cause.

Signs and symptoms associated with hyperchloremia are weakness, lethargy, and deep, rapid breathing. Proper interventions include treatments that correct the underlying cause.

INTERFERING FACTORS:
- Drugs that may cause an increase in chloride levels include acetazolamide, acetylsalicylic acid, ammonium chloride, androgens, bromide, chlorothiazide, cholestyramine, cyclosporine, estrogens, guanethidine, hydrochlorothiazide, lithium, methyldopa, nonsteroidal anti-inflammatory drugs, oxyphenbutazone, phenylbutazone, and triamterene.

- Drugs that may cause a decrease in chloride levels include aldosterone, bicarbonate, corticosteroids, corticotropin, cortisone, diuretics, ethacrynic acid, furosemide, hydroflumethiazide, laxatives (if chronic abuse occurs), mannitol, meralluride, mersalyl, methyclothiazide, metolazone, and triamterene. Many of these drugs can cause a diuretic action that inhibits the tubular reabsorption of chloride. *Note:* Triamterene has nephrotoxic and azotemic effects, and when organ damage has occurred, increased serum chloride levels result. Potassium chloride (found in salt substitutes) can lower blood chloride levels and raise urine chloride levels.

- Elevated triglyceride or protein levels may cause a volume-displacement error in the specimen, reflecting falsely decreased chloride values when chloride measurement methods employing predilution specimens are used (e.g., indirect ion-selective electrode, flame photometry).

- Specimens should never be collected above an intravenous (IV) line because of the potential for dilution when the specimen and the IV solution combine in the collection container, falsely decreasing the result. There is also the potential of contaminating the sample with the normal saline, contained in the IV solution, falsely increasing the result.

Nursing Implications and Procedure . . . .

Pretest:

➤ Inform the patient that the test is used to evaluate electrolytes, acid-base balance, and hydration level.

➤ Obtain a history of the patient's complaints, including a list of known allergens (especially allergies or sensitivities to latex), and inform the appropriate health care practitioner accordingly.

- Obtain a history of the patient's cardiovascular, endocrine, gastrointestinal, genitourinary, and respiratory systems, as well as results of previously performed laboratory tests, surgical procedures, and other diagnostic procedures. For related laboratory tests, refer to the Cardiovascular, Endocrine, Gastrointestinal, Genitourinary, and Respiratory System tables.

- Specimens should not be collected during hemodialysis.

- Obtain a list of medications the patient is taking, including herbs, nutritional supplements, and nutraceuticals. The requesting health care practitioner and laboratory should be advised if the patient regularly uses these products so that their effects can be taken into consideration when reviewing results.

- Review the procedure with the patient. Inform the patient that specimen collection takes approximately 5 to 10 minutes. Address concerns about pain related to the procedure. Explain to the patient that there may be some discomfort during the venipuncture.

- *Sensitivity to social and cultural issues,* as well as concern for modesty, is important in providing psychological support before, during, and after the procedure.

- There are no food, fluid, or medication restrictions unless by medical direction.

Intratest:

- If the patient has a history of severe allergic reaction to latex, care should be taken to avoid the use of equipment containing latex.

- Instruct the patient to cooperate fully and to follow directions. Direct the patient to breathe normally and to avoid unnecessary movement. Instruct the patient not to clench and unclench fist immediately before or during specimen collection.

- Observe standard precautions, and follow the general guidelines in Appendix A. Positively identify the patient, and label the appropriate tubes with the corresponding patient demographics, date, and time of collection. Perform a venipuncture; collect the specimen in a 5-mL red- or tiger-top tube.

- Remove the needle, and apply a pressure dressing over the puncture site.

- Promptly transport the specimen to the laboratory for processing and analysis.

- The results are recorded manually or in a computerized system for recall and postprocedure interpretation by the appropriate health care practitioner.

Post-test:

- Observe venipuncture site for bleeding or hematoma formation. Apply paper tape or other adhesive to hold pressure bandage in place, or replace with a plastic bandage.

- Observe the patient on saline IV fluid replacement therapy for signs of overhydration, especially in cases in which there is a history of cardiac or renal disease. Signs of overhydration include constant, irritable cough; chest rales; dyspnea; or engorgement of neck and hand veins.

- Evaluate the patient for signs and symptoms of dehydration. Check the patient's skin turgor, mucous membrane moisture, and ability to produce tears. Dehydration is a significant and common finding in geriatric and other patients in whom renal function has deteriorated.

- Monitor daily weights as well as intake and output to determine whether fluid retention is occurring because of sodium and chloride excess. Patients at risk for or with a history of fluid imbalance are also at risk for electrolyte imbalance.

- *Nutritional considerations:* Careful observation of the patient on IV fluid replacement therapy is important. A patient receiving a continuous 5% dextrose solution (D_5W) may not be taking in an adequate amount of chloride to meet the body's needs.

The patient, if allowed, should be encouraged to drink fluids such as broths, tomato juice, or colas and to eat foods such as meats, seafood, or eggs, which contain sodium and chloride. The use of table salt may also be appropriate.

➤ *Nutritional considerations:* Instruct patients with elevated chloride levels to avoid eating or drinking anything containing sodium chloride salt. The patient or caregiver should also be encouraged to read food labels to determine which products are suitable for a low-sodium diet.

➤ *Nutritional considerations:* Instruct patients with low chloride levels that a decrease in iron absorption may occur as a result of less chloride available to form gastric acid, which is essential for iron absorption. In prolonged periods of chloride deficit, iron-deficiency anemia could develop.

➤ A written report of the examination will be sent to the requesting health care practitioner, who will discuss the results with the patient.

➤ Reinforce information given by the patient's health care provider regarding further testing, treatment, or referral to another health care provider. Answer any questions or address any concerns voiced by the patient or family.

➤ Depending on the results of this procedure, additional testing may be performed to evaluate or monitor progression of the disease process and determine the need for a change in therapy. Evaluate test results in relation to the patient's symptoms and other tests performed.

Related laboratory tests:

➤ Related laboratory tests include anion gap, carbon dioxide, osmolality, potassium, and sodium.

CHLORIDE, SWEAT

SYNONYMS/ACRONYM: Sweat test, pilocarpine iontophoresis sweat test, sweat chloride.

SPECIMEN: Sweat (0.1 mL minimum) collected by pilocarpine iontophoresis.

REFERENCE VALUE: (Method: Ion-specific electrode or titration)

	Conventional Units	SI Units (Conventional Units × 1)
Normal	5–40 mEq/L	5–40 mmol/L
Intermediate	40–60 mEq/L	40–60 mmol/L

DESCRIPTION & RATIONALE: Cystic fibrosis (CF) is a genetic disease that affects normal functioning of the exocrine glands, causing them to excrete large amounts of electrolytes. Patients with CF have sweat electrolyte levels two to five times normal. Sweat test values, with family history and signs and symptoms, are required to establish a diagnosis of CF. CF is transmitted as an autosomal recessive trait and is characterized by abnormal exocrine secretions within the lungs, pancreas, small intestine, bile ducts, and skin. Clinical presentation may include chronic problems of the gastrointestinal and/or respiratory system. Testing of stool samples for decreased trypsin activity has been used as a screen for CF in infants and children, but this is a much less reliable method than the sweat test.

The sweat test is a noninvasive study done to assist in the diagnosis of CF when considered with other test results and physical assessments. This test is usually performed on children, although adults may also be tested; it is not usually ordered on adults because results can be highly variable and should be interpreted with caution. Sweat for specimen collection is induced by a small electrical current carrying the drug pilocarpine. The test measures the concentration of chloride produced by the sweat glands of the skin. A high concentration of chloride in the specimen indicates the presence of CF. The sweat test is used less commonly to measure the concentration of sodium ions for the same purpose. ∎

INDICATIONS:
- Assist in the diagnosis of CF
- Screen for CF in individuals with a family history of the disease
- Screen for suspected CF in children with recurring respiratory infections
- Screen for suspected CF in infants with failure to thrive and infants who pass meconium late
- Screen for suspected CF in individuals with malabsorption syndrome

RESULT

Increased in:
- Addison's disease
- Alcoholic pancreatitis
- CF
- Chronic pulmonary infections
- Congenital adrenal hyperplasia
- Diabetes insipidus
- Familial cholestasis
- Familial hypoparathyroidism
- Fucosidosis
- Glucose-6-phosphate dehydrogenase deficiency
- Hypothyroidism
- Mucopolysaccharidosis
- Nephrogenic diabetes insipidus
- Renal failure

Decreased in:
- Edema
- Hypoaldosteronism
- Hypoproteinemia
- Sodium depletion

CRITICAL VALUES:

20 years or younger: Greater than 60 mmol/L considered diagnostic of CF

Older than 20 years: Greater than 70 mmol/L considered diagnostic of CF

Note and immediately report to the health care practitioner any critically increased values and related symptoms. Values should be interpreted with consideration of family history and clinical signs and symptoms.

The validity of the test result is affected tremendously by proper specimen collection and handling. Before proceeding with appropriate patient education and counseling, it is important to perform duplicate testing on patients whose results are in the diagnostic or intermediate ranges. A negative test should be repeated if test results do not support the clinical picture.

INTERFERING FACTORS:

- An inadequate amount of sweat may produce inaccurate results. Sweat testing in infants less than 1 month old is not recommended because they are often incapable of producing an adequate amount of sweat sample.

- ⚠ This test should not be performed on patients with skin disorders (e.g., rash, erythema, eczema).

- Improper cleaning of the skin or improper application of gauze pad or filter paper for collection affects test results.

- Hot environmental temperatures may reduce the sodium chloride concentration in sweat; cool environmental temperatures may reduce the amount of sweat collected.

- If the specimen container that stores the gauze or filter paper is handled without gloves, the test results may show a false increase in the final weight of the collection container.

- Screening for CF can be performed using a silver nitrate test paper, and a positive test can be validated by pilocarpine iontophoresis.

Nursing Implications and Procedure . . . .

Pretest:

➤ Inform the patient that the test is used to assist in the diagnosis of cystic fibrosis.

➤ Obtain a history of the patient's complaints, including a list of known allergens (especially allergies or sensitivities to latex), and inform the appropriate health care practitioner accordingly.

➤ Obtain a history of the patient's endocrine and respiratory systems, especially failure to thrive or CF in other family members, as well as results of previously performed laboratory tests, surgical procedures, and other diagnostic procedures. For related laboratory tests, refer to the Endocrine and Respiratory System tables.

➤ Obtain a list of medications the patient is taking, including herbs, nutritional supplements, and nutraceuticals. The requesting health care practitioner and laboratory should be advised if the patient regularly uses these products so that their effects can be taken into consideration when reviewing results.

➤ Review the procedure with the patient and caregiver. Encourage the caregiver to stay with and support the child during the test. The iontophoresis and specimen collection usually takes approximately 75 to 90 minutes. Address concerns about pain related to the procedure. Inform the patient and caregiver there is no pain associated with the test, but a stinging sensation may be experienced when the low electrical current is applied at the site.

➤ *Sensitivity to social and cultural issues,* as well as concern for modesty, is important in providing psychological support before, during, and after the procedure.

➤ There are no food, fluid, or medication restrictions unless by medical direction.

Intratest: ▮

➤ Instruct the patient to cooperate fully and to follow directions.

➤ Observe standard precautions, and follow the general guidelines in Appendix A. Positively identify the patient, and label the appropriate collection container with the corresponding patient demographics, date, and time of collection.

➤ ⚠ The patient is placed in a position that will allow exposure of the site on the forearm or thigh. To ensure collection of an adequate amount of sweat in a small infant, two sites (right forearm and right thigh) can be used. The patient should be covered to prevent cool environmental temperatures from affecting sweat production. The site selected for iontophoresis should never be the chest or left side because of the risk of cardiac arrest from the electrical current.

➤ The site is washed with distilled water and dried. A positive electrode is attached to the site on the right forearm or right thigh and covered with a pad that is saturated with pilocarpine, a drug that stimulates sweating. A negative electrode is covered with a pad that is saturated with bicarbonate solution. Iontophoresis is achieved by supplying a low (4 to 5 mA) electrical current via the electrode for 12 to 15 minutes. Battery-powered equipment is preferred over an electrical outlet to supply the current.

➤ The electrodes are removed, revealing a red area at the site, and the site is washed with distilled water and dried to remove any possible contaminants on the skin.

➤ Preweighed disks made of filter paper are placed on the site with a forceps; to prevent evaporation of sweat collected at the site, the disks are covered with paraffin or plastic and sealed at the edges. The disks are left in place for about 1 hour. Distract the child with books or games to allay fears.

➤ After 1 hour, the paraffin covering is removed, and disks are placed in a preweighed container with a forceps. The container is sealed and sent immediately to the laboratory for weighing and analysis of chloride content. At least 100 mg of sweat is required for accurate results.

➤ Terminate the test if the patient complains of burning at the electrode site. Reposition the electrode before the test is resumed.

➤ Promptly transport the specimen to the laboratory for processing and analysis. Do not directly handle the preweighed specimen container or filter paper.

➤ The results are recorded manually or in a computerized system for recall and postprocedure interpretation by the appropriate health care practitioner.

Post-test: ▮

➤ Observe the site for unusual color, sensation, or discomfort.

➤ Inform the patient and caregiver that redness at the site fades in 2 to 3 hours.

➤ Instruct the patient to resume usual diet, fluids, medications, or activity, as directed by the health care practitioner.

➤ *Nutritional considerations:* If appropriate, instruct the patient and caregiver that nutrition may be altered because of impaired digestive processes associated with CF. Increased viscosity of exocrine gland secretion may lead to poor absorption of digestive enzymes and fat-soluble vitamins, necessitating supplementary oral intake of digestive enzymes with each meal and vitamin (A, D, E, and K) supplementation. Malnutrition also is seen commonly in patients with chronic, severe respiratory disease for many reasons, including fatigue, lack of appetite, and gastrointestinal distress. Research has estimated that the daily caloric intake for respiration in patients with chronic obstructive pulmonary disease is 10 times higher than normal individuals. Inadequate nutrition can result in hypophosphatemia, especially in a respirator-dependent patient. During periods of starvation, phosphorus leaves the intracellular space and moves outside the tissue, resulting in dangerously decreased phosphorus levels. To prevent pulmonary infection and decrease the extent of lung tissue damage, adequate intake of vitamins A and C is also important. Excessive loss of sodium chloride through the sweat glands of a patient with CF may necessitate increased salt intake, especially in environments where increased sweating is induced. The importance of following the prescribed diet should be stressed to the patient and caregiver.

➤ If appropriate, instruct the patient and caregiver that ineffective airway clearance related to excessive production of mucus and decreased ciliary action may result.

➤ A written report of the examination will be sent to the requesting health care practitioner, who will discuss the results with the patient.

➤ Recognize anxiety related to test results, and be supportive of impaired activity related to perceived loss of independence and fear of shortened life expectancy. Discuss the implications of abnormal test results on the patient's lifestyle. Provide teaching and information regarding the clinical implications of the test results, as appropriate.

Educate the patient regarding access to counseling services. Help the patient and caregiver to cope with long-term implications. Recognize that anticipatory anxiety and grief related to potential lifestyle changes may be expressed when someone is faced with a chronic disorder. Provide information regarding genetic counseling and possible screening of other family members if appropriate. Provide contact information, if desired, for the Cystic Fibrosis Foundation (*http://www.cff.org*).

➤ Reinforce information given by the patient's health care provider regarding further testing, treatment, or referral to another health care provider. Explain that a positive sweat test alone is not diagnostic of CF; repetition of borderline and positive tests is generally recommended. Answer any questions or address any concerns voiced by the patient or family.

➤ Depending on the results of this procedure, additional testing may be performed to evaluate or monitor progression of the disease process and determine the need for a change in therapy. Evaluate test results in relation to the patient's symptoms and other tests performed.

Related laboratory tests:

➤ Related laboratory tests include α_1-antitrypsin/phenotype, amylase, anion gap, electrolytes, fecal analysis, fecal fat, osmolality, and phosphorus.

CHOLANGIOGRAPHY, PERCUTANEOUS TRANSHEPATIC

· ·

SYNONYMS/ACRONYMS: Percutaneous cholecystogram, PTC, PTHC.

AREA OF APPLICATION: Biliary system.

CONTRAST: Radiopaque iodine-based contrast medium.

DESCRIPTION & RATIONALE: Percutaneous transhepatic cholangiography (PTC) is a test used to the visualize the biliary system in order to evaluate persistent upper abdominal pain after cholecystectomy and to determine the presence and cause of obstructive jaundice. The liver is punctured with a thin needle under fluoroscopic guidance, and contrast medium is injected as the needle is slowly withdrawn. This test visualizes the biliary ducts without depending on the gallbladder's concentrating ability. The intrahepatic and extrahepatic biliary ducts, and occasionally the gallbladder, can be visualized to determine possible obstruction. In obstruction of the extrahepatic ducts, a catheter can be placed in the duct to allow external drainage of bile. Endoscopic retrograde cholangiopancreatography (ERCP) and PTC are the only methods available to view the biliary tree in the presence of jaundice. ERCP poses less risk and is probably done more often. PTC is an invasive procedure and has potential risks, including bleeding, septicemia, bile peritonitis, and extravasation of the contrast medium. ∎

INDICATIONS:
- Aid in the diagnosis of obstruction caused by gallstones, benign strictures, malignant tumors, congenital cysts, and anatomic variations
- Determine the cause, extent, and location of mechanical obstruction
- Determine the cause of upper abdominal pain after cholecystectomy
- Distinguish between obstructive and nonobstructive jaundice

RESULT

Normal Findings:
- Biliary ducts are normal in diameter, with no evidence of dilation, filling defects, duct narrowing, or extravasation.
- Contrast medium fills the ducts and flows freely.
- Gallbladder appears normal in size and shape.

Abnormal Findings:
- Anatomic biliary or pancreatic duct variations
- Biliary sclerosis
- Cholangiocarcinoma
- Cirrhosis

- Common bile duct cysts
- Gallbladder carcinoma
- Gallstones
- Hepatitis
- Nonobstructive jaundice
- Pancreatitis
- Sclerosing cholangitis
- Tumors, strictures, inflammation, or gallstones of the common bile duct

CRITICAL VALUES: N/A

INTERFERING FACTORS:

This procedure is contraindicated for:

- ⚠ Patients with allergies to shellfish or iodinated dye. The contrast medium used may cause a life-threatening allergic reaction. Patients with a known hypersensitivity to the medium may benefit from premedication with corticosteroids or the use of nonionic contrast medium.

- Patients who are pregnant or suspected of being pregnant, unless the potential benefits of the procedure far outweigh the risks to the fetus and mother.

- ⚠ Patients with cholangitis. The injection of the contrast medium can increase biliary pressure, leading to bacteremia, septicemia, and shock.

- Patients with postoperative wound sepsis, hypersensitivity to iodine, or acute renal failure.

- ⚠ Patients with bleeding disorders, massive ascites, or acute renal failure.

Factors that may impair clear imaging:

- Gas or feces in the gastrointestinal tract resulting from inadequate cleansing or failure to restrict food intake before the study

- Retained barium from a previous radiologic procedure

- Metallic objects within the examination field (e.g., jewelry, body rings), which may inhibit organ visualization and can produce unclear images

- Improper adjustment of the radiographic equipment to accommodate obese or thin patients, which can cause overexposure or underexposure and a poor-quality study

- Patients who are very obese, who may exceed the weight limit for the equipment

- Incorrect positioning of the patient, which may produce poor visualization of the area to be examined

- Inability of the patient to cooperate or remain still during the procedure because of age, significant pain, or mental status

Other considerations:

- The procedure may be terminated if chest pain or severe cardiac arrhythmias occur.

- Failure to follow dietary restrictions and other pretesting preparations may cause the procedure to be canceled or repeated.

- Peritonitis may occur as a result of bile extravasation.

- Consultation with a physician should occur before the procedure for radiation safety concerns regarding younger patients or patients who are lactating.

- Risks associated with radiographic overexposure can result from frequent x-ray procedures. Personnel in the room with the patient should wear a protective lead apron, stand behind a shield, or leave the area while the examination is being done. Personnel working in the area where the examination is being done should wear badges that reveal their level of exposure to radiation.

Nursing Implications and Procedure • • • • • • • • • • •

➤ Inform the patient that the procedure assesses the biliary ducts.

➤ Obtain a history of the patient's complaints, including a list of known allergens, especially allergies or sensitivities to latex, iodine, seafood, contrast medium, and dyes.

➤ Obtain a history of results of previously performed diagnostic procedures, surgical procedures, and laboratory tests. For related diagnostic tests, refer to the Gastrointestinal and Hepatobiliary System tables.

➤ Ensure that this procedure is performed before an esophagogastroduodenoscopy (upper gastrointestinal study) or barium swallow.

➤ Record the date of the last menstrual period and determine the possibility of pregnancy in perimenopausal women.

➤ Obtain a list of the medications the patient is taking.

➤ Review the procedure with the patient. Explain to the patient that some pain may be experienced during the test, and there may be moments of discomfort. Explain the purpose of the test and how the procedure is performed. Inform the patient that there may be some abdominal discomfort from the needle insertion; however, the area will have received prior anesthesia. Inform the patient that the procedure is performed in a radiology department, usually by a health care practitioner and support staff, and takes approximately 30 to 60 minutes.

➤ *Sensitivity to cultural and social issues,* as well as concern for modesty, is important in providing psychological support before, during, and after the procedure.

➤ Type and screen the patient's blood for possible transfusion.

➤ Patients receiving metformin (Glucophage) for non–insulin-dependent (type 2) diabetes should discontinue the drug on the day of the test and continue to withhold it for 48 hours after the test. Failure to do so may result in lactic acidosis.

➤ Instruct the patient to fast and restrict fluids for 8 hours prior to the procedure.

➤ Inform the patient that a laxative and cleansing enema may be needed the day before the procedure, with cleansing enemas on the morning of the procedure depending on the institution's policy.

➤ *Make sure a written and informed consent has been signed prior to the procedure and before administering any medications.*

➤ Ensure that the patient has complied with dietary and medication restrictions and pretesting preparations for at least 6 hours prior to the procedure. Ensure that the patient has removed all external metallic objects prior to the procedure.

➤ Assess for completion of bowel preparation according to the institution's procedure.

➤ Instruct the patient to remove jewelry (including watches), credit cards, and other metallic objects.

➤ Obtain baseline vital signs.

➤ Have emergency equipment readily available.

➤ Patients are given a gown, robe, and foot coverings to wear and instructed to void prior to the procedure.

➤ Instruct the patient to cooperate fully and to follow directions. Instruct the patient to remain still throughout the procedure because movement produces unreliable results.

➤ Observe standard precautions, and follow the general guidelines in Appendix A.

➤ Place the patient in the supine position on an exam table.

➤ A kidney, ureter, and bladder (KUB) or plain film is taken to ensure that no barium or stool will obscure visualization of the biliary system.

➤ An area over the abdominal wall is anesthetized, and the needle is inserted and advanced under fluoroscopic guidance. Contrast medium is injected when placement is confirmed by the free flow of bile.

➤ A specimen of bile may be sent to the laboratory for culture and cytologic analysis.

➤ At the end of the procedure, the contrast medium is aspirated from the biliary ducts, relieving pressure on the dilated ducts.

➤ The results are recorded manually, on film, or by automated equipment, in a computerized system for recall and postprocedure interpretation by the appropriate health care practitioner.

➤ If an obstruction is found during the procedure, a catheter is inserted into the bile duct to allow drainage of bile.

➤ Maintain pressure over the needle insertion site for several hours if bleeding is persistent.

➤ Establish a closed and sterile drainage system if a catheter is left in place.

Post-test:

➤ Instruct the patient to resume usual diet, fluids, medications, or activity, as directed by the health care practitioner.

➤ Monitor vital signs and neurologic status every 15 minutes for 1 hour, then every 2 hours for 4 hours, and as ordered. Take temperature every 4 hours for 24 hours. Compare with baseline values. Notify the health care practitioner if temperature is elevated. Protocols may vary from facility to facility.

➤ Monitor for reaction to iodinated contrast medium, including rash, urticaria, tachycardia, hyperpnea, hypertension, palpitations, nausea, or vomiting.

➤ Renal function should be assessed before metformin is restarted.

➤ Observe the puncture site for signs of bleeding, hematoma formation, ecchymosis, or leakage of bile. Notify the health care practitioner if any of these is present.

➤ Advise the patient to watch for symptoms of infection, such as pain, fever, increased pulse rate, and muscle aches.

➤ A written report of the examination will be completed by a health care practitioner specializing in this branch of medicine. The report will be sent to the requesting health care practitioner, who will discuss the results with the patient.

➤ Depending on the results of this procedure, additional testing may be needed to evaluate or monitor progression of the disease process and determine the need for a change in therapy. Evaluate test results in relation to the patient's symptoms and other tests performed.

Related diagnostic tests:

➤ Related diagnostic tests include computed tomography of the abdomen, hepatobiliary scan, kidney, ureter, bladder (KUB) studies, and magnetic resonance imaging of the abdomen, and ultrasound of the liver and biliary tract.

CHOLANGIOGRAPHY, POSTOPERATIVE

· ·

SYNONYM/ACRONYM: T-tube cholangiography.

AREA OF APPLICATION: Gallbladder, bile ducts.

CONTRAST: Iodinated contrast medium.

DESCRIPTION & RATIONALE: After cholecystectomy, a self-retaining, T-shaped tube may be inserted into the common bile duct. Postoperative (T-tube) cholangiography is a fluoroscopic and radiographic examination of the biliary tract that involves the injection of a contrast medium through the T-tube inserted during surgery. This test may be performed at the time of surgery and 7 to 10 days after cholecystectomy to assess the patency of the common bile duct and to detect any remaining calculi. T-tube placement may also be done after a liver transplant because biliary duct obstruction or anastomotic leakage is possible. This test should be performed before any gastrointestinal studies using barium and after any studies involving the measurement of iodinated compounds. ∎

INDICATIONS:
* Determine biliary duct patency before T-tube removal

* Identify the cause, extent, and location of obstruction after surgery

RESULT

Normal Findings:
* Biliary ducts are normal in size.

* Contrast medium fills the ductal system and flows freely.

Abnormal Findings:
* Appearance of channels of contrast medium outside of the biliary ducts, indicating a fistula

* Filling defects, dilation, or shadows within the biliary ducts, indicating calculi or neoplasm

CRITICAL VALUES: N/A

INTERFERING FACTORS:

This procedure is contraindicated for:
* Patients who are pregnant or suspected of being pregnant, unless the potential benefits of the procedure far outweigh the risks to the fetus and mother.

* ⚠ Patients with cholangitis. The injection of the contrast medium can increase biliary pressure, leading to bacteremia, septicemia, and shock.

* ⚠ Patients with postoperative wound sepsis, hypersensitivity to iodine, or acute renal failure.

* ⚠ Patients with allergies to shellfish or iodinated dye. The contrast

medium used may cause a life-threatening allergic reaction. Patients with a known hypersensitivity to the medium may benefit from premedication with corticosteroids or the use of nonionic contrast medium.

Factors that may impair clear imaging:

- Gas or feces in the gastrointestinal tract resulting from inadequate cleansing or failure to restrict food intake before the study
- Retained barium from a previous radiologic procedure
- Metallic objects within the examination field (e.g., jewelry, body rings), which may inhibit organ visualization and can produce unclear images
- Improper adjustment of the radiographic equipment to accommodate obese or thin patients, which can cause overexposure or underexposure and a poor-quality study
- Patients who are very obese, who may exceed the weight limit for the equipment
- Incorrect positioning of the patient, which may produce poor visualization of the area to be examined
- Inability of the patient to cooperate or remain still during the procedure because of age, significant pain, or mental status

Other considerations:

- The procedure may be terminated if chest pain or severe cardiac arrhythmias occur.
- Air bubbles resembling calculi may be seen if there is inadvertent injection of air.
- Peritonitis may occur as a result of bile extravasation.
- Failure to follow dietary restrictions and other pretesting preparations may cause the procedure to be canceled or repeated.

- Consultation with a physician should occur before the procedure for radiation safety concerns regarding younger patients or patients who are lactating.
- Risks associated with radiographic overexposure can result from frequent x-ray procedures. Personnel in the room with the patient should wear a protective lead apron, stand behind a shield, or leave the area while the examination is being done. Personnel working in the area where the examination is being done should wear badges that reveal their level of exposure to radiation.

Nursing Implications and Procedure

Pretest:

▶ Inform the patient that the procedure assesses the biliary ducts.

▶ Obtain a history of the patient's complaints, including a list of known allergens, especially allergies or sensitivities to latex, iodine, seafood, contrast medium, and dyes.

▶ Obtain a history of results of previously performed diagnostic procedures, surgical procedures, and laboratory tests. For related diagnostic tests, refer to the Gastrointestinal and Hepatobiliary System tables.

▶ Ensure that this procedure is performed before an esophagogastroduodenoscopy (upper gastrointestinal study) or barium swallow.

▶ Record the date of the last menstrual period and determine the possibility of pregnancy in perimenopausal women.

▶ Obtain a list of the medications the patient is taking.

▶ Review the procedure with the patient. Explain to the patient that some pain may be experienced during the test, and there may be moments of discomfort. Explain the purpose of the test and how the procedure is performed. Inform the patient that the procedure is performed in a radiology department, usually by a health care practitioner and support staff, and takes approximately 30 to 60 minutes.

➤ *Sensitivity to cultural and social issues,* as well as concern for modesty, is important in providing psychological support before, during, and after the procedure.

➤ Instruct the patient to fast and restrict fluids for 8 hours prior to the procedure.

➤ *Make sure a written and informed consent has been signed prior to the procedure and before administering any medications.*

Intratest:

➤ Ensure that the patient has complied with dietary and medication restrictions and pretesting preparations for at least 6 hours prior to the procedure. Ensure that the patient has removed all external metallic objects prior to the procedure.

➤ Assess for completion of bowel preparation according to the institution's procedure.

➤ Instruct the patient to remove jewelry (including watches), credit cards, and other metallic objects.

➤ Have emergency equipment readily available.

➤ Patients are given a gown, robe, and foot coverings to wear and instructed to void prior to the procedure.

➤ Observe standard precautions, and follow the general guidelines in Appendix A.

➤ Instruct the patient to cooperate fully and to follow directions. Instruct the patient to remain still throughout the procedure because movement produces unreliable results.

➤ Clamp the T-tube 24 hours before and during the procedure, if ordered, to help prevent air bubbles from entering the ducts.

➤ An x-ray of the abdomen is obtained to determine if any residual contrast medium is present from previous studies.

➤ The patient is placed on an examination table in the supine position.

➤ The area around the T-tube is draped; the end of the T-tube is cleansed with 70% alcohol. If the T-tube site is inflamed and painful, a local anesthetic (e.g., lidocaine) may be injected around the site. A needle is inserted into the open end of the T-tube, and the clamp is removed.

➤ Contrast medium is injected, and fluoroscopy is performed to visualize contrast medium moving through the duct system.

➤ The patient may feel a bloating sensation in the upper right quadrant as the contrast medium is injected. The tube is clamped, and films are taken of the right upper quadrant in multiple positions. A delayed film may be taken 15 minutes later to visualize passage of the contrast medium into the duodenum.

➤ For procedures done after surgery, the T-tube is removed if findings are normal; a dry, sterile dressing is applied to the site.

➤ If retained calculi are identified, the T-tube is left in place for 4 to 6 weeks until the tract surrounding the T-tube is healed to perform a percutaneous removal.

➤ The results are recorded manually, on film, or by automated equipment, in a computerized system, for recall and postprocedure interpretation by the appropriate health care practitioner.

Post-test:

➤ Monitor T-tube site and change sterile dressing, as ordered. Instruct the patient on the care of the site and dressing changes.

➤ Instruct the patient to resume usual diet, fluids, medications, or activity, as directed by the health care practitioner.

➤ Monitor vital signs and neurologic status every 15 minutes for 1 hour, then every 2 hours for 4 hours, and as ordered. Take temperature every 4 hours for 24 hours. Compare with baseline values. Notify the health care practitioner if temperature is elevated. Protocols may vary from facility to facility.

➤ Monitor for reaction to iodinated contrast medium, including rash, urticaria, tachycardia, hyperpnea, hypertension, palpitations, nausea, or vomiting.

➤ Carefully monitor the patient for fatigue and fluid and electrolyte imbalance.

➤ A written report of the examination will be completed by a health care practitioner specializing in this branch of medicine. The report will be sent to the requesting health care practitioner, who will discuss the results with the patient.

➤ Depending on the results of this procedure, additional testing may be needed to evaluate or monitor progression of the disease process and determine the need for a change in therapy. Evaluate test results in relation to the patient's symptoms and other tests performed.

Related diagnostic tests:

➤ Related diagnostic tests include computed tomography of the abdomen; hepatobiliary scan; kidney, ureter, and bladder film; magnetic resonance imaging of the abdomen, and ultrasound of the liver and hepatobiliary system.

CHOLANGIOPANCREATOGRAPHY, ENDOSCOPIC RETROGRADE

SYNONYM/ACRONYM: ERCP.

AREA OF APPLICATION: Gallbladder, bile ducts, pancreatic ducts.

CONTRAST: Iodinated contrast medium.

DESCRIPTION & RATIONALE: Endoscopic retrograde cholangiopancreatography (ERCP) allows direct visualization of the pancreatic and biliary ducts with a flexible endoscope and, after injection of contrast material, with x-rays. It allows the physician to view the pancreatic, hepatic, and common bile ducts and the ampulla of Vater. ERCP and percutaneous transhepatic cholangiography (PTC) are the only procedures that allow direct visualization of the biliary and pancreatic ducts. ERCP is less invasive and has less morbidity than PTC. It is useful in the evaluation of patients with jaundice, because the ducts can be visualized even when the patient's bilirubin level is high. (In contrast, oral cholecystography and intravenous cholangiography are not able to visualize the biliary system when the patient has high bilirubin levels.) By endoscopy, the distal end of the common bile duct can be widened, and gallstones can be removed and stents placed in narrowed bile ducts to allow bile to be drained in jaundiced patients. During endoscopy, specimens of suspicious tissue can be taken for pathologic review, and manometry pressure readings can be obtained from the bile and pancreatic ducts. ERCP is used in the diagnosis and follow-up of pancreatic disease. ▪

INDICATIONS:

- Assess jaundice of unknown cause to differentiate biliary tract obstruction from liver disease

- Collect specimens for cytology

- Identify obstruction caused by calculi, cysts, ducts, strictures, stenosis, and anatomic abnormalities

- Retrieve calculi from the distal common bile duct and release strictures

- Perform therapeutic procedures, such as sphincterotomy and placement of biliary drains

RESULT

Normal Findings:
- Normal appearance of the duodenal papilla
- Patency of the pancreatic and common bile ducts

Abnormal Findings:
- Duodenal papilla tumors
- Pancreatic cancer
- Pancreatic fibrosis
- Pancreatitis
- Sclerosing cholangitis

CRITICAL VALUES: N/A

INTERFERING FACTORS:

This procedure is contraindicated for:

- Patients who are pregnant or suspected of being pregnant, unless the potential benefits of the procedure far outweigh the risks to the fetus and mother.

- ⚠ Patients with allergies to shellfish or iodinated dye. The contrast medium used may cause a life-threatening allergic reaction. Patients with a known hypersensitivity to the medium may benefit from premedication with corticosteroids or the use of nonionic contrast medium.

Factors that may impair clear imaging:

- Gas or feces in the gastrointestinal tract resulting from inadequate cleansing or failure to restrict food intake before the study

- Retained barium from a previous radiologic procedure

- Previous surgery involving the stomach or duodenum, which can make locating the duodenal papilla difficult

- A patient with Zenker's diverticulum involving the esophagus, who may be unable to undergo ERCP

- A patient with unstable cardiopulmonary status, blood coagulation defects, or cholangitis (test may have to be rescheduled unless the patient received antibiotic therapy before the test)

- A patient with known acute pancreatitis

- Improper adjustment of the radiographic equipment to accommodate obese or thin patients, which can cause overexposure or underexposure and a poor-quality study

- Patients who are very obese, who may exceed the weight limit for the equipment

- Incorrect positioning of the patient,

which may produce poor visualization of the area to be examined

- Inability of the patient to cooperate or remain still during the procedure because of age, significant pain, or mental status

Other considerations:
- The procedure may be terminated if chest pain or severe cardiac arrhythmias occur.

- Failure to follow dietary restrictions and other pretesting preparations may cause the procedure to be canceled or repeated.

- Consultation with a physician should occur before the procedure for radiation safety concerns regarding younger patients or patients who are lactating.

- Risks associated with radiographic overexposure can result from frequent x-ray procedures. Personnel in the room with the patient should wear a protective lead apron, stand behind a shield, or leave the area while the examination is being done. Personnel working in the area where the examination is being done should wear badges that reveal their level of exposure to radiation.

Nursing Implications and Procedure • • • • • • • • • • •

Pretest:

➤ Inform the patient that the procedure assesses the biliary ducts.

➤ Obtain a history of the patient's complaints, including a list of known allergens, especially allergies or sensitivities to latex, iodine, seafood, contrast medium, and dyes.

➤ Obtain a history of results of previously performed diagnostic procedures, surgical procedures, and laboratory tests. For related diagnostic tests, refer to the Gastrointestinal and Hepatobiliary System tables.

➤ Ensure that this procedure is performed before an upper gastrointestinal study or barium swallow.

➤ Record the date of the last menstrual period and determine the possibility of pregnancy in perimenopausal women.

➤ Obtain a list of the medications the patient is taking.

➤ Review the procedure with the patient. Explain to the patient that some pain may be experienced during the test, and there may be moments of discomfort. Explain the purpose of the test and how the procedure is performed. Inform the patient that the procedure is performed in a GI lab or radiology department, usually by a health care practitioner and support staff, and takes approximately 30 to 60 minutes.

➤ *Sensitivity to cultural and social issues, as well as concern for modesty, is important in providing psychological support before, during, and after the procedure.*

➤ Instruct the patient to fast and restrict fluids for 8 hours prior to the procedure.

➤ *Make sure a written and informed consent has been signed prior to the procedure and before administering any medications.*

Intratest:

➤ Ensure that the patient has complied with dietary, and medication restrictions and pretesting preparations for at least 6 hours prior to the procedure. Ensure that the patient has removed all external metallic objects prior to the procedure.

➤ Assess for completion of bowel preparation according to the institution's procedure.

➤ Instruct the patient to remove jewelry, including watches, credit cards, and other metallic objects.

➤ Have emergency equipment readily available.

➤ Patients are given a gown, robe, and foot coverings to wear and instructed to void prior to the procedure.

➤ Observe standard precautions, and follow the general guidelines in Appendix A. Positively identify the patient, and label the appropriate containers with the corresponding patient demographics, date, and time of collection, if cytology samples are collected.

➤ Instruct the patient to cooperate fully and to follow directions. Instruct the patient to remain still throughout the procedure because movement produces unreliable results.

➤ Insert an intravenous line for administration of drugs, as needed.

➤ Administer ordered sedation.

➤ An x-ray of the abdomen is obtained to determine if any residual contrast medium is present from previous studies.

➤ The oropharynx is sprayed or swabbed with a topical local anesthetic.

➤ The patient is placed on an examination table in the left lateral position with the left arm behind the back and right hand at the side with the neck slightly flexed. A protective guard is inserted into the mouth to cover the teeth. A bite block can also be inserted to maintain adequate opening of the mouth.

➤ The endoscope is passed through the mouth with a dental suction device in place to drain secretions. A side-viewing flexible fiberoptic endoscope is passed into the duodenum, and a small cannula is inserted into the duodenal papilla (ampulla of Vater).

➤ The patient is placed in the prone position. The duodenal papilla is visualized and cannulated with a catheter. Occasionally the patient can be turned slightly to the right side to aid in visualization of the papilla.

➤ Intravenous glucagon or anticholinergics can be administered to minimize duodenal spasm and to facilitate visualization of the ampulla of Vater.

➤ ERCP manometry can be done at this time to measure the pressure in the bile duct, pancreatic duct, and sphincter of Oddi at the papilla area via the catheter as it is placed in the area before the contrast medium is injected.

➤ When the catheter is in place, contrast medium is injected into the pancreatic and biliary ducts via the catheter, and fluoroscopic films are taken. Biopsy specimens for cytologic analysis can be obtained during the procedure.

➤ Place specimens in appropriate containers, label them properly, and promptly transport them to the laboratory.

➤ The results are recorded manually, on film, or by automated equipment, in a computerized system, for recall and postprocedure interpretation by the appropriate health care practitioner.

Post-test:

➤ Instruct the patient to resume usual diet, fluids, medications, or activity after 24 hours, or as directed by the health care practitioner.

➤ Do not allow the patient to eat or drink until the gag reflex returns, after which the patient is permitted to eat lightly for 12 to 24 hours.

➤ Monitor vital signs and neurologic status every 15 minutes for 1 hour, then every 2 hours for 4 hours, and as ordered. Take temperature every 4 hours for 24 hours. Compare with baseline values. Notify the health care practitioner if temperature is elevated. Protocols may vary from facility to facility.

➤ Monitor for reaction to iodinated contrast medium, including rash, urticaria, tachycardia, hyperpnea, hypertension, palpitations, nausea, or vomiting.

➤ Tell the patient to expect some throat soreness and possible hoarseness. Advise the patient to use warm gargles, lozenges, ice packs to the neck, or cool fluids to alleviate throat discomfort.

➤ Inform the patient that any belching, bloating, or flatulence is the result of air insufflation.

➤ Emphasize that any severe pain, fever, difficulty breathing, or expectoration of blood must be reported to the physician immediately.

➤ A written report of the examination will be completed by a health care practitioner specializing in this branch of medicine. The report will be sent to the requesting health care practitioner, who will discuss the results with the patient.

➤ Depending on the results of this procedure, additional testing may be needed to evaluate or monitor progression of the disease process and determine the need for a change in therapy. Evaluate test results in relation to the patient's symptoms and other tests performed.

Related diagnostic tests:

➤ Related diagnostic tests include computed tomography of the abdomen; hepatobiliary scan; kidney, ureter, and bladder film; magnetic resonance imaging of the abdomen, and ultrasound of the liver and hepatobiliary system.

CHOLESTEROL, HDL AND LDL

SYNONYMS/ACRONYMS: α_1-Lipoprotein cholesterol, high-density cholesterol, HDLC, β-lipoprotein cholesterol, low-density cholesterol, LDLC.

SPECIMEN: Serum (2 mL) collected in a red- or tiger-top tube.

REFERENCE VALUE: (Method: Spectrophotometry)

HDLC	Conventional Units	SI Units (Conventional Units × 0.0259)
Birth	6–56 mg/dL	0.16–1.45 mmol/L
Children and adults		
Desirable	Greater than 60 mg/dL	Greater than 1.56 mmol/L
Acceptable	40–60 mg/dL	0.9–1.56 mmol/L
Low	Less than 40 mg/dL	Less than 0.9 mmol/L

Risk	Units Conventional	SI Units (Conventional Factor × 0.0259)
Optimal	Less than 100 mg/dL	Less than 2.59 mmol/L
Near optimal	100–129 mg/dL	2.59–3.34 mmol/L
Borderline high	130–159 mg/dL	2.67–4.11 mmol/L
High	160–189 mg/dL	4.14–4.90 mmol/L
Very high	Greater than 190 mg/dL	Greater than 4.92 mmol/L

DESCRIPTION & RATIONALE: High-density lipoprotein cholesterol (HDLC) and low-density lipoprotein cholesterol (LDLC) are the major transport proteins for cholesterol in the body. It is believed that HDLC may have protective properties in that its role includes transporting cholesterol from the arteries to the liver. LDLC is the major transport protein for cholesterol to the arteries from the liver. LDLC can be calculated using total cholesterol, total triglycerides, and HDLC levels.

HDLC levels less than 40 mg/dL in men and women represent a coronary risk factor. There is an inverse relationship between HDLC and risk of coronary artery disease (CAD) (i.e., lower HDLC levels represent a higher risk of CAD). Levels of LDLC in terms of risk for CAD are directly proportional to risk and vary by age group. The LDLC can be estimated using the Friedewald formula:

$$LDLC = (Total\ Cholesterol) - (HDLC) - (VLDLC)$$

Very-low-density lipoprotein cholesterol (VLDLC) is estimated by dividing the triglycerides (conventional units) by 5. Triglycerides in SI units would be divided by 2.18 to estimate VLDLC. It is important to note that the formula is valid only if the triglycerides are less than 400 mg/dL or 4.52 mmol/L. ∎

INDICATIONS:
- Determine the risk of cardiovascular disease

- Evaluate the response to dietary and drug therapy for hypercholesterolemia
- Investigate hypercholesterolemia in light of family history of cardiovascular disease

RESULT

LDLC Recommended Levels

HDLC increased in:
- Alcoholism
- Biliary cirrhosis
- Chronic hepatitis
- Exercise
- Familial hyper-α-lipoproteinemia

HDLC decreased in:
- Abetalipoproteinemia
- Cholestasis
- Chronic renal failure
- Fish eye disease
- Genetic predisposition or enzyme/cofactor deficiency
- Hepatocellular disorders
- Hypertriglyceridemia
- Nephrotic syndrome
- Obesity
- Premature CAD
- Sedentary lifestyle
- Smoking
- Tangier disease
- Syndrome X (metabolic syndrome)
- Uncontrolled diabetes

LDLC increased in:
- Anorexia nervosa
- Chronic renal failure
- Corneal arcus
- Cushing's syndrome
- Diabetes
- Diet high in cholesterol and saturated fat
- Dysglobulinemias
- Hepatic disease
- Hepatic obstruction
- Hyperlipoproteinemia types IIA and IIB
- Hypothyroidism
- Nephrotic syndrome
- Porphyria
- Pregnancy
- Premature CAD
- Syndrome X (metabolic syndrome)
- Tendon and tuberous xanthomas

LDLC decreased in:
- Acute stress (severe burns, illness)
- Chronic anemias
- Chronic pulmonary disease
- Genetic predisposition or enzyme/cofactor deficiency
- Hyperthyroidism
- Hypolipoproteinemia and abetalipoproteinemia
- Inflammatory joint disease
- Myeloma
- Reye's syndrome
- Severe hepatocellular destruction or disease
- Tangier disease

CRITICAL VALUES: N/A

INTERFERING FACTORS:
- Drugs that may increase HDLC levels include albuterol, anticonvulsants, cholestyramine, cimetidine, clofibrate and other fibric acid derivatives, estrogens, ethanol (moderate use), lovastatin, niacin, oral contraceptives,

pindolol, pravastatin, prazosin, and simvastatin.

* Drugs that may decrease HDLC levels include acebutolol, atenolol, danazol, diuretics, etretinate, interferon, isotretinoin, linseed oil, metoprolol, neomycin, nonselective β-adrenergic blocking agents, probucol, progesterone, steroids, and thiazides.

* Drugs that may increase LDLC levels include androgens, catecholamines, chenodiol, cyclosporine, danazol, diuretics, etretinate, glucogenic corticosteroids, and progestins.

* Drugs that may decrease LDLC levels include aminosalicylic acid, cholestyramine, colestipol, estrogens, fibric acid derivatives, interferon, lovastatin, neomycin, niacin, pravastatin, prazosin, probucol, simvastatin, terazosin, and thyroxine.

* Some of the drugs used to lower total cholesterol and LDLC or increase HDLC may cause liver damage.

* Grossly elevated triglyceride levels invalidate the Friedewald formula for mathematical estimation of LDLC; if the triglyceride level is greater than 400 mg/dL, the formula should not be used.

* Fasting before specimen collection is highly recommended. Ideally, the patient should be on a stable diet for 3 weeks and fast for 12 hours before specimen collection.

* Failure to follow dietary restrictions before the procedure may cause the procedure to be canceled or repeated.

Nursing Implications and Procedure • • • • • • • • • •

Pretest:

➤ Inform the patient that the test is used to assess and monitor risk for coronary artery disease.

➤ Obtain a history of the patient's complaints, including a list of known allergens (especially allergies or sensitivities to latex), and inform the appropriate health care practitioner accordingly.

➤ Obtain a history of the patient's cardiovascular system and results of previously performed laboratory tests, surgical procedures, and other diagnostic procedures. The presence of other risk factors, such as family history of heart disease, smoking, obesity, diet, lack of physical activity, hypertension, diabetes, previous myocardial infarction, and previous vascular disease, should be investigated. For related laboratory tests, refer to the Cardiovascular System table.

➤ Obtain a list of medications the patient is taking, including herbs, nutritional supplements, and nutraceuticals. The requesting health care practitioner and laboratory should be advised if the patient regularly uses these products so that their effects can be taken into consideration when reviewing results.

➤ Review the procedure with the patient. Inform the patient that specimen collection takes approximately 5 to 10 minutes. Address concerns about pain related to the procedure. Explain to the patient that there may be some discomfort during the venipuncture.

➤ Instruct the patient to fast for 12 hours before specimen collection.

➤ Confirm with the requesting health care practitioner that the patient should withhold medications known to influence test results, and instruct the patient accordingly.

➤ There are no fluid restrictions unless by medical direction.

Intratest:

Ensure that the patient has complied with dietary and medication restrictions as well as other pretesting preparations; assure that food has been restricted for at least 12 hours prior to the procedure.

➤ If the patient has a history of severe allergic reaction to latex, care should be taken to avoid the use of equipment containing latex.

➤ Instruct the patient to cooperate fully and to follow directions. Direct the patient to breathe normally and to avoid unnecessary movement.

➤ Observe standard precautions, and follow the general guidelines in Appendix A. Positively identify the patient, and label the appropriate tubes with the corresponding patient demographics, date, and time of collection. Perform a venipuncture; collect the specimen in a 5-mL red- or tiger-top tube.

➤ Remove the needle and apply a pressure dressing over the puncture site.

➤ Promptly transport the specimen to the laboratory for processing and analysis.

➤ The results are recorded manually or in a computerized system for recall and postprocedure interpretation by the appropriate health care practitioner.

Post-test:

➤ Observe venipuncture site for bleeding or hematoma formation. Apply paper tape or other adhesive to hold pressure bandage in place, or replace with a plastic bandage.

➤ Instruct the patient to resume usual diet, fluids, and medications, as directed by the health care practitioner.

➤ *Nutritional considerations:* Decreased HDLC level and increased LDLC level may be associated with CAD. Nutritional therapy is recommended for the patient identified to be at high risk for developing CAD. If overweight, the patient should be encouraged to achieve a normal weight. The American Heart Association Step 1 and Step 2 diets may be helpful in achieving a goal of lowering total cholesterol and triglyceride levels. The Step 1 diet emphasizes a reduction in foods high in saturated fats and cholesterol. Red meats,

eggs, and dairy products are the major sources of saturated fats and cholesterol. If triglycerides also are elevated, the patient should be advised to eliminate or reduce alcohol and simple carbohydrates from the diet. The Step 2 diet recommends stricter reductions.

➤ *Social and cultural considerations:* Numerous studies point to the prevalence of excess body weight in American children and adolescents. Experts estimate that obesity is present in 25% of the population ages 6 to 11 years. The medical, social, and emotional consequences of excess body weight are significant. Special attention should be given to instructing the child and caregiver regarding health risks and weight-control education.

➤ A written report of the examination will be sent to the requesting health care practitioner, who will discuss the results with the patient.

➤ Recognize anxiety related to test results, and be supportive of fear of shortened life expectancy. Discuss the implications of abnormal test results on the patient's lifestyle. Provide teaching and information regarding the clinical implications of the test results, as appropriate. Educate the patient regarding access to counseling services. Provide contact information, if desired, for the American Heart Association *(http://www.americanheart.org)*.

➤ Reinforce information given by the patient's health care provider regarding further testing, treatment, or referral to another health care provider. Answer any questions or address any concerns voiced by the patient or family.

➤ Depending on the results of this procedure, additional testing may be performed to evaluate or monitor progression of the disease process and determine the need for a change in therapy. Evaluate test results in relation to the patient's symptoms and other tests performed.

Related laboratory tests:

➤ Related laboratory tests include antiarrhythmic drugs, apolipoprotein A, apolipoprotein B, aspartate aminotransferase, atrial natriuretic peptide, blood gases, B-type natriuretic peptide, calcium (blood and ionized), C-reactive protein, creatine kinase and isoenzymes, glucose, glycated hemoglobin, homocysteine, ketones, lactate dehydrogenase and isoenzymes, lipoprotein electrophoresis, magnesium, myoglobin, potassium, total cholesterol, triglycerides, and troponin.

CHOLESTEROL, TOTAL

. . . .

SYNONYM/ACRONYM: N/A.

SPECIMEN: Serum (1 mL) collected in a red- or tiger-top tube. Plasma (1 mL) collected in green-top (heparin) tube is also acceptable. It is important to use the same tube type when serial specimen collections are anticipated for consistency in testing.

REFERENCE VALUE: (Method: Spectrophotometry)

Serum

Risk	Conventional Units	SI Units (Conventional Units × 0.0259)
Desirable	Less than 200 mg/dL	Less than 5.18 mmol/L
Borderline	200–239 mg/dL	5.18–6.19 mmol/L
High	Greater than 240 mg/dL	Greater than 6.22 mmol/L

Plasma values may be 10% lower than serum values.

DESCRIPTION & RATIONALE: Cholesterol is a lipid needed to form cell membranes and a component of the materials that render the skin waterproof. It also helps form bile salts, adrenal corticosteroids, estrogen, and androgens. Cholesterol is obtained from the diet (exogenous cholesterol) and also synthesized in the body (endogenous cholesterol). Although most body cells can form some cholesterol, it is produced mainly by the liver and intestinal mucosa. Cholesterol is an integral component in cell membrane maintenance and hormone production. Very low cholesterol values, as are sometimes seen in critically ill patients, can be as life-threatening as very high levels.

According to the National Cholesterol Education Program, maintaining cholesterol levels less than 200 mg/dL significantly reduces the risk of coronary heart disease; no age and gender stratification is presented as part of its recommendation. Numerous studies have been done, and there are inconsistencies among the studies as to target "normals" segregated by age and gender. Beyond the total cholesterol and high-density lipoprotein cholesterol (HDLC) values, other important risk factors must be considered. Many myocardial infarctions occur even in patients whose cholesterol levels are considered to be within acceptable limits or who are in a moderate-risk category. The combination of risk factors and lipid values helps identify individuals at risk so that appropriate interventions can be taken. If the cholesterol level is greater than 200 mg/dL, repeat testing after a 12- to 24-hour fast is recommended. ■

INDICATIONS:

- Assist in determining risk of cardiovascular disease
- Assist in the diagnosis of nephrotic syndrome, hepatic disease, pancreatitis, and thyroid disorders
- Evaluate the response to dietary and drug therapy for hypercholesterolemia
- Investigate hypercholesterolemia in light of family history of cardiovascular disease

RESULT

Increased in:
- Acute intermittent porphyria
- Alcoholism
- Anorexia nervosa
- Cholestasis
- Chronic renal failure
- Diabetes (with poor control)
- Diets high in cholesterol and fats
- Familial hyperlipoproteinemia
- Glomerulonephritis
- Glycogen storage disease (von Gierke disease)
- Gout
- Hypothyroidism (primary)
- Ischemic heart disease
- Nephrotic syndrome
- Obesity
- Pancreatic and prostatic malignancy
- Pregnancy
- Syndrome X (metabolic syndrome)
- Werner's syndrome

Decreased in:
- Burns
- Chronic myelocytic leukemia
- Chronic obstructive pulmonary disease
- Hyperthyroidism
- Liver disease (severe)
- Malabsorption and malnutrition syndromes
- Myeloma
- Pernicious anemia
- Polycythemia vera
- Severe illness

- Sideroblastic anemias
- Tangier disease
- Thalassemia
- Waldenström's macroglobulinemia

CRITICAL VALUES: N/A

INTERFERING FACTORS:

- Drugs that may increase cholesterol levels include amiodarone, androgens, catecholamines, cyclosporine, danazol, diclofenac, disulfiram, glucogenic corticosteroids, ibuprofen, isotretinoin, levodopa, methyclothiazide, miconazole (owing to castor oil vehicle, not the drug), nafarelin, nandrolone, some oral contraceptives, oxymetholone, phenobarbital, phenothiazine, prochlorperazine, and sotalol.

- Drugs that may decrease cholesterol levels include acebutolol, amiloride, aminosalicylic acid, ascorbic acid, asparaginase, atenolol, atorvastatin, beclobrate, bezafibrate, carbutamide, cerivastatin, cholestyramine, ciprofibrate, clofibrate, clonidine, colestipol, dextrothyroxine, doxazosin, enalapril, estrogens, fenfluramine, fenofibrate, fluvastatin, gemfibrozil, haloperidol, hydralazine, interferon, lovastatin, neomycin, niacin, pravastatin, probucol, simvastatin, tamoxifen, terazosin, thyroxine, ursodiol, and verapamil.

- Ingestion of alcohol 12 to 24 hours before the test can falsely elevate results.

- Ingestion of drugs that alter cholesterol levels within 12 hours of the test may give a false impression of cholesterol levels, unless the test is done to evaluate such effects.

- Positioning can affect results; lower levels are obtained if the specimen is from a patient who has been supine for 20 minutes.

- Failure to follow dietary restrictions

before the procedure may cause the procedure to be canceled or repeated.

Nursing Implications and Procedure ● ● ● ● ● ● ● ● ● ● ●

Pretest:

➤ Inform the patient that the test is used to assess and monitor risk for coronary artery disease.

➤ Obtain a history of the patient's complaints, including a list of known allergens (especially allergies or sensitivities to latex), and inform the appropriate health care practitioner accordingly.

➤ Obtain a history of the patient's cardiovascular, gastrointestinal, hematopoietic, and hepatobiliary systems, as well as results of previously performed laboratory tests, surgical procedures, and other diagnostic procedures. The presence of other risk factors, such as family history of heart disease, smoking, obesity, diet, lack of physical activity, hypertension, diabetes, previous myocardial infarction, and previous vascular disease, should be investigated. For related laboratory tests, refer to the Cardiovascular, Gastrointestinal, Hematopoietic, and Hepatobiliary System tables.

➤ Obtain a list of medications the patient is taking, including herbs, nutritional supplements, and nutraceuticals. The requesting health care practitioner and laboratory should be advised if the patient regularly uses these products so that their effects can be taken into consideration when reviewing results.

➤ Review the procedure with the patient. Inform the patient that specimen collection takes approximately 5 to 10 minutes. Address concerns about pain related to the procedure. Explain to the patient that there may be some discomfort during the venipuncture.

➤ Instruct the patient to withhold alcohol and drugs known to alter cholesterol levels for 12 to 24 hours before specimen collection, at the direction of the health care practitioner.

➤ There are no fluid or medication restrictions unless by medical direction.

➤ Fasting 6 to 12 hours before specimen collection is required if triglyceride measurements are included; it is recommended if cholesterol levels alone are measured for screening.

Intratest:

➤ Ensure that the patient has complied with dietary restrictions and pretesting preparations; assure that food has been restricted for at least 6 to 12 hours prior to the procedure if triglycerides are to be measured.

➤ If the patient has a history of severe allergic reaction to latex, care should be taken to avoid the use of equipment containing latex.

➤ Instruct the patient to cooperate fully and to follow directions. Direct the patient to breathe normally and to avoid unnecessary movement.

➤ Observe standard precautions, and follow the general guidelines in Appendix A. Positively identify the patient, and label the appropriate tubes with the corresponding patient demographics, date, and time of collection. Perform a venipuncture; collect the specimen in a 5-mL red- or tiger-top tube.

➤ Remove the needle, and apply a pressure dressing over the puncture site.

➤ Promptly transport the specimen to the laboratory for processing and analysis.

➤ The results are recorded manually or in a computerized system for recall and postprocedure interpretation by the appropriate health care practitioner.

Post-test:

➤ Observe venipuncture site for bleeding or hematoma formation. Apply

paper tape or other adhesive to hold pressure bandage in place, or replace with a plastic bandage.

➤ Instruct the patient to resume usual diet as directed by the health care practitioner.

➤ Secondary causes for increased cholesterol levels should be ruled out before therapy to decrease levels is initiated by use of drugs.

➤ *Nutritional considerations:* Increases in total cholesterol levels may be associated with coronary artery disease (CAD). Nutritional therapy is recommended for patients identified to be at high risk for developing CAD. If overweight, the patient should be encouraged to achieve a normal weight. The American Heart Association Step 1 and Step 2 diets may be helpful in achieving a goal of lowering total cholesterol and triglyceride levels. The Step 1 diet emphasizes a reduction in foods high in saturated fats and cholesterol. Red meats, eggs, and dairy products are the major sources of saturated fats and cholesterol. If triglycerides are also elevated, the patient should be advised to eliminate or reduce alcohol and simple carbohydrates from the diet. The Step 2 diet recommends stricter reductions.

➤ *Social and cultural considerations:* Numerous studies point to the prevalence of excess body weight in American children and adolescents. Experts estimate that obesity is present in 25% of the population ages 6 to 11 years. The medical, social, and emotional consequences of excess body weight are significant. Special attention should be given to instructing the child and caregiver regarding health risks and weight-control education.

➤ A written report of the examination will be sent to the requesting health care practitioner, who will discuss the results with the patient.

➤ Recognize anxiety related to test results, and be supportive of fear of shortened life expectancy. Discuss the implications of abnormal test results on the patient's lifestyle. Provide teaching and information regarding the clinical implications of the test results, as appropriate. Educate the patient regarding access to counseling services. Provide contact information, if desired, for the American Heart Association *(http://www.americanheart.org)*.

➤ Reinforce information given by the patient's health care provider regarding further testing, treatment, or referral to another health care provider. Answer any questions or address any concerns voiced by the patient or family.

➤ Depending on the results of this procedure, additional testing may be performed to evaluate or monitor progression of the disease process and determine the need for a change in therapy. Evaluate test results in relation to the patient's symptoms and other tests performed.

Related laboratory tests:

➤ Related laboratory tests include antiarrhythmic drugs, apolipoprotein A, apolipoprotein B, aspartate aminotransferase, atrial natriuretic peptide, blood gases, B-type natriuretic peptide, calcium, cholesterol (HDL and LDL), C-reactive protein, creatine kinase and isoenzymes, glucose, glycated hemoglobin, homocysteine, ketones, lactate dehydrogenase and isoenzymes, lipoprotein electrophoresis, magnesium, myoglobin, potassium, triglycerides, and troponin.

CHROMOSOME ANALYSIS, BLOOD

SYNONYM/ACRONYM: N/A.

SPECIMEN: Whole blood (2 mL) collected in green-top (sodium heparin) tube.

REFERENCE VALUE: (Method: Tissue culture and microscopic analysis) No chromosomal abnormalities identified.

DESCRIPTION & RATIONALE: Testing for birth defects as well as mental and physical retardation can be accomplished through the use of several technologies. Chromosome analysis by phytohemagglutination assay is used to detect Down syndrome and abnormal sexual development. Fluorescence in situ hybridization (FISH) testing is useful in the detection of specific microdeletion syndromes (e.g., Prader-Willi, Angelman, Beckwith-Wiedemann, Smith-Magenis, DiGeorge, Williams,

Miller-Dieker) and other acquired chromosomal changes associated with hematologic disorders. Amniotic fluid, chorionic villus sampling, and cells from fetal tissue or products of conception can also be evaluated for chromosomal abnormalities. ■

INDICATIONS:
* Evaluate conditions related to cryptorchidism, hypogonadism, primary amenorrhea, and infertility

* Evaluate congenital anomaly, delayed development (physical or mental), mental retardation, and ambiguous sexual organs

* Investigate the carrier status of patients or relatives with known genetic abnormalities

* Investigate the cause of multiple miscarriages

* Provide prenatal care or genetic counseling

RESULT: The following tables list some common genetic defects:

Syndrome	Autosomal Chromosome Defect	Features
Beckwith-Wiedemann	Duplication 11p15	Macroglossia, omphalocele, earlobe creases
Cat's-eye	Trisomy 2q11	Anal atresia, coloboma
Cri du chat	Deletion 5p	Catlike cry, microcephaly, hypertelorism, mental retardation, retrognathia
Down	Trisomy 21	Epicanthal folds, simian crease of palm, flat nasal bridge, mental retardation, congenital heart disease
Edwards'	Trisomy 18	Micrognathia, clenched third/fourth fingers with the fifth finger overlapping, rocker-bottom feet, mental retardation, congenital heart disease
Pallister-Killian	Trisomy 12p	Psychomotor delay, sparse anterior scalp hair, micrognathia, hypotonia
Patau	Trisomy 13	Microcephaly, cleft palate or lip, polydactyly, mental retardation, congenital heart disease
Warkam	Mosaic trisomy 8	Malformed ears, bulbous nose, deep palm creases, absent or hypoplastic patellae
Wolf-Hirschhorn	Deletion 4p	Microcephaly, growth retardation, mental retardation, carp mouth

Syndrome	Sex-Chromosome Defect	Features
XYY	47,XYY	Tall, increased risk of behavior problems
Klinefelter's	47,XXY	Hypogonadism, infertility, underdeveloped secondary sex characteristics, learning disabilities
Triple X	47,XXX	Increased risk of infertility and learning disabilities
Ullrich-Turner	45,X	Short, gonadal dysgenesis, webbed neck, low posterior hairline, renal and cardiovascular abnormalities

CRITICAL VALUES: N/A

INTERFERING FACTORS: N/A

Nursing Implications and Procedure • • • • • • • • • • • •

Pretest:

> Inform the patient that the test is used to evaluate suspected chromosomal disorders.

> Obtain a history of the patient's complaints, including a list of known allergens (especially allergies or sensitivities to latex), and inform the appropriate health care practitioner accordingly.

> Obtain a history of the patient's reproductive system, family history of known or suspected genetic disorders, and results of previously performed laboratory tests, surgical procedures, and other diagnostic procedures. For related laboratory tests, refer to the Reproductive System table.

> Obtain a list of the medications the patient is taking, including herbs, nutritional supplements, and nutraceuticals. The requesting health care practitioner and laboratory should be advised if the patient regularly uses these products so that their effects can be taken into consideration when reviewing results.

> Review the procedure with the patient. Inform the patient that specimen collection takes approximately 5 to 10 minutes. Address concerns about pain related to the procedure. Explain to the patient that there may be some discomfort during the venipuncture.

> There are no food, fluid, or medication restrictions unless by medical direction.

Intratest:

> If the patient has a history of severe allergic reaction to latex, care should be taken to avoid the use of equipment containing latex.

> Instruct the patient to cooperate fully and to follow directions. Direct the patient to breathe normally and to avoid unnecessary movement.

> Observe standard precautions, and follow the general guidelines in Appendix A. Positively identify the patient, and label the appropriate tubes with the corresponding patient demographics, date, and time of collection. Perform a venipuncture; collect the specimen in a 5-mL green-top tube.

➤ Remove the needle, and apply a pressure dressing over the puncture site.

➤ Promptly transport the specimen to the laboratory for processing and analysis.

➤ The results are recorded manually or in a computerized system for recall and postprocedure interpretation by the appropriate health care practitioner.

Post-test:

➤ Observe venipuncture site for bleeding or hematoma formation. Apply paper tape or other adhesive to hold pressure bandage in place, or replace with a plastic bandage.

➤ A written report of the examination will be sent to the requesting health care practitioner, who will discuss the results with the patient.

➤ Recognize anxiety related to test results, and be supportive of the sensitive nature of the testing. Discuss the implications of abnormal test results on the patient's lifestyle. Provide teaching and information regarding the clinical implications of the test results, as appropriate. Educate the patient regarding access to counseling services.

➤ *Social and cultural considerations:* Encourage the family to seek counseling if they are contemplating pregnancy termination or to seek genetic counseling if a chromosomal abnormality is determined. Decisions regarding elective abortion should occur in the presence of both parents. Provide a nonjudgmental, nonthreatening atmosphere for discussing the risks and difficulties of delivering and raising a developmentally challenged infant, as well as exploring other options (termination of pregnancy or adoption). It is also important to discuss feelings the mother and father may experience (e.g., guilt, depression, anger) if fetal abnormalities are detected. Educate the patient and family regarding access to counseling services, as appropriate.

➤ Reinforce information given by the patient's health care provider regarding further testing, treatment, or referral to another health care provider. Answer any questions or address any concerns voiced by the patient or family.

➤ Depending on the results of this procedure, additional testing may be performed to evaluate or monitor progression of the disease process and determine the need for a change in therapy. Evaluate test results in relation to the patient's symptoms and other tests performed.

Related laboratory tests:

➤ Related laboratory tests include amniotic fluid analysis, chorionic villus biopsy, and α_1-fetoprotein.

CLOT RETRACTION

SYNONYM/ACRONYM: N/A.

SPECIMEN: Whole blood collected in a full 5-mL red-top tube.

REFERENCE VALUE: (Method: Macroscopic observation of sample) A normal clot, gently separated from the side of the test tube and incubated at 37°C, shrinks to about half of its original size within 1 hour. The result is a firm, cylindrical fibrin clot that contains red blood cells and is sharply demarcated from the clear serum. Complete clot retraction can take 6 to 24 hours.

DESCRIPTION & RATIONALE: The clot retraction test measures the adequacy of platelet function by measuring the speed and extent of clot retraction. Normally, when blood clots in a test tube, it retracts away from the sidewalls of the tube. Platelets play a major role in the clot retraction process. When platelets are decreased or function is impaired, scant serum and a soft, plump, poorly demarcated clot form in the tube. In addition to normal platelets, clot retraction depends on the contractile protein thrombosthenin, magnesium, adenosine triphosphate (ATP), and pyruvate kinase. Clot retraction is also influenced by hematocrit and by fibrinogen structure and concentration. ■

INDICATIONS:
• Evaluate the adequacy of platelet function
• Evaluate thrombocytopenia of unknown origin
• Investigate the possibility of Glanzmann's disease
• Investigate suspected abnormalities of fibrinogen or fibrinolytic activity

RESULT

Increased in: N/A

Decreased in: Glanzmann's thrombasthenia

CRITICAL VALUES: N/A

INTERFERING FACTORS:
• Drugs that may produce a decreased result include apronalide, carbenicillin, and plicamycin.
• Platelet count less than 100,000/μL, acetylsalicylic acid therapy, altered fibrinogen/fibrin structure, hypofibrinogenemia, polycythemia or hemoconcentration, and multiple myeloma are conditions in which abnormal clot retraction may occur, limiting the ability to form a valid assessment of platelet function.
• Prompt and proper specimen processing, storage, and analysis are important to achieve accurate results. Specimens received in the laboratory more than 1 hour after collection should be rejected.

Nursing Implications and Procedure • • • • • • • • • • •

Pretest:

➤ Inform the patient that the test is used to assist in the diagnosis of bleeding disorders.

➤ Obtain a history of the patient's complaints, including a list of known allergens (especially allergies or sensitivities to latex), and inform the appropriate health care practitioner accordingly.

➤ Obtain a history of the patient's hematopoietic system and results of previously performed laboratory tests, surgical procedures, and other diagnostic procedures. For related laboratory tests, refer to the Hematopoietic System table.

➤ Note any recent procedures that can interfere with test results.

➤ Obtain a list of medications the

patient is taking, including herbs, nutritional supplements, and nutraceuticals. The requesting health care practitioner and laboratory should be advised if the patient regularly uses these products so that their effects can be taken into consideration when reviewing results.

➤ Review the procedure with the patient. Inform the patient that specimen collection takes approximately 5 to 10 minutes. Address concerns about pain related to the procedure. Explain to the patient that there may be some discomfort during the venipuncture.

➤ There are no food, fluid, or medication restrictions unless by medical direction.

Intratest:

➤ If the patient has a history of severe allergic reaction to latex, care should be taken to avoid the use of equipment containing latex.

➤ Instruct the patient to cooperate fully and to follow directions. Direct the patient to breathe normally and to avoid unnecessary movement.

➤ Observe standard precautions, and follow the general guidelines in Appendix A. Positively identify the patient, and label the appropriate tubes with the corresponding patient demographics, date, and time of collection. Perform a venipuncture; collect the specimen in a 5-mL red-top tube.

➤ Remove the needle, and apply a pressure dressing over the puncture site.

➤ Promptly transport the specimen to the laboratory within 1 hour of collection for processing and analysis.

➤ The results are recorded manually or in a computerized system for recall and postprocedure interpretation by the appropriate health care practitioner.

Post-test:

➤ Observe venipuncture site for bleeding or hematoma formation. Apply paper tape or other adhesive to hold pressure bandage in place, or replace with a plastic bandage.

➤ Inform the patient with abnormal clot retraction of the importance of taking precautions against bruising and bleeding. These precautions may include the use of a soft bristle toothbrush, use of an electric razor, avoidance of constipation, avoidance of acetylsalicylic acid and similar products, and avoidance of intramuscular injections.

➤ A written report of the examination will be sent to the requesting health care practitioner, who will discuss the results with the patient.

➤ Reinforce information given by the patient's health care provider regarding further testing, treatment, or referral to another health care provider. Answer any questions or address any concerns voiced by the patient or family.

➤ Depending on the results of this procedure, additional testing may be performed to evaluate or monitor progression of the disease process and determine the need for a change in therapy. Evaluate test results in relation to the patient's symptoms and other tests performed.

Related laboratory tests:

➤ Related laboratory tests include bleeding time, coagulation factor XIII, complete blood count, fibrinogen, hematocrit, hemoglobin, and platelet count.

COAGULATION FACTORS

SYNONYMS/ACRONYMS: See table.

SPECIMEN: Whole blood in a completely filled 5-mL blue-top (sodium citrate) tube.

REFERENCE VALUE: (Method: Photo-optical clot detection) Activity from 50% to 150%.

	Preferred Name	Synonym
Factor I	Fibrinogen	—
Factor II	Prothrombin	Prethrombin
Factor III	Tissue factor	Tissue thromboplastin
Factor IV	Calcium	Ca^{2+}
Factor V	Proaccelerin	Labile factor, accelerator globulin (AcG)
Factor VII	Proconvertin	Stabile factor, serum prothrombin conversion accelerator, autoprothrombin I
Factor VIII:C	Antihemophilic factor (AHF)	Antihemophilic globulin (AHG), antihemophilic factor A, platelet cofactor 1
Factor IX	Plasma thromboplastin component (PTC)	Christmas factor, antihemophilic factor B, platelet cofactor 2
Factor X	Stuart-Prower factor	Autoprothrombin III, thrombokinase
Factor XI	Plasma thromboplastin antecedent (PTA)	Antihemophilic factor C
Factor XII	Hageman factor	Glass factor, contact factor
Factor XIII	Fibrin-stabilizing factor (FSF)	Laki-Lorand factor (LLF), fibrinase, plasma transglutinase
	Prekallikrein	Fletcher factor
	High-molecular-weight kininogen (HMWK)	Fitzgerald factor, contact activation cofactor, Williams factor, Flaujeac factor

DESCRIPTION & RATIONALE: The coagulation proteins respond to blood vessel injury in a chain of events. The intrinsic and extrinsic pathways of secondary hemostasis are a series of reactions involving the substrate protein fibrinogen, the coagulation factors (also known as *enzyme precursors* or *zymogens*), nonenzymatic cofactors (Ca^{2+}), and phospholipid. The factors were assigned Roman numerals in the order of their discovery, not their place in the coagulation sequence. Factor VI was originally thought to be a separate clotting factor. It was subsequently proved to be the same as a modified form of Factor V, and therefore the number is no longer used.

The coagulation factors are formed in the liver. They can be divided into three groups based on their common properties:

1. The contact group is activated in vitro by a surface such as glass and is activated in vivo by collagen. The contact group includes factor XI, factor XII, prekallikrein, and high-molecular-weight kininogen.
2. The prothrombin or vitamin K–dependent group includes factors II, VII, IX, and X.
3. The fibrinogen group includes factors I, V, VIII, and XIII. They are the most labile of the factors and are consumed during the coagulation process. The factors listed in the table are the ones most commonly measured. ■

INDICATIONS:
• Identify the presence of inherited bleeding disorders

• Identify the presence of qualitative or quantitative factor deficiency

RESULT

Increased in: N/A

Decreased in:
• Congenital deficiency
• Disseminated intravascular coagulation
• Liver disease

CRITICAL VALUES: N/A

INTERFERING FACTORS:
• Drugs that may increase factor II levels include fluoxymesterone, methandrostenolone, nandrolone, and oxymetholone.

• Drugs that may decrease factor II levels include warfarin.

• Drugs that may increase factor V, VII, and X levels include anabolic steroids, fluoxymesterone, methandrostenolone, nandrolone, oral contraceptives, and oxymetholone.

• Drugs that may decrease factor V levels include streptokinase.

• Drugs that may decrease factor VII levels include acetylsalicylic acid, asparaginase, cefamandole, ceftriaxone, dextran, dicumarol, gemfibrozil, oral contraceptives, and warfarin.

• Drugs that may increase factor VIII levels include chlormadinone.

• Drugs that may decrease factor VIII levels include asparaginase.

• Drugs that may increase factor IX levels include chlormadinone and oral contraceptives.

• Drugs that may decrease factor IX levels include asparaginase and warfarin.

• Drugs that may decrease factor X levels include chlormadinone, dicumarol, oral contraceptives, and warfarin.

• Drugs that may decrease factor XI levels include asparaginase and captopril.

- Drugs that may decrease factor XII levels include captopril.

- Test results of patients on anticoagulant therapy are unreliable.

- Placement of tourniquet for longer than 1 minute can result in venous stasis and changes in the concentration of plasma proteins to be measured. Platelet activation may also occur under these conditions, causing erroneous results.

- Vascular injury during phlebotomy can activate platelets and coagulation factors, causing erroneous results.

- Hemolyzed specimens must be rejected because hemolysis is an indication of platelet and coagulation factor activation.

- Icteric or lipemic specimens interfere with optical testing methods, producing erroneous results.

- Incompletely filled collection tubes, specimens contaminated with heparin, clotted specimens, or unprocessed specimens not delivered to the laboratory within 1 hour of collection should be rejected.

Nursing Implications and Procedure • • • • • • • • • • •

Pretest:

➤ Inform the patient that the test is used to detect factor deficiencies and related coagulopathies.

➤ Obtain a history of the patient's complaints, including a list of known allergens (especially allergies or sensitivities to latex), and inform the appropriate health care practitioner accordingly.

➤ Obtain a history of the patient's hematopoietic and hepatobiliary systems, any bleeding disorders, and results of previously performed laboratory tests (especially bleeding time, clotting time, complete blood count, partial thromboplastin time, platelets, and prothrombin time), surgical procedures, and other diagnostic procedures. For related laboratory tests, refer to the Hematopoietic and Hepatobiliary System tables.

➤ Obtain a list of medications the patient is taking, including anticoagulant therapy, acetylsalicylic acid, herbals, and nutraceuticals known to affect coagulation. It is recommended that use of these substances be discontinued 14 days before dental or surgical procedures. The requesting health care practitioner and laboratory should be advised if the patient regularly uses these products so that their effects can be taken into consideration when reviewing results.

➤ Review the procedure with the patient. Inform the patient that specimen collection takes approximately 5 to 10 minutes. Address concerns about pain related to the procedure. Explain to the patient that there may be some discomfort during the venipuncture.

➤ There are no food, fluid, or medication restrictions unless by medical direction.

Intratest:

➤ If the patient has a history of severe allergic reaction to latex, care should be taken to avoid the use of equipment containing latex.

➤ Instruct the patient to cooperate fully and to follow directions. Direct the patient to breathe normally and to avoid unnecessary movement.

➤ Observe standard precautions, and follow the general guidelines in Appendix A. Positively identify the patient, and label the appropriate tubes with the corresponding patient demographics, date, and time of collection. Perform a venipuncture; collect the specimen in a 5-mL blue-top tube. *Important note:* Two different concentrations of sodium citrate preservative are currently added to blue-top tubes for coagulation studies: 3.2% and 3.8%. The Clinical and Laboratory Standards Institute/CLSI (formerly the National Committee for Clinical Laboratory Standards/NCCLS) guideline for sodium citrate is 3.2%. Laboratories establish reference ranges for coagulation testing based on numerous factors, including sodium citrate concentration, test equipment, and test reagents. It is important to inquire from the laboratory which concentration it recommends, because each concentration will have its own specific reference range. When multiple specimens are drawn, the blue-top tube should be collected after sterile (i.e., blood culture) and red-top tubes. When coagulation testing is the only work to be done, an extra red-top tube should be collected before the blue-top tube to avoid contaminating the specimen with tissue thromboplastin.

➤ Remove the needle and apply a pressure dressing over the puncture site.

➤ Promptly transport the specimen to the laboratory for processing and analysis. The CLSI recommendation for processed and unprocessed samples stored in unopened tubes is that testing should be completed within 1 to 4 hours of collection.

➤ The results are recorded manually or in a computerized system for recall and postprocedure interpretation by the appropriate health care practitioner.

Post-test:

➤ Observe venipuncture site for bleeding or hematoma formation. Apply paper tape or other adhesive to hold pressure bandage in place, or replace with a plastic bandage.

➤ Instruct the patient to report immediately any signs of unusual bleeding or bruising.

➤ Inform the patient with decreased factor levels of the importance of taking precautions against bruising and bleeding. These precautions may include the use of a soft bristle toothbrush, use of an electric razor, avoidance of constipation, avoidance of acetylsalicylic acid and similar products, and avoidance of intramuscular injections.

➤ A written report of the examination will be sent to the requesting health care practitioner, who will discuss the results with the patient.

➤ Reinforce information given by the patient's health care provider regarding further testing, treatment, or referral to another health care provider. Answer any questions or address any concerns voiced by the patient or family.

➤ Depending on the results of this procedure, additional testing may be performed to evaluate or monitor progression of the disease process and determine the need for a change in therapy. Evaluate test results in relation to the patient's symptoms and other tests performed.

Related laboratory tests:

➤ Related laboratory tests include alanine aminotransferase, alkaline phosphatase, aspartate aminotransferase, clot retraction, copper, activated partial thromboplastin time, plasminogen, protein C, prothrombin time, and vitamin K.

COLD AGGLUTININ TITER

SYNONYM/ACRONYM: Mycoplasma serology.

SPECIMEN: Serum (2 mL) collected in a red-top tube. The tube must be placed in a water bath or heat block at 37°C for 1 hour and allowed to clot before the serum is separated from the red blood cells (RBCs).

REFERENCE VALUE: (Method: Patient serum containing autoantibodies titered against type O RBCs at 2°C to 8°C. Type O cells are used because they have no antigens on the cell membrane surface. Agglutination with patient sera would not occur because of reaction between RBC blood type antigens and patient blood type antibodies.) Negative: Single titer less than 1:32 or less than a fourfold increase in titer over serial samples.

DESCRIPTION & RATIONALE: Cold agglutinins are antibodies that cause clumping or agglutination of RBCs at cold temperatures in individuals with certain conditions or who are infected by particular organisms. Cold agglutinins are associated with *Mycoplasma pneumoniae* infection. *M. pneumoniae* has I antigen specificity to human RBC membranes. Fetal cells largely contain i antigens, but by 18 months most cells carry the I antigen. The agglutinins are usually immunoglobulin M (IgM) antibodies and cause agglutination of cells at temperatures in the range of 0°C to 10°C. The temperature of circulating blood in the extremities may be lower than core temperatures. RBCs of affected individuals may agglutinate and obstruct blood vessels in fingers, toes, and ears, or they may initiate the complement cascade. Affected cells may be lysed immediately within the capillaries and blood vessels as a result of the action of complement on the cell wall, or they may return to the circulatory system and be lysed in the spleen by macrophages.

The titer endpoint is the highest dilution of serum that shows a specific antigen-antibody reaction. Single titers greater than 1:64, or a fourfold increase in titer between specimens collected 5 or more days apart, are clinically significant. Patients affected with primary atypical viral pneumonia exhibit a rise in titer 8 to 10 days after the onset of illness. IgM antibodies peak in 12 to 25 days and begin to diminish 30 days after onset. ∎

INDICATIONS:

• Assist in the confirmation of primary atypical pneumonia, influenza, or pulmonary embolus

• Provide additional diagnostic support for cold agglutinin disease associated with viral infections or lymphoreticular cancers

RESULT

Increased in:

• Infectious mononucleosis

• Malaria

• *M. pneumoniae* (primary atypical pneumonia)

• Multiple myeloma

• Raynaud's disease (severe)

• Systemic lupus erythematosus

• Trypanosomiasis

Decreased in: N/A

CRITICAL VALUES: N/A

INTERFERING FACTORS:

• Antibiotic use may interfere with or decrease antibody production.

• A high antibody titer may interfere with blood typing and crossmatching procedures.

• High titers may appear spontaneously in elderly patients and persist for many years.

• Prompt and proper specimen processing, storage, and analysis are important to achieve accurate results. Specimens should always be transported to the laboratory as quickly as possible after collection. The specimen must clot in a 37°C water bath for 1 hour before separation. Refrigeration of the sample before serum separates from the RBCs may falsely decrease the titer.

Nursing Implications and Procedure • • • • • • • • • • •

Pretest:

➤ Inform the patient that the test is used to assist in the diagnosis of primary atypical pneumonia and other viral/infectious diseases.

➤ Obtain a history of the patient's complaints, including a list of known allergens (especially allergies or sensitivities to latex), and inform the appropriate health care practitioner accordingly.

➤ Obtain a history of the patient's immune and respiratory systems, as well as results of previously performed laboratory tests, surgical procedures, and other diagnostic procedures. For related laboratory tests, refer to the Immune and Respiratory System tables.

➤ Obtain a list of medications the patient is taking, including herbs, nutritional supplements, and nutraceuticals. The requesting health care practitioner and laboratory should be advised if the patient regularly uses these products so that their effects can be taken into consideration when reviewing results.

➤ Note any recent medications that can interfere with test results.

➤ Review the procedure with the patient. Inform the patient that multiple specimens may be required. Inform the patient that specimen collection takes approximately 5 to 10 minutes. Address concerns about pain related to the procedure. Explain to the patient that there may be some discomfort during the venipuncture.

➤ There are no food, fluid, or medication restrictions (except antibiotics) unless by medical direction.

Intratest:

➤ Ensure that the patient has complied with medication restrictions prior to the procedure.

➤ If the patient has a history of severe allergic reaction to latex, care should be taken to avoid the use of equipment containing latex.

➤ Instruct the patient to cooperate fully and to follow directions. Direct the patient to breathe normally and to avoid unnecessary movement.

➤ Observe standard precautions, and follow the general guidelines in Appendix A. Positively identify the patient, and label the appropriate tubes with the corresponding patient

demographics, date, and time of collection. Perform a venipuncture; collect the specimen in a 5-mL red-top tube.

➤ Remove the needle, and apply a pressure dressing over the puncture site.

➤ Promptly transport the specimen to the laboratory for processing and analysis.

➤ Inform the laboratory if the patient is receiving antibiotics.

➤ The results are recorded manually or in a computerized system for recall and postprocedure interpretation by the appropriate health care practitioner.

Post-test:

➤ Observe venipuncture site for bleeding or hematoma formation. Apply paper tape or other adhesive to hold pressure bandage in place, or replace with a plastic bandage.

➤ Instruct the patient to resume antibiotics as directed by the health care practitioner.

➤ A written report of the examination will be sent to the requesting health care practitioner, who will discuss the results with the patient.

➤ Reinforce information given by the patient's health care provider regarding further testing, treatment, or referral to another health care provider. Emphasize the need for the patient to return in 7 to 14 days for a convalescent blood sample. Answer any questions or address any concerns voiced by the patient or family.

➤ Depending on the results of this procedure, additional testing may be performed to evaluate or monitor progression of the disease process and determine the need for a change in therapy. Evaluate test results in relation to the patient's symptoms and other tests performed.

Related laboratory tests:

➤ Related laboratory tests include arterial/alveolar oxygen ratio, blood gases, and complete blood count.

COLLAGEN CROSSLINKED N-TELOPEPTIDE

SYNONYM/ACRONYM: NT_x.

SPECIMEN: Urine (2 mL) from a random specimen collected in a clean plastic container.

REFERENCE VALUE: (Method: Immunoassay)

Male	0–85 nmol bone collagen equivalents/mmol creatinine
Female (premenopausal)	14–76 nmol bone collagen equivalents/mmol creatinine

DESCRIPTION & RATIONALE: Osteoporosis is the most common bone disease in the West. It is often called the "silent disease" because bone loss occurs without symptoms. The formation and maintenance of bone mass is dependent on a combination of factors that include genetics, nutrition, exercise, and hormone function. Normally the rate of bone formation is equal to the rate of bone resorption. After midlife, the rate of bone loss begins to increase. Osteoporosis is more commonly identified in women than in men. Other risk factors include thin, small-framed body structure; family history of osteoporosis; diet low in calcium; white or Asian race; excessive use of alcohol; cigarette smoking; sedentary lifestyle; long-term use of corticosteroids, thyroid replacement medications, or antiepileptics; history of bulimia, anorexia nervosa, chronic liver disease, or malabsorption disorders; and postmenopausal state. Osteoporosis is a major consequence of menopause in women owing to the decline of estrogen production. Osteoporosis is rare in premenopausal women. Estrogen replacement therapy (after menopause) is one strategy that has been commonly employed to prevent osteoporosis, although its exact protective mechanism is unknown. Results of some recently published studies indicate that there may be significant adverse side effects to estrogen replacement therapy; more research is needed to understand the long-term effects (positive and negative) of this therapy. Other treatments include raloxifene (selectively modulates estrogen receptors), calcitonin (interacts directly with osteoclasts), and bisphosphates (inhibit osteoclast-mediated bone resorption).

A noninvasive test to detect the presence of collagen cross-linked N-telopeptide (NT_x) is used to follow the progress of patients who have begun treatment for osteoporosis. NT_x is formed when collagenase acts on bone. Small NT_x fragments are excreted in the urine after bone resorption. A desirable response, 2 to 3 months after therapy is initiated, is a 30% reduction in NT_x and a reduction of 50% below baseline by 12 months. ∎

INDICATIONS:
• Assist in the evaluation of osteoporosis
• Assist in the management and treatment of osteoporosis
• Monitor effects of estrogen replacement therapy

RESULT

Increased in:
• Hyperparathyroidism
• Osteomalacia
• Osteoporosis
• Paget's disease

Decreased in:
• Effective therapy for osteoporosis

CRITICAL VALUES: N/A

INTERFERING FACTORS:
• NT_x levels are affected by urinary excretion, and values may be influenced by the presence of renal impairment or disease.

Nursing Implications and Procedure ....

Pretest:

▶ Inform the patient that the test is used to assist in the diagnosis of osteoporosis and evaluation of therapy.

➤ Obtain a history of the patient's complaints, including a list of known allergens, and inform the appropriate health care practitioner accordingly.

➤ Obtain a history of the patient's musculoskeletal and reproductive systems and results of previously performed laboratory tests, surgical procedures, and other diagnostic procedures. For related laboratory tests, refer to the Musculoskeletal and Reproductive System tables.

➤ Obtain a list of medications the patient is taking, including herbs, nutritional supplements, and nutraceuticals. The requesting health care practitioner and laboratory should be advised if the patient is regularly using these products so that their effects can be taken into consideration when reviewing results.

➤ Review the procedure with the patient. Inform the patient that specimen collection takes approximately 5 to 10 minutes. Address concerns about pain related to the procedure. Explain to the patient that there should be no discomfort during the procedure.

➤ *Sensitivity to social and cultural issues*, as well as concern for modesty, is important in providing psychological support before, during, and after the procedure.

➤ There are no food, fluid, or medication restrictions unless by medical direction.

Intratest:

➤ Instruct the patient to cooperate fully and to follow directions.

➤ Observe standard precautions, and follow the general guidelines in Appendix A. Positively identify the patient, and label the appropriate collection container with the corresponding patient demographics, date, and time of collection.

➤ Instruct the patient to collect a second-void morning specimen as follows: (1) void and then drink a glass of water; (2) wait 30 minutes, and then try to void again.

➤ Promptly transport the specimen to the laboratory for processing and analysis.

➤ The results are recorded manually or in a computerized system for recall and postprocedure interpretation by the appropriate health care practitioner.

Post-test:

➤ Instruct the patient to resume usual diet, fluids, medications, or activity, as directed by the health care practitioner.

➤ *Dietary considerations:* Increased NT_x levels may be associated with osteoporosis. Nutritional therapy may be indicated for patients identified as being at high risk for developing osteoporosis. Educate the patient about the National Osteoporosis Foundation's guidelines regarding a regular regimen of weight-bearing exercises, limited alcohol intake, avoidance of tobacco products, and adequate dietary intake of vitamin D (400 to 800 IU/d) and calcium (1200 to 1500 mg/d). Dietary calcium can be obtained in animal or plant sources. Milk and milk products, sardines, clams, oysters, salmon, rhubarb, spinach, beet greens, broccoli, kale, tofu, legumes, and fortified orange juice are high in calcium. Milk and milk products also contain vitamin D and lactose to assist in absorption. Cooked vegetables yield more absorbable calcium than raw vegetables. Patients should also be informed of the substances that can inhibit calcium absorption by irreversibly binding to some of the calcium and making it unavailable for absorption, such as oxalates, which naturally occur in some vegetables; phytic acid, found in some cereals; and excessive intake of insoluble dietary fiber. Excessive protein intake also can affect calcium absorption negatively, especially if it is combined with foods high in phosphorus. Vitamin D is synthesized by the skin and is available in fortified dairy foods and cod liver oil.

➤ A written report of the examination will be sent to the requesting health

care practitioner, who will discuss the results with the patient.

➤ Recognize anxiety related to test results, and be supportive of impaired activity related to lack of muscular control, perceived loss of independence, and fear of shortened life expectancy. Discuss the implications of abnormal test results on the patient's lifestyle. Provide teaching and information regarding the clinical implications of the test results, as appropriate. Educate the patient regarding access to counseling services. Provide contact information, if desired, for the National Osteoporosis Foundation *(http://www.nof.org)*.

➤ Reinforce information given by the patient's health care provider regarding further testing, treatment, or referral to another health care provider. Answer any questions or address any concerns voiced by the patient or family.

➤ Depending on the results of this procedure, additional testing may be performed to evaluate or monitor progression of the disease process and determine the need for a change in therapy. Evaluate test results in relation to the patient's symptoms and other tests performed.

Related laboratory tests:

➤ Related laboratory tests include alkaline phosphatase, calcitonin, calcium (blood and urine), creatinine, creatinine clearance, parathyroid hormone, phosphorus, and vitamin D.

COLONOSCOPY

· ·

SYNONYMS/ACRONYM: Full colonoscopy, lower endoscopy, lower panendoscopy.

AREA OF APPLICATION: Colon.

CONTRAST: Air.

DESCRIPTION & RATIONALE: Colonoscopy allows inspection of the mucosa of the entire colon, ileocecal valve, and terminal ileum using a flexible fiberoptic colonoscope inserted through the anus and advanced to the terminal ileum. The colonoscope is a multichannel instrument that allows viewing of the gastrointestinal (GI) tract lining, insufflation of air, aspiration of fluid, obtaining of tissue biopsy samples, and passage of a laser beam for obliteration of tissue and control of bleeding. Mucosal surfaces of the lower GI tract are examined for ulcerations, polyps, chronic diarrhea, hemorrhagic sites, neoplasms, and strictures. During the procedure, tissue samples may be obtained for cytology, and some therapeutic procedures may be performed, such as excision of small tumors or polyps, coagulation of bleeding sites, and removal of foreign bodies. ▪

INDICATIONS:

- Assess GI function in a patient with a personal or family history of colon cancer, polyps, or ulcerative colitis

- Confirm diagnosis of colon cancer and inflammatory bowel disease

- Detect Hirschsprung's disease and determine the areas affected by the disease

- Determine cause of lower GI disorders, especially when barium enema and proctosigmoidoscopy are inconclusive

- Determine source of rectal bleeding and perform hemostasis by coagulation

- Evaluate postsurgical status of colon resection

- Evaluate stools that show a positive occult blood test, lower GI bleeding, or change in bowel habits

- Follow up on previously diagnosed and treated colon cancer

- Investigate iron-deficiency anemia of unknown origin

- Reduce volvulus and intussusception in children

- Remove colon polyps

- Remove foreign bodies and sclerosing strictures by laser

RESULT

Normal Findings:

- Normal intestinal mucosa with no abnormalities of structure, function, or mucosal surface in the colon or terminal ileum

Abnormal Findings:

- Benign lesions
- Bleeding sites
- Bowel distention
- Bowel infection or inflammation
- Colitis
- Colon cancer

- Crohn's disease
- Diverticula
- Foreign bodies
- Hemorrhoids
- Polyps
- Proctitis
- Tumors
- Vascular abnormalities

CRITICAL VALUES: N/A

INTERFERING FACTORS:

This procedure is contraindicated for:

- Patients with bleeding disorders or cardiac conditions

- Patients with bowel perforation, acute peritonitis, acute colitis, ischemic bowel necrosis, toxic colitis, recent bowel surgery, advanced pregnancy, severe cardiac or pulmonary disease, recent myocardial infarction, known or suspected pulmonary embolus, and large abdominal aortic or iliac aneurysm

- Patients who have had a colon anastomosis within the past 14 to 21 days, because an anastomosis may break down with gas insufflation

Factors that may impair clear imaging:

- Gas or feces in the gastrointestinal tract resulting from inadequate cleansing or failure to restrict food intake before the study

- Retained barium from a previous radiologic procedure

- Metallic objects within the examination field (e.g., jewelry, body rings), which may inhibit organ visualization and can produce unclear images

- Improper adjustment of the radiographic equipment to accommodate obese or thin patients, which can cause overexposure or underexposure and a poor-quality study

- Patients who are very obese, who may exceed the weight limit for the equipment

- Incorrect positioning of the patient, which may produce poor visualization of the area to be examined

- Inability of the patient to cooperate or remain still during the procedure because of age, significant pain, or mental status

- Severe lower GI bleeding or the presence of feces, barium, blood, or blood clots, which can interfere with visualization

- Spasm of the colon, which can mimic the radiographic signs of cancer (*Note:* the use of intravenous [IV] glucagon minimizes spasm)

- Inability of the patient to tolerate introduction of or retention of barium, air, or both in the bowel

Other considerations:

- Complications of the procedure may include hemorrhage and cardiac arrhythmias.

- The procedure may be terminated if chest pain or severe cardiac arrhythmias occur.

- Failure to follow dietary restrictions and other pretesting preparations may cause the procedure to be canceled or repeated.

- Bowel preparations that include laxatives or enemas should be avoided in pregnant patients or patients with inflammatory bowel disease, unless specifically directed by a health care practitioner.

- Consultation with a physician should occur before the procedure for radiation safety concerns regarding younger patients or patients who are lactating.

- Risks associated with radiographic overexposure can result from frequent x-ray procedures. Personnel in the room with the patient should wear a protective lead apron, stand behind a shield, or leave the area while the examination is being done. Personnel working in the area where the examination is being done should wear badges that reveal their level of exposure to radiation.

Nursing Implications and Procedure • • • • • • • • • •

Pretest:

➤ Inform the patient that the procedure assesses the colon.

➤ Obtain a history of the patient's complaints.

➤ Obtain a history of results of previously performed diagnostic procedures, surgical procedures, and laboratory tests. For related diagnostic tests, refer to the Gastrointestinal System table.

➤ Ensure that this procedure is performed before an upper gastrointestinal study or barium swallow.

➤ Record the date of the last menstrual period and determine the possibility of pregnancy in perimenopausal women.

➤ Obtain a list of the medications the patient is taking, including drugs that affect bleeding, such as aspirin and other salicylates.

➤ Note intake of oral iron preparations within 1 week before the procedure because these cause black, sticky feces that are difficult to remove with bowel preparation.

➤ Review the procedure with the patient. Explain to the patient that some pain may be experienced during the test, and there may be moments of discomfort. Explain the purpose of the test and how the procedure is performed. Inform the patient that the procedure is performed in a GI lab, usually by a health care practitioner and support staff, and takes approximately 30 to 60 minutes.

➤ *Sensitivity to cultural and social*

issues, as well as concern for modesty, is important in providing psychological support before, during, and after the procedure.

➤ Instruct the patient to eat a low-residue diet for several days before the procedure and to consume only clear liquids the evening before the test. The patient should fast and restrict fluids for 8 hours prior to the procedure.

➤ Ensure that ordered laxatives have been administered late in the afternoon of the day before the procedure.

➤ Inform the patient that it is important that the bowel be cleaned thoroughly so that the physician can visualize the colon. Inform the patient that a laxative and cleansing enema may be needed the day before the procedure, with cleansing enemas on the morning of the procedure, depending on the institution's policy.

➤ *Make sure a written and informed consent has been signed prior to the procedure and before administering any medications.*

Intratest:

➤ Ensure that the patient has complied with dietary, and medication restrictions and pretesting preparations for at least 6 hours prior to the procedure.

➤ Assess for completion of bowel preparation according to the institution's procedure.

➤ Instruct the patient to remove jewelry, including watches, credit cards, and other metallic objects.

➤ Have emergency equipment readily available.

➤ Patients are given a gown, robe, and foot coverings to wear and instructed to void prior to the procedure.

➤ Observe standard precautions, and follow the general guidelines in Appendix A. Positively identify the patient, and label the appropriate containers with the corresponding patient demographics, date, and time of collection.

➤ Instruct the patient to cooperate fully and to follow directions. Instruct the patient to remain still throughout the procedure because movement produces unreliable results.

➤ Obtain and record baseline vital signs.

➤ An intravenous (IV) line may be started to allow infusion of a sedative or IV fluids.

➤ Administer medications, as ordered, to reduce discomfort and to promote relaxation and sedation.

➤ The patient is placed on an examination table in the left lateral decubitus position and draped with the buttocks exposed.

➤ The physician performs a visual inspection of the perianal area and a digital rectal examination.

➤ The patient is requested to bear down as if having a bowel movement as the fiberoptic tube is inserted through the rectum.

➤ The scope is advanced through the sigmoid. The patient's position is changed to supine to facilitate passage into the transverse colon. Air is insufflated through the tube during passage to aid in visualization.

➤ The patient is instructed to take deep breaths to aid in movement of the scope downward through the ascending colon to the cecum and into the terminal portion of the ileum.

➤ Air is insufflated to distend the GI tract, as needed. Biopsies, cultures, or any endoscopic surgery is performed.

➤ Foreign bodies or polyps are removed and placed in appropriate specimen containers, labelled, and sent to the laboratory.

➤ Photographs are obtained for future reference.

➤ At the end of the procedure, excess air and secretions are aspirated through the scope, and the colonoscope is removed.

Post-test:

➤ Monitor the patient for signs of respiratory depression.

➤ Monitor vital signs and neurologic status every 15 minutes for 1 hour, then every 2 hours for 4 hours, and as ordered. Take temperature every 4 hours for 24 hours. Compare with baseline values. Notify the health care practitioner if temperature is elevated. Protocols may vary from facility to facility.

➤ Observe the patient until the effects of the sedation have worn off.

➤ Instruct the patient to resume usual diet, fluids, medications, or activity, as directed by the health care practitioner.

➤ Monitor for any rectal bleeding. Instruct the patient to expect slight rectal bleeding for 2 days after removal of polyps or biopsy specimens, but that an increasing amount of bleeding or sustained bleeding should be reported to the physician immediately.

➤ Observe the patient for indications of chest pain, abdominal pain or tenderness, or breathing problems. If these symptoms are present or increase in frequency or severity, the change should be reported to a physician immediately.

➤ Inform the patient that belching, bloating, or flatulence is the result of air insufflation.

➤ Emphasize that any severe pain, fever, difficulty breathing, or GI bleeding must be reported to the physician immediately.

➤ Encourage the patient to drink several glasses of water to help replace fluids lost during the preparation for the test.

➤ Carefully monitor the patient for fatigue and fluid and electrolyte imbalance.

➤ A written report of the examination will be completed by a health care practitioner specializing in this branch of medicine. The report will be sent to the requesting health care practitioner, who will discuss the results with the patient.

➤ Reinforce information given by the patient's health care provider regarding further testing, treatment, or referral to another health care provider. Answer any questions or address any concerns voiced by the patient or family.

➤ Depending on the results of this procedure, additional testing may be needed to evaluate or monitor progression of the disease process and determine the need for a change in therapy. Evaluate test results in relation to the patient's symptoms and other tests performed.

Related diagnostic tests:

➤ Related diagnostic tests include barium enema, computed tomography of the abdomen, magnetic resonance imaging of the abdomen, and proctosigmoidoscopy.

COLOR PERCEPTION TEST

SYNONYM/ACRONYM: Color blindness test.

AREA OF APPLICATION: Eyes.

CONTRAST: N/A.

DESCRIPTION & RATIONALE: Defects in color perception can be hereditary or aquired. The congenital defect for color blindness is carried by the female, who is generally unaffected, and expressed dominantly in males. Color blindness occurs in 8% of males and 0.4% of females. Aquired color blindness may occur as a result of diseases of the optic nerve or retina. Color blindness may be partial or complete. The partial form is the hereditary form, and in the majority of patients the color deficiency is in the red-green area of the spectrum. Color perception tests are performed to determine the acuity of color discrimination. The most common test uses pseudoisochromic plates with numbers or letters buried in a maze of dots. Misreading the numbers or letters indicates a color perception deficiency and may indicate color blindness, a genetic dysfunction, or retinal pathology. ■

INDICATIONS:
• Detect deficiencies in color perception

• Evaluate because of family history of color visual defects

• Investigate suspected retinal pathology affecting the cones

RESULT

Normal Findings:
• Normal visual color discrimination. No difficulty in identification of color combinations.

Abnormal Findings:
• Identification of some but not all colors.

CRITICAL VALUES: N/A

INTERFERING FACTORS:
• Inability of the patient to cooperate or remain still during the procedure because of age, significant pain, or mental status

• Inability of the patient to read

• Poor visual acuity or poor lighting

• Failure of the patient to wear corrective lenses (glasses or contact lenses)

• Damaged or discolored test plates

Nursing Implications and Procedure ● ● ● ● ● ● ● ● ● ● ●

Pretest:

➤ Inform the patient that the procedure detects color vision impairment.

➤ Obtain a history of the patient's complaints, including a list of known allergens.

➤ Obtain a history of the patient's known or suspected vision loss, changes in visual acuity, including type and cause; use of glasses or contact lenses; eye conditions with treatment regimens; eye surgery; and other tests and procedures to assess and diagnose visual deficit.

➤ Obtain a history of results of previously performed laboratory tests, surgical procedures, and other diagnostic procedures.

➤ Obtain a list of the medications the patient is taking, including herbs, nutritional supplements, and nutraceuticals. The requesting health care practitioner should be advised if the patient regularly uses these products so that their effects can be taken into consideration when reviewing results.

➤ Review the procedure with the patient. Ask the patient if he or she wears corrective lenses; also inquire about the importance of color discrimination in his or her work, as applicable. Address concerns about pain related to the procedure. Explain to the patient that no discomfort will be experienced during the test. Inform the patient that a technician, optometrist, or physician performs the test, in a quiet, darkened room, and that to evaluate both eyes, the test can take 5 to 15 or up to 30 minutes, depending on the complexity of testing required.

➤ There are no food, fluid, or medication restrictions unless by medical direction.

Intratest:

➤ Instruct the patient to cooperate fully and to follow directions.

➤ Seat the patient comfortably. Occlude one eye and hold test booklet 12 to 14 inches in front of the exposed eye.

➤ Ask the patient to identify the numbers or letters buried in the maze of dots or to trace the objects with a hand-held pointed object.

➤ Repeat on the other eye.

➤ The results are recorded manually for recall and postprocedure interpretation by the appropriate health care practitioner.

Post-test:

➤ A written report of the examination will be completed by a health care practitioner specializing in this branch of medicine. The report will be sent to the requesting health care practitioner, who will discuss the results with the patient.

➤ Recognize anxiety related to test results and be supportive of impaired activity related to color vision loss. Discuss the implications of abnormal test results on the patient's lifestyle. Provide teaching and information regarding the clinical implications of the test results, as appropriate.

➤ Reinforce information given by the patient's health care provider regarding further testing, treatment, or referral to another health care provider. Answer any questions or address any concerns voiced by the patient or family.

➤ Depending on the results of this procedure, additional testing may be performed to evaluate or monitor progression of the disease process and determine the need for a change in therapy. Evaluate test results in relation to the patient's symptoms and other tests performed.

Related diagnostic tests:

➤ Related diagnostic tests include refraction and slit-lamp biomicroscopy.

COLPOSCOPY

. . . .

SYNONYMS/ACRONYM: Endometrial biopsy, cervical biopsy.

AREA OF APPLICATION: Vagina and cervix.

CONTRAST: None.

DESCRIPTION & RATIONALE: In this procedure, the vagina and cervix are viewed using a colposcope, a special binocular microscope and light system that magnifies the mucosal surfaces. Colposcopy is usually performed after suspicious Papanicolaou (Pap) test results or when suspected lesions cannot be visualized fully by the naked eye. The procedure is useful for identifying areas of cellular dysplasia and diagnosing cervical cancer because it provides the best view of the suspicious lesion, ensuring that the most representative area of the lesion is obtained for cytologic analysis to confirm malignant changes. Colposcopy is also valuable for assessing women with a history of exposure to diethylstilbestrol (DES) in utero. The goal is to identify precursor changes in cervical tissue before the changes advance from benign or atypical cells to cervical cancer. Photographs (cervicography) can also be taken of the cervix. ■

INDICATIONS:
- Evaluate the cervix after abnormal Pap smear
- Evaluate vaginal lesions
- Localize the area from which cervical biopsy samples should be obtained because such areas may not be visible to the naked eye
- Monitor conservatively treated cervical intraepithelial neoplasia
- Monitor women whose mothers took DES during pregnancy

RESULT

Normal Findings:
- Normal appearance of the vagina and cervix
- No abnormal cells or tissues

Abnormal Findings:
- Atrophic changes
- Cervical erosion
- Cervical intraepithelial neoplasia
- Infection
- Inflammation
- Invasive carcinoma
- Leukoplakia
- Papilloma, including condyloma

CRITICAL VALUES: N/A

INTERFERING FACTORS:

This procedure is contraindicated for:
- Patients who are pregnant or suspected of being pregnant, unless the potential benefits of the procedure far outweigh the risks to the fetus and mother
- Patients with cardiac conditions
- Patients with bleeding disorders, especially if cervical biopsy specimens are to be obtained
- Women who are currently menstruating

Factors that may impair clear imaging:
- Inadequate cleansing of the cervix of secretions and medications
- Scarring of the cervix
- Patients who are very obese, who may exceed the weight limit for the equipment
- Incorrect positioning of the patient, which may produce poor visualization of the area to be examined
- Inability of the patient to cooperate or remain still during the procedure because of age, significant pain, or mental status

- Severe bleeding or the presence of feces, blood, or blood clots, which can interfere with visualization

Other considerations:

- Complications of the procedure may include hemorrhage and cardiac arrhythmias.

- The procedure may be terminated if chest pain or severe cardiac arrhythmias occur.

- Failure to follow dietary restrictions and other pretesting preparations may cause the procedure to be canceled or repeated.

Nursing Implications and Procedure • • • • • • • • • • •

Pretest:

➤ Inform the patient that the procedure assesses the uterus and cervix.

➤ Obtain a history of the patient's complaints.

➤ Obtain a history of results of previously performed diagnostic procedures, surgical procedures, and laboratory tests. For related diagnostic tests, refer to the Reproductive System table.

➤ Record the date of the last menstrual period and determine the possibility of pregnancy in perimenopausal women.

➤ Obtain a list of the medications the patient is taking, including drugs that affect bleeding, such as aspirin and other salicylates.

➤ Review the procedure with the patient. Explain to the patient that some pain may be experienced during the test, and there may be moments of discomfort. Oral solution may be ordered. Explain the purpose of the test and how the procedure is performed. Inform the patient that the procedure is performed in a GI lab or medical office

setting, usually by a health care practitioner and support staff, and takes approximately 30 to 60 minutes.

➤ *Sensitivity to cultural and social issues,* as well as concern for modesty, is important in providing psychological support before, during, and after the procedure.

➤ There are no food, fluid, or medication restrictions unless by medical direction.

➤ Explain to the patient that if a biopsy is performed, she may feel menstrual-like cramping during the procedure and experience a minimal amount of bleeding.

➤ *Make sure a written and informed consent has been signed prior to the procedure and before administering any medications.*

Intratest:

➤ Instruct the patient to remove jewelry (including watches), credit cards, and other metallic objects.

➤ Have emergency equipment readily available.

➤ Patients are given a gown, robe, and foot coverings to wear and instructed to void prior to the procedure.

➤ Observe standard precautions, and follow the general guidelines in Appendix A. Positively identify the patient, and label the appropriate containers with the corresponding patient demographics, date, and time of collection.

➤ Instruct the patient to cooperate fully and to follow directions. Instruct the patient to remain still throughout the procedure because movement produces unreliable results.

➤ Obtain and record baseline vital signs.

➤ An intravenous (IV) line may be started to allow infusion of a sedative or IV fluids.

➤ Administer medications, as ordered, to reduce discomfort and to promote relaxation and sedation.

➤ Place the patient in the lithotomy position on the examining table and drape. Cleanse the external genitalia with an antiseptic solution.

➤ If a Pap smear is performed, the vaginal speculum is inserted, using water as a lubricant.

➤ The cervix is swabbed with 3% acetic acid to remove mucus or any cream medication and to improve the contrast between tissue types. The scope is positioned at the speculum and is focused on the cervix. The area is examined carefully, using light and magnification. Photographs can be taken for future reference.

➤ Tissues that appear abnormal or atypical undergo biopsy using a forceps inserted through the speculum. Bleeding, which is common after cervical biopsy, may be controlled by cautery, suturing, or application of silver nitrate or ferric subsulfate (Monsel's solution) to the site.

➤ The vagina is rinsed with sterile saline or water to remove the acetic acid and prevent burning after the procedure. If bleeding persists, a tampon may be inserted after removal of the speculum.

➤ Biopsy samples are placed in appropriate labelled containers with special preservative solution, and promptly transported to the laboratory.

Post-test:

➤ Monitor the patient for signs of respiratory depression.

➤ Monitor vital signs and neurologic status every 15 minutes for 1 hour, then every 2 hours for 4 hours, and as ordered. Take temperature every 4 hours for 24 hours. Compare with baseline values. Notify the health care practitioner if temperature is elevated. Protocols may vary from facility to facility.

➤ Observe the patient until the effects of the sedation if ordered have worn off.

➤ Instruct the patient to remove the vaginal tampon, if inserted, within 8 to 24 hours; after that time, the patient should wear pads if there is bleeding or drainage.

➤ If a biopsy was performed, inform the patient that a discharge may persist for a few days to a few weeks.

➤ Advise the patient to avoid strenuous exercise 8 to 24 hours after the procedure, and to avoid douching and intercourse for about 2 weeks or as directed by the health care practitioner.

➤ Monitor for any bleeding. Instruct the patient to expect slight bleeding for 2 days after removal of biopsy specimens, but emphasize that persistent vaginal bleeding or abnormal vaginal discharge, an increasing amount of bleeding, abdominal pain, and fever must be reported to the health care practitioner immediately.

➤ Observe the patient for indications of chest pain, abdominal pain or tenderness, or breathing problems. If these symptoms are present or increase in frequency or severity, the change should be reported to the health care practitioner immediately.

➤ A written report of the examination will be completed by a health care practitioner specializing in this branch of medicine. The report will be sent to the requesting health care practitioner, who will discuss the results with the patient.

➤ Reinforce information given by the patient's health care provider regarding further testing, treatment, or referral to another health care provider. Answer any questions or address any concerns voiced by the patient or family.

➤ Depending on the results of this procedure, additional testing may be needed to evaluate or monitor progression of the disease process and determine the need for a change in therapy. Evaluate test results in relation to the patient's symptoms and other tests performed.

Related diagnostic tests:

➤ Related diagnostic tests include computed tomography of the abdomen, magnetic resonance imaging of the abdomen, and ultrasound of the pelvis.

COMPLEMENT C3 AND COMPLEMENT C4

. . . .

SYNONYMS/ACRONYM: C3 and C4.

SPECIMEN: Serum (1 mL) collected in a red-top tube.

REFERENCE VALUE: (Method: Nephelometry)

C3

Age	Conventional Units	SI Units (Conventional Units × 10)
Newborn	57–116 mg/dL	570–1160 mg/L
6 mo–adult	74–166 mg/dL	740–1660 mg/L
Adult	83–177 mg/dL	830–1770 mg/L

C4

Age	Conventional Units	SI Units (Conventional Units × 10)
Newborn	10–31 mg/dL	100–310 mg/L
6 mo–6 y	15–52 mg/dL	150–520 mg/L
7–12 y	19–40 mg/dL	190–400 mg/L
13–15 y	19–57 mg/dL	190–570 mg/L
16–18 y	19–42 mg/dL	190–420 mg/L
Adult	12–36 mg/dL	120–360 mg/L

DESCRIPTION & RATIONALE: Complement proteins act as enzymes that aid in the immunologic and inflammatory response. The complement system is an important mechanism for the destruction and removal of foreign materials. Serum complement levels are used to detect autoimmune diseases. C3 and C4 are the most frequently assayed complement proteins, along with total complement.

Circulating C3 is synthesized in the liver and comprises 70% of the complement system, but cells in other tissues can also produce C3. C3 is an essential activating protein in the classic and alternate complement cascades. It is decreased in patients with immunologic diseases, in whom it is consumed at an increased rate. C4 is produced primarily in the liver but can also be produced by monocytes, fibroblasts, and macrophages. C4 participates in the classic complement pathway. ∎

* Detect genetic deficiencies
* Evaluate immunologic diseases

RESULT

Normal C4 and decreased C3	Acute glomerulonephritis, membranous glomerulonephritis, immune complex diseases, SLE, C3 deficiency
Decreased C4 and normal C3	Immune complex diseases, cryoglobulinemia, C4 deficiency, hereditary angioedema
Decreased C4 and decreased C3	Immune complex diseases

Increased in:
* C3 and C4
  Acute-phase reactions

* C3
  Amyloidosis
  Cancer
  Diabetes
  Myocardial infarction
  Pneumococcal pneumonia
  Pregnancy
  heumatic disease
  Thyroiditis
  Viral hepatitis

* C4
  Certain malignancies

Decreased in:
* C3 and C4
  Hereditary deficiency
  Liver disease
  Systemic lupus erythematosus (SLE)

* C3
  Chronic infection (bacterial, parasitic, viral)
  Post–membranoproliferative glomerulonephritis

  Post–streptococcal infection
  Rheumatic arthritis

* C4
  Angioedema (hereditary and acquired)
  Autoimmune hemolytic anemia
  Autoimmune thyroiditis
  Cryoglobulinemia
  Glomerulonephritis
  Juvenile dermatomyositis
  Meningitis (bacterial, viral)
  Pneumonia
  Streptococcal or staphylococcal sepsis

CRITICAL VALUES: N/A

INTERFERING FACTORS:
* Drugs that may increase C3 levels include cimetidine and cyclophosphamide.

* Drugs that may decrease C3 levels include danazol and phenytoin.

* Drugs that may increase C4 levels include cimetidine, cyclophosphamide, and danazol.

* Drugs that may decrease C4 levels include dextran and penicillamine.

Nursing Implications and Procedure • • • • • • • • • •

Pretest:

➤ Inform the patient that the test is used to assist in the diagnosis of immunologic diseases in which complement is consumed at an increased rate or to detect inborn deficiency.

➤ Obtain a history of the patient's complaints, including a list of known allergens (especially allergies or sensitivities to latex), and inform the appropriate health care practitioner accordingly.

➤ Obtain a history of the patient's immune system and results of previously performed laboratory tests, surgical procedures, and other diagnostic procedures. For related laboratory tests, refer to the Immune System table.

➤ Obtain a list of medications the patient is taking, including herbs, nutritional supplements, and nutraceuticals. The requesting health care practitioner and laboratory should be advised if the patient regularly uses these products so that their effects can be taken into consideration when reviewing results.

➤ Review the procedure with the patient. Inform the patient that specimen collection takes approximately 5 to 10 minutes. Address concerns about pain related to the procedure. Explain to the patient that there may be some discomfort during the venipuncture.

➤ There are no food, fluid, or medication restrictions unless by medical direction.

Intratest:

➤ If the patient has a history of severe allergic reaction to latex, care should be taken to avoid the use of equipment containing latex.

➤ Instruct the patient to cooperate fully and to follow directions. Direct the patient to breathe normally and to avoid unnecessary movement.

➤ Observe standard precautions, and follow the general guidelines in Appendix A. Positively identify the patient, and label the appropriate tubes with the corresponding patient demographics, date, and time of collection. Perform a venipuncture; collect the specimen in a 5-mL red-top tube.

➤ Remove the needle, and apply a pressure dressing over the puncture site.

➤ Promptly transport the specimen to the laboratory for processing and analysis.

➤ The results are recorded manually or in a computerized system for recall and postprocedure interpretation by the appropriate health care practitioner.

Post-test:

➤ Observe venipuncture site for bleeding or hematoma formation. Apply paper tape or other adhesive to hold pressure bandage in place, or replace with a plastic bandage.

➤ A written report of the examination will be sent to the requesting health care practitioner, who will discuss the results with the patient.

➤ Reinforce information given by the patient's health care provider regarding further testing, treatment, or referral to another health care provider. Answer any questions or address any concerns voiced by the patient or family.

➤ Depending on the results of this procedure, additional testing may be performed to evaluate or monitor progression of the disease process and determine the need for a change in therapy. Evaluate test results in relation to the patient's symptoms and other tests performed.

Related laboratory tests:

➤ Related laboratory tests include anticardiolipin antibody, antinuclear antibodies, erythrocyte sedimentation rate, and total complement.

COMPLEMENT, TOTAL

. . . .

Synonym/Acronym: Total hemolytic complement, CH_{50}, CH_{100}.

Specimen: Serum (1 mL) collected in a red-top tube.

Reference Value: (Method: Quantitative hemolysis)

Conventional Units	SI Units (Conventional Units × 1)
40–100 CH_{50} U/mL	40–100 CH_{50} kU/L

Description & Rationale: The complement system comprises proteins that become activated and interact in a sequential cascade. The complement system is an important part of the body's natural defense against allergic and immune reactions. It is activated by plasmin and is interrelated with the coagulation and fibrinolytic systems. Activation of the complement system results in cell lysis, release of histamine, chemotaxis of white blood cells, increased vascular permeability, and contraction of smooth muscle. The activation of this system can sometimes occur with uncontrolled self-destructive effects on the body. In the serum complement assay, a patient's serum is mixed with sheep red blood cells coated with antibodies. If complement is present in sufficient quantities, 50% of the red blood cells are lysed. Lower amounts of lysed cells are associated with decreased complement levels. ∎

Indications:
- Assist in the diagnosis of hereditary angioedema
- Evaluate complement activity in autoimmune disorders
- Evaluate and monitor therapy for systemic lupus erythematosus
- Screen for complement deficiency

Result

Increased in:
- Acute-phase immune response

Decreased in:
- Autoimmune diseases
- Autoimmune hemolytic anemia
- Burns
- Cryoglobulinemia
- Hereditary deficiency
- Infections (bacterial, parasitic, viral)
- Liver disease
- Malignancy

- Membranous glomerulonephritis
- Rheumatoid arthritis
- Systemic lupus erythematosus
- Trauma
- Vasculitis

CRITICAL VALUES: N/A

INTERFERING FACTORS:
- Drugs that may increase total complement levels include cyclophosphamide and danazol.

- Specimen should not remain at room temperature longer than 1 hour.

Nursing Implications and Procedure • • • • • • • • • • •

Pretest:

➤ Inform the patient that the test is used to evaluate immune dieases related to complement activity and follow up on a patient's response to therapy.

➤ Obtain a history of the patient's complaints, including a list of known allergens (especially allergies or sensitivities to latex), and inform the appropriate health care practitioner accordingly.

➤ Obtain a history of the patient's immune system and results of previously performed laboratory tests, surgical procedures, and other diagnostic procedures. For related laboratory tests, refer to the Immune System table.

➤ Obtain a list of medications the patient is taking, including herbs, nutritional supplements, and nutraceuticals. The requesting health care practitioner and laboratory should be advised if the patient regularly uses these products so that their effects can be taken into consideration when reviewing results.

➤ Review the procedure with the patient. Inform the patient that specimen collection takes approximately 5 to 10 minutes. Address concerns about pain related to the procedure. Explain to the patient that there may be some discomfort during the venipuncture.

➤ There are no food, fluid, or medication restrictions unless by medical direction.

Intratest:

➤ If the patient has a history of severe allergic reaction to latex, care should be taken to avoid the use of equipment containing latex.

➤ Instruct the patient to cooperate fully and to follow directions. Direct the patient to breathe normally and to avoid unnecessary movement.

➤ Observe standard precautions, and follow the general guidelines in Appendix A. Positively identify the patient, and label the appropriate tubes with the corresponding patient demographics, date, and time of collection. Perform a venipuncture; collect the specimen in a 5-mL red-top tube.

➤ Remove the needle, and apply a pressure dressing over the puncture site.

➤ Promptly transport the specimen to the laboratory for processing and analysis.

➤ The results are recorded manually or in a computerized system for recall and postprocedure interpretation by the appropriate health care practitioner.

Post-test:

➤ Observe venipuncture site for bleeding or hematoma formation. Apply paper tape or other adhesive to hold pressure bandage in place, or replace with a plastic bandage.

➤ A written report of the examination will be sent to the requesting health care practitioner, who will discuss the results with the patient.

➤ Reinforce information given by the patient's health care provider regarding further testing, treatment, or referral to another health care provider. Answer any questions or address any concerns voiced by the patient or family.

➤ Depending on the results of this pro-cedure, additional testing may be performed to evaluate or monitor progression of the disease process and determine the need for a change in therapy. Evaluate test results in relation to the patient's symptoms and other tests performed.

Related laboratory tests:

➤ Related laboratory tests include anti-nuclear antibodies, complement C3 and C4, and erythrocyte sedimentation rate.

COMPLETE BLOOD COUNT

. . . .

SYNONYM/ACRONYM: CBC.

SPECIMEN: Whole blood from one full lavender-top (EDTA) tube or Microtainer. Whole blood from a green-top (lithium or sodium heparin) tube may be submitted, but the following automated values may not be reported: white blood cell (WBC) count, WBC differential, platelet count, and mean platelet volume.

REFERENCE VALUE: (Method: Automated, computerized multichannel analyzers that sort and size cells on the basis of changes in either electrical impedance or light pulses as the cells pass in front of a laser. Many of these analyzers are capable of determining a five-part WBC differential.) This battery of tests includes hemoglobin, hematocrit, red blood cell (RBC) count, RBC morphology, RBC indices, RBC distribution width index (RDW), platelet count, platelet size, WBC count, and WBC differential. The five-part automated WBC differential identifies and enumerates neutrophils, lymphocytes, monocytes, eosinophils, and basophils.

Hemoglobin (See "Hemoglobin" monograph for more detailed information)

Age	Conventional Units	SI Units (Conventional Units × 10)
Cord blood	13.5–20.5 g/dL	135–205 mmol/L
2 wk	13.4–19.8 g/dL	134–198 mmol/L
1 mo	10.7–17.1 g/dL	107–171 mmol/L
6 mo	11.1–14.4 g/dL	111–144 mmol/L
1 y	11.3–14.1 g/dL	113–141 mmol/L
9–14 y	12.0–14.4 g/dL	120–144 mmol/L
Adult		
Male	13.2–17.3 g/dL	132–173 mmol/L
Female	11.7–15.5 g/dL	117–155 mmol/L
Older adult (65–74 y)		
Male	12.6–17.4 g/dL	126–174 mmol/L
Female	11.7–16.1 g/dL	117–161 mmol/L

Hematocrit (See "Hematocrit" monograph for more detailed information)

Age	Conventional Units(%)	SI Units (Conventional Units × 0.01*)
Cord blood	47–57	0.47–0.57
1 d	51–65	0.51–0.65
2 wk	47–57	0.47–0.57
1 mo	38–52	0.38–0.52
6 mo	35–41	0.35–0.41
1 y	37–41	0.37–0.41
10 y	36–42	0.36–0.42
Adult		
Male	43–49	0.43–0.49
Female	38–44	0.38–0.44

*Volume fraction.

White Blood Cell Count and Differential (See "White Blood Cell Count and Cell Differential" monograph for more detailed information)

Age	SI Units (Conventional Units × 1) WBC × 10³/mm³ or cells/µL	Neutrophils			Lymphocytes	Monocytes	Eosinophils	Basophils
		Total (Absolute) and %	Bands (Absolute) and %	Segments (Absolute) and %	(Absolute) and %	(Absolute) and %	(Absolute) and %	(Absolute) and %
Birth	0.0–30.0	(6.0–26.0) 61%	(1.65) 9.1%	(9.4) 52%	(2.0–11) 31%	(0.4–3.1) 5.8%	(0.02–0.85) 2.2%	(0–0.64) 0.6%
1 d	9.4–34.0	(5.0–21.0) 61%	(1.75) 9.2%	(9.8) 52%	(2.0–11.5) 31%	(0.2–3.1) 5.8%	(0.02–0.95) 2.0%	(0–0.30) 0.5%
2 wk	5.0–20.0	(1.0–9.5) 40%	(0.63) 5.5%	(3.9) 34%	(2.0–17.0) 48%	(0.2–2.4) 8.8%	(0.07–1.0) 3.1%	(0–0.23) 0.4%
1 mo	5.0–19.5	(1.0–9.0) 35%	(0.49) 4.5%	(3.3) 30%	(2.5–16.5) 56%	(0.15–2.0) 6.5%	(0.07–0.90) 2.8%	(0–0.20) 0.5%
6 mo	6.0–17.5	(1.0–8.5) 32%	(0.45) 3.8%	(3.3) 28%	(4.0–13.5) 61%	(0.1–1.3) 4.8%	(0.07–0.75) 2.5%	(0–0.20) 0.4%
1 y	6.0–17.5	(1.5–8.5) 31%	(0.35) 3.1%	(3.2) 28%	(4.0–10.5) 61%	(0.05–1.1) 4.8%	(0.05–0.70) 2.6%	(0–0.20) 0.4%
10 y	4.5–13.5	(1.8–8.0) 54%	(1.8–7.0) 3.0%	(1.8–7.0) 51%	(1.5–6.5) 38%	(0–0.8) 4.3%	(0–0.60) 2.4%	(0–0.20) 0.5%
Adult	4.5–11.0	(1.8–7.7) 59%	(0–0.7) 3.0%	(1.8–7.0) 56%	(1.0–4.8) 34%	(0–0.8) 4.0%	(0–0.45) 2.7%	(0–0.20) 0.5%

Red Blood Cell Count (See "Red Blood Cell Count" monograph for more detailed information)

Age	Conventional Units	SI Units (Conventional Units × 1)
Cord blood	4.14–4.69×10^6 cells/mm^3	4.14–4.69×10^{12} cells /L
1 d	5.33–5.47×10^6 cells/mm^3	5.33–5.47×10^{12} cells /L
2 wk	4.32–4.98×10^6 cells/mm^3	4.32–4.98×10^{12} cells /L
1 mo	3.75–4.95×10^6 cells/mm^3	3.75–4.95×10^{12} cells /L
6 mo	3.71–4.25×10^6 cells/mm^3	3.71–4.25×10^{12} cells /L
1 y	4.40–4.48×10^6 cells/mm^3	4.40–4.48×10^{12} cells /L
10 y	4.75–4.85×10^6 cells/mm^3	4.75–4.85×10^{12} cells /L
Adult		
Male	4.71–5.14×10^6 cells/mm^3	4.71–5.14×10^{12} cells /L
Female	4.20–4.87×10^6 cells/mm^3	4.20–4.87×10^{12} cells /L

Red Blood Cell Indices (See "Red Blood Cell Indices" monograph for more detailed information)

Age	MCV (fl)	MCH (pg/cell)	MCHC (g/dL)	RDW
Cord blood	107–119	35–39	32–34	14.9–18.7
1 d	104–116	35–39	32–34	14.9–18.7
2 wk	95–117	29–35	28–32	14.9–18.7
1 mo	93–115	29–35	28–34	14.9–18.7
6 mo	82–100	24–30	28–32	14.9–18.7
1 y	81–95	25–29	29–31	11.6–14.8
10 y	75–87	25–31	33–35	11.6–14.8
Adult				
Male	85–95	28–32	33–35	11.6–14.8
Female	85–95	28–32	33–35	11.6–14.8

MCV = mean corpuscular volume; MCH = mean corpuscular hemoglobin; MCHC = mean corpuscular hemoglobin concentration; RDW = RBC distribution width index.

Red Blood Cell Morphology (See "Red Blood Cell Morphology and Inclusions" monograph for more detailed information)

Morphology	Within Normal Limits	1+	2+	3+	4+
			Size		
Anisocytosis	0–5+	5–10	10–20	20–50	Greater than 50
Macrocytes	0–5+	5–10	10–20	20–50	Greater than 50
Microcytes	0–5+	5–10	10–20	20–50	Greater than 50

Morphology	Within Normal Limits	1+	2+	3+	4+
Shape					
Poikilocytes	0–2+	3–10	10–20	20–50	Greater than 50
Burr cells	0–2+	3–10	10–20	20–50	Greater than 50
Acanthocytes	Less than 1+	2–5	5–10	10–20	Greater than 20
Schistocytes	Less than 1+	2–5	5–10	10–20	Greater than 20
Dacryocytes (teardrop cells)	0–2+	2–5	5–10	10–20	Greater than 20
Codocytes (target cells)	0–2+	2–10	10–20	20–50	Greater than 50
Spherocytes	0–2+	2–10	10–20	20–50	Greater than 50
Ovalocytes	0–2+	2–10	10–20	20–50	Greater than 50
Stomatocytes	0–2+	2–10	10–20	20–50	Greater than 50
Drepanocytes (sickle cells)	Absent	Reported as present or absent			
Helmet cells	Absent	Reported as present or absent			
Agglutination	Absent	Reported as present or absent			
Rouleaux	Absent	Reported as present or absent			
Hemoglobin Content					
Hypochromia	0–2+	3–10	10–50	50–75	Greater than 75
Polychromasia					
Adult	Less than 1+	2–5	5–10	10–20	Greater than 20
Newborn	1–6+	7–15	15–20	20–50	Greater than 50

Red Blood Cell Inclusions (See "Red Blood Cell Morphology and Inclusions" monograph for more detailed information)

Inclusions	Within Normal Limits	1+	2+	3+	4+
Cabot's rings	Absent	Reported as present or absent			
Basophilic stippling	0–1+	1–5	5–10	10–20	Greater than 20

(Continued on the following page)

Inclusions	Within Normal Limits	1+	2+	3+	4+
Howell-Jolly bodies	Absent	1–2	3–5	5–10	Greater than 10
Heinz bodies	Absent	Reported as present or absent			
Hemoglobin C crystals	Absent	Reported as present or absent			
Pappenheimer bodies	Absent	Reported as present or absent			
Intracellular parasites (e.g., *Plasmodium*, *Babesia*, trypanosomes)	Absent	Reported as present or absent			

Platelet Count (See "Platelet Count" monograph for more detailed information)

Age	Conventional Units	SI Units (Conventional Units × 1)	MPV (fl)
1–5 y	217–497 × 10³/µL/ mm³	217–497 × 10⁹/L	7.2–10.0
Adult	150–450 × 10³/µL/ mm³	181–521 × 10⁹/L	7.0–10.2

DESCRIPTION & RATIONALE: A complete blood count (CBC) is a group of tests used for basic screening purposes. It is probably the most widely ordered laboratory test. Results provide the enumeration of the cellular elements of the blood, measurement of RBC indices, and determination of cell morphology by automation and evaluation of stained smears. The results can provide valuable diagnostic information regarding the overall health of the patient and the patient's response to disease and treatment. ■

INDICATIONS:

• Detect hematologic disorder, neoplasm, leukemia, or immunologic abnormality

• Determine the presence of hereditary hematologic abnormality

• Evaluate known or suspected anemia and related treatment

• Monitor blood loss and response to blood replacement

• Monitor the effects of physical or emotional stress

• Monitor fluid imbalances or treatment for fluid imbalances

• Monitor hematologic status during pregnancy

• Monitor progression of nonhematologic disorders, such as chronic obstructive pulmonary disease, malabsorption syndromes, cancer, and renal disease

• Monitor response to chemotherapy and evaluate undesired reactions to drugs that may cause blood dyscrasias

• Provide screening as part of a general physical examination, especially on admission to a health care facility or before surgery

RESULT: See monographs titled "Hemoglobin," "Hematocrit," "Red Blood Cell Indices," "Red Blood Cell Morphology and Inclusions," "Red Blood Cell Count,"

"Platelet Count," and "White Blood Cell Count and Cell Differential."

Increased in: See above-listed monographs.

Decreased in: See above-listed monographs.

CRITICAL VALUES

Hemoglobin:
* Less than 6 g/dL
* Greater than 18 g/dL

Hematocrit:
* Less than 18%
* Greater than 54%

WBC count (on admission):
* Less than 2500/mm^3
* Greater than 30,000/mm^3

Platelet count:
* Less than 20,000/mm^3
* Greater than 1,000,000/mm^3

Note and immediately report to the health care practitioner any critically increased or decreased values and related symptoms.

The presence of abnormal cells, other morphologic characteristics, or cellular inclusions may signify a potentially life-threatening or serious health condition and should be investigated. Examples are the presence of sickle cells, moderate numbers of spherocytes, marked schistocytosis, oval macrocytes, basophilic stippling, eosinophil count greater than 10%, monocytosis greater than 15%, nucleated RBCs (if patient is not an infant), malarial organisms, hypersegmented neutrophils, agranular neutrophils, blasts or other immature cells, Auer rods, Döhle bodies, marked toxic granulation, or plasma cells.

INTERFERING FACTORS:
* Failure to fill the tube sufficiently (less than three-fourths full) may yield inadequate sample volume for automated analyzers and may be a reason for specimen rejection.

* Hemolyzed or clotted specimens should be rejected for analysis.

* Elevated serum glucose or sodium levels may produce elevated mean corpuscular volume values because of swelling of erythrocytes.

* Recent transfusion history should be considered when evaluating the CBC.

Nursing Implications and Procedure • • • • • • • • • • •

Pretest:

➤ Inform the patient that the test is used to evaluate numerous conditions involving red blood cells, white blood cells, and platelets. The test is also used to indicate inflammation, infection, and response to chemotherapy.

➤ Obtain a history of the patient's complaints, including a list of known allergens (especially allergies or sensitivities to latex), and inform the appropriate health care practitioner accordingly.

➤ Obtain a history of the patient's gastrointestinal, hematopoietic, immune, and respiratory systems, as well as results of previously performed laboratory tests, surgical procedures, and other diagnostic procedures. For related laboratory tests, refer to the Gastrointestinal, Genitourinary, Hematopoietic, Immune, and Respiratory System tables.

➤ Obtain a list of medications the patient is taking, including herbs, nutritional supplements, and nutraceuticals. The requesting health care practitioner and laboratory should be advised if the patient regularly uses these products so that their effects can be taken into consideration when reviewing results.

➤ Review the procedure with the patient. Inform the patient that specimen collection takes approximately 5 to 10 minutes. Address concerns about pain related to the procedure. Explain to the patient that there may be some discomfort during the venipuncture.

➤ *Sensitivity to social and cultural issues*, as well as concern for modesty, is important in providing psychological support before, during, and after the procedure.

➤ There are no food, fluid, or medication restrictions unless by medical direction.

Intratest:

➤ If the patient has a history of severe allergic reaction to latex, care should be taken to avoid the use of equipment containing latex.

➤ Instruct the patient to cooperate fully and to follow directions. Direct the patient to breathe normally and to avoid unnecessary movement.

➤ Observe standard precautions, and follow the general guidelines in Appendix A. Positively identify the patient, and label the appropriate tubes with the corresponding patient demographics, date, and time of collection. Perform a venipuncture; collect the specimen in a 5-mL lavender-top (EDTA) tube. An EDTA Microtainer sample may be obtained from infants, children, and adults for whom venipuncture may not be feasible. The specimen should be analyzed within 6 hours when stored at room temperature or within 24 hours if stored at refrigerated temperature. If it is anticipated that the specimen will not be analyzed within 4 to 6 hours, two blood smears should be made immediately after the venipuncture and submitted with the blood sample. Smears made from specimens older than 6 hours will contain an unacceptable number of misleading artifactual abnormalities of the RBCs, such as echinocytes and spherocytes, as well as necrobiotic WBCs.

➤ Remove the needle, and apply a pressure dressing over the puncture site.

➤ Promptly transport the specimen to the laboratory for processing and analysis.

➤ The results are recorded manually or in a computerized system for recall and postprocedure interpretation by the appropriate health care practitioner.

Post-test:

➤ Observe venipuncture site for bleeding or hematoma formation. Apply paper tape or other adhesive to hold pressure bandage in place, or replace with a plastic bandage.

➤ *Nutritional considerations:* Instruct patients to consume a variety of foods within the basic food groups, maintain a healthy weight, be physically active, limit salt intake, limit alcohol intake, and be a nonsmoker.

➤ A written report of the examination will be sent to the requesting health care practitioner, who will discuss the results with the patient.

➤ Reinforce information given by the patient's health care provider regarding further testing, treatment, or referral to another health care provider. Answer any questions or address any concerns voiced by the patient or family.

➤ Depending on the results of this procedure, additional testing may be performed to evaluate or monitor progression of the disease process and determine the need for a change in therapy. Evaluate test results in relation to the patient's symptoms and other tests performed.

Related laboratory tests:

➤ Related laboratory tests include erythropoietin, ferritin, hematocrit, hemoglobin, iron/total iron-binding capacity, platelet count, RBC count, RBC indices, RBC morphology and inclusions, reticulocyte count, and WBC count and cell differential.

COMPUTED TOMOGRAPHY, ABDOMEN

. . . .

SYNONYMS/ACRONYMS: Computed axial tomography (CAT), computed transaxial tomography (CTT), abdominal CT.

AREA OF APPLICATION: Abdomen.

CONTRAST: Can be done with or without oral or intravenous (IV) iodinated contrast medium.

DESCRIPTION & RATIONALE: Abdominal computed tomography (CT) is a noninvasive procedure used to enhance certain anatomic views of the abdominal structures, but it becomes invasive when a contrast medium is used. The patient lies on a table and is moved in and out of a doughnut-like device called a *gantry*, which houses the x-ray tube and associated electronics. The scanner uses multiple x-ray beams and a series of detectors that rotate around the patient to produce cross-sectional views in a three-dimensional fashion by detecting and recording differences in tissue density after having an x-ray beam passed through the tissues. These density measurements are sent to a computer that produces a digital image of the anatomy, enabling a physician to look at slices or thin sections of certain anatomic views of the liver, biliary tract, pancreas, kidneys, spleen, intestines, and vascular system. Differentiations can be made among solid, cystic, inflammatory, or vascular lesions, and suspected hematomas and aneurysms can be identified. Iodinated contrast medium is given intravenously for blood vessel and vascular evaluation or orally for bowel and adjacent structure evaluation. Images can be recorded on photographic or x-ray film or stored in digital format as digitized computer data. Cine scanning is used to produce a series of moving images of the area scanned. The CT scan can be used to guide biopsy needles into areas of abdominal tumors to obtain tissue for laboratory analysis and to guide placement of catheters for drainage of intra-abdominal abscesses. Tumors, before and after therapy, may be monitored with CT scanning. ■

INDICATIONS:
- Assist in differentiating between benign and malignant tumors
- Detect aortic aneurysms
- Detect tumor extension of masses and metastasis into the abdominal area
- Differentiate aortic aneurysms from tumors near the aorta
- Differentiate between infectious and inflammatory processes
- Evaluate cysts, masses, abscesses, renal calculi, gastrointestinal (GI) bleeding and obstruction, and trauma
- Evaluate retroperitoneal lymph nodes

• Monitor and evaluate the effectiveness of medical, radiation, or surgical therapies

RESULT

Normal Findings:
• Normal size, position, and shape of abdominal organs and vascular system

Abnormal Findings:
• Abdominal abscess

• Abdominal aortic aneurysm

• Adrenal tumor or hyperplasia

• Dilation of the common hepatic duct, common bile duct, or gallbladder

• Hematomas, diverticulitis, gallstones

• Hemoperitoneum

• Hepatic cysts or abscesses

• Pancreatic pseudocyst

• Primary and metastatic neoplasms

• Renal calculi, bowel perforation, and GI bleeding and obstruction

• Splenic laceration, tumor, infiltration, and trauma

CRITICAL VALUES: N/A

INTERFERING FACTORS:

This procedure is contraindicated for:
• ⚠ Patients with allergies to shellfish or iodinated dye. The contrast medium used may cause a life-threatening allergic reaction. Patients with a known hypersensitivity to the medium may benefit from premedication with corticosteroids or the use of nonionic contrast medium.

• Patients who are claustrophobic.

• Patients who are pregnant or suspected of being pregnant, unless the potential benefits of the procedure far outweigh the risks to the fetus and mother.

• ⚠ Elderly and other patients who are chronically dehydrated before the test, because of their risk of contrast-induced renal failure.

• ⚠ Patients who are in renal failure.

• Young patients (17 years old and younger), unless the benefits of the x-ray diagnosis outweigh the risks of exposure to high levels of radiation.

Factors that may impair clear imaging:
• Gas or feces in the gastrointestinal tract resulting from inadequate cleansing or failure to restrict food intake before the study

• Retained barium from a previous radiologic procedure

• Metallic objects within the examination field (e.g., jewelry, body rings), which may inhibit organ visualization and can produce unclear images

• Improper adjustment of the radiographic equipment to accommodate obese or thin patients, which can cause overexposure or underexposure and a poor-quality study

• Patients who are very obese, who may exceed the weight limit for the equipment

• Patients with extreme claustrophobia unless sedation is given before the study

• Incorrect positioning of the patient, which may produce poor visualization of the area to be examined

• Inability of the patient to cooperate or remain still during the procedure because of age, significant pain, or mental status

Other considerations:
• Complications of the procedure include hemorrhage, infection at the IV needle insertion site, and cardiac arrhythmias.

- The procedure may be terminated if chest pain or severe cardiac arrhythmias occur.

- Failure to follow dietary restrictions and other pretesting preparations may cause the procedure to be canceled or repeated.

- Consultation with a health care provider should occur before the procedure for radiation safety concerns regarding younger patients or patients who are lactating.

- Risks associated with radiographic overexposure can result from frequent x-ray procedures. Personnel in the room with the patient should wear a protective lead apron, stand behind a shield, or leave the area while the examination is being done. Personnel working in the area where the examination is being done should wear badges that reveal their level of exposure to radiation.

Nursing Implications and Procedure • • • • • • • • • • •

Pretest:

➤ Inform the patient that the procedure assesses the abdomen.

➤ Obtain a history of the patient's complaints, including a list of known allergens, especially allergies or sensitivities to iodine, seafood, or other contrast mediums.

➤ Obtain a history of results of previously performed diagnostic procedures, surgical procedures, and laboratory tests. Include specific tests as they apply (e.g., blood urea nitrogen [BUN], creatinine, coagulation tests, platelets, bleeding time). Ensure that the results of blood tests are obtained and recorded before the procedure, especially BUN and creatinine, if contrast medium is to be used. For related diagnostic tests, refer to the Gastrointestinal, Hepatobiliary, and Genitourinary System tables.

➤ Note any recent barium or other radiologic contrast procedures. Ensure that barium studies were performed more than 4 days before the CT scan.

➤ Record the date of the last menstrual period and determine the possibility of pregnancy in perimenopausal women.

➤ Obtain a list of the medications the patient is taking.

➤ When contrast is used, patients receiving metformin (glucophage) for non–insulin-dependent (type 2) diabetes should discontinue the drug on the day of the test and continue to withhold it for 48 hours after the test. Failure to do so may result in lactic acidosis.

➤ Review the procedure with the patient. Explain to the patient that some pain may be experienced during the test, and there may be moments of discomfort. Explain the purpose of the test and how the procedure is performed. Inform the patient that the procedure is performed in a radiology department, usually by a health care practitioner and support staff, and takes approximately 30 to 60 minutes.

➤ *Sensitivity to cultural and social issues,* as well as concern for modesty, is important in providing psychological support before, during, and after the procedure.

➤ Explain that an IV line may be inserted to allow infusion of IV fluids, contrast medium, dye, or sedatives. Usually contrast medium and normal saline are infused.

➤ Inform the patient that he or she may experience nausea, a feeling of warmth, a salty or metallic taste, or a transient headache after injection of contrast medium, if given.

➤ The patient may be requested to drink approximately 450 mL of a dilute barium solution (approximately 1% barium) beginning 1 hour before the examination. This is administered to distinguish gastrointestinal organs from the other abdominal organs.

➤ The patient should fast and restrict

fluids for 8 hours prior to the procedure. Instruct the patient to avoid taking anticoagulant medication or to reduce dosage as ordered prior to the procedure.

➤ Instruct the patient to remove jewelry (including watches), credit cards, keys, coins, cell phones, pagers, and other metallic objects.

➤ *Make sure a written and informed consent has been signed prior to the procedure and before administering any medications.*

Intratest:

➤ Ensure that the patient has complied with dietary, fluids, and medication restrictions and pretesting preparations; assure that food has been restricted for at least 8 hours prior to the procedure. Ensure that the patient has removed all external metallic objects (jewelry, dentures, etc.) prior to the procedure.

➤ Have emergency equipment readily available.

➤ If the patient has a history of severe allergic reactions to any substance or drug, administer ordered prophylactic steroids or antihistamines before the procedure. Use nonionic contrast medium for the procedure.

➤ Patients are given a gown, robe, and foot coverings to wear and instructed to void prior to the procedure.

➤ Observe standard precautions, and follow the general guidelines in Appendix A.

➤ Instruct the patient to cooperate fully and to follow directions. Instruct the patient to remain still throughout the procedure because movement produces unreliable results.

➤ Establish an IV fluid line for the injection of contrast, emergency drugs, and sedatives.

➤ Administer an antianxiety agent as ordered, if the patient has claustrophobia. Administer a sedative to a child or to an uncooperative adult, as ordered.

➤ Place the patient in the supine position on an exam table.

➤ If contrast is used, the contrast medium is injected, and a rapid series of images is taken during and after the filling of the vessels to be examined. Delayed images may be taken to examine the vessels after a time and to monitor the venous phase of the procedure.

➤ Ask the patient to inhale deeply and hold his or her breath while the x-ray images are taken, and then to exhale after the images are taken.

➤ Instruct the patient to take slow, deep breaths if nausea occurs during the procedure. Monitor and administer an antiemetic agent if ordered. Ready an emesis basin for use.

➤ Monitor the patient for complications related to the procedure (e.g., allergic reaction, anaphylaxis, bronchospasm) if contrast is used.

➤ The needle or vascular catheter is removed, and a pressure dressing is applied over the puncture site.

➤ The results are recorded on film or by automated equipment in a computerized system for recall and postprocedure interpretation by the appropriate health care practitioner.

Post-test:

➤ Instruct the patient to resume usual diet, fluids, medications, or activity, as directed by the health care practitioner. Renal function should be assessed before metformin is resumed, if contrast was used.

➤ Monitor vital signs and neurologic status every 15 minutes for 30 minutes. Compare with baseline values. Protocols may vary from facility to facility.

➤ If contrast was used, observe for delayed allergic reactions, such as rash, urticaria, tachycardia, hyperpnea, hypertension, palpitations, nausea, or vomiting.

➤ If contrast was used, advise the patient to immediately report symptoms such as fast heart rate, difficulty breathing, skin rash, itching or decreased urinary output.

➤ Observe the needle/catheter insertion site for bleeding, inflammation, or hematoma formation.

➤ Instruct the patient to apply cold compresses to the puncture site, as needed, to reduce discomfort or edema.

➤ Instruct the patient to increase fluid intake to help eliminate the contrast medium, if used.

➤ Inform the patient that diarrhea may occur after ingestion of oral contrast medium.

➤ A written report of the examination will be completed by a health care practitioner specializing in this branch of medicine. The report will be sent to the requesting health care practitioner, who will discuss the results with the patient.

➤ Depending on the results of this procedure, additional testing may be needed to evaluate or monitor progression of the disease process and determine the need for a change in therapy. Evaluate test results in relation to the patient's symptoms and other tests performed.

Related diagnostic tests:

➤ Related diagnostic tests include angiography of the abdomen; kidney, ureter, and bladder film; magnetic resonance imaging of the abdomen; and ultrasound of the pelvis.

COMPUTED TOMOGRAPHY, ANGIOGRAPHY

SYNONYM/ACRONYM: Computed axial tomography (CAT) angiography, CTA.

AREA OF APPLICATION: Vessels.

CONTRAST: Intravenous (IV) iodinated contrast medium.

DESCRIPTION & RATIONALE: Computed tomography angiography (CTA) is a noninvasive procedure that enhances certain anatomic views of vascular structures. This procedure complements traditional angiography and allows reconstruction of the images in different planes and removal of surrounding structures, leaving only the vessels to be studied. While lying on a table, the patient moves in and out of a doughnut-like device called a *gantry,* which houses the x-ray tube and associated electronics. The scanner uses multiple x-ray beams and a series of detectors that rotate around the patient to produce cross-sectional views in a three-dimensional fashion by detecting and recording differences in tissue density after having an x-ray beam passed through the tissues. CTA uses spiral CT technology and collects large amounts of data with each scan. Retrospectively, the data can be manipulated to produce the desired image without exposure to additional radiation or contrast medium. Multiplanar reconstruction images are reviewed by the physician at a computerized workstation. These images are helpful when there are heavily calcified vessels. The axial images give the most precise information regarding the true percentage of stenosis, and they can also evaluate intracerebral aneurysms. Small ulcerations and plaque irregularity are readily seen with CTA; the degree of stenosis can be estimated better with CTA because of the increased number of imaging planes. Density measurements are sent to a computer that produces a digital image of the anatomy, enabling a physician to look at slices or thin sections of certain anatomic views of the vessels. Iodinated contrast medium is given intravenously for vascular evaluation. Images can be recorded on photographic or x-ray film or stored in digital format as digitized computer data. ■

INDICATIONS:
- Detect aneurysms
- Detect embolism or other occlusions
- Detect fistula
- Detect stenosis
- Detect vascular disease
- Differentiate aortic aneurysms from tumors near the aorta
- Differentiate between vascular and nonvascular tumors
- Evaluate atherosclerosis
- Evaluate hemorrhage or trauma
- Monitor and evaluate the effectiveness of medical or surgical therapies

RESULT

Normal Findings:
- Normal size, position, and shape of vascular structures

Abnormal Findings:
- Aortic aneurysm
- Cysts or abscesses
- Emboli
- Hemorrhage
- Neoplasm
- Occlusion
- Shunting
- Stenosis

CRITICAL VALUES: N/A

INTERFERING FACTORS:

This procedure is contraindicated for:
- ⚠ Patients with allergies to shellfish or iodinated dye. The contrast medium used may cause a life-threatening allergic reaction. Patients with a known hypersensitivity to the medium may benefit from premedication with corticosteroids or the use of nonionic contrast medium.

- Patients who are claustrophobic.

- Patients who are pregnant or suspected of being pregnant, unless the potential benefits of the procedure far outweigh the risks to the fetus and mother.

- ⚠ Elderly and other patients who are chronically dehydrated before the test, because of their risk of contrast-induced renal failure.

- ⚠ Patients who are in renal failure.

- Young patients (17 years old and younger), unless the benefits of the x-ray diagnosis outweigh the risks of exposure to high levels of radiation.

Factors that may impair clear imaging:

- Gas or feces in the gastrointestinal tract resulting from inadequate cleansing or failure to restrict food intake before the study

- Retained barium from a previous radiologic procedure

- Metallic objects within the examination field (e.g., jewelry, body rings), which may inhibit organ visualization and can produce unclear images

- Improper adjustment of the radiographic equipment to accommodate obese or thin patients, which can cause overexposure or underexposure and a poor-quality study

- Patients who are very obese, who may exceed the weight limit for the equipment

- Patients with extreme claustrophobia unless sedation is given before the study

- Incorrect positioning of the patient, which may produce poor visualization of the area to be examined

- Inability of the patient to cooperate or remain still during the procedure because of age, significant pain, or mental status

Other considerations:

- Complications of the procedure include hemorrhage, infection at the IV needle insertion site, and cardiac arrhythmias.

- The procedure may be terminated if chest pain or severe cardiac arrhythmias occur.

- Failure to follow dietary restrictions and other pretesting preparations may cause the procedure to be canceled or repeated.

- Consultation with a health care provider should occur before the procedure for radiation safety concerns regarding younger patients or patients who are lactating.

- Risks associated with radiographic overexposure can result from frequent x-ray procedures. Personnel in the room with the patient should wear a protective lead apron, stand behind a shield, or leave the area while the examination is being done. Personnel working in the area where the examination is being done should wear badges that reveal their level of exposure to radiation.

Nursing Implications and Procedure • • • • • • • • • • •

Pretest:

➤ Inform the patient that the procedure assesses the cardiovascular system.

➤ Obtain a history of the patient's complaints or clinical symptoms, including a list of known allergens, especially allergies or sensitivities to iodine, seafood, or other contrast mediums.

➤ Obtain a history of results of previously performed diagnostic procedures, surgical procedures, and laboratory tests. Include specific tests as they apply (e.g., blood urea nitrogen [BUN], creatinine, coagulation tests, platelets, bleeding time). Ensure that the results of blood tests are obtained and recorded before the procedure, especially BUN and creatinine, if contrast medium is to be used. For related diagnostic tests, refer to the Cardiovascular System table.

➤ Note any recent barium or other radiologic contrast procedures. Ensure that barium studies were performed more than 4 days before the CT scan.

➤ Record the date of the last menstrual period and determine the possibility of pregnancy in perimenopausal women.

➤ Obtain a list of the medications the patient is taking.

➤ Patients receiving metformin (glucophage) for non–insulin-dependent (type 2) diabetes should discontinue the drug on the day of the test and continue to withhold it for 48 hours after the test. Failure to do so may result in lactic acidosis.

➤ Review the procedure with the patient. Explain to the patient that some pain may be experienced during the test, and there may be moments of discomfort. Explain the purpose of the test and how the procedure is performed. Inform the patient that the procedure is performed in a radiology department, usually by a health care practitioner and support staff, and takes approximately 30 to 60 minutes.

➤ *Sensitivity to cultural and social issues,* as well as concern for modesty, is important in providing psychological support before, during, and after the procedure.

➤ Explain that an IV line may be inserted to allow infusion of IV fluids, contrast medium, dye, or sedatives. Usually contrast medium and normal saline are infused.

➤ Inform the patient that he or she may experience nausea, a feeling of warmth, a salty or metallic taste, or a transient headache after injection of contrast medium, if given.

➤ The patient should fast and restrict fluids for 8 hours prior to the procedure. Instruct the patient to avoid taking anticoagulant medication or to reduce dosage as ordered prior to the procedure.

➤ Instruct the patient to remove jewelry (including watches), credit cards, keys, coins, cell phones, pagers, and other metallic objects.

➤ *Make sure a written and informed consent has been signed prior to the procedure and before administering any medications.*

Intratest:

➤ Ensure that the patient has complied with dietary, fluids, and medication restrictions and pretesting prepara-

tions. Ensure that the patient has removed all external metallic objects (jewelry, dentures, etc.) prior to the procedure.

➤ Have emergency equipment readily available.

➤ If the patient has a history of severe allergic reactions to any substance or drug, administer ordered prophylactic steroids or antihistamines before the procedure. Use nonionic contrast medium for the procedure.

➤ Patients are given a gown, robe, and foot coverings to wear and instructed to void prior to the procedure.

➤ Observe standard precautions, and follow the general guidelines in Appendix A.

➤ Instruct the patient to cooperate fully and to follow directions. Instruct the patient to remain still throughout the procedure because movement produces unreliable results.

➤ Establish an IV fluid line for the injection of contrast, emergency drugs, and sedatives.

➤ Administer an antianxiety agent, as ordered, if the patient has claustrophobia. Administer a sedative to a child or to an uncooperative adult, as ordered.

➤ Place the patient in the supine position on an exam table.

➤ The contrast medium is injected, and a rapid series of images is taken during and after the filling of the vessels to be examined. Delayed images may be taken to examine the vessels after a time and to monitor the venous phase of the procedure.

➤ Ask the patient to inhale deeply and hold his or her breath while the x-ray images are taken, and then to exhale after the images are taken.

➤ Instruct the patient to take slow, deep breaths if nausea occurs during the procedure. Monitor and administer an antiemetic agent if ordered. Ready an emesis basin for use.

➤ Monitor the patient for complications related to the procedure (e.g., allergic reaction, anaphylaxis, bronchospasm).

➤ The needle or vascular catheter is removed, and a pressure dressing is applied over the puncture site.

➤ The results are recorded on film or by automated equipment in a computerized system, for recall and postprocedure interpretation by the appropriate health care practitioner.

Post-test:

➤ Instruct the patient to resume usual diet, fluids, medications, or activity, as directed by the health care practitioner. Renal function should be assessed before metformin is resumed.

➤ Monitor vital signs and neurologic status every 15 minutes for 30 minutes. Compare with baseline values. Protocols may vary from facility to facility.

➤ Observe for delayed allergic reactions, such as rash, urticaria, tachycardia, hyperpnea, hypertension, palpitations, nausea, or vomiting.

➤ Advise the patient to immediately report symptoms such as fast heart rate, difficulty breathing, skin rash, itching or decreased urinary output.

➤ Observe the needle/catheter insertion site for bleeding, inflammation, or hematoma formation.

➤ Instruct the patient to apply cold compresses to the puncture site, as needed, to reduce discomfort or edema.

➤ Instruct the patient to increase fluid intake to help eliminate the contrast medium.

➤ A written report of the examination will be completed by a health care practitioner specializing in this branch of medicine. The report will be sent to the requesting health care practitioner, who will discuss the results with the patient.

➤ Depending on the results of this procedure, additional testing may be needed to evaluate or monitor progression of the disease process and determine the need for a change in therapy. Evaluate test results in relation to the patient's symptoms and other tests performed.

Related diagnostic tests:

➤ Related diagnostic tests include angiography of the specific area, magnetic resonance angiography, and ultrasound venous Doppler.

COMPUTED TOMOGRAPHY, BILIARY TRACT AND LIVER

. . . .

SYNONYMS/ACRONYMS: Computed axial tomography (CAT), computed transaxial tomography (CTT), abdominal CT.

AREA OF APPLICATION: Liver, biliary tract, and adjacent structures.

CONTRAST: Can be done with or without intravenous (IV) iodinated contrast medium.

DESCRIPTION & RATIONALE: Computed tomography (CT) of the liver and biliary tract is a noninvasive procedure that enhances certain anatomic views of these structures, but it becomes invasive with the use of contrast medium. The patient lies on a table that moves in and out of a doughnut-like device called a *gantry*, which houses the x-ray tube and associated electronics. The scanner uses multiple x-ray beams and a series of detectors that rotate around the patient to produce cross-sectional views in a three-dimensional fashion by detecting and recording differences in tissue density after having an x-ray beam passed through the tissues. These density measurements are sent to a computer that produces a digital image of the anatomy, enabling a physician to look at slices or thin sections of certain anatomic views of the liver, biliary tract, and vascular system. Differentiations can be made among solid, cystic, inflammatory, or vascular lesions, and suspected hematomas and aneurysms can be identified. Iodinated contrast medium is given intravenously for blood vessel and vascular evaluation. Images can be recorded on photographic or x-ray film or stored in digital format as digitized computer data. Cine scanning produces a series of moving images of the area scanned. The CT scan can be used to guide biopsy needles into areas of suspected tumors to obtain tissue for laboratory analysis and to guide placement of catheters for drainage of abscesses. Tumors, before and after therapy, may be monitored with CT scanning. ∎

INDICATIONS:
- Assist in differentiating between benign and malignant tumors

- Detect dilation or obstruction of the biliary ducts with or without calcification or gallstone
- Detect liver abnormalities, such as cirrhosis with ascites and fatty liver
- Detect tumor extension of masses and metastasis into the hepatic area
- Differentiate aortic aneurysms from tumors near the aorta
- Differentiate between obstructive and nonobstructive jaundice
- Differentiate infectious from inflammatory processes
- Evaluate hepatic cysts, masses, abscesses, or hematomas, or hepatic trauma
- Monitor and evaluate effectiveness of medical, radiation, or surgical therapies

RESULT

Normal Findings:
- Normal size, position, and contour of the liver and biliary ducts

Abnormal Findings:
- Dilation of the common hepatic duct, common bile duct, or gallbladder
- Gallstones
- Hematomas
- Hepatic cysts or abscesses
- Jaundice (obstructive or nonobstructive)
- Primary and metastatic neoplasms

CRITICAL VALUES: N/A

INTERFERING FACTORS:

This procedure is contraindicated for:
- ⚠ Patients with allergies to shellfish or iodinated dye. The contrast medium used may cause a life-threatening allergic reaction. Patients with a known hypersensitivity to the medium

may benefit from premedication with corticosteroids or the use of nonionic contrast medium.

- Patients who are claustrophobic.

- Patients who are pregnant or suspected of being pregnant, unless the potential benefits of the procedure far outweigh the risks to the fetus and mother.

- ⚠ Elderly and other patients who are chronically dehydrated before the test, because of their risk of contrast-induced renal failure.

- ⚠ Patients who are in renal failure.

- Young patients (17 years old and younger), unless the benefits of the x-ray diagnosis outweigh the risks of exposure to high levels of radiation.

Factors that may impair clear imaging:

- Gas or feces in the gastrointestinal tract resulting from inadequate cleansing or failure to restrict food intake before the study

- Retained barium from a previous radiologic procedure

- Metallic objects within the examination field (e.g., jewelry, body rings), which may inhibit organ visualization and can produce unclear images

- Improper adjustment of the radiographic equipment to accommodate obese or thin patients, which can cause overexposure or underexposure and a poor-quality study

- Patients who are very obese, who may exceed the weight limit for the equipment

- Patients with extreme claustrophobia unless sedation is given before the study

- Incorrect positioning of the patient, which may produce poor visualization of the area to be examined

- Inability of the patient to cooperate or remain still during the procedure because of age, significant pain, or mental status

Other considerations:

- Complications of the procedure include hemorrhage, infection at the IV needle insertion site, and cardiac arrhythmias.

- The procedure may be terminated if chest pain or severe cardiac arrhythmias occur.

- Failure to follow dietary restrictions and other pretesting preparations may cause the procedure to be canceled or repeated.

- Consultation with a health care provider should occur before the procedure for radiation safety concerns regarding younger patients or patients who are lactating.

- Risks associated with radiographic overexposure can result from frequent x-ray procedures. Personnel in the room with the patient should wear a protective lead apron, stand behind a shield, or leave the area while the examination is being done. Personnel working in the area where the examination is being done should wear badges that reveal their level of exposure to radiation.

Nursing Implications and Procedure • • • • • • • • • • •

Pretest:

➤ Inform the patient that the procedure assesses the liver, biliary tract and adjacent structures.

➤ Obtain a history of the patient's complaints or clinical symptoms, including a list of known allergens, especially allergies or sensitivities to iodine, seafood, or other contrast mediums.

➤ Obtain a history of results of previously performed diagnostic procedures, surgical procedures, and laboratory tests. Include specific tests as they apply (e.g., blood urea nitrogen [BUN], creatinine, coagulation tests, platelets, bleeding time). Ensure that the results of blood tests are obtained and recorded before the procedure, especially BUN and creatinine, if contrast medium is to be used. For related diagnostic tests, refer to the Gastrointestinal, Hepatobiliary, and Genitourinary System tables.

➤ Note any recent barium or other radiologic contrast procedures. Ensure that barium studies were performed more than 4 days before the CT scan.

➤ Record the date of the last menstrual period and determine the possibility of pregnancy in perimenopausal women.

➤ Obtain a list of the medications the patient is taking.

➤ When contrast is used, patients receiving metformin (glucophage) for non–insulin-dependent (type 2) diabetes should discontinue the drug on the day of the test and continue to withhold it for 48 hours after the test. Failure to do so may result in lactic acidosis.

➤ Review the procedure with the patient. Explain to the patient that some pain may be experienced during the test, and there may be moments of discomfort. Explain the purpose of the test and how the procedure is performed. Inform the patient that the procedure is performed in a radiology department, usually by a health care practitioner and support staff, and takes approximately 30 to 60 minutes.

➤ *Sensitivity to cultural and social issues,* as well as concern for modesty, is important in providing psychological support before, during, and after the procedure.

➤ Explain that an IV line may be inserted to allow infusion of IV fluids, contrast medium, dye, or sedatives. Usually contrast medium and normal saline are infused.

➤ Inform the patient that he or she may experience nausea, a feeling of warmth, a salty or metallic taste, or a transient headache after injection of contrast medium, if given.

➤ The patient should fast and restrict fluids for 6 to 8 hours prior to the procedure. Instruct the patient to avoid taking anticoagulant medication or to reduce dosage as ordered prior to the procedure.

➤ Instruct the patient to remove jewelry (including watches), credit cards, keys, coins, cell phones, pagers, and other metallic objects.

➤ *Make sure a written and informed consent has been signed prior to the procedure and before administering any medications.*

Intratest:

➤ Ensure that the patient has complied with dietary, fluids, and medication restrictions and pretesting preparations; assure that food has been restricted for at least 6 hours prior to the procedure. Ensure that the patient has removed all external metallic objects (jewelry, dentures, etc.) prior to the procedure.

➤ Have emergency equipment readily available.

➤ If the patient has a history of severe allergic reactions to any substance or drug, administer ordered prophylactic steroids or antihistamines before the procedure. Use nonionic contrast medium for the procedure.

➤ Patients are given a gown robe, and foot coverings to wear and instructed to void prior to the procedure.

➤ Observe standard precautions, and follow the general guidelines in Appendix A.

➤ Instruct the patient to cooperate fully and to follow directions. Instruct the patient to remain still throughout the procedure because movement produces unreliable results.

➤ Establish an IV fluid line for the injection of contrast, emergency drugs, and sedatives.

➤ Administer an antianxiety agent, as ordered, if the patient has claustrophobia. Administer a sedative to a child or to an uncooperative adult, as ordered.

➤ Place the patient in the supine position on an exam table.

➤ If contrast is used, the contrast medium is injected, and a rapid series of images is taken during and after the filling of the vessels to be examined. Delayed images may be taken to examine the vessels after a time and to monitor the venous phase of the procedure.

➤ Ask the patient to inhale deeply and hold his or her breath while the x-ray images are taken, and then to exhale after the images are taken.

➤ Instruct the patient to take slow, deep breaths if nausea occurs during the procedure. Monitor and administer an antiemetic agent if ordered. Ready an emesis basin for use.

➤ Monitor the patient for complications related to the procedure (e.g., allergic reaction, anaphylaxis, bronchospasm) if contrast is used.

➤ The needle or vascular catheter is removed, and a pressure dressing is applied over the puncture site.

➤ The results are recorded on film or by automated equipment in a computerized system, for recall and postprocedure interpretation by the appropriate health care practitioner.

Post-test:

➤ Instruct the patient to resume usual diet, fluids, medications, or activity, as directed by the health care practitioner. Renal function should be assessed before metformin is resumed, if contrast was used,.

➤ Monitor vital signs and neurologic status every 15 minutes for 30 minutes. Compare with baseline values. Protocols may vary from facility to facility.

➤ If contrast was used, observe for delayed allergic reactions, such as rash, urticaria, tachycardia, hyperpnea, hypertension, palpitations, nausea, or vomiting, if contrast medium was used.

➤ If contrast was used, advise the patient to immediately report symptoms such as fast heart rate, difficulty breathing, skin rash, itching or decreased urinary output.

➤ Observe the needle/catheter insertion site for bleeding, inflammation, or hematoma formation.

➤ Instruct the patient to apply cold compresses to the puncture site, as needed, to reduce discomfort or edema.

➤ Instruct the patient to increase fluid intake to help eliminate the contrast medium, if used.

➤ Inform the patient that diarrhea may occur after ingestion of oral contrast media.

➤ A written report of the examination will be completed by a health care practitioner specializing in this branch of medicine. The report will be sent to the requesting health care practitioner, who will discuss the results with the patient.

➤ Depending on the results of this procedure, additional testing may be needed to evaluate or monitor progression of the disease process and determine the need for a change in therapy. Evaluate test results in relation to the patient's symptoms and other tests performed.

Related diagnostic tests:

➤ Related diagnostic tests include hepatobiliary scan; kidney, ureter, and bladder film; magnetic resonance imaging of the abdomen, and ultrasound of the liver.

COMPUTED TOMOGRAPHY, BRAIN

· ·

SYNONYMS/ACRONYMS: Computed axial tomography (CAT) of the head, computed transaxial tomography (CTT) of the head, brain CT.

AREA OF APPLICATION: Brain.

CONTRAST: Can be done with or without intravenous (IV) iodinated contrast medium.

DESCRIPTION & RATIONALE: Computed tomography (CT) of the brain is a noninvasive procedure used to assist in diagnosing abnormalities of the head, brain tissue, cerebrospinal fluid, and blood circulation. Brain CT becomes invasive if contrast medium is used for image enhancement when pathology causing destruction of the blood-brain barrier is suspected. CT is useful for evaluating suspected brain tumors, infarction, intracranial hemorrhage, hematomas, arteriovenous malformations, ventricular abnormalities, aneurysms, and other vascular abnormalities. The patient lies on a table and is moved in and out of a doughnut-like device called a *gantry*, which houses the x-ray tube and associated electronics. The scanner uses multiple x-ray beams and a series of detectors that rotate around the patient to produce cross-sectional views in a three-dimensional fashion by detecting and recording differences in tissue density after having an x-ray beam passed through the tissues. Low-density tissue appears black on the images, medium-density tissue appears in shades of gray, and high-density tissue appears nearly white. These density measurements are sent to a computer that produces a digital image of the anatomy, enabling a physician to look at slices or thin sections of certain anatomic views of the brain and associated vascular system. Differentiations can be made among solid, cystic, inflammatory, or vascular lesions, and suspected hematomas or aneurysms can be identified. The procedure may be repeated after iodinated contrast medium is given intravenously for blood vessel and vascular evaluation. Images can be recorded on photographic or x-ray film or stored in digital format as digitized computer data. Cine scanning is used to produce a series of moving images of the area scanned. Tumor progression, before and after therapy, and effectiveness of medical interventions may be monitored by CT scanning. ■

INDICATIONS:
• Detect the presence of a brain infection or inflammatory condition, such as abscess or necrosis, as evidenced by decreased density on the image

• Detect ventricular enlargement or displacement by increased cerebrospinal fluid

• Determine benign and cancerous intracranial tumors and cyst formation, as evidenced by changes in tissue densities (white indicating increased density, darker areas indicating decreased density)

• Determine the cause of increased intracranial pressure

• Determine the presence and type of hemorrhage in infants and children experiencing signs and symptoms of intracranial trauma, or of congenital conditions such as hydrocephalus and arteriovenous malformations

• Determine the presence of multiple sclerosis, as evidenced by sclerotic plaques 3 to 4 mm in diameter

• Determine the size and location of a lesion causing a stroke, such as an infarct or hemorrhage

• Differentiate among hematoma locations after trauma (e.g., subdural, epidural, cerebral), and determine the extent of edema resulting from injury, as evidenced by higher blood densities compared with normal tissue

• Differentiate between cerebral infarction and hemorrhage

• Evaluate abnormalities of the middle ear ossicles, auditory nerve, and optic nerve

• Monitor and evaluate the effectiveness of medical, radiation, or surgical therapies

RESULT

Normal Findings:
• Normal size, position, and shape of intracranial contents and vascular system

Abnormal Findings:
• Abscess
• Aneurysm
• Arteriovenous malformations
• Cerebral atrophy
• Cerebral edema
• Cerebral infarction
• Congenital abnormalities
• Craniopharyngioma
• Cysts
• Hematomas (e.g., epidural, subdural, intracerebral)
• Hemorrhage
• Hydrocephaly
• Increased intracranial pressure or trauma
• Infection
• Sclerotic plaques suggesting multiple sclerosis
• Tumor
• Ventricular or tissue displacement or enlargement

CRITICAL VALUES: N/A

INTERFERING FACTORS:

This procedure is contraindicated for:

• ⚠ Patients with allergies to shellfish or iodinated dye. The contrast medium used may cause a life-threatening allergic reaction. Patients with a known hypersensitivity to the medium may benefit from premedication with corticosteroids or the use of nonionic contrast medium.

• Patients who are claustrophobic.

• Patients who are pregnant or suspected of being pregnant, unless the potential benefits of the procedure far outweigh the risks to the fetus and mother.

• ⚠ Elderly and other patients who are chronically dehydrated before the test, because of their risk of contrast-induced renal failure.

- ⚠️ Patients who are in renal failure.

- Young patients (17 years old and younger), unless the benefits of the x-ray diagnosis outweigh the risks of exposure to high levels of radiation.

Factors that may impair clear imaging:

- Gas or feces in the gastrointestinal tract resulting from inadequate cleansing or failure to restrict food intake before the study

- Retained barium from a previous radiologic procedure

- Metallic objects within the examination field (e.g., jewelry, dentures, body rings), which may inhibit organ visualization and can produce unclear images

- Improper adjustment of the radiographic equipment to accommodate obese or thin patients, which can cause overexposure or underexposure and a poor-quality study

- Patients who are very obese, who may exceed the weight limit for the equipment

- Patients with extreme claustrophobia unless sedation is given before the study

- Incorrect positioning of the patient, which may produce poor visualization of the area to be examined

- Inability of the patient to cooperate or remain still during the procedure because of age, significant pain, or mental status

Other considerations:

- Complications of the procedure include hemorrhage, infection at the IV needle insertion site, and cardiac arrhythmias.

- The procedure may be terminated if chest pain or severe cardiac arrhythmias occur.

- Failure to follow dietary restrictions and other pretesting preparations may cause the procedure to be canceled or repeated.

- Consultation with a health care provider should occur before the procedure for radiation safety concerns regarding younger patients or patients who are lactating.

- Risks associated with radiographic overexposure can result from frequent x-ray procedures. Personnel in the room with the patient should wear a protective lead apron, stand behind a shield, or leave the area while the examination is being done. Personnel working in the area where the examination is being done should wear badges that reveal their level of exposure to radiation.

Nursing Implications and Procedure

Pretest:

➤ Inform the patient that the procedure assesses the brain.

➤ Obtain a history of the patient's complaints or clinical symptoms, including a list of known allergens, especially allergies or sensitivities to iodine, seafood, or other contrast mediums.

➤ Obtain a history of results of previously performed diagnostic procedures, surgical procedures, and laboratory tests. Include specific tests as they apply (e.g., blood urea nitrogen [BUN], creatinine, coagulation tests, bleeding time). Ensure that the results of blood tests are obtained and recorded before the procedure, especially BUN and creatinine, if contrast medium is to be used. For related diagnostic tests, refer to the Cardiovascular and Endocrine Systems tables.

➤ Note any recent barium or other radiologic contrast procedures. Ensure that barium studies were performed more than 4 days before the CT scan.

➤ Record the date of the last menstrual period and determine the possibility of pregnancy in perimenopausal women.

➤ Obtain a list of the medications the patient is taking.

➤ In case contrast is used, patients receiving metformin (glucophage) for non–insulin-dependent (type 2) diabetes should discontinue the drug on the day of the test and continue to withhold it for 48 hours after the test. Failure to do so may result in lactic acidosis.

➤ Review the procedure with the patient. Explain to the patient that some pain may be experienced during the test, and there may be moments of discomfort. Explain the purpose of the test and how the procedure is performed. Inform the patient that the procedure is performed in a radiology department, usually by a health care practitioner and support staff, and takes approximately 30 to 60 minutes.

➤ *Sensitivity to cultural and social issues,* as well as concern for modesty, is important in providing psychological support before, during, and after the procedure.

➤ Explain that an IV line may be inserted to allow infusion of IV fluids, contrast medium, dye, or sedatives. Usually contrast medium and normal saline are infused.

➤ Inform the patient that he or she may experience nausea, a feeling of warmth, a salty or metallic taste, or a transient headache after injection of contrast medium, if given.

➤ The patient should not fast or restrict fluids prior to the procedure. Instruct the patient to avoid taking anticoagulant medication or to reduce dosage as ordered prior to the procedure.

➤ Instruct the patient to remove jewelry, including watches, dentures, credit cards, keys, coins, cell phones, pagers, and other metallic objects.

➤ *Make sure a written and informed consent has been signed prior to the procedure and before administering any medications.*

Intratest:

➤ Ensure that the patient has complied with medication restrictions and pretesting preparations. Ensure that the patient has removed all external metallic objects (jewelry, dentures, etc.) prior to the procedure.

➤ Have emergency equipment readily available.

➤ If the patient has a history of severe allergic reactions to any substance or drug, administer ordered prophylactic steroids or antihistamines before the procedure. Use nonionic contrast medium for the procedure.

➤ Observe standard precautions, and follow the general guidelines in Appendix A.

➤ Instruct the patient to cooperate fully and to follow directions. Instruct the patient to remain still throughout the procedure because movement produces unreliable results.

➤ Establish an IV fluid line for the injection of contrast, emergency drugs, and sedatives.

➤ Administer an antianxiety agent, as ordered, if the patient has claustrophobia. Administer a sedative to a child or to an uncooperative adult, as ordered.

➤ Place the patient in the supine position on an exam table.

➤ If contrast is used, the contrast medium is injected, and a rapid series of images is taken during and after the filling of the vessels to be examined. Delayed images may be taken to examine the vessels after a time and to monitor the venous phase of the procedure.

➤ Ask the patient to inhale deeply and hold his or her breath while the x-ray images are taken, and then to exhale after the images are taken.

➤ Instruct the patient to take slow, deep breaths if nausea occurs during the procedure. Monitor and administer an antiemetic agent if ordered. Ready an emesis basin for use.

➤ Monitor the patient for complications related to the procedure (e.g., allergic reaction, anaphylaxis, bronchospasm) if contrast is used.

➤ The needle or vascular catheter is removed, and a pressure dressing is applied over the puncture site.

➤ The results are recorded on film or by automated equipment in a computerized system for recall and postprocedure interpretation by the appropriate health care practitioner.

Post-test:

➤ Instruct the patient to resume medications and activity, as directed by the health care practitioner. Renal function should be assessed before metformin is resumed, if contrast was used.

➤ Monitor vital signs and neurologic status every 15 minutes for 30 minutes. Compare with baseline values. Protocols may vary from facility to facility.

➤ If contrast was used, observe for delayed allergic reactions, such as rash, urticaria, tachycardia, hyperpnea, hypertension, palpitations, nausea, or vomiting.

➤ If contrast was used, advise the patient to immediately report symp-toms such as fast heart rate, difficulty breathing, skin rash, itching or decreased urinary output.

➤ Observe the needle/catheter insertion site for bleeding, inflammation, or hematoma formation.

➤ Instruct the patient to apply cold compresses to the puncture site, as needed, to reduce discomfort or edema.

➤ Instruct the patient to increase fluid intake to help eliminate the contrast medium, if used.

➤ A written report of the examination will be completed by a health care practitioner specializing in this branch of medicine. The report will be sent to the requesting health care practitioner who will discuss the results with the patient.

➤ Depending on the results of this procedure, additional testing may be needed to evaluate or monitor progression of the disease process and determine the need for a change in therapy. Evaluate test results in relation to the patient's symptoms and other tests performed.

Related diagnostic tests:

➤ Related diagnostic tests include angiography of the carotids, computed tomography angiography, magnetic resonance angiography, and magnetic resonance imaging of the brain.

COMPUTED TOMOGRAPHY, CARDIAC SCORING

SYNONYMS/ACRONYMS: Computed axial tomography (CAT), computed transaxial tomography (CTT), heart vessel calcium CT, cardiac plaque CT.

AREA OF APPLICATION: Heart.

CONTRAST: None.

DESCRIPTION & RATIONALE: Cardiac scoring is a noninvasive test for quantifying coronary artery calcium content. Coronary artery disease (CAD) occurs when the arteries that carry blood and oxygen to the heart muscle become clogged or built up with plaque. Plaque buildup slows the flow of blood to the heart muscle, causing ischemia and increasing the risk of heart failure. The procedure begins with a computed tomography (CT) scan of the heart. The patient lies on a table and is moved in and out of a doughnut-like device called a *gantry*, which houses the x-ray tube and associated electronics. The scanner uses multiple x-ray beams and a series of detectors that rotate around the patient to produce cross-sectional views in a three-dimensional fashion by detecting and recording differences in plaque density after having an x-ray beam passed through the tissues. The scanner takes an image of the beating heart while the patient holds his or her breath for approximately 20 seconds. The procedure requires no contrast medium injections. These density measurements are sent to a computer that produces a digital analysis of the anatomy, enabling a physician to look at the quantified amount of calcium (cardiac plaque score) in the coronary arteries. The data can be recorded on photographic or x-ray film or stored in digital format as digitized computer data. ∎

INDICATIONS:

- Detect and quantify coronary artery calcium content
  CAD is the leading cause of death in most industrialized nations
  Cardiac scoring is a more powerful predictor of CAD than cholesterol screening
  Of all myocardial infarctions (MIs), 45% occur in people younger than age 65
  Of women who have had MIs, 44% will die within 1 year after the attack
  Women are more likely to die of heart disease than of breast cancer

- Family history of heart disease

- Screening for coronary artery calcium in patients with:
  Diabetes
  High blood pressure
  High cholesterol
  High-stress lifestyle
  Overweight by 20% or more
  Personal history of smoking
  Sedentary lifestyle

- Screening for coronary artery plaque in patients with chest pain of unknown cause

RESULT

Normal Findings:

- If the score is 100 or less, the probability of having significant CAD is minimal or is unlikely to be causing a narrowing at the time of the examination.

Abnormal Findings:

- If the score is between 101 and 400, a significant amount of calcified plaque was found in the coronary arteries. There is an increased risk of a future MI, and a medical assessment of cardiac risk factors needs to be done. Additional testing may be needed.

- If the score is greater than 400, the procedure has detected extensive calcified plaque in the coronary arteries, which may have caused a critical narrowing of the vessels. A full medical assessment is needed as soon as possible. Further testing may be needed, and treatment may be needed to reduce the risk of MI.

CRITICAL VALUES: N/A

INTERFERING FACTORS:

This procedure is contraindicated for:

• Patients who are claustrophobic.

• Patients who are pregnant or suspected of being pregnant, unless the potential benefits of the procedure far outweigh the risks to the fetus and mother.

• Young patients (17 years old and younger), unless the benefits of the x-ray diagnosis outweigh the risks of exposure to high levels of radiation.

Factors that may impair clear imaging:

• Retained barium or radiologic contrast from a previous radiologic procedure

• Metallic objects within the examination field (e.g., jewelry, body rings), which may inhibit organ visualization and can produce unclear images

• Improper adjustment of the radiographic equipment to accommodate obese or thin patients, which can cause overexposure or underexposure and a poor-quality study

• Patients who are very obese, who may exceed the weight limit for the equipment

• Patients with extreme claustrophobia unless sedation is given before the study

• Incorrect positioning of the patient, which may produce poor visualization of the area to be examined

• Inability of the patient to cooperate or remain still during the procedure because of age, significant pain, or mental status

Other considerations:

• The procedure may be terminated if chest pain or severe cardiac arrhythmias occur.

• Consultation with a health care provider should occur before the procedure for radiation safety concerns regarding younger patients or patients who are lactating.

• Risks associated with radiographic overexposure can result from frequent x-ray procedures. Personnel in the room with the patient should wear a protective lead apron, stand behind a shield, or leave the area while the examination is being done. Personnel working in the area where the examination is being done should wear badges that reveal their level of exposure to radiation.

Nursing Implications and Procedure • • • • • • • • • • •

Pretest:

➤ Inform the patient that the procedure assesses the coronary arteries.

➤ Obtain a history of the patient's complaints or clinical symptoms.

➤ Obtain a history of results of previously performed diagnostic procedures and surgical procedures. For related diagnostic tests, refer to the Cardiovascular System table.

➤ Note any recent barium or other radiologic contrast procedures. Ensure that barium studies were performed more than 4 days before the CT scan.

➤ Record the date of the last menstrual period and determine the possibility of pregnancy in perimenopausal women.

➤ Obtain a list of the medications the patient is taking.

➤ Review the procedure with the patient. Explain to the patient that some pain may be experienced during the test, and there may be moments of discomfort. Explain the purpose of the test and how the procedure is performed. Inform the patient that the procedure is performed in a radiology department, usually by a health care practitioner and support staff, and takes approximately 15 to 30 minutes.

➤ *Sensitivity to cultural and social issues,* as well as concern for modesty, is important in providing psychological support before, during, and after the procedure.

➤ The patient should not fast or restrict fluids prior to the procedure.

➤ Instruct the patient to remove jewelry (including watches), credit cards, keys, coins, cell phones, pagers, and other metallic objects.

Intratest:

➤ Ensure that the patient has removed all external metallic objects (jewelry, dentures, etc.) prior to the procedure.

➤ Have emergency equipment readily available.

➤ Patients are given a gown, robe, and foot coverings to wear and instructed to void prior to the procedure.

➤ Observe standard precautions, and follow the general guidelines in Appendix A.

➤ Instruct the patient to cooperate fully and to follow directions. Instruct the patient to remain still throughout the procedure because movement produces unreliable results.

➤ Administer an antianxiety agent, as ordered, if the patient has claustrophobia. Administer a sedative to a child or to an uncooperative adult, as ordered.

➤ Place the patient in the supine position on an exam table.

➤ A rapid series of images is taken of the vessels to be examined. Ask the patient to inhale deeply and hold his or her breath while the x-ray images are taken, and then to exhale after the images are taken.

➤ The results are recorded on film or by automated equipment in a computerized system for recall and postprocedure interpretation by the appropriate health care practitioner.

Post-test:

➤ A written report of the examination will be completed by a health care practitioner specializing in this branch of medicine. The report will be sent to the requesting health care practitioner, who will discuss the results with the patient.

➤ Depending on the results of this procedure, additional testing may be needed to evaluate or monitor progression of the disease process and determine the need for a change in therapy. Evaluate test results in relation to the patient's symptoms and other tests performed.

Related diagnostic tests:

➤ Related diagnostic tests include chest x-ray, coronary angiography, computed tomography of the thorax, echocardiogram, electrocardiography, lung scan, and magnetic resonance imaging of the chest.

COMPUTED TOMOGRAPHY, COLONOSCOPY

· ·

SYNONYMS/ACRONYMS: Computed axial tomography (CAT), computed transaxial tomography (CTT), CT virtual colonoscopy, CT colonography.

AREA OF APPLICATION: Colon.

CONTRAST: Screening examinations are done without intravenous (IV) iodinated contrast medium. Examinations done to clarify questionable or abnormal areas may require IV iodinated contrast medium.

DESCRIPTION & RATIONALE: Computed tomography (CT) colonoscopy is a noninvasive technique that involves examining the colon by taking multiple CT scans of the patient's colon and rectum and using computer software to create three-dimensional images. The procedure is used to detect polyps, which are growths of tissue in the colon or rectum. Some types of polyps increase the risk of colon cancer, especially if they are large or if a patient has several polyps. Compared to conventional colonoscopy, CT colonoscopy is less effective in detecting polyps smaller than 5 mm, more effective when the polyps are between 5 and 9.9 mm, and most effective when the polyps are 10 mm or larger. This test may be valuable for patients who have diseases rendering them unable to undergo conventional colonoscopy (e.g., bleeding disorders, lung or heart disease) and for patients who are unable to undergo the sedation required for traditional colonoscopy.

The procedure is less invasive than conventional colonoscopy, with little risk of complications and no recovery time. CT colonoscopy can be done as an outpatient procedure, and the patient may return to work or usual activities the same day.

CT colonoscopy and conventional colonoscopy require the bowel to be cleansed before the examination. The patient lies on a table and is moved in and out of a doughnut-like device called a *gantry*, which houses the x-ray tube and associated electronics. The scanner uses multiple x-ray beams and a series of detectors that rotate around the patient to produce cross-sectional views in a three-dimensional fashion by detecting and recording differences in densities in the colon after having an x-ray beam passed through it. The scanner takes an image of the colon while the patient holds his or her breath for approximately 10 to 30 seconds. The screening procedure requires no contrast medium injections, but if a suspicious area or abnormality is detected, a repeat series of images may be completed after IV contrast medium is given. These density measurements are sent to a computer that produces a digital analysis of the anatomy, enabling a physician to look at slices or thin sections of certain anatomic views of the colon and vascular system. The data can be recorded on photographic or x-ray film or stored in digital format as digitized computer data. A drawback of CT colonoscopy is that polyp removal and biopsies of tissue in the colon must be done using conventional colonoscopy. Therefore, if polyps are discovered during CT colonoscopy and biopsy becomes necessary, the patient must undergo bowel preparation a second time. ■

INDICATIONS:

- Detect polyps in the colon
- Evaluate the colon for metachronous lesions
- Evaluate the colon in patients with obstructing rectosigmoid disease
- Evaluate polyposis syndromes
- Evaluate the site of resection for local recurrence of lesions
- Examine the colon in patients with heart or lung disease, patients unable to be sedated, and patients unable to undergo colonoscopy
- Failure to visualize the entire colon during conventional colonoscopy
- Identify metastases
- Investigate cause of positive occult blood test
- Investigate further after an abnormal barium enema
- Investigate further when flexible sigmoidoscopy is positive for polyps

RESULT

Normal Findings:
- Normal colon and rectum, with no evidence of polyps or growths

Abnormal Findings:
- Abnormal endoluminal wall of the colon
- Extraluminal extension of primary cancer
- Mesenteric and retroperitoneal lymphadenopathy
- Metachronous lesions
- Metastases of cancer
- Polyps or growths in colon or rectum
- Tumor recurrence after surgery

CRITICAL VALUES: N/A

INTERFERING FACTORS:

This procedure is contraindicated for:
- ⚠ Patients with allergies to shellfish or iodinated dye. The contrast medium used may cause a life-threatening allergic reaction. Patients with a known hypersensitivity to the medium may benefit from premedication with corticosteroids or the use of nonionic contrast medium, if contrast is used.

- Patients who are claustrophobic.

- Patients who are pregnant or suspected of being pregnant, unless the potential benefits of the procedure far outweigh the risks to the fetus and mother.

- ⚠ Elderly and other patients who are chronically dehydrated before the test, because of their risk of contrast-induced renal failure, if contrast is used.

- ⚠ Patients who are in renal failure, if contrast is used.

- Young patients (17 years old and younger), unless the benefits of the x-ray diagnosis outweigh the risks of exposure to high levels of radiation.

Factors that may impair clear imaging:

- Gas or feces in the gastrointestinal tract resulting from inadequate cleansing or failure to restrict food intake before the study

- Retained barium from a previous radiologic procedure

- Metallic objects within the examination field (e.g., jewelry, body rings), which may inhibit organ visualization and can produce unclear images

- Improper adjustment of the radiographic equipment to accommodate obese or thin patients, which can cause overexposure or underexposure and a poor-quality study

- Patients who are very obese, who may exceed the weight limit for the equipment

- Patients with extreme claustrophobia unless sedation is given before the study

- Incorrect positioning of the patient, which may produce poor visualization of the area to be examined

- Inability of the patient to cooperate or remain still during the procedure because of age, significant pain, or mental status

Other considerations:

- Complications of the procedure include hemorrhage, infection at the IV needle insertion site, and cardiac arrhythmias.

- The procedure may be terminated if chest pain or severe cardiac arrhythmias occur.

- Failure to follow dietary restrictions and other pretesting preparations may

cause the procedure to be canceled or repeated.

- Consultation with a health care provider should occur before the procedure for radiation safety concerns regarding younger patients or patients who are lactating.

- Risks associated with radiographic overexposure can result from frequent x-ray procedures. Personnel in the room with the patient should wear a protective lead apron, stand behind a shield, or leave the area while the examination is being done. Personnel working in the area where the examination is being done should wear badges that reveal their level of exposure to radiation.

Nursing Implications and Procedure

Pretest:

➤ Inform the patient that the procedure assesses the colon.

➤ Obtain a history of the patient's complaints or clinical symptoms, including a list of known allergens, especially allergies or sensitivities to iodine, seafood, or other contrast mediums.

➤ Obtain a history of results of previously performed diagnostic procedures, surgical procedures, and laboratory tests. Include specific tests as they apply (e.g., blood urea nitrogen [BUN], creatinine, coagulation tests, bleeding time). Ensure that the results of blood tests are obtained and recorded before the procedure, especially BUN and creatinine, if contrast medium is to be used. For related diagnostic tests, refer to the Gastrointestinal System table.

➤ Note any recent barium or other radiologic contrast procedures. Ensure that barium studies were performed more than 4 days before the CT scan.

➤ Record the date of the last menstrual

period and determine the possibility of pregnancy in perimenopausal women.

➤ Obtain a list of the medications the patient is taking.

➤ If contrast is used, patients receiving metformin (glucophage) for non–insulin-dependent (type 2) diabetes should discontinue the drug on the day of the test and continue to withhold it for 48 hours after the test. Failure to do so may result in lactic acidosis.

➤ Review the procedure with the patient. Explain to the patient that some pain may be experienced during the test, and there may be moments of discomfort. Explain the purpose of the test and how the procedure is performed. Inform the patient that the procedure is performed in a radiology department, usually by a health care practitioner and support staff, and takes approximately 30 to 60 minutes.

➤ *Sensitivity to cultural and social issues,* as well as concern for modesty, is important in providing psychological support before, during, and after the procedure.

➤ Explain that an IV line may be inserted to allow infusion of IV fluids, contrast medium, dye, or sedatives.

➤ Inform the patient that he or she may experience nausea, a feeling of warmth, a salty or metallic taste, or a transient headache after injection of contrast medium, if given.

➤ The patient should fast and restrict fluids for 6 to 8 hours prior to the procedure. Instruct the patient to avoid taking anticoagulant medication or to reduce dosage as ordered prior to the procedure.

➤ Instruct the patient to remove jewelry (including watches), credit cards, keys, coins, cell phones, pagers, and other metallic objects.

➤ *Make sure a written and informed consent has been signed prior to the procedure and before administering any medications.*

Intratest:

➤ Ensure that the patient has complied with dietary, fluids, and medication restrictions and pretesting preparations; assure that food has been restricted for at least 6 hours prior to the procedure. Ensure that the patient has removed all external metallic objects (jewelry, dentures, etc.) prior to the procedure.

➤ Have emergency equipment readily available.

➤ If the patient has a history of severe allergic reactions to any substance or drug, administer ordered prophylactic steroids or antihistamines before the procedure. Use nonionic contrast medium for the procedure.

➤ Patients are given a gown, robe, and foot coverings to wear and instructed to void prior to the procedure.

➤ Observe standard precautions, and follow the general guidelines in Appendix A.

➤ Instruct the patient to cooperate fully and to follow directions. Instruct the patient to remain still throughout the procedure because movement produces unreliable results.

➤ Establish an IV fluid line for the injection of contrast (if used), emergency drugs, and sedatives.

➤ Administer an antianxiety agent, as ordered, if the patient has claustrophobia. Administer a sedative to a child or to an uncooperative adult, as ordered.

➤ Place the patient in the supine position on an exam table.

➤ The colon is distended with room air or carbon dioxide by means of a rectal tube and balloon retention device. Maximal colonic distention is guided by patient tolerance.

➤ If contrast is used, the contrast medium is injected, and a rapid series of images is taken during and after the filling of the vessels to be examined. Delayed images may be taken to examine the vessels after a time and to monitor the venous phase of the procedure.

➤ Ask the patient to inhale deeply and hold his or her breath while the x-ray images are taken, and then to exhale after the images are taken.

➤ The sequence of images is repeated in the prone position.

➤ Instruct the patient to take slow, deep breaths if nausea occurs during the procedure. Monitor and administer an antiemetic agent if ordered. Ready an emesis basin for use.

➤ Monitor the patient for complications related to the procedure (e.g., allergic reaction, anaphylaxis, bronchospasm) if contrast is used.

➤ The needle or vascular catheter is removed, and a pressure dressing is applied over the puncture site.

➤ The results are recorded on film or by automated equipment in a computerized system for recall and postprocedure interpretation by the appropriate health care practitioner.

Post-test:

➤ Instruct the patient to resume usual diet, fluids, medications, or activity, as directed by the health care practitioner. Renal function should be assessed before metformin is resumed, if contrast was used.

➤ Monitor vital signs and neurologic status every 15 minutes for 30 minutes. Compare with baseline values. Protocols may vary from facility to facility.

➤ If contrast was used, observe for delayed allergic reactions, such as rash, urticaria, tachycardia, hyperpnea, hypertension, palpitations, nausea, or vomiting, if contrast medium was used.

➤ If contrast was used, advise the patient to immediately report symptoms such as fast heart rate, difficulty breathing, skin rash, itching or decreased urinary output.

➤ Observe the needle/catheter insertion site for bleeding, inflammation, or hematoma formation.

➤ Instruct the patient to apply cold compresses to the puncture site, as needed, to reduce discomfort or edema.

➤ Instruct the patient to increase fluid intake to help eliminate the contrast medium, if used.

➤ Inform the patient that diarrhea may occur after ingestion of oral contrast media.

➤ A written report of the examination will be completed by a health care practitioner specializing in this branch of medicine. The report will be sent to the requesting health care practitioner, who will discuss the results with the patient.

➤ Depending on the results of this procedure, additional testing may be needed to evaluate or monitor progression of the disease process and determine the need for a change in therapy. Evaluate test results in relation to the patient's symptoms and other tests performed.

Related diagnostic tests:

➤ Related diagnostic tests include barium enema; colonoscopy; computed tomography of the abdomen; kidney, ureter, and bladder (KUB) film; magnetic resonance imaging of the abdomen; proctosigmoidoscopy, and ultrasound of the pelvis.

COMPUTED TOMOGRAPHY, PANCREAS

SYNONYMS/ACRONYMS: Computed axial tomography (CAT), computed transaxial tomography (CTT).

AREA OF APPLICATION: Pancreas.

CONTRAST: Can be done with or without oral or intravenous (IV) iodinated contrast medium.

DESCRIPTION & RATIONALE: Computed tomography (CT) is a noninvasive procedure used to enhance certain anatomic views of the abdominal structures, but it becomes an invasive procedure when contrast medium is used. CT of the pancreas aids in the diagnosis or evaluation of pancreatic cysts, pseudocysts, inflammation, tumors, masses, metastases, abscesses, and trauma. In all but the thinnest or most emaciated patients, the pancreas is surrounded by fat that clearly defines its margins. While lying on a table, the patient is moved in and out of a doughnut-like device called a *gantry*, which houses the x-ray tube and associated electronics. The scanner uses multiple x-ray beams and a series of detectors that rotate around the patient to produce cross-sectional views in a three-dimensional fashion by detecting and recording differences in tissue density after having an x-ray beam passed through the tissues. These density measurements are sent to a computer that produces a digital image of the anatomy, enabling the radiologist to look at slices or thin sections of certain anatomic views of the pancreas and associated vascular system. Differentiations can be made among solid, cystic, inflammatory, or vascular lesions. CT scanning can detect the swelling that accompanies acute inflammation of the gland and, in chronic cases, the calcium deposits missed on other examinations. Intravenous iodinated contrast medium is given for blood vessel and vascular evaluation, and oral contrast medium is given for bowel and adjacent structure evaluation. Images can be recorded on photographic or x-ray film or stored in digital format as digitized computer data. Cine scanning produces a series of moving images of the scanned area. The CT scan can be used to guide biopsy needles into areas of pancreatic masses to obtain tissue for laboratory analysis and for placement of needles to aspirate cysts or abscesses. CT scanning can monitor mass, cyst, or tumor growth and post-therapy response. ■

INDICATIONS:
• Detect dilation or obstruction of the pancreatic ducts

• Differentiate between pancreatic disorders and disorders of the retroperitoneum

• Evaluate benign or cancerous tumors or metastasis to the pancreas

• Evaluate pancreatic abnormalities (e.g., bleeding, pancreatitis, pseudocyst, abscesses)

• Evaluate unexplained weight loss, jaundice, and epigastric pain

• Monitor and evaluate effectiveness of medical or surgical therapies

RESULT

Normal Findings:
• Normal size, position, and contour of the pancreas, which lies obliquely in the upper abdomen

Abnormal Findings:
• Acute or chronic pancreatitis

• Obstruction of the pancreatic ducts

• Pancreatic abscesses

• Pancreatic carcinoma

• Pancreatic pseudocyst

• Pancreatic tumor

CRITICAL VALUES: N/A

INTERFERING FACTORS:

This procedure is contraindicated for:
• ⚠ Patients with allergies to shellfish or iodinated dye. The contrast medium used may cause a life-threatening allergic reaction. Patients with a known hypersensitivity to the medium may benefit from premedication with corticosteroids or the use of nonionic contrast medium.

• Patients who are claustrophobic.

• Patients who are pregnant or suspected of being pregnant, unless the potential benefits of the procedure far outweigh the risks to the fetus and mother.

• ⚠ Elderly and other patients who are chronically dehydrated before the test, because of their risk of contrast-induced renal failure.

• ⚠ Patients who are in renal failure.

• Young patients (17 years old and younger), unless the benefits of the x-ray diagnosis outweigh the risks of exposure to high levels of radiation.

Factors that may impair clear imaging:
• Gas or feces in the gastrointestinal tract resulting from inadequate cleansing or failure to restrict food intake before the study

• Retained barium from a previous radiologic procedure

• Metallic objects within the examination field (e.g., jewelry, body rings), which may inhibit organ visualization and can produce unclear images

• Improper adjustment of the radiographic equipment to accommodate obese or thin patients, which can cause overexposure or underexposure and a poor-quality study

• Patients who are very obese, who may exceed the weight limit for the equipment

• Patients with extreme claustrophobia unless sedation is given before the study

• Incorrect positioning of the patient, which may produce poor visualization of the area to be examined

- Inability of the patient to cooperate or remain still during the procedure because of age, significant pain, or mental status

Other considerations:

- Complications of the procedure include hemorrhage, infection at the IV needle insertion site, and cardiac arrhythmias.

- The procedure may be terminated if chest pain or severe cardiac arrhythmias occur.

- Failure to follow dietary restrictions and other pretesting preparations may cause the procedure to be canceled or repeated.

- Consultation with a health care provider should occur before the procedure for radiation safety concerns regarding younger patients or patients who are lactating.

- Risks associated with radiographic overexposure can result from frequent x-ray procedures. Personnel in the room with the patient should wear a protective lead apron, stand behind a shield, or leave the area while the examination is being done. Personnel working in the area where the examination is being done should wear badges that reveal their level of exposure to radiation.

Nursing Implications and Procedure ....

Pretest:

➤ Inform the patient that the procedure assesses the abdomen and pancreatic area.

➤ Obtain a history of the patient's complaints or clinical symptoms, including a list of known allergens, especially allergies or sensitivities to iodine, seafood, or other contrast mediums.

➤ Obtain a history of results of previously performed diagnostic procedures, surgical procedures, and laboratory tests. Include specific tests as they apply (e.g., blood urea nitrogen [BUN], creatinine, coagulation tests, bleeding time). Ensure that the results of blood tests are obtained and recorded before the procedure, especially BUN and creatinine, if contrast medium is to be used. For related diagnostic tests, refer to the Gastrointestinal, Hepatobiliary, and Genitourinary Systems tables.

➤ Note any recent barium or other radiologic contrast procedures. Ensure that barium studies were performed more than 2 days before the CT scan.

➤ Record the date of the last menstrual period and determine the possibility of pregnancy in perimenopausal women.

➤ Obtain a list of the medications the patient is taking.

➤ In case contrast is used, patients receiving metformin (glucophage) for non–insulin-dependent (type 2) diabetes should discontinue the drug on the day of the test and continue to withhold it for 48 hours after the test. Failure to do so may result in lactic acidosis.

➤ Review the procedure with the patient. Explain to the patient that some pain may be experienced during the test, and there may be moments of discomfort. Explain the purpose of the test and how the procedure is performed. Inform the patient that the procedure is performed in a radiology department, usually by a health care practitioner and support staff, and takes approximately 30 to 60 minutes.

➤ *Sensitivity to cultural and social issues,* as well as concern for modesty, is important in providing psychological support before, during, and after the procedure.

➤ Explain that an IV line may be inserted to allow infusion of IV fluids, contrast medium, dye, or sedatives. Usually contrast medium and normal saline are infused.

➤ Inform the patient that he or she may experience nausea, a feeling of warmth, a salty or metallic taste, or a transient headache after injection of contrast medium, if given.

➤ The patient may be requested to drink approximately 450 mL of a dilute barium solution (approximately 1% barium) beginning 1 hour before the examination. This is administered to distinguish GI organs from the other abdominal organs.

➤ The patient should fast and restrict fluids for 8 hours prior to the procedure. Instruct the patient to avoid taking anticoagulant medication or to reduce dosage as ordered prior to the procedure.

➤ Instruct the patient to remove jewelry (including watches), credit cards, keys, coins, cell phones, pagers, and other metallic objects.

➤ *Make sure a written and informed consent has been signed prior to the procedure and before administering any medications.*

Intratest:

➤ Ensure that the patient has complied with dietary, fluids, and medication restrictions and pretesting preparations; assure that food has been restricted for at least 8 hours prior to the procedure. Ensure that the patient has removed all external metallic objects (jewelry, dentures, etc.) prior to the procedure.

➤ Have emergency equipment readily available.

➤ If the patient has a history of severe allergic reactions to any substance or drug, administer ordered prophylactic steroids or antihistamines before the procedure. Use nonionic contrast medium for the procedure.

➤ Patients are given a gown, robe, and foot coverings to wear and instructed to void prior to the procedure.

➤ Observe standard precautions, and follow the general guidelines in Appendix A.

➤ Instruct the patient to cooperate fully and to follow directions. Instruct the patient to remain still throughout the procedure because movement produces unreliable results.

➤ Establish intravenous fluid line for the injection of contrast, emergency drugs, and sedatives.

➤ Administer an antianxiety agent, as ordered, if the patient has claustrophobia. Administer a sedative to a child or to an uncooperative adult, as ordered.

➤ Place the patient in the supine position on an exam table.

➤ If contrast is used, the contrast medium is injected, and a rapid series of images is taken during and after the filling of the vessels to be examined. Delayed images may be taken to examine the vessels after a time and to monitor the venous phase of the procedure.

➤ Ask the patient to inhale deeply and hold his or her breath while the x-ray images are taken, and then to exhale after the images are taken.

➤ Instruct the patient to take slow, deep breaths if nausea occurs during the procedure. Monitor and administer an antiemetic agent if ordered. Ready an emesis basin for use.

➤ Monitor the patient for complications related to the procedure (e.g., allergic reaction, anaphylaxis, bronchospasm) if contrast is used.

➤ The needle or vascular catheter is removed, and a pressure dressing is applied over the puncture site.

➤ The results are recorded on film or by automated equipment in a computerized system for recall and postprocedure interpretation by the appropriate health care practitioner.

Post-test:

➤ Instruct the patient to resume usual diet, fluids, medications or activity, as directed by the health care practitioner. Renal function should be assessed before metformin is resumed, if contrast was used.

➤ Monitor vital signs and neurologic status every 15 minutes for 30 minutes. Compare with baseline values.

Protocols may vary from facility to facility.

➤ If contrast was used, observe for delayed allergic reactions, such as rash, urticaria, tachycardia, hyperpnea, hypertension, palpitations, nausea, or vomiting.

➤ If contrast was used, advise the patient to immediately report symptoms such as fast heart rate, difficulty breathing, skin rash, itching or decreased urinary output.

➤ Observe the needle/catheter insertion site for bleeding, inflammation, or hematoma formation.

➤ Instruct the patient to apply cold compresses to the puncture site, as needed, to reduce discomfort or edema.

➤ Instruct the patient to increase fluid intake to help eliminate the contrast medium, if used.

➤ Inform the patient that diarrhea may occur after ingestion of oral contrast medium.

➤ A written report of the examination will be completed by a health care practitioner specializing in this branch of medicine. The report will be sent to the requesting health care practitioner, who will discuss the results with the patient.

➤ Depending on the results of this procedure, additional testing may be needed to evaluate or monitor progression of the disease process and determine the need for a change in therapy. Evaluate test results in relation to the patient's symptoms and other tests performed.

Related diagnostic tests:

➤ Related diagnostic tests include angiography of the abdomen, magnetic resonance imaging of the abdomen, and ultrasound of the pancreas.

COMPUTED TOMOGRAPHY, PELVIS

· ·

SYNONYMS/ACRONYMS: Computed axial tomography (CAT), computed transaxial tomography (CTT), pelvic CT.

AREA OF APPLICATION: Pelvis.

CONTRAST: Can be done with or without oral or intravenous (IV) iodinated contrast medium.

DESCRIPTION & RATIONALE: Computed tomography (CT) of the pelvis is a noninvasive procedure used to enhance certain anatomic views of the pelvic structures, but it becomes an invasive procedure when intravenous contrast medium is used. The patient lies on a table and moves in and out of a doughnut-like device called a *gantry*, which houses the x-ray tube and associated electronics. The scanner uses multiple x-ray beams and a series of detectors that rotate around the patient to produce cross-sectional views in a three-dimensional fashion by detecting and recording differences in tissue density after having an x-ray beam pass through them. These density measurements are sent to a computer that produces a digital image of the anatomy, enabling a physician to look at slices or thin sections of certain anatomic views, as appropriate depending on gender, of the ovaries, uterus, fallopian tubes, bladder, rectum, sigmoid colon, prostate, seminal vesicles, cervix, and associated vascular system and to determine the presence and extent of malignancy. Differentiations can be made among solid, cystic, inflammatory, or vascular lesions, and suspected hematomas or aneurysms can be identified. Iodinated contrast medium is given intravenously for blood vessel and vascular evaluation or orally for bowel and adjacent structure evaluation. Images can be recorded on photographic or x-ray film or stored in digital format as digitized computer data. Cine scanning produces a series of moving images of the scanned area. The CT scan can be used to guide biopsy needles into areas of suspected tumor to obtain tissue for laboratory analysis and to place catheters for drainage of abscesses. Tumor size, progression, and changes before and after therapy may be monitored with CT scanning. In rare cases, CT pelvimetry may be performed on a pregnant woman whose fetus is in a breech position. CT pelvimetry measurements are accurate, and less radiation exposure occurs to the mother and the fetus than with radiographic pelvimetry. ∎

INDICATIONS:
• Assist in differentiating between benign and malignant tumors

• Detect tumor extension of masses and metastasis into the pelvic area

• Differentiate infectious from inflammatory processes

• Evaluate pelvic lymph nodes

• Evaluate cysts, masses, abscesses, ureteral and bladder calculi, gastrointestinal bleeding and obstruction, and trauma

• Monitor and evaluate effectiveness of medical, radiation, or surgical therapies

RESULT

Normal Findings:
• Normal size, position, and shape of pelvic organs and vascular system

Abnormal Findings:
• Bladder calculi

• Ectopic pregnancy

• Fibroid tumors

• Hydrosalpinx

• Ovarian cyst or abscess

• Primary and metastatic neoplasms

CRITICAL VALUES: N/A

INTERFERING FACTORS:

This procedure is contraindicated for:
• ⚠ Patients with allergies to shellfish or iodinated dye. The contrast medium used may cause a life-threatening allergic reaction. Patients with a known hypersensitivity to the medium may benefit from premedication with corticosteroids or the use of nonionic contrast medium.

• Patients who are claustrophobic.

• Patients who are pregnant or suspected of being pregnant, unless the potential benefits of the procedure far outweigh the risks to the fetus and mother.

- ⚠ Elderly and other patients who are chronically dehydrated before the test, because of their risk of contrast-induced renal failure.

- ⚠ Patients who are in renal failure.

- Young patients (17 years old and younger), unless the benefits of the x-ray diagnosis outweigh the risks of exposure to high levels of radiation.

Factors that may impair clear imaging:

- Gas or feces in the gastrointestinal tract resulting from inadequate cleansing or failure to restrict food intake before the study

- Retained barium from a previous radiologic procedure

- Metallic objects within the examination field (e.g., jewelry, body rings), which may inhibit organ visualization and can produce unclear images

- Improper adjustment of the radiographic equipment to accommodate obese or thin patients, which can cause overexposure or underexposure and a poor-quality study

- Patients who are very obese, who may exceed the weight limit for the equipment

- Patients with extreme claustrophobia unless sedation is given before the study

- Incorrect positioning of the patient, which may produce poor visualization of the area to be examined

- Inability of the patient to cooperate or remain still during the procedure because of age, significant pain, or mental status

Other considerations:

- Complications of the procedure include hemorrhage, infection at the IV needle insertion site, and cardiac arrhythmias.

- The procedure may be terminated if chest pain or severe cardiac arrhythmias occur.

- Failure to follow dietary restrictions and other pretesting preparations may cause the procedure to be canceled or repeated.

- Consultation with a health care provider should occur before the procedure for radiation safety concerns regarding younger patients or patients who are lactating.

- Risks associated with radiographic overexposure can result from frequent x-ray procedures. Personnel in the room with the patient should wear a protective lead apron, stand behind a shield, or leave the area while the examination is being done. Personnel working in the area where the examination is being done should wear badges that reveal their level of exposure to radiation.

Nursing Implications and Procedure • • • • • • • • • • •

Pretest:

▶ Inform the patient that the procedure assesses the pelvis.

▶ Obtain a history of the patient's complaints or clinical symptoms, including a list of known allergens, especially allergies or sensitivities to iodine, seafood, or other contrast mediums.

▶ Obtain a history of results of previously performed diagnostic procedures, surgical procedures, and laboratory tests. Include specific tests as they apply (e.g., blood urea nitrogen [BUN], creatinine, coagulation tests, bleeding time). Ensure that the results of blood tests are obtained and recorded before the procedure, especially BUN and creatinine, if contrast medium is to be used. For related diagnostic tests, refer to the Gastrointestinal, Reproductive, and Genitourinary System tables.

➤ Note any recent barium or other radiologic contrast procedures. Ensure that barium studies were performed more than 4 days before the CT scan.

➤ Record the date of the last menstrual period and determine the possibility of pregnancy in perimenopausal women.

➤ Obtain a list of the medications the patient is taking.

➤ In case contrast is used, patients receiving metformin (glucophage) for non–insulin-dependent (type 2) diabetes should discontinue the drug on the day of the test and continue to withhold it for 48 hours after the test. Failure to do so may result in lactic acidosis.

➤ Review the procedure with the patient. Explain to the patient that some pain may be experienced during the test, and there may be moments of discomfort. Explain the purpose of the test and how the procedure is performed. Inform the patient that the procedure is performed in a radiology department, usually by a health care practitioner and support staff, and takes approximately 30 to 60 minutes.

➤ *Sensitivity to cultural and social issues,* as well as concern for modesty, is important in providing psychological support before, during, and after the procedure.

➤ Explain that an IV line may be inserted to allow infusion of IV fluids, contrast medium, dye, or sedatives. Usually contrast medium and normal saline are infused.

➤ Inform the patient that he or she may experience nausea, a feeling of warmth, a salty or metallic taste, or a transient headache after injection of contrast medium, if given.

➤ The patient may be requested to drink approximately 450 mL of a dilute barium solution (approximately 1% barium) beginning 1 hour before the examination. This is administered to distinguish gastrointestinal organs from the other abdominal organs.

➤ The patient should fast and restrict fluids for 6 to 8 hours prior to the procedure. Instruct the patient to avoid taking anticoagulant medication or to reduce dosage as ordered prior to the procedure.

➤ Instruct the patient to remove jewelry (including watches), credit cards, keys, coins, cell phones, pagers, and other metallic objects.

➤ *Make sure a written and informed consent has been signed prior to the procedure and before administering any medications.*

Intratest:

➤ Ensure that the patient has complied with dietary, fluids, and medication restrictions and pretesting preparations; assure that food has been restricted for at least 6 hours prior to the procedure. Ensure that the patient has removed all external metallic objects (jewelry, dentures, etc.) prior to the procedure.

➤ Have emergency equipment readily available.

➤ If the patient has a history of severe allergic reactions to any substance or drug, administer ordered prophylactic steroids or antihistamines before the procedure. Use nonionic contrast medium for the procedure.

➤ Patients are given a gown, robe, and foot coverings to wear and instructed to void prior to the procedure.

➤ Observe standard precautions, and follow the general guidelines in Appendix A.

➤ Instruct the patient to cooperate fully and to follow directions. Instruct the patient to remain still throughout the procedure because movement produces unreliable results.

➤ Establish an IV fluid line for the injection of contrast, emergency drugs, and sedatives.

➤ Administer an antianxiety agent, as ordered, if the patient has claustrophobia. Administer a sedative to a child or to an uncooperative adult, as ordered.

➤ Place the patient in the supine position on an exam table.

➤ If contrast is used, the contrast medium is injected, and a rapid series of images is taken during and after the filling of the vessels to be examined. Delayed images may be taken to examine the vessels after a time and to monitor the venous phase of the procedure.

➤ Ask the patient to inhale deeply and hold his or her breath while the x-ray images are taken, and then to exhale after the images are taken.

➤ Instruct the patient to take slow, deep breaths if nausea occurs during the procedure. Monitor and administer an antiemetic agent if ordered. Ready an emesis basin for use.

➤ Monitor the patient for complications related to the procedure (e.g., allergic reaction, anaphylaxis, bronchospasm) if contrast is used.

➤ The needle or vascular catheter is removed, and a pressure dressing is applied over the puncture site.

➤ The results are recorded on film or by automated equipment in a computerized system for recall and postprocedure interpretation by the appropriate healthcare practitioner.

Post-test:

➤ Instruct the patient to resume usual diet, fluids, medications, or activity, as directed by the health care practitioner. Renal function should be assessed before metformin is resumed, if contrast was used.

➤ Monitor vital signs and neurologic status every 15 minutes for 30 minutes. Compare with baseline values. Protocols may vary from facility to facility.

➤ If contrast was used, observe for delayed allergic reactions, such as rash, urticaria, tachycardia, hyperpnea, hypertension, palpitations, nausea, or vomiting.

➤ If contrast was used, advise the patient to immediately report symptoms such as fast heart rate, difficulty breathing, skin rash, itching or decreased urinary output.

➤ Observe the needle/catheter insertion site for bleeding, inflammation, or hematoma formation.

➤ Instruct the patient to apply cold compresses to the puncture site, as needed, to reduce discomfort or edema.

➤ Instruct the patient to increase fluid intake to help eliminate the contrast medium, if used.

➤ Inform the patient that diarrhea may occur after ingestion of oral contrast medium.

➤ A written report of the examination will be completed by a health care practitioner specializing in this branch of medicine. The report will be sent to the requesting health care practitioner, who will discuss the results with the patient.

➤ Depending on the results of this procedure, additional testing may be needed to evaluate or monitor progression of the disease process and determine the need for a change in therapy. Evaluate test results in relation to the patient's symptoms and other tests performed.

Related diagnostic tests:

➤ Related diagnostic tests include angiogram of the pelvis; kidney, ureter, and bladder film; magnetic resonance imaging of the abdomen, and ultrasound of the pelvis.

COMPUTED TOMOGRAPHY, PITUITARY

SYNONYMS/ACRONYMS: Computed axial tomography (CAT), computed transaxial tomography (CTT), pituitary CT.

AREA OF APPLICATION: Pituitary/brain.

CONTRAST: Can be done with or without intravenous (IV) iodinated contrast medium.

DESCRIPTION & RATIONALE: Computed tomography (CT) of the pituitary is a noninvasive procedure that enhances certain anatomic views of the pituitary gland and perisellar region, but it becomes an invasive procedure when a contrast medium is used. CT scanning is a safe and rapid method for pituitary gland evaluation. This procedure aids in the evaluation of pituitary adenoma, craniopharyngioma, meningioma, aneurysm, metastatic disease, exophthalmos, and cysts. It provides unique cross-sectional anatomic information; it is also unsurpassed in evaluating lesions containing calcium. Visualization of bony septa in the sphenoid sinus and evaluation for nonpneumatization of the sphenoid sinus are best performed with this procedure. The patient lies on a table and moves in and out of a doughnut-like device called a *gantry*, which houses the x-ray tube and associated electronics. The scanner uses multiple x-ray beams and a series of detectors that rotate around the patient to produce cross-sectional views in a three-dimensional fashion by detecting and recording differences in tissue density after having an x-ray beam passed through the tissues. These density measurements are sent to a computer that produces a digital image of the anatomy, enabling a physician to look at slices or thin sections of certain anatomic views of the pituitary and associated vascular system. Differentiations can be made among solid, cystic, inflammatory, or vascular lesions, and suspected hematomas and aneurysms can be identified. The procedure may be repeated after iodinated contrast medium is given intravenously for blood vessel and vascular evaluation. Images can be recorded on photographic or x-ray film or stored in digital format as digitized computer data. Cine scanning produces a series of moving images of the scanned area. Tumors, before and after therapy, may be monitored by CT scanning. ■

INDICATIONS:
- Assist in differentiating between benign and malignant tumors
- Detect aneurysms and vascular abnormalities

- Detect congenital anomalies, such as partially empty sella

- Detect tumor extension of masses and metastasis

- Determine pituitary size and location in relation to surrounding structures

- Evaluate cysts, masses, abscesses, and trauma

- Monitor and evaluate effectiveness of medical, radiation, or surgical therapies

RESULT

Normal Findings:
- Normal size, position, and shape of the pituitary fossa, cavernous sinuses, and vascular system

Abnormal Findings:
- Abscess
- Adenoma
- Aneurysm
- Chordoma
- Craniopharyngioma
- Cyst
- Meningioma
- Metastasis
- Pituitary hemorrhage

CRITICAL VALUES: N/A

INTERFERING FACTORS:

This procedure is contraindicated for:
- ⚠ Patients with allergies to shellfish or iodinated dye. The contrast medium used may cause a life-threatening allergic reaction. Patients with a known hypersensitivity to the medium may benefit from premedication with corticosteroids or the use of nonionic contrast medium.

- Patients who are claustrophobic.

- Patients who are pregnant or suspected of being pregnant, unless the potential benefits of the procedure far outweigh the risks to the fetus and mother.

- ⚠ Elderly and other patients who are chronically dehydrated before the test, because of their risk of contrast-induced renal failure.

- ⚠ Patients who are in renal failure.

- Young patients (17 years old and younger), unless the benefits of the x-ray diagnosis outweigh the risks of exposure to high levels of radiation.

Factors that may impair clear imaging:
- Retained contrast from a previous radiologic procedure

- Metallic objects within the examination field (e.g., jewelry, dentures, body rings), which may inhibit organ visualization and can produce unclear images

- Improper adjustment of the radiographic equipment to accommodate obese or thin patients, which can cause overexposure or underexposure and a poor-quality study

- Patients who are very obese, who may exceed the weight limit for the equipment

- Patients with extreme claustrophobia unless sedation is given before the study

- Incorrect positioning of the patient, which may produce poor visualization of the area to be examined

- Inability of the patient to cooperate or remain still during the procedure because of age, significant pain, or mental status

Other considerations:
- Complications of the procedure include hemorrhage, infection at the IV needle insertion site, and cardiac arrhythmias.

- The procedure may be terminated if chest pain or severe cardiac arrhythmias occur.

- Failure to follow dietary restrictions and other pretesting preparations may cause the procedure to be canceled or repeated.

- Consultation with a health care provider should occur before the procedure for radiation safety concerns regarding younger patients or patients who are lactating.

- Risks associated with radiographic overexposure can result from frequent x-ray procedures. Personnel in the room with the patient should wear a protective lead apron, stand behind a shield, or leave the area while the examination is being done. Personnel working in the area where the examination is being done should wear badges that reveal their level of exposure to radiation.

Nursing Implications and Procedure • • • • • • • • • •

Pretest:

➤ Inform the patient that the procedure assesses the brain and pituitary.

➤ Obtain a history of the patient's complaints or clinical symptoms, including a list of known allergens, especially allergies or sensitivities to iodine, seafood, or other contrast mediums.

➤ Obtain a history of results of previously performed diagnostic procedures, surgical procedures, and laboratory tests. Include specific tests as they apply (e.g., blood urea nitrogen [BUN], creatinine, coagulation tests, bleeding time). Ensure that the results of blood tests are obtained and recorded before the procedure, especially BUN and creatinine, if contrast medium is to be used. For related diagnostic tests, refer to the Endocrine System table.

➤ Record the date of the last menstrual period and determine the possibility of pregnancy in perimenopausal women.

➤ Obtain a list of the medications the patient is taking.

➤ In case contrast is used, patients receiving metformin (glucophage) for non–insulin-dependent (type 2) diabetes should discontinue the drug on the day of the test and continue to withhold it for 48 hours after the test. Failure to do so may result in lactic acidosis.

➤ Review the procedure with the patient. Explain to the patient that some pain may be experienced during the test, and there may be moments of discomfort. Explain the purpose of the test and how the procedure is performed. Inform the patient that the procedure is performed in a radiology department, usually by a health care practitioner and support staff, and takes approximately 30 to 60 minutes.

➤ *Sensitivity to cultural and social issues,* as well as concern for modesty, is important in providing psychological support before, during and after the procedure.

➤ Explain that an IV line may be inserted to allow infusion of IV fluids, contrast medium, dye, or sedatives. Usually contrast medium and normal saline are infused.

➤ Inform the patient that he or she may experience nausea, a feeling of warmth, a salty or metallic taste, or a transient headache after injection of contrast medium, if given.

➤ The patient should not fast or restrict fluids prior to the procedure. Instruct the patient to avoid taking anticoagulant medication or to reduce dosage as ordered prior to the procedure.

➤ Instruct the patient to remove jewelry (including watches), credit cards, keys, coins, cell phones, pagers, and other metallic objects.

➤ *Make sure a written and informed consent has been signed prior to the procedure and before administering any medications.*

Intratest:

➤ Ensure that the patient has complied with medication restrictions and pretesting preparations. Ensure that the patient has removed all external metallic objects (jewelry, dentures, etc.) prior to the procedure.

▶ Have emergency equipment readily available.

▶ If the patient has a history of severe allergic reactions to any substance or drug, administer ordered prophylactic steroids or antihistamines before the procedure. Use nonionic contrast medium for the procedure.

▶ Patients are given a gown, robe, and foot coverings to wear and instructed to void prior to the procedure.

▶ Observe standard precautions, and follow the general guidelines in Appendix A.

▶ Instruct the patient to cooperate fully and to follow directions. Instruct the patient to remain still throughout the procedure because movement produces unreliable results.

▶ Establish an IV fluid line for the injection of contrast, emergency drugs, and sedatives.

▶ Administer an antianxiety agent, as ordered, if the patient has claustrophobia. Administer a sedative to a child or to an uncooperative adult, as ordered.

▶ Place the patient in the supine position on an exam table.

▶ If contrast is used, the contrast medium is injected, and a rapid series of images is taken during and after the filling of the vessels to be examined. Delayed images may be taken to examine the vessels after a time and to monitor the venous phase of the procedure.

▶ Ask the patient to inhale deeply and hold his or her breath while the x-ray images are taken, and then to exhale after the images are taken.

▶ Instruct the patient to take slow, deep breaths if nausea occurs during the procedure. Monitor and administer an antiemetic agent if ordered. Ready an emesis basin for use.

▶ Monitor the patient for complica-

tions related to the procedure (e.g., allergic reaction, anaphylaxis, bronchospasm) if contrast is used.

▶ The needle or vascular catheter is removed, and a pressure dressing is applied over the puncture site.

▶ The results are recorded on film or by automated equipment in a computerized system for recall and postprocedure interpretation by the appropriate health care practitioner.

Post-test:

▶ Instruct the patient to resume usual medications and activity, as directed by the health care practitioner. Renal function should be assessed before metformin is resumed, if contrast was used.

▶ Monitor vital signs and neurologic status every 15 minutes for 30 minutes. Compare with baseline values. Protocols may vary from facility to facility.

▶ If contrast was used, observe for delayed allergic reactions, such as rash, urticaria, tachycardia, hyperpnea, hypertension, palpitations, nausea, or vomiting.

▶ If contrast was used, advise the patient to immediately report symptoms such as fast heart rate, difficulty breathing, skin rash, itching or decreased urinary output.

▶ Observe the needle/catheter insertion site for bleeding, inflammation, or hematoma formation.

▶ Instruct the patient to apply cold compresses to the puncture site, as needed, to reduce discomfort or edema.

▶ Instruct the patient to increase fluid intake to help eliminate the contrast medium, if used.

▶ A written report of the examination will be completed by a health care practitioner specializing in this branch of medicine. The report will be sent to the requesting health care practitioner, who will discuss the results with the patient.

➤ Depending on the results of this procedure, additional testing may be needed to evaluate or monitor progression of the disease process and determine the need for a change in therapy. Evaluate test results in relation to the patient's symptoms and other tests performed.

Related diagnostic tests:

➤ Related diagnostic tests include CT angiography, CT of the brain, positron emission tomography of the brain, magnetic resonance angiography, and magnetic resonance imaging of the brain.

COMPUTED TOMOGRAPHY, RENAL

SYNONYMS/ACRONYM: Computed axial tomography (CAT), computed transaxial tomography (CTT), kidney CT.

AREA OF APPLICATION: Kidney.

CONTRAST: Can be done with or without oral or intravenous (IV) iodinated contrast medium.

DESCRIPTION & RATIONALE: Renal computed tomography (CT) is a non-invasive procedure used to enhance certain anatomic views of the renal structures, but it becomes an invasive procedure when a contrast medium is used. CT scanning is a safe and rapid method for renal evaluation that is independent of renal function. It provides unique cross-sectional anatomic information and is unsurpassed in evaluating lesions containing fat or calcium. The patient lies on a table and is moved in and out of a doughnut-like device called a *gantry*, which houses the x-ray tube and associated electronics. The scanner uses multiple x-ray beams and a series of detectors that rotate around the patient to produce cross-sectional views in a three-dimensional fashion by detecting and recording differences in tissue density after having an x-ray beam passed through the tissues. These density measurements are sent to a computer that produces a digital image of the anatomy, enabling a physician to look at slices or thin sections of certain anatomic views of the kidneys and associated vascular system. Differentiations can be made among solid, cystic, inflammatory, or vascular lesions, and suspected hematomas and aneurysms can be identified. The procedure is repeated after iodinated contrast medium is given intravenously for blood vessel and vascular evaluation or orally for bowel and adjacent structure evaluation. Images can be recorded on photographic or x-ray film or stored in digital format as digitized computer data. Cine scanning produces a series of moving images of the area scanned. The CT scan can be used to guide biopsy needles into areas of suspected tumors to obtain tissue for laboratory analysis and to guide placement of catheters for drainage of renal abscesses. Tumors, before and after therapy, may be monitored with CT scanning. ■

INDICATIONS:

- Aid in the diagnosis of congenital anomalies, such as polycystic kidney disease, horseshoe kidney, absence of one kidney, or kidney displacement

- Aid in the diagnosis of perirenal hematomas and abscesses and assist in localizing for drainage

- Assist in differentiating between benign and malignant tumors

- Assist in differentiating between an infectious and an inflammatory process

- Detect aneurysms and vascular abnormalities

- Detect bleeding or hyperplasia of the adrenal glands

- Detect tumor extension of masses and metastasis into the renal area

- Determine kidney size and location in relation to the bladder in post-transplant patients

- Determine presence and type of adrenal tumor, such as benign adenoma, cancer, or pheochromocytoma

- Evaluate abnormal fluid accumulation around the kidney

- Evaluate cysts, masses, abscesses, renal calculi, obstruction, and trauma

- Evaluate spread of a tumor or invasion of nearby retroperitoneal organs

- Monitor and evaluate effectiveness of medical, radiation, or surgical therapies

RESULT

Normal Findings:

- Normal size, position, and shape of kidneys and vascular system

Abnormal Findings:

- Adrenal tumor or hyperplasia

- Congenital anomalies, such as polycystic kidney disease, horseshoe kidney, absence of one kidney, or kidney displacement

- Dilation of the common hepatic duct, common bile duct, or gallbladder

- Renal artery aneurysm

- Renal calculi and ureteral obstruction

- Renal cell carcinoma

- Renal cysts or abscesses

- Renal laceration, fracture, tumor, and trauma

- Perirenal abscesses and hematomas

- Primary and metastatic neoplasms

CRITICAL VALUES: N/A

INTERFERING FACTORS:

This procedure is contraindicated for:

- ⚠ Patients with allergies to shellfish or iodinated dye. The contrast medium used may cause a life-threatening allergic reaction. Patients with a known hypersensitivity to the medium may benefit from premedication with corticosteroids or the use of nonionic contrast medium.

- Patients who are claustrophobic.

- Patients who are pregnant or suspected of being pregnant, unless the potential benefits of the procedure far outweigh the risks to the fetus and mother.

- ⚠ Elderly and other patients who are chronically dehydrated before the test, because of their risk of contrast-induced renal failure.

- ⚠️ Patients who are in renal failure.

- Young patients (17 years old and younger), unless the benefits of the x-ray diagnosis outweigh the risks of exposure to high levels of radiation.

Factors that may impair clear imaging:

- Gas or feces in the gastrointestinal tract resulting from inadequate cleansing or failure to restrict food intake before the study

- Retained barium from a previous radiologic procedure

- Metallic objects within the examination field (e.g., jewelry, body rings), which may inhibit organ visualization and can produce unclear images

- Improper adjustment of the radiographic equipment to accommodate obese or thin patients, which can cause overexposure or underexposure and a poor-quality study

- Patients who are very obese, who may exceed the weight limit for the equipment

- Patients with extreme claustrophobia unless sedation is given before the study

- Incorrect positioning of the patient, which may produce poor visualization of the area to be examined

- Inability of the patient to cooperate or remain still during the procedure because of age, significant pain, or mental status

Other considerations:

- Complications of the procedure include hemorrhage, infection at the IV needle insertion site, and cardiac arrhythmias.

- The procedure may be terminated if chest pain or severe cardiac arrhythmias occur.

- Failure to follow dietary restrictions and other pretesting preparations may cause the procedure to be canceled or repeated.

- Consultation with a health care provider should occur before the procedure for radiation safety concerns regarding younger patients or patients who are lactating.

- Risks associated with radiographic overexposure can result from frequent x-ray procedures. Personnel in the room with the patient should wear a protective lead apron, stand behind a shield, or leave the area while the examination is being done. Personnel working in the area where the examination is being done should wear badges that reveal their level of exposure to radiation.

Nursing Implications and Procedure

Pretest:

➤ Inform the patient that the procedure assesses the kidney.

➤ Obtain a history of the patient's complaints or clinical symptoms, including a list of known allergens, especially allergies or sensitivities to iodine, seafood, or other contrast mediums.

➤ Obtain a history of results of previously performed diagnostic procedures, surgical procedures, and laboratory tests. Include specific tests as they apply (e.g., blood urea nitrogen [BUN], creatinine, coagulation tests, bleeding time). Ensure that the results of blood tests are obtained and recorded before the procedure, especially BUN and creatinine, if contrast medium is to be used. For related diagnostic tests, refer to the Gastrointestinal and Genitourinary System tables.

➤ Note any recent barium or other radiologic contrast procedures. Ensure that barium studies were performed more than 4 days before the CT scan.

- Record the date of the last menstrual period and determine the possibility of pregnancy in perimenopausal women.

- Obtain a list of the medications the patient is taking.

- In case contrast is used, patients receiving metformin (glucophage) for non–insulin-dependent (type 2) diabetes should discontinue the drug on the day of the test and continue to withhold it for 48 hours after the test. Failure to do so may result in lactic acidosis.

- Review the procedure with the patient. Explain to the patient that some pain may be experienced during the test, and there may be moments of discomfort. Explain the purpose of the test and how the procedure is performed. Inform the patient that the procedure is performed in a radiology department, usually by a health care practitioner and support staff, and takes approximately 30 to 60 minutes.

- *Sensitivity to cultural and social issues,* as well as concern for modesty, is important in providing psychological support before, during, and after the procedure.

- Explain that an IV line may be inserted to allow infusion of IV fluids, contrast medium, dye, or sedatives. Usually contrast medium and normal saline are infused.

- Inform the patient that he or she may experience nausea, a feeling of warmth, a salty or metallic taste, or a transient headache after injection of contrast medium, if given.

- The patient may be requested to drink approximately 450 mL of a dilute barium solution (approximately 1% barium) beginning 1 hour before the examination. This is administered to distinguish gastrointestinal organs from the other abdominal organs.

- The patient should fast and restrict fluids for 6 to 8 hours prior to the procedure. Instruct the patient to avoid taking anticoagulant medication or to reduce dosage as ordered prior to the procedure.

- Instruct the patient to remove jewelry (including watches), credit cards, keys, coins, cell phones, pagers, and other metallic objects.

- *Make sure a written and informed consent has been signed prior to the procedure and before administering any medications.*

Intratest:

- Ensure that the patient has complied with dietary, fluids, and medication restrictions and pretesting preparations; assure that food has been restricted for at least 6 hours prior to the procedure. Ensure that the patient has removed all external metallic objects (jewelry, dentures, etc.) prior to the procedure.

- Have emergency equipment readily available.

- If the patient has a history of severe allergic reactions to any substance or drug, administer ordered prophylactic steroids or antihistamines before the procedure. Use nonionic contrast medium for the procedure.

- Patients are given a gown, robe, and foot coverings to wear and instructed to void prior to the procedure.

- Observe standard precautions, and follow the general guidelines in Appendix A.

- Instruct the patient to cooperate fully and to follow directions. Instruct the patient to remain still throughout the procedure because movement produces unreliable results.

- Establish an IV fluid line for the injection of contrast, emergency drugs, and sedatives.

- Administer an antianxiety agent, as ordered, if the patient has claustrophobia. Administer a sedative to a child or to an uncooperative adult, as ordered.

- Place the patient in the supine position on an exam table.

- If contrast is used, the contrast medium is injected and a rapid series of images is taken during and after the filling of the vessels to be examined. Delayed images may be taken to examine the vessels after a time and to monitor the venous phase of the procedure.

➤ Ask the patient to inhale deeply and hold his or her breath while the x-ray images are taken, and then to exhale after the images are taken.

➤ Instruct the patient to take slow, deep breaths if nausea occurs during the procedure. Monitor and administer an antiemetic agent if ordered. Ready an emesis basin for use.

➤ Monitor the patient for complications related to the procedure (e.g., allergic reaction, anaphylaxis, bronchospasm) if contrast is used.

➤ The needle or vascular catheter is removed, and a pressure dressing is applied over the puncture site.

➤ The results are recorded on film or by automated equipment in a computerized system for recall and postprocedure interpretation by the appropriate health care practitioner.

Post-test:

➤ Instruct the patient to resume usual diet, fluids, medications, or activity, as directed by the health care practitioner. Renal function should be assessed before metformin is resumed, if contrast was used.

➤ Monitor vital signs and neurologic status every 15 minutes for 30 minutes. Compare with baseline values. Protocols may vary from facility to facility.

➤ If contrast was used, observe for delayed allergic reactions, such as rash, urticaria, tachycardia, hyperpnea, hypertension, palpitations, nausea, or vomiting.

➤ If contrast was used, advise the patient to immediately report symptoms such as fast heart rate, difficulty breathing, skin rash, itching or decreased urinary output.

➤ Observe the needle/catheter insertion site for bleeding, inflammation, or hematoma formation.

➤ Instruct the patient to apply cold compresses to the puncture site, as needed, to reduce discomfort or edema.

➤ Instruct the patient to increase fluid intake to help eliminate the contrast medium, if used.

➤ Inform the patient that diarrhea may occur after ingestion of oral contrast medium.

➤ A written report of the examination will be completed by a health care practitioner specializing in this branch of medicine. The report will be sent to the requesting health care practitioner, who will discuss the results with the patient.

➤ Depending on the results of this procedure, additional testing may be needed to evaluate or monitor progression of the disease process and determine the need for a change in therapy. Evaluate test results in relation to the patient's symptoms and other tests performed.

Related diagnostic tests:

➤ Related diagnostic tests include CT of the abdomen; intravenous pyelography; kidney, ureter, and bladder film; magnetic resonance imaging of the pelvis; and ultrasound of the kidney.

COMPUTED TOMOGRAPHY, SPINE

SYNONYMS/ACRONYMS: Computed axial tomography (CAT), computed transaxial tomography (CTT), spine CT, CT myelogram.

AREA OF APPLICATION: Spine.

CONTRAST: Can be done with or without oral or intravenous (IV) iodinated contrast medium.

DESCRIPTION & RATIONALE: Computed tomography (CT) of the spine is a noninvasive procedure that enhances certain anatomic views of the spinal structures, but it becomes an invasive procedure when intravenous contrast medium is used. CT scanning is more versatile than conventional radiography and can easily detect and identify tumors and their types. The patient lies on a table and is moved in and out of a doughnut-like device called a *gantry,* which houses the x-ray tube and associated electronics. The scanner uses multiple x-ray beams and a series of detectors that rotate around the patient to produce cross-sectional views in a three-dimensional fashion by detecting and recording differences in tissue density after having an x-ray beam passed through the tissues. These density measurements are sent to a computer that produces a digital image of the anatomy, enabling a physician to look at slices or thin sections of certain anatomic views of the spine and associated vascular system and to determine the extent of malignancy.

Differentiations can be made among solid, cystic, inflammatory, or vascular lesions, and suspected hematomas and aneurysms can be identified. Iodinated contrast medium is given intravenously for blood vessel and vascular evaluation or orally for bowel and adjacent structure evaluation. Images can be recorded on photographic or x-ray film or stored in digital format as digitized computer data. Cine scanning produces a series of moving images of the scanned area. CT scanning can be used to guide biopsy needles into areas of suspected tumor to obtain tissue for laboratory analysis and to guide placement of catheters for drainage of abscesses. Tumor size, progression, and pretherapy and post-therapy changes may be monitored with CT scanning. ∎

INDICATIONS:

- Assist in differentiating between benign and malignant tumors

- Detect congenital spinal anomalies, such as spina bifida, meningocele, and myelocele

- Detect herniated intervertebral disks

- Detect paraspinal cysts
- Detect vascular malformations
- Monitor and evaluate effectiveness of medical, radiation, or surgical therapies

RESULT

Normal Findings:
- Normal density, size, position, and shape of spinal structures

Abnormal Findings:
- Congenital spinal malformations, such as meningocele, myelocele, or spina bifida
- Herniated intervertebral disks
- Paraspinal cysts
- Spinal tumors
- Spondylosis (cervical or lumbar)
- Vascular malformations

CRITICAL VALUES: N/A

INTERFERING FACTORS:

This procedure is contraindicated for:
- ⚠ Patients with allergies to shellfish or iodinated dye. The contrast medium used may cause a life-threatening allergic reaction. Patients with a known hypersensitivity to the medium may benefit from premedication with corticosteroids or the use of nonionic contrast medium.

- Patients who are claustrophobic.

- Patients who are pregnant or suspected of being pregnant, unless the potential benefits of the procedure far outweigh the risks to the fetus and mother.

- ⚠ Elderly and other patients who are chronically dehydrated before the test, because of their risk of contrast-induced renal failure.

- ⚠ Patients who are in renal failure.

- Young patients (17 years old and younger), unless the benefits of the x-ray diagnosis outweigh the risks of exposure to high levels of radiation.

Factors that may impair clear imaging:
- Gas or feces in the gastrointestinal tract resulting from inadequate cleansing or failure to restrict food intake before the study
- Retained barium from a previous radiologic procedure
- Metallic objects within the examination field (e.g., jewelry, body rings), which may inhibit organ visualization and can produce unclear images
- Improper adjustment of the radiographic equipment to accommodate obese or thin patients, which can cause overexposure or underexposure and a poor-quality study
- Patients who are very obese, who may exceed the weight limit for the equipment
- Patients with extreme claustrophobia unless sedation is given before the study
- Incorrect positioning of the patient, which may produce poor visualization of the area to be examined
- Inability of the patient to cooperate or remain still during the procedure because of age, significant pain, or mental status

Other considerations:
- Complications of the procedure include hemorrhage, infection at the IV needle insertion site, and cardiac arrhythmias.
- The procedure may be terminated if chest pain or severe cardiac arrhythmias occur.
- Failure to follow dietary restrictions and other pretesting preparations may cause the procedure to be canceled or repeated.

- Consultation with a health care provider should occur before the procedure for radiation safety concerns regarding younger patients or patients who are lactating.

- Risks associated with radiographic overexposure can result from frequent x-ray procedures. Personnel in the room with the patient should wear a protective lead apron, stand behind a shield, or leave the area while the examination is being done. Personnel working in the area where the examination is being done should wear badges that reveal their level of exposure to radiation.

Nursing Implications and Procedure • • • • • • • • • •

Pretest:

▶ Inform the patient that the procedure assesses the spine.

▶ Obtain a history of the patient's complaints or clinical symptoms, including a list of known allergens, especially allergies or sensitivities to iodine, seafood, or other contrast mediums.

▶ Obtain a history of results of previously performed diagnostic procedures, surgical procedures, and laboratory tests. Include specific tests as they apply (e.g., blood urea nitrogen [BUN], creatinine, coagulation tests, bleeding time). Ensure that the results of blood tests are obtained and recorded before the procedure, especially BUN and creatinine, if contrast medium is to be used. For related diagnostic tests, refer to the Musculoskeletal System table.

▶ Note any recent barium or other radiologic contrast procedures. Ensure that barium studies were performed more than 4 days before the CT scan.

▶ Record the date of the last menstrual period and determine the possibility of pregnancy in perimenopausal women.

▶ Obtain a list of the medications the patient is taking.

▶ In case contrast is used, patients receiving metformin (glucophage) for non–insulin-dependent (type 2) diabetes should discontinue the drug on the day of the test and continue to withhold it for 48 hours after the test. Failure to do so may result in lactic acidosis.

▶ Review the procedure with the patient. Explain to the patient that some pain may be experienced during the test, and there may be moments of discomfort. Explain the purpose of the test and how the procedure is performed. Inform the patient that the procedure is performed in a radiology department, usually by a health care practitioner and support staff, and takes approximately 30 to 60 minutes.

▶ *Sensitivity to cultural and social issues,* as well as concern for modesty, is important in providing psychological support before, during, and after the procedure.

▶ Explain that an IV line may be inserted to allow infusion of IV fluids, contrast medium, dye, or sedatives. Usually contrast medium and normal saline are infused.

▶ Inform the patient that he or she may experience nausea, a feeling of warmth, a salty or metallic taste, or a transient headache after injection of contrast medium, if given.

▶ The patient may be requested to drink approximately 450 mL of a dilute barium solution (approximately 1% barium) beginning 1 hour before the examination. This is administered to distinguish gastrointestinal organs from the other abdominal organs.

▶ The patient should fast and restrict fluids for 6 to 8 hours prior to the procedure. Instruct the patient to avoid taking anticoagulant medication or to reduce dosage as ordered prior to the procedure.

▶ Instruct the patient to remove jewelry (including watches), credit cards, keys, coins, cell phones, pagers, and other metallic objects.

➤ Make sure a written and informed consent has been signed prior to the procedure and before administering any medications.

Intratest:

➤ Ensure that the patient has complied with dietary, fluids, and medication restrictions and pretesting preparations; assure that food has been restricted for at least 6 hours prior to the procedure. Ensure that the patient has removed all external metallic objects (jewelry, dentures, etc.) prior to the procedure.

➤ Have emergency equipment readily available.

➤ If the patient has a history of severe allergic reactions to any substance or drug, administer ordered prophylactic steroids or antihistamines before the procedure. Use nonionic contrast medium for the procedure.

➤ Patients are given a gown, robe, and foot coverings to wear and instructed to void prior to the procedure.

➤ Observe standard precautions, and follow the general guidelines in Appendix A.

➤ Instruct the patient to cooperate fully and to follow directions. Instruct the patient to remain still throughout the procedure because movement produces unreliable results.

➤ Establish an IV fluid line for the injection of contrast, emergency drugs, and sedatives.

➤ Administer an antianxiety agent, as ordered, if the patient has claustrophobia. Administer a sedative to a child or to an uncooperative adult, as ordered.

➤ Place the patient in the supine position on an exam table.

➤ If contrast is used, the contrast medium is injected, and a rapid series of images is taken during and after the filling of the vessels to be examined. Delayed images may be taken to examine the vessels after a time and to monitor the venous phase of the procedure.

➤ Ask the patient to inhale deeply and hold his or her breath while the x-ray images are taken, and then to exhale after the images are taken.

➤ Instruct the patient to take slow, deep breaths if nausea occurs during the procedure. Monitor and administer an antiemetic agent if ordered. Ready an emesis basin for use.

➤ Monitor the patient for complications related to the procedure (e.g., allergic reaction, anaphylaxis, bronchospasm) if contrast is used.

➤ The needle or vascular catheter is removed, and a pressure dressing is applied over the puncture site.

➤ The results are recorded on film or by automated equipment in a computerized system for recall and post-procedure interpretation by the appropriate health care practitioner.

Post-test:

➤ Instruct the patient to resume usual diet, fluids, medications, or activity, as directed by the health care practitioner. Renal function should be assessed before metformin is resumed, if contrast was used.

➤ Monitor vital signs and neurologic status every 15 minutes for 30 minutes. Compare with baseline values. Protocols may vary from facility to facility.

➤ If contrast was used, observe for delayed allergic reactions, such as rash, urticaria, tachycardia, hyperpnea, hypertension, palpitations, nausea, or vomiting.

➤ If contrast was used, advise the patient to immediately report symptoms such as fast heart rate, difficulty breathing, skin rash, itching or decreased urinary output.

➤ Observe the needle/catheter insertion site for bleeding, inflammation, or hematoma formation.

➤ Instruct the patient to apply cold compresses to the puncture site, as needed, to reduce discomfort or edema.

➤ Instruct the patient to increase fluid

intake to help eliminate the contrast medium, if used.

➤ Inform the patient that diarrhea may occur after ingestion of oral contrast medium.

➤ A written report of the examination will be completed by a health care practitioner specializing in this branch of medicine. The report will be sent to the requesting health care practitioner, who will discuss the results with the patient.

➤ Depending on the results of this procedure, additional testing may be needed to evaluate or monitor progression of the disease process and determine the need for a change in therapy. Evaluate test results in relation to the patient's symptoms and other tests performed.

Related diagnostic tests:

➤ Related diagnostic tests include radiography of the bones.

COMPUTED TOMOGRAPHY, SPLEEN

SYNONYMS/ACRONYMS: Computed axial tomography (CAT), computed transaxial tomography (CTT), splenic CT.

AREA OF APPLICATION: Abdomen/spleen.

CONTRAST: Can be done with or without oral or intravenous (IV) iodinated contrast medium.

DESCRIPTION & RATIONALE: Computed tomography (CT) of the spleen is a noninvasive procedure that enhances certain anatomic views of the splenic structures, but it becomes an invasive procedure with the use of contrast medium. The spleen is not often the organ of interest when abdominal CT scans are obtained. However, a wide variety of splenic variations and abnormalities may be detected on abdominal scans designed to evaluate the liver, pancreas, or retroperitoneum. The patient lies on a table and is moved in and out of a doughnut-like device called a *gantry,* which houses the x-ray tube and associated electronics. The scanner uses multiple x-ray beams and a series of detectors that rotate around the patient to produce cross-sectional views in a three-dimensional fashion by detecting and recording differences in tissue density after having an x-ray beam passed through the tissues. These density measurements are sent to a computer that produces a digital image of the anatomy, enabling a physician to look at slices or thin sections of certain anatomic views of the spleen and vascular system. Differentiations can be made among solid, cystic, inflammatory, or vascular lesions, and suspected hematomas and aneurysms can be identified. CT is the first choice in the evaluation of abdominal trauma because of its diagnostic accuracy. Iodinated contrast medium is given intravenously for blood vessel and vascular evaluation or orally for bowel and adjacent structure evaluation. Images can be recorded on photographic or x-ray film or stored in digital format as digitized computer data. Cine scanning produces a series of moving images of the scanned area. CT scanning can be used to guide biopsy needles into areas of tumor to obtain tissue for laboratory analysis and to guide placement of catheters for drainage of abscesses. Tumors, before and after medical or surgical therapy, may be monitored with CT scanning. ■

INDICATIONS:

• Assist in differentiating between benign and malignant tumors

• Detect tumor extension of masses and metastasis

• Differentiate infectious from inflammatory processes

• Evaluate cysts, masses, abscesses, and trauma

• Evaluate the presence of an accessory spleen, polysplenia, or asplenia

• Evaluate splenic vein thrombosis

• Monitor and evaluate effectiveness of medical, radiation, or surgical therapies

RESULT

Normal Findings:
• Normal size, position, and shape of the spleen and associated vascular system

Abnormal Findings:
• Abdominal aortic aneurysm

• Hematomas

• Hemoperitoneum

• Primary and metastatic neoplasms

• Splenic cysts or abscesses

• Splenic laceration, tumor, infiltration, and trauma

CRITICAL VALUES: N/A

INTERFERING FACTORS:

This procedure is contraindicated for:
• ⚠ Patients with allergies to shellfish or iodinated dye. The contrast medium used may cause a life-threatening allergic reaction. Patients with a known hypersensitivity to the medium may benefit from premedication with corticosteroids or the use of nonionic contrast medium.

• Patients who are claustrophobic.

• Patients who are pregnant or suspected of being pregnant, unless the potential benefits of the procedure far outweigh the risks to the fetus and mother.

• ⚠ Elderly and other patients who are chronically dehydrated before the test, because of their risk of contrast-induced renal failure.

• ⚠ Patients who are in renal failure.

• Young patients (17 years old and younger), unless the benefits of the x-ray diagnosis outweigh the risks of exposure to high levels of radiation.

Factors that may impair clear imaging:
• Gas or feces in the gastrointestinal tract resulting from inadequate cleansing or failure to restrict food intake before the study

- Retained barium from a previous radiologic procedure

- Metallic objects within the examination field (e.g., jewelry, body rings), which may inhibit organ visualization and can produce unclear images

- Improper adjustment of the radiographic equipment to accommodate obese or thin patients, which can cause overexposure or underexposure and a poor-quality study

- Patients who are very obese, who may exceed the weight limit for the equipment

- Patients with extreme claustrophobia unless sedation is given before the study

- Incorrect positioning of the patient, which may produce poor visualization of the area to be examined

- Inability of the patient to cooperate or remain still during the procedure because of age, significant pain, or mental status

Other considerations:
- Complications of the procedure include hemorrhage`, infection at the IV needle insertion site, and cardiac arrhythmias.

- The procedure may be terminated if chest pain or severe cardiac arrhythmias occur.

- Failure to follow dietary restrictions and other pretesting preparations may cause the procedure to be canceled or repeated.

- Consultation with a health care provider should occur before the procedure for radiation safety concerns regarding younger patients or patients who are lactating.

- Risks associated with radiographic overexposure can result from frequent x-ray procedures. Personnel in the room with the patient should wear a protective lead apron, stand behind a shield, or leave the area while the examination is being done. Personnel working in the area where the examination is being done should wear badges that reveal their level of exposure to radiation.

Nursing Implications and Procedure • • • • • • • • • • •

Pretest:

➤ Inform the patient that the procedure assesses the abdomen and spleen.

➤ Obtain a history of the patient's complaints or clinical symptoms, including a list of known allergens, especially allergies or sensitivities to iodine, seafood, or other contrast mediums.

➤ Obtain a history of results of previously performed diagnostic procedures, surgical procedures, and laboratory tests. Include specific tests as they apply (e.g., blood urea nitrogen [BUN], creatinine, coagulation tests, bleeding time). Ensure that the results of blood tests are obtained and recorded before the procedure, especially BUN and creatinine, if contrast medium is to be used. For related diagnostic tests, refer to the Gastrointestinal, Hepatobiliary, and Genitourinary System tables.

➤ Note any recent barium or other radiologic contrast procedures. Ensure that barium studies were performed more than 4 days before the CT scan.

➤ Record the date of the last menstrual period and determine the possibility of pregnancy in perimenopausal women.

➤ Obtain a list of the medications the patient is taking.

➤ In case contrast is used, patients receiving metformin (glucophage) for non–insulin-dependent (type 2) diabetes should discontinue the drug on the day of the test and continue to withhold it for 48 hours after the test. Failure to do so may result in lactic acidosis.

➤ Review the procedure with the patient. Explain to the patient that some pain may be experienced during the test, and there may be moments of discomfort. Explain the purpose of the test and how the procedure is performed. Inform the patient that the procedure is performed in a radiology department, usually by a health care practitioner and support staff, and takes approximately 30 to 60 minutes.

➤ *Sensitivity to cultural and social issues,* as well as concern for modesty, is important in providing psychological support before, during, and after the procedure.

➤ Explain that an IV line may be inserted to allow infusion of IV fluids, contrast medium, dye, or sedatives. Usually contrast medium and normal saline are infused.

➤ Inform the patient that he or she may experience nausea, a feeling of warmth, a salty or metallic taste, or a transient headache after injection of contrast medium, if given.

➤ The patient may be requested to drink approximately 900 mL of a dilute barium solution (approximately 1% barium) beginning 1 hour before the examination. This is administered to distinguish gastrointestinal organs from the other abdominal organs.

➤ The patient should fast and restrict fluids for 6 to 8 hours prior to the procedure. Instruct the patient to avoid taking anticoagulant medication or to reduce dosage as ordered prior to the procedure.

➤ Instruct the patient to remove jewelry (including watches), credit cards, keys, coins, cell phones, pagers, and other metallic objects.

➤ *Make sure a written and informed consent has been signed prior to the procedure and before administering any medications.*

Intratest:

➤ Ensure that the patient has complied with dietary, fluids, and medication restrictions and pretesting preparations; assure that food has been restricted for at least 6 hours prior to the procedure. Ensure that the patient has removed all external metallic objects (jewelry, dentures, etc.) prior to the procedure.

➤ Have emergency equipment readily available.

➤ If the patient has a history of severe allergic reactions to any substance or drug, administer ordered prophylactic steroids or antihistamines before the procedure. Use nonionic contrast medium for the procedure.

➤ Patients are given a gown, robe, and foot coverings to wear and instructed to void prior to the procedure.

➤ Observe standard precautions, and follow the general guidelines in Appendix A.

➤ Instruct the patient to cooperate fully and to follow directions. Instruct the patient to remain still throughout the procedure because movement produces unreliable results.

➤ Establish an IV fluid line for the injection of contrast, emergency drugs, and sedatives.

➤ Administer an antianxiety agent, as ordered, if the patient has claustrophobia. Administer a sedative to a child or to an uncooperative adult, as ordered.

➤ Place the patient in the supine position on an exam table.

➤ If contrast is used, the contrast medium is injected, and a rapid series of images is taken during and after the filling of the vessels to be examined. Delayed images may be taken to examine the vessels after a time and to monitor the venous phase of the procedure.

➤ Ask the patient to inhale deeply and hold his or her breath while the x-ray images are taken, and then to exhale after the images are taken.

➤ Instruct the patient to take slow, deep breaths if nausea occurs during the procedure. Monitor and administer an antiemetic agent if ordered. Ready an emesis basin for use.

➤ Monitor the patient for complications related to the procedure (e.g., allergic reaction, anaphylaxis, bronchospasm) if contrast is used.

➤ The needle or vascular catheter is removed, and a pressure dressing is applied over the puncture site.

➤ The results are recorded on film or by automated equipment in a computerized system for recall and post-procedure interpretation by the appropriate health care practitioner.

Post-test:

➤ Instruct the patient to resume usual diet, fluids, medications or activity, as directed by the health care practitioner. Renal function should be assessed before metformin is resumed, if contrast was used.

➤ Monitor vital signs and neurologic status every 15 minutes for 30 minutes. Compare with baseline values. Protocols may vary from facility to facility.

➤ If contrast was used, observe for delayed allergic reactions, such as rash, urticaria, tachycardia, hyperpnea, hypertension, palpitations, nausea, or vomiting.

➤ If contrast was used, advise the patient to immediately report symptoms such as fast heart rate, difficulty breathing, skin rash, itching or decreased urinary output.

➤ Observe the needle/catheter insertion site for bleeding, inflammation, or hematoma formation.

➤ Instruct the patient to apply cold compresses to the puncture site, as needed, to reduce discomfort or edema.

➤ Instruct the patient to increase fluid intake to help eliminate the contrast medium, if used.

➤ Inform the patient that diarrhea may occur after ingestion of oral contrast medium.

➤ A written report of the examination will be completed by a health care practitioner specializing in this branch of medicine. The report will be sent to the requesting health care practitioner who will discuss the results with the patient.

➤ Depending on the results of this procedure, additional testing may be needed to evaluate or monitor progression of the disease process and determine the need for a change in therapy. Evaluate test results in relation to the patient's symptoms and other tests performed.

Related diagnostic tests:

➤ Related diagnostic tests include angiography of the abdomen; kidney, ureter, and bladder film; magnetic resonance imaging of the abdomen; and ultrasound of the liver.

COMPUTED TOMOGRAPHY, THORACIC

SYNONYMS/ACRONYMS: Computed axial tomography (CAT), computed transaxial tomography (CTT), chest CT.

AREA OF APPLICATION: Thorax.

CONTRAST: Can be done with or without oral or intravenous (IV) iodinated contrast medium.

DESCRIPTION & RATIONALE: Computed tomography (CT) of the thorax is more detailed than a chest x-ray. It is a noninvasive procedure used to enhance certain anatomic views of the lungs, heart, and mediastinal structures. The patient lies on a table and is moved in and out of a doughnut-like device called a *gantry*, which houses the x-ray tube and associated electronics. The scanner uses multiple x-ray beams and a series of detectors that rotate around the patient to produce cross-sectional views in a three-dimensional fashion by detecting and recording differences in tissue density after having an x-ray beam passed through the tissues. These density measurements are sent to a computer that produces a digital image of the anatomy, enabling a physician to look at slices or thin sections of certain anatomic views of the spine, spinal cord, and lung areas. Iodinated contrast medium is given intravenously for blood vessel and vascular evaluation or orally for esophageal evaluation. Images can be recorded on photographic or x-ray film or stored in digital format as digitized computer data. Cine scanning is used to produce moving images of the heart. ▪

INDICATIONS:
- Detect aortic aneurysms
- Detect bronchial abnormalities, such as stenosis, dilation, or tumor
- Detect lymphomas, especially Hodgkin's disease
- Detect mediastinal and hilar lymphadenopathy
- Detect primary and metastatic pulmonary, esophageal, or mediastinal tumors
- Detect tumor extension of neck mass to thoracic area
- Determine blood, fluid, or fat accumulation in tissues, pleuritic space, or vessels
- Differentiate aortic aneurysms from tumors near the aorta
- Differentiate between benign tumors (granulomas) and malignancies
- Differentiate infectious from inflam-

matory processes (abscess, nodules, or pneumonitis)

- Differentiate tumor from tuberculosis (which appears as coin-sized, calcified lesions)

- Evaluate cardiac chambers and pulmonary vessels

- Evaluate the presence of plaque in cardiac vessels

- Monitor and evaluate effectiveness of medical or surgical therapeutic regimen

RESULT

Normal Findings:
- Normal size, position, and shape of chest organs, tissues, and structures

Abnormal Findings:
- Aortic aneurysm

- Chest lesions (benign lesions, neoplastic tumors, or metastatic mediastinal lesions to ribs or spine)

- Cysts or abscesses

- Enlarged lymph nodes

- Esophageal pathology, including tumors

- Hodgkin's disease

- Pleural effusion

- Pneumonitis

CRITICAL VALUES: N/A

INTERFERING FACTORS:

This procedure is contraindicated for:
- ⚠ Patients with allergies to shellfish or iodinated dye. The contrast medium used may cause a life-threatening allergic reaction. Patients with a known hypersensitivity to the medium may benefit from premedication with corticosteroids or the use of nonionic contrast medium.

- Patients who are claustrophobic.

- Patients who are pregnant or suspected of being pregnant, unless the potential benefits of the procedure far outweigh the risks to the fetus and mother.

- ⚠ Elderly and other patients who are chronically dehydrated before the test, because of their risk of contrast-induced renal failure.

- ⚠ Patients who are in renal failure.

- Young patients (17 years old and younger), unless the benefits of the x-ray diagnosis outweigh the risks of exposure to high levels of radiation.

Factors that may impair clear imaging:
- Retained barium from a previous radiologic procedure

- Metallic objects within the examination field (e.g., jewelry, body rings), which may inhibit organ visualization and can produce unclear images

- Improper adjustment of the radiographic equipment to accommodate obese or thin patients, which can cause overexposure or underexposure and a poor-quality study

- Patients who are very obese, who may exceed the weight limit for the equipment

- Patients with extreme claustrophobia unless sedation is given before the study

- Incorrect positioning of the patient, which may produce poor visualization of the area to be examined

- Inability of the patient to cooperate or remain still during the procedure because of age, significant pain, or mental status

Other considerations:
- Complications of the procedure include hemorrhage, infection at the IV needle insertion site, and cardiac arrhythmias.

- The procedure may be terminated if chest pain or severe cardiac arrhythmias occur.

- Failure to follow dietary restrictions and other pretesting preparations may cause the procedure to be canceled or repeated.

- Consultation with a health care provider should occur before the procedure for radiation safety concerns regarding younger patients or patients who are lactating.

- Risks associated with radiographic overexposure can result from frequent x-ray procedures. Personnel in the room with the patient should wear a protective lead apron, stand behind a shield, or leave the area while the examination is being done. Personnel working in the area where the examination is being done should wear badges that reveal their level of exposure to radiation.

Nursing Implications and Procedure • • • • • • • • • • •

Pretest:

➤ Inform the patient that the procedure assesses the chest.

➤ Obtain a history of the patient's complaints or clinical symptoms, including a list of known allergens, especially allergies or sensitivities to iodine, seafood, or other contrast mediums.

➤ Obtain a history of results of previously performed diagnostic procedures, surgical procedures, and laboratory tests. Include specific tests as they apply (e.g., blood urea nitrogen [BUN], creatinine, coagulation tests, bleeding time). Ensure that the results of blood tests are obtained and recorded before the procedure, especially BUN and creatinine, if contrast medium is to be used. For related diagnostic tests, refer to the Respiratory System table.

➤ Note any recent barium or other radiologic contrast procedures. Ensure that barium studies were performed more than 4 days before the CT scan.

➤ Record the date of the last menstrual period and determine the possibility of pregnancy in perimenopausal women.

➤ Obtain a list of the medications the patient is taking.

➤ In case contrast is used, patients receiving metformin (glucophage) for non–insulin-dependent (type 2) diabetes should discontinue the drug on the day of the test and continue to withhold it for 48 hours after the test. Failure to do so may result in lactic acidosis.

➤ Review the procedure with the patient. Explain to the patient that some pain may be experienced during the test, and there may be moments of discomfort. Explain the purpose of the test and how the procedure is performed. Inform the patient that the procedure is performed in a radiology department, usually by a health care practitioner and support staff, and takes approximately 30 to 60 minutes.

➤ *Sensitivity to cultural and social issues,* as well as concern for modesty, is important in providing psychological support before, during, and after the procedure.

➤ Explain that an IV line may be inserted to allow infusion of IV fluids, contrast medium, dye, or sedatives. Usually contrast medium and normal saline are infused.

➤ Inform the patient that he or she may experience nausea, a feeling of warmth, a salty or metallic taste, or a transient headache after injection of contrast medium, if given.

➤ The patient should fast and restrict fluids for 6 to 8 hours prior to the procedure. Instruct the patient to avoid taking anticoagulant medication or to reduce dosage as ordered prior to the procedure.

➤ Instruct the patient to remove jewelry (including watches), credit cards, keys, coins, cell phones, pagers, and other metallic objects.

➤ *Make sure a written and informed consent has been signed prior to the procedure and before administering any medications.*

Intratest:

➤ Ensure that the patient has complied with dietary, fluids, and medication restrictions and pretesting preparations; assure that food has been restricted for at least 6 hours prior to the procedure. Ensure that the patient has removed all external metallic objects (jewelry, dentures, etc.) prior to the procedure.

➤ Have emergency equipment readily available.

➤ If the patient has a history of severe allergic reactions to any substance or drug, administer ordered prophylactic steroids or antihistamines before the procedure. Use nonionic contrast medium for the procedure.

➤ Patients are given a gown, robe, and foot coverings to wear and instructed to void prior to the procedure.

➤ Observe standard precautions, and follow the general guidelines in Appendix A.

➤ Instruct the patient to cooperate fully and to follow directions. Instruct the patient to remain still throughout the procedure because movement produces unreliable results.

➤ Establish an IV fluid line for the injection of contrast, emergency drugs, and sedatives.

➤ Administer an antianxiety agent, as ordered, if the patient has claustrophobia. Administer a sedative to a child or to an uncooperative adult, as ordered.

➤ Place the patient in the supine position on an exam table.

➤ If contrast is used, the contrast medium is injected, and a rapid series of images is taken during and after the filling of the vessels to be examined. Delayed images may be taken to examine the vessels after a time and to monitor the venous phase of the procedure.

➤ Ask the patient to inhale deeply and hold his or her breath while the x-ray images are taken, and then to exhale after the images are taken.

➤ Instruct the patient to take slow, deep breaths if nausea occurs during the procedure. Monitor and administer an antiemetic agent if ordered. Ready an emesis basin for use.

➤ Monitor the patient for complications related to the procedure (e.g., allergic reaction, anaphylaxis, bronchospasm) if contrast is used.

➤ The needle or vascular catheter is removed, and a pressure dressing is applied over the puncture site.

➤ The results are recorded on film, or by automated equipment in a computerized system for recall and postprocedure interpretation by the appropriate health care practitioner.

Post-test:

➤ Instruct the patient to resume usual diet, fluids, medications, or activity, as directed by the health care practitioner. Renal function should be assessed before metformin is resumed, if contrast was used.

➤ Monitor vital signs and neurologic status every 15 minutes for 30 minutes. Compare with baseline values. Protocols may vary from facility to facility.

➤ If contrast was used, observe for delayed allergic reactions, such as rash, urticaria, tachycardia, hyperpnea, hypertension, palpitations, nausea, or vomiting.

➤ If contrast was used, advise the patient to immediately report symptoms such as fast heart rate, difficulty breathing, skin rash, itching or decreased urinary output.

➤ Observe the needle/catheter insertion site for bleeding, inflammation, or hematoma formation.

➤ Instruct the patient to apply cold compresses to the puncture site, as needed, to reduce discomfort or edema.

➤ Instruct the patient to increase fluid intake to help eliminate the contrast medium, if used.

➤ Inform the patient that diarrhea may occur after ingestion of oral contrast medium.

➤ A written report of the examination will be completed by a health care practitioner specializing in this branch of medicine. The report will be sent to the requesting health care practitioner, who will discuss the results with the patient.

➤ Depending on the results of this procedure, additional testing may be needed to evaluate or monitor progression of the disease process and determine the need for a change in therapy. Evaluate test results in relation to the patient's symptoms and other tests performed.

Related diagnostic tests:

➤ Related diagnostic tests include chest x-ray, lung scan, and magnetic resonance imaging of the chest.

COOMBS' ANTIGLOBULIN, DIRECT

SYNONYM/ACRONYM: Direct antiglobulin testing (DAT).

SPECIMEN: Serum (1 mL) collected in a red-top tube and whole blood (1 mL) collected in lavender-top (EDTA) tube.

REFERENCE VALUE: (Method: Agglutination) Negative (no agglutination).

DESCRIPTION & RATIONALE: Direct antiglobulin testing (DAT) detects in vivo antibody sensitization of red blood cells (RBCs). Immunoglobulin G (IgG) produced in certain disease states or in response to certain drugs can coat the surface of RBCs, resulting in cellular damage and hemolysis. When DAT is performed, RBCs are taken from the patient's blood sample, washed with saline to remove residual globulins, and mixed with anti–human globulin reagent. If the anti–human globulin reagent causes agglutination of the patient's RBCs,

specific antiglobulin reagents can be used to determine whether the patient's RBCs are coated with IgG, complement, or both. (See monograph titled "Blood Groups and Antibodies" for more information regarding transfusion reactions.) ▪

INDICATIONS:
• Detect autoimmune hemolytic anemia or hemolytic disease of the newborn

• Evaluate suspected drug-induced hemolytic anemia

• Evaluate transfusion reaction

RESULT

Positive in:

- Anemia (autoimmune hemolytic, drug-induced)
- Hemolytic disease of the newborn
- Infectious mononucleosis
- Lymphomas
- *Mycoplasma* pneumonia
- Paroxysmal cold hemoglobinuria (idiopathic or disease related)
- Passively acquired antibodies from plasma products
- Post–cardiac vascular surgery
- Systemic lupus erythematosus and other connective tissue immune disorders
- Transfusion reactions (blood incompatibility)

Negative in:

- Samples in which sensitization of erythrocytes has not occurred

CRITICAL VALUES: N/A

INTERFERING FACTORS:

- Drugs and substances that may cause a positive DAT include acetaminophen, aminopyrine, aminosalicylic acid, ampicillin, antihistamines, aztreonam, cephalosporins, chlorinated hydrocarbon insecticides, chlorpromazine, chlorpropamide, cisplatin, clonidine, dipyrone, ethosuximide, fenfluramine, hydralazine, hydrochlorothiazide, ibuprofen, insulin, isoniazid, levodopa, mefenamic acid, melphalan, methadone, methicillin, methyldopa, moxalactam, penicillin, phenytoin, probenecid, procainamide, quinidine, quinine, rifampin, stibophen, streptomycin, sulfonamides, and tetracycline.
- Wharton's jelly may cause a false-positive DAT.

- Cold agglutinins and large amounts of paraproteins in the specimen may cause false-positive results.
- Newborns' cells may give negative results in ABO hemolytic disease.

Nursing Implications and Procedure

Pretest:

▶ Inform the patient that the test is used to detect associated conditions or drug therapies that can result in cell hemolysis.

▶ Obtain a history of the patient's complaints, including a list of known allergens (especially allergies or sensitivities to latex), and inform the appropriate health care practitioner accordingly.

▶ Obtain a history of the patient's hematopoietic system as well as results of previously performed laboratory tests, surgical procedures, and other diagnostic procedures. For related laboratory tests, refer to the Hematopoietic System table.

▶ Obtain a list of all medications the patient is taking, including herbs, nutritional supplements, and nutraceuticals. The requesting health care practitioner and laboratory should be advised if the patient is regularly using these products so that their effects can be taken into consideration when reviewing results.

▶ Review the procedure with the patient. Inform the patient that specimen collection takes approximately 5 to 10 minutes. Address concerns about pain related to the procedure. Explain to the patient that there may be some discomfort during the venipuncture. If a cord sample is to be taken from a newborn, inform parents that the sample will be obtained at the time of delivery and will not result in blood loss to the infant.

▶ There are no food, fluid, or medication restrictions unless by medical direction.

Intratest:

➤ If the patient has a history of severe allergic reaction to latex, care should be taken to avoid the use of equipment containing latex.

➤ Instruct the patient to cooperate fully and to follow directions. Direct the patient to breathe normally and to avoid unnecessary movement.

➤ Observe standard precautions, and follow the general guidelines in Appendix A. Positively identify the patient, and label the appropriate tubes with the corresponding patient demographics, date, and time of collection. Perform a venipuncture; collect the specimen in a 5-mL red-top (serum) and lavender-top (whole blood) tube. Cord specimens are obtained by inserting a needle attached to a syringe into the umbilical vein. The specimen is drawn into the syringe and gently expressed into the appropriate collection container.

➤ Remove the needle, and apply a pressure dressing over the puncture site.

➤ Promptly transport the specimen to the laboratory for processing and analysis.

➤ The results are recorded manually or in a computerized system for recall and postprocedure interpretation by the appropriate health care practitioner.

Post-test:

➤ Observe venipuncture site for bleeding or hematoma formation. Apply paper tape or other adhesive to hold pressure bandage in place, or replace with a plastic bandage.

➤ Note positive test results in cord blood of neonate; also assess newborn's bilirubin and hematocrit levels. Results may indicate the need for immediate exchange transfusion of fresh whole blood that has been typed and crossmatched with the mother's serum.

➤ Inform the postpartum patient of the implications of positive test results in cord blood. Prepare the newborn for exchange transfusion, on medical direction.

➤ A written report of the examination will be sent to the requesting health care practitioner, who will discuss the results with the patient.

➤ Reinforce information given by the patient's health care provider regarding further testing, treatment, or referral to another health care provider. Answer any questions or address any concerns voiced by the patient or family.

➤ Depending on the results of this procedure, additional testing may be performed to evaluate or monitor progression of the disease process and determine the need for a change in therapy. Evaluate test results in relation to the patient's symptoms and other tests performed.

Related laboratory tests:

➤ Related laboratory tests include bilirubin, blood group and type, Coombs' indirect antiglobulin (IAT), Ham's test, haptoglobin, hematocrit, and hemoglobin.

COOMBS' ANTIGLOBULIN, INDIRECT

SYNONYMS/ACRONYM: Indirect antiglobulin test (IAT), antibody screen.

SPECIMEN: Serum (1 mL) collected in a red-top tube.

REFERENCE VALUE: (Method: Agglutination) Negative (no agglutination).

DESCRIPTION & RATIONALE: The indirect antiglobulin test (IAT) detects and identifies unexpected circulating complement molecules or antibodies in the patient's serum. The first use of this test was for the detection and identification of anti-D using an indirect method. The test is now commonly used to screen a patient's serum for the presence of antibodies that may react against transfused red blood cells (RBCs). During testing, the patient's serum is allowed to incubate with reagent RBCs. The reagent RBCs used are from group O donors and have most of the clinically significant antigens present (D, C, E c, e, K, M, N, S, s, Fy^a, Fy,^{b} Jk,^{a} and Jk^b). Antibodies present in the patient's serum coat antigenic sites on the RBC membrane. The reagent cells are washed with saline to remove any unbound antibody. Antihuman globulin is added in the final step of the test. If the patient's serum contained antibodies, the antihuman globulin would cause the antibody-coated RBCs to stick together or agglutinate. (See monograph titled "Blood Groups and Antibodies" for more information regarding transfusion reactions.) ∎

INDICATIONS:
- Detect other antibodies in maternal blood that can be potentially harmful to the fetus
- Determine antibody titers in Rh-negative women sensitized by an Rh-positive fetus
- Screen for antibodies before blood transfusions
- Test for the weak Rh-variant antigen D^u.

RESULT

Positive in:
- Hemolytic anemia (drug-induced or autoimmune)
- Hemolytic disease of the newborn
- Incompatible crossmatch
- Maternal-fetal Rh incompatibility

Negative in:
- Samples in which the patient's antibodies exhibit dosage effects (i.e., stronger

reaction with homozygous than with heterozygous expression of an antigen) and reagent erythrocyte antigens contain single-dose expressions of the corresponding antigen (heterozygous)

• Samples in which reagent erythrocyte antigens are unable to detect low-prevalence antibodies

• Samples in which sensitization of erythrocytes has not occurred (complete absence of antibodies)

CRITICAL VALUES: N/A

INTERFERING FACTORS:
• Drugs that may cause a positive IAT include penicillin, phenacetin, quinidine, and rifampin.

• Recent administration of dextran, whole blood or fractions, or intravenous contrast media can result in a false-positive reaction.

Nursing Implications and Procedure • • • • • • • • • • • •

Pretest:

➤ Inform the patient that the test is used to check donor and recipient blood cells for antibodies prior to blood transfusion.

➤ Obtain a history of the patient's complaints, including a list of known allergens (especially allergies or sensitivities to latex), and inform the appropriate health care practitioner accordingly.

➤ Obtain a history of the patient's hematopoietic system as well as results of previously performed laboratory tests, surgical procedures, and other diagnostic procedures. For related laboratory tests, refer to the Hematopoietic System table.

➤ Note any recent procedures that can interfere with test results.

➤ Obtain a list of all the medications the patient is taking, including herbs, nutritional supplements, and nutraceuticals. The requesting health care practitioner and laboratory should be advised if the patient regularly uses these products so that their effects can be taken into consideration when reviewing results.

➤ Review the procedure with the patient. Inform the patient that specimen collection takes approximately 5 to 10 minutes. Address concerns about pain related to the procedure. Explain to the patient that there may be some discomfort during the venipuncture.

➤ There are no food, fluid, or medication restrictions unless by medical direction.

Intratest:

➤ If the patient has a history of severe allergic reaction to latex, care should be taken to avoid the use of equipment containing latex.

➤ Instruct the patient to cooperate fully and to follow directions. Direct the patient to breathe normally and to avoid unnecessary movement.

➤ Observe standard precautions, and follow the general guidelines in Appendix A. Positively identify the patient, and label the appropriate tubes with the corresponding patient demographics, date, and time of collection. Perform a venipuncture; collect the specimen in a 5-mL red-top tube.

➤ Remove the needle, and apply a pressure dressing over the puncture site.

➤ Promptly transport the specimen to the laboratory for processing and analysis.

➤ The results are recorded manually or in a computerized system for recall and postprocedure interpretation by the appropriate health care practitioner.

Post-test:

➤ Observe venipuncture site for bleeding or hematoma formation. Apply

paper tape or other adhesive to hold pressure bandage in place, or replace with a plastic bandage.

➤ Inform pregnant women that negative tests during the first 12 weeks' gestation should be repeated at 28 weeks to rule out the presence of an antibody.

➤ Positive test results in pregnant women after 28 weeks' gestation indicate the need for antibody identification testing.

➤ A written report of the examination will be sent to the requesting health care practitioner, who will discuss the results with the patient.

➤ Reinforce information given by the patient's health care provider regarding further testing, treatment, or referral to another health care provider. Answer any questions or address any concerns voiced by the patient or family.

➤ Depending on the results of this procedure, additional testing may be performed to evaluate or monitor progression of the disease process and determine the need for a change in therapy. Evaluate test results in relation to the patient's symptoms and other tests performed.

Related laboratory tests:

➤ Related laboratory tests include bilirubin, blood group and type, Coombs' direct antiglobulin (DAT), haptoglobin, hematocrit, and hemoglobin.

COPPER

. . . .

SYNONYM/ACRONYM: Cu.

SPECIMEN: Serum (1 mL) collected in a royal blue–top, trace element–free tube.

REFERENCE VALUE: (Method: Atomic absorption spectrophotometry)

Age	Conventional Units	SI Units (Conventional Units × 0.157)
Newborn–5 d	9–46 μg/dL	1.4–7.2 μmol/L
1–5 y	80–150 μg/dL	12.6–23.6 μmol/L
6–9 y	84–136 μg/dL	13.2–21.4 μmol/L
10–14 y	80–121 μg/dL	12.6–19.0 μmol/L
15–19 y	80–171 μg/dL	10.1–18.4 μmol/L
Adult		
Men	70–140 μg/dL	11.0–22.0 μmol/L
Women	80–155 μg/dL	12.6–24.3 μmol/L
Pregnant women	118–302 μg/dL	18.5–47.4 μmol/L

Values for African Americans are 8% to 12% higher.

DESCRIPTION & RATIONALE: Copper is an important cofactor for the enzymes that participate in the formation of hemoglobin and collagen. Copper is also a component of coagulation factor V, assists in the oxidation of glucose, is required for melanin pigment formation, is used to synthesize ceruloplasmin, and is necessary for maintenance of myelin sheaths. Copper levels vary with intake. This mineral is absorbed in the stomach and duodenum, stored in the liver, and excreted in urine and in feces with bile salts. Copper deficiency results in neutropenia and a hypochromic, microcytic anemia that is not responsive to iron therapy. Other signs and symptoms of copper deficiency include osteoporosis, depigmentation of skin and hair, impaired immune system response, and possible neurologic and cardiac abnormalities. ∎

INDICATIONS:
- Assist in establishing a diagnosis of Menkes disease
- Assist in establishing a diagnosis of Wilson's disease
- Monitor patients receiving long-term parenteral nutrition therapy

RESULT

Increased in:
- Anemias
- Ankylosing spondylitis
- Biliary cirrhosis
- Collagen diseases
- Complications of renal dialysis
- Hodgkin's disease
- Infections
- Inflammation

- Leukemia
- Malignant neoplasms
- Myocardial infarction
- Pellagra
- Poisoning from copper-contaminated solutions or insecticides
- Pregnancy
- Pulmonary tuberculosis
- Rheumatic fever
- Rheumatoid arthritis
- Systemic lupus erythematosus
- Thalassemias
- Thyroid disease (hypothyroid or hyperthyroid)
- Trauma
- Typhoid fever
- Use of copper intrauterine device

Decreased in:
- Burns
- Chronic ischemic heart disease
- Cystic fibrosis
- Dysproteinemia
- Infants (especially premature infants) receiving milk deficient in copper
- Iron-deficiency anemias (some)
- Long-term total parenteral nutrition
- Malabsorption disorders (celiac disease, tropical sprue)
- Malnutrition
- Menkes disease
- Nephrotic syndrome
- Wilson's disease

CRITICAL VALUES: N/A

INTERFERING FACTORS:
- Drugs that may increase copper levels include anticonvulsants and oral contraceptives.

- Drugs that may decrease copper levels include citrates, penicillamine, and valproic acid.
- Excessive therapeutic intake of zinc may interfere with intestinal absorption of copper.

Nursing Implications and Procedure • • • • • • • • • • •

Pretest:

➤ Inform the patient that the test is used to monitor exposure to copper.

➤ Obtain a history of the patient's complaints, including a list of known allergens (especially allergies or sensitivities to latex), and inform the appropriate health care practitioner accordingly.

➤ Obtain a history of the patient's hematopoietic, hepatobiliary, and immune systems, as well as results of previously performed laboratory tests, surgical procedures, and other diagnostic procedures. For related laboratory tests, refer to the Hematopoietic, Hepatobiliary, and Immune System tables.

➤ Obtain a list of medications the patient is taking, including herbs, nutritional supplements, and nutraceuticals. The requesting health care practitioner and laboratory should be advised if the patient regularly uses these products so that their effects can be taken into consideration when reviewing results.

➤ Review the procedure with the patient. Inform the patient that specimen collection takes approximately 5 to 10 minutes. Address concerns about pain related to the procedure. Explain to the patient that there may be some discomfort during the venipuncture.

➤ There are no food, fluid, or medication restrictions unless by medical direction.

Intratest:

➤ If the patient has a history of severe allergic reaction to latex, care should be taken to avoid the use of equipment containing latex.

➤ Instruct the patient to cooperate fully and to follow directions. Direct the patient to breathe normally and to avoid unnecessary movement.

➤ Observe standard precautions, and follow the general guidelines in Appendix A. Positively identify the patient, and label the appropriate tubes with the corresponding patient demographics, date, and time of collection. Perform a venipuncture; collect the specimen in a 5-mL royal blue–top, trace element–free tube.

➤ Remove the needle, and apply a pressure dressing over the puncture site.

➤ Promptly transport the specimen to the laboratory for processing and analysis.

➤ The results are recorded manually or in a computerized system for recall and postprocedure interpretation by the appropriate health care practitioner.

Post-test:

➤ Observe venipuncture site for bleeding or hematoma formation. Apply paper tape or other adhesive to hold pressure bandage in place, or replace with a plastic bandage.

➤ *Nutritional considerations:* Instruct the patient with increased copper levels to avoid foods rich in copper or increase intake of elements that interfere with copper absorption, as appropriate. Organ meats, shellfish, nuts, and legumes are good sources of dietary copper. High intake of zinc, iron, calcium, and manganese interferes with copper absorption. Copper deficiency does not normally occur in adults, but patients receiving long-term total parenteral nutrition should be evaluated if signs and symptoms of copper deficiency appear.

➤ A written report of the examination will be sent to the requesting health care practitioner, who will discuss the results with the patient.

➤ Reinforce information given by the patient's health care provider regarding further testing, treatment, or referral to another health care provider. Answer any questions or address any concerns voiced by the patient or family.

➤ Depending on the results of this procedure, additional testing may be performed to evaluate or monitor progression of the disease process and determine the need for a change in therapy. Evaluate test results in relation to the patient's symptoms and other tests performed.

Related laboratory tests:

➤ Related laboratory tests include ceruloplasmin, complete blood count, liver biopsy, and zinc.

CORTISOL AND CHALLENGE TESTS

· ·

SYNONYMS/ACRONYM: Hydrocortisone, compound F.

SPECIMEN: Serum (1 mL) collected in a red- or tiger-top tube. Plasma (1 mL) collected in green-top (heparin) tube is also acceptable. Care must be taken to use the same type of collection container if serial measurements are to be taken.

Procedure	Medication Administered	Recommended Collection Times
ACTH stimulation, rapid test	1 μg (low-dose protocol) cosyntropin IM	3 cortisol levels: baseline immediately before bolus, 30 min after bolus, and 60 min after bolus
CRH stimulation	IV dose of 1 μg/kg ovine CRH at 9 a.m. or 8 p.m.	8 cortisol and 8 ACTH levels: baseline collected 15 min before injection, 0 minutes before injection, and then 5, 15, 30, 60, 120, and 180 min after injection
Dexamethasone suppression (overnight)	Oral dose of 1 mg dexamethasone (Decadron) at 11 p.m.	Collect cortisol at 8 a.m. on the morning after the dexamethasone dose
Metyrapone stimulation (overnight)	Oral dose of 30 mg/kg metyrapone with snack at midnight	Collect cortisol and ACTH at 8 a.m. on the morning after the metyrapone dose

ACTH = adrenocorticotropic hormone; CRH = corticotropin-releasing hormone; IM = intramuscular; IV = intravenous.

REFERENCE VALUE: (Method: Immunoassay)

	Conventional Units	SI Units
Cortisol		
		(*Conventional Units × 27.6*)
8 a.m.	5–25 µg/dL	138–690 nmol/L
4 p.m.	3–16 µg/dL	83–442 nmol/L
ACTH Challenge Tests		
CRH stimulation	2–4 fold increase over baseline ACTH or cortisol level	2–4 fold increase over baseline value
Dexamethasone Suppressed		
		(*Conventional Units × 27.6*)
	Cortisol less than 3 µg/dL next day	Less than 83 nmol/L
ACTH (Cosyntropin) Stimulated, Rapid Test		
		(*Conventional Units × 27.6*)
	Cortisol greater than 20 µg/dL	Greater than 552 nmol/L
Metyrapone Stimulated		
		(*Conventional Units × 0.22*)
	ACTH greater than 75 pg/mL	Greater than 16.5 pmol/L
		(*Conventional Units × 27.6*)
	Cortisol less than 3 µg/dL next day	Less than 83 nmol/L

ACTH = adrenocorticotropic hormone; CRH = corticotropin-releasing hormone.

DESCRIPTION & RATIONALE: Cortisol (hydrocortisone) is the predominant glucocorticoid secreted in response to stimulation by the hypothalamus and pituitary adrenocorticotropic hormone (ACTH). Cortisol stimulates gluconeogenesis, mobilizes fats and proteins, antagonizes insulin, and suppresses inflammation. Measuring levels of cortisol in blood is the best indicator of adrenal function. Cortisol secretion varies diurnally, with highest levels occurring on awakening and lowest levels occurring late in the day. Bursts of cortisol excretion can occur at night. Cortisol and ACTH test results are evaluated together because they each control the other's concentrations (i.e., any change in one causes a change in the other). ACTH levels exhibit a diurnal variation, peaking between 6 and 8 a.m. and reaching the lowest point between 6 and 11 p.m. Evening levels are generally one-half to two-thirds lower than morning levels. (See monograph titled "Adrenocorticotropic Hormone [and Challenge Tests].") ▪

INDICATIONS:
* Detect adrenal hyperfunction (Cushing's syndrome)
* Detect adrenal hypofunction (Addison's disease)

RESULT: The dexamethasone suppression test is useful in differentiating the causes for increased cortisol levels. Dexamethasone is a synthetic steroid that suppresses secretion of ACTH. With this test, a baseline morning cortisol level is collected, and the patient is given a 1-mg dose of dexamethasone at bedtime. A second specimen is collected the following morning. If cortisol levels have not been suppressed, adrenal adenoma may be suspected. The dexamethasone suppression test also produces abnormal results in patients with psychiatric illnesses.

The corticotropin-releasing hormone (CRH) stimulation test works as well as the dexamethasone suppression test in distinguishing Cushing's disease from conditions in which ACTH is secreted ectopically. In this test, cortisol levels are measured after an injection of CRH. A fourfold increase in cortisol levels above baseline is seen in Cushing's disease. No increase in cortisol is seen if ectopic ACTH secretion is the cause.

The cosyntropin test is used when adrenal insufficiency is suspected. Cosyntropin is a synthetic form of ACTH. A baseline cortisol level is collected before the injection of cosyntropin. Specimens are subsequently collected at 30- and 60-minute intervals. If the adrenal glands are functioning normally, cortisol levels rise significantly after administration of cosyntropin.

The metyrapone stimulation test is used to distinguish corticotropin-dependent (pituitary Cushing's disease and ectopic Cushing's disease) from corticotropin-independent (carcinoma of the lung or thyroid) causes of increased cortisol levels. Metyrapone inhibits the conversion of 11-deoxycortisol to cortisol. Cortisol levels should decrease to less than 3 μg/dL if normal pituitary stimulation by ACTH occurs after an oral dose of metyrapone. Specimen collection and administration of the medication are performed as with the overnight dexamethasone test.

Increased in:
* Adrenal adenoma
* Cushing's syndrome
* Ectopic ACTH production
* Hyperglycemia
* Pregnancy
* Stress

Decreased in:
* Addison's disease
* Adrenogenital syndrome
* Hypopituitarism

CRITICAL VALUES: N/A

INTERFERING FACTORS:
* Drugs and substances that may increase cortisol levels include amphetamines, anticonvulsants, clomipramine, corticotropin, cortisone, CRH, cyclic AMP, ether, fenfluramine, hydrocortisone, insulin, lithium, methadone, metoclopramide, naloxone, opiates, oral contraceptives, prednisolone, ranitidine, spironolactone, tetracosactrin, and vasopressin.

* Drugs and substances that may decrease cortisol levels include barbiturates, beclomethasone, betamethasone, clonidine, danazol, desoximetasone, desoxycorticosterone, dexamethasone, ephedrine, etomidate, fluocinolone, ketoconazole, levodopa, lithium, methylprednisolone, metyrapone, midazolam, morphine, nitrous oxide,

oxazepam, phenytoin, ranitidine, and trimipramine.

- Test results are affected by the time this test is done because cortisol levels vary diurnally.

- Stress and excessive physical activity can produce elevated levels.

- Normal values can be obtained in the presence of partial pituitary deficiency.

- Recent radioactive scans within 1 week of the test can interfere with test results.

- ⚠ The metyrapone stimulation test is contraindicated in patients with suspected adrenal insufficiency.

- ⚠ Metyrapone may cause gastrointestinal distress and/or confusion. Administer oral dose of metyrapone with milk and snack.

Nursing Implications and Procedure • • • • • • • • • • •

Pretest:

➤ Inform the patient that the test is used to asssit in the diagnosis of adrenocortical insufficiency.

➤ Obtain a history of the patient's complaints, including a list of known allergens (especially allergies or sensitivities to latex), and inform the appropriate health care practitioner accordingly.

➤ Obtain a history of the patient's endocrine system, as well as results of previously performed laboratory tests, surgical procedures, and other diagnostic procedures. For related laboratory tests, refer to the Endocrine System table.

➤ Obtain a list of medications the patient is taking, including herbs, nutritional supplements, and nutraceuticals. The requesting health care practitioner and laboratory should be advised if the patient regularly uses these products so that their effects can be taken into consideration when reviewing results.

➤ Review the procedure with the patient. Inform the patient that multiple specimens may be required. Inform the patient that specimen collection takes approximately 5 to 10 minutes. Address concerns about pain related to the procedure. Explain to the patient that there may be some discomfort during the venipuncture.

➤ *Sensitivity to social and cultural issues,* as well as concern for modesty, is important in providing psychological support before, during, and after the procedure.

➤ There are no food, fluid, or medication restrictions unless by medical direction.

➤ Drugs that enhance steroid metabolism may be withheld by medical direction prior to metyrapone stimulation testing.

➤ Instruct the patient to minimize stress to avoid raising cortisol levels.

Intratest:

➤ Have emergency equipment readily available.

➤ If the patient has a history of severe allergic reaction to latex, care should be taken to avoid the use of equipment containing latex.

➤ Instruct the patient to cooperate fully and to follow directions. Direct the patient to breathe normally and to avoid unnecessary movement.

➤ Observe standard precautions, and follow the general guidelines in Appendix A. Positively identify the patient, and label the appropriate tubes with the corresponding patient demographics, date, and time of collection. Collect specimen between 6 and 8 a.m., when cortisol levels are highest. Perform a venipuncture; collect the specimen in a 5-mL red- or tiger-top tube.

➤ Adverse reactions to metyrapone include nausea and vomiting (N/V), abdominal pain, headache, dizziness, sedation, allergic rash, decreased white blood cell count, or bone marrow depression. Signs and symptoms of overdose or acute adreno-cortical insuffiency include cardiac arrhythmias, hypotension, dehydration, anxiety, confusion, weakness, impairment of consciousness, N/V, epigastric pain, diarrhea, hyponatremia, and hyperkalemia.

➤ Remove the needle, and apply a pressure dressing over the puncture site.

➤ Promptly transport the specimen to the laboratory for processing and analysis.

➤ The results are recorded manually or in a computerized system for recall and postprocedure interpretation by the appropriate health care practitioner.

Post-test:

➤ Instruct the patient to resume usual medications, as directed by the health care practitioner.

➤ Observe venipuncture site for bleeding or hematoma formation. Apply paper tape or other adhesive to hold pressure bandage in place, or replace with a plastic bandage.

➤ A written report of the examination will be sent to the requesting health care practitioner, who will discuss the results with the patient.

➤ Recognize anxiety related to test results. Discuss the implications of abnormal test results on the patient's lifestyle. Provide teaching and information regarding the clinical implications of the test results, as appropriate. Educate the patient regarding access to counseling services.

➤ Reinforce information given by the patient's health care provider regarding further testing, treatment, or referral to another health care provider. Answer any questions or address any concerns voiced by the patient or family.

➤ Depending on the results of this procedure, additional testing may be performed to evaluate or monitor progression of the disease process and determine the need for a change in therapy. Evaluate test results in relation to the patient's symptoms and other tests performed.

Related laboratory tests:

➤ Related laboratory tests include ACTH, glucose, and glucose tolerance test.

C-PEPTIDE

SYNONYMS/ACRONYM: Connecting peptide insulin, insulin C-peptide, proinsulin C-peptide.

SPECIMEN: Serum (1 mL) collected in a red-top tube.

REFERENCE VALUE: (Method: Immunochemiluminometric assay, ICMA)

Conventional Units	SI Units (Conventional Units × 0.333)
0.78–1.8 ng/mL	0.26–0.63 nmol/L

DESCRIPTION & RATIONALE: C-peptide is a biologically inactive peptide formed when beta cells of the pancreas convert proinsulin to insulin. Most of C-peptide is secreted by the kidneys. C-peptide levels usually correlate with insulin levels and provide a reliable indication of how well the beta cells secrete insulin. Release of C-peptide is not affected by exogenous insulin administration. C-peptide values double after stimulation with glucose or glucagon. An insulin/C-peptide ratio less than 1.0 indicates endogenous insulin secretion, whereas a ratio of greater than 1.0 indicates an excess of exogenous insulin. ■

INDICATIONS:
- Assist in the diagnosis of insulinoma: Serum levels of insulin and C-peptide are elevated.

- Detect suspected factitious cause of hypoglycemia (excessive insulin administration): C-peptide levels do not increase with serum insulin levels.

- Determine beta cell function when insulin antibodies preclude accurate measurement of serum insulin production.

- Distinguish between insulin-dependent (type 1) and non–insulin-dependent (type 2) diabetes (with C-peptide–stimulating test): Patients with diabetes whose C-peptide stimulation level is greater than 18 ng/mL can be managed without insulin treatment.

- Evaluate hypoglycemia.

RESULT

Increased in:
- Endogenous hyperinsulinism
- Islet cell tumor
- Non–insulin-dependent (type 2) diabetes

- Oral hypoglycemic medication
- Pancreas or beta cell transplants
- Renal failure

Decreased in:
- Factitious hypoglycemia
- Insulin-dependent (type 1) diabetes
- Pancreatectomy

CRITICAL VALUES: N/A

INTERFERING FACTORS:
- Drugs that may increase C-peptide levels include betamethasone, chloroquine, danazol, deferoxamine, ethinyl estradiol, oral contraceptives, prednisone, and rifampin.

- Drugs that may decrease C-peptide levels include atenolol and calcitonin.

- C-peptide and endogenous insulin levels do not always correlate in obese patients.

- Failure to follow dietary restrictions before the procedure may cause the procedure to be canceled or repeated.

Nursing Implications and Procedure • • • • • • • • • • •

Pretest:

➤ Inform the patient that the test is primarily used in the evaluation of hypoglycemia.

➤ Obtain a history of the patient's complaints, including a list of known allergens (especially allergies or sensitivities to latex), and inform the appropriate health care practitioner accordingly.

➤ Obtain a history of the patient's endocrine system and results of previously performed laboratory tests, surgical procedures, and other diagnostic procedures. For related laboratory tests, refer to the Endocrine System table.

➤ Obtain a list of the medications the patient is taking, including herbs, nutritional supplements, and nutraceuticals. The requesting health care practitioner and laboratory should be advised if the patient is regularly using these products so that their effects can be taken into consideration when reviewing results.

➤ Review the procedure with the patient. Inform the patient that specimen collection takes approximately 5 to 10 minutes. Address concerns about pain related to the procedure. Explain to the patient that there may be some discomfort during the venipuncture.

➤ The patient should fast for at least 10 hours before specimen collection.

➤ There are no fluid or medication restrictions unless by medical direction.

Intratest:

➤ Ensure that the patient has complied with dietary restrictions and pretesting preparations; assure that food has been restricted for at least 10 hours prior to the procedure.

➤ If the patient has a history of severe allergic reaction to latex, care should be taken to avoid the use of equipment containing latex.

➤ Instruct the patient to cooperate fully and to follow directions. Direct the patient to breathe normally and to avoid unnecessary movement.

➤ Observe standard precautions, and follow the general guidelines in Appendix A. Positively identify the patient, and label the appropriate tubes with the corresponding patient demographics, date, and time of collection. Perform a venipuncture; collect the specimen in a 5-mL redtop tube.

➤ Remove the needle, and apply a pressure dressing over the puncture site.

➤ Promptly transport the specimen to the laboratory for processing and analysis.

➤ The results are recorded manually or in a computerized system for recall and postprocedure interpretation by the appropriate health care practitioner.

Post-test:

➤ Observe venipuncture site for bleeding or hematoma formation. Apply paper tape or other adhesive to hold pressure bandage in place, or replace with a plastic bandage.

➤ Instruct the patient to resume usual diet as directed by the health care practitioner.

➤ *Nutritional considerations:* Abnormal C-peptide levels may be associated with diabetes. Instruct the diabetic patient, as appropriate, in nutritional management of the disease. Patients who adhere to dietary recommendations report a better general feeling of health, better weight management, greater control of glucose and lipid values, and improved use of insulin. There is no "diabetic diet"; however, there are many meal-planning approaches with nutritional goals endorsed by the American Dietetic Association. The nutritional requirements of each diabetic patient need to be determined individually with the appropriate health care professionals, particularly health care workers trained in nutrition.

➤ Instruct the patient and caregiver to report signs and symptoms of hypoglycemia (weakness, confusion, diaphoresis, rapid pulse) or hyperglycemia (thirst, polyuria, hunger, lethargy). Emphasize, as appropriate, that good control of glucose levels delays the onset and slows the progression of diabetic retinopathy, nephropathy, and neuropathy.

➤ A written report of the examination will be sent to the requesting health care practitioner, who will discuss the results with the patient.

➤ Reinforce information given by the patient's health care provider regarding further testing, treatment, or referral to another health care provider. Answer any questions or address any concerns voiced by the patient or family.

▶ Depending on the results of this procedure, additional testing may be performed to evaluate or monitor progression of the disease process and determine the need for a change in therapy. Evaluate test results in relation to the patient's symptoms and other tests performed.

Related laboratory tests:

▶ Related laboratory tests include cortisol, creatinine, creatinine clearance, fructose, glucagon, glucose, glucose tolerance tests, glycated hemoglobin, insulin, insulin antibodies, microalbumin, and urea nitrogen.

C-REACTIVE PROTEIN

SYNONYM/ACRONYM: CRP.

SPECIMEN: Serum (1 mL) collected in a red- or tiger-top tube.

REFERENCE VALUE: (Method: High-sensitivity immunoassay, nephelometry)

High-sensitivity immunoassay (cardiac applications)	1.0–3.0 mg/L

Nephelometry	Conventional Units
Adult	0–4.9 mg/L

DESCRIPTION & RATIONALE: C-reactive protein (CRP) is a glycoprotein produced by the liver in response to acute inflammation. The CRP assay is a nonspecific test that determines the presence (not the cause) of inflammation; it is often ordered in conjunction with erythrocyte sedimentation rate (ESR). CRP assay is a more sensitive and rapid indicator of the presence of an inflammatory process than ESR. CRP disappears from the serum rapidly when inflammation has subsided. The inflammatory process and its association with atherosclerosis make the presence of CRP, as detected by highly sensitive CRP assays, a potential marker for coronary artery disease. It is believed that the inflammatory process may instigate the conversion of a stable plaque to a weaker one that can rupture and occlude an artery. Several major studies are in progress to confirm the correlation and to establish standardized reference ranges for this purpose. ■

INDICATIONS:

- Assist in the differential diagnosis of appendicitis and acute pelvic inflammatory disease
- Assist in the differential diagnosis of Crohn's disease and ulcerative colitis
- Assist in the differential diagnosis of rheumatoid arthritis and uncomplicated systemic lupus erythematosus (SLE)
- Assist in the evaluation of coronary artery disease
- Detect the presence or exacerbation of inflammatory processes
- Monitor response to therapy for autoimmune disorders such as rheumatoid arthritis

RESULT

Increased in:
- Acute bacterial infections
- Crohn's disease
- Inflammatory bowel disease
- Myocardial infarction
- Pregnancy (second half)
- Rheumatic fever
- Rheumatoid arthritis
- SLE
- Syndrome X (metabolic syndrome)

Decreased in: N/A

CRITICAL VALUES: N/A

INTERFERING FACTORS:
- Drugs that may decrease CRP levels include aurothiomalate, methotrexate, nonsteroidal anti-inflammatory drugs, oral contraceptives (progestogen effect), penicillamine, pentopril, and sulfasalazine.

- Nonsteroidal anti-inflammatory drugs, salicylates, and steroids may cause false-negative results because of suppression of inflammation.

- Falsely elevated levels may occur with the presence of an intrauterine device.

- Lipemic samples that are turbid in appearance may be rejected for analysis when nephelometry is the test method.

Nursing Implications and Procedure

Pretest:

➤ Inform the patient that the test is used to indicate nonspecific inflammatory response; the highly sensitive CRP is used to assess risk for cardiovascular and peripheral vascular disease.

➤ Obtain a history of the patient's complaints, including a list of known allergens (especially allergies or sensitivities to latex), and inform the appropriate health care practitioner accordingly. The patient may complain of pain related to the inflammatory process in connective or other tissues.

➤ Obtain a history of the patient's cardiovascular and immune systems, as well as results of previously performed laboratory tests, surgical procedures, and other diagnostic procedures. For related laboratory tests, refer to the Cardiovascular and Immune System tables.

➤ Obtain a list of the medications the patient is taking, including herbs, nutritional supplements, and nutraceuticals. The requesting health care practitioner and laboratory should be advised if the patient regularly uses these products so that their effects can be taken into consideration when reviewing results.

➤ Review the procedure with the patient. Inform the patient that specimen collection takes approximately 5 to 10 minutes. Address concerns about pain related to the procedure. Explain to the patient that there may be some discomfort during the venipuncture.

➤ There are no food, fluid, or medication restrictions unless by medical direction.

Intratest:

➤ If the patient has a history of severe allergic reaction to latex, care should be taken to avoid the use of equipment containing latex.

➤ Instruct the patient to cooperate fully and to follow directions. Direct the patient to breathe normally and to avoid unnecessary movement.

➤ Observe standard precautions, and follow the general guidelines in Appendix A. Positively identify the patient, and label the appropriate tubes with the corresponding patient demographics, date, and time of collection. Perform a venipuncture; collect the specimen in a 5-mL red- or tiger-top tube.

➤ Remove the needle, and apply a pressure dressing over the puncture site.

➤ Promptly transport the specimen to the laboratory for processing and analysis.

➤ The results are recorded manually or in a computerized system for recall and postprocedure interpretation by the appropriate health care practitioner.

Post-test:

➤ Observe venipuncture site for bleeding or hematoma formation. Apply paper tape or other adhesive to hold pressure bandage in place, or replace with a plastic bandage.

➤ A written report of the examination will be sent to the requesting health care practitioner, who will discuss the results with the patient.

➤ Reinforce information given by the patient's health care provider regarding further testing, treatment, or referral to another health care provider. Answer any questions or address any concerns voiced by the patient or family.

➤ Depending on the results of this procedure, additional testing may be performed to evaluate or monitor progression of the disease process and determine the need for a change in therapy. Evaluate test results in relation to the patient's symptoms and other tests performed.

Related laboratory tests:

➤ Related laboratory tests include antiarrhythmic drugs, apolipoprotein A, apolipoprotein B, aspartate aminotransferase, atrial natriuretic peptide, blood gases, B-type natriuretic peptide, calcium (blood and ionized), cholesterol (total, HDL, and LDL), C-reactive protein, creatine kinase and isoenzymes, ESR, glucose, glycated hemoglobin, homocysteine, ketones, lactate dehydrogenase and isoenzymes, myoglobin, potassium, triglycerides, troponin, and white blood cell count.

CREATINE KINASE AND ISOENZYMES

SYNONYM/ACRONYM: CK and isos.

SPECIMEN: Serum (1 mL) collected in a red- or tiger-top tube. Serial specimens are highly recommended. Care must be taken to use the same type of collection container if serial measurements are to be taken.

REFERENCE VALUE: (Method: Enzymatic for CK, electrophoresis for isoenzymes; enzyme immunoassay techniques are in common use for CK-MB)

	Conventional & SI Units
Total CK	
Newborn	3 × adult values
Male (children and adult)	38–174 U/L
Female (children and adult)	26–140 U/L
CK isoenzymes by electrophoresis	
CK-BB	Absent
CK-MB	Less than 4–6%
CK-MM	94–96%
CK-MB by immunoassay	Less than 10 ng/mL

CK = creatine kinase; CK-BB = CK isoenzyme in brain; CK-MB = CK isoenzyme in heart; CK-MM = CK isoenzyme in skeletal muscle.

DESCRIPTION & RATIONALE: Creatine kinase (CK) is an enzyme that exists almost exclusively in skeletal muscle, heart muscle, and, in smaller amounts, in the brain. This enzyme is important in intracellular storage and energy release. Three isoenzymes, based on primary location, have been identified by electrophoresis: brain CK-BB, cardiac CK-MB, and skeletal muscle CK-MM. When injury to these tissues occurs, the enzymes are released into the bloodstream. Levels increase and decrease in a predictable time frame. Measuring the serum levels can help determine the extent and timing of the damage. Noting the presence of the specific isoenzyme helps determine the location of the tissue damage.

Acute myocardial infarction (MI) releases CK into the serum within the first 48 hours; values return to normal in about 3 days. The isoenzyme CK-MB appears in the first 6 to 24 hours and is usually gone in 72 hours. Recurrent elevation of CK suggests reinfarction or extension of ischemic damage. Significant elevations of CK are expected in early phases of muscular dystrophy, even before the clinical signs and symptoms appear. CK elevation diminishes as the disease progresses and muscle mass decreases. Differences in total CK with age and gender relate to the fact that the predominant isoenzyme is muscular in origin. Body builders have higher values, whereas older individuals have lower values because of deterioration of muscle mass.

The use of the mass assay for CK-MB with cardiac troponin T, myoglobin, and serial electrocardiograms in the assessment of MI has largely replaced the use of CK isoenzyme assay by electrophoresis. CK-MB mass assays are more sensitive and rapid than electrophoresis. The evaluation of serial samples for CK-MB is highly recommended. ■

INDICATIONS:
* Assist in the diagnosis of acute MI and evaluate cardiac ischemia (CK-MB)

* Detect musculoskeletal disorders that do not have a neurologic basis, such as dermatomyositis or Duchenne's muscular dystrophy (CK-MM)

* Determine the success of coronary artery reperfusion after streptokinase infusion or percutaneous transluminal angioplasty, as evidenced by a decrease in CK-MB

RESULT

Increased in:
* Alcoholism
* Brain infarction (extensive)
* Congestive heart failure
* Delirium tremens
* Dermatomyositis
* Head injury
* Hypothyroidism
* Hypoxic shock
* Infectious diseases
* Gastrointestinal (GI) tract infarction
* Loss of blood supply to any muscle
* Malignant hyperthermia
* MI
* Muscular dystrophies
* Myocarditis
* Neoplasms of the prostate, bladder, and GI tract
* Polymyositis
* Pregnancy
* Prolonged hypothermia
* Pulmonary edema
* Pulmonary embolism
* Reye's syndrome
* Rhabdomyolysis
* Surgery
* Tachycardia
* Tetanus
* Trauma

Decreased in:
* Small stature
* Sedentary lifestyle

CRITICAL VALUES: N/A

INTERFERING FACTORS:
* Drugs that may increase total CK levels include any intramuscularly injected preparations because of tissue trauma caused by injection.

* Drugs that may decrease total CK levels include dantrolene and statins.

Nursing Implications and Procedure • • • • • • • • • •

Pretest:

> Inform the patient that the test is primarily used to assist in monitoring MI and some disorders of the musculoskeletal system.

> Obtain a history of the patient's complaints, including a list of known allergens (especially allergies or sensitivities to latex), and inform the appropriate health care practitioner accordingly.

> Obtain a history of the patient's cardiovascular and musculoskeletal systems, as well as results of previously performed laboratory tests, surgical procedures, and other diagnostic procedures. For related laboratory tests, refer to the Cardiovascular and Musculoskeletal System tables.

> Obtain a list of the medications the patient is taking, including herbs, nutritional supplements, and nutraceuticals. The requesting health care practitioner and laboratory should be advised if the patient is regularly using these products so that their effects can be taken into consideration when reviewing results.

> Review the procedure with the patient. Inform the patient that a series of samples will be required. (Samples at time of admission and 2 to 4 hours, 6 to 8 hours, and 12 hours after admission are the minimal recommendations. Additional samples may be requested.) Inform the patient that specimen collection takes approximately 5 to 10 minutes. Address concerns about pain related to the procedure. Explain to the patient that there may be some discomfort during the venipuncture.

> There are no food, fluid, or medication restrictions unless by medical direction.

Intratest:

> If the patient has a history of severe allergic reaction to latex, care should be taken to avoid the use of equipment containing latex.

> Instruct the patient to cooperate fully and to follow directions. Direct the patient to breathe normally and to avoid unnecessary movement.

> Observe standard precautions, and follow the general guidelines in Appendix A. Positively identify the patient, and label the appropriate tubes with the corresponding patient demographics, date, and time of collection. Perform a venipuncture; collect the specimen in a 5-mL red- or tiger-top tube.

> Remove the needle, and apply a pressure dressing over the puncture site.

> Promptly transport the specimen to the laboratory for processing and analysis.

> The results are recorded manually or in a computerized system for recall and postprocedure interpretation by the appropriate health care practitioner.

Post-test:

> Observe venipuncture site for bleeding or hematoma formation. Apply paper tape or other adhesive to hold pressure bandage in place, or replace with a plastic bandage.

> *Nutritional considerations:* Increased CK levels may be associated with coronary artery disease (CAD). Nutritional therapy is recommended for individuals identified to be at high risk for developing CAD. If overweight, the patient should be encouraged to achieve a normal weight. The American Heart Association Step 1 and Step 2 diets may be helpful in achieving a goal of lowering total cholesterol and triglyceride levels. The Step 1 diet emphasizes a reduction in foods high in saturated fats and cholesterol. Red meats, eggs, and dairy products are the major sources of saturated fats and cholesterol. If triglycerides are also elevated, the patient should be advised to eliminate or reduce alcohol and simple

carbohydrates from the diet. The Step 2 diet recommends stricter reductions.

➤ A written report of the examination will be sent to the requesting health care practitioner, who will discuss the results with the patient.

➤ Recognize anxiety related to test results, and be supportive of fear of shortened life expectancy. Discuss the implications of abnormal test results on the patient's lifestyle. Provide teaching and information regarding the clinical implications of the test results, as appropriate. Educate the patient regarding access to counseling services. Provide contact information, if desired, for the American Heart Association (http:// www.americanheart.org).

➤ Reinforce information given by the patient's health care provider regarding further testing, treatment, or referral to another health care provider. Answer any questions or address any concerns voiced by the patient or family.

➤ Depending on the results of this procedure, additional testing may be performed to evaluate or monitor progression of the disease process and determine the need for a change in therapy. Evaluate test results in relation to the patient's symptoms and other tests performed.

Related laboratory tests:

➤ Related laboratory tests include antiarrhythmic drugs, apolipoprotein A, apolipoprotein B, aspartate aminotransferase, atrial natriuretic peptide, blood gases, B-type natriuretic peptide, calcium (blood and ionized), cholesterol (total, HDL and LDL), C-reactive protein, glucose, glycated hemoglobin, homocysteine, ketones, lactate dehydrogenase and isoenzymes, lipoprotein electrophoresis, magnesium, myoglobin, pericardial fluid, potassium, triglycerides, and troponin.

CREATININE, BLOOD

SYNONYM/ACRONYM: N/A.

SPECIMEN: Serum (1 mL) collected in a red- or tiger-top tube. Plasma (1 mL) collected in green-top (heparin) tube is also acceptable.

REFERENCE VALUE: (Method: Spectrophotometry)

Age	Conventional Units	SI Units (Conventional Units × 88.4)
1–5 y	0.3–0.5 mg/dL	27–44 μmol/L
6–10 y	0.5–0.8 mg/dL	44–71 μmol/L
Adult male	0.6–1.2 mg/dL	53–106 μmol/L
Adult female	0.5–1.1 mg/dL	44–97 μmol/L

DESCRIPTION & RATIONALE: Creatinine is the end product of creatine metabolism. Creatine resides almost exclusively in skeletal muscle, where it participates in energy-requiring metabolic reactions. In these processes, a small amount of creatine is irreversibly converted to creatinine, which then circulates to the kidneys and is excreted. The amount of creatinine generated in an individual is proportional to the mass of skeletal muscle present and remains fairly constant, unless there is massive muscle damage resulting from crushing injury or degenerative muscle disease. Creatinine values also decrease with age owing to diminishing muscle mass. Blood urea nitrogen (BUN) is often ordered with creatinine for comparison. The BUN/creatinine ratio is also a useful indicator of disease. The ratio should be between 10:1 and 20:1. Creatinine is the ideal substance for determining renal clearance because a fairly constant quantity is produced within the body. The creatinine clearance test measures a blood sample and a urine sample to determine the rate at which the kidneys are clearing creatinine from the blood; this accurately reflects the glomerular filtration rate. (See monograph titled "Creatinine, Urine, and Creatinine Clearance, Urine" for additional information.) ∎

INDICATIONS:
- Assess a known or suspected disorder involving muscles in the absence of renal disease
- Evaluate known or suspected impairment of renal function

RESULT

Increased in:

- Acromegaly
- Congestive heart failure
- Dehydration
- Gigantism
- Hyperthyroidism
- Poliomyelitis
- Renal calculi
- Renal disease, acute and chronic renal failure
- Rhabdomyolysis
- Shock

Decreased in:
- Decreased muscle mass owing to debilitating disease or increasing age
- Inadequate protein intake
- Liver disease (severe)
- Muscular dystrophy
- Pregnancy
- Small stature

CRITICAL VALUES: ⚠

Potential critical value is greater than 7.4 mg/dL (nondialysis patient).

Note and immediately report to the health care practitioner any critically increased values and related symptoms. Chronic renal insufficiency is identified by creatinine levels between 1.5 and 3.0 mg/dL; chronic renal failure is present at levels greater than 3.0 mg/dL.

Possible interventions may include renal or peritoneal dialysis and organ transplant, but early discovery of the cause of elevated creatinine levels might avoid such drastic interventions.

INTERFERING FACTORS:
- Drugs and substances that may increase creatinine levels include acebutolol, acetaminophen (overdose), acetylsalicylic acid, aldatense, amikacin, amiodarone, amphotericin B, arginine,

arsenicals, ascorbic acid, asparaginase, barbiturates, capreomycin, captopril, carbutamide, carvedilol, cephalothin, chlorthalidone, cimetidine, cisplatin, clofibrate, colistin, corn oil (Lipomul), cyclosporine, dextran, doxycycline, enalapril, ethylene glycol, gentamicin, indomethacin, ipodate, kanamycin, levodopa, mannitol, methicillin, methoxyflurane, mitomycin, neomycin, netilmycin, nitrofurantoin, nonteroidal anti-inflammatory drugs, oxyphenbutazone, paromomycin, penicillin, pentamidine, phosphorus, plicamycin, radiographic agents, semustine, streptokinase, streptozocin, tetracycline, thiazides, tobramycin, triamterene, vancomycin, vasopressin, viomycin, and vitamin D.

- Drugs that may decrease creatinine levels include citrates, dopamine, ibuprofen, and lisinopril.

- High blood levels of bilirubin and glucose can cause false decreases in creatinine.

- A diet high in meat can cause increased creatinine levels.

- Ketosis can cause a significant increase in creatinine.

- Hemolyzed specimens are unsuitable for analysis.

Nursing Implications and Procedure . . . .

Pretest:

▷ Inform the patient that the test is used to assess kidney function.

▷ Obtain a history of the patient's complaints, including a list of known allergens (especially allergies or sensitivities to latex), and inform the appropriate health care practitioner accordingly.

▷ Obtain a history of the patient's genitourinary and musculoskeletal systems, as well as results of previously performed laboratory tests, surgical procedures, and other diagnostic procedures. For related laboratory tests, refer to the Genitourinary and Musculoskeletal System tables.

▷ Obtain a list of medications the patient is taking, including herbs, nutritional supplements, and nutraceuticals. The requesting health care practitioner and laboratory should be advised if the patient is regularly using these products so that their effects can be taken into consideration when reviewing results.

▷ Review the procedure with the patient. Inform the patient that specimen collection takes approximately 5 to 10 minutes. Address concerns about pain related to the procedure. Explain to the patient that there may be some discomfort during the venipuncture.

▷ *Sensitivity to social and cultural issues,* as well as concern for modesty, is important in providing psychological support before, during, and after the procedure.

▷ There are no food, fluid, or medication restrictions unless by medical direction.

▷ Instruct the patient to refrain from excessive exercise for 8 hours before the test.

Intratest:

▷ Ensure that the patient has complied with activity restrictions; assure that activity has been restricted for at least 8 hours prior to the procedure.

▷ If the patient has a history of severe allergic reaction to latex, care should be taken to avoid the use of equipment containing latex.

▷ Instruct the patient to cooperate fully and to follow directions. Direct the patient to breathe normally and to avoid unnecessary movement.

▷ Observe standard precautions, and follow the general guidelines in Appendix A. Positively identify the patient, and label the appropriate tubes with the corresponding patient demographics, date, and time of collection. Perform a venipuncture; collect the specimen in a 5-mL red- or tiger-top tube.

▶ Remove the needle, and apply a pressure dressing over the puncture site.

▶ Promptly transport the specimen to the laboratory for processing and analysis.

▶ The results are recorded manually or in a computerized system for recall and postprocedure interpretation by the appropriate health care practitioner.

Post-test:

▶ Observe venipuncture site for bleeding or hematoma formation. Apply paper tape or other adhesive to hold pressure bandage in place, or replace with a plastic bandage.

▶ Instruct the patient to resume usual activity as directed by the health care practitioner.

▶ *Nutritional considerations:* Increased creatinine levels may be associated with kidney disease. The nutritional needs of patients with kidney disease vary widely and are in constant flux. Anorexia, nausea, and vomiting commonly occur, prompting the need for continuous nutritional monitoring for malnutrition, especially among patients receiving long-term hemodialysis therapy.

▶ A written report of the examination will be sent to the requesting health care practitioner, who will discuss the results with the patient.

▶ Reinforce information given by the patient's health care provider regarding further testing, treatment, or referral to another health care provider. Answer any questions or address any concerns voiced by the patient or family.

▶ Depending on the results of this procedure, additional testing may be performed to evaluate or monitor progression of the disease process and determine the need for a change in therapy. Evaluate test results in relation to the patient's symptoms and other tests performed.

Related laboratory tests:

▶ Related laboratory tests include anion gap, BUN/creatinine ratio, creatinine clearance, electrolytes (blood and urine), gentamicin, kidney stone analysis, microalbumin, osmolality (blood and urine), tobramycin, urea nitrogen (blood and urine), uric acid (blood and urine), urine creatinine, and vancomycin.

CREATININE, URINE, AND CREATININE CLEARANCE, URINE

• •

SYNONYM/ACRONYM: N/A.

SPECIMEN: Urine (5 mL) from an unpreserved random or timed specimen collected in a clean plastic collection container.

REFERENCE VALUE: (Method: Spectrophotometry)

Age	Conventional Units	SI Units
Urine Creatinine (Conventional Units × 8.84)		
2–3 y	6–22 mg/kg/24 h	53–194 µmol/kg/24 h
4–18 y	12–30 mg/kg/24 h	106–265 µmol/kg/24 h
Adult male	14–26 mg/kg/24 h	124–230 µmol/kg/24 h
Adult female	11–20 mg/kg/24 h	97–177 µmol/kg/24 h
Creatinine Clearance (Conventional Units × 0.0167)		
Children	70–140 mL/min/1.73 m^2	1.17–2.33 mL/s/1.73 m^2
Adult male	85–125 mL/min/1.73 m^2	1.42–2.08 mL/s/1.73 m^2
Adult female	75–115 mL/min/1.73 m^2	1.25–1.92 mL/s/1.73 m^2
For each decade after 40 y	Decrease of 6–7 mL/min/ 1.73 m^2	Decrease of 0.06–0.07 mL/s/1.73 m^2

DESCRIPTION & RATIONALE: Creatinine is the end product of creatine metabolism. Creatine resides almost exclusively in skeletal muscle, where it participates in energy-requiring metabolic reactions. In these processes, a small amount of creatine is irreversibly converted to creatinine, which then circulates to the kidneys and is excreted. The amount of creatinine generated in an individual is proportional to the mass of skeletal muscle present and remains fairly constant, unless there is massive muscle damage resulting from crushing injury or degenerative muscle disease. Creatinine values decrease with advancing age owing to diminishing muscle mass. Although the measurement of urine creatinine is an effective indicator of renal function, the creatinine clearance test is more precise. The creatinine clearance test measures a blood sample and a urine sample to determine the rate at which the kidneys are clearing creatinine from the blood; this accurately reflects the glomerular filtration rate and is based on an estimate of body surface. ■

INDICATIONS:
- Determine the extent of nephron damage in known renal disease (at least 50% of functioning nephrons must be lost before values are decreased)

- Determine renal function before administering nephrotoxic drugs

- Evaluate accuracy of a 24-hour urine collection, based on the constant level of creatinine excretion

- Evaluate glomerular function

- Monitor effectiveness of treatment in renal disease

RESULT

Increased in:
- Acromegaly

- Acute tubular necrosis

- Carnivorous diets

- Congestive heart failure

- Dehydration

- Diabetes

- Exercise

- Exposure to nephrotoxic drugs and chemicals

- Gigantism
- Glomerulonephritis
- Hypothyroidism
- Infections
- Neoplasms (bilateral renal)
- Nephrosclerosis
- Polycystic kidney disease
- Pyelonephritis
- Renal artery atherosclerosis
- Renal artery obstruction
- Renal disease
- Renal vein thrombosis
- Shock and hypovolemia
- Tuberculosis

Decreased in:

- Acute or chronic glomerulonephritis
- Anemia
- Chronic bilateral pyelonephritis
- Hyperthyroidism
- Leukemia
- Muscle wasting diseases
- Paralysis
- Polycystic kidney disease
- Shock
- Urinary tract obstruction (e.g., from calculi)
- Vegetarian diets

CRITICAL VALUES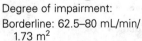

Degree of impairment:
Borderline: 62.5–80 mL/min/ 1.73 m²
Slight: 52–62.5 mL/min/1.73 m²
Mild: 42–52 mL/min/1.73 m²
Moderate: 28–42 mL/min/1.73 m²
Marked: Less than 28 mL/min/ 1.73 m²

Note and immediately report to the health care practitioner any critically increased values and related symptoms.

INTERFERING FACTORS:

- Drugs that may increase urine creatinine levels include ascorbic acid, cefoxitin, cephalothin, corticosteroids, fluoxymesterone, levodopa, methandrostenolone, methotrexate, methyldopa, nitrofurans (including nitrofurazone), oxymetholone, phenolphthalein, and prednisone.

- Drugs that may increase urine creatinine clearance include enalapril, oral contraceptives, prednisone, and ramipril.

- Drugs that may decrease urine creatinine levels include anabolic steroids, androgens, captopril, and thiazides.

- Drugs that may decrease the urine creatinine clearance include acetylsalicylic acid, amphotericin B, carbenoxolone, chlorthalidone, cimetidine, cisplatin, cyclosporine, guancidine, ibuprofen, indomethacin, mitomycin, oxyphenbutazone, paromycin, probenecid (coadministered with digoxin), and thiazides.

- Excessive ketones in urine may cause falsely decreased values.

- Failure to follow proper technique in collecting 24-hour specimen may invalidate test results.

- Failure to refrigerate specimen throughout urine collection period allows decomposition of creatinine, causing falsely decreased values.

- Consumption of large amounts of meat, excessive exercise, and stress should be avoided for 24 hours before the test.

- Failure to follow dietary restrictions before the procedure may cause the procedure to be canceled or repeated.

Nursing Implications and Procedure • • • • • • • • • • •

Pretest:

➤ Inform the patient that the test is used to assess renal function.

➤ Obtain a history of the patient's complaints, including a list of known allergens (especially allergies or sensitivities to latex), and inform the appropriate health care practitioner accordingly.

➤ Obtain a history of the patient's genitourinary system and results of previously performed laboratory tests, surgical procedures, and other diagnostic procedures. For related laboratory tests, refer to the Genitourinary System table.

➤ Obtain a list of medications the patient is taking, including herbs, nutritional supplements, and nutraceuticals. The requesting health care practitioner and laboratory should be advised if the patient regularly uses these products so that their effects can be taken into consideration when reviewing results.

➤ Review the procedure with the patient. Provide a nonmetallic urinal, bedpan, or toilet-mounted collection device. Address concerns about pain related to the procedure. Explain to the patient that there should be no discomfort during the procedure.

➤ Usually a 24-hour time frame for urine collection is ordered. Inform the patient that all urine must be saved during that 24-hour period. Instruct the patient not to void directly into the laboratory collection container. Instruct the patient to avoid defecating in the collection device and to keep toilet tissue out of the collection device to prevent contamination of the specimen. Place a sign in the bathroom to remind the patient to save all urine.

➤ Instruct the patient to void all urine into the collection device and then to pour the urine into the laboratory collection container. Alternatively, the specimen can be left in the collection device for a health care staff member to add to the laboratory collection container.

➤ *Sensitivity to social and cultural issues,* as well as concern for modesty, is important in providing psychological support before, during, and after the procedure.

➤ There are no fluid or medication restrictions unless by medical direction.

➤ Instruct the patient to refrain from eating meat during the test.

Intratest:

➤ Ensure that the patient has complied with dietary and activity restrictions for 24 hours prior to the procedure; assure that ingestion of meat has been restricted during the test.

➤ If the patient has a history of severe allergic reaction to latex, care should be taken to avoid the use of equipment containing latex.

➤ Instruct the patient to cooperate fully and to follow directions.

➤ Observe standard precautions, and follow the general guidelines in Appendix A. Positively identify the patient, and label the appropriate collection container with the corresponding patient demographics, date, and time of collection.

Random specimen (collect in early morning)

Clean-catch specimen:

➤ Instruct the male patient to (1) thoroughly wash his hands, (2) cleanse the meatus, (3) void a small amount into the toilet, and (4) void directly into the specimen container.

➤ Instruct the female patient to (1) thoroughly wash her hands; (2) cleanse the labia from front to back; (3) while keeping the labia separated, void a small amount into the toilet; and (4) without interrupting the urine stream, void directly into the specimen container.

Pediatric urine collector:

➤ Put on gloves. Appropriately cleanse the genital area and allow the area to dry. Remove the covering over the adhesive strips on the collector bag and apply over the genital area. Diaper the child. When specimen is obtained, place the entire collection bag in a sterile urine container.

Indwelling catheter:

➤ Put on gloves. Empty drainage tube of urine. It may be necessary to clamp off the catheter for 15 to 30 minutes before specimen collection. Cleanse specimen port with antiseptic swab, and then aspirate 5 mL of urine with a 21- to 25-gauge needle and syringe. Transfer urine to a sterile container.

Urinary catheterization:

➤ Place female patient in lithotomy position or male patient in supine position. Using sterile technique, open the straight urinary catheterization kit and perform urinary catheterization. Place the retained urine in a sterile specimen container.

Suprapubic aspiration:

➤ Place the patient in a supine position. Cleanse the area with antiseptic and drape with sterile drapes. A needle is inserted through the skin into the bladder. A syringe attached to the needle is used to aspirate the urine sample. The needle is then removed and a sterile dressing is applied to the site. Place the sterile sample in a sterile specimen container.

➤ Do not collect urine from the pouch from the patient with a urinary diversion (e.g., ilieal conduit). Instead, perform catheterization through the stoma.

Timed specimen:

➤ Obtain a clean 3-L urine specimen container, toilet-mounted collection device, and plastic bag (for transport of the specimen container). The specimen must be refrigerated or kept on ice throughout the entire collection period. If an indwelling urinary catheter is in place, the drainage bag must be kept on ice.

➤ Begin the test between 6 and 8 a.m., if possible. Collect first voiding and discard. Record the time the specimen was discarded as the beginning of the timed collection period. The next morning, ask the patient to void at the same time the collection was started and add this last voiding to the container.

➤ If an indwelling catheter is in place, replace the tubing and container system at the start of the collection time. Keep the container system on ice during the collection period, or empty the urine into a larger container periodically during the collection period; monitor to ensure continued drainage, and conclude the test the next morning at the same hour the collection was begun.

➤ At the conclusion of the test, compare the quantity of urine with the urinary output record for the collection; if the specimen contains less than what was recorded as output, some urine may have been discarded, invalidating the test.

➤ Include on the collection container's label the amount of urine, test start and stop times, and any foods or medications that can affect test results.

➤ Promptly transport the specimen to the laboratory for processing and analysis.

➤ The results are recorded manually or in a computerized system for recall and postprocedure interpretation by the appropriate health care practitioner.

Post-test:

➤ Instruct the patient to resume usual diet, medications, or activity, as directed by the health care practitioner.

➤ A written report of the examination will be sent to the requesting health care practitioner, who will discuss the results with the patient.

➤ Recognize anxiety related to test results. Discuss the implications of abnormal test results on the patient's lifestyle. Provide teaching and information regarding the clinical implications of the test results, as appropriate. Educate the patient regarding access to counseling services. Provide contact information, if desired, for the National Kidney Foundation *(http://www.kidney.org)*.

➤ Reinforce information given by the patient's health care provider regarding further testing, treatment, or referral to another health care provider. Answer any questions or address any concerns voiced by the patient or family.

➤ Depending on the results of this procedure, additional testing may be performed to evaluate or monitor progression of the disease process and determine the need for a change in therapy. Evaluate test results in relation to the patient's symptoms and other tests performed.

Related laboratory tests:

➤ Related laboratory tests include anion gap, blood urea nitrogen (BUN), BUN/creatinine ratio, creatinine, electrolytes (blood and urine), gentamicin, kidney stone analysis, microalbumin, osmolality (blood and urine), tobramycin, urea nitrogen (blood and urine), uric acid (blood and urine), and vancomycin.

CRYOGLOBULIN

. . . .

SYNONYMS/ACRONYM: Cryo.

SPECIMEN: Serum (1 mL) collected in a red-top tube.

REFERENCE VALUE: (Method: Visual observation for changes in appearance) Negative.

DESCRIPTION & RATIONALE: Cryoglobulins are abnormal serum proteins that cannot be detected by protein electrophoresis. Cryoglobulins cause vascular problems because they can precipitate in the blood vessels of the fingers when exposed to cold, causing Raynaud's phenomenon. They are usually associated with immunologic disease. The laboratory procedure to detect cryoglobulins is a two-step process. The serum sample is observed

for cold precipitation after 72 hours of storage at 4°C. True cryoglobulins disappear on warming to room temperature, so in the second step of the procedure, the sample is rewarmed to confirm reversibility of the reaction. ∎

INDICATIONS:

• Assist in diagnosis of neoplastic diseases, acute and chronic infections, and collagen diseases

• Detect cryoglobulinemia in patients

with symptoms indicating or mimicking Raynaud's disease

- Monitor course of collagen and rheumatic disorders

RESULT

Increased in:

- Type I cryoglobulin (monoclonal)
  Chronic lymphocytic leukemia
  Lymphoma
  Multiple myeloma

- Type II cryoglobulin (mixtures of monoclonal immunoglobulin [Ig] M and polyclonal IgG)
  Autoimmune hepatitis
  Rheumatoid arthritis
  Sjögren's syndrome
  Waldenström's macroglobulinemia

- Type III cryoglobulin (mixtures of polyclonal IgM and IgG)
  Acute poststreptococcal glomerulonephritis
  Chronic infection (especially hepatitis C)
  Cirrhosis
  Endocarditis
  Infectious mononucleosis
  Polymyalgia rheumatica
  Rheumatoid arthritis
  arcoidosis
  Systemic lupus erythematosus

Decreased in: N/A

CRITICAL VALUES: N/A

INTERFERING FACTORS:

- Testing the sample prematurely (before total precipitation) may yield incorrect results.

- Failure to maintain sample at normal body temperature before centrifugation can affect results.

- A recent fatty meal can increase turbidity of the blood, decreasing visibility.

Nursing Implications and Procedure • • • • • • • • • • •

Pretest:

➤ Inform the patient that the test is primarily used to assist in identification the presence of certain immunologic disorders.

➤ Obtain a history of the patient's complaints, including a list of known allergens (especially allergies or sensitivities to latex), and inform the appropriate health care practitioner accordingly.

➤ Obtain a history of the patient's immune system as well as results of previously performed laboratory tests, surgical procedures, and other diagnostic procedures. For related laboratory tests, refer to the Immune System table.

➤ Obtain a list of the medications the patient is taking, including herbs, nutritional supplements, and nutraceuticals. The requesting health care practitioner and laboratory should be advised if the patient regularly uses these products so that their effects can be taken into consideration when reviewing results.

➤ Review the procedure with the patient. Inform the patient that specimen collection takes approximately 5 to 10 minutes. Address concerns about pain related to the procedure. Explain to the patient that there may be some discomfort during the venipuncture.

➤ There are no food, fluid, or medication restrictions unless by medical direction.

Intratest:

➤ If the patient has a history of severe allergic reaction to latex, care should be taken to avoid the use of equipment containing latex.

➤ Instruct the patient to cooperate fully and to follow directions. Direct the patient to breathe normally and to avoid unnecessary movement.

➤ Observe standard precautions, and follow the general guidelines in

Appendix A. Positively identify the patient, and label the appropriate tubes with the corresponding patient demographics, date, and time of collection. Perform a venipuncture; collect the specimen in a 5-mL red-top tube.

➤ Remove the needle, and apply a pressure dressing over the puncture site.

➤ Promptly transport the specimen to the laboratory for processing and analysis.

➤ The results are recorded manually or in a computerized system for recall and postprocedure interpretation by the appropriate health care practitioner.

➤ Observe venipuncture site for bleeding or hematoma formation. Apply paper tape or other adhesive to hold pressure bandage in place, or replace with a plastic bandage.

➤ A written report of the examination will be sent to the requesting health care practitioner, who will discuss the results with the patient.

➤ Reinforce information given by the patient's health care provider regarding further testing, treatment, or referral to another health care provider. Answer any questions or address any concerns voiced by the patient or family.

➤ Depending on the results of this procedure, additional testing may be performed to evaluate or monitor progression of the disease process and determine the need for a change in therapy. Evaluate test results in relation to the patient's symptoms and other tests performed.

Related laboratory tests: ▮

➤ Related laboratory tests include antinuclear antibody, hepatitis C antibody, IgA, IgG, IgM, immunofixation electrophoresis, protein, protein electrophoresis, and rheumatoid factor.

CULTURE AND SMEAR, MYCOBACTERIA

. . . .

SYNONYMS/ACRONYMS: Acid-fast bacilli (AFB) culture and smear, tuberculosis (TB) culture and smear, *Mycobacterium* culture and smear.

SPECIMEN: Sputum (5 to 10 mL), bronchopulmonary lavage, tissue, material from fine-needle aspiration.

REFERENCE VALUE: (Method: Culture on selected media, microscopic examination of sputum by acid-fast or auramine-rhodamine fluorochrome stain) Rapid methods include: chemiluminescent-labeled DNA probes that target ribosomal RNA of the *Mycobacterium*, radiometric carbon dioxide detection from ^{14}C-labeled media, polymerase chain reaction/amplification techniques.

Culture: No growth
Smear: Negative for AFB

DESCRIPTION & RATIONALE: A culture and smear test is used primarily to detect *Mycobacterium tuberculosis,* which is a tubercular bacillus. The cell wall of this mycobacterium contains complex lipids and waxes that do not take up ordinary stains. Cells that resist decolorization by acid alcohol are termed acid fast. There are only a few groups of *acid-fast* bacilli (AFB); this characteristic is helpful in rapid identification so that therapy can be initiated in a timely manner. Smears may be negative 50% of the time even though the culture develops positive growth 3 to 8 weeks later. AFB cultures are used to confirm positive and negative AFB smears. *M. tuberculosis* grows in culture slowly. Automated liquid culture systems, such as the Bactec and MGIT (Becton Dickinson and Company, 1 Becton Drive, Franklin Lakes, NJ, 07417), have a turnaround time of approximately 10 days. Results of tests by polymerase chain reaction culture methods are available in 36 to 48 hours.

M. tuberculosis is transmitted via the airborne route to the lungs. It causes areas of granulomatous inflammation, cough, fever, and hemoptysis. It can remain dormant in the lungs for long periods. The incidence of tuberculosis has increased since the late 1980s in depressed inner-city areas, among prison populations, and among human immunodeficiency virus (HIV)–positive patients. Of great concern is the increase in antibiotic-resistant strains of *M. tuberculosis.* HIV-positive patients often become ill from concomitant infections caused by *M. tuberculosis* and *Mycobacterium avium intracellulare. M. avium intracellulare* is acquired via the gastrointestinal tract through ingestion of contaminated food or water. The organism's waxy cell wall protects it from acids in the human digestive tract. Isolation of mycobacteria in the stool does not mean the patient has tuberculosis of the intestines because mycobacteria in stool are most often present in sputum that has been swallowed. ∎

INDICATIONS:

- Assist in the diagnosis of mycobacteriosis

- Assist in the diagnosis of suspected pulmonary tuberculosis secondary to acquired immunodeficiency syndrome (AIDS)

- Assist in the differentiation of tuberculosis from carcinoma or bronchiectasis

- Investigate suspected pulmonary tuberculosis

- Monitor the response to treatment for pulmonary tuberculosis

RESULT

Identified Organism	Primary Specimen Source	Condition
Mycobacterium avium intracellulare	Sputum	Opportunistic pulmonary infection
M. fortuitum	Surgical wound, sputum	Opportunistic infection (usually pulmonary)

Identified Organism	Primary Specimen Source	Condition
M. kansasii	Sputum	Pulmonary tuberculosis
M. tuberculosis	Sputum	Pulmonary tuberculosis
M. xenopi	Sputum	Pulmonary tuberculosis

CRITICAL VALUES:

Smear: Positive for AFB

Culture: Growth of pathogenic bacteria

Note and immediately report to the health care practitioner positive results and related symptoms.

INTERFERING FACTORS:

• Specimen collection after initiation of treatment with antituberculosis drug therapy may result in inhibited or no growth of organisms.

• Contamination of the sterile container with organisms from an exogenous source may produce misleading results.

• Specimens received on a dry swab should be rejected: A dry swab indicates that the sample is unlikely to have been collected properly or unlikely to contain a representative quantity of significant organisms for proper evaluation.

• Inadequate or improper (e.g., saliva) samples should be rejected.

• Failure to follow dietary restrictions before the procedure may cause the procedure to be canceled or repeated.

Nursing Implications and Procedure ● ● ● ● ● ● ● ● ● ● ●

Pretest:

➤ Inform the patient that the test is primarily used to assist in the diagnosis of tuberculosis.

➤ Obtain a history of the patient's complaints, including a list of known allergens (especially allergies or sensitivities to latex), and inform the appropriate health care practitioner accordingly. Obtain a history of the patient's exposure to tuberculosis.

➤ Obtain a history of the patient's immune and respiratory systems, and results of previously performed laboratory tests, surgical procedures, and other diagnostic procedures. For related laboratory tests, refer to the Immune and Respiratory System tables.

➤ Obtain a list of medications the patient is taking, including herbs, nutritional supplements, and nutraceuticals. The requesting health care practitioner and laboratory should be advised if the patient is regularly using these products so that their effects can be taken into consideration when reviewing results.

➤ Note any recent procedures that can interfere with test results.

➤ Review the procedure with the patient. Reassure the patient that he or she will be able to breathe during the procedure if specimen collected is accomplished via suction method. Ensure that oxygen has been administered 20 to 30 minutes before the procedure if the specimen is to be obtained by tracheal suctioning. Address concerns about pain related to the procedure. Atropine is usually given before bronchoscopy examinations to reduce bronchial secretions and prevent vagally induced bradycardia. Meperidine (Demerol) or morphine may be given as a sedative. Lidocaine is sprayed in the patient's throat to reduce discomfort caused by the presence of the tube.

➤ Explain to the patient that the time it takes to collect a proper specimen varies according to the level of cooperation of the patient and the specimen collection site. Emphasize that sputum and saliva are not the same. Inform the patient that multiple specimens may be required at timed intervals. Inform the patient that the culture results will not be reported for 3 to 8 weeks.

➤ *Sensitivity to social and cultural issues,* as well as concern for modesty, is important in providing psychological support before, during, and after the procedure.

Bronchoscopy:

➤ *Make sure a written and informed consent has been signed prior to the procedure and before administering any medications.*

➤ Other than antimicrobial drugs, there are no medication restrictions, unless by medical direction.

➤ The patient should fast and refrain from drinking liquids beginning at midnight the night before the procedure.

Expectorated specimen:

➤ Additional liquids the night before may assist in liquefying secretions during expectoration the following morning.

➤ Assist the patient with oral cleaning before sample collection to reduce the amount of sample contamination by organisms that normally inhabit the mouth.

➤ Instruct the patient not to touch the edge or inside of the container with the hands or mouth.

➤ Other than antimicrobial drugs, there are no medication restrictions, unless by medical direction.

➤ There are no food or fluid restrictions, unless by medical direction.

Tracheal Suctioning:

➤ Assist in providing extra fluids, unless contraindicated, and proper humidification to decrease tenacious secretions. Inform the patient that increasing fluid intake before retiring on the night before the test aids in liquefying secretions and may make it easier to expectorate in the morning. Also explain that humidifying inspired air also helps liquefy secretions.

➤ Other than antimicrobial drugs, there are no medication restrictions, unless by medical direction.

➤ There are no food or fluid restrictions, unless by medical direction.

Intratest:

➤ Ensure that the patient has complied with dietary and medication restrictions; assure that food and fluids have been restricted for at least 12 hours prior to the bronchoscopy procedure.

➤ Have patient remove dentures, contact lenses, eyeglasses, and jewelry. Notify the physician if the patient has permanent crowns on teeth. Have the patient remove clothing and change into a gown for the procedure.

➤ Have emergency equipment readily available. Keep resuscitation equipment on hand in case of respiratory impairment or laryngospasm after the procedure.

➤ Avoid using morphine sulfate in patients with asthma or other pulmonary disease. This drug can further exacerbate bronchospasms and respiratory impairment.

➤ If the patient has a history of severe allergic reaction to latex, care should be taken to avoid the use of equipment containing latex.

➤ Assist the patient to a comfortable position, and direct the patient to breath normally during the beginning of the local anesthesia. Instruct the patient to cooperate fully and to follow directions. Direct the patient to breathe normally and to avoid unnecessary movement during the local anesthetic and the procedure.

➤ Observe standard precautions, and follow the general guidelines in Appendix A. Positively identify the patient, and label the appropriate collection container with the corresponding patient demographics, date and time of collection, and any medication the patient is taking that may interfere with test results (e.g., antibiotics).

Bronchoscopy:

➤ Record baseline vital signs.

➤ The patient is positioned in relation to the type of anesthesia being used. If local anesthesia is used, the patient is seated and the tongue and oropharynx are sprayed and swabbed with anesthetic before the bronchoscope is inserted. For general anesthesia, the patient is placed in a supine position with the neck hyperextended. After anesthesia, the patient is kept in supine or shifted to a side-lying position and the bronchoscope is inserted. After inspection, the samples are collected from suspicious sites by bronchial brush or biopsy forceps.

Expectorated specimen:

➤ Ask the patient to sit upright, with assistance and support (e.g., with an overbed table) as needed.

➤ Ask the patient to take two or three deep breaths and cough deeply. Any sputum raised should be expectorated directly into a sterile sputum collection container.

➤ If the patient is unable to produce the desired amount of sputum, several strategies may be attempted. One approach is to have the patient drink two glasses of water, and then assume the position for postural drainage of the upper and middle lung segments. Effective coughing may be assisted by placing either the hands or a pillow over the diaphragmatic area and applying slight pressure.

➤ Another approach is to place a vaporizer or other humidifying device at the bedside. After sufficient exposure to adequate humidification, postural drainage of the upper and middle lung segments may be repeated before attempting to obtain the specimen.

➤ Other methods may include obtaining an order for an expectorant to be administered with additional water approximately 2 hours before attempting to obtain the specimen. Chest percussion and postural drainage of all lung segments may also be employed. If the patient is still unable to raise sputum, the use of an ultrasonic nebulizer ("induced sputum") may be necessary; this is usually done by a respiratory therapist.

Tracheal suctioning:

➤ Obtain the necessary equipment, including a suction device, suction kit, and Lukens tube or in-line trap.

➤ Position the patient with head elevated as high as tolerated.

➤ Put on sterile gloves. Maintain the dominant hand as sterile and the nondominant hand as clean.

➤ Using the sterile hand, attach the suction catheter to the rubber tubing of the Lukens tube or in-line trap. Then attach the suction tubing to the male adapter of the trap with the clean hand. Lubricate the suction catheter with sterile saline.

➤ Tell nonintubated patients to protrude the tongue and to take a deep breath as the suction catheter is passed through the nostril. When the catheter enters the trachea, a reflex cough is stimulated; immediately advance the catheter into the trachea and apply suction. Maintain suction for approximately 10 seconds, but never longer than 15 seconds. Withdraw the catheter without applying suction. Separate the suction catheter and suction tubing from the trap, and place the rubber tubing over the male adapter to seal the unit.

➤ For intubated patients or patients with a tracheostomy, the previous procedure is followed except that the suction catheter is passed through the existing endotracheal or tracheostomy tube rather than through the nostril. The patient should be hyperoxygenated before and after the procedure in accordance with standard protocols for suctioning these patients.

➤ Generally, a series of three to five early morning sputum samples are collected in sterile containers. If leprosy is suspected, obtain a smear from nasal scrapings or a biopsy specimen from lesions in a sterile container.

General:

➤ Monitor the patient for complications related to the procedure (e.g., allergic reaction, anaphylaxis, bronchospasm).

➤ Promptly transport the specimen to the laboratory for processing and analysis.

➤ The results are recorded manually or in a computerized system for recall and postprocedure interpretation by the appropriate health care practitioner.

Post-test:

➤ Instruct the patient to resume preoperative diet, as directed by the health care practitioner. Assess the patient's ability to swallow before allowing the patient to attempt liquids or solid foods.

➤ Inform the patient that he or she may experience some throat soreness and hoarseness. Instruct patient to treat throat discomfort with lozenges and warm gargles when the gag reflex returns.

➤ Monitor vital signs and compare with baseline values every 15 minutes for 1 hour, then every 2 hours for 4 hours, and then as ordered by the health care practitioner. Monitor temperature every 4 hours for 24 hours. Notify the health care practitioner if temperature is elevated. Protocols may vary from facility to facility.

➤ Emergency resuscitation equipment should be readily available if the vocal cords become spastic after intubation.

➤ Observe for delayed allergic reactions, such as rash, urticaria, tachycardia, hyperpnea, hypertension, palpitations, nausea, or vomiting.

➤ Observe the patient for hemoptysis, difficulty breathing, cough, air hunger, excessive coughing, pain, or absent breathing sounds over the affected area. Report any symptoms to the health care provider.

➤ Evaluate the patient for symptoms indicating the development of pneumothorax, such as dyspnea, tachypnea, anxiety, decreased breathing sounds, or restlessness. A chest x-ray may be ordered to check for the presence of this complication.

➤ Evaluate the patient for symptoms of empyema, such as fever, tachycardia, malaise, or elevated white blood cell count.

➤ Administer antibiotic therapy if ordered. Remind the patient of the importance of completing the entire course of antibiotic therapy, even if signs and symptoms disappear before completion of therapy.

➤ *Nutritional considerations:* Malnutrition is commonly seen in patients with severe respiratory disease for numerous reasons, including fatigue, lack of appetite, and gastrointestinal distress. Adequate intake of vitamins A and C are also important to prevent pulmonary infection and to decrease the extent of lung tissue damage.

➤ A written report of the examination will be completed by a health care practitioner specializing in this branch of medicine. The report will be sent to the requesting health care practitioner, who will discuss the results with the patient.

➤ Recognize anxiety related to test results. Discuss the implications of abnormal test results on the patient's lifestyle. Provide teaching and information regarding the clinical implications of the test results, as appropriate. Educate the patient regarding access to counseling services.

▶ Reinforce information given by the patient's health care provider regarding further testing, treatment, or referral to another health care provider. Instruct the patient to use lozenges or gargle for throat discomfort. Inform the patient of smoking cessation programs as appropriate. The importance of following the prescribed diet should be stressed to the patient/caregiver. Educate the patient regarding access to counseling services, as appropriate. Answer any questions or address any concerns voiced by the patient or family.

▶ Instruct the patient in the use of any ordered medications. Explain the importance of adhering to the therapy regimen. As appropriate, instruct the patient in significant side effects and systemic reactions associated with the prescribed medication. Encourage him or her to review corresponding literature provided by a pharmacist.

▶ Depending on the results of this procedure, additional testing may be needed to evaluate or monitor progression of the disease process and determine the need for a change in therapy. Evaluate test results in relation to the patient's symptoms and other tests performed.

Related laboratory tests:

▶ Related laboratory tests include anti–glomerular basement membrane antibody, arterial/alveolar oxygen ratio, blood gases, chest x-ray, complete blood count, computed tomography of the thorax, lung scan, magnetic resonance imaging of the chest, culture, Gram/acid-fast stain, cytology, and sputum findings.

CULTURE, BACTERIAL, ANAL/GENITAL, EAR, EYE, SKIN, AND WOUND

• •

SYNONYM/ACRONYM: N/A.

SPECIMEN: Sterile fluid or swab from affected area placed in transport media tube provided by laboratory.

REFERENCE VALUE: (Method: Culture aerobic and/or anaerobic on selected media; DNA probe assays are available for identification of *Neisseria gonorrhoeae*.) Negative: no growth of pathogens.

DESCRIPTION & RATIONALE: When indicated by patient history, anal cultures may be performed to isolate the organism responsible for sexually transmitted disease.

Ear and eye cultures are performed to isolate the organism responsible for chronic or acute infectious disease of the ear and eye.

Skin and soft tissue samples from infected sites must be collected carefully to avoid contamination from the surrounding normal skin flora. Skin and tissue infections may be caused by both aerobic and anaerobic organisms. Therefore, a portion of the sample should be placed in aerobic and a portion in anaerobic transport media. Care must be taken to use transport media that are approved by the laboratory performing the testing.

A wound culture involves collecting a specimen of exudates, drainage, or tissue so that the causative organism can be isolated and pathogens identified. Specimens can be obtained from superficial and deep wounds.

Optimally, specimens should be obtained before antibiotic use. The method used to culture and grow the organism depends on the suspected infectious organism. There are transport media specifically for bacterial agents. The laboratory will select the appropriate media for suspect organisms. The laboratory will initiate antibiotic sensitivity testing if indicated by test results. Sensitivity testing identifies the antibiotics to which organisms are susceptible to ensure an effective treatment plan. ▪

INDICATIONS

Anal/genital:

- Assist in the diagnosis of sexually transmitted diseases

- Determine the cause of genital itching or purulent drainage

- Determine effective antimicrobial therapy specific to the identified pathogen

Ear:

- Isolate and identify organisms responsible for ear pain, drainage, or changes in hearing

- Isolate and identify organisms responsible for outer-, middle-, or inner-ear infection

- Determine effective antimicrobial therapy specific to the identified pathogen

Eye:

- Isolate and identify pathogenic microorganisms responsible for infection of the eye

- Determine effective antimicrobial therapy specific to identified pathogen

Skin:

- Isolate and identify organisms responsible for skin eruptions, drainage, or other evidence of infection

- Determine effective antimicrobial therapy specific to the identified pathogen

Sterile fluids:

- Isolate and identify organisms before surrounding tissue becomes infected

- Determine effective antimicrobial therapy specific to the identified pathogen

Wound:

- Detect abscess or deep-wound infectious process

- Determine if an infectious agent is the cause of wound redness, warmth, or edema with drainage at a site

- Determine presence of infectious agents in a stage 3 and stage 4 decubitus ulcer

- Isolate and identify organisms responsible for the presence of pus or other exudate in an open wound

• Determine effective antimicrobial therapy specific to the identified pathogen

RESULT

Positive findings in:

Anal/Endocervical/Genital

Infections or carrier states are caused by the following organisms: *Gardnerella vaginalis, N. gonorrhoeae,* toxin-producing strains of *Staphylococcus aureus,* and *Treponema pallidum.*

Ear

Commonly identified organisms include *Escherichia coli, Proteus* spp., *Pseudomonas aeruginosa, Staphylococcus aureus,* and β-hemolytic streptococci.

Eye

Commonly identified organisms include *Haemophilus influenzae, H. aegyptius, N. gonorrhoeae, Pseudomonas aeruginosa, Staphylococcus aureus,* and *Streptococcus pneumoniae.*

Skin

Commonly identified organisms include *Bacteroides, Clostridium, Corynebacterium, Pseudomonas,* staphylococci, and group A streptococci.

Sterile fluids

Commonly identified pathogens include *Bacteroides, Enterococcus* spp., *E. coli, Pseudomonas aeruginosa,* and *Peptostreptococcus* spp.

Wound

Aerobic and anaerobic microorganisms can be identified in wound culture specimens. Commonly identified organisms include *Clostridium perfringens, Klebsiella, Proteus, Pseudomonas, Staphylococcus aureus,* and group A streptococci.

CRITICAL VALUES: N/A

INTERFERING FACTORS:

• Failure to collect adequate specimen, improper collection or storage technique, and failure to transport specimen in a timely fashion are causes for specimen rejection.

• Pretest antimicrobial therapy will delay or inhibit the growth of pathogens.

• Testing specimens more than 1 hour after collection may result in decreased growth or nongrowth of organisms.

Nursing Implications and Procedure • • • • • • • • • • •

Pretest:

➤ Inform the patient that the test is used to identify pathogenic bacterial organisms.

➤ Obtain a history of the patient's complaints, including a list of known allergens, and inform the appropriate health care practitioner accordingly.

➤ Obtain a history of the patient's immune system and results of previously performed laboratory tests, surgical procedures, and other diagnostic procedures. Obtain, as appropriate, a history of sexual activity. For related laboratory tests, refer to the Immune System table.

➤ Obtain a list of the medications the patient is taking, including herbs, nutritional supplements, and nutraceuticals. The requesting health care practitioner and laboratory should be advised if the patient regularly uses these products so that their effects can be taken into consideration when reviewing results.

➤ Note any recent medications that can interfere with test results.

➤ Review the procedure with the patient. Inform the patient that specimen collection takes approximately 5 minutes. Address concerns about pain related to the procedure. Explain to the patient that there may be some discomfort during the specimen collection. Instruct female patients not to douche for 24 hours before a cervical or vaginal specimen is to be obtained.

➤ *Sensitivity to social and cultural issues,* as well as concern for modesty, is important in providing psychological support before, during, and after the procedure.

➤ There are no food or fluid restrictions unless by medical direction.

Intratest:

➤ Ensure that the patient has complied with medication restrictions prior to the procedure.

➤ Instruct the patient to cooperate fully and to follow directions. Direct the patient to breathe normally and to avoid unnecessary movement.

➤ Observe standard precautions, and follow the general guidelines in Appendix A. Positively identify the patient, and label the appropriate specimen containers with the corresponding patient demographics, specimen source (left or right as appropriate), patient age and gender, date and time of collection, and any medication the patient is taking that may interfere with the test results (e.g. antibiotics). Do not freeze the specimen or allow it to dry.

Anal

➤ Place the patient in a lithotomy or side-lying position and drape for privacy. Insert the swab 1 inch into the anal canal and rotate, moving it from side to side to allow it to come into contact with the microorganisms. Remove the swab. Place the swab in the Culturette tube, and squeeze the bottom of the tube to release the transport medium. Ensure that the end of the swab is immersed in the medium. Repeat with a clean swab if the swab is pushed into feces.

Genital

Female patient

➤ Position the patient on the gynecologic examination table with the feet up in stirrups. Drape the patient's legs to provide privacy and reduce chilling.

➤ Cleanse the external genitalia and perineum from front to back with towelettes provided in culture kit. Using a Culturette swab, obtain a sample of the lesion or discharge from the urethra or vulva. Place the swab in the Culturette tube, and squeeze the bottom of the tube to release the transport medium. Ensure that the end of the swab is immersed in the medium.

➤ To obtain a vaginal and endocervical culture, insert a water-lubricated vaginal speculum. Insert the swab into the cervical orifice and rotate the swab to collect the secretions containing the microorganisms. Remove and place in the appropriate culture medium. Material from the vagina can be collected by moving a swab along the sides of the vaginal mucosa. The swab is removed and then placed in a tube of saline medium.

Male patient

➤ To obtain a urethral culture, cleanse the penis (retracting the foreskin), have the patient milk the penis to express discharge from the urethra. Insert a swab into the urethral orifice to obtain a sample of the discharge. Place the swab in the Culturette tube, and squeeze the bottom of the tube to release the transport medium. Ensure that the end of the swab is immersed in the medium.

Ear

➤ Cleanse the area surrounding the site with a swab containing cleaning solution to remove any contaminating material or flora that have collected in the ear canal. If needed, assist the appropriate heath care practitioner in removing any cerumen that has collected.

➤ Insert a Culturette swab approximately 1/4 inch into the external ear canal. Rotate the swab in the area containing the exudate. Carefully remove the swab, ensuring that it does not touch the side or opening of the ear canal.

➤ Place the swab in the Culturette tube, and squeeze the bottom of the tube to release the transport medium. Ensure that the end of the swab is immersed in the medium.

Eye

➤ Pass a moistened swab over the appropriate site, avoiding eyelid and eyelashes unless those areas are selected for study. Collect any visible pus or other exudate. Place the swab in the Culturette tube, and squeeze the bottom of the tube to release the transport medium. Ensure that the end of the swab is immersed in the medium.

➤ An appropriate health care practitioner should perform procedures requiring eye scrapings.

Skin

➤ Assist the appropriate health care practitioner in obtaining a skin sample from several areas of the affected site. If indicated, the dark, moist areas of the folds of the skin and outer growing edges of the infection where microorganisms are most likely to flourish should be selected. Place the scrapings in a collection container or spread on a slide. Aspirate any fluid from a pustule or vesicle using a sterile needle and tuberculin syringe. The exudate will be flushed into a sterile collection tube. If the lesion is not fluid filled, open the lesion with a scalpel and swab the area with a sterile cotton-tipped swab. Place the swab in the Culturette tube, and squeeze the bottom of the tube to release the transport medium. Ensure that the end of the swab is immersed in the medium.

Sterile fluid

➤ Refer to related body fluid monographs (i.e., amniotic fluid, cerebrospinal fluid, pericardial fluid, peritoneal fluid, pleural fluid, synovial fluid) for specimen collection.

Wound

➤ Place the patient in a comfortable position, and drape the site to be cultured. Cleanse the area around the wound to remove flora indigenous to the skin.

➤ Place a Culturette swab in a superficial wound where the exudate is the most excessive without touching the wound edges. Place the swab in the Culturette tube, and squeeze the bottom of the tube to release the transport medium. Ensure that the end of the swab is immersed in the medium. Use more than one swab and Culturette tube to obtain specimens from other areas of the wound.

➤ To obtain a deep wound specimen, insert a sterile syringe and needle into the wound and aspirate the drainage. Following aspiration, inject the material into a tube containing an anaerobic culture medium.

General:

➤ Promptly transport the specimen to the laboratory for processing and analysis.

➤ The results are recorded manually or in a computerized system for recall and postprocedure interpretation by the appropriate health care practitioner.

Post-test:

➤ Instruct the patient to resume usual medication as directed by the health care practitioner.

➤ Instruct the patient to report symptoms such as pain related to tissue inflammation or irritation.

➤ Instruct the patient to begin antibiotic therapy, as prescribed. Instruct the patient in the importance of completing the entire course of antibiotic therapy even if no symptoms are present.

➤ Inform the patient that a repeat culture may be needed in 1 week after completion of the antimicrobial regimen.

➤ Advise the patient that final test results may take 24 to 72 hours depending on the organism suspected, but that antibiotic therapy may be started immediately.

Anal/endocervical/genital

➤ Inform the patient that final results may take from 24 hours to 4 weeks, depending on the test performed.

➤ Advise the patient to avoid sexual contact until test results are available.

➤ Instruct the patient in vaginal suppository and medicated cream installation and administration of topical medication to treat specific conditions, as indicated.

➤ Inform infected patients that all sexual partners must be tested for the microorganism.

➤ Inform the patient that positive culture findings for certain organisms must be reported to a local health department official, who will question him or her regarding sexual partners.

➤ *Social and cultural considerations:* Offer support, as appropriate, to patients who may be the victims of rape or sexual assault. Educate the patient regarding access to counseling services. Provide a nonjudgmental, nonthreatening atmosphere for discussing the risks of sexually transmitted diseases. It is also important to address problems the patient may experience (e.g., guilt, depression, anger).

Wound

➤ Instruct the patient in wound care and nutritional requirements (e.g., protein, vitamin C) to promote wound healing.

General

➤ A written report of the examination will be sent to the requesting health care practitioner, who will discuss the results with the patient.

➤ Recognize anxiety related to test results. Discuss the implications of abnormal test results on the patient's lifestyle. Provide teaching and information regarding the clinical implications of the test results, as appropriate.

➤ Reinforce information given by the patient's health care provider regarding further testing, treatment, or referral to another health care provider. Emphasize the importance of reporting continued signs and symptoms of the infection. Answer any questions or address any concerns voiced by the patient or family.

➤ Depending on the results of this procedure, additional testing may be performed to evaluate or monitor progression of the disease process and determine the need for a change in therapy. Evaluate test results in relation to the patient's symptoms and other tests performed.

Related laboratory tests:

➤ Related laboratory tests include relevant tissue biopsies, Gram stain, vitamin C, and zinc.

CULTURE, BACTERIAL, BLOOD

SYNONYM/ACRONYM: N/A.

SPECIMEN: Whole blood collected in bottles containing standard aerobic and anaerobic culture media; 10 to 20 mL for adult patients or 1 to 5 mL for pediatric patients.

REFERENCE VALUE: (Method: Growth of organisms in standard culture media identified by radiometric or infrared automation, or by manual reading of subculture.) Negative: no growth of pathogens.

DESCRIPTION & RATIONALE: Blood cultures are collected whenever bacteremia or septicemia is suspected. Although mild bacteremia is found in many infectious diseases, a persistent, continuous, or recurrent bacteremia indicates a more serious condition that may require immediate treatment. Early detection of pathogens in the blood may aid in making clinical and etiologic diagnoses.

Blood culture involves the introduction of a specimen of blood into artificial aerobic and anaerobic growth culture medium. The culture is incubated for a specific length of time, at a specific temperature, and under other conditions suitable for the growth of pathogenic microorganisms. Pathogens enter the bloodstream from soft-tissue infection sites, contaminated intravenous lines, or invasive procedures (e.g., surgery, tooth extraction, cystoscopy). A blood culture may also be done with an antimicrobial removal device (ARD). This involves transferring some of the blood sample into a special vial containing absorbent resins that remove antibiotics from the sample before the culture is performed. The laboratory will initiate antibiotic sensitivity testing if indicated by test results. Sensitivity testing identifies the antibiotics to which the organisms are susceptible to ensure an effective treatment plan. ■

INDICATIONS:
- Determine sepsis in the newborn as a result of prolonged labor, early rupture of membranes, maternal infection, or neonatal aspiration
- Evaluate chills and fever in patients with infected burns, urinary tract infections, rapidly progressing tissue infection, postoperative wound sepsis, and indwelling venous or arterial catheter
- Evaluate intermittent or continuous temperature elevation of unknown origin
- Evaluate persistent, intermittent fever associated with a heart murmur
- Evaluate a sudden change in pulse and temperature with or without chills and diaphoresis
- Evaluate suspected bacteremia after invasive procedures
- Identify the cause of shock in the postoperative period

RESULT

Positive findings in:
- Bacteremia or septicemia: *Aerobacter, Bacteroides, Brucella, Clostridium perfringens,* enterococci, *Escherichia coli* and other coliform bacilli, *Haemophilus influenzae, Klebsiella, Listeria monocytogenes, Pseudomonas aeruginosa, Salmonella, Staphylococcus aureus, Staphylococcus epidermidis,* and β-hemolytic streptococci.
- Plague
- Malaria (by special request, a stained capillary smear would be examined)
- Typhoid fever

Note: *Candida albicans* is a yeast that can cause disease and can be isolated by blood culture.

CRITICAL VALUES:

Note and immediately report to the health care practitioner positive results and related symptoms.

INTERFERING FACTORS:

• Pretest antimicrobial therapy will delay or inhibit growth of pathogens.

• Contamination of the specimen by the skin's resident flora may invalidate interpretation of test results.

• An inadequate amount of blood or number of blood specimens drawn for examination may invalidate interpretation of results.

• Testing specimens more than 1 hour after collection may result in decreased growth or nongrowth of organisms.

• Negative findings do not ensure the absence of infection.

Nursing Implications and Procedure ....

Pretest:

➤ Inform the patient that the test is used to identify pathogenic bacterial organisms.

➤ Obtain a history of the patient's complaints, including a list of known allergens (especially allergies or sensitivities to iodine), and inform the appropriate health care practitioner accordingly.

➤ Obtain a history of the patient's immune system and results of previously performed laboratory tests, surgical procedures, and other diagnostic procedures. For related laboratory tests, refer to the Immune System table.

➤ Obtain a list of the medications the patient is taking, including herbs, nutritional supplements, and nutraceuticals. The requesting health care

practitioner and laboratory should be advised if the patient regularly uses these products so that their effects can be taken into consideration when reviewing results.

➤ Note any recent medications that can interfere with test results.

➤ Review the procedure with the patient. Inform the patient that specimen collection takes approximately 5 minutes. Inform the patient that multiple specimens may be required at timed intervals. Address concerns about pain related to the procedure. Explain to the patient that there may be some discomfort during the venipuncture.

➤ There are no food or fluid restrictions unless by medical direction.

Intratest:

➤ Ensure that the patient has complied with medication prior to the procedure.

➤ If the patient has a history of severe allergic reaction to iodine, care should be taken to avoid the use of iodine.

➤ Instruct the patient to cooperate fully and to follow directions. Direct the patient to breathe normally and to avoid unnecessary movement.

➤ Observe standard precautions, and follow the general guidelines in Appendix A. Positively identify the patient, and label the appropriate specimen containers with the corresponding patient demographics, date and time of collection, and any medication the patient is taking that may interfere with test results (e.g. antibiotics). Perform a venipuncture; collect the specimen in the appropriate blood culture collection container.

➤ The high risk for infecting a patient by venipuncture can be decreased by using an aseptic technique during specimen collection.

➤ The contamination of blood cultures by skin and other flora can also be dramatically reduced by careful preparation of the puncture site and collection containers before specimen collection. Cleanse the rubber stoppers of the collection containers with the appropriate disinfectant as recommended by the laboratory, allow to air-dry, and cleanse with 70% alcohol. Once the vein has been located by palpation, cleanse the site with 70% alcohol followed by swabbing with an iodine solution. The iodine should be swabbed in a circular concentric motion, moving outward or away from the puncture site. The iodine should be allowed to completely dry before the sample is collected. If the patient is sensitive to iodine, a double alcohol scrub or green soap may be substituted.

➤ If collection is performed by directly drawing the sample into a culture tube, fill the aerobic culture tube first.

➤ If collection is performed using a syringe, transfer the blood sample directly into each culture bottle.

➤ Remove the needle, and apply a pressure dressing over the puncture site.

➤ Promptly transport the specimen to the laboratory for processing and analysis.

➤ The results are recorded manually or in a computerized system for recall and postprocedure interpretation by the appropriate health care practitioner.

➤ More than three sets of cultures per day do not significantly add to the likelihood of pathogen capture. Capture rates are more likely affected by obtaining a sufficient volume of blood per culture.

➤ The use of ARDs or resin bottles is costly and controversial with respect to their effectiveness versus standard culture techniques. They may be useful in selected cases, such as when septicemia or bacteremia is suspected after antimicrobial therapy has been initiated.

Disease Suspected	Recommended Collection
Bacterial pneumonia, fever of unknown origin, meningitis, osteomyelitis, sepsis	2 sets of cultures; each collected from a separate site, 30 minutes apart
Acute or subacute endocarditis	3 sets of cultures; each collected from a separate site, 60 minutes apart. If cultures are negative after 24 to 48 hours, repeat collections
Septicemia, fungal or mycobacterial infection in immunocompromised patient	2 sets of cultures; each collected from a separate site, 30 to 60 minutes apart (laboratory may use a lysis concentration technique to enhance recovery)
Septicemia, bacteremia after therapy has been initiated or request to monitor effectiveness of antimicrobial therapy	2 sets of cultures; each collected from a separate site, 30 to 60 minutes apart (consider use of ARD to enhance recovery)

Post-test:

➤ Instruct the patient to resume usual medication as directed by the health care practitioner.

➤ Cleanse the iodine from the collection site.

➤ Observe the venipuncture site for bleeding or hematoma formation. Apply paper tape or other adhesive to hold pressure bandage in place, or replace with a plastic bandage.

➤ Instruct the patient to report symptoms such as pain related to tissue inflammation or irritation.

➤ Instruct the patient to report fever,

chills, and other signs and symptoms of acute infection to the health care practitioner.

➤ Instruct the patient to begin antibiotic therapy, as prescribed. Instruct the patient in the importance of completing the entire course of antibiotic therapy even if no symptoms are present.

➤ Inform the patient that preliminary results should be available in 24 to 72 hours, but final results are not available for 5 to 7 days.

➤ A written report of the examination will be sent to the requesting health care practitioner, who will discuss the results with the patient.

➤ Recognize anxiety related to test results. Discuss the implications of abnormal test results on the patient's lifestyle. Provide teaching and information regarding the clinical implications of the test results, as appropriate.

➤ Reinforce information given by the patient's health care provider regarding further testing, treatment, or referral to another health care provider. Emphasize the importance of reporting continued signs and symptoms of the infection. Answer any questions or address any concerns voiced by the patient or family.

➤ Depending on the results of this procedure, additional testing may be performed to evaluate or monitor progression of the disease process and determine the need for a change in therapy. Evaluate test results in relation to the patient's symptoms and other tests performed.

Related laboratory tests:

➤ A related laboratory test is the complete blood count.

CULTURE, BACTERIAL, SPUTUM

SYNONYM/ACRONYM: Routine culture of sputum.

SPECIMEN: Sputum (10 to 15 mL).

REFERENCE VALUE: (Method: Aerobic culture on selective and enriched media; microscopic examination of sputum by Gram stain.) The presence of normal upper respiratory tract flora should be expected. Tracheal aspirates and bronchoscopy samples can be contaminated with normal flora, but transtracheal aspiration specimens should show no growth. Normal respiratory flora include *Neisseria catarrhalis, Candida albicans,* diphtheroids, α-hemolytic streptococci, and some staphylococci. The presence of normal flora does not rule out infection. A normal Gram stain of sputum contains polymorphonuclear leukocytes, alveolar macrophages, and a few squamous epithelial cells.

DESCRIPTION & RATIONALE: This test involves collecting a sputum specimen so the pathogen can be isolated and identified. The test results will reflect the type and number of organisms present in the specimen, as well as the antibiotics to which the identified pathogenic organisms are susceptible. Sputum collected by expectoration or suctioning with catheters and by bronchoscopy cannot be cultured for anaerobic organisms; instead, transtracheal aspiration or lung biopsy must be used. The laboratory will initiate antibiotic sensitivity testing if indicated by test results. Sensitivity testing identifies antibiotics to which the organisms are susceptible to ensure an effective treatment plan. ▪

INDICATIONS:

Culture:

• Assist in the diagnosis of respiratory infections, as indicated by the presence or absence of organisms in culture

Gram Stain:

• Assist in the differentiation of gram-positive from gram-negative bacteria in respiratory infection

• Assist in the differentiation of sputum from upper respiratory tract secretions, the latter being indicated by excessive squamous cells or absence of polymorphonuclear leukocytes

RESULT

• The major difficulty in evaluating results is in distinguishing organisms infecting the lower respiratory tract from organisms that have colonized but not infected the lower respiratory tract. Review of the Gram stain assists in this process. The presence of greater than 25 squamous epithelial cells per low-power field (lpf) indicates oral contamination, and the specimen should be rejected. The presence of many polymorphonuclear neutrophils and few squamous epithelial cells indicates that the specimen was collected from an area of infection and is satisfactory for further analysis.

• Bacterial pneumonia can be caused by *Streptococcus pneumoniae, Haemophilus influenzae,* staphylococci, and some gram-negative bacteria. Other pathogens that can be identified by culture are *Corynebacterium diphtheriae, Klebsiella pneumoniae,* and *Pseudomonas aeruginosa.* Some infectious agents, such as *C. diphtheriae,* are more fastidious in their growth requirements and cannot be cultured and identified without special treatment. Suspicion of infection by less commonly identified and/or fastidious organisms must be communicated to the laboratory to ensure selection of the proper procedure required for identification.

CRITICAL VALUES: N/A

INTERFERING FACTORS:

• Contamination with oral flora may invalidate results.

• Specimen collection after antibiotic therapy has been initiated may result in inhibited or no growth of organisms.

Nursing Implications and Procedure • • • • • • • • • • •

Pretest:

➤ Inform the patient that the test is used to identify pathogenic bacterial organisms.

➤ Obtain a history of the patient's complaints, including a list of known allergens (especially allergies or sensitivities to latex), and inform the appropriate health care practitioner accordingly.

➤ Obtain a history of the patient's immune and respiratory systems, and results of previously performed laboratory tests, surgical procedures, and other diagnostic procedures. For related laboratory tests, refer to the Immune and Respiratory System tables.

➤ Obtain a list of the medications the patient is taking, including herbs, nutritional supplements, and nutraceuticals. The requesting health care practitioner and laboratory should be advised if the patient regularly uses these products so that their effects can be taken into consideration when reviewing results.

➤ Note any recent medications that can interfere with test results.

➤ Review the procedure with the patient. Reassure the patient that he or she will be able to breathe during the procedure if specimen collected is accomplished via suction method. Ensure that oxygen has been administered 20 to 30 minutes before the procedure if the specimen is to be obtained by tracheal suctioning. Address concerns about pain related to the procedure. Atropine is usually given before bronchoscopy examinations to reduce bronchial secretions and prevent vagally induced bradycardia. Meperidine (Demerol) or morphine may be given as a sedative. Lidocaine is sprayed in the patient's throat to reduce discomfort caused by the presence of the tube.

➤ Explain to the patient that the time it takes to collect a proper specimen varies according to the level of cooperation of the patient and the specimen collection site. Emphasize that sputum and saliva are not the same. Inform the patient that multiple specimens may be required at timed intervals.

➤ *Sensitivity to social and cultural issues,* as well as concern for modesty, is important in providing psychological support before, during, and after the procedure.

Bronchoscopy:

➤ *Make sure a written and informed consent has been signed prior to the bronchoscopy/biopsy procedure and before administering any medications.*

➤ Other than antimicrobial drugs, there are no medication restrictions, unless by medical direction.

➤ The patient should fast and refrain from drinking liquids beginning at midnight the night before the procedure.

Expectorated specimen:

➤ Additional liquids the night before may assist in liquefying secretions during expectoration the following morning.

➤ Assist the patient with oral cleaning before sample collection to reduce the amount of sample contamination by organisms that normally inhabit the mouth.

➤ Instruct the patient not to touch the edge or inside of the container with the hands or mouth.

➤ Other than antimicrobial drugs, there are no medication restrictions, unless by medical direction.

➤ There are no food or fluid restrictions, unless by medical direction.

Tracheal suctioning:

➤ Assist in providing extra fluids, unless contraindicated, and proper humidification to decrease tenacious secretions. Inform the patient that increasing fluid intake before retiring on the night before the test aids in liquefying secretions and may make it easier to expectorate in the morning. Also explain that humidifying inspired air also helps liquefy secretions.

➤ Other than antimicrobial drugs, there are no medication restrictions, unless by medical direction.

➤ There are no food or fluid restrictions, unless by medical direction.

➤ If the specimen is collected by

expectoration or tracheal suctioning, there are no food, fluid, or medication restrictions (except antibiotics), unless by medical direction.

Intratest:

> Ensure that the patient has complied with dietary and medication restrictions; assure that food and fluids have been restricted for at least 12 hours prior to the bronchoscopy procedure.

> Have patient remove dentures, contact lenses, eyeglasses, and jewelry. Notify the physician if the patient has permanent crowns on teeth. Have the patient remove clothing and change into a gown for the procedure.

> Have emergency equipment readily available. Keep resuscitation equipment on hand in case of respiratory impairment or laryngospasm after the procedure.

> Avoid using morphine sulfate in patients with asthma or other pulmonary disease. This drug can further exacerbate bronchospasms and respiratory impairment.

> If the patient has a history of severe allergic reaction to latex, care should be taken to avoid the use of equipment containing latex.

> Assist the patient to a comfortable position and direct the patient to breath normally during the beginning of the general anesthesia. Instruct the patient to cooperate fully and to follow directions. Direct the patient to breathe normally and to avoid unnecessary movement during the local anesthetic and the procedure.

> Observe standard precautions and follow the general guidelines in Appendix A. Positively identify the patient, and label the appropriate tubes with the corresponding patient demographics, date and time of collection, and any medication the patient is taking that may interfere with test results (e.g., antibiotics).

Collect the specimen in the appropriate sterile collection container.

Bronchoscopy:

> Record baseline vital signs.

> The patient is positioned in relation to the type of anesthesia being used. If local anesthesia is used, the patient is seated and the tongue and oropharynx are sprayed and swabbed with anesthetic before the bronchoscope is inserted. For general anesthesia, the patient is placed in a supine position with the neck hyperextended. After anesthesia, the patient is kept in supine or shifted to a side-lying position and the bronchoscope is inserted. After inspection, the samples are collected from suspicious sites by bronchial brush or biopsy forceps.

Expectorated specimen:

> Ask the patient to sit upright, with assistance and support (e.g., with an overbed table) as needed.

> Ask the patient to take two or three deep breaths and cough deeply. Any sputum raised should be expectorated directly into a sterile sputum collection container.

> If the patient is unable to produce the desired amount of sputum, several strategies may be attempted. One approach is to have the patient drink two glasses of water, and then assume the position for postural drainage of the upper and middle lung segments. Effective coughing may be assisted by placing either the hands or a pillow over the diaphragmatic area and applying slight pressure.

> Another approach is to place a vaporizer or other humidifying device at the bedside. After sufficient exposure to adequate humidification, postural drainage of the upper and middle lung segments may be repeated before attempting to obtain the specimen.

> Other methods may include obtaining an order for an expectorant to be administered with additional

water approximately 2 hours before attempting to obtain the specimen. Chest percussion and postural drainage of all lung segments may also be employed. If the patient is still unable to raise sputum, the use of an ultrasonic nebulizer ("induced sputum") may be necessary; this is usually done by a respiratory therapist.

Tracheal suctioning:

➤ Obtain the necessary equipment, including a suction device, suction kit, and Lukens tube or in-line trap.

➤ Position the patient with head elevated as high as tolerated.

➤ Put on sterile gloves. Maintain the dominant hand as sterile and the nondominant hand as clean.

➤ Using the sterile hand, attach the suction catheter to the rubber tubing of the Lukens tube or in-line trap. Then attach the suction tubing to the male adapter of the trap with the clean hand. Lubricate the suction catheter with sterile saline.

➤ Tell nonintubated patients to protrude the tongue and to take a deep breath as the suction catheter is passed through the nostril. When the catheter enters the trachea, a reflex cough is stimulated; immediately advance the catheter into the trachea and apply suction. Maintain suction for approximately 10 seconds, but never longer than 15 seconds. Withdraw the catheter without applying suction. Separate the suction catheter and suction tubing from the trap, and place the rubber tubing over the male adapter to seal the unit.

➤ For intubated patients or patients with a tracheostomy, the previous procedure is followed except that the suction catheter is passed through the existing endotracheal or tracheostomy tube rather than through the nostril. The patient should be hyperoxygenated before and after the procedure in accordance with standard protocols for suctioning these patients.

➤ Generally, a series of three to five early morning sputum samples are collected in sterile containers.

General:

➤ Monitor the patient for complications related to the procedure (e.g., allergic reaction, anaphylaxis, bronchospasm).

➤ Promptly transport the specimen to the laboratory for processing and analysis.

➤ The results are recorded manually or in a computerized system for recall and postprocedure interpretation by the appropriate health care practitioner.

Post-test:

➤ Instruct the patient to resume preoperative diet, as directed by the health care practitioner. Assess the patient's ability to swallow before allowing the patient to attempt liquids or solid foods.

➤ Inform the patient that he or she may experience some throat soreness and hoarseness. Instruct patient to treat throat discomfort with lozenges and warm gargles when the gag reflex returns.

➤ Monitor vital signs and compare with baseline values every 15 minutes for 1 hour, then every 2 hours for 4 hours, and then as ordered by the health care practitioner. Monitor temperature every 4 hours for 24 hours. Notify the health care practitioner if temperature is elevated. Protocols may vary from facility to facility.

➤ Emergency resuscitation equipment should be readily available if the vocal cords become spastic after intubation.

➤ Observe for delayed allergic reactions, such as rash, urticaria, tachycardia, hyperpnea, hypertension, palpitations, nausea, or vomiting.

➤ Observe the patient for hemoptysis, difficulty breathing, cough, air hunger, excessive coughing, pain, or absent breathing sounds over the affected area. Report any symptoms to the health care provider.

➤ Evaluate the patient for symptoms indicating the development of pneumothorax, such as dyspnea, tachypnea, anxiety, decreased breathing sounds, or restlessness. A chest x-ray may be ordered to check for the presence of this complication.

➤ Evaluate the patient for symptoms of empyema, such as fever, tachycardia, malaise, or elevated white blood cell count.

➤ Administer antibiotic therapy if ordered. Remind the patient of the importance of completing the entire course of antibiotic therapy, even if signs and symptoms disappear before completion of therapy.

➤ *Nutritional considerations:* Malnutrition is commonly seen in patients with severe respiratory disease for numerous reasons including fatigue, lack of appetite, and gastrointestinal distress. Adequate intake of vitamins A and C are also important to prevent pulmonary infection and to decrease the extent of lung tissue damage.

➤ A written report of the examination will be completed by a health care practitioner specializing in this branch of medicine. The report will be sent to the requesting health care practitioner, who will discuss the results with the patient.

➤ Recognize anxiety related to test results. Discuss the implications of abnormal test results on the patient's lifestyle. Provide teaching and information regarding the clinical implications of the test results, as appropriate. Educate the patient regarding access to counseling services.

➤ Reinforce information given by the patient's health care provider regarding further testing, treatment, or referral to another health care provider. Instruct the patient to use lozenges or gargle for throat discomfort. Inform the patient of smoking cessation programs as appropriate. The importance of following the prescribed diet should be stressed to the patient/caregiver. Educate the patient regarding access to counseling services, as appropriate. Answer any questions or address any concerns voiced by the patient or family.

➤ Instruct the patient in the use of any ordered medications. Explain the importance of adhering to the therapy regimen. As appropriate, instruct the patient in significant side effects and systemic reactions associated with the prescribed medication. Encourage him or her to review corresponding literature provided by a pharmacist.

➤ Depending on the results of this procedure, additional testing may be needed to evaluate or monitor progression of the disease process and determine the need for a change in therapy. Evaluate test results in relation to the patient's symptoms and other tests performed.

Related laboratory tests:

➤ Related laboratory tests include anti–glomerular basement membrane antibody, arterial/alveolar oxygen ratio, blood gases, chest x-ray, complete blood count, computed tomography of the thorax, lung scan, magnetic resonance imaging of the chest, culture, Gram/acid-fast stain, cytology, and sputum findings.

CULTURE, BACTERIAL, STOOL

SYNONYM/ACRONYM: N/A.

SPECIMEN: Fresh random stool collected in a clean plastic container.

REFERENCE VALUE: (Method: Culture on selective media for identification of pathogens usually to include *Salmonella, Shigella, Escherichia coli* O157:H7, *Yersinia enterocolitica,* and *Campylobacter;* latex agglutination or enzyme immunoassay for *Clostridium* A and B toxins) Negative: No growth of pathogens. Normal fecal flora is 96% to 99% anaerobes and 1% to 4% aerobes. Normal flora present may include *Bacteroides, Candida albicans, Clostridium, Enterococcus, E. coli, Proteus, Pseudomonas,* and *Staphylococcus aureus.*

DESCRIPTION & RATIONALE: Stool culture involves collecting a sample of feces so that organisms present can be isolated and identified. Certain bacteria are normally found in feces. However, when overgrowth of these organisms occurs or pathologic organisms are present, diarrhea or other signs and symptoms of systemic infection occur. These symptoms are the result of damage to the intestinal tissue by the pathogenic organisms. Routine stool culture normally screens for a small number of common pathogens, such as *Campylobacter, Salmonella,* and *Shigella.* Identification of other bacteria is initiated by special request or upon consultation with a microbiologist when there is knowledge of special circumstances. The laboratory will initiate antibiotic sensitivity testing if indicated by test results. Sensitivity testing identifies the antibiotics to which organisms are susceptible to ensure an effective treatment plan. ∎

INDICATIONS:
• Assist in establishing a diagnosis for diarrhea of unknown etiology
• Identify pathogenic organisms causing gastrointestinal disease and carrier states

RESULT

Positive findings in:
• Bacterial infection: *Aeromonas* spp., *Bacillus cereus, Campylobacter, Clostridium, E. coli,* including serotype O157:H7, *Plesiomonas shigelloides, Salmonella, Shigella, Yersinia,* and *Vibrio.* Isolation of *Staphylococcus aureus* may indicate infection or a carrier state.

• Botulism: *Clostridium botulinum* (the bacteria must also be isolated from the food or the presence of toxin confirmed in the stool specimen).

CRITICAL VALUES: Note and immediately report to the health care practitioner positive results for *Salmonella, Shigella,* or *Campylobacter* and related symptoms.

INTERFERING FACTORS:

- A rectal swab does not provide an adequate amount of specimen for evaluating the carrier state and should be avoided in favor of a standard stool specimen.

- A rectal swab should never be submitted for *Clostridium* toxin studies. Specimens for *Clostridium* toxins should be refrigerated if they are not immediately transported to the laboratory as toxins degrade rapidly.

- A rectal swab should never be submitted for *Campylobacter* culture. Excessive exposure of the sample to air or room temperature may damage this bacterium so that it will not grow in the culture.

- Therapy with antibiotics before specimen collection may decrease the type and the amount of bacteria.

- Failure to transport the culture within 1 hour of collection or urine contamination of the sample may affect results.

- Barium and laxatives used less than 1 week before the test may reduce bacterial growth.

Nursing Implications and Procedure ● ● ● ● ● ● ● ● ● ● ● ●

Pretest:

➤ Inform the patient that the test is used to identify pathogenic bacterial organisms.

➤ Obtain a history of the patient's complaints, including a list of known allergens, and inform the appropriate health care practitioner accordingly.

➤ Obtain a history of the patient's gastrointestinal and immune system and results of previously performed laboratory tests, surgical procedures, and other diagnostic procedures. For related laboratory tests, refer to the Gastrointestinal and Immune System tables.

➤ Obtain a history of the patient's travel to foreign countries.

➤ Obtain a list of the medications the patient is taking, including herbs, nutritional supplements, and nutraceuticals. The requesting health care practitioner and laboratory should be advised if the patient regularly uses these products so that their effects can be taken into consideration when reviewing results.

➤ Note any recent medications that can interfere with test results.

➤ Review the procedure with the patient. Address concerns about pain related to the procedure. Explain to the patient that there may be some discomfort during the specimen collection. Inform the patient that specimen collection takes approximately 5 minutes.

➤ There are no food or fluid restrictions, unless by medical direction.

Intratest:

➤ Ensure that the patient has complied with medication restrictions prior to the procedure.

➤ Instruct the patient to cooperate fully and to follow directions. Direct the patient to breathe normally and to avoid unnecessary movement.

➤ Observe standard precautions, and follow the general guidelines in Appendix A. Positively identify the patient, and label the appropriate collection containers with the corresponding patient demographics, date and time of collection, and any medication the patient is taking that may interfere with test results (e.g., antibiotics).

➤ Collect a stool specimen directly into a clean container. If the patient requires a bedpan, make sure it is clean and dry, and use a tongue blade to transfer the specimen to the container. Make sure representative portions of the stool are sent for analysis. Note specimen appearance on collection container label.

➤ Promptly transport the specimen to the laboratory for processing and analysis.

➤ The results are recorded manually or in a computerized system for recall and postprocedure interpretation by the appropriate health care practitioner.

Post-test:

➤ Instruct the patient to resume usual medication as directed by the health care practitioner.

➤ Instruct the patient to report symptoms such as pain related to tissue inflammation or irritation.

➤ Advise the patient that final test results may take up to 72 hours but that antibiotic therapy may be started immediately. Instruct the patient about the importance of completing the entire course of antibiotic therapy even if no symptoms are present. *Note:* Antibiotic therapy is frequently contraindicated for *Salmonella* infection unless the infection has progressed to a systemic state.

➤ A written report of the examination will be sent to the requesting health care practitioner, who will discuss the results with the patient.

➤ Recognize anxiety related to test results. Discuss the implications of abnormal test results on the patient's lifestyle. Provide teaching and information regarding the clinical implications of the test results, as appropriate.

➤ Reinforce information given by the patient's health care provider regarding further testing, treatment, or referral to another health care provider. Emphasize the importance of reporting continued signs and symptoms of the infection. Answer any questions or address any concerns voiced by the patient or family.

➤ Depending on the results of this procedure, additional testing may be performed to evaluate or monitor progression of the disease process and determine the need for a change in therapy. Evaluate test results in relation to the patient's symptoms and other tests performed.

Related laboratory tests:

➤ Related laboratory tests include fecal analysis and ova and parasites.

CULTURE, BACTERIAL, THROAT OR NASOPHARYNGEAL

. . . .

SYNONYM/ACRONYM: Routine throat culture.

SPECIMEN: Throat or nasopharyngeal swab.

REFERENCE VALUE: (Method: Aerobic culture) No growth.

DESCRIPTION & RATIONALE: The routine throat culture is a commonly ordered test to screen for the presence of group A β-hemolytic streptococci.

S. pyogenes is the organism that most commonly causes acute pharyngitis. The more dangerous sequelae of scarlet fever, rheumatic heart disease, and glomerulonephritis are less frequently seen because of the early treatment of infection at the pharyngitis stage. There are a number of other bacterial agents responsible for pharyngitis. Specific cultures can be set up to detect other pathogens such as *Bordetella, Corynebacteria, Haemophilus,* or *Neisseria* if they are suspected or by special request from the health care practitioner. *Corynebacterium diphtheriae* is the causative agent of diphtheria. *Neisseria gonorrhoeae* is a sexually transmitted pathogen. In children, a positive throat culture for *Neisseria* usually indicates sexual abuse. The laboratory will initiate antibiotic sensitivity testing if indicated by test results. Sensitivity testing identifies the antibiotics to which the organisms are susceptible to ensure an effective treatment plan. ■

INDICATIONS:
• Assist in the diagnosis of bacterial infections such as tonsillitis, diphtheria, gonorrhea, or pertussis

• Assist in the diagnosis of upper respiratory infections resulting in bronchitis, pharyngitis, croup, and influenza

• Isolate and identify group A β-hemolytic streptococci as the cause of strep throat, acute glomerulonephritis, scarlet fever, or rheumatic fever

RESULT: Reports on cultures that are positive for group A β-hemolytic streptococci are generally available within 24 to 48 hours. Cultures that report on normal respiratory flora are issued after 48 hours. Culture results of no growth for *Corynebacterium* require 72 hours to report; 48 hours are required to report negative *Neisseria* cultures.

CRITICAL VALUES: N/A

INTERFERING FACTORS:
• Contamination with oral flora may invalidate results.

• Specimen collection after antibiotic therapy has been initiated may result in inhibited or nongrowth of organisms.

Nursing Implications and Procedure . . . .

Pretest:

➤ Inform the patient that the test is used to identify pathogenic bacterial organisms.

➤ Obtain a history of the patient's complaints, including a list of known allergens (especially allergies or sensitivities to latex), and inform the appropriate health care practitioner accordingly.

➤ Obtain a history of the patient's immune and respiratory systems and results of previously performed laboratory tests, surgical procedures, and other diagnostic procedures. For related laboratory tests, refer to the Immune and Respiratory System tables.

➤ Obtain a list of the medications the patient is taking, including herbs, nutritional supplements, and nutraceuticals. The requesting health care practitioner and laboratory should be advised if the patient regularly uses these products so that their effects can be taken into consideration when reviewing results.

➤ Note any recent medications that can interfere with test results.

➤ Review the procedure with the patient. In cases of acute epiglottitis, do not swab the throat! This can cause a laryngospasm resulting in a loss of airway. A patient with epiglottitis will be sitting up and leaning forward in the tripod position with the head and jaw thrusted forward to breathe. Address concerns about pain related to the procedure. Explain to the patient that there may be some discomfort during the specimen collection. The time it takes to collect a proper specimen varies according to the level of cooperation of the patient. Inform the patient that specimen collection takes approximately 5 minutes.

➤ There are no food or fluid restrictions unless by medical direction.

➤ *Sensitivity to social and cultural issues,* as well as concern for modesty, is important in providing psychological support before, during, and after the procedure.

Intratest:

➤ Ensure that the patient has complied with medication restrictions prior to the procedure.

➤ Have emergency equipment readily available. Keep resuscitation equipment on hand in case of respiratory impairment or laryngospasm after the procedure.

➤ Instruct the patient to cooperate fully and to follow directions. Direct the patient to breathe normally and to avoid unnecessary movement.

➤ Observe standard precautions, and follow the general guidelines in Appendix A. Positively identify the patient, and label the appropriate collection containers with the corresponding patient demographics, date and time of collection, and any medication the patient is taking that may interfere with test results (e.g., antibiotics).

➤ To collect the throat culture, tilt the patient's head back. Swab both tonsillar pillars and oropharynx with the sterile Culturette. A tongue depressor can be used to ensure that contact with the tongue and uvula is avoided.

➤ A nasopharyngeal specimen is collected through the use of a flexible probe inserted through the nose and directed toward the back of the throat.

➤ Place the swab in the Culturette tube and squeeze the bottom of the Culturette tube to release the liquid transport medium. Ensure that the

end of the swab is immersed in the liquid transport medium.

➤ Promptly transport the specimen to the laboratory for processing and analysis.

➤ The results are recorded manually or in a computerized system for recall and postprocedure interpretation by the appropriate health care practitioner.

Post-test:

➤ Instruct the patient to resume usual medication as directed by the health care practitioner.

➤ Instruct the patient to notify the health care practitioner immediately if difficulty in breathing or swallowing occurs or if bleeding occurs.

➤ Instruct the patient to perform mouth care after the specimen has been obtained.

➤ Provide comfort measures and treatment such as antiseptic gargles, inhalants, and warm, moist applications as needed. A cool beverage may aid in relieving throat irritation caused by coughing or suctioning.

➤ Administer antibiotic therapy if ordered. Remind the patient of the importance of completing the entire course of antibiotic therapy, even if signs and symptoms disappear before completion of therapy.

➤ *Nutritional considerations:* Dehydration can been seen in patients with a bacterial throat infection due to pain with swallowing. Pain medications reduce patient's dysphagia and allow for adequate intake of fluids and foods.

➤ A written report of the examination will be sent to the requesting health care practitioner, who will discuss the results with the patient.

➤ Recognize anxiety related to test results. Discuss the implications of abnormal test results on the patient's lifestyle. Provide teaching and information regarding the clinical implications of the test results, as appropriate.

➤ Reinforce information given by the

patient's health care provider regarding further testing, treatment, or referral to another health care provider. Instruct the patient to use lozenges or gargle for throat discomfort. Inform the patient of smoking cessation programs as appropriate. Emphasize the importance of reporting continued signs and symptoms of the infection. Answer any questions or address any concerns voiced by the patient or family.

▶ Depending on the results of this

procedure, additional testing may be performed to evaluate or monitor progression of the disease process and determine the need for a change in therapy. Evaluate test results in relation to the patient's symptoms and other tests performed

Related laboratory tests:

▶ Related laboratory tests include complete blood count and group A streptococcal screen.

CULTURE, BACTERIAL, URINE

SYNONYM/ACRONYM: Routine urine culture.

SPECIMEN: Urine (5 mL) collected in a sterile plastic collection container.

REFERENCE VALUE: (Method: Culture on selective and enriched media) Negative: no growth.

DESCRIPTION & RATIONALE: A urine culture involves collecting a urine specimen so that the organism causing disease can be isolated and identified. Urine can be collected by clean catch, urinary catheterization, or suprapubic aspiration. The severity of the infection or contamination of the specimen can be determined by knowing the type and number of organisms (colonies) present in the specimen. The laboratory will initiate sensitivity testing if indicated by test results. Sensitivity testing identifies the antibiotics to which the organisms are susceptible to ensure an effective treatment plan. ▪

Commonly detected organisms are those normally found in the genitourinary tract, including enterococci, *Escherichia coli, Klebsiella, Proteus,* and *Pseudomonas.* A culture showing multiple organisms indicates a contaminated specimen.

Colony counts of 100,000/mL or more indicate urinary tract infection (UTI).

Colony counts of 1000/mL or less suggest contamination resulting from poor collection technique.

Colony counts between 1000 and 10,000/mL may be significant depending on a variety of factors, including patient's age, gender, number of types of organisms present, method of specimen collection, and presence of antibiotics.

INDICATIONS:
• Assist in the diagnosis of suspected UTI

• Determine the sensitivity of significant organisms to antibiotics

• Monitor the response to UTI treatment

RESULT

Positive findings in: UTIs

Negative findings in: N/A

CRITICAL VALUES: N/A

INTERFERING FACTORS:
• Antibiotic therapy initiated before specimen collection may produce false-negative results.

• Improper collection techniques may result in specimen contamination.

• Specimen storage for longer than 30 minutes at room temperature or 24 hours at refrigerated temperature may result in overgrowth of bacteria and false-positive results.

• Results of urine culture are often interpreted along with routine urinalysis findings.

• Discrepancies between culture and urinalysis may be reason to recollect the specimen.

Nursing Implications and Procedure

Pretest:

➤ Inform the patient that the test is used to identify pathogenic bacterial organisms.

➤ Obtain a history of the patient's complaints, including a list of known allergens, and inform the appropriate health care practitioner accordingly.

➤ Obtain a history of the patient's genitourinary and immune systems and results of previously performed laboratory tests, surgical procedures, and other diagnostic procedures. For related laboratory tests, refer to the Genitourinary and Immune System tables.

➤ Obtain a list of the medications the patient is taking, including herbs, nutritional supplements, and nutraceuticals. The requesting health care practitioner and laboratory should be advised if the patient regularly uses these products so that their effects can be taken into consideration when reviewing results.

➤ Note any recent medications that can interfere with test results.

➤ Review the procedure with the patient. Address concerns about pain related to the procedure. Explain to the patient that there may be some discomfort during the specimen collection. Inform the patient that specimen collection depends on patient cooperation and usually takes approximately 5 to 10 minutes.

➤ *Sensitivity to social and cultural issues,* as well as concern for modesty, is important in providing psychological support before, during, and after the procedure.

➤ There are no food or fluid restrictions, unless by medical direction.

➤ Instruct the patient on clean-catch procedure and provide necessary supplies.

Intratest:

➤ Ensure that the patient has complied with medication restrictions prior to the procedure.

➤ Instruct the patient to cooperate fully and to follow directions. Direct the patient to breathe normally and to avoid unnecessary movement.

➤ Observe standard precautions, and follow the general guidelines in Appendix A. Positively identify the patient, and label the appropriate collection containers with the corresponding patient demographics, date and time of collection, method of specimen collection, and any medications the patient has taken that may interfere with test results (e.g. antibiotics).

Clean-catch specimen:

➤ Instruct the male patient to (1) thoroughly wash his hands, (2) cleanse the meatus, (3) void a small amount into the toilet, and (4) void directly into the specimen container.

➤ Instruct the female patient to (1) thoroughly wash her hands; (2) cleanse the labia from front to back; (3) while keeping the labia separated, void a small amount into the toilet; and (4) without interrupting the urine stream, void directly into the specimen container.

Pediatric urine collector:

➤ Put on gloves. Appropriately cleanse the genital area, and allow the area to dry. Remove the covering over the adhesive strips on the collector bag and apply over the genital area. Diaper the child. When specimen is obtained, place the entire collection bag in a sterile urine container.

Indwelling catheter:

➤ Put on gloves. Empty drainage tube of urine. It may be necessary to clamp off the catheter for 15 to 30 minutes before specimen collection. Cleanse specimen port with antiseptic swab, and then aspirate 5 mL of urine with a 21- to 25-gauge needle and syringe. Transfer urine to a sterile container.

Urinary catheterization:

➤ Place female patient in lithotomy position or male patient in supine position. Using sterile technique, open the straight urinary catheterization kit and perform urinary catheterization. Place the retained urine in a sterile specimen container.

Suprapubic aspiration:

➤ Place the patient in supine position. Cleanse the area with antiseptic, and drape with sterile drapes. A needle is inserted through the skin into the bladder. A syringe attached to the needle is used to aspirate the urine sample. The needle is then removed and a sterile dressing is applied to the site. Place the sterile sample in a sterile specimen container.

➤ Do not collect urine from the pouch from a patient with a urinary diversion (e.g., ileal conduit). Instead, perform catheterization through the stoma.

General:

➤ Promptly transport the specimen to the laboratory for processing and analysis. If a delay in transport is expected, add an equal volume of 50% alcohol to the specimen as a preservative.

➤ The results are recorded manually or in a computerized system for recall and postprocedure interpretation by the appropriate health care practitioner.

Post-test:

➤ Instruct the patient to resume usual medication as directed by the health care practitioner.

➤ Instruct the patient to report symptoms such as pain related to tissue inflammation, pain or irritation during void, bladder spasms, or alterations in urinary elimination.

➤ Observe for signs of inflammation if the specimen is obtained by suprapubic aspiration.

➤ Administer antibiotic therapy as ordered. Remind the patient of the importance of completing the entire course of antibiotic therapy, even if signs and symptoms disappear before completion of therapy.

➤ *Nutritional considerations:* Instruct the patient to increase water consumption by drinking 8 to 12 glasses of water to assist in flushing the urinary tract. Instruct the patient to avoid alcohol, caffeine, and carbonated beverages, which can cause bladder irritation.

➤ Prevention of UTIs includes increasing daily water consumption, urinating when urge occurs, wiping the perineal area from front to back after urination/defecation, and urinating immediately after intercourse. Prevention also includes maintaining the normal flora of the body. Patients should avoid using spermicidal creams with diaphragms or condoms (when recommended by a health care practitioner), becoming constipated, douching, taking bubble baths, wearing tight- fitting garments, and using deodorizing feminine hygiene products that alter the body's normal flora and increase susceptibility to UTIs.

➤ A written report of the examination will be sent to the requesting health care practitioner, who will discuss the results with the patient.

➤ Recognize anxiety related to test results. Discuss the implications of abnormal test results on the patient's lifestyle. Provide teaching and information regarding the clinical implications of the test results, as appropriate.

➤ Reinforce information given by the patient's health care provider regarding further testing, treatment, or referral to another health care provider. Emphasize the importance of reporting continued signs and symptoms of the infection. Instruct patient on the proper technique for wiping the perineal area (front to back) after a bowel movement. Answer any questions or address any concerns voiced by the patient or family.

➤ Depending on the results of this procedure, additional testing may be performed to evaluate or monitor progression of the disease process and determine the need for a change in therapy. Evaluate test results in relation to the patient's symptoms and other tests performed.

Related laboratory tests:

➤ Related laboratory tests include Gram stain, urinalysis, and white blood cell count.

CULTURE, FUNGAL

SYNONYM/ACRONYM: N/A.

SPECIMEN: Hair, skin, nail, pus, sterile fluids, blood, bone marrow, stool, bronchial washings, sputum, or tissue samples collected in a sterile plastic, tightly capped container.

REFERENCE VALUE: (Method: Culture on selective media; macroscopic and microscopic examination) No presence of fungi.

DESCRIPTION & RATIONALE: Fungi, organisms that normally live in soil, can be introduced into humans through the accidental inhalation of spores or inoculation of spores into tissue through trauma. Individuals most susceptible to fungal infection usually are debilitated by chronic disease, are receiving prolonged antibiotic therapy, or have impaired immune systems. Fungal diseases may be classified according to the involved tissue type: dermatophytoses involve superficial and cutaneous tissue; there are also subcutaneous and systemic mycoses. ▪

INDICATIONS:
• Determine antimicrobial sensitivity of the organism
• Isolate and identify organisms responsible for nail infections or abnormalities
• Isolate and identify organisms responsible for skin eruptions, drainage, or other evidence of infection

RESULT

Positive findings in:
• Blood
  Candida albicans
  Histoplasma capsulatum
• Cerebrospinal fluid
  Coccidioides immitis
  Cryptococcus neoformans
  Members of the order Mucorales
  Paracoccidioides brasiliensis
  Sporothrix schenckii
• Hair
  Epidermophyton
  Microsporum
  Trichophyton
• Nails
  Candida albicans
  Cephalosporium

  Epidermophyton
  Trichophyton
• Skin
  Actinomyces israelii
  Candida albicans
  Coccidioides immitis
  Epidermophyton
  Microsporum
  Trichophyton
• Tissue
  A. israelii
  Aspergillus
  Candida albicans
  Nocardia
  P. brasiliensis

CRITICAL VALUES: N/A

INTERFERING FACTORS: Prompt and proper specimen processing, storage, and analysis are important to achieve accurate results.

Nursing Implications and Procedure • • • • • • • • • • •

Pretest:

➤ Inform the patient that the test is used to identify pathogenic fungal organisms.

➤ Obtain a history of the patient's complaints, including a list of known allergens, and inform the appropriate health care practitioner accordingly.

➤ Obtain a history of the patient's immune system and results of previously performed laboratory tests, surgical procedures, and other diagnostic procedures. For related laboratory tests, refer to the Immune System table.

➤ Obtain a list of the medications the patient is taking, including herbs, nutritional supplements, and nutraceuticals. The requesting health care practitioner and laboratory should be

advised if the patient regularly uses these products so that their effects can be taken into consideration when reviewing results.

➤ Note any recent medications that can interfere with test results.

➤ Review the procedure with the patient. Inform the patient that specimen collection takes approximately 5 minutes. Address concerns about pain related to the procedure. Explain to the patient that there may be some discomfort during the specimen collection.

➤ There are no food or fluid restrictions unless by medical direction.

Intratest:

➤ Instruct the patient to cooperate fully and to follow directions. Direct the patient to breathe normally and to avoid unnecessary movement.

➤ Observe standard precautions, and follow the general guidelines in Appendix A. Instructions regarding the appropriate transport materials for blood, bone marrow, bronchial washings, sputum, sterile fluids, stool, and tissue samples should be obtained from the laboratory. Positively identify the patient, and label the appropriate collection containers with the corresponding patient demographics, date, and time of collection.

➤ Promptly transport the specimen to the laboratory for processing and analysis.

➤ The results are recorded manually or in a computerized system for recall and postprocedure interpretation by the appropriate health care practitioner.

Skin:

➤ Clean the collection site with 70% alcohol. Scrape the peripheral margin of the collection site with a sterile scalpel or wooden spatula. Place the scrapings in a sterile collection container.

Hair:

➤ Fungi usually grow at the base of the hair shaft. Infected hairs can be identified by using a Wood's lamp in a darkened room. A Wood's lamp provides rays of ultraviolet light at a wavelength of 366 nm, or 3660 Å. Infected hairs fluoresce a bright yellow-green when exposed to light from the Wood's lamp. Using tweezers, pluck hair from skin.

Nails:

➤ Ideally, softened material from the nail bed is sampled from beneath the nail plate. Alternatively, shavings from the deeper portions of the nail itself can be collected.

➤ The potassium hydroxide (KOH) test is used to indicate the presence of mycelium, mycelial fragments, spores, or budding yeast cells. A portion of the specimen is mixed with 15% KOH on a glass slide, and then the slide is covered and gently heated briefly. The slide is examined under a microscope for the presence of fungal elements.

Post-test:

➤ Instruct patient to begin antibiotic therapy, as prescribed. Instruct the patient in the importance of completing the entire course of antibiotic therapy even if no symptoms are present.

➤ A written report of the examination will be sent to the requesting health care practitioner, who will discuss the results with the patient.

➤ Recognize anxiety related to test results. Discuss the implications of abnormal test results on the patient's lifestyle. Provide teaching and information regarding the clinical implications of the test results, as appropriate.

➤ Reinforce information given by the patient's health care provider regarding further testing, treatment, or referral to another health care provider. Emphasize the importance of reporting continued signs and symptoms of the infection. Answer any questions or address any concerns voiced by the patient or family.

➤ Depending on the results of this procedure, additional testing may be performed to evaluate or monitor progression of the disease process and determine the need for a change in therapy. Evaluate test results in relation to the patient's symptoms and other tests performed.

➤ Related laboratory tests include relevant bacterial cultures, tissue biopsies, and body fluid analysis.

CULTURE, VIRAL

SYNONYM/ACRONYM: N/A.

SPECIMEN: Urine, semen, blood, body fluid, stool, tissue, or swabs from the affected site.

REFERENCE VALUE: (Method: Culture in special media, enzyme-linked immunoassays, direct fluorescent antibody techniques, latex agglutination, immunoperoxidase techniques) No virus isolated.

DESCRIPTION & RATIONALE: Viruses, the most common cause of human infection, are submicroscopic organisms that invade living cells. They can be classified as either RNA- or DNA-type viruses. Viral titers are highest in the early stages of disease before the host has begun to manufacture significant antibodies against the invader. Specimens need to be collected as early in the disease process as possible. ■

INDICATIONS: Assist in the identification of viral infection

RESULT

Positive findings in:
• Acquired immunodeficiency syndrome
  Human immunodeficiency virus (HIV)

• Acute respiratory failure
  Hantavirus

• Anorectal infections
  Herpes simplex virus (HSV)
  Human papillomavirus

• Bronchitis
  Parainfluenza virus
  Respiratory syncytial virus (RSV)

• Condylomata
  Human papilloma DNA virus

• Conjunctivitis/keratitis
  Adenovirus
  Epstein-Barr virus
  HSV
  Measles virus
  Parvovirus
  Rubella virus
  Varicella-zoster virus

- Croup
  Parainfluenza virus
  RSV

- Cutaneous infection with rash
  Enteroviruses
  HSV
  Varicella-zoster virus

- Encephalitis
  Enteroviruses
  Flaviviruses
  HSV
  HIV
  Measles virus
  Rabies virus
  Togaviruses

- Febrile illness with rash
  Coxsackieviruses
  Echovirus

- Gastroenteritis
  Norwalk virus
  Rotavirus

- Genital herpes
  HSV-1
  HSV-2

- Hemorrhagic cystitis
  Adenovirus

- Hemorrhagic fever
  Ebola virus
  Hantavirus
  Lassa virus
  Marburg virus

- Herpangina
  Coxsackievirus (group A)

- Infectious mononucleosis
  Cytomegalovirus
  Epstein-Barr virus

- Meningitis
  Coxsackieviruses
  Echovirus
  HSV-2
  Lymphocytic choriomeningitis virus

- Myocarditis/pericarditis
  Coxsackievirus
  Echovirus

- Parotitis
  Mumps virus
  Parainfluenza virus

- Pharyngitis
  Adenovirus
  Coxsackievirus (group A)
  Epstein-Barr virus
  HSV
  Influenza virus
  Parainfluenza virus
  Rhinovirus

- Pleurodynia
  Coxsackievirus (group B)

- Pneumonia
  Adenovirus
  Influenza virus
  Parainfluenza virus
  RSV

- Upper respiratory tract infection
  Adenovirus
  Coronavirus
  Influenza virus
  Parainfluenza virus
  RSV
  Rhinovirus

CRITICAL VALUES: Positive RSV culture should be reported immediately to the requesting health care practitioner.

INTERFERING FACTORS: Viral specimens are unstable. Prompt and proper specimen processing, storage, and analysis are important to achieve accurate results.

Nursing Implications and Procedure

Pretest:

➤ Inform the patient that the test is used to identify pathogenic viral organisms.

➤ Obtain a history of the patient's complaints, including a list of known allergens (especially allergies or sensitivities to latex), and inform the appropriate health care practitioner accordingly.

➤ Obtain a history of the patient's gastrointestinal, genitourinary, immune, reproductive, and respiratory systems and results of previously performed laboratory tests, surgical procedures, and other diagnostic procedures. For related laboratory tests, refer to the Gastrointestinal, Genitourinary, Immune, Reproductive, and Respiratory System tables.

➤ Obtain a list of the medications the patient is taking, including herbs, nutritional supplements, and nutraceuticals. The requesting health care practitioner and laboratory should be advised if the patient regularly uses these products so that their effects can be taken into consideration when reviewing results.

➤ Note any recent medications that can interfere with test results.

➤ Review the procedure with the patient. Inform the patient that specimen collection takes approximately 5 minutes. Address concerns about pain related to the procedure. Explain to the patient that there may be some discomfort during the specimen collection.

➤ There are no food, fluid, or medication restrictions, unless by medical direction.

➤ *Sensitivity to social and cultural issues,* as well as concern for modesty, is important in providing psychological support before, during, and after the procedure.

Intratest:

➤ Instruct the patient to cooperate fully and to follow directions. Direct the patient to breathe normally and to avoid unnecessary movement.

➤ Observe standard precautions, and follow the general guidelines in Appendix A. Positively identify the patient, and label the appropriate collection containers with the corresponding patient demographics, date and time of collection, exact site, contact person for notification of results, and other pertinent information (e.g., patient immunocompromised owing to organ transplant, radiation, or chemotherapy).

➤ Instructions regarding the appropriate transport materials for blood, bronchial washings, sputum, sterile fluids, stool, and tissue samples should be obtained from the laboratory. The type of applicator used to obtain swabs should be verified by consultation with the testing laboratory personnel.

➤ The appropriate viral transport material should be obtained from the laboratory. Nasopharyngeal washings or swabs for RSV testing should be immediately placed in cold viral transport media.

➤ Promptly transport the specimen to the laboratory for processing and analysis.

➤ The results are recorded manually or in a computerized system for recall and postprocedure interpretation by the appropriate health care practitioner.

Post-test:

➤ *Nutritional considerations:* Dehydration can been seen in patients with viral infections due to loss of fluids through fever, diarrhea, and/or vomiting. Antipyretic medication includes acetaminophen to decrease fever and allow for adequate intake of fluids and foods. Do not give acetylsalicylic acid to patients with a viral illness as there is an increase risk of Reye's syndrome.

➤ A written report of the examination will be sent to the requesting health care practitioner, who will discuss the results with the patient.

➤ Recognize anxiety related to test results. Discuss the implications of abnormal test results on the patient's lifestyle. Provide teaching and information regarding the clinical implications of the test results, as appropriate.

Reinforce information given by the patient's health care provider regarding further testing, treatment, or referral to another health care provider. Answer any questions or address any concerns voiced by the patient or family.

Depending on the results of this procedure, additional testing may be performed to evaluate or monitor progression of the disease process and determine the need for a change in therapy. Evaluate test results in relation to the patient's symptoms and other tests performed.

Related laboratory tests:

Related laboratory tests include relevant tissue biopsy, bacterial cultures, and viral serology tests.

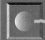

CYSTOMETRY

SYNONYM/ACRONYM: Urodynamic testing of bladder function, CMG.

AREA OF APPLICATION: Bladder, urethra.

CONTRAST: None.

DESCRIPTION & RATIONALE: Cystometry evaluates the motor and sensory function of the bladder when incontinence is present or neurological bladder dysfunction is suspected, and monitors the effects of treatment for the abnormalities. This noninvasive manometric study measures the bladder pressure and volume characteristics in centimeters of water (cm H_2O) during the filling and emptying phases. The test provides information about bladder structure and function that can lead to uninhibited bladder contractions, sensations of bladder fullness and need to void, and ability to inhibit voiding. These abnormalities cause incontinence and other impaired patterns of micturition. Cystometry can be performed with cystoscopy and sphincter electromyography. ■

INDICATIONS:
• Detect congenital urinary abnormalities

• Determine cause of bladder dysfunction and pathology

• Determine cause of recurrent urinary tract infections (UTIs)

• Determine cause of urinary retention

• Determine type of incontinence: *functional* (involuntary and unpredictable), *reflex* (involuntary when a specific volume is reached), *stress* (weak pelvic muscles), *total* (continuous and unpredictable), *urge* (involuntary when urgency is sensed), and *psychological*

(e.g., dementia, confusion affecting awareness)

- Determine type of neurogenic bladder (motor or sensory)

- Evaluate the management of neurological bladder before surgical intervention

- Evaluate postprostatectomy incontinence

- Evaluate signs and symptoms of urinary elimination pattern dysfunction

- Evaluate urinary obstruction in male patients experiencing urinary retention

- Evaluate the usefulness of drug therapy on detrusor muscle function and tonicity and on internal and external sphincter function

- Evaluate voiding disorders associated with spinal cord injury

RESULT

Normal Findings:
- Absence of residual urine (0 mL)

- Normal sensory perception of bladder fullness, desire to void, and ability to inhibit urination; appropriate response to temperature (hot and cold)

- Normal bladder capacity: 350 to 750 mL for men and 250 to 550 mL for women

- Normal functioning bladder pressure: 8 to 15 cm H_2O

- Normal sensation of fullness: 40 to 100 cm H_2O or 300 to 500 mL

- Normal bladder pressure during voiding: 30 to 40 cm H_2O

- Normal detrusor pressure: less than 10 cm H_2O

- Normal urge to void: 150 to 450 mL

- Normal filling pattern

- Urethral pressure that is higher than bladder pressure, ensuring continence

Abnormal Findings:
- Flaccid bladder that fills without contracting

- Inability to perceive bladder fullness

- Inability to initiate or maintain urination without applying external pressure

- Sensory or motor paralysis of bladder

- Total loss of conscious sensation and vesical control or uncontrollable micturition (incontinence)

CRITICAL VALUES: N/A

INTERFERING FACTORS:

This procedure is contraindicated for:
- Patients with acute UTIs because the study can cause infection to spread to the kidneys

- Patients who are pregnant or suspected of being pregnant, unless the potential benefits of the procedure far outweigh the risks to the fetus and mother

- Patients with urethral obstruction

- Patients with cervical cord lesions because they may exhibit autonomic dysreflexia, as seen by bradycardia, flushing, hypertension, diaphoresis, and headache

- Inability to catheterize the patient

Factors that may impair examination results:
- Inability of the patient to cooperate or remain still during the procedure because of age, significant pain, or mental status

- Inability of the patient to void in a supine position or straining to void during the study

- A high level of patient anxiety or embarrassment, which may interfere with the study, making it difficult to distinguish whether the results are due to stress or organic pathology

• Administration of drugs that affect bladder function, such as muscle relaxants or antihistamines

Nursing Implications and Procedure • • • • • • • • • • •

Pretest:

➤ Inform the patient that the procedure assesses bladder function.

➤ Obtain a history of the patient's complaints or symptoms, including a list of known allergens, especially allergies or sensitivities to latex, iodine, seafood, contrast medium, and dyes. Determine the patient's allergies or sensitivities to anesthetics, analgesics, or antibiotics.

➤ Obtain a history of the patient's genitourinary and renal systems as well as results of previously performed medical and surgical therapeutic interventions. Assess hematologic status, blood-clotting ability, and urinalysis findings for abnormalities. For related diagnostic tests, refer to the Genitourinary and Renal System tables.

➤ Record the date of the last menstrual period and determine the possibility of pregnancy in perimenopausal women.

➤ Obtain a list of the medications the patient is taking (e.g., antihistamines and muscle relaxants).

➤ Review the procedure with the patient. Address concerns about pain related to the procedure. Inform the patient that the only discomfort he or she will experience is the insertion of the urethral catheter, and that there may be some sensation of pressure and/or having to void. Explain that patient cooperation with positioning and activity before and during the test is crucial for achieving accurate results. Inform the patient that the procedure is performed in a special urology room or in a clinic setting by the health care practitioner. Inform

the patient that the procedure takes approximately 30 to 45 minutes.

➤ *Sensitivity to cultural and social issues,* as well as concern for modesty, is important in providing psychological support before, during, and after the procedure.

➤ Instruct the patient to report pain, sweating, nausea, headache, and the urge to void during the study.

➤ There are no food, fluid, or medication restrictions, unless by medical direction.

➤ *Make sure a written and informed consent has been signed prior to the procedure and before administering any medications.*

Intratest:

➤ Give the patient a gown and robe to wear; ensure that the patient is draped during the procedure to avoid unnecessary exposure.

➤ Position the patient in a supine or lithotomy position on the examining table. If spinal cord injury is present, the patient can remain on a stretcher in a supine position and be draped appropriately.

➤ Ask the patient to void prior to the procedure. During voiding, note characteristics such as start time; force and continuity of the stream; volume voided; presence of dribbling, straining, or hesitancy; and stop time.

➤ Instruct the patient to cooperate fully and to follow directions. Instruct the patient to remain still during the procedure.

➤ Observe standard precautions, and follow the general guidelines in Appendix A.

➤ A urinary catheter is inserted into the bladder under sterile conditions, and residual urine is measured and recorded. A test for sensory response to temperature is done by instilling 30 mL of room-temperature sterile water followed by 30 mL of warm sterile water. Sensations are assessed and recorded.

Fluid is removed from the bladder, and the catheter is connected to a cystometer that measures the pressure. Sterile normal saline, distilled water, or carbon dioxide gas is instilled in controlled amounts into the bladder. When the client indicates the urge to void, the bladder is considered full. The patient is instructed to void, and urination amounts as well as start and stop times are then recorded.

Pressure and volume readings are recorded and graphed for response to heat, full bladder, urge to void, and ability to inhibit voiding. The patient is requested to void without straining, and pressures are taken and recorded during this activity.

After completion of voiding, the bladder is emptied of any other fluid, and the catheter is withdrawn, unless further testing is planned.

If further testing is done to determine if abnormal bladder function is being caused by muscle incompetence or interruption in innervation, anticholinergic medication (e.g., atropine) or cholinergic medication (e.g., bethanechol [Urecholine]) can be injected and the study repeated in 20 or 30 minutes.

The results are recorded manually or in a computerized system for recall and postprocedure interpretation by the appropriate health care practitioner.

Post-test:

Inform the patient that further examinations may be necessary.

Monitor fluid intake and urinary output for 24 hours after the procedure.

Monitor vital signs after the procedure every 15 minutes for 2 hours or as directed. Elevated temperature may indicate infection. Notify the health care practitioner if temperature is elevated. Protocols may vary from facility to facility.

Inform the patient that he or she may experience burning or discomfort on urination for a few voidings after the procedure.

Emphasize that persistent flank or suprapubic pain, fever, chills, blood in the urine, difficulty urinating, or change in urinary pattern must be reported immediately to the health care practitioner.

A written report of the examination will be completed by a health care practitioner specializing in this branch of medicine. The report will be sent to the requesting health care practitioner, who will discuss the results with the patient.

Reinforce information given by the patient's health care provider regarding further testing, treatment, or referral to another health care provider. Answer any questions or address any concerns voiced by the patient or family.

Depending on the results of this procedure, additional testing may be needed to evaluate or monitor progression of the disease process and determine the need for a change in therapy. Evaluate test results in relation to the patient's symptoms and other tests performed.

Related diagnostic tests:

Related diagnostic tests include computed tomography of the pelvis, intravenous pyelography, magnetic resonance imaging of the pelvis, and ultrasound of the pelvis.

CYSTOSCOPY

SYNONYMS/ACRONYM: Cystoureterography, cystourethrography, prostatography.

AREA OF APPLICATION: Bladder, urethra, ureteral orifices.

CONTRAST: None.

DESCRIPTION & RATIONALE: Cystoscopy provides direct visualization of the urethra, urinary bladder, and ureteral orifices—areas not usually visible with x-ray procedures. This procedure is also used to obtain specimens and treat pathology associated with the aforementioned structures. Cystoscopy is accomplished by transurethral insertion of a cystoscope into the bladder. Rigid cystoscopes contain an obturator and a telescope with a lens and light system; there are also flexible cystoscopes, which use fiberoptic technology. The procedure may be performed during or after ultrasonography or radiography, or during urethroscopy or retrograde pyelography. ∎

INDICATIONS:
- Coagulate bleeding areas
- Determine the possible source of persistent urinary tract infections
- Determine the source of hematuria of unknown cause
- Differentiate, through tissue biopsy, between benign and cancerous lesions involving the bladder
- Dilate the urethra and ureters
- Evacuate blood clots and perform fulguration of bleeding sites within the lower urinary tract
- Evaluate changes in urinary elimination patterns
- Evaluate the extent of prostatic hyperplasia and degree of obstruction
- Evaluate the function of each kidney by obtaining urine samples via ureteral catheters
- Evaluate urinary tract abnormalities such as dysuria, frequency, retention, inadequate stream, urgency, and incontinence
- Identify and remove polyps and small tumors (including by fulguration) from the bladder
- Identify congenital anomalies, such as duplicate ureters, ureteroceles, urethral or ureteral strictures, diverticula, and areas of inflammation or ulceration
- Implant radioactive seeds
- Place ureteral catheters to drain urine from the renal pelvis or for retrograde pyelography
- Place ureteral stents and resect prostate gland tissue (transurethral resection of the prostate)

- Remove renal calculi from the bladder or ureters

- Resect small tumors

RESULT

Normal Findings:
- Normal ureter, bladder, and urethral structure

Abnormal Findings:
- Diverticulum of the bladder, fistula, stones, and strictures

- Inflammation or infection

- Obstruction

- Polyps

- Prostatic hypertrophy or hyperplasia

- Renal calculi

- Tumors

- Ureteral or urethral stricture

- Urinary tract malformation and congenital anomalies

CRITICAL VALUES: N/A

INTERFERING FACTORS:

This procedure is contraindicated for:
- Patients who are pregnant or suspected of being pregnant, unless the potential benefits of the procedure far outweigh the risks to the fetus and mother

- Patients with bleeding disorders because instrumentation may lead to excessive bleeding from the lower urinary tract

- Patients with acute cystitis or urethritis because instrumentation could allow bacteria to enter the bloodstream, resulting in septicemia

Factors that may impair examination results:
- Inability of the patient to cooperate or remain still during the procedure

because of age, significant pain, or mental status

Other considerations:
- Failure to follow dietary restrictions before the procedure may cause the procedure to be canceled or repeated.

Nursing Implications and Procedure • • • • • • • • • • •

Pretest:

➤ Inform the patient that the procedure is used to evaluate and treat conditions in the urinary tract.

➤ Obtain a history of the patient's complaints or symptoms, including a list of known allergens, especially allergies or sensitivities to latex, iodine, seafood, contrast medium, and dyes. Determine the patient's allergies or sensitivities to anesthetics, analgesics, or antibiotics.

➤ Obtain a history of results of previously performed diagnostic procedures, surgical procedures, and laboratory tests. Assess hematologic status and blood-clotting ability and urinalysis findings for abnormalities. For related diagnostic tests, refer to the Genitourinary System table.

➤ Review the procedure with the patient. Address concerns about pain related to the procedure. Inform the patient that the procedure is generally performed under general, spinal, or local anesthesia. Explain to the patient that no pain will be experienced during the test when general or spinal anesthesia is used, and that any discomfort will be minimized with local anesthetics. Inform the patient that he or she may feel some sensation of pressure and/or having to void. Inform the patient that the procedure is performed by a health care practitioner in a special cystoscopy suite near or in the operating room (or in a health care practitioner's office) and takes approximately 30 to 60 minutes.

➤ Record the date of the last menstrual period and determine the possibility of pregnancy in perimenopausal women.

➤ Restrict food and fluids for 8 hours if the patient is having general or spinal anesthesia. For local anesthesia, allow only clear liquids 8 hours before the procedure.

➤ *Sensitivity to cultural and social issues*, as well as concern for modesty, is important in providing psychological support before, during, and after the procedure.

➤ Obtain and record the patient's vital signs.

➤ *Make sure a written and informed consent has been signed prior to the procedure and before administering any medications.*

Intratest:

➤ Ensure that the patient has complied with dietary restrictions; assure that food has been restricted for at least 8 hours depending on the anesthetic chosen for the procedure.

➤ Administer ordered preoperative sedation.

➤ Give the patient a gown and robe to wear; ensure that the patient is draped during the procedure to avoid unnecessary exposure.

➤ Instruct the patient to void prior to the procedure.

➤ Observe standard precautions, and follow the general guidelines in Appendix A. Positively identify the patient, and label the appropriate collection container with the corresponding patient demographics, date, and time of collection.

➤ Position patient on the examination table draped and with legs in stirrups. If general or spinal anesthesia is to be used, it is administered before positioning the patient on the table.

➤ Cleanse external genitalia with antiseptic solution. If local anesthetic is used, it is instilled into the urethra and retained for 5 to 10 minutes. A penile clamp may be used for male patients to aid in retention of anesthetic.

➤ The physician inserts a cystoscope or a urethroscope to examine the urethra before cystoscopy. The urethroscope has a sheath that may be left in place, and the cystoscope is inserted through it, avoiding multiple instrumentations.

➤ After insertion of the cystoscope, a sample of residual urine may be obtained for culture or other analysis.

➤ The bladder is irrigated via an irrigation system attached to the scope. The irrigant is usually sterile water, unless an isotonic solution, such as mannitol, is used during transurethral resection procedures. The irrigation fluid aids in bladder visualization.

➤ If a prostatic tumor is found, a biopsy specimen may be obtained by means of a cytology brush or biopsy forceps inserted through the scope. If the tumor is small and localized, it can be excised and fulgurated. This procedure is termed *transurethral resection of the bladder*. Polyps can also be identified and excised.

➤ Ulcers or bleeding sites can be fulgurated using electrocautery.

➤ Renal calculi can be crushed and removed from the ureters and bladder.

➤ Ureteral catheters can be inserted via the scope to obtain urine samples from each kidney for comparative analysis and radiographic studies.

➤ Ureteral and urethral strictures can also be dilated during this procedure.

➤ Upon completion of the examination and related procedures, the cystoscope is withdrawn.

➤ Place obtained specimens in proper containers, label them properly, and immediately transport them to the laboratory.

➤ The results are recorded manually or in a computerized system for recall and postprocedure interpretation by the appropriate health care practitioner.

Post-test:

> Inform the patient that further examinations may be necessary to evaluate progression of the disease process or to determine the need for a change in therapy.

> Instruct the patient to resume his or her usual diet and medications, as directed by the health care provider.

> Encourage the patient to drink increased amounts of fluids (125 mL/h for 24 hours) after the procedure.

> Monitor vital signs and neurologic status every 15 minutes for 1 hour, then every 2 hours for 4 hours, and then as ordered by the health care practitioner. Take the temperature every 4 hours for 24 hours. Compare with baseline values. Notify the health care practitioner if temperature is elevated. Protocols may vary from facility to facility.

> Monitor fluid intake and urinary output for 24 hours after the procedure. Decreased urine output may indicate bladder edema or perforation caused by forceful advancement of instrumentation.

> Inform the patient that burning or discomfort on urination can be experienced for a few voidings after the procedure and that the urine may be blood-tinged for the first and second voidings after the procedure.

> Emphasize that persistent flank or suprapubic pain, fever, chills, blood in the urine, difficulty urinating, or change in urinary pattern must be reported immediately to the health care practitioner.

> A written report of the examination will be completed by a health care practitioner specializing in this branch of medicine. The report will be sent to the requesting health care practitioner, who will discuss the results with the patient.

> Reinforce information given by the patient's health care provider regarding further testing, treatment, or referral to another health care provider. Answer any questions or address any concerns voiced by the patient or family.

> Depending on the results of this procedure, additional testing may be needed to evaluate or monitor progression of the disease process and determine the need for a change in therapy. Evaluate test results in relation to the patient's symptoms and other tests performed.

Related diagnostic tests:

> Related diagnostic tests include computed tomography of the pelvis, intravenous pyelography, magnetic resonance imaging of the pelvis, and ultrasound of the pelvis.

CYSTOURETHROGRAPHY, VOIDING

SYNONYM/ACRONYM: Voiding cystography (VCU).

AREA OF APPLICATION: Bladder, urethra.

CONTRAST: Radiopaque iodine–based contrast medium.

DESCRIPTION & RATIONALE: Voiding cystourethrography involves visualization of the bladder filled with contrast medium instilled through a catheter by use of a syringe or gravity, and, after the catheter is removed, the excretion of the contrast medium. Excretion or micturition is recorded electronically or on videotape for confirmation or exclusion of ureteral reflux and evaluation of the urethra. Fluoroscopic films or plain radiographs may also be taken to record bladder filling and emptying. This procedure is often used to evaluate chronic urinary tract infections (UTIs). ■

INDICATIONS:
- Assess the degree of compromise of a stenotic prostatic urethra
- Assess hypertrophy of the prostate lobes
- Assess ureteral stricture
- Confirm the diagnosis of congenital lower urinary tract anomaly
- Evaluate abnormal bladder emptying and incontinence
- Evaluate the effects of bladder trauma
- Evaluate possible cause of frequent UTIs
- Evaluate the presence and extent of ureteral reflux
- Evaluate the urethra for obstruction and strictures

RESULT

Normal Findings:
- Normal bladder and urethra structure and function

Abnormal Findings:
- Bladder trauma
- Bladder tumors
- Hematomas
- Neurogenic bladder
- Pelvic tumors
- Prostatic enlargement
- Ureteral stricture
- Ureterocele
- Urethral diverticula
- Vesicoureteral reflux

CRITICAL VALUES: N/A

INTERFERING FACTORS:

This procedure is contraindicated for:
- ⚠ Patients with allergies to shellfish or iodinated dye. The contrast medium used may cause a life-threatening allergic reaction. Patients with a known hypersensitivity to the contrast medium may benefit from premedication with corticosteroids or the use of nonionic contrast medium.
- Patients with bleeding disorders.
- Patients who are pregnant or suspected of being pregnant, unless the potential benefits of the procedure far outweigh the risks to the fetus and mother.
- Patients with UTI, obstruction, or injury.
- ⚠ Elderly and other patients who are chronically dehydrated before the test, because of their risk of contrast-induced renal failure.
- ⚠ Patients who are in renal failure.

Factors that may impair clear imaging:
- Inability of the patient to cooperate or remain still during the procedure because of age, significant pain, or mental status
- Improper adjustment of the radiographic equipment to accommodate

obese or thin patients, which can cause overexposure or underexposure and a poor-quality study

- Patients who are very obese, who may exceed the weight limit for the equipment

- Incorrect positioning of the patient, which may produce poor visualization of the area to be examined

- Gas or feces in the gastrointestinal tract resulting from inadequate cleansing or failure to restrict food intake before the study

- Retained barium from a previous radiologic procedure

- Metallic objects within the examination field (e.g., jewelry, body rings), which may inhibit organ visualization and can produce unclear images

Other considerations:

- Consultation with a physician should occur before the procedure for radiation safety concerns regarding younger patients or patients who are lactating.

- Risks associated with radiographic overexposure can result from frequent x-ray procedures. Personnel in the room with the patient should wear a protective lead apron, stand behind a shield, or leave the area while the examination is being done. Personnel working in the area where the examination is being done should wear badges that reveal their level of exposure to radiation.

Nursing Implications and Procedure • • • • • • • • • •

Pretest:

▶ Inform the patient that the procedure assesses the urinary tract.

▶ Obtain a history of the patient's complaints or symptoms, including a list of known allergens, especially allergies or sensitivities to latex, iodine, seafood, contrast medium, and dyes.

▶ Obtain a history of results of previously performed diagnostic procedures, surgical procedures, and laboratory tests. For related diagnostic tests, refer to the Genitourinary System table.

▶ Ensure that this procedure is performed before an upper gastrointestinal study or barium swallow.

▶ Record the date of the last menstrual period and determine the possibility of pregnancy in perimenopausal women.

▶ Obtain a list of the medications the patient is taking.

▶ Review the procedure with the patient. Explain to the patient that some pain may be experienced during the test, and there may be moments of discomfort. Explain the purpose of the test and how the procedure is performed. Inform the patient that the procedure is performed in a radiology department, usually by a technologist and support staff, and takes approximately 30 to 60 minutes.

▶ *Sensitivity to cultural and social issues, as well as concern for modesty, is important in providing psychological support before, during, and after the procedure.*

▶ Instruct the patient to increase fluid intake the day before the test, but to have only clear fluids 8 hours before the test.

▶ Inform the patient that he or she may receive a laxative the night before the test or an enema or a cathartic the morning of the test, as ordered.

▶ *Make sure a written and informed consent has been signed prior to the procedure and before administering any medications.*

Intratest:

▶ Ensure that the patient has complied with fluid restrictions. Assess for completion of bowel preparation if ordered.

➤ Remove patient's clothing and any metallic objects from the lower abdominal area.

➤ Give the patient a gown and robe to wear; ensure that the patient is draped during the procedure to avoid unnecessary exposure.

➤ Have the patient void before the procedure.

➤ Observe standard precautions, and follow the general guidelines in Appendix A. Instruct the patient to cooperate fully and to follow directions.

➤ Insert a Foley catheter before the procedure, if ordered. Inform the patient that he or she may feel some pressure when the catheter is inserted and when the contrast medium is instilled through the catheter.

➤ Administer an antihistamine or steroid, as ordered by a physician, for patients with a known significant allergic reaction to the intravenous contrast medium.

➤ Place the patient on the table in a supine or lithotomy position.

➤ A kidney, ureter, and bladder film or plain radiograph is taken to ensure that no barium or stool obscures visualization of the urinary system.

➤ A catheter is filled with contrast medium to eliminate air pockets and is inserted until the balloon reaches the meatus. The patient is placed in the right posterior oblique position with the thigh drawn up to a 90° angle and, in men, the penis placed along its axis.

➤ When three-fourths of the contrast medium has been injected, another radiographic exposure is made while the remainder of the contrast medium is injected.

➤ Left lateral and oblique views may be necessary to visualize the area in question.

➤ If the patient is able to void, the catheter is removed and the patient is asked to urinate while films are taken or radiographic images of the bladder and urethra are recorded.

➤ The procedure may be done on women using a double balloon to occlude the bladder neck from above and below the external meatus.

➤ Monitor the patient for complications related to the procedure (e.g., allergic reaction, anaphylaxis, bronchospasm).

➤ The results are recorded manually, on film, or by automated equipment in a computerized system for recall and postprocedure interpretation by the appropriate health care practitioner.

Post-test:

➤ Inform the patient that further examinations may be necessary to evaluate progression of the disease process or to determine the need for a change in therapy.

➤ Instruct the patient to resume usual diet and medications, as directed by the health care provider.

➤ Monitor vital signs and neurologic status every 15 minutes for 1 hour, then every 2 hours for 4 hours, and as ordered. Take temperature every 4 hours for 24 hours. Compare with baseline values. Notify the health care practitioner if temperature is elevated. Protocols may vary from facility to facility.

➤ Monitor for reaction to iodinated contrast medium, including rash, urticaria, tachycardia, hyperpnea, hypertension, palpitations, nausea, or vomiting.

➤ Maintain the patient on adequate hydration after the procedure. Encourage the patient to drink increased amounts of fluids (125 mL/h for 24 h) after the procedure to prevent stasis and bacterial buildup.

➤ Monitor fluid intake and urinary output for 24 hours after the procedure. Decreased urinary output may indicate impending renal failure or edema caused by instrumentation.

➤ Monitor for signs of sepsis: fever, chills, and severe pelvic pain.

➤ A written report of the examination will be completed by a health care practitioner specializing in this branch of medicine. The report will be sent to the requesting health care practitioner, who will discuss the results with the patient.

➤ Reinforce information given by the patient's health care provider regarding further testing, treatment, or referral to another health care provider. Answer any questions or address any concerns voiced by the patient or family.

➤ Depending on the results of this procedure, additional testing may be needed to evaluate or monitor progression of the disease process and determine the need for a change in therapy. Evaluate test results in relation to the patient's symptoms and other tests performed.

Related diagnostic tests:

➤ Related diagnostic tests include computed tomography of the pelvis, intravenous pyelography, magnetic resonance imaging of the pelvis, and ultrasound of the pelvis.

CYTOLOGY, SPUTUM

SYNONYM/ACRONYM: N/A.

SPECIMEN: Sputum (10 to 15 mL) collected on 3 to 5 consecutive first-morning, deep-cough expectorations.

REFERENCE VALUE: (Method: Macroscopic and microscopic examination) Negative for abnormal cells, fungi, ova, and parasites.

DESCRIPTION & RATIONALE: Cytology is the study of the origin, structure, function, and pathology of cells. In clinical practice, cytologic examinations are generally performed to detect cell changes resulting from neoplastic or inflammatory conditions. Sputum specimens for cytologic examinations may be collected by expectoration alone, by suctioning, by lung biopsy, during bronchoscopy, or by expectoration after bronchoscopy.

A description of the method of specimen collection by bronchoscopy and biopsy is found in the monograph titled "Biopsy, Lung." ■

INDICATIONS:
• Assist in the diagnosis of lung cancer

• Assist in the identification of *Pneumocystis carinii* in persons with acquired immunodeficiency syndrome

• Detect known or suspected fungal or parasitic infection involving the lung

- Detect known or suspected viral disease involving the lung

- Screen cigarette smokers for neoplastic (nonmalignant) cellular changes

- Screen patients with history of acute or chronic inflammatory or infectious lung disorders, which may lead to benign atypical or metaplastic changes

RESULT: (Method: Microscopic examination) The method of reporting results of cytology examinations varies according to the laboratory performing the test. Terms used to report results may include *negative* (no abnormal cells seen), *inflammatory, benign atypical, suspect for neoplasm,* and *positive for neoplasm.*

Positive findings in:

- Infections caused by fungi, ova, or parasites

- Lipoid or aspiration pneumonia, as seen by lipid droplets contained in macrophages

- Neoplasms

- Viral infections and lung disease

CRITICAL VALUES:

If the patient becomes hypoxic or cyanotic, remove catheter immediately and administer oxygen.

If patient has asthma or chronic bronchitis, watch for aggravated bronchospasms with use of normal saline or acetylcysteine in an aerosol.

INTERFERING FACTORS:

- Improper specimen fixation may be cause for specimen rejection.

- Improper technique used to obtain bronchial washing may be cause for specimen rejection.

- Failure to follow dietary restrictions before the procedure may cause the procedure to be canceled or repeated.

Nursing Implications and Procedure ....

➤ Inform the patient that the test helps identify cellular changes associated with neoplasms or organisms that result in respiratory tract infections. When the actual infectious organisms are identified by cytology, tell the patient that the findings will be confirmed by culture.

➤ Obtain a history of the patient's complaints, including a list of known allergens (especially allergies or sensitivities to latex), and inform the appropriate health care practitioner accordingly.

➤ Obtain a history of the patient's immune and respiratory systems, and results of previously performed laboratory tests, surgical procedures, and other diagnostic procedures. For related laboratory tests, refer to the Immune and Respiratory System tables.

➤ Obtain a list of the medications the patient is taking, including herbs, nutritional supplements, and nutraceuticals. The requesting health care practitioner and laboratory should be advised if the patient is regularly using these products so that their effects can be taken into consideration when reviewing results.

➤ Note any recent procedures that can interfere with test results.

➤ Review the procedure with the patient. If the laboratory has provided a container with fixative, instruct the patient that the fixative contents of the specimen collection container should not be ingested or otherwise removed. Instruct the patient not to touch the edge or inside of the specimen container with the hands or mouth. Inform the patient that three samples may be required, on three separate mornings, either by passing a small tube (tracheal catheter) and adding suction or by expectoration. The time it takes to collect a proper specimen varies according to the level of cooperation of the patient and the specimen collection procedure. Address concerns about pain related to the procedure. Atropine is usually given before bronchoscopy examinations to reduce bronchial secretions and to prevent vagally induced bradycardia. Meperidine (Demerol) or morphine may be given as a sedative. Lidocaine is sprayed in the patient's throat to reduce discomfort caused by the presence of the tube.

> Reassure the patient that he or she will be able to breathe during the procedure if specimen collected is accomplished via suction method. Ensure that oxygen has been administered 20 to 30 minutes before the procedure if the specimen is to be obtained by tracheal suctioning.

> Assist in providing extra fluids, unless contraindicated, and proper humidification to decrease tenacious secretions. Inform the patient that increasing fluid intake before retiring on the night before the test aids in liquefying secretions and may make it easier to expectorate in the morning. Also explain that humidifying inspired air also helps to liquefy secretions.

> Assist with mouth care (brushing teeth or rinsing mouth with water), if needed, before collection so as not to contaminate the specimen by oral secretions.

> *Sensitivity to social and cultural issues,* as well as concern for modesty, is important in providing psychological support before, during and after the procedure.

> For specimens collected by suctioning or expectoration without bronchoscopy, there are no food, fluid, or medication restrictions unless by medical direction.

> Instruct the patient to fast and refrain from taking liquids from midnight the night before if bronchoscopy or biopsy is to be performed.

> *Make sure a written and informed consent has been signed prior to the*

bronchoscopy or biopsy procedure and before administering any medications.

Intratest:

> Ensure that the patient has complied with dietary restrictions; assure that food and liquids have been restricted for at least 6 to 8 hours prior to the procedure.

> Have patient remove dentures, contact lenses, eyeglasses, and jewelry. Notify the physician if the patient has permanent crowns on teeth. Have the patient remove clothing and change into a gown for the procedure.

> Have emergency equipment readily available. Keep resuscitation equipment on hand in the case of respiratory impairment or laryngospasm after the procedure.

> Avoid using morphine sulfate in those with asthma or other pulmonary disease. This drug can further exacerbate bronchospasms and respiratory impairment.

> If the patient has a history of severe allergic reaction to latex, care should be taken to avoid the use of equipment containing latex.

> Assist the patient to a comfortable position, and direct the patient to breath normally during the beginning of the general anesthesia. Instruct the patient to cooperate fully and to follow directions. Direct the patient to breathe normally and to avoid unnecessary movement during the local anesthetic and the procedure.

> Observe standard precautions, and follow the general guidelines in Appendix A. Positively identify the patient, and label the appropriate collection container with the corresponding patient demographics, date and time of collection, and any medication the patient is taking that may interfere with tes results (e.g., antibiotics). Cytology specimens may also be expressed onto a glass slide and sprayed with a fixative or 95% alcohol.

Bronchoscopy:

➤ Record baseline vital signs.

➤ The patient is positioned in relation to the type of anesthesia being used. If local anesthesia is used, the patient is seated, and the tongue and oropharynx are sprayed and swabbed with anesthetic before the bronchoscope is inserted. For general anesthesia, the patient is placed in a supine position with the neck hyperextended. After anesthesia, the patient is kept in supine or shifted to side-lying position, and the bronchoscope is inserted. After inspection, the samples are collected from suspicious sites by bronchial brush or biopsy forceps.

Expectorated specimen:

➤ Ask the patient to sit upright, with assistance and support (e.g., with an overbed table) as needed.

➤ Ask the patient to take two or three deep breaths and cough deeply. Any sputum raised should be expectorated directly into a sterile sputum collection container.

➤ If the patient is unable to produce the desired amount of sputum, several strategies may be attempted. One approach is to have the patient drink two glasses of water, and then assume the position for postural drainage of the upper and middle lung segments. Effective coughing may be assisted by placing either the hands or a pillow over the diaphragmatic area and applying slight pressure.

➤ Another approach is to place a vaporizer or other humidifying device at the bedside. After sufficient exposure to adequate humidification, postural drainage of the upper and middle lung segments may be repeated before attempting to obtain the specimen.

➤ Other methods may include obtaining an order for an expectorant to be administered with additional water approximately 2 hours before attempting to obtain the specimen.

Chest percussion and postural drainage of all lung segments may also be employed. If the patient is still unable to raise sputum, the use of an ultrasonic nebulizer ("induced sputum") may be necessary; this is usually done by a respiratory therapist.

Tracheal suctioning:

➤ Obtain the necessary equipment, including a suction device, suction kit, and Lukens tube or in-line trap.

➤ Position the patient with head elevated as high as tolerated.

➤ Put on sterile gloves. Maintain the dominant hand as sterile and the nondominant hand as clean.

➤ Using the sterile hand, attach the suction catheter to the rubber tubing of the Lukens tube or in-line trap. Then attach the suction tubing to the male adapter of the trap with the clean hand. Lubricate the suction catheter with sterile saline.

➤ Tell nonintubated patients to protrude the tongue and to take a deep breath as the suction catheter is passed through the nostril. When the catheter enters the trachea, a reflex cough is stimulated; immediately advance the catheter into the trachea and apply suction. Maintain suction for approximately 10 seconds, but never longer than 15 seconds. Withdraw the catheter without applying suction. Separate the suction catheter and suction tubing from the trap, and place the rubber tubing over the male adapter to seal the unit.

➤ For intubated patients or patients with a tracheostomy, the previous procedure is followed except that the suction catheter is passed through the existing endotracheal or tracheostomy tube rather than through the nostril. The patient should be hyperoxygenated before and after the procedure in accordance with standard protocols for suctioning these patients.

➤ Generally, a series of three to five early morning sputum samples are collected in sterile containers.

General:

➤ Monitor the patient for complications related to the procedure (e.g., allergic reaction, anaphylaxis, bronchospasm).

➤ Promptly transport the specimen to the laboratory for processing and analysis.

➤ The results are recorded manually or in a computerized system for recall and postprocedure interpretation by the appropriate health care practitioner.

Post-test:

➤ Instruct the patient to resume usual diet, as directed by the health care practitioner. Assess the patient's ability to swallow before allowing the patient to attempt liquids or solid foods.

➤ Inform the patient that he or she may experience some throat soreness and hoarseness. Instruct patient to treat throat discomfort with lozenges and warm gargles when the gag reflex returns.

➤ Monitor vital signs and compare with baseline values every 15 minutes for 1 hour, then every 2 hours for 4 hours, and then as ordered by the health care practitioner. Monitor temperature every 4 hours for 24 hours. Notify the health care practitioner if temperature is elevated. Protocols may vary from facility to facility.

➤ Emergency resuscitation equipment should be readily available if the vocal cords become spastic after intubation.

➤ Observe for delayed allergic reactions, such as rash, urticaria, tachycardia, hyperpnea, hypertension, palpitations, nausea, or vomiting.

➤ Observe the patient for hemoptysis, difficulty breathing, cough, air hunger, excessive coughing, pain, or absent breathing sounds over the affected area. Report any symptoms to the health care provider.

➤ Evaluate the patient for symptoms indicating the development of pneumothorax, such as dyspnea, tachypnea, anxiety, decreased breathing sounds, or restlessness. A chest x-ray may be ordered to check for the presence of this complication.

➤ Evaluate the patient for symptoms of empyema, such as fever, tachycardia, malaise, or elevated white blood cell count.

➤ Administer antibiotic therapy if ordered. Remind the patient of the importance of completing the entire course of antibiotic therapy, even if signs and symptoms disappear before completion of therapy.

➤ *Nutritional considerations:* Malnutrition is commonly seen in patients with severe respiratory disease for numerous reasons including fatigue, lack of appetite, and gastrointestinal distress. Adequate intake of vitamins A and C are also important to prevent pulmonary infection and to decrease the extent of lung tissue damage.

➤ A written report of the examination will be completed by a health care practitioner specializing in this branch of medicine. The report will be sent to the requesting health care practitioner, who will discuss the results with the patient.

➤ Recognize anxiety related to test results, and be supportive of impaired activity related to perceived loss of independence and fear of shortened life expectancy. Discuss the implications of abnormal test results on the patient's lifestyle. Provide teaching and information regarding the clinical implications of the test results, as appropriate. Educate the patient regarding access to counseling services. Provide contact information, if desired, for the American Lung Association (*http://www.lungusa. org*).

➤ Reinforce information given by the patient's health care provider regarding further testing, treatment, or referral to another health care provider. Inform the patient of smoking cessation programs, as appropriate. Inform the patient with abnormal findings of the importance of medical follow-up, and suggest ongoing support resources to assist in coping with chronic illness and possible early death. Answer any questions or address any concerns voiced by the patient or family.

➤ Instruct the patient in the use of any ordered medications. Explain the importance of adhering to the therapy regimen. As appropriate, instruct the patient in significant side effects and systemic reactions associated with the prescribed medication. Encourage him or her to review corresponding literature provided by a pharmacist.

➤ Depending on the results of this procedure, additional testing may be performed to evaluate or monitor progression of the disease process and determine the need for a change in therapy. Evaluate test results in relation to the patient's symptoms and other tests performed.

Related laboratory tests:

➤ Related laboratory tests include arterial/alveolar oxygen ratio, blood gases, complete blood count, computed tomography of the thorax, lung scan, magnetic resonance imaging of the chest, Gram/acid-fast stain, and relevant cultures.

CYTOLOGY, URINE

SYNONYM/ACRONYM: N/A.

SPECIMEN: Urine (180 mL for an adult or at least 10 mL for a child) collected in a clean wide-mouth plastic container.

REFERENCE VALUE: (Method: Microscopic examination) No abnormal cells or inclusions seen.

DESCRIPTION & RATIONALE: Cytology is the study of the origin, structure, function, and pathology of cells. In clinical practice, cytologic examinations are generally performed to detect cell changes resulting from neoplastic or inflammatory conditions. Cells from the epithelial lining of the urinary tract can be found in the urine. Examination of these cells for abnormalities is useful with suspected infection, inflammatory conditions, or malignancy. ■

INDICATIONS:
• Assist in the diagnosis of urinary tract diseases, such as cancer, cytomegalovirus infection, and other inflammatory conditions

RESULT

Positive findings in:
• Cancer of the urinary tract

• Cytomegalic inclusion disease

• Inflammatory disease of the urinary tract

Negative findings in: N/A

CRITICAL VALUES: N/A

INTERFERING FACTORS: N/A

Nursing Implications and Procedure • • • • • • • • • • •

Pretest:

➤ Inform the patient that the test is used to identify the presence of neoplasms of the urinary tract and assist in the diagnosis of urinary tract infections.

➤ Obtain a history of the patient's complaints, including a list of known allergens (especially allergies or sensitivities to latex), and inform the appropriate health care practitioner accordingly.

➤ Obtain a history of the patient's genitourinary and immune systems, as well as results of previously performed laboratory tests, surgical procedures, and other diagnostic procedures. For related laboratory tests, refer to the Genitourinary and Immune System tables.

➤ Obtain a list of medications the patient is taking, including herbs, nutritional supplements, and nutraceuticals. The requesting health care practitioner and laboratory should be advised if the patient regularly uses these products so that their effects can be taken into consideration when reviewing results.

➤ Note any recent procedures that can interfere with test results.

➤ Review the procedure with the patient. If a catheterized specimen is to be collected, explain this procedure to the patient and obtain a catheterization tray. Address concerns about pain related to the procedure. Explain to the patient that there may be some discomfort during the catheterization.

➤ *Sensitivity to social and cultural issues*, as well as concern for modesty, is important in providing psychological support before, during, and after the procedure.

➤ There are no food, fluid, or medication restrictions, unless by medical direction.

➤ Instruct the patient on clean-catch procedure and provide necessary supplies.

Intratest:

➤ If the patient has a history of severe allergic reaction to latex, care should be taken to avoid the use of equipment containing latex.

➤ Instruct the patient to cooperate fully and to follow directions.

➤ Observe standard precautions, and follow the general guidelines in Appendix A. Positively identify the patient, and label the appropriate tubes with the corresponding patient demographics, date and time of collection, method of specimen collection, and any medications the patient has taken that may interfere with test results (e.g., antibiotics).

Clean-catch specimen:

➤ Instruct the male patient to (1) thoroughly wash his hands, (2) cleanse the meatus, (3) void a small amount into the toilet, and (4) void directly into the specimen container.

➤ Instruct the female patient to (1) thoroughly wash her hands; (2) cleanse the labia from front to back; (3) while keeping the labia separated, void a small amount into the toilet; and (4) without interrupting the urine stream, void directly into the specimen container.

Pediatric urine collector:

➤ Put on gloves. Appropriately cleanse the genital area, and allow the area to dry. Remove the covering over the adhesive strips on the collector bag and apply over the genital area. Diaper the child. After obtaining the specimen, place the entire collection bag in a sterile urine container.

Indwelling catheter:

➤ Put on gloves. Empty drainage tube of urine. It may be necessary to clamp off the catheter for 15 to 30 minutes before specimen collection. Cleanse specimen port with antiseptic swab, and then aspirate 5 mL of urine with a 21- to 25-gauge needle and syringe. Transfer urine to a sterile container.

Urinary catheterization:

➤ Place female patient in lithotomy position or male patient in supine position. Using sterile technique, open the straight urinary catheterization kit and perform urinary catheterization. Place the retained urine in a sterile specimen container.

Suprapubic aspiration:

➤ Place the patient in supine position. Cleanse the area with antiseptic, and drape with sterile drapes. A needle is inserted through the skin into the bladder. A syringe attached to the needle is used to aspirate the urine sample. The needle is then removed and a sterile dressing is applied to the site. Place the sterile sample in a sterile specimen container.

➤ Do not collect urine from the pouch from a patient with a urinary diversion (e.g., ileal conduit). Instead perform catheterization through the stoma.

General:

➤ Promptly transport the specimen to the laboratory for processing and analysis. If a delay in transport is expected, add an equal volume of 50% alcohol to the specimen as a preservative.

➤ The results are recorded manually or in a computerized system for recall and postprocedure interpretation by the appropriate health care practitioner.

Post-test:

➤ Instruct the patient to resume usual medication as directed by the health care practitioner.

➤ Instruct the patient to report symptoms such as pain related to tissue inflammation, pain or irritation during void, bladder spasms, or alterations in urinary elimination.

➤ Observe for signs of inflammation if the specimen is obtained by suprapubic aspiration.

➤ Administer antibiotic therapy as ordered. Remind the patient of the importance of completing the entire course of antibiotic therapy, even if signs and symptoms disappear before completion of therapy.

➤ A written report of the examination will be sent to the requesting health care practitioner, who will discuss the results with the patient.

➤ Recognize anxiety related to test results, and be supportive of fear of shortened life expectancy. Discuss the implications of abnormal test results on the patient's lifestyle. Provide teaching and information regarding the clinical implications of the test results, as appropriate. Educate the patient regarding access to counseling services.

➤ Reinforce information given by the patient's health care provider regarding further testing, treatment, or referral to another health care provider. Answer any questions or address any concerns voiced by the patient or family.

➤ Depending on the results of this procedure, additional testing may be performed to evaluate or monitor progression of the disease process and determine the need for a change in therapy. Evaluate test results in relation to the patient's symptoms and other tests performed.

Related laboratory tests:

➤ Related laboratory tests include bladder cancer markers, kidney biopsy, and Papanicolaou smear.

CYTOMEGALOVIRUS, IMMUNOGLOBULIN G AND IMMUNOGLOBULIN M

· ·

SYNONYM/ACRONYM: CMV.

SPECIMEN: Serum (1 mL) collected in a plain red-top tube.

REFERENCE VALUE: (Method: Indirect fluorescent antibody) Negative or less than a fourfold increase in titer.

DESCRIPTION & RATIONALE: Cytomegalovirus (CMV) is a double-stranded DNA herpesvirus. The incubation period for primary infection is 4 to 8 weeks. Transmission may occur by direct contact with oral, respiratory, or venereal secretions and excretions. CMV infection is of primary concern in pregnant or immunocompromised patients or patients who have recently received an organ transplant. Blood units are sometimes tested for the presence of CMV if patients in these high-risk categories are the transfusion recipients. CMV serology is part of the TORCH (*t*oxoplasmosis, *o*ther [congenital syphilis and viruses], *r*ubella, *C*MV, and *h*erpes simplex type 2) panel used to test pregnant women. CMV, as well as these other infectious agents, can cross the placenta and result in congenital malformations, abortion, or stillbirth. The presence of immunoglobulin (Ig) M antibodies indicates acute infection. The presence of IgG antibodies indicates current or past infection. ■

INDICATIONS:
• Assist in the diagnosis of congenital CMV infection in newborns

• Determine susceptibility, particularly in pregnant women, immunocompromised patients, and patients who recently have received an organ transplant

• Screen blood for high-risk-category transfusion recipients

RESULT

Positive findings in: CMV infection

Negative findings in: N/A

CRITICAL VALUES: N/A

INTERFERING FACTORS:
• False-positive results may occur in the presence of rheumatoid factor.

• False-negative results may occur if treatment was begun before antibodies developed or if the test was done less than 6 days after exposure to the virus.

Nursing Implications and Procedure · · · · · · · · · · · ·

Pretest:

➤ Inform the patient that the test is used to assist in the diagnosis of CMV infection.

➤ Obtain a history of the patient's complaints and history of exposure. Obtain a list of known allergens, especially allergies or sensitivities to latex, and inform the appropriate health care practitioner accordingly.

➤ Obtain a history of the patient's immune and reproductive systems, as well as results of previously performed laboratory tests, surgical procedures, and other diagnostic procedures. For related laboratory tests, refer to the Immune and Reproductive System tables.

➤ Obtain a list of the medications the patient is taking, including herbs, nutritional supplements, and nutraceuticals. The requesting health care practitioner and laboratory should be advised if the patient is regularly using these products so that their effects can be taken into consideration when reviewing results.

➤ Review the procedure with the patient. Inform the patient that multiple specimens may be required. Any individual positive result should be repeated in 7 to 14 days to monitor a change in titer. Inform the patient that specimen collection takes approximately 5 to 10 minutes. Address concerns about pain related to the procedure. Explain to the patient that there may be some discomfort during the venipuncture.

➤ There are no food, fluid, or medication restrictions, unless by medical direction.

Intratest:

➤ If the patient has a history of severe allergic reaction to latex, care should be taken to avoid the use of equipment containing latex.

➤ Instruct the patient to cooperate fully and to follow directions. Direct the patient to breathe normally and to avoid unnecessary movement.

➤ Observe standard precautions, and follow the general guidelines in Appendix A. Positively identify the patient, and label the appropriate tubes with the corresponding patient demographics, date, and time of collection. Perform a venipuncture; collect the specimen in a 5-mL red-top tube.

➤ Remove the needle, and apply a pressure dressing over the puncture site.

➤ Promptly transport the specimen to the laboratory for processing and analysis.

➤ The results are recorded manually or in a computerized system for recall and postprocedure interpretation by the appropriate health care practitioner.

Post-test:

➤ Observe venipuncture site for bleeding or hematoma formation. Apply paper tape or other adhesive to hold pressure bandage in place, or replace with a plastic bandage.

➤ Instruct the patient in isolation precautions during time of communicability or contagion.

➤ Emphasize the need to return to have a convalescent blood sample taken in 7 to 14 days.

➤ Warn the patient that there is a possibility of false-negative or false-positive results.

➤ A written report of the examination will be sent to the requesting health care practitioner, who will discuss the results with the patient.

➤ Recognize anxiety related to test results if the patient is pregnant, and offer support. Discuss the implications of abnormal test results on the patient's lifestyle. Provide teaching and information regarding the clinical implications of the test results, as appropriate. Educate the patient regarding access to counseling services.

➤ Reinforce information given by the patient's health care provider regarding further testing, treatment, or referral to another health care provider. Answer any questions or

address any concerns voiced by the patient or family.

> Depending on the results of this procedure, additional testing may be performed to evaluate or monitor progression of the disease process and determine the need for a change in therapy. Evaluate test results in relation to the patient's symptoms and other tests performed.

> Related laboratory tests include herpesvirus viral culture, rubella antibody, and *Toxoplasma* antibody.

D-DIMER

SYNONYMS/ACRONYM: Dimer, fibrin degradation fragment.

SPECIMEN: Plasma (1 mL) collected in a completely filled blue-top (sodium citrate) tube.

REFERENCE VALUE: (Method: Latex semiquantitative screen or quantitative enzyme-linked immunosorbent assay [ELISA])
Semiquantitative: No fragments detected
Quantitative: Less than 250 ng/mL

DESCRIPTION & RATIONALE: The D-dimer is an asymmetric carbon compound formed by a cross-link between two identical fibrin molecules. The test is specific for secondary fibrinolysis because the cross-linkage occurs with fibrin and not fibrinogen. A positive test is presumptive evidence of disseminated intravascular coagulation (DIC). ■

INDICATIONS:
- Assist in the detection of DIC and deep venous thrombosis (DVT)
- Assist in the evaluation of myocardial infarction (MI) and unstable angina
- Assist in the evaluation of possible veno-occlusive disease associated with sequelae of bone marrow transplant
- Assist in the evaluation of pulmonary embolism

RESULT: The sensitivity and specificity of the assay varies among test kits and between test methods (e.g., latex vs. ELISA).

Increased in:
- Arterial or venous thrombosis
- DVT
- DIC
- Neoplastic disease
- Pre-eclampsia
- Pregnancy (late and postpartum)
- Pulmonary embolism
- Recent surgery (within 2 days)
- Secondary fibrinolysis

Decreased in: N/A

CRITICAL VALUES: N/A

INTERFERING FACTORS:

- High rheumatoid factor titers can cause a false-positive result.

- Increased CA 125 levels can cause a false-positive result.

- Drugs that may cause an increase in plasma D-dimer include those administered for antiplatelet therapy.

- Drugs that may cause a decrease in plasma D-dimer include pravastatin and warfarin.

- Placement of tourniquet for longer than 1 minute can result in venous stasis and changes in the concentration of plasma proteins to be measured. Platelet activation may also occur under these conditions, causing erroneous results.

- Vascular injury during phlebotomy can activate platelets and coagulation factors, causing erroneous results.

- Hemolyzed specimens must be rejected because hemolysis is an indication of platelet and coagulation factor activation.

- Incompletely filled tubes contaminated with heparin or clotted specimens must be rejected.

- Icteric or lipemic specimens interfere with optical testing methods, producing erroneous results.

Nursing Implications and Procedure • • • • • • • • • • •

Pretest:

➤ Inform the patient that the test is used in the evaluation of acute MI and DIC and to detect DVT.

➤ Obtain a history of the patient's complaints, including a list of known allergens (especially allergies or sensitivities to latex), and inform the appropriate health care practitioner accordingly.

➤ Obtain a history of hematologic diseases and recent surgery.

➤ Obtain a history of the patient's cardiovascular, hematopoietic, and respiratory systems, as well as results of previously performed laboratory tests, surgical procedures, and other diagnostic procedures. For related laboratory tests, refer to the Cardiovascular, Hematopoietic, and Respiratory System tables.

➤ Obtain a list of the medications the patient is taking, including herbs, nutritional supplements, and nutraceuticals. The requesting health care practitioner and laboratory should be advised if the patient is regularly using these products so that their effects can be taken into consideration when reviewing results.

➤ Review the procedure with the patient. Inform the patient that specimen collection takes approximately 5 to 10 minutes. Address concerns about pain related to the procedure. Explain to the patient that there may be some discomfort during the venipuncture.

➤ There are no food, fluid, or medication restrictions, unless by medical direction.

Intratest:

➤ If the patient has a history of severe allergic reaction to latex, care should be taken to avoid the use of equipment containing latex.

➤ Instruct the patient to cooperate fully and to follow directions. Direct the patient to breathe normally and to avoid unnecessary movement.

➤ Observe standard precautions, and follow the general guidelines in Appendix A. Positively identify the patient, and label the appropriate tubes with the corresponding patient demographics, date, and time of collection. Perform a venipuncture; collect the specimen in a 5-mL blue-top tube. Fill the tube completely. *Important note:* Two different concentrations of sodium citrate preservative are currently added to blue-top tubes for coagulation studies: 3.2% and 3.8%. The Clinical and Laboratory Standards Institute/CLSI (formerly the National Committee for Clinical Laboratory Standards/NCCLS) guideline for sodium citrate is 3.2%. Laboratories establish reference ranges for coagulation testing based on numerous factors, including sodium citrate concentration, test equipment, and test reagents. It is important to inquire from the laboratory which concentration it recommends, because each concentration will have its own specific reference range.

➤ When multiple specimens are drawn, the blue-top tube should be collected after sterile (i.e., blood culture) and nonadditive red-top tubes. When coagulation testing is the only work to be done, an extra red-top tube should be collected before the blue-top tube to avoid contaminating the specimen with tissue thromboplastin, which can falsely decrease values.

➤ Remove the needle, and apply a pressure dressing over the puncture site.

➤ Promptly transport the specimen to the laboratory for processing and analysis. The CLSI recommendation for processed and unprocessed samples stored in unopened tubes is that testing should be completed within 1 to 4 hours.

➤ The results are recorded manually or in a computerized system for recall and postprocedure interpretation by the appropriate health care practitioner.

Post-test:

➤ Observe venipuncture site for bleeding or hematoma formation. Apply paper tape or other adhesive to hold pressure bandage in place, or replace with a plastic bandage.

➤ A written report of the examination will be sent to the requesting health care practitioner, who will discuss the results with the patient.

➤ Reinforce information given by the patient's health care provider regarding further testing, treatment, or referral to another health care provider. Answer any questions or address any concerns voiced by the patient or family.

➤ Depending on the results of this procedure, additional testing may be performed to evaluate or monitor progression of the disease process and determine the need for a change in therapy. Evaluate test results in relation to the patient's symptoms and other tests performed.

Related laboratory tests:

➤ Related laboratory tests include activated partial thromboplastin time, fibrin split products, fibrinogen, platelet count, and prothrombin time.

DEHYDROEPIANDROSTERONE SULFATE

· ·

SYNONYM/ACRONYM: DHEAS.

SPECIMEN: Serum (1 mL) collected in a red- or tiger-top tube. Plasma (1 mL) collected in lavender-top (ethylenediaminetetra-acetic [EDTA]) tube is also acceptable.

REFERENCE VALUE: (Method: Radioimmunoassay)

Age	Conventional Units	SI Units (Conversion Factor × 0.027)
Newborn		
Male	108–406 μg/dL	2.9–10.9 μmol/L
Female	10–248 μg/dL	0.3–6.7 μmol/L
6–9 y	25–145 mg/dL	0.07–3.9 mmol/L
10–11 y		
Male	15–115 μg/dL	0.4–3.1 μmol/L
Female	15–260 μg/dL	0.4–7.0 μmol/L
12–17 y		
Male	20–555 μg/dL	0.5–15.0 μmol/L
Female	20–535 μg/dL	0.5–14.4 μmol/L
19–30 y		
Male	125–619 μg/dL	3.4–16.7 μmol/L
Female	29–781 μg/dL	0.8–21.1 μmol/L
31–50 y		
Male	59–452 μg/dL	1.6–12.2 μmol/L
Female	12–379 μg/dL	0.8–10.2 μmol/L
51–60 y		
Male	20–413 μg/dL	0.5–11.1 μmol/L
61–83 y		
Male	10–285 μg/dL	0.3–7.7 μmol/L
Postmenopausal		
woman	30–260 mg/dL	0.8–7.0 mmol/L

DESCRIPTION & RATIONALE: Dehydroepiandrosterone sulfate (DHEAS) is the major precursor of 17-ketosteroids. DHEAS is a metabolite of DHEA, the principal adrenal androgen. DHEAS is primarily synthesized in the adrenal gland, with a small amount secreted by the ovaries. It is secreted in concert with cortisol, under the control of adrenocorticotropic hormone (ACTH) and prolactin. Excessive production causes masculinization in women and children. DHEAS has replaced measurement of urinary 17-ketosteroids in the estimation of adrenal androgen production. ■

INDICATIONS:

* Assist in the evaluation of androgen excess, including congenital adrenal hyperplasia, adrenal tumor, and Stein-Leventhal syndrome

* Evaluate women with infertility, amenorrhea, or hirsutism

RESULT

Increased in:

* Anovulation

* Cushing's syndrome

* Ectopic ACTH-producing tumors

* Hirsutism

* Hyperprolactinemia

* Polycystic ovary

* Stein-Leventhal syndrome

* Virilizing adrenal tumors

Decreased in:

* Addison's disease

* Adrenal insufficiency (primary or secondary)

* Aging adults

* Hyperlipidemia

* Pregnancy

* Psoriasis

* Psychosis

CRITICAL VALUES: N/A

INTERFERING FACTORS:

* Drugs that may increase DHEAS levels include clomiphene, corticotropin, danazol, DHEA, mifepristone, and nitrendipine.

* Drugs that may decrease DHEAS levels include carbamazepine, dexamethasone, ketoconazole, oral contraceptives, and phenytoin.

* Recent radioactive scans or radiation within 1 week before the test can interfere with test results when radioimmunoassay is the test method.

Nursing Implications and Procedure • • • • • • • • • • •

Pretest:

➤ Inform the patient that the test is used to assist in identifying the cause for infertility, amenorrhea, or hirsutism.

➤ Obtain a history of the patient's complaints, including a list of known allergens (especially allergies or sensitivities to latex), and inform the appropriate health care practitioner accordingly.

➤ Obtain a history of the patient's endocrine system, as well as phase of menstrual cycle and results of previously performed laboratory tests, surgical procedures, and other diagnostic procedures. For related laboratory tests, refer to the Endocrine System table.

➤ Note any recent procedures that can interfere with test results.

➤ Obtain a list of the medications the patient is taking, including herbs, nutritional supplements, and nutraceuticals. The requesting health care practitioner and laboratory should be advised if the patient regularly uses these products so that their effects can be taken into consideration when reviewing results.

➤ Review the procedure with the patient. Inform the patient that specimen collection takes approximately 5 to 10 minutes. Address concerns about pain related to the procedure. Explain to the patient that there may be some discomfort during the venipuncture.

➤ There are no food, fluid, or medication restrictions, unless by medical direction.

Intratest:

➤ If the patient has a history of severe allergic reaction to latex, care should be taken to avoid the use of equipment containing latex.

➤ Instruct the patient to cooperate fully and to follow directions. Direct the patient to breathe normally and to avoid unnecessary movement.

➤ Observe standard precautions, and follow the general guidelines in Appendix A. Positively identify the patient, and label the appropriate tubes with the corresponding patient demographics, date, and time of collection. Perform a venipuncture; collect the specimen in a 5-mL red- or tiger-top tube.

➤ Remove the needle, and apply a pressure dressing over the puncture site.

➤ Promptly transport the specimen to the laboratory for processing and analysis.

➤ The results are recorded manually or in a computerized system for recall and postprocedure interpretation by the appropriate health care practitioner.

Post-test:

➤ Observe venipuncture site for bleeding or hematoma formation. Apply paper tape or other adhesive to hold pressure bandage in place, or replace with a plastic bandage.

➤ A written report of the examination will be sent to the requesting health care practitioner, who will discuss the results with the patient.

➤ Reinforce information given by the patient's health care provider regarding further testing, treatment, or referral to another health care provider. Answer any questions or address any concerns voiced by the patient or family.

➤ Depending on the results of this procedure, additional testing may be performed to evaluate or monitor progression of the disease process and determine the need for a change in therapy. Evaluate test results in relation to the patient's symptoms and other tests performed.

Related laboratory tests:

➤ Related laboratory tests include ACTH, cortisol, prolactin, and testosterone.

DRUGS OF ABUSE

Amphetamines
Barbiturates
Benzodiazepines
Cannabinoids
Cocaine

Ethanol
Opiates
Phencyclidine
Tricyclic Antidepressants

SYNONYMS/ACRONYMS: Amphetamines, barbiturates, benzodiazepines (tranquilizers), cannabinoids (THC), cocaine, ethanol (alcohol, ethyl alcohol, ETOH), phencyclidine (PCP), opiates (heroin), tricyclic antidepressants (TCA)

SPECIMEN: For ethanol, serum (1 mL) collected in a red-top tube; plasma (1 mL) collected in gray-top (sodium fluoride/potassium oxalate) tube is also acceptable. For drug screen, urine (15 mL) collected in a clean plastic container. Gastric contents (20 mL) may also be submitted for testing.

Workplace drug-screening programs, because of the potential medicolegal consequences associated with them, require collection of urine and blood specimens using a *chain of custody protocol*. The protocol provides securing the sample in a sealed transport device in the presence of the donor and a representative of the donor's employer, such that tampering would be obvious. The protocol also provides a written document of specimen transfer from donor to specimen collection personnel, to storage, to analyst, and to disposal.

REFERENCE VALUE: (Method: Spectrophotometry for ethanol; immunoassay for drugs of abuse)
Ethanol: None detected
Drug screen: None detected

DESCRIPTION & RATIONALE: Drug abuse continues to be one of the most significant social and economic problems in the United States. The National Institute for Drug Abuse (NIDA) has identified opiates, cocaine, cannabinoids, amphetamines, and phencyclidines (PCPs) as the most commonly abused illicit drugs. Ethanol is the most commonly encountered legal substance of abuse. Chronic alcohol abuse can lead to liver disease, high blood pressure, cardiac disease, and birth defects. ■

INDICATIONS:
- Differentiate alcohol intoxication from diabetic coma, cerebral trauma, or drug overdose
- Investigate suspected drug abuse
- Investigate suspected drug overdose
- Investigate suspected noncompliance with drug or alcohol treatment program
- Monitor ethanol levels when administered to treat methanol intoxication
- Routine workplace screening

Cutoff Concentrations for Drugs of Abuse Recommended by NIDA	
Amphetamines	1000 ng/mL
Barbiturates	300 ng/mL
Benzodiazepines	300 ng/mL
Cannabinoids	50 ng/mL
Cocaine	300 ng/mL
Opiates	300 ng/mL
Phencyclidine	25 ng/mL
Tricyclic antidepressants	1000 ng/mL

RESULT: A urine screen merely identifies the presence of these substances in urine; it does not indicate time of exposure, amount used, quality of the source used, or level of impairment. Positive screens should be considered presumptive. Drug-specific confirmatory methods should be used to investigate questionable results of a positive urine screen.

CRITICAL VALUES:

Note and immediately report to the health care practitioner any critically increased values and related symptoms.

The legal limit for ethanol intoxication varies from state to state, but in most states greater than 100 mg/dL (0.1G%) is considered impaired for driving. Levels greater than 300 mg/dL are associated with amnesia, vomiting, double vision, and hypothermia. Levels of 400 to 700 mg/dL are associated with coma and may be fatal. Possible interventions for ethanol toxicity include administration of tap water or 3% sodium bicarbonate lavage, breathing support, and hemodialysis (usually indicated only if levels exceed 300 mg/dL).

Barbiturate and benzodiazepine intoxication causes central nervous system (CNS) depression, which may progress to respiratory failure, hypotension, coma, and death. Do not induce emesis because of the risk of aspiration. Possible interventions include airway protection, administration of oxygen, gastric lavage with water or saline (up to 24 hours after ingestion), administration of activated charcoal, and monitoring CNS depression.

PCP intoxication causes a variety of symptoms depending on the stage of intoxication. Stage I includes psychiatric signs, muscle spasms, fever, tachycardia, flushing, small pupils, salivation, nausea, and vomiting. Stage II includes stupor, convulsions, hallucinations, increased heart rate, and increased blood pressure. Stage III includes further increases of heart rate and blood pressure that may culminate in cardiac and respiratory failure. Possible interventions may include providing respiratory support, administration of activated charcoal with a cathartic such as sorbitol, gastric lavage and suction, administration of intravenous nutrition and electrolytes, and acidification of the urine to promote PCP excretion.

Cocaine intoxication causes short-term symptoms of CNS stimulation, hypertension, tachypnea, mydriasis, and tachycardia. Possible interventions include emesis (if orally ingested and if the patient has a gag reflex and normal CNS function), gastric lavage (if orally ingested), whole-bowel irrigation (if packs of the drug were ingested), airway protection, cardiac support, and administration of diazepam or phenobarbital for convulsions. The use of β-blockers is contraindicated.

Amphetamine intoxication causes psychoses, tremors, convulsions, insomnia, tachycardia, dysrhythmias, impotence, cerebrovascular accident, and respiratory failure. Possible interventions include emesis (if orally ingested and if the patient has a gag reflex and normal CNS function), administration of activated charcoal followed by magnesium citrate cathartic, acidification of the urine to promote excretion, and administration of liquids to promote urinary output.

Heroin is an opiate that at toxic levels causes bradycardia, flushing, itching, hypotension, hypothermia, and respiratory depression. Possible interventions include airway protection and the administration of naloxone (Narcan).

Tricyclic antidepressant intoxication causes confusion, agitation, hallucinations, seizures, dysrhythmias, hyperthermia, dilation of the pupils, and coma. Possible interventions may include administration of activated charcoal; gastric lavage with saline; intravenous administration of physostigmine (to counteract coma, hypertension, respiratory depression, and seizures); administration of bicarbonate (to control dysrhythmia); administration of propranolol, lidocaine, or phenytoin to control convulsions; and monitoring cardiac function.

INTERFERING FACTORS:

- Codeine-containing cough medicines and antidiarrheal preparations, as well as ingestion of large amounts of poppy seeds, may produce a false-positive opiate result.

- Adulterants such as bleach or other strong oxidizers can produce erroneous urine drug screen results.

- Ethanol is a volatile substance, and specimens should be stored in a tightly stoppered container to avoid falsely decreased values.

Nursing Implications and Procedure • • • • • • • • • • •

Pretest:

- Inform the patient that the test is used to rapidly identify commonly abused drugs in suspected drug overdose or for routine workplace drug screening.

- Obtain a history of the patient's complaints, including a list of known allergens (especially allergies or sensitivities to latex), and inform the appropriate health care practitioner accordingly.

- Obtain a history of previously performed laboratory tests, surgical procedures, and other diagnostic procedures. For related laboratory tests, refer to the Therapeutic/Toxicology table.

- Obtain a list of the medications the patient is taking, including herbs, nutritional supplements, and nutraceuticals. The requesting health care practitioner and laboratory should be advised if the patient regularly uses these products so that their effects can be taken into consideration when reviewing results.

- Review the entire procedure with the patient, especially if the circumstances require collection of urine and blood specimens using a chain of custody protocol. Inform the patient that specimen collection takes approximately 5 to 10 minutes but may vary depending on the level of patient cooperation. Address concerns about pain related to the procedure. Explain to the patient that there may be some discomfort during the venipuncture but there should be no discomfort during urine specimen collection.

- *Sensitivity to social and cultural issues,* as well as concern for modesty, is important in providing psychological support before, during, and after the procedure.

- There are no food, fluid, or medication restrictions.

- *Make sure a written and informed consent has been signed prior to the procedure.*

Intratest:

- If the patient has a history of severe allergic reaction to latex, care should be taken to avoid the use of equipment containing latex.

- Instruct the patient to cooperate fully and to follow directions. Direct the patient receiving venipuncture to breathe normally and to avoid unnecessary movement.

- Observe standard precautions, and follow the general guidelines in Appendix A. Positively identify the patient, and label the appropriate collection containers with the corresponding patient demographics, date, and time of collection. For ethanol level, use a non–alcohol-containing solution to cleanse the venipuncture site before specimen collection. Perform a venipuncture, as appropriate; collect the specimen in a 5-mL red-top tube. Cadaver blood is taken from the aorta. For a urine drug screen, instruct the patient to obtain a clean-catch urine specimen.

- Remove the needle, as appropriate, and apply a pressure dressing over the puncture site.

Clean-catch specimen:

- Instruct the male patient to (1) thoroughly wash his hands, (2) cleanse

the meatus, (3) void a small amount into the toilet, and (4) void directly into the specimen container.

➤ Instruct the female patient to (1) thoroughly wash her hands; (2) cleanse the labia from front to back; (3) while keeping the labia separated, void a small amount into the toilet; and (4) without interrupting the urine stream, void directly into the specimen container.

➤ Follow the chain of custody protocol, if required. Monitor specimen collection, labeling, and packaging to prevent tampering. This protocol may vary by institution.

➤ Promptly transport the specimen to the laboratory for processing and analysis.

➤ The results are recorded manually or in a computerized system for recall and postprocedure interpretation by the appropriate health care practitioner.

Post-test:

➤ Observe venipuncture site for bleeding or hematoma formation. Apply paper tape or other adhesive to hold pressure bandage in place, or replace with a plastic bandage.

➤ A written report of the examination will be sent to the requesting health care practitioner, who will discuss the results with the patient. Ensure that results are communicated to the proper individual, as indicated in the chain of custody protocol.

➤ Recognize anxiety related to test results. Discuss the implications of abnormal test results on the patient's lifestyle. Provide teaching and information regarding the clinical implications of the test results, as appropriate. Educate the patient regarding access to counseling services. Provide support and information regarding detoxification programs, as appropriate.

➤ Reinforce information given by the patient's health care provider regarding further testing, treatment, or referral to another health care provider. Answer any questions or address any concerns voiced by the patient or family.

➤ Depending on the results of this procedure, additional testing may be performed to evaluate or monitor progression of the disease process or determine the need for a change in therapy. Evaluate test results in relation to the patient's symptoms and other tests performed.

D-XYLOSE TOLERANCE TEST

SYNONYM/ACRONYM: N/A.

SPECIMEN: Plasma (1 mL) collected in gray-top (fluoride/oxalate) tube and urine (10 mL from a 5-hour collection) from a timed collection in a clean amber plastic container.

REFERENCE VALUE: (Method: Spectrophotometry)

Dose by Age	Conventional Units	SI Units
Plasma		*(Conventional Units × 0.0666)*
Adult dose		
25 g	Greater than 25 mg/dL	Greater than 1.7 mmol/L
5 g	Greater than 20 mg/dL	Greater than 1.3 mmol/L
Pediatric dose		
0.5 g/kg (max. 25 g)	Greater than 30 mg/dL	Greater than 2.0 mmol/L
Urine		*(Conventional Units × 6.66)*
Adult dose		
25 g	Greater than 4 g/5 h collection	Greater than 26.6 mmol/5 h
5 g	Greater than 1.2 g/5 h collection	Greater than 8 mmol/5 h
Pediatric dose		
0.5 g/kg (max. 25 g)	Greater than 16%–33% of dose	Greater than 16%–33% of dose

DESCRIPTION & RATIONALE: The D-xylose tolerance test is used to screen for intestinal malabsorption of carbohydrates. D-Xylose is a pentose sugar not normally present in the blood in significant amounts. It is partially absorbed when ingested and normally passes unmetabolized in the urine. ■

INDICATIONS: Assist in the diagnosis of malabsorption syndromes

RESULT

Increased in: N/A

Decreased in:
• Amyloidosis
• Bacterial overgrowth
• Eosinophilic gastroenteritis
• Lymphoma
• Nontropical sprue (celiac disease, gluten-induced enteropathy)
• Parasitic infestations (*Giardia,* schistosomiasis, hookworm)
• Postoperative period after massive resection of the intestine
• Radiation enteritis
• Scleroderma
• Small bowel ischemia
• Tropical sprue
• Whipple's disease
• Zollinger-Ellison syndrome

CRITICAL VALUES: N/A

INTERFERING FACTORS:
• Drugs that may increase urine D-xylose levels include phenazopyridine.
• Drugs and substances that may decrease urine D-xylose levels include acetylsalicylic acid, aminosalicylic acid, arsenicals, colchicine, digitalis, ethionamide, gold, indomethacin, isocarboxazid, kanamycin, monoamine oxidase inhibitors, neomycin, and phenelzine.

• Poor renal function or vomiting may cause low urine values.

Nursing Implications and Procedure • • • • • • • • • • •

Pretest:

➤ Inform the patient that the test is used to assist in the diagnosis of intestinal malabsorption syndromes.

➤ Obtain a history of the patient's complaints, including a list of known allergens (especially allergies or sensitivities to latex), and inform the appropriate health care practitioner accordingly.

➤ Obtain a history of the patient's gastrointestinal system and results of previously performed laboratory tests, surgical procedures, and other diagnostic procedures. For related laboratory tests, refer to the Gastrointestinal System table.

➤ Obtain a list of the medications the patient is taking, including herbs, nutritional supplements, and nutraceuticals. The requesting health care practitioner and laboratory should be advised if the patient regularly uses these products so that their effects can be taken into consideration when reviewing results.

➤ Review the procedure with the patient. Inform the patient that activity will be restricted during the test. Obtain the pediatric patient's weight to calculate dose of D-xylose to be administered. Inform the patient that blood specimen collection takes approximately 5 to 10 minutes. Address concerns about pain related to the procedure. Explain to the patient that there may be some discomfort during the venipuncture.

➤ Inform the patient that all urine for a 5-hour period must be saved. Provide a nonmetallic urinal, bedpan, or toilet-mounted collection device.

➤ Instruct the patient not to void directly into the laboratory collection container. Instruct the patient to avoid defecating in the collection device and to keep toilet tissue out of the collection device to prevent contamination of the specimen. Place a sign in the bathroom to remind the patient to save all urine.

➤ Instruct the patient to void all urine into the collection device and then to pour the urine into the laboratory collection container. Alternatively, the specimen can be left in the collection device for a health care staff member to add to the laboratory collection container.

➤ *Sensitivity to social and cultural issues,* as well as concern for modesty, is important in providing psychological support before, during, and after the procedure.

➤ Numerous medications (e.g., acetylsalicylic acid, indomethacin, neomycin) interfere with the test and should be withheld, by medical direction, for 24 hours before testing.

➤ There are no fluid restrictions, unless by medical direction.

➤ The patient should fast for at least 12 hours before the test. In addition, the patient should refrain from eating foods containing pentose sugars such as fruits, jams, jellies, and pastries.

Intratest:

➤ Ensure that the patient has complied with dietary and medication restrictions; assure that food has been restricted for at least 12 hours prior to the procedure and medications have been withheld, by medical direction, for 24 hours prior to the procedure.

➤ If the patient has a history of severe allergic reaction to latex, care should be taken to avoid the use of equipment containing latex.

➤ Instruct the patient to cooperate fully and to follow directions. Direct the patient to breathe normally and to avoid unnecessary movement.

➤ Observe standard precautions, and follow the general guidelines in Appendix A. Positively identify the patient, and label the appropriate tubes with the corresponding patient

demographics, date, and time of collection. Perform a venipuncture; collect the specimen in a 5-mL red- or tiger-top tube.

➤ Remove the needle, and apply a pressure dressing over the puncture site.

Timed specimen:

➤ Obtain a clean 3-L urine specimen container, toilet-mounted collection device, and plastic bag (for transport of the specimen container). The specimen must be refrigerated or kept on ice throughout the entire collection period. If an indwelling urinary catheter is in place, the drainage bag must be kept on ice.

➤ Begin the test between 6 a.m. and 8 a.m., if possible. Remind the patient to remain supine and at rest throughout the duration of the test. Instruct the patient to collect all urine for a 5-hour period after administration of the D-xylose.

➤ Adults are given a 25-g dose of D-xylose dissolved in 250 mL of water to take orally. The dose for pediatric patient is calculated by weight up to a maximum of 25 g. The patient should drink an additional 250 mL of water as soon as the D-xylose solution has been taken. Some adult patients with severe symptoms may be given a 5-g dose, but the test results are less sensitive at the lower dose.

➤ If an indwelling catheter is in place, replace the tubing and container system at the start of the collection time. Keep the container system on ice during the collection period or empty the urine into a larger container periodically during the collection period; monitor to ensure continued drainage.

➤ Blood samples are collected 1 hour postdose for pediatric patients and 2 hours postdose for adults.

➤ Direct the patient to breathe normally and to avoid unnecessary movement. Perform a venipuncture, and collect the specimen in a 5-mL gray-top tube.

➤ At the conclusion of the test, compare the quantity of urine with the urinary output record for the collection; if the specimen contains less than what was recorded as output, some urine may have been discarded, thus invalidating the test.

➤ Include on the collection container's label the amount of urine, test start and stop times, and ingestion of any foods or medications that could affect test results.

➤ Promptly transport the specimens to the laboratory for processing and analysis.

➤ The results are recorded manually or in a computerized system for recall and postprocedure interpretation by the appropriate health care practitioner.

Post-test:

➤ Observe venipuncture site for bleeding or hematoma formation. Apply paper tape or other adhesive to hold pressure bandage in place, or replace with a plastic bandage.

➤ Instruct the patient to resume usual medications, as directed by the health care practitioner.

➤ *Nutritional considerations:* Decreased D-Xylose levels may be associated with gastrointestinal disease. Nutritional therapy may be indicated in the presence of malabsorption disorders. Encourage the patient, as appropriate, to consult with a qualified nutrition specialist to plan a lactose- and gluten-free diet. This dietary planning is complex because patients are often malnourished and have related nutritional problems.

➤ A written report of the examination will be sent to the requesting health care practitioner, who will discuss the results with the patient.

➤ Recognize anxiety related to test results. Discuss the implications of abnormal test results on the patient's lifestyle. Provide teaching and information regarding the clinical implications of the test results, as appropriate. Offer support to help the patient and/or caregiver cope with the long-term implications of a chronic disorder and related lifestyle changes. Educate the patient regarding access to counseling services, as appropriate.

➤ Reinforce information given by the patient's health care provider regarding further testing, treatment, or referral to another health care provider. Answer any questions or address any concerns voiced by the patient or family.

➤ Depending on the results of this procedure, additional testing may be performed to evaluate or monitor progression of the disease process and determine the need for a change in therapy. Evaluate test results in relation to the patient's symptoms and other tests performed.

Related laboratory tests:

➤ Related laboratory tests include fecal analysis, fecal fat, intestinal biopsy, lactose tolerance, and sweat chloride.

ECHOCARDIOGRAPHY

SYNONYMS/ACRONYM: Doppler echo, Doppler ultrasound of the heart, echo.

AREA OF APPLICATION: Chest/thorax.

CONTRAST: Can be done with or without noniodinated contrast medium (microspheres).

DESCRIPTION & RATIONALE: Echocardiography, a noninvasive ultrasound procedure, uses high-frequency sound waves of various intensities to assist in diagnosing cardiovascular disorders. The procedure records the echoes created by the deflection of an ultrasonic beam off the cardiac structures and allows visualization of the size, shape, position, thickness, and movement of all four valves, atria, ventricular and atria septa, papillary muscles, chordae tendineae, and ventricles. This study can also determine blood-flow velocity and direction and the presence of pericardial effusion during the movement of the trans-

ducer over areas of the chest. Electrocardiography and phonocardiography can be done simultaneously to correlate the findings with the cardiac cycle. These procedures can be done at the bedside or in a specialized department, health care practitioner's office, or clinic.

Included in the study are the M-mode method, which produces a linear tracing of timed motions of the heart, its structures, and associated measurements over time; and the two-dimensional method, using real-time Doppler color-flow imaging with pulsed and continuous-wave Doppler spectral tracings, which produces a cross-section of the structures of the heart and their relationship to one another, including changes in the coronary vasculature, velocity and direction of blood flow, and areas of eccentric blood flow. Doppler color-flow imaging may also be helpful in depicting the function of biological and prosthetic valves.

Cardiac contrast medium is used to aid in the diagnosis of intracardiac shunt and tricuspid valve regurgitation. The contrast agent is injected intravenously and outlines the chambers of the heart. ■

INDICATIONS:

- Detect atrial tumors (myxomas)

- Detect subaortic stenosis as evidenced either by displacement of the anterior atrial leaflet or by a reduction in aortic valve flow, depending on the obstruction

- Detect ventricular or atrial mural thrombi and evaluate cardiac wall motion after myocardial infarction

- Determine the presence of pericardial effusion, tamponade, and pericarditis

- Determine the severity of valvular abnormalities such as stenosis, prolapse, and regurgitation

- Evaluate congenital heart disorders

- Evaluate endocarditis

- Evaluate or monitor prosthetic valve function

- Evaluate the presence of shunt flow and continuity of the aorta and pulmonary artery

- Evaluate unexplained chest pain, electrocardiographic changes, and abnormal chest x-ray (e.g., enlarged cardiac silhouette)

- Evaluate ventricular aneurysms and/or thrombus

- Measure the size of the heart's chambers and determine if hypertrophic cardiomyopathy or congestive heart failure is present

RESULT

Normal Findings:

- Normal appearance in the size, position, structure, and movements of the heart valves visualized and recorded in a combination of ultrasound modes; and normal heart muscle walls of both ventricles and left atrium, with adequate blood filling. Established values for the measurement of heart activities obtained by the study may vary by health care practitioner and institution.

Abnormal Findings:

- Aortic valve abnormalities
- Cardiac neoplasm
- Cardiomyopathy
- Congenital heart defect
- Congestive heart failure
- Coronary artery disease
- Endocarditis
- Mitral valve abnormalities
- Myxoma
- Pericardial effusion, tamponade, and pericarditis
- Pulmonary hypertension
- Pulmonary valve abnormalities
- Septal defects
- Ventricular hypertrophy
- Ventricular or atrial mural thrombi

CRITICAL VALUES: N/A

INTERFERING FACTORS:

Factors that may impair clear imaging:

- Incorrect placement of the transducer over the desired test site

- Retained barium from a previous radiologic procedure

- Patients who are dehydrated, resulting in failure to demonstrate the boundaries between organs and tissue structures

- Metallic objects within the examination field (e.g., jewelry, body rings), which may inhibit organ visualization and can produce unclear images

- Improper adjustment of the ultrasound equipment to accommodate obese or thin patients, which can cause a poor-quality study

- The presence of chronic obstructive pulmonary disease or use of mechanical ventilation, which increases the air between the heart and chest wall (hyperinflation) and can attenuate the ultrasound waves

- The presence of arrhythmias

- Patients who are very obese, who may exceed the weight limit for the equipment

- Incorrect positioning of the patient, which may produce poor visualization of the area to be examined

- Inability of the patient to cooperate or remain still during the procedure because of age, significant pain, or mental status

Nursing Implications and Procedure • • • • • • • • • • •

Pretest:

➤ Inform the patient that the procedure assesses cardiac function.

➤ Obtain a history of the patient's complaints or clinical symptoms.

➤ Obtain a history of results of previously performed diagnostic procedures, surgical procedures, and laboratory tests. For related diagnostic tests, refer to the Cardiovascular System table.

➤ Note any recent procedures that can interfere with test results (i.e., barium procedures, surgery, or biopsy). There should be 24 hours between administration of barium and this test.

➤ Record the date of the last menstrual period and determine the possibility of pregnancy in perimenopausal women.

➤ Obtain a list of the medications the patient is taking.

➤ Review the procedure with the patient. Address concerns about pain related to the procedure. Explain to the patient that some pain may be experienced during the test, and there may be moments of discomfort. Explain the purpose of the test and how the procedure is performed. Inform the patient that the procedure is performed in an ultrasound or cardiology department, usually by a technologist, and takes approximately 30 to 60 minutes.

➤ Explain that an IV line may be inserted to allow infusion of IV fluids, contrast medium, dye, or sedatives.

➤ *Sensitivity to social and cultural issues,* as well as concern for modesty, is important in providing psychological support before, during, and after the procedure.

➤ Instruct the patient to remove jewelry, body rings, and other metallic objects.

➤ There are no food or fluid restrictions, unless by medical direction.

Intratest:

➤ Have emergency equipment readily available.

➤ Patients are given a gown, robe, and foot coverings to wear and instructed to void prior to the procedure.

➤ Observe standard precautions, and follow the general guidelines in Appendix A.

➤ Instruct the patient to cooperate fully and to follow directions. Instruct the patient to remain still throughout the procedure because movement produces unreliable results. Ask the patient to breathe normally during the examination.

➤ Place the patient in a supine position on a flat table with foam wedges to help maintain position and immobilization.

➤ Expose the chest, and attach electrocardiogram leads for simultaneous tracings, if desired.

➤ Apply conductive gel to the chest slightly to the left of the sternum. Place the transducer on the chest surface along the left sternal border, the subxiphoid area, suprasternal notch, and supraclavicular areas to obtain views and tracings of the portions of the heart. Scan the areas by systematically moving the probe in a perpendicular position to direct the ultrasound waves to each part of the heart. These can be viewed immediately and recorded on moving graph paper (M-mode) or videotape (two-dimensional).

➤ To obtain different views or information about heart function, position the patient on the left side and/or sitting up, or request that the patient breathe slowly or hold the breath during the procedure. To evaluate heart function changes, the patient may be asked to inhale amyl nitrate (vasodilator).

➤ Administer contrast medium, if ordered. A second series of images is obtained.

➤ The results are recorded on x-ray film or in a computerized system for recall and postprocedure interpreta-

tion by the appropriate health care practitioner.

Post-test:

➤ When the study is completed, remove the gel from the skin.

➤ A written report of the examination will be completed by a health care practitioner specializing in this branch of medicine. The report will be sent to the requesting health care practitioner, who will discuss the results with the patient.

➤ Reinforce information given by the patient's health care provider regarding further testing, treatment, or referral to another health care provider. Answer any questions or address any concerns voiced by the patient or family.

➤ Depending on the results of this procedure, additional testing may be needed to evaluate or monitor progression of the disease process and determine the need for a change in therapy. Evaluate test results in relation to the patient's symptoms and other tests performed.

Related diagnostic tests:

➤ Related diagnostic tests include chest x-ray, computed tomography scan of the thorax, magnetic resonance imaging of the chest, myocardial perfusion scan, and positron emission tomography of the heart.

ECHOCARDIOGRAPHY, TRANSESOPHAGEAL

· ·

SYNONYM/ACRONYM: Echo, TEE.

AREA OF APPLICATION: Chest/thorax.

CONTRAST: Can be done with or without noniodinated contrast medium (microspheres).

DESCRIPTION & RATIONALE: Transesophageal echocardiography (TEE) is performed to assist in the diagnosis of cardiovascular disorders when non-invasive echocardiography is contraindicated or does not reveal enough information to confirm a diagnosis. Noninvasive echocardiography may be an inadequate procedure for patients who are obese, have chest wall structure abnormalities, or have chronic obstructive pulmonary disease (COPD). TEE provides a better view of the posterior aspect of the heart, including the atrium and aorta. It is done with a transducer attached to a gastroscope that is inserted into the esophagus. The transducer and the ultrasound instrument allow the beam to be directed to the back of the heart. The echoes are amplified and recorded on a screen for visualization, and recorded on graph paper or videotape. The depth of the endoscope and movement of the transducer is controlled to obtain various images of the heart structures. TEE is usually performed during surgery; it is also used on patients who are in the intensive care unit, in whom the transmission of waves to and from the chest has been compromised and more definitive information is needed. The images obtained by TEE have better resolution than those obtained by routine transthoracic echocardiography because TEE uses higher frequency sound waves and offers closer proximity of the transducer to the cardiac structures. Cardiac contrast medium is used to improve the visualization of viable myocardial tissue within the heart. ■

INDICATIONS:

• Confirm diagnosis if conventional echocardiography does not correlate with other findings

• Detect and evaluate congenital heart disorders

• Detect atrial tumors (myxomas)

• Detect or determine the severity of valvular abnormalities and regurgitation

• Detect subaortic stenosis as evidenced by displacement of the anterior atrial leaflet and reduction in aortic valve flow, depending on the obstruction

- Detect thoracic aortic dissection and coronary artery disease (CAD)

- Detect ventricular or atrial mural thrombi and evaluate cardiac wall motion after myocardial infarction

- Determine the presence of pericardial effusion

- Evaluate aneurysms and ventricular thrombus

- Evaluate or monitor biological and prosthetic valve function

- Evaluate septal defects

- Measure the size of the heart's chambers and determine if hypertrophic cardiomyopathy or congestive heart failure is present

- Monitor cardiac function during open heart surgery (most sensitive method for monitoring ischemia)

- Re-evaluate after inadequate visualization with conventional echocardiography as a result of obesity, trauma to or deformity of the chest wall, or lung hyperinflation associated with COPD

RESULT

Normal Findings:
- Normal appearance of the size, position, structure, movements of the heart valves and heart muscle walls, and chamber blood filling; and no evidence of valvular stenosis or insufficiency, cardiac tumor, foreign bodies, or CAD. The established values for the measurement of heart activities obtained by the study may vary by health care practitioner and institution.

Abnormal Findings:
- Aneurysm
- Aortic valve abnormalities
- CAD
- Cardiomyopathy
- Congenital heart defects

- Congestive heart failure
- Mitral valve abnormalities
- Myocardial infarction
- Myxoma
- Pericardial effusion
- Pulmonary hypertension
- Pulmonary valve abnormalities
- Septal defects
- Shunting of blood flow
- Thrombus
- Ventricular hypertrophy
- Ventricular or atrial mural thrombi

CRITICAL VALUES: N/A

INTERFERING FACTORS:

This procedure is contraindicated for:
- Patients with significant esophageal pathology (procedure may cause bleeding)

Factors that may impair clear imaging:
- Incorrect placement of the transducer over the desired test site

- Retained barium from a previous radiologic procedure

- Patients who are dehydrated, resulting in failure to demonstrate the boundaries between organs and tissue structures

- Laryngospasm, dysrhythmias, or esophageal bleeding

- Known upper esophageal pathology

- Conditions such as esophageal dysphagia and irradiation of the mediastinum

- Improper adjustment of the ultrasound equipment to accommodate obese or thin patients, which can cause a poor-quality study

- The presence of COPD or use of mechanical ventilation, which increases the air between the heart and chest wall (hyperinflation) and can attenuate the ultrasound waves

- The presence of arrhythmias

- Patients who are very obese, who may exceed the weight limit for the equipment

- Inability of the patient to cooperate or remain still during the procedure because of age, significant pain, or mental status

Other considerations:
- Failure to follow dietary restrictions before the procedure may cause the procedure to be canceled or repeated.

Nursing Implications and Procedure • • • • • • • • • • •

Pretest:

➤ Inform the patient that the procedure assesses cardiac function.

➤ Obtain a history of the patient's complaints or clinical symptoms.

➤ Obtain a history of results of previously performed diagnostic procedures, surgical procedures, and laboratory tests. For related diagnostic tests, refer to the Cardiovascular System table.

➤ Note any recent procedures that can interfere with test results (i.e., barium procedures, surgery, or biopsy). There should be 24 hours between administration of barium and this test.

➤ Record the date of the last menstrual period and determine the possibility of pregnancy in perimenopausal women.

➤ Obtain a list of the medications the patient is taking.

➤ Review the procedure with the patient. Address concerns about pain related to the procedure. Explain to the patient that some pain may be experienced during the test, and there may be moments of discomfort during insertion of the scope. Lidocaine is sprayed in the patient's throat to reduce discomfort caused by the presence of the endoscope. Explain the purpose of the test and how the procedure is performed. Inform the patient that the procedure is performed in a ultrasound or cardiology department, usually by a technologist, and takes approximately 30 to 60 minutes.

➤ Explain that an intravenous (IV) line may be inserted to allow infusion of IV fluids, contrast medium, dye, or sedatives.

➤ *Sensitivity to social and cultural issues, as well as concern for modesty, is important in providing psychological support before, during and after the procedure.*

➤ The patient should fast and refrain from drinking liquids for 8 hours before the procedure.

➤ Obtain and record the patient's vital signs.

➤ *Make sure a written and informed consent has been signed prior to the procedure and before administering any medications.*

Intratest:

➤ Ensure that the patient has complied with dietary restrictions; assure that food has been restricted for at least 8 hours depending on the anesthetic chosen for the procedure.

➤ Have emergency equipment readily available.

➤ Patients are given a gown, robe, and foot coverings to wear and instructed to void prior to the procedure.

➤ Observe standard precautions, and follow the general guidelines in Appendix A.

➤ Instruct the patient to cooperate fully and to follow directions. Instruct the patient to remain still throughout the procedure because movement produces unreliable results.

➤ Remove dentures from the patient's mouth.

➤ Monitor pulse oximetry to determine oxygen saturation in sedated patients.

➤ Expose the chest, and attach electrocardiogram leads for simultaneous tracings, if desired.

➤ Spray or swab the patient's throat with a local anesthetic, and place the oral bridge device in the mouth to prevent biting of the endoscope.

➤ Place the patient in a left side-lying position on a flat table with foam wedges that will help maintain position and immobilization. The pharyngeal area is anesthetized and the endoscope with the ultrasound device attached to its tip is inserted 30 to 50 cm to the posterior area of the heart, as in any esophagogastroduodenoscopy procedure.

➤ Ask the patient to swallow as the scope is inserted. When the transducer is in place, the scope is manipulated by controls on the handle to obtain scanning that provides real-time images of the heart motion and recordings of the images for viewing. Actual scanning is usually limited to 15 minutes or until the desired number of image planes is obtained at different depths of the scope.

➤ Administer contrast medium, if ordered. A second series of images is obtained.

➤ The results are recorded on x-ray film or in a computerized system for recall and postprocedure interpretation by the appropriate health care practitioner.

Post-test:

➤ Instruct the patient to resume usual diet and activity 4 to 6 hours after the test, as directed by the health care practitioner.

➤ Instruct patient to treat throat discomfort with lozenges and warm gargles when the gag reflex returns.

➤ Monitor vital signs and neurologic status every 15 minutes for 1 hour, then every 2 hours for 4 hours, and as ordered. Take temperature every 4 hours for 24 hours. Compare with baseline values. Notify the health care practitioner if temperature is elevated. Protocols may vary from facility to facility.

➤ A written report of the examination will be completed by a health care practitioner specializing in this branch of medicine. The report will be sent to the requesting health care practitioner, who will discuss the results with the patient.

➤ Reinforce information given by the patient's health care provider regarding further testing, treatment, or referral to another health care provider. Answer any questions or address any concerns voiced by the patient or family.

➤ Depending on the results of this procedure, additional testing may be needed to evaluate or monitor progression of the disease process and determine the need for a change in therapy. Evaluate test results in relation to the patient's symptoms and other tests performed.

Related diagnostic tests:

➤ Related diagnostic tests include chest x-ray, computed tomography of the thorax, magnetic resonance imaging of the chest, myocardial perfusion scan, and positron emission tomography of the heart.

ELECTROCARDIOGRAM

· ·

SYNONYMS/ACRONYMS: ECG, VCG, EKG.

AREA OF APPLICATION: Heart.

CONTRAST: None.

DESCRIPTION & RATIONALE: The cardiac muscle consists of three layers of cells—the inner layer called the *endocardium*, the middle layer called the *myocardium*, and the outer layer called the *epicardium*. The systolic phase of the cardiac cycle reflects the contraction of the myocardium, whereas the diastolic phase takes place when the heart relaxes to allow blood to rush in. All muscle cells have a characteristic rate of contraction called *depolarization*. Therefore, the heart will maintain a predetermined heart rate unless other stimuli are received.

The monitoring of pulse and blood pressure evaluates only the mechanical activity of the heart. The electrocardiogram (ECG), a noninvasive study, measures the electrical currents or impulses that the heart generates during a cardiac cycle (see figure of a normal ECG at end of monograph). Electrical impulses travel through a conduction system beginning with the sinoatrial (SA) node and moving to the atrioventricular (AV) node via internodal pathways. From the AV node, the impulses travel to the bundle of His and onward to the right and left bundle branches. These bundles are located within the right and left ventricles. The impulses continue to the cardiac muscle cells by terminal fibers called *Purkinje fibers*. The ECG is a graphic display of the electrical activity of the heart, which is analyzed by time intervals and segments. Continuous tracing of the cardiac cycle activities is captured as heart cells are electrically stimulated, causing depolarization and movement of the activity through the cells of the myocardium.

The ECG study is completed by using 12 electrodes attached to the skin surface to obtain the total electrical activity of the heart. Each lead records the electrical potential between the limbs or between the heart and limbs. The ECG machine records and marks the 12 leads on the strip of paper in the machine in proper sequence, usually 6 inches of the strip for each lead. The ECG pattern, called a *heart rhythm*, is recorded by a machine as a series of waves, intervals, and segments, each of which pertains to a specific occurrence during the contraction of the heart. The ECG tracings are recorded on graph paper using vertical and horizontal lines for analysis and calculations of time, measured by the vertical lines (1 mm apart and 0.04 seconds per line), and of voltage, measured by the horizontal lines (1 mm apart and 0.5 mV per 5 squares). A pulse rate can be calculated from the ECG strip to obtain the beats per minute. The P wave represents the depolarization of the atrial myocardium; the QRS complex represents the depolarization of the ventricular myocardium; the P-R interval represents the time from beginning of the excitation of the atrium to the beginning of the ventricular excitation; and the ST segment has no deflection from baseline, but in an abnormal state may be elevated or depressed. An abnormal rhythm is called an *arrhythmia*. ∎

INDICATIONS:

- Assess the extent of congenital heart disease

- Assess the extent of myocardial infarction (MI) or ischemia, as indicated by abnormal ST segment, interval times, and amplitudes

- Assess the function of heart valves

- Assess global cardiac function

- Detect arrhythmias, as evidenced by abnormal wave deflections

- Detect pericarditis, shown by ST segment changes or shortened P-R interval

- Determine electrolyte imbalances, as evidenced by short or prolonged Q-T interval

- Determine hypertrophy of the chamber of the heart or heart hypertrophy, as evidenced by P or R wave deflections

- Evaluate and monitor cardiac pacemaker function

- Evaluate and monitor the effect of drugs, such as digitalis, antiarrhythmics, or vasodilating agents

- Monitor ECG changes during an exercise test

- Monitor rhythm changes during the recovery phase after an MI

RESULT

Normal Findings:

- Normal heart rate according to age: range of 60 to 100 beats/min in adults

- Normal, regular rhythm and wave deflections with normal measurement of ranges of cycle components and height, depth, and duration of complexes as follows:

  P wave: 0.12 seconds or 3 small blocks with amplitude of 2.5 mm

  Q wave: less than 0.04 mm

  R wave: 5 to 27 mm amplitude, depending on lead

  T wave: 1 to 13 mm amplitude, depending on lead

  QRS complex: 0.12 seconds or 3 small blocks

  ST segment: 1 mm

Abnormal Findings:

- Arrhythmias.

- Atrial or ventricular hypertrophy.

- Bundle branch block.

- Electrolyte imbalances.

- MI or ischemia.

- Pericarditis.

- Pulmonary infarction.

- P wave: An enlarged P wave deflection could indicate atrial enlargement. An absent or altered P wave could suggest that the electrical impulse did not come from the SA node.

- P-R interval: An increased interval could imply a conduction delay in the AV node.

- QRS complex: An enlarged Q wave may indicate an old infarction; an enlarged deflection could indicate ventricular hypertrophy. Increased time duration may indicate a bundle branch block.

- ST segment: A depressed ST segment indicates myocardial ischemia. An elevated ST segment may indicate an acute MI or pericarditis. A prolonged ST segment may indicate hypocalcemia or hypokalemia (short segment).

- T wave: A flat or inverted T wave may indicate myocardial ischemia, infarction, or hypokalemia. A tall T wave may indicate hyperkalemia.

CRITICAL VALUES: N/A

INTERFERING FACTORS:

Factors that may impair the results of the examination:

- Anatomic variation of the heart (i.e., the heart may be rotated in both the horizontal and frontal planes)

- Distortion of cardiac cycles due to age, sex, weight, or a medical condition (e.g., infants, women [may exhibit slight ST segment depression], obese patients, pregnant patients, patients with ascites)

- High intake of carbohydrates or electrolyte imbalances of potassium or calcium

- Improper placement of electrodes or inadequate contact between skin and electrodes because of insufficient conductive gel or poor placement, which can cause ECG tracing problems

- ECG machine malfunction or interference from electromagnetic waves in the vicinity

- Inability of the patient to remain still during the procedure, because movement, muscle tremor, or twitching can affect accurate test recording

- Increased patient anxiety, causing hyperventilation or deep respirations

- Medications such as barbiturates and digitalis

- Strenuous exercise before the procedure

Nursing Implications and Procedure

Pretest:

> Inform the patient that the procedure assesses cardiac function.

> Obtain a history of the patient's complaints or symptoms, including cardiac disease and present cardiovascular status. Ask if the patient has had a heart transplant or pacemaker implanted.

> Obtain a history of results of previously performed diagnostic procedures, surgical procedures, and laboratory tests. For related diagnostic tests, refer to the Cardiovascular System table.

> Obtain a list of the medications the patient is taking.

> Review the procedure with the patient. Address concerns about pain related to the procedure. Explain to the patient that there should be no discomfort during the procedure. Inform the patient that the procedure takes approximately 15 minutes.

> Record baseline vital signs.

> No food, fluid, or medication restrictions exist, unless by medical direction.

> *Sensitivity to cultural and social issues,* as well as concern for modesty, is important in providing psychological support before, during and after the procedure.

Intratest:

> Have the patient remove clothing to the waist and shoes and any hosiery. Patients may want to wear a gown (open to the front).

> Observe standard precautions, and follow the general guidelines in Appendix A.

> Instruct the patient to lie very still in a relaxed position during the study and to refrain from tensing muscles after electrode placement. Direct the patient to breathe normally and to avoid touching the bed or couch.

- Place patient in a supine position. Expose and appropriately drape the chest, arms, and legs.
- Prepare the skin surface with alcohol and remove excess hair. Shaving may be necessary. Dry skin sites.
- Apply the electrodes in the proper position. When placing the six unipolar chest leads, place V_1 at the fourth intercostal space at the border of the right sternum, V_2 at the fourth intercostal space at the border of the left sternum, V_3 between V_2 and V_4, V_4 at the fifth intercostal space at the midclavicular line, V_5 at the left anterior axillary line at the level of V_4 horizontally, and V_6 at the level of V_4 horizontally and at the left midaxillary line. The wires are connected to the matched electrodes and the ECG machine. Chest leads (V_1, V_2, V_3, V_4, V_5, and V_6) record data from the horizontal plane of the heart.
- Place three limb bipolar leads (two electrodes combined for each) on the arms and legs. Lead I is the combination of two arm electrodes, lead II is the combination of right arm and left leg electrodes, and lead III is the combination of left arm and left leg electrodes. Limb leads (I, II, III, aV L, aVF, and aVR) record data from the frontal plane of the heart.
- The machine is set and turned on after the electrodes, grounding, connections, paper supply, computer, and data storage device are checked.
- If the patient has any chest discomfort or pain during the procedure, mark the ECG strip indicating that occurrence.
- The results are recorded on a paper strip for postprocedure interpretation by the appropriate health care practitioner.

Post-test:

- When the procedure is complete, remove the electrodes and clean the skin where the electrode pads were applied.
- Evaluate the results in relation to previously performed ECGs. Denote cardiac rhythm abnormalities on the strip.

- Monitor vital signs and compare with baseline values. Protocols may vary from facility to facility.
- Instruct the patient to immediately notify a health care practitioner of chest pain, changes in pulse rate, or shortness of breath.
- A written report of the examination will be completed by a health care practitioner specializing in this branch of medicine. The report will be sent to the requesting health care practitioner, who will discuss the results with the patient.
- Recognize anxiety related to the test results and be supportive of perceived loss of independence and fear of shortened life expectancy. Discuss the implications of abnormal test results on the patient's lifestyle. Provide teaching and information regarding the clinical implications of the test results, as appropriate.
- Reinforce information given by the patient's health care provider regarding further testing, treatment, or referral to another health care provider. Answer any questions or address any concerns voiced by the patient or family.
- Instruct the patient or caregiver in the use of any ordered medications. Explain the importance of adhering to the therapy regimen. As appropriate, instruct the patient in significant side effects and systemic reactions associated with the prescribed medication. Encourage him or her to review corresponding literature provided by a pharmacist.
- Depending on the results of this procedure, additional testing may be performed to evaluate or monitor progression of the disease process and determine the need for a change in therapy. Evaluate test results in relation to the patient's symptoms and other tests performed.

Related diagnostic tests:

- Related diagnostic tests include coronary angiography, echocardiogram, myocardial perfusion scan of the heart, and positron emission tomography scan of the heart.

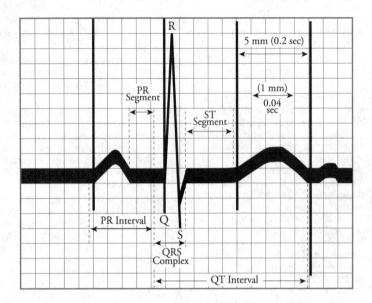

ELECTROENCEPHALOGRAPHY

. . . .

SYNONYM/ACRONYM: Sonogram (for sleep disturbances), EEG.

AREA OF APPLICATION: Brain.

CONTRAST: None.

DESCRIPTION & RATIONALE: Electroencephalography (EEG) is a noninvasive study that measures the brain's electrical activity and records that activity on graph paper. These electrical impulses arise from the brain cells of the cerebral cortex. Electrodes, placed at 8 to 20 sites (or pairs of sites) on the patient's scalp, transmit the different frequencies and amplitudes of the brain's electrical activity to the EEG machine, which records the results in graph form on a moving paper strip. This procedure can evaluate responses to various stimuli, such as flickering light, hyperventilation, auditory signals, or somatosensory signals generated by skin electrodes. The procedure is usually performed in a room designed to eliminate electrical interference and minimize distractions. EEG can be done at the bedside, especially to confirm brain death. A physician analyzes the waveforms. The test is used to detect epilepsy, intracranial abscesses, or tumors; to evaluate cerebral involvement due to head injury or meningitis; and to monitor for cerebral tissue ischemia during surgery when cerebral vessels must be occluded. EEG is also used to confirm brain death, which can be defined as absence of electrical activity in the brain. To evaluate abnormal EEG waves further, the patient may be connected to an ambulatory EEG system similar to a Holter monitor for the heart. Patients keep a journal of their activities and any symptoms that occur during the monitoring period. ■

INDICATIONS:

- Confirm brain death
- Confirm suspicion of increased intracranial pressure caused by trauma or disease
- Detect cerebral ischemia during endarterectomy
- Detect intracranial cerebrovascular lesions, such as hemorrhages and infarcts
- Detect seizure disorders and identify focus of seizure and seizure activity, as evidenced by abnormal spikes and waves recorded on the graph
- Determine the presence of tumors, abscesses, or infection
- Evaluate the effect of drug intoxication on the brain
- Evaluate sleeping disorders, such as sleep apnea and narcolepsy
- Identify area of abnormality in dementia

RESULT

Normal Findings:

- Normal occurrences of alpha, beta, theta, and delta waves (rhythms varying depending on the patent's age)
- Normal frequency, amplitude, and characteristics of brain waves

Abnormal Findings:

- Abscess
- Brain death
- Cerebral infarct
- Encephalitis
- Glioblastoma and other brain tumors
- Head injury
- Hypocalcemia or hypoglycemia
- Intracranial hemorrhage
- Meningitis
- Migraine headaches
- Narcolepsy
- Seizure disorders (grand mal, focal, temporal lobe, myoclonic, petit mal)
- Sleep apnea

CRITICAL VALUES: N/A

INTERFERING FACTORS:

Factors that may impair the results of the examination:

- Inability of the patient to cooperate or remain still during the procedure because of age, significant pain, or mental status
- Drugs and substances such as sedatives, anticonvulsants, anxiolytics, and alcohol, and stimulants such as caffeine and nicotine
- Hypoglycemic or hypothermic states
- Hair that is dirty, oily, or sprayed or treated with hair preparations

Nursing Implications and Procedure • • • • • • • • • •

➤ Inform the patient that the procedure is performed to measure electrical activity of the brain.

➤ Obtain a history of the patient's neurologic system, known or suspected seizure conditions, intracranial abnormalities, traumatic incidents to head, and sleep disorders, as well as the results of previously performed laboratory tests, surgical procedures, and other diagnostic procedures. For related diagnostic tests, refer to the Musculoskeletal System table.

➤ Obtain a list of the medications the patient is taking, including herbs, nutritional supplements, and nutraceuticals. The requesting health care practitioner and laboratory should be advised if the patient regularly uses these products so that their effects can be taken into consideration when reviewing results.

➤ Review the procedure with the patient. Address concerns about pain related to the procedure. Assure the patient that there is no discomfort during the procedure, but that, if needle electrodes are used, a slight pinch may be felt. Explain the purpose of the test and how the procedure is performed. Explain that electricity flows from the patient's body, not into the body, during the procedure. Explain that the procedure reveals brain activity only, not thoughts, feelings, or intelligence. Inform the patient that the procedure is performed in a neurodiagnostic department, usually by a technologist and support staff, and takes approximately 30 to 60 minutes.

➤ Inform the patient that he or she may be asked to alter breathing pattern; be asked to follow simple commands such as opening or closing eyes, blinking, or swallowing; be stimulated with bright light; or be given a drug to induce sleep during the study.

➤ Instruct the patient to clean the hair and to refrain from using hair sprays, creams, or solutions before the test.

➤ Instruct the patient to refrain from drinking caffeine-containing beverages for 8 hours before the procedure, and to eat a meal before the study.

➤ Under medical direction, the patient should avoid sedatives, anticonvulsants, anxiolytics, alcohol, and stimulants such as caffeine and nicotine for 24 to 48 hours before the test.

➤ Instruct the patient to limit sleep to 5 hours for an adult and 7 hours for a child the night before the study. Young infants and children should not be allowed to nap before the study.

➤ *Sensitivity to cultural and social issues,* as well as concern for modesty, is important in providing psychological support before, during and after the procedure.

➤ *Make sure a written and informed consent has been signed prior to the procedure and before administering any medications.*

➤ Ensure that caffeine-containing beverages were withheld for 8 hours before the procedure, and that a meal was ingested before the study.

➤ Ensure that all substances with the potential to interfere with test results are withheld for 24 to 48 hours before the test.

➤ Ensure that the patient is able to relax; report any extreme anxiety or restlessness.

➤ Ensure that hair is clean and free of hair sprays, creams, or solutions.

➤ Observe standard precautions, and follow the general guidelines in Appendix A.

➤ Place the patient in the supine position in a bed or in a semi-Fowler's position on a recliner in a special room protected from any noise or electrical interferences that could affect the tracings.

> Remind the patient to relax and not to move any muscles or parts of the face or head. The technician should be able to observe the patient for movements or other interferences through a window into the test room.

> The electrodes are prepared and applied to the scalp. Electrodes are placed in as many as 16 locations over the frontal, temporal, parietal, and occipital areas, and amplifier wires are attached. An electrode is also attached to each earlobe as grounding electrodes. At this time, a baseline recording can be made with the patient at rest.

> Recordings are made with the patient at rest and with eyes closed. The test recordings are stopped about every 5 minutes to allow the patient to move. Recordings are also made during a drowsy and sleep period, depending on the patient's clinical condition and symptoms.

> Procedures (e.g., stroboscopic light stimulation, hyperventilation to induce alkalosis, and sleep induction by administration of sedative to detect abnormalities that occur only during sleep) may be done to bring out abnormal electrical activity or other brain abnormalities.

> Observations for seizure activity are carried out during the study, and a description and time of activity is noted by the technician.

> The results are recorded on a paper strip for postprocedure interpretation by the appropriate health care practitioner.

Post-test:

> When the procedure is complete, remove electrodes from the hair and remove paste by cleansing with oil or witch hazel.

> If a sedative was given during the test, allow the patient to recover.

Bedside rails are put in the raised position for safety.

> Instruct the patient to resume medications, as directed by the health care practitioner.

> Instruct the patient to report any seizure activity.

> A written report of the examination will be completed by a health care practitioner specializing in this branch of medicine. The report will be sent to the requesting health care practitioner, who will discuss the results with the patient.

> Recognize anxiety related to test results, and be supportive of perceived loss of independent function. Discuss the implications of abnormal test results on the patient's lifestyle. Provide teaching and information regarding the clinical implications of the test results, as appropriate.

> Reinforce information given by the patient's health care provider regarding further testing, treatment, or referral to another health care provider. Answer any questions or address any concerns voiced by the patient or family.

> Instruct the patient in the use of any ordered medications. Explain the importance of adhering to the therapy regimen. As appropriate, instruct the patient in significant side effects and systemic reactions associated with the prescribed medication. Encourage him or her to review corresponding literature provided by a pharmacist.

> Depending on the results of this procedure, additional testing may be performed to evaluate or monitor progression of the disease process and determine the need for a change in therapy. Evaluate test results in relation to the patient's symptoms and other tests performed.

Related diagnostic tests:

> Related diagnostic tests include computed tomography of the brain and magnetic resonance imaging of the brain.

ELECTROMYOGRAPHY

· ·

SYNONYMS/ACRONYM: Electrodiagnostic study, neuromuscular junction testing, EMG.

AREA OF APPLICATION: Muscles.

CONTRAST: None.

DESCRIPTION & RATIONALE: Electromyography (EMG) measures skeletal muscle activity during rest, voluntary contraction, and electrical stimulation. Percutaneous extracellular needle electrodes containing fine wires are inserted into selected muscle groups to detect neuromuscular abnormalities and measure nerve and electrical conduction properties of skeletal muscles. The electrical potentials are amplified, displayed on a screen in waveforms, and electronically recorded, similar to electrocardiography. Comparison and analysis of the amplitude, duration, number, and configuration of the muscle activity provide diagnostic information about the extent of nerve and muscle involvement in the detection of primary muscle diseases, including lower motor neuron, anterior horn cell, or neuromuscular junction diseases; defective transmission at the neuromuscular junction; and peripheral nerve damage or disease. Responses of a relaxed muscle are electrically silent, but spontaneous muscle movement such as fibrillation and fasciculation can be detected in a relaxed, denervated muscle. Muscle action potentials are detected with minimal or maximal muscle contractions. The differences in the size and numbers of activity potentials during voluntary contractions determine whether the muscle weakness is a disease of the striated muscle fibers or cell membranes (myogenic), or a disease of the lower motor neuron (neurogenic). Nerve conduction studies (electroneurography) are commonly done in conjunction with electromyelography; the combination of the procedures is known as electromyoneurography. The examination's major use lies in differentiating among the following disease classes: primary myopathy, peripheral motor neuron disease, and disease of the neuromuscular junction. ▪

INDICATIONS:
• Assess primary muscle diseases affecting striated muscle fibers or cell membrane, such as muscular dystrophy or myasthenia gravis

• Detect muscle disorders caused by diseases of the lower motor neuron involving the motor neuron on the anterior horn of the spinal cord, such as anterior poliomyelitis, amyotrophic lateral sclerosis, amyotonia, and spinal tumors

- Detect muscle disorders caused by diseases of the lower motor neuron involving the nerve root, such as Guillain-Barré syndrome, herniated disc, or spinal stenosis

- Detect neuromuscular disorders, such as peripheral neuropathy caused by diabetes or alcoholism, and locate the site of the abnormality

- Determine if a muscle abnormality is caused by the toxic effects of drugs (e.g., antibiotics, chemotherapy) or toxins (e.g., *Clostridium botulinum,* snake venom, heavy metals)

- Differentiate between primary and secondary muscle disorders or between neuropathy and myopathy

- Differentiate secondary muscle disorders caused by polymyositis, sarcoidosis, hypocalcemia, thyroid toxicity, tetanus, and other disorders

- Monitor and evaluate progression of myopathies or neuropathies, including confirmation of diagnosis of carpal tunnel syndrome

RESULT

Normal Findings:
- Normal muscle electrical activity during rest and contraction states

Abnormal findings and possible meanings:
- Evidence of neuromuscular disorders or primary muscle disease (*note:* findings must be correlated with the patient's history, clinical features, and results of other neurodiagnostic tests):
  Amyotrophic lateral sclerosis
  Bell's palsy
  Beriberi
  Carpal tunnel syndrome
  Dermatomyositis
  Diabetic peripheral neuropathy
  Eaton-Lambert syndrome
  Guillain-Barré syndrome

Multiple sclerosis
Muscular dystrophy
Myasthenia gravis
Myopathy
Polymyositis
Radiculopathy
Traumatic injury

CRITICAL VALUES: N/A

INTERFERING FACTORS:

This procedure is contraindicated for:
- Patients with extensive skin infection

- Patients receiving anticoagulant therapy

- Patients with an infection at the sites of electrode placement

Factors that may impair the results of the examination:
- Inability of the patient to cooperate or remain still during the procedure because of age, significant pain, or mental status

- Age-related decreases in electrical activity

- Medications such as muscle relaxants, cholinergics, and anticholinergics

- Improper placement of surface or needle electrodes

Nursing Implications and Procedure • • • • • • • • • •

Pretest:

▶ Inform the patient that the procedure is performed to measure electrical activity of the muscles.

▶ Obtain a history of neuromuscular and neurosensory status, diseases or conditions that affect muscle function, level of muscular function and range of motion, and traumatic events, as well as the results of previously performed laboratory tests, surgical procedures, and other diagnostic procedures. For related diagnostic tests, refer to the Musculoskeletal System table.

➤ Obtain a list of the medications the patient is taking, especially medications known to affect bleeding including anticoagulants, aspirin and other salicylates, etc.

➤ Review the procedure with the patient. Address concerns about pain related to the procedure. Inform the patient that as many as 10 electrodes may be inserted at various locations on the body. Warn the patient that the procedure may be uncomfortable, but that an analgesic or sedative will be administered. Inform the patient that the procedure is performed in a special laboratory by a health care practitioner and takes approximately 1 hour to complete, but can take up to 3 hours depending on the patient's condition.

➤ Instruct the patient to refrain from smoking and drinking caffeine-containing beverages for 3 hours before the procedure.

➤ Under medical direction, the patient should avoid muscle relaxants, cholinergics, and anticholinergics for 3 to 6 days before the test.

➤ Assess for the ability to comply with directions given for exercising during the test.

➤ *Make sure a written and informed consent has been signed prior to the procedure and before administering any medications.*

Intratest:

➤ Ensure that the patient has refrained from smoking and drinking caffeine-containing beverages for 3 hours before the procedure.

➤ Ensure that medications such as muscle relaxants, cholinergics, and anticholinergics have been withheld, as ordered.

➤ Have patient remove clothing and any hosiery. Patients are given a gown to wear and instructed to void prior to the procedure.

➤ Ask the patient to remain very still and relaxed and to cooperate with instructions given to contract muscles during the procedure.

➤ Place the patient in a supine or sitting position depending on the location of the muscle to be tested. Ensure that the area or room is protected from noise or metallic interference that may affect the test results.

➤ Observe standard precautions, and follow the general guidelines in Appendix A.

➤ Administer mild analgesic (adult) or sedative (children), as ordered, to promote a restful state before the procedure.

➤ Cleanse the skin thoroughly with alcohol pads, as necessary.

➤ An electrode is applied to the skin to ground the patient, and then 24-gauge needles containing a fine-wire electrode are inserted into the muscle. The electrical potentials of the muscle are amplified, displayed on a screen, and electronically recorded.

➤ During the test, muscle activity is tested while the patient is at rest, during incremental needle insertion, and during varying degrees of muscle contraction.

➤ Ask the patient to alternate between a relaxed and a contracted muscle state, or to perform progressive muscle contractions while the potentials are being measured.

➤ The results are recorded manually or in a computerized system for recall and postprocedure interpretation by the appropriate health care practitioner.

Post-test:

➤ When the procedure is complete, remove the electrodes and clean the skin where the electrode was applied.

➤ Monitor electrode sites for bleeding, hematoma or inflammation.

➤ If residual pain is noted after the procedure, instruct the patient to apply warm compresses and to take analgesics, as ordered.

➤ Instruct the patient to resume usual

diet, medication, and activity, as directed by the health care practitioner.

➤ A written report of the examination will be completed by a health care practitioner specializing in this branch of medicine. The report will be sent to the requesting health care practitioner, who will discuss the results with the patient.

➤ Recognize anxiety related to test results, and be supportive of perceived loss of independent function. Discuss the implications of abnormal test results on the patient's lifestyle. Provide teaching and information regarding the clinical implications of the test results, as appropriate.

➤ Reinforce information given by the patient's health care provider regarding further testing, treatment, or referral to another health care provider. Answer any questions or address any concerns voiced by the patient or family.

➤ Depending on the results of this procedure, additional testing may be performed to evaluate or monitor progression of the disease process and determine the need for a change in therapy. Evaluate test results in relation to the patient's symptoms and other tests performed.

Related diagnostic tests:

➤ Related diagnostic tests include computed tomography of the brain and magnetic resonance imaging of the brain.

ELECTROMYOGRAPHY, PELVIC FLOOR SPHINCTER

· ·

SYNONYMS/ACRONYM: Electrodiagnostic study, rectal electromyography.

AREA OF APPLICATION: Sphincter muscles.

CONTRAST: None.

DESCRIPTION & RATIONALE: Pelvic floor sphincter electromyography, also known as rectal electromyography, is performed to measure electrical activity of the external urinary sphincter. This procedure, often done in conjunction with cystometry and voiding urethrography as part of a full urodynamic study, helps to diagnose neuromuscular dysfunction and incontinence. ■

INDICATIONS: Evaluate neuromuscular dysfunction and incontinence

CRITICAL VALUES: N/A

INTERFERING FACTORS:

This procedure is contraindicated for:
• Patients who are pregnant or suspected of being pregnant, unless the potential benefits of the procedure far outweigh the risks to the fetus and mother.

Factors that may impair the results of the examination:

- Inability of the patient to cooperate or remain still during the procedure because of age, significant pain, or mental status

- Age-related decreases in electrical activity

- Medications such as muscle relaxants, cholinergics, and anticholinergics

Other considerations:

- Failure to follow dietary restrictions before the procedure may cause the procedure to be canceled or repeated.

Nursing Implications and Procedure • • • • • • • • • • • •

Pretest:

➤ Inform the patient that the procedure is performed to measure electrical activity of the pelvic floor muscles.

➤ Obtain a history of neuromuscular and neurosensory status, diseases or conditions that affect muscle function, level of muscular function and range of motion, and traumatic events, as well as the results of previously performed laboratory tests, surgical procedures, and other diagnostic procedures. For related diagnostic tests, refer to the Genitourinary and Musculoskeletal System tables.

➤ Obtain a list of the medications the patient is taking, especially medications known to affect bleeding including anticoagulants, aspirin and other salicylates, etc.

➤ Ensure that the patient has refrained from smoking and drinking caffeine-containing beverages for 3 hours before the procedure.

➤ Review the procedure with the patient. Address concerns about pain related to the procedure. Warn the patient that the procedure may be uncomfortable, but that an analgesic or sedative will be administered. Assure the patient that the pain is

minimal during the catheter insertion. Inform the patient that the procedure is performed in a special laboratory by a health care practitioner and takes about 30 minutes to complete.

➤ Under medical direction, the patient should avoid muscle relaxants, cholinergics, and anticholinergics for 3 to 6 days before the test.

➤ Assess for ability to comply with directions given for exercising during the test.

➤ The patient should fast and refrain from drinking liquids for 8 hours prior to the procedure.

➤ *Make sure a written and informed consent has been signed prior to the procedure and before administering any medications.*

Intratest:

➤ Ensure that the patient has complied with dietary, fluids, and medication restrictions and pretesting preparations.

➤ Ask the patient to void immediately before the test.

➤ Place the patient in a supine position on the examining table and place a drape over the patient, exposing the perineal area.

➤ Ask the patient to remain very still and relaxed and to cooperate with instructions given to contract muscles during the procedure.

➤ Observe standard precautions, and follow the general guidelines in Appendix A.

➤ Two skin electrodes are positioned slightly to the left and right of the perianal area and a grounding electrode is placed on the thigh.

➤ If needle electrodes are used, they are inserted into the muscle surrounding the urethra.

➤ Muscle activity signals are recorded as waves, which are interpreted for number and configurations in diagnosing urinary abnormalities.

➤ An indwelling urinary catheter is inserted, and the bulbocavernosus reflex is tested; the patient is instructed to cough while the catheter is gently pulled.

➤ Voluntary control is tested by requesting the patient to contract and relax the muscle. Electrical activity is recorded during this period of relaxation with the bladder empty.

➤ The bladder is filled with sterile water at a rate of 100 mL/min while the electrical activity during filling is recorded.

➤ The catheter is removed; the patient is then placed in a position to void and is asked to urinate and empty the full bladder. This voluntary urination is then recorded until completed. The complete procedure includes recordings of electrical signals before, during, and at the end of urination.

➤ The results are recorded manually or in a computerized system for recall and postprocedure interpretation by the appropriate health care practitioner.

Post-test:

➤ Instruct the patient to resume usual diet, fluids, medications or activity, as directed by the health care practitioner.

➤ Monitor vital signs and neurologic status every 15 minutes for 1 hour, then every 2 hours for 4 hours, and as ordered. Take temperature every 4 hours for 24 hours. Compare with baseline values. Protocols may vary from facility to facility.

➤ Instruct the patient to increase fluid intake unless contraindicated.

➤ If tested with needle electrodes, warn female patients to expect hematuria after the first voiding.

➤ Advise the patient to report symptoms of urethral irritation, such as dysuria, persistent or prolonged hematuria, and urinary frequency.

➤ A written report of the examination will be completed by a health care practitioner specializing in this branch of medicine. The report will be sent to the requesting health care practitioner, who will discuss the results with the patient.

➤ Recognize anxiety related to test results, and be supportive of perceived loss of independent function. Discuss the implications of abnormal test results on the patient's lifestyle. Provide teaching and information regarding the clinical implications of the test results, as appropriate.

➤ Reinforce information given by the patient's health care provider regarding further testing, treatment, or referral to another health care provider. Answer any questions or address any concerns voiced by the patient or family.

➤ Depending on the results of this procedure, additional testing may be needed to evaluate or monitor progression of the disease process and determine the need for a change in therapy. Evaluate test results in relation to the patient's symptoms and other tests performed.

Related diagnostic tests:

➤ Related diagnostic tests include cystometry, cystoscopy, and intravenous pyelography.

ELECTRONEUROGRAPHY

· ·

SYNONYMS/ACRONYM: Electrodiagnostic study, nerve conduction study, ENG.

AREA OF APPLICATION: Muscles.

CONTRAST: None.

DESCRIPTION & RATIONALE: Electroneurography (ENG) is performed to identify peripheral nerve injury, to differentiate primary peripheral nerve pathology from muscular injury, and to monitor response of the nerve injury to treatment. A stimulus is applied through a surface electrode over a nerve. After a nerve is electrically stimulated proximally, the time for the impulse to travel to a second or distal site is measured. Because the conduction study of a nerve can vary from nerve to nerve, it is important to compare the results of the affected side to those of the contralateral side. The results of the stimulation are shown on a monitor, but the actual velocity must be calculated by dividing the distance in meters between the stimulation point and the response point, by the time between the stimulus and response. Traumatic nerve transection, contusion, or neuropathy will usually cause maximal slowing of conduction velocity in the affected side compared with that in the normal side. A velocity greater than normal does not indicate a pathologic condition. This test is usually performed in conjunction with electromyography in a combined test called *electromyoneurography.* ∎

INDICATIONS: Confirm diagnosis of peripheral nerve damage or trauma

RESULT

Normal Findings:
- No evidence of peripheral nerve injury or disease. Variable readings depend on the nerve being tested. For patients age 3 years and older, the maximum conduction velocity is 40 to 80 milliseconds; for infants and the elderly, the values are divided by 2.

Abnormal Findings:
- Carpal tunnel syndrome
- Diabetic neuropathy
- Guillain-Barré syndrome
- Herniated disk disease
- Muscular dystrophy
- Myasthenia gravis
- Poliomyelitis
- Tarsal tunnel syndrome
- Thoracic outlet syndrome

CRITICAL VALUES: N/A

INTERFERING FACTORS:

Factors that may impair the results of the examination:

- Inability of the patient to cooperate or remain still during the procedure because of age, significant pain, or mental status

- Age-related decreases in electrical activity

- Poor electrode conduction or failure to obtain contralateral value for comparison

Nursing Implications and Procedure • • • • • • • • • • •

Pretest:

▶ Inform the patient that the procedure is performed to measure electrical activity of the muscles.

▶ Obtain a history of neuromuscular and neurosensory status, diseases or conditions that affect muscle function, level of muscular function and range of motion, and traumatic events, as well as the results of previously performed laboratory tests, surgical procedures, and other diagnostic procedures. For related diagnostic tests, refer to the Musculoskeletal System table.

▶ Obtain a list of the medications the patient is taking.

▶ Review the procedure with the patient. Address concerns about pain related to the procedure. Inform the patient that the procedure may be uncomfortable because of a mild electrical shock, but that the electrical shock is brief and is not harmful. Inform the patient that the procedure is performed in a special laboratory by a physiatrist or neurologist and takes approximately 15 minutes to complete, but can take longer depending on the patient's condition.

▶ There are no food, fluid, or medica-

tion restrictions unless by medical direction.

▶ *Make sure a written and informed consent has been signed prior to the procedure and before administering any medications.*

Intratest:

▶ Have patient remove clothing and any hosiery. Patients are given a gown to wear and instructed to void prior to the procedure.

▶ Place the patient in a supine or sitting position, depending on the location of the muscle to be tested.

▶ Observe standard precautions, and follow the general guidelines in Appendix A.

▶ Shave the extremity in the area to be stimulated, and cleanse the skin thoroughly with alcohol pads.

▶ Apply electrode gel and place a recording electrode at a known distance from the stimulation point. Measure the distance between the stimulation point and the site of the recording electrode in centimeters.

▶ Place a reference electrode nearby on the skin surface.

▶ The nerve is electrically stimulated by a shock-emitter device; the time between nerve impulse and electrical contraction, measured in milliseconds (distal latency), is shown on a monitor.

▶ The nerve is also electrically stimulated at a location proximal to the area of suspected injury or disease.

▶ The time required for the impulse to travel from the stimulation site to location of the muscle contraction (total latency) is recorded in milliseconds.

▶ Calculate the conduction velocity. The conduction velocity is converted to meters per second and computed using the following equation:

$$\text{Conduction velocity (in meters per second)} = \frac{[\text{distance (in meters)}]}{[\text{total latency} - \text{distal latency}]}$$

Post-test:

▶ When the procedure is complete, remove the electrodes and clean the skin where the electrodes were applied.

▶ Monitor electrode sites for inflammation.

▶ If residual pain is noted after the procedure, instruct the patient to apply warm compresses and to take analgesics, as ordered.

▶ Instruct the patient to resume usual diet, medication, and activity, as directed by the health care practitioner.

▶ A written report of the examination will be completed by a health care practitioner specializing in this branch of medicine. The report will be sent to the requesting health care practitioner, who will discuss the results with the patient.

▶ Recognize anxiety related to test results, and be supportive of perceived loss of independent function. Discuss the implications of abnormal test results on the patient's lifestyle. Provide teaching and information regarding the clinical implications of the test results, as appropriate.

▶ Reinforce information given by the patient's health care provider regarding further testing, treatment, or referral to another health care provider. Answer any questions or address any concerns voiced by the patient or family.

▶ Depending on the results of this procedure, additional testing may be performed to evaluate or monitor progression of the disease process and determine the need for a change in therapy. Evaluate test results in relation to the patient's symptoms and other tests performed.

Related diagnostic tests:

▶ Related diagnostic tests include electromyography.

EOSINOPHIL COUNT

SYNONYMS/ACRONYM: Eos count, total eosinophil count.

SPECIMEN: Whole blood (1 mL) collected in a lavender-top (EDTA) tube.

REFERENCE VALUE: (Method: Manual count using eosinophil stain and hemocytometer or automated analyzer)
   Absolute count: 50 to 350/mm^3
   Relative percentage: 1% to 4%

DESCRIPTION & RATIONALE: Eosinophils are white blood cells whose function is phagocytosis of antigen-antibody complexes and response to allergy-inducing substances and parasites. Eosinophils have granules that contain histamine used to kill foreign cells in the body. Eosinophils also contain proteolytic substances that damage parasitic worms. The binding of histamine to receptor sites on cells results in smooth muscle contraction in the bronchioles and upper respiratory tract, constriction of pulmonary vessels, increased mucus production, and secretion of acid by the cells that line the stomach. Eosinophil counts can increase to greater than 30% of normal in parasitic infections; however, a significant percentage of children with visceral larva migrans infestations have normal eosinophil counts. ∎

INDICATIONS: Assist in the diagnosis of conditions such as allergies, parasitic infections, drug reactions, collagen diseases, Hodgkin's disease, and myeloproliferative disorders

RESULT

Increased in:
* Addison's disease
* Allergy
* Asthma
* Cancer
* Dermatitis
* Drug reactions
* Eczema
* Hay fever
* Hodgkin's disease
* Hypereosinophilic syndrome
* Löffler's syndrome
* Myeloproliferative disorders
* Parasitic infection (visceral larva migrans)
* Pernicious anemia

* Polycythemia vera
* Rheumatoid arthritis
* Rhinitis
* Sarcoidosis
* Splenectomy
* Tuberculosis

Decreased in:
* Aplastic anemia
* Eclampsia
* Infections (shift to the left)
* Stress

CRITICAL VALUES: N/A

INTERFERING FACTORS:
* Numerous drugs and substances can cause an increase in eosinophil levels as a result of an allergic response or hypersensitivity reaction. These include acetophenazine, allopurinol, aminosalicylic acid, ampicillin, butaperazine, capreomycin, carisoprodol, cephaloglycin, cephaloridine, cephalosporins, cephapirin, cephradine, chloramphenicol, clindamycin, cloxacillin, dapsone, epicillin, erythromycin, fluorides, gold, imipramine, iodides, kanamycin, mefenamic acid, methicillin, methyldopa, minocycline, nalidixic acid, niridazole, nitrofurans (including nitrofurantoin), nonsteroidal anti-inflammatory drugs, nystatin, oxamniquine, penicillin, penicillin G, procainamide, ristocetin, streptokinase, streptomycin, tetracycline, triamterene, tryptophan, and viomycin.

* Drugs that can cause a decrease in eosinophil levels include acetylsalicylic acid, amphotericin B, corticotropin, desipramine, glucocorticoids, hydrocortisone, interferon, niacin, prednisone, and procainamide.

* Clotted specimens should be rejected for analysis.

• Specimens more than 4 hours old should be rejected for analysis.

• There is a diurnal variation in eosinophil counts. The count is lowest in the morning and continues to rise throughout the day until midnight. Therefore, serial measurements should be performed at the same time of day for purposes of continuity.

Nursing Implications and Procedure • • • • • • • • • • •

Pretest:

➤ Inform the patient that the test is used to assist in the diagnosis of conditions related to immune response, such as allergy or parasitic infection.

➤ Obtain a history of the patient's complaints, including a list of known allergens (especially allergies or sensitivities to latex), and inform the appropriate health care practitioner accordingly.

➤ Obtain a history of the patient's hematopoietic, immune, and respiratory systems, as well as results of previously performed laboratory tests, surgical procedures, and other diagnostic procedures. For related laboratory tests, refer to the Hematopoietic, Immune, and Respiratory System tables.

➤ Obtain a list of the medications the patient is taking, including herbs, nutritional supplements, and nutraceuticals. The requesting health care practitioner and laboratory should be advised if the patient regularly uses these products so that their effects can be taken into consideration when reviewing results.

➤ Review the procedure with the patient. Inform the patient that specimen collection takes approximately 5 to 10 minutes. Address concerns about pain related to the procedure. Explain to the patient that there may be some discomfort during the venipuncture.

➤ There are no food, fluid, or medication restrictions, unless by medical direction.

Intratest:

➤ If the patient has a history of severe allergic reaction to latex, care should be taken to avoid the use of equipment containing latex.

➤ Instruct the patient to cooperate fully and to follow directions. Direct the patient to breathe normally and to avoid unnecessary movement.

➤ Observe standard precautions, and follow the general guidelines in Appendix A. Positively identify the patient, and label the appropriate tubes with the corresponding patient demographics, date, and time of collection. Perform a venipuncture; collect the specimen in a 5-mL lavender-top (EDTA) tube.

➤ Remove the needle, and apply a pressure dressing over the puncture site.

➤ Promptly transport the specimen to the laboratory for processing and analysis.

➤ The results are recorded manually or in a computerized system for recall and postprocedure interpretation by the appropriate health care practitioner.

Post-test:

➤ Observe venipuncture site for bleeding or hematoma formation. Apply paper tape or other adhesive to hold pressure bandage in place, or replace with a plastic bandage.

➤ *Nutritional considerations:* Consideration should be given to diet if food allergies are present.

➤ Instruct the patient with an elevated eosinophil count to report any signs or symptoms of infection, such as fever.

➤ Instruct the patient with an elevated count to rest and take medications as prescribed, to increase fluid intake as appropriate, and to monitor temperature.

➤ A written report of the examination will be sent to the requesting health care practitioner, who will discuss the results with the patient.

➤ Reinforce information given by the patient's health care provider regarding further testing, treatment, or referral to another health care provider. Answer any questions or address any concerns voiced by the patient or family.

➤ Depending on the results of this procedure, additional testing may be performed to evaluate or monitor progression of the disease process and determine the need for a change in therapy. Evaluate test results in relation to the patient's symptoms and other tests performed.

Related laboratory tests:

➤ Related laboratory tests include allergen-specific immunoglobulin E (IgE), complete blood count, fecal analysis, hypersensitivity pneumonitis screen, IgE, ova and parasites, and stool culture.

ERYTHROCYTE PROTOPORPHYRIN, FREE

. . . .

SYNONYM/ACRONYM: Free erythrocyte protoporphyrin (FEP).

SPECIMEN: Whole blood (1 mL) collected in lavender-top (ethylenediaminetetra-acetic acid [EDTA]) or green-top (heparin) tube.

REFERENCE VALUE: (Method: Fluorometry)

Conventional Units	SI Units (Conventional Units × 0.0178)
17–77 μg/dL of packed cells	0.3–1.37 μmol/L of packed cells

DESCRIPTION & RATIONALE: The free erythrocyte protoporphyrin test measures the concentration of protoporphyrin in red blood cells. Protoporphyrin comprises the predominant porphyrin in red blood cells, which combines with iron to form the heme portion of hemoglobin. Protoporphyrin converts to bilirubin, combines with albumin, and remains unconjugated in the circulation after hemoglobin breakdown. Increased amounts of protoporphyrin can be detected in erythrocytes, urine, and stool in conditions interfering with heme synthesis. Protoporphyria is an autosomal dominant disorder in which increased amounts of protoporphyrin are secreted and excreted; the disorder is thought to be the result of an enzyme deficiency. Protoporphyria causes photosensitivity and may lead to cirrhosis of the liver and cholelithiasis as a result of protoporphyrin deposits. ■

INDICATIONS:

- Assist in the diagnosis of erythropoietic protoporphyrias
- Assist in the differential diagnosis of iron deficiency in pediatric patients
- Evaluate lead poisoning

RESULT

Increased in:
- Anemia of chronic disease
- Conditions with marked erythropoiesis (e.g., hemolytic anemias)
- Erythropoietic protoporphyria
- Iron-deficiency anemias
- Lead poisoning
- Some sideroblastic anemias

Decreased in: N/A

CRITICAL VALUES: N/A

INTERFERING FACTORS:

- Drugs that may increase erythrocyte protoporphyrin levels include barbiturates, chlorpropamide, oral contraceptives, sulfomethane, and tolbutamide.
- The test is unreliable in infants less than 6 months of age.

Nursing Implications and Procedure . . . .

Pretest:

▶ Inform the patient that the test is used to detect lead toxicity and to monitor chronic lead exposure. It is also used to differentiate disorders in heme and globin production.

▶ Obtain a history of the patient's complaints, including a list of known allergens (especially allergies or sensitivities to latex), and inform the appropriate health care practitioner accordingly.

▶ Obtain a history of the patient's hematopoietic system, as well as results of previously performed laboratory tests, surgical procedures, and other diagnostic procedures. For related laboratory tests, refer to the Hematopoietic System table.

▶ Obtain a list of the medications the patient is taking, including herbs, nutritional supplements, and nutraceuticals. The requesting health care practitioner and laboratory should be advised if the patient regularly uses these products so that their effects can be taken into consideration when reviewing results.

▶ Review the procedure with the patient. Inform the patient that specimen collection takes approximately 5 to 10 minutes. Address concerns about pain related to the procedure. Explain to the patient that there may be some discomfort during the venipuncture.

▶ There are no food, fluid, or medication restrictions, unless by medical direction.

Intratest:

▶ If the patient has a history of severe allergic reaction to latex, care should be taken to avoid the use of equipment containing latex.

▶ Instruct the patient to cooperate fully and to follow directions. Direct the patient to breathe normally and to avoid unnecessary movement.

▶ Observe standard precautions, and follow the general guidelines in Appendix A. Positively identify the patient, and label the appropriate tubes with the corresponding patient demographics, date, and time of collection. Perform a venipuncture; collect the specimen in a 5-mL lavender-top tube. Specimens should be protected from light.

▶ Remove the needle, and apply a pressure dressing over the puncture site.

- Promptly transport the specimen to the laboratory for processing and analysis.

- The results are recorded manually or in a computerized system for recall and postprocedure interpretation by the appropriate health care practitioner.

Post-test:

- Observe venipuncture site for bleeding or hematoma formation. Apply paper tape or other adhesive to hold pressure bandage in place, or replace with a plastic bandage.

- A written report of the examination will be sent to the requesting health care practitioner, who will discuss the results with the patient.

- Reinforce information given by the patient's health care provider regarding further testing, treatment, or referral to another health care provider. Answer any questions or address any concerns voiced by the patient or family.

- Depending on the results of this procedure, additional testing may be performed to evaluate or monitor progression of the disease process and determine the need for a change in therapy. Evaluate test results in relation to the patient's symptoms and other tests performed.

Related laboratory tests:

- Related laboratory tests include hematocrit, hemoglobin, iron/total iron-binding capacity, lead, and urine porphyrins.

ERYTHROCYTE SEDIMENTATION RATE

SYNONYM/ACRONYM: Sed rate, ESR.

SPECIMEN: Whole blood (5 mL) collected in a lavender-top (ethylenediaminetetra-acetic acid [EDTA]) tube for the modified Westergren method or gray-top (3.8% sodium citrate) tube for the original Westergren method.

REFERENCE VALUE: (Method: Westergren)

Age	Male	Female
Newborn	0–2 mm/h	0–2 mm/h
Less than 50 y	0–15 mm/h	0–25 mm/h
50 y and older	0–20 mm/h	0–30 mm/h

DESCRIPTION & RATIONALE: The erythrocyte sedimentation rate (ESR) is a measure of the rate of sedimentation of red blood cells (RBCs) in an anticoagulated whole blood sample over a specified period of time. The basis of the ESR test is the alteration of blood proteins by inflammatory and necrotic processes that cause the RBCs to stick together, become heavier, and rapidly settle at the bottom of a vertically held, calibrated tube over time. In general, relatively little settling occurs in normal blood because normal RBCs do not form rouleaux and would not stack together, increasing their mass and rate of sedimentation. The sedimentation rate is proportional to the size or mass of the falling RBCs and is inversely proportional to plasma viscosity. The test is a nonspecific indicator of disease but is fairly sensitive and is frequently the earliest indicator of widespread inflammatory reaction due to infection or autoimmune disorders. Prolonged elevations are also present in malignant disease. The ESR can also be used to monitor the course of a disease and the effectiveness of therapy. The two most commonly used methods to measure the ESR are the Westergren (or modified Westergren) method and the Wintrobe hematocrit method. ■

INDICATIONS:

- Assist in the diagnosis of acute infection, such as tuberculosis or tissue necrosis

- Assist in the diagnosis of acute inflammatory processes

- Assist in the diagnosis of chronic infections

- Assist in the diagnosis of rheumatoid or autoimmune disorders

- Assist in the diagnosis of temporal arthritis and polymyalgia rheumatica

- Monitor inflammatory and malignant disease

RESULT

Increased in:

- Acute myocardial infarction
- Anemia
- Carcinoma
- Cat scratch fever
- Collagen diseases, including systemic lupus erythematosus (SLE)
- Crohn's disease
- Endocarditis
- Heavy metal poisoning
- Increased plasma protein level
- Infections (e.g., pneumonia, syphilis)
- Inflammatory diseases
- Lymphoma
- Lymphosarcoma
- Multiple myeloma
- Nephritis
- Pregnancy
- Pulmonary embolism
- Rheumatic fever
- Rheumatoid arthritis
- Subacute bacterial endocarditis
- Temporal arteritis
- Toxemia
- Tuberculosis
- Waldenström's macroglobulinemia

Normal in:

- Congestive heart failure
- Glucose-6-phosphate dehydrogenase deficiency
- Hemoglobin C disease
- Hypofibrinogenemia
- Polycythemia

- Sickle cell anemia
- Spherocytosis

Decreased in:
- Conditions resulting in high hemoglobin and RBC count
- Elevated blood glucose

CRITICAL VALUES: N/A

INTERFERING FACTORS:
- Some drugs cause an SLE-like syndrome that results in a physiologic increase in ESR. These include anticonvulsants, hydrazine derivatives, nitrofurantoin, procainamide, and quinidine. Other drugs that may cause an increased ESR include acetylsalicylic acid, cephalothin, cephapirin, cyclosporin A, dextran, and oral contraceptives.
- Drugs that may cause a decrease in ESR include aurothiomalate, corticotropin, cortisone, and quinine.
- Menstruation may cause falsely increased test results.
- Prolonged tourniquet constriction around the arm may cause hemoconcentration and falsely low values.
- The Westergren and modified Westergren methods are affected by heparin, which causes a false elevation in values.
- Bubbles in the Westergren tube or pipette, or tilting the measurement column more than 3° from vertical, will falsely increase the values.
- Movement or vibration of the surface on which the test is being conducted will affect the results.
- Inaccurate timing will invalidate test results.
- Specimens that are clotted, hemolyzed, or insufficient in volume should be rejected for analysis.
- The test should be performed within 4 hours of collection when the specimen has been stored at room temperature; delays in testing may result in decreased values. If a delay in testing is anticipated, refrigerate the sample at 2°C to 4°C; stability at refrigerated temperature is reported to be extended up to 12 hours. Refrigerated specimens should be brought to room temperature before testing.

Nursing Implications and Procedure . . . .

Pretest:

➤ Inform the patient that the test is a nonspecific indicator of inflammation.

➤ Obtain a history of the patient's complaints, including a list of known allergens (especially allergies or sensitivities to latex), and inform the appropriate health care practitioner accordingly.

➤ Obtain a history of infectious, autoimmune, or neoplastic diseases.

➤ Obtain a history of the patient's hematopoietic, immune, and respiratory systems, as well as results of previously performed laboratory tests, surgical procedures, and other diagnostic procedures. For related laboratory tests, refer to the Hematopoietic, Immune, and Respiratory System tables.

➤ Obtain a list of the medications the patient is taking, including herbs, nutritional supplements, and nutraceuticals. The requesting health care practitioner and laboratory should be advised if the patient regularly uses these products so that their effects can be taken into consideration when reviewing results.

➤ Review the procedure with the patient. Inform the patient that specimen collection takes approximately 5 to 10 minutes. Address concerns about pain related to the procedure. Explain to the patient that there may be some discomfort during the venipuncture.

> There are no food, fluid, or medication restrictions, unless by medical direction.

Intratest:

> If the patient has a history of severe allergic reaction to latex, care should be taken to avoid the use of equipment containing latex.

> Instruct the patient to cooperate fully and to follow directions. Direct the patient to breathe normally and to avoid unnecessary movement.

> Observe standard precautions, and follow the general guidelines in Appendix A. Positively identify the patient, and label the appropriate tubes with the corresponding patient demographics, date, and time of collection. Perform a venipuncture; collect the specimen in a 5-mL gray-top (sodium citrate) tube if the Westergren method will be used. Collect the specimen in a 5-mL purple-top (EDTA) tube if the modified Westergren method will be used.

> Remove the needle, and apply a pressure dressing over the puncture site.

> Promptly transport the specimen to the laboratory for processing and analysis.

> The results are recorded manually or in a computerized system for recall and postprocedure interpretation by the appropriate health care practitioner.

Post-test:

> Observe venipuncture site for bleeding or hematoma formation. Apply paper tape or other adhesive to hold pressure bandage in place, or replace with a plastic bandage.

> A written report of the examination will be sent to the requesting health care practitioner, who will discuss the results with the patient.

> Reinforce information given by the patient's health care provider regarding further testing, treatment, or referral to another health care provider. Answer any questions or address any concerns voiced by the patient or family.

> Depending on the results of this procedure, additional testing may be performed to evaluate or monitor progression of the disease process and determine the need for a change in therapy. Evaluate test results in relation to the patient's symptoms and other tests performed.

Related laboratory tests:

> Related laboratory tests include complete blood count, C-reactive protein, rheumatoid factor, microorganism-specific serologies, and related cultures.

ERYTHROPOIETIN

SYNONYM/ACRONYM: EPO.

SPECIMEN: Serum (2 mL) collected in a red- or tiger-top tube.

REFERENCE VALUE: (Method: Radioimmunoassay)

Conventional Units	SI Units (Conventional Units × 1)
5–36 mU/mL	5–36 U/L

DESCRIPTION & RATIONALE: Erythropoietin (EPO) is a glycoprotein produced mainly by the kidney. Its function is to stimulate the bone marrow to make red blood cells. EPO levels fall after removal of the kidney but do not disappear completely. It is thought that small amounts of EPO may be produced by the liver. Erythropoiesis is regulated by EPO and tissue PO_2. When PO_2 is normal, EPO levels decrease; when PO_2 falls, EPO secretion occurs and EPO levels increase. ■

INDICATIONS:
• Assist in assessment of anemia of end-stage renal disease
• Assist in the diagnosis of EPO-producing tumors
• Evaluate the presence of rare anemias
• Monitor patients receiving EPO therapy

RESULT

Increased in:
• After moderate bleeding in an otherwise healthy patient
• Anemias
• Hepatoma
• Kidney transplant rejection
• Nephroblastoma
• Pheochromocytoma
• Polycystic kidney disease
• Pregnancy

• Secondary polycythemia (high-altitude hypoxia, chronic obstructive pulmonary disease, pulmonary fibrosis)

Decreased in:
• Chemotherapy
• Primary polycythemia
• Renal failure

CRITICAL VALUES: N/A

INTERFERING FACTORS:
• Drugs that may increase EPO levels include anabolic steroids.
• Drugs that may decrease EPO levels include amphotericin B, cisplatin, enalapril, estrogens, and theophylline.
• Blood transfusions may also decrease EPO levels.
• Recent radioactive scans or radiation within 1 week before the test can interfere with test results when radioimmunoassay is the test method.

Nursing Implications and Procedure • • • • • • • • • • • •

Pretest:

➤ Inform the patient that the test is used in the evaluation of anemias.

➤ Obtain a history of the patient's complaints, including a list of known allergens (especially allergies or sensitivities to latex), and inform the appropriate health care practitioner accordingly.

➤ Obtain a history of the patient's hematopoietic and genitourinary systems, as well as results of previously performed laboratory tests, surgical procedures, and other diagnostic procedures. For related laboratory tests, refer to the Hematopoietic and Genitourinary System tables.

➤ Note any recent procedures that can interfere with test results.

➤ Obtain a list of the medications the

patient is taking, including herbs, nutritional supplements, and nutraceuticals. The requesting health care practitioner and laboratory should be advised if the patient regularly uses these products so that their effects can be taken into consideration when reviewing results.

➤ Review the procedure with the patient. Inform the patient that specimen collection takes approximately 5 to 10 minutes. Address concerns about pain related to the procedure. Explain to the patient that there may be some discomfort during the venipuncture.

➤ There are no food, fluid, or medication restrictions, unless by medical direction.

Intratest:

➤ If the patient has a history of severe allergic reaction to latex, care should be taken to avoid the use of equipment containing latex.

➤ Instruct the patient to cooperate fully and to follow directions. Direct the patient to breathe normally and to avoid unnecessary movement.

➤ Observe standard precautions, and follow the general guidelines in Appendix A. Positively identify the patient, and label the appropriate tubes with the corresponding patient demographics, date, and time of collection. Perform a venipuncture; collect the specimen in a 5-mL red- or tiger-top tube.

➤ Remove the needle, and apply a pressure dressing over the puncture site.

➤ Promptly transport the specimen to the laboratory for processing and analysis.

➤ The results are recorded manually or in a computerized system for recall and postprocedure interpretation by the appropriate health care practitioner.

Post-test:

➤ Observe venipuncture site for bleeding or hematoma formation. Apply paper tape or other adhesive to hold pressure bandage in place, or replace with a plastic bandage.

➤ A written report of the examination will be sent to the requesting health care practitioner, who will discuss the results with the patient.

➤ Reinforce information given by the patient's health care provider regarding further testing, treatment, or referral to another health care provider. Answer any questions or address any concerns voiced by the patient or family.

➤ Depending on the results of this procedure, additional testing may be performed to evaluate or monitor progression of the disease process and determine the need for a change in therapy. Evaluate test results in relation to the patient's symptoms and other tests performed.

Related laboratory tests:

➤ Related laboratory tests include bone marrow biopsy, complete blood count, creatinine, creatinine clearance, ferritin, hemoglobin, hematocrit, iron/total iron-binding capacity, microalbumin, red blood cell count, red blood cell indices, red blood cell morphology and inclusions, urea nitrogen, and vitamin B_{12}.

ESOPHAGEAL MANOMETRY

SYNONYMS/ACRONYM: Esophageal function study, esophageal acid study (Tuttle test), acid reflux test, Bernstein test (aid perfusion), esophageal motility study.

AREA OF APPLICATION: Esophagus.

CONTRAST: Done with or without noniodinated contrast medium.

DESCRIPTION & RATIONALE: Esophageal manometry (EM) consists of a group of invasive studies performed to assist in diagnosing abnormalities of esophageal muscle function and esophageal structure. These studies measure esophageal pressure, the effects of gastric acid in the esophagus, lower esophageal sphincter pressure, and motility patterns that result during swallowing. EM can be used to document and quantify gastroesophageal reflux (GER). It is indicated when a patient is experiencing difficulty swallowing, heartburn, regurgitation, or vomiting; or has chest pain for which no diagnosis has been found. Tests performed in combination with EM include the acid reflux, acid clearing, and acid perfusion (Bernstein) tests. ■

INDICATIONS:
- Aid in the diagnosis of achalasia, evidenced by increased pressure in EM
- Aid in the diagnosis of chalasia in children, evidenced by decreased pressure in EM
- Aid in the diagnosis of esophageal scleroderma, evidenced by decreased pressure in EM

- Aid in the diagnosis of esophagitis, evidenced by decreased motility
- Aid in the diagnosis of GER, evidenced by low pressure in EM, decreased pH in acidity test, and pain in acid reflux and perfusion tests
- Differentiate between esophagitis or cardiac condition as the cause of epigastric pain
- Evaluate pyrosis and dysphagia to determine if the cause is GER or esophagitis

RESULT

Normal Findings:
- Acid clearing: fewer than 10 swallows
- Acid perfusion: no GER
- Acid reflux: no regurgitation into the esophagus
- Bernstein test: negative
- Esophageal secretions: pH 5 to 6
- Esophageal sphincter pressure: 10 to 20 mm Hg

Abnormal Findings:
- Achalasia (sphincter pressure of 50 mm Hg)
- Chalasia

- Esophageal scleroderma

- Esophagitis

- GER (sphincter pressure of 0 to 5 mm Hg, pH of 1 to 3)

- Hiatal hernia

- Progressive systemic sclerosis (scleroderma)

- Spasms

CRITICAL VALUES: N/A

INTERFERING FACTORS:

This procedure is contraindicated for:

- Patients with unstable cardiopulmonary status, blood coagulation defects, recent gastrointestinal surgery, esophageal varices, or bleeding

Factors that may impair the results of the examination:

- Inability of the patient to cooperate or remain still during the procedure because of age, significant pain, or mental status

- Administration of medications (e.g., sedatives, antacids, anticholinergics, cholinergics, corticosteroids) that can change pH or relax the sphincter muscle, causing inaccurate results

Other considerations:

- Failure to follow dietary restrictions before the procedure may cause the procedure to be canceled or repeated.

Nursing Implications and Procedure • • • • • • • • • • •

Pretest:

➤ Inform the patient that the procedure assesses the esophagus.

➤ Obtain a history of the patient's complaints, including a list of known allergens, especially allergies or sensitivities to latex, iodine, seafood, contrast medium, and dyes.

➤ Obtain a history of the patient's respiratory and gastrointestinal systems, and results of previously performed diagnostic procedures, surgical procedures, and laboratory tests. For related diagnostic tests, refer to the Respiratory and Gastrointestinal System tables.

➤ Ensure that this procedure is performed before an upper gastrointestinal study or barium swallow.

➤ Record the date of the last menstrual period and determine the possibility of pregnancy in perimenopausal women.

➤ Obtain a list of the medications the patient is taking.

➤ Review the procedure with the patient. Address concerns about pain related to the procedure. Explain to the patient that some pain may be experienced during the test, and there may be moments of discomfort and gagging when the scope is inserted, but there are no complications resulting from the procedure and the throat will be anesthetized with a spray or swab. Explain the purpose of the test and how the procedure is performed. Inform the patient that the procedure is performed in an endoscopy suite by a health care practitioner, under local anesthesia, and takes approximately 30 to 45 minutes.

➤ Inform the patient that dentures and eyewear will be removed before the test.

➤ Inform the patient that he or she will not be able to speak during the procedure, but that breathing will not be affected.

➤ Explain that an intravenous (IV) line may be started to allow for the infusion of a sedative or IV fluids.

➤ *Sensitivity to cultural and social issues,* as well as concern for modesty, is important in providing psychological support before, during and after the procedure.

➤ The patient should fast and refrain from drinking liquids for 6 to 8 hours before the test.

➤ Under medical direction, the patient should withhold medications for 24 hours before the study; special arrangements may be necessary for diabetic patients.

➤ Obtain and record baseline vital signs.

➤ *Make sure a written and informed consent has been signed prior to the procedure and before administering any medications.*

➤ Ensure that the patient has complied with dietary, fluids, and medication restrictions and pretesting preparations.

➤ Keep resuscitation equipment on hand in the case of respiratory impairment or laryngospasm after the procedure.

➤ Avoid using morphine sulfate in patients with asthma or other pulmonary disease. This drug can further exacerbate bronchospasms and respiratory impairment.

➤ Have patient remove dentures, contact lenses, eyeglasses, and jewelry. Notify the physician if the patient has permanent crowns on teeth. Have the patient remove clothing and change into a gown for the procedure.

➤ Have the patient void before the procedure begins.

➤ Instruct the patient to cooperate fully and to follow directions. Instruct the patient to remain still throughout the procedure because movement produces unreliable results.

➤ Observe standard precautions, and follow the general guidelines in Appendix A.

➤ Start an IV line and administer ordered sedation.

➤ Spray or swab the oropharynx with a topical local anesthetic.

➤ Provide an emesis basin for the increased saliva and encourage the patient to spit out the saliva because the gag reflex may be impaired.

➤ During the procedure, monitor the patient to prevent aspiration of stomach contents into the lungs. Note any change in respirations (dyspnea, tachypnea, adventitious sounds).

➤ Suction the mouth, pharynx, and trachea, and administer oxygen as ordered.

Esophageal manometry:

➤ One or more small tubes are inserted through the nose into the esophagus and stomach.

➤ A small transducer is attached to the ends of the tubes; pressures are measured at the lower esophageal sphincter, and intraluminal pressures as well as regularity and duration of peristaltic contractions are measured.

➤ The patient is asked to swallow small amounts of water or flavored gelatin.

➤ Pressures are taken and recorded, and a motility pattern is recorded on a graph.

Esophageal acid and clearing (Tuttle test):

➤ With the tube in place, a pH electrode probe is inserted into the esophagus with Valsalva maneuvers performed to stimulate reflux of stomach contents into the esophagus.

➤ If acid reflux is absent, 100 mL of 0.1% hydrochloric acid is instilled into the stomach during a 3-minute period, and then the pH measurement is repeated.

➤ To determine acid clearing, hydrochloric acid is instilled into the esophagus and the patient is asked to swallow while the probe measures the pH.

Acid perfusion (Bernstein test):

➤ A catheter is inserted through the nose into the esophagus and the patient is asked to inform the technician when pain is experienced.

➤ Normal saline solution is allowed to drip into the catheter at about 10 mL/min. Then hydrochloric acid is allowed to drip into the catheter.

➤ Pain experienced when the hydrochloric acid is instilled determines the presence of an esophageal abnormality. If no pain is experienced, symptoms are the result of some other condition.

General:

➤ The results are recorded manually or in a computerized system for recall and postprocedure interpretation by the appropriate health care practitioner.

Post-test:

➤ Do not allow the patient to eat or drink until the gag reflex returns; then allow the patient to eat lightly for 12 to 24 hours.

➤ Instruct the patient to resume usual activity, medication, and diet 24 hours after the examination or as tolerated, as directed by the health care practitioner.

➤ Tell the patient to expect some throat soreness and possible hoarseness. Advise the patient to use warm gargles, lozenges, or ice packs to the neck; or to drink cool fluids to alleviate throat discomfort.

➤ Monitor the patient for signs of respiratory depression (less than 15 respirations per minute) every 15 minutes for 2 hours. Resuscitation equipment should be available.

➤ Observe the patient for indications of perforation: painful swallowing with neck movement, substernal pain with respiration, shoulder pain, dyspnea, abdominal or back pain, cyanosis, and fever.

➤ Emphasize that any severe pain, fever, difficulty breathing, or expectoration of blood must be reported to the health care practitioner immediately.

➤ A written report of the examination will be completed by a health care practitioner specializing in this branch of medicine. The report will be sent to the requesting health care practitioner, who will discuss the results with the patient.

➤ Reinforce information given by the patient's health care provider regarding further testing, treatment, or referral to another health care provider. Answer any questions or address any concerns voiced by the patient or family.

➤ Depending on the results of this procedure, additional testing may be needed to evaluate or monitor progression of the disease process and determine the need for a change in therapy. Evaluate test results in relation to the patient's symptoms and other tests performed.

Related diagnostic tests:

➤ Related diagnostic tests include chest x-ray, computed tomography of the thorax, lung scan, and magnetic resonance imaging of the chest.

ESOPHAGOGASTRODUODENOSCOPY

SYNONYMS/ACRONYMS: Esophagoscopy, gastroscopy, upper GI endoscopy, EGD.

AREA OF APPLICATION: Esophagus, stomach, and upper duodenum.

CONTRAST: Done without contrast.

DESCRIPTION & RATIONALE: Esophagogastroduodenoscopy (EGD) allows direct visualization of the upper gastrointestinal (GI) tract mucosa, which includes the esophagus, stomach, and upper portion of the duodenum, by means of a flexible endoscope. The standard flexible fiberoptic endoscope contains three channels that allow passage of the instruments needed to perform therapeutic or diagnostic procedures, such as biopsies or cytology washings. The endoscope, a multichannel instrument, allows visualization of the GI tract linings, insufflation of air, aspiration of fluid, removal of foreign bodies by suction or by snare or forceps, and passage of a laser beam for obliteration of abnormal tissue or control of bleeding. Direct visualization yields greater diagnostic data than is possible through radiologic procedures, and therefore EGD is rapidly replacing upper GI series as the diagnostic procedure of choice. ∎

INDICATIONS:
- Assist in differentiating between benign and neoplastic tumors
- Detect gastric or duodenal ulcers
- Detect upper GI inflammatory disease
- Determine the presence and location of acute upper GI bleeding
- Evaluate the extent of esophageal injury after ingestion of chemicals
- Evaluate stomach or duodenum after surgical procedures
- Evaluate suspected gastric outlet obstruction
- Identify tissue abnormalities and obtain biopsy specimens
- Investigate the cause of dysphagia, dyspepsia, and epigastric pain

RESULT

Normal Findings:
- Esophageal mucosa is normally yellow-pink. At about 9 inches from the incisor teeth, a pulsation indicates the location of the aortic arch. The gastric mucosa is orange-red and contains rugae. The proximal duodenum is reddish and contains a few longitudinal folds, whereas the distal duodenum has circular folds lined with villi. No abnormal structures or functions are observed in the esophagus, stomach, or duodenum.

Abnormal Findings:
- Acute and chronic gastric and duodenal ulcers

- Diverticular disease
- Duodenitis
- Esophageal varices
- Esophageal or pyloric stenosis
- Esophagitis or strictures
- Gastritis
- Hiatal hernia
- Mallory-Weiss syndrome
- Tumors (benign or malignant)

CRITICAL VALUES: N/A

INTERFERING FACTORS:

This procedure is contraindicated for:
- Patients who have had surgery involving the stomach or duodenum, which can make locating the duodenal papilla difficult
- Patients with a bleeding disorder
- Patients with unstable cardiopulmonary status, blood coagulation defects, or cholangitis, unless the patient received prophylactic antibiotic therapy before the test (otherwise the examination must be rescheduled)
- Patients with unstable cardiopulmonary status, blood coagulation defects, known aortic arch aneurysm, large esophageal Zenker's diverticulum, recent GI surgery, esophageal varices, or known esophageal perforation

Factors that may impair clear imaging:
- Gas or food in the gastrointestinal tract resulting from inadequate cleansing or failure to restrict food intake before the study
- Retained barium from a previous radiologic procedure
- Patients who are very obese, who may exceed the weight limit for the equipment

- Incorrect positioning of the patient, which may produce poor visualization of the area to be examined
- Inability of the patient to cooperate or remain still during the procedure because of age, significant pain, or mental status

Other considerations:
- The procedure may be terminated if chest pain or severe cardiac arrhythmias occur.
- Failure to follow dietary restrictions and other pretesting preparations may cause the procedure to be canceled or repeated.

Nursing Implications and Procedure ....

Pretest:

▶ Inform the patient that the procedure assesses the esophagus and upper gastrointestinal tract.

▶ Obtain a history of the patient's complaints, including a list of known allergens, especially allergies or sensitivities to latex, iodine, seafood, contrast medium, and dyes.

▶ Obtain a history of the patient's gastrointestinal system, and results of previously performed diagnostic procedures, surgical procedures, and laboratory tests. For related diagnostic tests, refer to the Gastrointestinal System table.

▶ Ensure that this procedure is performed before an upper gastrointestinal study or barium swallow.

▶ Record the date of the last menstrual period and determine the possibility of pregnancy in perimenopausal women.

▶ Obtain a list of the medications the patient is taking.

▶ Review the procedure with the patient. Address concerns about pain related to the procedure. Explain to the patient that some pain may be experienced during the test, and there may be moments of discomfort, but that the throat will be anesthetized with a spray or swab. Explain the purpose of the test and how the procedure is performed. Inform the patient that the procedure is performed in a GI Lab or radiology department, usually by a health care practitioner and support staff, and takes approximately 30 to 60 minutes.

➤ Inform the patient that dentures and eyewear will be removed before the test.

➤ Inform the patient that he or she will not be able to speak during the procedure, but that breathing will not be affected.

➤ Explain that an intravenous (IV) line may be started to allow for the infusion of a sedative or IV fluids.

➤ *Sensitivity to cultural and social issues,* as well as concern for modesty, is important in providing psychological support before, during and after the procedure.

➤ The patient should fast and refrain from drinking liquids for 8 hours prior to the procedure.

➤ Inform the patient that a laxative and cleansing enema may be needed the day before the procedure, with cleansing enemas on the morning of the procedure, depending on the institution's policy.

➤ Instruct the patient to remove jewelry, including watches, credit cards, and other metallic objects.

➤ Obtain and record baseline vital signs.

➤ *Make sure a written and informed consent has been signed prior to the procedure and before administering any medications.*

Intratest:

➤ Assess for completion of bowel preparation according to the institution's procedure.

➤ Ensure that the patient has complied with dietary, fluids, and medication restrictions and pretesting preparations for at least 6 hours prior to the procedure. Ensure that the patient has removed all external metallic objects (jewelry, dentures, etc.) prior to the procedure.

➤ Have emergency equipment readily available.

➤ Patients are given a gown, robe, and foot coverings to wear and instructed to void prior to the procedure.

➤ Instruct the patient to cooperate fully and to follow directions. Instruct the patient to remain still throughout the procedure because movement produces unreliable results.

➤ Observe standard precautions, and follow the general guidelines in Appendix A. Positively identify the patient, and label the appropriate collection container with the corresponding patient demographics, date, and time of collection.

➤ Start an IV line and administer ordered sedation.

➤ Spray or swab the oropharynx with a topical local anesthetic.

➤ Provide an emesis basin for the increased saliva and encourage the patient to spit out the saliva because the gag reflex may be impaired.

➤ Place the patient on an examination table in the left lateral decubitus position with the neck slightly flexed forward.

➤ The endoscope is passed through the mouth with a dental suction device in place to drain secretions. A side-viewing flexible, fiberoptic endoscope is advanced, and visualization of the GI tract is started.

➤ Air is insufflated to distend the upper GI tract, as needed. Biopsy specimens are obtained and/or endoscopic surgery is performed.

➤ Promptly transport the specimens to the laboratory for processing and analysis.

➤ At the end of the procedure, excess air and secretions are aspirated through the scope and the endoscope is removed.

➤ The results are recorded manually or in a computerized system for recall and postprocedure interpretation by the appropriate health care practitioner.

➤ Do not allow the patient to eat or drink until the gag reflex returns; then allow the patient to eat lightly for 12 to 24 hours.

➤ Instruct the patient to resume usual activity and diet in 24 hours or as tolerated after the examination, as directed by the health care practitioner.

➤ Inform the patient that he or she may experience some throat soreness and hoarseness. Instruct patient to treat throat discomfort with lozenges and warm gargles when the gag reflex returns.

➤ Monitor vital signs and neurologic status every 15 minutes for 1 hour, then every 2 hours for 4 hours, and as ordered by the health care practitioner. Take temperature every 4 hours for 24 hours. Compare with baseline values. Notify the health care practitioner if temperature is elevated. Protocols may vary from facility to facility.

➤ Observe the patient for indications of esophageal perforation (i.e., painful swallowing with neck movement, substernal pain with respiration, shoulder pain or dyspnea, and abdominal or back pain, cyanosis, fever).

➤ Inform the patient that any belching, bloating, or flatulence is the result of air insufflation and is temporary.

➤ Emphasize that any severe pain, fever, difficulty breathing, or expectoration of blood must be immediately reported to the health care practitioner.

➤ A written report of the examination will be completed by a health care practitioner specializing in this branch of medicine. The report will be sent to the requesting health care practitioner. who will discuss the results with the patient.

➤ Reinforce information given by the patient's health care provider regarding further testing, treatment, or referral to another health care provider. Answer any questions or address any concerns voiced by the patient or family.

➤ Depending on the results of this procedure, additional testing may be needed to evaluate or monitor progression of the disease process and determine the need for a change in therapy. Evaluate test results in relation to the patient's symptoms and other tests performed.

➤ Related diagnostic tests include computed tomography of the abdomen; hepatobiliary scan; hepatobiliary ultrasound; kidney, ureter, and bladder film; and magnetic resonance imaging of the abdomen.

ESTRADIOL

SYNONYM/ACRONYM: E2.

SPECIMEN: Serum (1 mL) collected in a red- or tiger-top tube. Plasma (1 mL) collected in green-top (heparin) tube is also acceptable.

REFERENCE VALUE: (Method: Immunoassay)

Age	Conventional Units	SI Units (Conventional Units × 3.67)
6 m–10 y	Less than 15 pg/mL	Less than 55 pmol/L
11–15 y		
Male	Less than 40 pg/mL	Less than 147 pmol/L
Female	10–300 pg/mL	37–1100 pmol/L
Adult male	10–50 pg/mL	37–184 pmol/L
Adult female		
Early follicular phase	20–150 pg/mL	73–551 pmol/L
Late follicular phase	40–350 pg/mL	147–1285 pmol/L
Midcycle peak	150–750 pg/mL	551–2753 pmol/L
Luteal phase	30–450 pg/mL	110–1652 pmol/L
Postmenopause	Less than 20 pg/mL	Less than 73 pmol/L

DESCRIPTION & RATIONALE: Estrogens are hormones secreted in large amounts by the ovaries and during pregnancy by the placenta. Estradiol is also secreted in minute amounts by the adrenal cortex and the testes. Only three types of estrogen are present in the blood in measurable amounts: estrone, estradiol, and estriol. Estradiol is the most active of the estrogens. Estrone (E_1) is the immediate precursor of estradiol (E_2). Estriol (E_3) is secreted in large amounts from the placenta during pregnancy from precursors produced by the fetal liver. ■

INDICATIONS:
* Assist in determining the presence of gonadal dysfunction.

* Evaluate menstrual abnormalities, fertility problems, and estrogen-producing tumors in women, and testicular or adrenal tumors and feminization disorders in men.

* Monitor menotropins (Pergonal) therapy. Menotropins is a preparation of follicle-stimulating hormone (FSH) and luteinizing hormone (LH) used to induce ovulation and increase the chance of pregnancy.

RESULT

Increased in:
* Adrenal tumors
* Estrogen-producing tumors
* Feminization in children
* Gynecomastia
* Hepatic cirrhosis
* Hyperthyroidism

Decreased in:
* Ovarian failure
* Primary and secondary hypogonadism
* Turner's syndrome

CRITICAL VALUES: N/A

INTERFERING FACTORS:
* Drugs that may increase estradiol levels include cimetidine, clomiphene, dehydroepiandrosterone, diazepam, estrogen/progestin therapy, ketoconazole, mifepristone (some patients with meningiomas and not receiving any other drugs), nafarelin, nilutamide, phenytoin, tamoxifen, and troleandomycin.

* Drugs that may decrease estradiol levels include aminoglutethimide, chemotherapy drugs, cimetidine, danazol,

fadrozole, formestane, goserelin, leuprolide, megestrol, mepartricin, mifepristone (pregnant women with expulsion of fetus), nafarelin (women being treated for endometriosis), and oral contraceptives.

• Estradiol is secreted in a biphasic pattern during normal menstruation. Knowledge of the phase of the menstrual cycle may assist interpretation of estradiol levels.

Nursing Implications and Procedure • • • • • • • • • • •

Pretest:

▶ Inform the patient that the test is used to assist in the evaluation of fertility or postmenopausal status.

▶ Obtain a history of the patient's complaints, including a list of known allergens (especially allergies or sensitivities to latex), and inform the appropriate health care practitioner accordingly.

▶ Obtain a history of the patient's endocrine and reproductive systems, as well as phase of menstrual cycle and results of previously performed laboratory tests, surgical procedures, and other diagnostic procedures. For related laboratory tests, refer to the Endocrine and Reproductive System tables.

▶ Record the date of the last menstrual period and determine the possibility of pregnancy in perimenopausal women.

▶ Obtain a list of the medications the patient is taking, including herbs, nutritional supplements, and nutraceuticals. Note the last time and dose of medication taken. The requesting health care practitioner and laboratory should be advised if the patient regularly uses these products so that their effects can be taken into consideration when reviewing results.

▶ Review the procedure with the patient. Inform the patient that specimen collection takes approximately 5 to 10 minutes. Address concerns about pain related to the procedure. Explain to the patient that there may be some discomfort during the venipuncture.

▶ *Sensitivity to cultural and social issues,* as well as concern for modesty, is important in providing psychological support before, during, and after the procedure.

▶ There are no food, fluid, or medication restrictions, unless by medical direction.

Intratest:

▶ If the patient has a history of severe allergic reaction to latex, care should be taken to avoid the use of equipment containing latex.

▶ Instruct the patient to cooperate fully and to follow directions. Direct the patient to breathe normally and to avoid unnecessary movement.

▶ Observe standard precautions, and follow the general guidelines in Appendix A. Positively identify the patient, and label the appropriate tubes with the corresponding patient demographics, date, and time of collection. Perform a venipuncture; collect the specimen in a 5-mL red- or tiger-top tube.

▶ Remove the needle, and apply a pressure dressing over the puncture site.

▶ Promptly transport the specimen to the laboratory for processing and analysis.

▶ The results are recorded manually or in a computerized system for recall and postprocedure interpretation by the appropriate health care practitioner.

Post-test:

▶ Observe venipuncture site for bleeding or hematoma formation. Apply paper tape or other adhesive to hold pressure bandage in place, or replace with a plastic bandage.

▶ A written report of the examination will be sent to the requesting health

care practitioner, who will discuss the results with the patient.

➤ Reinforce information given by the patient's health care provider regarding further testing, treatment, or referral to another health care provider. Explain to the patient the importance of following the medication regimen and instructions regarding drug interactions. Answer any questions or address any concerns voiced by the patient or family.

➤ Instruct the patient to be prepared to provide the pharmacist with a list of other medications he or she is already taking in the event that the requesting health care practitioner prescribes a medication.

➤ Depending on the results of this procedure, additional testing may be performed to evaluate or monitor progression of the disease process and determine the need for a change in therapy. Evaluate test results in relation to the patient's symptoms and other tests performed.

Related laboratory tests:

➤ Related laboratory tests include FSH, LH, progesterone, and prolactin.

ESTROGEN AND PROGESTERONE RECEPTOR ASSAYS

. . . .

SYNONYMS/ACRONYMS: Estrogen receptor protein (ERP), progesterone receptor protein (PRP).

SPECIMEN: Breast tissue.

REFERENCE VALUE: (Method: Cytochemical or immunocytochemical) Interpretation of results is subjective depending on the intensity of staining and the number of cells classified as positive. More recently, immunoperoxidase methods employing monoclonal antibodies have been introduced. These antibodies have greater specificity and are not subject to interference by exogenous hormones.

Cytochemical Findings	Values
Favorable findings	Greater than 20% of cell nuclei are stained
Borderline findings	11–20% of cell nuclei are stained
Unfavorable findings	Less than 10% of cell nuclei are stained

DESCRIPTION & RATIONALE: Estrogen and progesterone receptor assays are used to identify patients with a type of breast cancer that may be more responsive than other types of tumors to estrogen-deprivation (antiestrogen) therapy or removal of the ovaries. Patients with these types of tumors generally have a better prognosis. DNA ploidy testing by flow cytometry may also be performed on suspicious tissue. Cancer cells contain abnormal amounts of DNA. The higher the grade of tumor cells, the more likely abnormal DNA will be detected. The ploidy, or number of chromosome sets in the nucleus, is an indication of the speed of cell replication and tumor growth. ■

INDICATIONS:

• Identify patients with breast or other types of cancer that may respond to hormone or antihormone therapy

• Monitor responsiveness to hormone or antihormone therapy

RESULT

Positive findings in:
• Hormonal therapy

• Receptor-positive tumors

Negative findings in:
• Receptor-negative tumors

CRITICAL VALUES: N/A

INTERFERING FACTORS:

• Antiestrogen preparations (e.g., tamoxifen) ingested 2 months before tissue sampling will affect test results.

• Tissue specimens contaminated with formalin or failure to freeze the specimen adequately using liquid nitrogen or dry ice will falsely decrease results.

• Massive tumor necrosis or tumors with low cellular composition falsely decrease results.

• Failure to transport specimen to the laboratory immediately can result in degradation of receptor sites. Prompt and proper specimen processing, stor-

age, and analysis are important to achieve accurate results.

Nursing Implications and Procedure • • • • • • • • • •

Pretest: ■

➤ Inform the patient that the test is primarily used to assist in the prognosis and in the management of response to therapy for breast and endometrial cancer.

➤ Obtain a history of the patient's complaints, including a list of known allergens (especially allergies or sensitivities to latex), and inform the appropriate health care practitioner accordingly.

➤ Obtain a history of the patient's endocrine, immune, and reproductive systems and results of previously performed laboratory tests, surgical procedures, and other diagnostic procedures. For related laboratory tests, refer to the Endocrine, Immune, and Reproductive System tables.

➤ Record the date of the last menstrual period and determine the possibility of pregnancy in perimenopausal women.

➤ Note any recent procedures that can interfere with test results. Ensure that the patient has not received antiestrogen therapy within 2 months of the test.

➤ Obtain a list of the medications the patient is taking, including anticoagulant therapy, acetylsalicylic acid, herbs, nutritional supplements, and nutraceuticals, especially those known to affect coagulation. It is recommended that use be discontinued 14 days before dental or surgical procedures. The requesting health care practitioner and laboratory should be advised if the patient regularly uses these products so that their effects can be taken into consideration when reviewing results.

➤ Review the procedure with the patient. Inform the patient that it may be necessary to shave the site before the procedure. Instruct that prophylactic antibiotics may be administered prior to the procedure. Address concerns about pain related to the procedure. Explain that a sedative and/or analgesia will be administered to promote relaxation and reduce discomfort prior to the percutaneous biopsy; a general anesthesia will be administered prior to the open biopsy. Explain to the patient that no pain will be experienced during the test when general anesthesia is used, but that any discomfort with a needle biopsy will be minimized with local anesthetics and systemic analgesics. Inform the patient that the biopsy is performed under sterile conditions by a health care practitioner specializing in this procedure. The surgical procedure usually takes about 20 to 30 minutes to complete, and that sutures may be necessary to close the site. A needle biopsy usually takes about 15 minutes to complete.

➤ *Sensitivity to cultural and social issues,* as well as concern for modesty, is important in providing psychological support before, during, and after the procedure.

➤ Explain that an intravenous (IV) line will be inserted to allow infusion of IV fluids, antibiotics, anesthetics, and analgesics.

➤ Ensure that anticoagulant therapy has been withheld for the appropriate amount of days prior to the procedure. Amount of days to withhold medication is dependant on the type of anticoagulant. Notify health care practitioner if patient anticoagulant therapy has not been withheld.

Open biopsy:

➤ Instruct the patient that nothing should be taken by mouth for 6 to 8 hours prior to a general anesthetic.

Needle biopsy:

➤ Instruct the patient that nothing should be taken by mouth for at least 4 hours prior to the procedure

to reduce the risk of nausea and vomiting.

General:

➤ *Make sure a written and informed consent has been signed prior to the procedure and before administering any medications.*

Intratest:

➤ Ensure that the patient has complied with dietary restrictions; assure that food has been restricted for at least 4 to 8 hours prior to the procedure, depending on the anesthetic chosen for the procedure.

➤ Have emergency equipment readily available.

➤ Have the patient void before the procedure.

➤ Observe standard precautions, and follow the general guidelines in Appendix A. Positively identify the patient, and label the appropriate collection containers with the corresponding patient demographics, date and time of collection, and site location, especially left or right breast.

➤ Assist the patient to the desired position depending on the test site to be used, and direct the patient to breath normally during the beginning of the general anesthesic. Instruct the patient to cooperate fully and to follow directions. Direct the patient to breathe normally and to avoid unnecessary movement during the local anesthetic and the procedure.

➤ Record baseline vital signs and continue to monitor throughout the procedure. Protocols may vary from facility to facility.

➤ After the administration of general or local anesthesia, cleanse the site with an antiseptic solution, and drape the area with sterile towels.

Open biopsy:

➤ After administration of general anesthesia and surgical prep is completed, an incision is made, suspicious area(s) are located, and tissue samples are collected. Using needle biopsy or resection, suspicious areas are located and a tissue specimen weighing at least 200 mg is collected.

Needle biopsy:

➤ Direct the patient to take slow deep breaths when the local anesthetic is injected. Protect the site with sterile drapes. Instruct the patient to take a deep breath, exhale forcefully, and hold the breath while the biopsy needle is inserted and rotated to obtain a core of breast tissue. Once the needle is removed, the patient may breathe. Pressure is applied to the site for 3 to 5 minutes, then a sterile pressure dressing is applied.

General:

➤ Monitor the patient for complications related to the procedure (e.g., allergic reaction, anaphylaxis).

➤ Place tissue samples in a formalin-free specimen container. Label the specimen, indicating site location, and promptly transport the specimen to the laboratory for processing and analysis.

➤ The results are recorded manually or in a computerized system for recall and postprocedure interpretation by the appropriate health care practitioner.

Post-test:

➤ Instruct the patient to resume preoperative diet, as directed by the health care practitioner.

➤ Monitor vital signs and neurologic status every 15 minutes for 1 hour, and then every 2 hours for 4 hours, and then as ordered by the health care practitioner. Monitor temperature every 4 hours for 24 hours. Compare with baseline values. Notify the health care practitioner if temperature is elevated. Protocols may vary from facility to facility.

➤ Observe for delayed allergic reactions, such as rash, urticaria, tachycardia, hyperpnea, hypertension, palpitations, nausea, or vomiting.

➤ Observe the biopsy site for bleeding, inflammation, or hematoma formation.

➤ Instruct the patient in the care and assessment of the site. Instruct the patient to report any redness, edema, bleeding, or pain at the biopsy site. Instruct the patient to immediately report chills or fever. Instruct the patient to keep the site clean and change the dressing as needed.

➤ Assess for nausea and pain. Administer antiemetic and analgesic medications as needed and as directed by the health care practitioner.

➤ Administer antibiotic therapy if ordered. Remind the patient of the importance of completing the entire course of antibiotic therapy, even if signs and symptoms disappear before completion of therapy.

➤ A written report of the examination will be completed by a health care practitioner specializing in this branch of medicine. The report will be sent to the requesting health care practitioner, who will discuss the results with the patient.

➤ Recognize anxiety related to test results, and offer support. Discuss the implications of abnormal test results on the patient's lifestyle. Provide teaching and information regarding the clinical implications of the test results, as appropriate. Inform the patient about hormone therapy, as appropriate based on test results. Educate the patient regarding access to counseling services.

➤ Reinforce information given by the patient's health care provider regarding further testing, treatment, or referral to another health care provider. Inform the patient of a follow-up appointment for removal of sutures, if indicated. Instruct and educate the patient on how to perform monthly breast self-examination and emphasize, as appropriate, the importance of having a mammogram performed annually. Answer any questions or address any concerns voiced by the patient or family.

➤ Instruct the patient in the use of any ordered medications. Explain the importance of adhering to the therapy regimen. As appropriate, instruct the patient in significant side effects and systemic reactions associated with the prescribed medication. Encourage him or her to review corresponding literature provided by a pharmacist.

➤ Depending on the results of this procedure, additional testing may be performed to evaluate or monitor progression of the disease process and determine the need for a change in therapy. Evaluate test results in relation to the patient's symptoms and other tests performed.

Related laboratory tests:

➤ Related laboratory tests include breast biopsy, CA 15-3, carcinoembryonic antigen, and HER-2/neu oncoprotein.

EVOKED BRAIN POTENTIALS

∙ ∙

SYNONYMS/ACRONYMS: EP studies, brainstem auditory evoked potentials (BAEP), brainstem auditory evoked responses (BAER).

AREA OF APPLICATION: Brain.

CONTRAST: None.

DESCRIPTION & RATIONALE: Evoked brain potentials, also known as evoked potential (EP) responses, are electrophysiologic studies performed to measure the brain's electrical responses to various visual, auditory, and somatosensory stimuli. EP studies help diagnose lesions of the nervous system by evaluating the integrity of the visual, somatosensory, and auditory nerve pathways. Three response types are measured: visual evoked response (VER), auditory brainstem response (ABR), and somatosensory evoked response (SER). The stimuli activate the nerve tracts that connect the stimulated (receptor) area with the cortical (visual and somatosensory) or midbrain (auditory) sensory area. A number of stimuli are given and then responses are electronically displayed in waveforms, recorded, and computer analyzed. Abnormalities are determined by a delay in time, measured in milliseconds, between the stimulus and the response. This is known as *increased latency.* VER provides information about visual pathway function to identify lesions of the optic nerves, optic tracts, and demyelinating diseases such as multiple sclerosis. ABR provides information about auditory pathways to identify hearing loss and lesions of the brainstem. SER provides information about the somatosensory pathways to identify lesions at various levels of the central nervous system (spinal cord and brain) and peripheral nerve disease. EP studies are especially useful in patients with problems and those unable to speak or respond to instructions during the test, because these studies do not require voluntary cooperation or participation in the activity. This allows collection of objective diagnostic information about visual or auditory disorders affecting infants and children, and allows differentiation between organic brain and psychological disorders in adults. EP studies are also used to monitor the progression of or the effectiveness of treatment for deteriorating neurologic diseases such as multiple sclerosis. ■

INDICATIONS

VER (potentials):

- Detect cryptic or past retrobulbar neuritis
- Detect lesions of the eye or optic nerves
- Detect neurologic disorders such as multiple sclerosis, Parkinson's disease, and Huntington's chorea
- Evaluate binocularity in infants
- Evaluate optic pathway lesions and visual cortex defects

ABR (potentials):

- Detect abnormalities or lesions in the brainstem or auditory nerve areas
- Detect brainstem tumors and acoustic neuromas
- Screen or evaluate neonates, infants, children, and adults for auditory problems (EP studies may be indicated when a child falls below growth chart norms)

SER (potentials):

- Detect multiple sclerosis and Guillain-Barré syndrome
- Detect sensorimotor neuropathies and cervical pathology
- Evaluate spinal cord and brain injury and function
- Monitor sensory potentials to determine spinal cord function during a surgical procedure or medical regimen

ERP (potentials):

- Detect suspected psychosis or dementia
- Differentiate between organic brain disorder and cognitive function abnormality

RESULT

Normal Findings:

VER and ABR: Normal latency in recorded cortical and brainstem waveforms depending on age, sex, and stature

ERP: Normal recognition and attention span

SER: No loss of consciousness or presence of weakness

Abnormal Findings:

- VER (potentials):

P100 latencies (extended) confined to one eye suggest a lesion anterior to the optic chiasm.

Bilateral abnormal P100 latencies indicate multiple sclerosis, optic neuritis, retinopathies, spinocerebellar degeneration, sarcoidosis, Parkinson's disease, adrenoleukodystrophy, Huntington's chorea, and amblyopias.

- ABR (potentials):

Normal response at high intensities; wave V may occur slightly later. Earlier wave distortions suggest cochlear lesion.

Absent or late waves at high intensities; increased amplitude of wave V suggests retrocochlear lesion.

- SER (potentials):

  Abnormal upper limb latencies suggest cervical spondylosis or intracerebral lesions.

  Abnormal lower limb latencies suggest peripheral nerve root disease such as Guillain-Barré syndrome, multiple sclerosis, transverse myelitis, or traumatic spinal cord injuries.

CRITICAL VALUES: N/A

INTERFERING FACTORS

Factors that may impair the results of the examination:

- Inability of the patient to cooperate or remain still during the procedure because of age, significant pain, or mental status (*note:* significant behavioral problems may limit the ability to complete the test)

- Improper placement of electrodes

- Patient stress, which can affect brain chemistry, thus making it difficult to distinguish whether the results are due to the patient's emotional reaction or to organic pathology

- Extremely poor visual acuity, which can hinder accurate determination of VER

- Severe hearing loss, which can interfere with accurate determination of ABR

Nursing Implications and Procedure ● ● ● ● ● ● ● ● ● ● ●

Pretest:

➤ Inform the patient that this procedure measures electrical activity in the nervous system.

➤ Obtain a history of the patient's neu-

rologic system, known or suspected neurologic conditions, and trauma to the head or spinal cord, as well as the results of previously performed laboratory tests, surgeries, treatments, and procedures. For related diagnostic tests, refer to the Musculoskeletal System table.

➤ Obtain a list of the medications the patient is taking, including herbs, nutritional supplements, and nutraceuticals. The requesting health care practitioner and laboratory should be advised if the patient regularly uses these products so that their effects can be taken into consideration when reviewing results.

➤ Review the procedure with the patient. Inform the patient that the procedure is painless and harmless. Inform the patient that the procedure is performed in a special laboratory by a technologist and takes approximately 30 minutes to 2 hours, depending on the test.

➤ Instruct the patient to clean the hair and to refrain from using hair sprays, creams, or solutions before the test.

➤ There are no food, fluid, or medication restrictions, unless by medical direction.

➤ *Make sure a written and informed consent has been signed prior to the procedure and before administering any medications.*

Intratest:

➤ Ensure that the patient is able to relax; report any extreme anxiety or restlessness.

➤ Ensure that hair is clean and free of hair sprays, creams, or solutions.

➤ Have the patient remove any jewelry or metallic objects above the neck.

➤ Observe standard precautions, and follow the general guidelines in Appendix A.

Visual evoked potentials:

➤ Place the patient in a comfortable position about 1 m from the stimulation source. Attach electrodes to the occipital and vertex lobe areas and a reference electrode to the ear. A light-emitting stimulation or a checkerboard pattern is projected on a screen at a regulated speed. This procedure is done for each eye (with the opposite eye covered) as the patient looks at a dot on the screen without any change in the gaze while the stimuli are delivered. A computer interprets the brain's responses to the stimuli and records them in waveforms.

Auditory evoked potentials:

➤ Place the patient in a comfortable position, and place the electrodes on the scalp at the vertex lobe area and on each earlobe. Earphones are placed on the patient's ears, and a clicking noise stimulus is delivered into one ear while a continuous tone is delivered to the opposite ear. Responses to the stimuli are recorded as waveforms for analysis.

Somatosensory evoked potentials:

➤ Place the patient in a comfortable position, and place the electrodes at the nerve sites of the wrist, knee, and ankle and on the scalp at the sensory cortex of the hemisphere on the opposite side (the electrode that picks up the response and delivers it to the recorder). Additional electrodes can be positioned at the cervical or lumbar vertebrae for upper or lower limb stimulation. The rate at which the electric shock stimulus is delivered to the nerve electrodes and travels to the brain is measured, computer analyzed, and recorded in waveforms for analysis. Both sides of the area being examined can be tested by switching the electrodes and repeating the procedure.

Event-related potentials:

➤ Place the patient in a sitting position in a chair in a quiet room. Earphones are placed on the patient's ears and auditory cues administered. The patient is asked to push a button when the tones are recognized. Flashes of light are also used as visual cues, with the client pushing a button when cues are noted. Results are compared to normal EP waveforms for correct, incorrect, or absent responses.

Post-test:

➤ When the procedure is complete, remove the electrodes and clean the skin where the electrodes were applied.

➤ A written report of the examination will be completed by a health care practitioner specializing in this branch of medicine. The report will be sent to the requesting health care practitioner, who will discuss the results with the patient.

➤ Reinforce information given by the patient's health care provider regarding further testing, treatment, or referral to another health care provider. Answer any questions or address any concerns voiced by the patient or family.

➤ Depending on the results of this procedure, additional testing may be needed to evaluate or monitor progression of the disease process and determine the need for a change in therapy. Evaluate test results in relation to the patient's symptoms and other tests performed.

Related diagnostic tests:

➤ Related diagnostic tests include computed tomography of the brain, electroencephalography, and magnetic resonance imaging of the brain.

EXERCISE STRESS TEST

SYNONYMS/ACRONYMS: Exercise electrocardiogram (ECG, EKG), graded exercise tolerance test, stress testing, treadmill test.

AREA OF APPLICATION: Heart.

CONTRAST: None.

DESCRIPTION & RATIONALE: The exercise stress test is a noninvasive study to measure cardiac function during physical stress. Exercise electrocardiography is primarily useful in determining the extent of coronary artery occlusion by the heart's ability to meet the need for additional oxygen in response to the stress of exercising in a safe environment. The patient exercises on a treadmill or pedals a stationary bicycle to increase the heart rate to 80% to 90% of maximal heart rate determined by age and sex, known as the *target heart rate*. Every 2 to 3 minutes the speed and/or grade of the treadmill is increased to yield an increment of stress. The patient's electrocardiogram (ECG) and blood pressure are monitored during the test. The test proceeds until the patient reaches the target heart rate or experiences chest pain or fatigue. The risks involved in the procedure are possible myocardial infarction (1 in 500) and death (1 in 10,000) in patients experiencing frequent angina episodes before the test. Although useful, this procedure is not as accurate as cardiac nuclear scans for diagnosing coronary artery disease (CAD).

For patients unable to complete the test, pharmacologic stress testing can be done. Medications used to increase the patient's heart include vasodilators such as dipyridamole and β-agonists such as dobutamine. ■

INDICATIONS:
- Detect dysrhythmias during exercising, as evidenced by ECG changes

- Detect peripheral arterial occlusive disease (intermittent claudication), as evidenced by leg pain or cramping during exercising

- Determine exercise-induced hypertension

- Evaluate cardiac function after myocardial infarction or cardiac surgery to determine safe exercise levels for cardiac rehabilitation as well as work limitations

- Evaluate effectiveness of medication regimens, such as antianginals or antiarrhythmics

- Evaluate suspected CAD in the presence of chest pain and other symptoms

• Screen for CAD in the absence of pain and other symptoms in patients at risk

RESULT

Normal Findings:
• Normal heart rate during physical exercise. Heart rate and systolic blood pressure rise in direct proportion to workload and to metabolic oxygen demand, which is based on age and exercise protocol. Maximal heart rate for adults is normally 150 to 200 beats/min.

Abnormal Findings:
• Activity intolerance related to oxygen supply and demand imbalance

• Bradycardia

• CAD

• Chest pain related to ischemia or inflammation

• Decreased cardiac output

• Dysrhythmias

• Hypertension

• Peripheral arterial occlusive disease

• S-T segment depression of 1 mm (considered a positive test), indicating myocardial ischemia

• Tachycardia

CRITICAL VALUES: N/A

INTERFERING FACTORS: The following factors may impair interpretation of examination results because they create an artificial state that makes it difficult to determine true physiologic function:

• Improper electrode placement

• High food intake or smoking before testing

• Drugs such as β-blockers, cardiac glycosides, calcium channel blockers, coronary vasodilators, and barbiturates

• Potassium or calcium imbalance

• Hypertension, hypoxia, left bundle branch block, and ventricular hypertrophy

• Wolff-Parkinson-White syndrome (anomalous atrioventricular excitation)

• Anxiety or panic attack

Nursing Implications and Procedure

Pretest:

➤ Inform the patient that the test assesses the heart's ability to respond to an increasing workload.

➤ Obtain a pertinent history of the results of previously performed cardiac tests and procedures, present cardiac conditions or abnormalities, and therapies received for the cardiac conditions. For related diagnostic tests, refer to the Cardiovascular System table.

➤ Obtain a list of medications the patient is taking, including herbs, nutritional supplements, and nutraceuticals. The requesting health care practitioner and laboratory should be advised if the patient regularly uses these products so that their effects can be taken into consideration when reviewing results.

➤ Review the procedure with the patient. Address concerns about pain related to the procedure. Assure the patient that the test has very few risks and that exercising can be terminated if extreme symptoms occur. Inform the patient that the procedure is performed in a special department by a technician and takes approximately 30 to 60 minutes.

➤ Ask the patient if he or she has had any chest pain within the prior 48 hours, or has a history of anginal attacks several times a day; if either of these is the case, inform the health care practitioner immediately because the stress test may be too risky and should be rescheduled in 4 to 6 weeks.

➤ *Sensitivity to cultural and social issues,* as well as concern for modesty, is important in providing psychological support before, during and after the procedure.

➤ Record a baseline 12-lead ECG and vital signs, if these recordings were not already obtained or are not available.

➤ The patient should fast and refrain from drinking liquids and smoking for at least 4 hours prior to the test.

➤ Advise the patient to wear comfortable shoes and clothing for the exercise.

➤ *Make sure a written and informed consent has been signed prior to the procedure and before administering any medications.*

Intratest:

➤ Ensure that the patient has abstained from food, fluids, and smoking for at least 4 hours before the test and that the patient has discontinued specific medications that can interfere with test results, as ordered.

➤ Have emergency equipment readily available.

➤ An intravenous access may be established for emergency use.

➤ Ask the patient to remove clothing from the waist up (give women a hospital gown that opens in the front).

➤ Observe standard precautions, and follow the general guidelines in Appendix A.

➤ Electrodes are placed in appropriate positions on the patient, a blood pressure cuff connected to a monitoring device is applied, and if the patient's oxygen consumption is to be continuously monitored, the patient is connected to a machine via a mouthpiece or to a pulse oximeter via a finger lead.

➤ The patient is asked to walk on a treadmill (most commonly used) or

to peddle a bicycle. As the stress is increased, the patient is asked to report any symptoms, such as chest or leg pain, dyspnea, or fatigue.

➤ The patient is asked to step onto the treadmill and is instructed to use the handrails to maintain balance.

➤ The treadmill is turned on to a slow speed, but is increased in speed and elevation to increase the patient's heart rate. Stress is increased until the patient's predicted target heart rate is reached.

➤ Instruct the patient to report symptoms such as dizziness, sweating, breathlessness, or nausea, which can be normal as speed increases. The test is terminated if pain or fatigue is severe; maximum heart rate under stress is attained; signs of ischemia are present; maximum effort has been achieved; or dyspnea, hypertension (systolic blood pressure greater than 250 mm Hg), tachycardia (greater than 200 beats/minute minus person's age), new dysrhythmias, chest pain that begins or worsens, faintness, extreme dizziness, or confusion develops.

➤ After the exercise period, a 3- to 15-minute rest period is given with the patient in a sitting position. During this period, the ECG, blood pressure, and heart rate monitoring is continued.

➤ The results are recorded on a paper strip for postprocedure interpretation by the appropriate health care practitioner.

Post-test:

➤ Remove the electrodes and cleanse the skin of any remaining gel or ECG electrode adhesive.

➤ Instruct the patient to contact the health care practitioner to report any anginal pain or other discomforts experienced after the test.

➤ Instruct the patient regarding special dietary intake and medication regimen, as needed.

> Instruct the patient to resume activities discontinued before the test.
> A written report of the examination will be completed by a health care practitioner specializing in this branch of medicine. The report will be sent to the requesting health care practitioner, who will discuss the results with the patient.
> Reinforce information given by the patient's health care provider regarding further testing, treatment, or referral to another health care provider. Answer any questions or address any concerns voiced by the patient or family.

> Depending on the results of this procedure, additional testing may be performed to evaluate or monitor progression of the disease process and determine the need for a change in therapy. Evaluate test results in relation to the patient's symptoms and other tests performed.

Related diagnostic tests:

> Related diagnostic tests include electrocardiogram (ECG), myocardial perfusion scan of the heart, and positron emission tomography scan of the heart.

FECAL ANALYSIS

SYNONYM/ACRONYM: N/A.

SPECIMEN: Stool.

REFERENCE VALUE: (Method: Macroscopic examination, for appearance and color; microscopic examination, for cell count and presence of meat fibers; leukocyte esterase, for leukocytes; Clinitest [Bayer Corporation, Pittsburgh, Pennsylvania] for reducing substances; guaiac, for occult blood; x-ray paper, for trypsin)

Characteristic	Normal Result
Appearance	Solid and formed
Color	Brown
Epithelial cells	Few to moderate
Fecal fat	See "Fecal Fat" monograph
Leukocytes (white blood cells)	Negative
Meat fibers	Negative
Occult blood	Negative
Reducing substances	Negative
Trypsin	2+ to 4+

DESCRIPTION & RATIONALE: Feces consist mainly of cellulose and other undigested foodstuffs, bacteria, and water. Other substances normally found in feces include epithelial cells shed from the gastrointestinal (GI) tract, small amounts of fats, bile pigments in the form of urobilinogen, GI and pancreatic secretions, electrolytes, and trypsin. Trypsin is a proteolytic enzyme produced in the pancreas. The average adult excretes 100 to 300 g of fecal material per day, the residue of approximately 10 L of liquid material that enters the GI tract each day. The laboratory analysis of feces includes macroscopic examination (volume, odor, shape, color, consistency, presence of mucus), microscopic examination (leukocytes, epithelial cells, meat fibers), and chemical tests for specific substances (occult blood, trypsin, estimation of carbohydrate). ∎

INDICATIONS:

- Assist in diagnosing disorders associated with GI bleeding or drug therapy that leads to bleeding
- Assist in the diagnosis of pseudomembranous enterocolitis after use of broad-spectrum antibiotic therapy
- Assist in the diagnosis of suspected inflammatory bowel disorder
- Detect altered protein digestion
- Detect intestinal parasitic infestation, as indicated by diarrhea of unknown cause
- Investigate diarrhea of unknown cause
- Monitor effectiveness of therapy for intestinal malabsorption or pancreatic insufficiency
- Screen for cystic fibrosis

RESULT

Unusual Appearance:

- Bloody: Excessive intestinal wall irritation or malignancy
- Bulky or frothy: Malabsorption
- Mucous: Inflammation of intestinal walls
- Slender or ribbonlike: Obstruction

Unusual Color:

- Black: Bismuth (antacid) or charcoal ingestion, iron therapy, upper GI bleed
- Grayish white: Barium ingestion, bile duct obstruction
- Green: Antibiotics, biliverdin, green vegetables
- Red: Beets and food coloring, lower GI bleed, phenazopyridine hydrochloride compounds, rifampin
- Yellow: Rhubarb

Increased:

- Carbohydrates/reducing substances: Malabsorption syndromes
- Epithelial cells: Inflammatory bowel disorders
- Leukocytes: Bacterial infections of the intestinal wall, salmonellosis, shigellosis, and ulcerative colitis
- Meat fibers: Altered protein digestion
- Occult blood: Anal fissure, diverticular disease, esophageal varices, esophagitis, gastritis, hemorrhoids, infectious diarrheas, inflammatory bowel disease, Mallory-Weiss tears, polyps, tumors, ulcers

Decreased:

- Leukocytes: Amebic colitis, cholera, disorders resulting from toxins, parasites, viral diarrhea
- Trypsin: Cystic fibrosis, malabsorption syndromes, pancreatic deficiency

CRITICAL VALUES: N/A

INTERFERING FACTORS:

- Drugs that can cause positive results for occult blood include acetylsalicylic acid, anticoagulants, colchicine, corticosteroids, iron preparations, and phenylbutazone.

- Ingestion of a diet high in red meat, certain vegetables, and bananas can cause false-positive results for occult blood.

- Large doses of vitamin C can cause false-negative occult blood.

- Constipated stools may not indicate any trypsin activity owing to extended exposure to intestinal bacteria.

Nursing Implications and Procedure • • • • • • • • • • •

Pretest:

➤ Inform the patient that the test is used to assist in the diagnosis of intestinal disorders.

➤ Obtain a history of the patient's complaints, including a list of known allergens, and inform the appropriate health care practitioner accordingly.

➤ Obtain a history of the patient's gastrointestinal system and results of previously performed laboratory tests, surgical procedures, and other diagnostic procedures. For related laboratory tests, refer to the Gastrointestinal System table.

➤ Obtain a list of medications the patient is taking, including herbs, nutritional supplements, and nutraceuticals. The requesting health care practitioner and laboratory should be advised if the patient regularly uses these products so that their effects can be taken into consideration when reviewing results.

➤ Review the procedure with the patient. Inform the patient of the procedure for collecting a stool sample, including the importance of good handwashing techniques. The patient should place the sample in a tightly covered container. Instruct the

patient not to contaminate the specimen with urine, water, or toilet tissue. Address concerns about pain related to the procedure. Explain to the patient that there should be no discomfort during the procedure.

➤ *Sensitivity to social and cultural issues,* as well as concern for modesty, is important in providing psychological support before, during, and after the procedure.

➤ Instruct the patient not to use laxatives, enemas, or suppositories for 3 days before the test.

➤ Instruct the patient to follow a normal diet for several days before the test.

Intratest:

➤ Ensure that the patient has complied with medication restrictions; assure laxatives, enemas, or suppositories have been restricted for at least 3 days prior to the procedure.

➤ Instruct the patient to cooperate fully and to follow directions.

➤ Observe standard precautions, and follow the general guidelines in Appendix A. Positively identify the patient, and label the appropriate collection container with the corresponding patient demographics, date and time of collection, and suspected cause of enteritis; note any current or recent antibiotic therapy.

➤ Collect a stool specimen in a half-pint waterproof container with a tight-fitting lid; if the patient is not ambulatory, collect it in a clean, dry bedpan. Use a tongue blade to transfer the specimen to the container, and include any mucoid and bloody portions. Collect specimen from the first, middle, and last portion of the stool. The specimen should be refrigerated if it will not be transported to the laboratory within 4 hours after collection.

➤ To collect specimen by rectal swab, insert the swab past the anal sphincter, rotate gently, and withdraw. Place the swab in the appropriate container.

➤ Promptly transport the specimen to the laboratory for processing and analysis.

> The results are recorded manually or in a computerized system for recall and postprocedure interpretation by the appropriate health care practitioner.

Post-test:

> A written report of the examination will be sent to the requesting health care practitioner, who will discuss the results with the patient.

> Recognize anxiety related to test results. Discuss the implications of abnormal test results on the patient's lifestyle. Provide teaching and information regarding the clinical implications of the test results, as appropriate.

> Reinforce information given by the patient's health care provider regarding further testing, treatment, or referral to another health care provider. Answer any questions or address any concerns voiced by the patient or family.

> Depending on the results of this procedure, additional testing may be performed to evaluate or monitor progression of the disease process and determine the need for a change in therapy. Evaluate test results in relation to the patient's symptoms and other tests performed.

Related laboratory tests:

> Related laboratory tests include α_1-antitrypsin/phenotyping, sweat chloride, D-xylose tolerance, fecal fat, gliadin antibody, intestinal biopsy, lactose tolerance, ova and parasites, and stool culture.

FECAL FAT

SYNONYMS/ACRONYM: Stool fat, fecal fat stain.

SPECIMEN: Stool (80 mL) aliquot from an unpreserved and homogenized 24- to 72-hour timed collection. Random specimens may also be submitted.

REFERENCE VALUE: (Method: Stain with Sudan black or oil red O. Treatment with ethanol identifies neutral fats; treatment with acetic acid identifies fatty acids.)

Random, Semiquantitative	
Neutral fat	Less than 50 fat globules/hpf
Fatty acids	Less than 100 fat globules/hpf
Age (diet)	*72-hour, Quantitative*
Infant (breast milk)	Less than 1 g/24 h
0–6 y	Less than 2 g/24 h
Adult	2–7 g/24 h; less than 20% of total solids
Adult (fat-free)	Less than 4 g/24 h

hpf = high-power field.

DESCRIPTION & RATIONALE: Fecal fat primarily consists of triglycerides (neutral fats), fatty acids, and fatty acid salts. Through microscopic examination, the number and size of fat droplets can be determined as well as the type of fat present. Excretion of greater than 7 g of fecal fat in a 24-hour period is abnormal but nonspecific for disease. Increases in excretion of neutral fats are associated with pancreatic exocrine insufficiency, whereas decreases are related to small bowel disease. An increase in triglycerides indicates that insufficient pancreatic enzymes are available to convert the triglycerides into fatty acids. Patients with malabsorption conditions have normal amounts of triglycerides but an increase in total fecal fat because the fats are not absorbed through the intestine. Malabsorption disorders (e.g., cystic fibrosis) cause blockage of the pancreatic ducts by mucus, which prevents the enzymes from reaching the duodenum and results in lack of fat digestion. Without digestion, the fats cannot be absorbed, and steatorrhea results. The appearance and odor of stool from patients with steatorrhea is typically foamy, greasy, soft, and foul-smelling. The semiquantitative test is used to screen for the presence of fecal fat. The quantitative method, which requires a 72-hour stool collection, measures the amount of fat present in grams. ∎

INDICATIONS:
• Assist in the diagnosis of malabsorption or pancreatic insufficiency, as indicated by elevated fat levels
• Monitor the effectiveness of therapy

RESULT

Increased in:

• Abetalipoprotein deficiency
• Addison's disease
• Amyloidosis
• Bile salt deficiency
• Carcinoid syndrome
• Celiac disease
• Crohn's disease
• Cystic fibrosis
• Diabetes
• Enteritis
• Malnutrition
• Multiple sclerosis
• Pancreatic insufficiency or obstruction
• Peptic ulcer disease
• Pernicious anemia
• Progressive systemic sclerosis
• Thyrotoxicosis
• Tropical sprue
• Viral hepatitis
• Whipple's disease
• Zollinger-Ellison syndrome

Decreased in: N/A

CRITICAL VALUES: N/A

INTERFERING FACTORS:
• Cimetidine has been associated with decreased fecal fat in some patients with cystic fibrosis who are also receiving pancreatic enzyme therapy.

• Some drugs cause steatorrhea as a result of mucosal damage. These include colchicine, kanamycin, lincomycin, methotrexate, and neomycin. Other drugs that can cause an increase in fecal fat include aminosalicylic acid, bisacodyl and phenolphthalein (observed in laxative abusers), and cholestyramine (in high doses).

- Use of suppositories, oily lubricants, or mineral oil in the perianal area for 3 days before the test can falsely increase neutral fats.

- Use of herbals with laxative effects, including cascara, psyllium, and senna, for 3 days before the test can falsely increase neutral fats.

- Barium interferes with test results.

- Failure to collect all stools may reflect falsely decreased results.

- Ingestion of a diet too high or low in fats may alter the results.

Nursing Implications and Procedure • • • • • • • • • • •

Pretest:

▶ Inform the patient that the test is used to assist in the diagnosis of malabsorption syndromes.

▶ Obtain a history of the patient's complaints that indicate a gastrointestinal (GI) disorder, diarrhea related to GI dysfunction, pain related to tissue inflammation or irritation, alteration in diet resulting from an inability to digest certain foods, or fluid volume deficit related to active loss. Obtain a history of known allergens and inform the appropriate health care practitioner accordingly.

▶ Obtain a history of the patient's GI and respiratory systems, and results of previously performed laboratory tests, surgical procedures, and other diagnostic procedures. For related laboratory tests, refer to the Gastrointestinal and Respiratory System tables.

▶ Note any recent procedures that can interfere with test results.

▶ Obtain a list of the medications the patient is taking, including herbs, nutritional supplements, and nutraceuticals. The requesting health care practitioner and laboratory should be advised if the patient regularly uses these products so that their effects can be taken into consideration when reviewing results.

▶ Review the procedure with the patient. Stress the importance of collecting all stools for the quantitative test, including diarrhea, over the timed specimen-collection period. Inform the patient not to urinate in the stool-collection container and not to put toilet paper in the container. Address concerns about pain related to the procedure. Explain to the patient that there should be no discomfort during the procedure.

▶ *Sensitivity to social and cultural issues,* as well as concern for modesty, is important in providing psychological support before, during and after the procedure.

▶ Instruct the patient not to use laxatives, enemas, or suppositories for 3 days before the test.

▶ There are no fluid restrictions, unless by medical direction.

▶ Instruct the patient to ingest a diet containing 50 to 150 g of fat for at least 3 days before beginning specimen collection. This approach does not work well with children; instruct the caregiver to record the child's dietary intake to provide a basis from which an estimate of fat intake can be made.

Intratest:

▶ Ensure that the patient has complied with dietary and other pretesting preparations prior to the procedure.

▶ Instruct the patient to cooperate fully and to follow directions.

▶ Observe standard precautions, and follow the general guidelines in Appendix A. Positively identify the patient, and label the appropriate collection container with the corresponding patient demographics, date, and the start and stop times of collection.

▶ Obtain the appropriate-sized specimen container, toilet-mounted collection container to aid in specimen collection, and plastic bag for specimen transport. A large, clean, preweighed container should be used for the timed test. A smaller, clean container can be used for the collection of the random sample.

> For the quantitative procedure, instruct the patient to collect each stool and place it in the 500-mL container during the timed collection period. Keep the container refrigerated in the plastic bag throughout the entire collection period.

> Promptly transport the specimen to the laboratory for processing and analysis.

> The results are recorded manually or in a computerized system for recall and postprocedure interpretation by the appropriate health care practitioner.

Post-test:

> Instruct the patient to resume usual diet and medication, as directed by the health care practitioner.

> A written report of the examination will be sent to the requesting health care practitioner, who will discuss the results with the patient.

> Recognize anxiety related to test results. Discuss the implications of abnormal test results on the patient's lifestyle. Instruct the patient with abnormal values on the importance of fluid intake and proper diet specific to his or her condition. Provide teaching and information regarding the clinical implications of the test results, as appropriate. Educate the patient regarding access to counseling services.

> Reinforce information given by the patient's health care provider regarding further testing, treatment, or referral to another health care provider. Answer any questions or address any concerns voiced by the patient or family.

> Depending on the results of this procedure, additional testing may be performed to evaluate or monitor progression of the disease process and determine the need for a change in therapy. Evaluate test results in relation to the patient's symptoms and other tests performed.

Related laboratory tests:

> Related laboratory tests include α_1-antitrypsin/phenotyping, complete blood count, D-xylose tolerance test, fecal analysis, and sweat chloride.

FERRITIN

. . . .

SYNONYM/ACRONYM: N/A.

SPECIMEN: Serum (1 mL) collected in a red- or tiger-top tube.

REFERENCE VALUE: (Method: Immunoassay)

Age	Conventional Units	SI Units (Conventional Units × 1)
Newborn	25–200 ng/mL	25–200 µg/L
1 mo	200–600 ng/mL	200–600 µg/L
2–5 mo	50–200 ng/mL	50–200 µg/L
6 mo–15 y	7–140 ng/mL	7–140 µg/L
Adult		
Men	20–250 ng/mL	20–250 µg/L
Women younger than 40 y	10–120 ng/mL	10–120 µg/L
Women 40 y and older	12–263 ng/mL	12–263 µg/L

DESCRIPTION & RATIONALE: Ferritin, a protein manufactured in the liver, spleen, and bone marrow, consists of a protein shell, apoferritin, and an iron core. The amount of ferritin in the circulation is usually proportional to the amount of stored iron (ferritin and hemosiderin) in body tissues. Levels vary according to age and gender, but they are not affected by exogenous iron intake or subject to diurnal variations. Compared to iron and total iron-binding capacity, ferritin is a more sensitive and specific test for diagnosing iron-deficiency anemia. Iron-deficiency anemia in adults is indicated at ferritin levels less than 10 ng/mL; hemochromatosis or hemosiderosis is indicated at levels greater than 400 ng/mL. ■

INDICATIONS:
- Assist in the diagnosis of iron-deficiency anemia

- Assist in the differential diagnosis of microcytic, hypochromic anemias

- Monitor hematologic responses during pregnancy, when serum iron is usually decreased and ferritin may be decreased

- Support diagnosis of hemochromatosis or other disorders of iron metabolism and storage

RESULT

Increased in:
- Alcoholism (active abusers)
- Breast cancer
- Fasting
- Hemochromatosis
- Hemolytic anemia
- Hemosiderosis
- Hepatocellular disease (acute or chronic)
- Hodgkin's disease
- Hyperthyroidism
- Infection (acute or chronic)
- Inflammatory diseases
- Leukemias
- Oral or parenteral administration of iron
- Thalassemia

Decreased in:
- Hemodialysis
- Iron-deficiency anemia

CRITICAL VALUES: N/A

INTERFERING FACTORS:
- Drugs that may increase ferritin levels include ethanol, ferric polymaltose, iron, and oral contraceptives.

- Drugs that may decrease ferritin levels

include erythropoietin, methimazole, propylthiouracil, and thiamazole.

• Recent transfusion can elevate serum ferritin.

Nursing Implications and Procedure . . . .

Pretest:

> Inform the patient that the test is used to assist in the diagnosis of hypochromic, microcytic anemias.

> Obtain a history of the patient's complaints, including a list of known allergens (especially allergies or sensitivities to latex), and inform the appropriate health care practitioner accordingly.

> Obtain a history of the patient's hematopoietic system as well as results of previously performed laboratory tests, surgical procedures, and other diagnostic procedures. For related laboratory tests, refer to the Hematopoietic System table.

> Note any recent procedures that can interfere with test results.

> Obtain a list of the medications the patient is taking, including herbs, nutritional supplements, and nutraceuticals. The requesting health care practitioner and laboratory should be advised if the patient regularly uses these products so that their effects can be taken into consideration when reviewing results.

> Review the procedure with the patient. Inform the patient that specimen collection takes approximately 5 to 10 minutes. Address concerns about pain related to the procedure. Explain to the patient that there may be some discomfort during the venipuncture.

> There are no food, fluid, or medication restrictions, unless by medical direction.

Intratest:

> If the patient has a history of severe allergic reaction to latex, care should be taken to avoid the use of equipment containing latex.

> Instruct the patient to cooperate fully and to follow directions. Direct the patient to breathe normally and to avoid unnecessary movement.

> Observe standard precautions, and follow the general guidelines in Appendix A. Positively identify the patient, and label the appropriate tubes with the corresponding patient demographics, date, and time of collection. Perform a venipuncture; collect the specimen in a 5-mL red- or tiger-top tube.

> Remove the needle, and apply a pressure dressing over the puncture site.

> Promptly transport the specimen to the laboratory for processing and analysis.

> The results are recorded manually or in a computerized system for recall and postprocedure interpretation by the appropriate health care practitioner.

Post-test:

> Observe venipuncture site for bleeding or hematoma formation. Apply paper tape or other adhesive to hold pressure bandage in place, or replace with a plastic bandage.

> *Nutritional considerations:* Nutritional therapy may be indicated for patients with decreased ferritin values because this may indicate corresponding iron deficiency. Instruct these patients in the dietary inclusion of iron-rich foods and in the administration of iron supplements, including side effects, as appropriate.

> A written report of the examination will be sent to the requesting health care practitioner, who will discuss the results with the patient.

> Reinforce information given by the patient's health care provider regarding further testing, treatment, or referral to another health care provider. Answer any questions or

address any concerns voiced by the patient or family.

➤ Depending on the results of this procedure, additional testing may be performed to evaluate or monitor progression of the disease process and determine the need for a change in therapy. Evaluate test results in relation to the patient's symptoms and other tests performed.

➤ Related laboratory tests include bone marrow biopsy, complete blood count, erythropoietin, hematocrit, hemoglobin, iron/total iron-binding capacity, liver biopsy, platelet count, red blood cell count, red blood cell indices, red blood cell morphology and inclusions, and white blood cell count and differential.

FETAL FIBRONECTIN

SYNONYM/ACRONYM: fFN.

SPECIMEN: Swab of vaginal secretions.

REFERENCE VALUE: (Method: Immunoassay) Negative.

DESCRIPTION & RATIONALE: Fibronectin is a protein found in the vaginal secretions of pregnant women. It is first secreted early in pregnancy and is believed to help implantation of the fertilized egg to the uterus. Fibronectin is not detectable again until 22 to 34 weeks of gestation; if it is detected in vaginal secretions at this gestational age, delivery may happen prematurely. The test is a useful marker for impending membrane rupture within 7 to 14 days if the level rises to greater than 0.05 μg/mL. ▪

INDICATIONS: Investigate signs of premature labor

RESULT

Positive in: Premature labor

Negative in: N/A

CRITICAL VALUES: N/A

INTERFERING FACTORS: If signs and symptoms persist in light of negative test results, repeat testing may be necessary.

Nursing Implications and Procedure • • • • • • • • • •

Pretest:

➤ Inform the patient that the test is used to assess the risk of preterm delivery.

➤ Obtain a history of the patient's complaints, including a list of known allergens (especially allergies or sensitivities to latex), and inform the appropriate health care practitioner accordingly.

➤ Obtain a history of the patient's

reproductive system and results of previously performed laboratory tests, surgical procedures, and other diagnostic procedures. For related laboratory tests, refer to the Reproductive System table.

➤ Ensure that the patient knows the symptoms of premature labor, which include uterine contractions (with or without pain) lasting 20 seconds or longer or increasing in frequency, menstrual-like cramping (intermittent or continuous), pelvic pressure, lower back pain that does not dissipate with a change in position, persistent diarrhea, intestinal cramps, changes in vaginal discharge, or a feeling that something is wrong.

➤ The health care practitioner should be informed if contractions occur more frequently than 4 times per hour.

➤ Obtain a list of the medications the patient is taking, including herbs, nutritional supplements, and nutraceuticals. The requesting health care practitioner and laboratory should be advised if the patient regularly uses these products so that their effects can be taken into consideration when reviewing results.

➤ Review the procedure with the patient. Inform the patient that specimen collection takes approximately 5 to 10 minutes and will be performed by a health care practitioner specializing in this branch of medicine. Address concerns about pain related to the procedure. Explain to the patient that there should be minimal to no discomfort during the procedure.

➤ *Sensitivity to social and cultural issues,* as well as concern for modesty, is important in providing psychological support before, during, and after the procedure.

➤ There are no food, fluid, or medication restrictions, unless by medical direction.

Intratest:

➤ If the patient has a history of severe allergic reaction to latex, care should be taken to avoid the use of equipment containing latex.

➤ Instruct the patient to cooperate fully and to follow directions. Direct the patient to breathe normally and to avoid unnecessary movement.

➤ Observe standard precautions, and follow the general guidelines in Appendix A. Positively identify the patient, and label the appropriate collection container with the corresponding patient demographics, date, and time of collection.

➤ Position the patient on the gynecologic examination table with the feet up in stirrups. Drape the patient's legs to provide privacy and to reduce chilling. Collect a small amount of vaginal secretion using a special swab from a fetal fibronectin kit.

➤ Promptly transport the specimen to the laboratory for processing and analysis.

➤ The results are recorded manually or in a computerized system for recall and postprocedure interpretation by the appropriate health care practitioner.

Post-test:

➤ A written report of the examination will be sent to the requesting health care practitioner, who will discuss the results with the patient.

➤ Recognize anxiety related to test results. Discuss the implications of abnormal test results on the patient's lifestyle. Provide teaching and information regarding the clinical implications of the test results, as appropriate. Educate the patient regarding access to counseling services.

➤ Reinforce information given by the patient's health care provider regarding further testing, treatment, or referral to another health care provider. Explain the possible causes and increased risks associated with premature labor and delivery. Reinforce education on signs and symptoms of labor, as appropriate. Inform the patient that hospitalization or more frequent prenatal checks may be ordered. Other therapies may also be administered, such as antibiotics, corticosteroids, and intravenous tocolytics. Instruct the patient in the importance of completing the entire course of antibiotic therapy, if ordered, even if no symptoms are present. Answer any questions or address any concerns voiced by the patient or family.

➤ Depending on the results of this procedure, additional testing may be performed to evaluate or monitor progression of the disease process and determine the need for a change in therapy. Evaluate test results in relation to the patient's symptoms and other tests performed.

Related laboratory tests:

➤ Related laboratory tests include amniotic fluid analysis, chorionic villus biopsy, chromosome analysis, estradiol, α₁-fetoprotein, human chorionic gonadotropin, and lecithin/sphingomyelin ratio.

α₁-FETOPROTEIN

SYNONYM/ACRONYM: AFP.

SPECIMEN: Serum (1 mL for tumor marker in men and nonpregnant women; 3 mL for maternal triple-marker testing), collected in a red- or tiger-top tube. For maternal triple-marker testing, include human chorionic gonadotropin and free estriol measurement.

REFERENCE VALUE: (Method: Immunoassay for tumor marker, radioimmunoassay for maternal triple-marker testing)

Tumor Marker, Men and Women

AFP	
Fetus, first-trimester peak	200–400 mg/dL
Cord blood	Less than 5 mg/dL

AFP in Maternal Serum	White AFP (Median)	Black AFP (Median)	Hispanic AFP (Median)	Asian AFP (Median)
Low risk	Less than 2 MoM	Less than 2 MoM	Less than 2 MoM	Less than 2 MoM

(*Continued on the following page*)

AFP in Maternal Serum	White AFP (Median)	Black AFP (Median)	Hispanic AFP (Median)	Asian AFP (Median)
Gestational Age (wk)				
14	19.9 ng/mL	23.2 ng/mL	18.3 ng/mL	22.4 ng/mL
15	23.2 ng/mL	26.9 ng/mL	22.6 ng/mL	28.3 ng/mL
16	27.0 ng/mL	31.1 ng/mL	27.3 ng/mL	32.7 ng/mL
17	31.5 ng/mL	35.9 ng/mL	32.3 ng/mL	37.9 ng/mL
18	36.7 ng/mL	41.6 ng/mL	38.1 ng/mL	44.8 ng/mL
19	42.7 ng/mL	48.0 ng/mL	45.0 ng/mL	52.0 ng/mL
20	49.8 ng/mL	55.6 ng/mL	52.2 ng/mL	62.2 ng/mL
21	58.1 ng/mL	64.2 ng/mL	61.9 ng/mL	79.5 ng/mL
22	67.8 ng/mL	74.2 ng/mL	64.3 ng/mL	78.2 ng/mL

MoM = multiples of the median.

HCG and Estriol in Maternal Serum	HCG	Free Estriol
Gestational Age (wk)	Median Value	Median Value
14	41.5 IU/mL	0.5 ng/mL
15	36.0 IU/mL	0.7 ng/mL
16	31.0 IU/mL	0.9 ng/mL
17	27.0 IU/mL	1.1 ng/mL
18	24.0 IU/mL	1.4 ng/mL
19	21.0 IU/mL	1.8 ng/mL
20	18.0 IU/mL	2.3 ng/mL
21	16.0 IU/mL	2.8 ng/mL
22	14.0 IU/mL	3.6 ng/mL

Results vary widely from laboratory to laboratory and method to method.
HCG = human chorionic gonadotropin.

DESCRIPTION & RATIONALE: α_1-Fetoprotein (AFP) is a glycoprotein produced in the fetal liver, gastrointestinal tract, and yolk sac. AFP is the major serum protein produced for 10 weeks in early fetal life. (See "Amniotic Fluid Analysis" monograph for measurement of AFP levels in amniotic fluid.) After 10 weeks of gestation, levels of fetal AFP can be detected in maternal blood, with peak levels occurring at 16 to 18 weeks. Elevated maternal levels of AFP on two tests taken 1 week apart suggest further investigation into fetal well-being by ultrasound or amniocentesis. Human chorionic gonadotropin (HCG), a hormone secreted by the placenta, stimulates secretion of progesterone by the corpus luteum. (The use of HCG as a triple marker is also discussed in the monograph titled "Human Chorionic Gonadotropin.") During intrauterine development, the normal fetus and placenta produce estriol, a portion of which passes into maternal circulation. Decreased estriol levels are an independent indicator of neural tube defects. The incidence of neural tube defects is about 1 in 1000 births.

The presence of AFP in excessive amounts is abnormal in adults. AFP measurements are used as a tumor marker to assist in the diagnosis of cancer. ■

INDICATIONS:

* Assist in the diagnosis of primary hepatocellular carcinoma or metastatic lesions involving the liver, as indicated by highly elevated levels (30% to 50% of Americans with liver cancer do not have elevated AFP levels)

* Investigate suspected hepatitis or cirrhosis, indicated by slightly to moderately elevated levels

* Monitor response to treatment for hepatic carcinoma, with successful treatment indicated by an immediate decrease in levels

* Monitor for recurrence of hepatic carcinoma, with elevated levels occurring 1 to 6 months before the patient becomes symptomatic

* Investigate suspected intrauterine fetal death, as indicated by elevated levels

* Routine prenatal screening at 13 to 16 weeks of pregnancy for fetal neural tube defects and other disorders, as indicated by elevated levels in maternal serum and amniotic fluid

* Support diagnosis of embryonal gonadal teratoblastoma, hepatoblastoma, and testicular or ovarian carcinomas

RESULT: Maternal serum AFP test results report actual values and multiples of the median (MoM) by gestational age (in weeks). MoM are calculated by dividing the patient's AFP by the midpoint (or median) of values expected for a large population of unaffected women at the same gestational age in weeks. MoM should be corrected for maternal weight.

The MoM should also be corrected for maternal insulin requirement (achieved by dividing MoM by 1.1 for diabetic African American patients and by 0.8 for diabetic patients of other races) and multiple fetuses (multiply by 2.13 for twins). Some laboratories also provide additional statistical information regarding Down's syndrome risk.

Increased in:

* Pregnant women:
  Congenital nephrosis
  Fetal abdominal wall defects
  Fetal distress
  Fetal neural tube defects (e.g., anencephaly, spina bifida, myelomeningocele)
  Low birth weight
  Multiple pregnancy
  Polycystic kidneys
  Underestimation of gestational age

* Men or nonpregnant women:
  Cirrhosis
  Hepatic carcinoma
  Hepatitis
  Metastatic lesions involving the liver

Decreased in:

* Pregnant women:
  Down's syndrome (trisomy 21)
  Edwards' syndrome (trisomy 18)
  Fetal demise (undetected over a lengthy period of time)
  Hydatidiform moles
  Overestimation of gestational age
  Pseudopregnancy
  Spontaneous abortion

CRITICAL VALUES: N/A

INTERFERING FACTORS:

* Drugs that may decrease AFP levels in pregnant women include acetaminophen, acetylsalicylic acid, and phenacetin.

* Recent radioactive scans or radiation

within 1 week before the test can interfere with test results when radioimmunoassay is the test method.

- Multiple fetuses can cause increased levels.

- Gestational age must be between 15 and 22 weeks for initial and follow-up testing. The most common cause of an abnormal MoM is inaccurate estimation of gestational age (defined as weeks from the first day of the last menstrual period).

- Maternal AFP levels vary by race.

Nursing Implications and Procedure . . . .

Pretest:

▶ Inform the patient that the test is primarily used to screen for neural tube defects.

▶ Obtain a history of the patient's complaints and known or suspected malignancy. Obtain a list of known allergens, especially allergies or sensitivities to latex, and inform the appropriate health care practitioner accordingly.

▶ Obtain a history of the patient's immune and reproductive systems, gestational age, and results of previously performed laboratory tests, surgical procedures, and other diagnostic procedures. For related laboratory tests, refer to the Immune and Reproductive System tables.

▶ Note any recent procedures that can interfere with test results.

▶ Provide required information to laboratory for triple-marker testing, including maternal birth date, weight, age, race, calculated gestational age, gestational age by ultrasound, gestational date by physical examination, first day of last menstrual period, estimated date of delivery, and whether the patient has insulin-dependent (type 1) diabetes.

▶ Obtain a list of the medications the

patient is taking, including herbs, nutritional supplements, and nutraceuticals. The requesting health care practitioner and laboratory should be advised if the patient is regularly using these products so that their effects can be taken into consideration when reviewing results.

▶ Review the procedure with the patient. Inform the patient that specimen collection takes approximately 5 to 10 minutes. Address concerns about pain related to the procedure. Explain to the patient that there may be some discomfort during the venipuncture.

▶ There are no food, fluid, or medication restrictions, unless by medical direction.

▶ *Make sure a written and informed consent has been signed prior to the procedure and before administering any medications.*

Intratest:

▶ If the patient has a history of severe allergic reaction to latex, care should be taken to avoid the use of equipment containing latex.

▶ Instruct the patient to cooperate fully and to follow directions. Direct the patient to breathe normally and to avoid unnecessary movement.

▶ Observe standard precautions, and follow the general guidelines in Appendix A. Positively identify the patient, and label the appropriate tubes with the corresponding patient demographics, date, and time of collection. Perform a venipuncture; collect the specimen in a 5-mL red-top tube.

▶ The sample may be collected directly from the cord using a syringe and transferred to a red-top tube.

▶ Remove the needle, and apply a pressure dressing over the puncture site.

▶ Promptly transport the specimen to the laboratory for processing and analysis.

▶ The results are recorded manually or in a computerized system for recall and postprocedure interpretation by the appropriate health care practitioner.

Post-test:

> Observe venipuncture site for bleeding or hematoma formation. Apply paper tape or other adhesive to hold pressure bandage in place, or replace with a plastic bandage.

> *Nutritional considerations:* Hyperhomocysteinemia resulting from folate deficiency in pregnant women is believed to increase the risk of neural tube defects. Elevated levels of homocysteine are thought to chemically damage the exposed neural tissue of the developing fetus. As appropriate, instruct pregnant women to eat foods rich in folate, such as liver, salmon, eggs, asparagus, green leafy vegetables, broccoli, sweet potatoes, beans, and whole wheat.

> A written report of the examination will be sent to the requesting health care practitioner, who will discuss the results with the patient.

> *Social and cultural considerations:* In pregnant patients, recognize anxiety related to test results, and encourage the family to seek counseling if concerned with pregnancy termination or to seek genetic counseling if a chromosomal abnormality is determined. Discuss the implications of abnormal test results on the patient's lifestyle. Provide teaching and information regarding the clinical implications of the test results, as appropriate. Decisions regarding elective abortion should take place in the presence of both parents. Provide a nonjudgmental, nonthreatening atmosphere for discussing the risks and difficulties of delivering and raising a developmentally challenged infant, as well as exploring other options (termination of pregnancy or adoption). It is also important to discuss feelings the mother and father may experience (e.g., guilt, depression, anger) if fetal abnormalities are detected. Educate the patient regarding access to counseling services.

> In patients with carcinoma, recognize anxiety related to test results, and offer support. Discuss the implications of abnormal test results on the patient's lifestyle. Provide teaching and information regarding the clinical implications of the test results, as appropriate. Educate the patient regarding access to counseling services, as appropriate.

> Reinforce information given by the patient's health care provider regarding further testing, treatment, or referral to another health care provider. Answer any questions or address any concerns voiced by the patient or family.

> Depending on the results of this procedure, additional testing may be performed to evaluate or monitor progression of the disease process and determine the need for a change in therapy. Inform the pregnant patient that an ultrasound may be performed and AFP levels in amniotic fluid may be analyzed if maternal blood levels are elevated in two samples obtained 1 week apart. Evaluate test results in relation to the patient's symptoms and other tests performed.

Related laboratory tests:

> Related laboratory tests include amniotic fluid analysis, chorionic villus biopsy, carcinoembryonic antigen, estradiol, fetal fibronectin, folic acid, hexosamidase, homocysteine, human chorionic gonadotropin, and lecithin/sphingomyelin ratio.

FIBRIN DEGRADATION PRODUCTS

SYNONYMS/ACRONYMS: Fibrin split products, fibrin breakdown products, FDP, FSP, FBP.

SPECIMEN: Plasma (1 mL) collected in special blue-top tube containing thrombin and a protease inhibitor.

REFERENCE VALUE: (Method: Latex agglutination)

Conventional Units	SI Units (Conventional Units × 1)
Less than 10 µg/mL	Less than 10 mg/dL

DESCRIPTION & RATIONALE: This coagulation test evaluates fibrin split products or fibrin/fibrinogen degradation products that interfere with normal coagulation and formation of the hemostatic platelet plug. After a fibrin clot has formed, the fibrinolytic system prevents excessive clotting. In the fibrinolytic system, plasmin digests fibrin. Fibrinogen also can be degraded if there is a disproportion among plasmin, fibrin, and fibrinogen. Seven substances labeled *A, B, C, D, E, X,* and *Y* result from this degradation, which can indicate abnormal coagulation. Under normal conditions, the liver and reticuloendothelial system remove fibrin split products from the circulation. ■

INDICATIONS:
• Assist in the diagnosis of suspected disseminated intravascular coagulation (DIC)

• Evaluate response to therapy with fibrinolytic drugs

• Monitor the effects on hemostasis of trauma, extensive surgery, obstetric complications, and disorders such as liver or renal disease

RESULT

Increased in:
• DIC

• Excessive bleeding

• Liver disease

• Myocardial infarction

• Obstetric complications, such as pre-eclampsia, abruptio placentae, intrauterine fetal death

• Post–cardiothoracic surgery period

• Pulmonary embolism

• Renal disease

• Renal transplant rejection

CRITICAL VALUES:

Greater than 40 µg/mL.

Note and immediately report to the health care practitioner any critically increased values and related symptoms.

INTERFERING FACTORS:

- Traumatic venipunctures and excessive agitation of the sample can alter test results.

- Drugs that may increase fibrin degradation product levels include heparin and fibrinolytic drugs such as streptokinase and urokinase.

- The presence of rheumatoid factor may falsely elevate results with some test kits.

- The test should not be ordered on patients receiving heparin therapy.

Nursing Implications and Procedure ● ● ● ● ● ● ● ● ● ● ●

Pretest:

▶ Inform the patient that the test is used to evaluate conditions associated with abnormal fibrinolytic and fibrinogenolytic activity, such as DIC, deep vein thrombosis, and pulmonary embolism.

▶ Obtain a history of the patient's complaints, including a list of known allergens (especially allergies or sensitivities to latex), and inform the appropriate health care practitioner accordingly.

▶ Obtain a history of the patient's cardiovascular and hematopoietic systems, any bleeding disorders, and results of previously performed laboratory tests (especially bleeding time, clotting time, complete blood count, D-dimer, partial thromboplastin time, platelets, and prothrombin time), surgical procedures, and other diagnostic procedures. For related laboratory tests, refer to the Cardiovascular and Hematopoietic System tables.

▶ Note any recent procedures that can interfere with test results.

▶ Obtain a list of medications the patient takes, including anticoagulant therapy, acetylsalicylic acid, herbs, nutritional supplements, and nutraceuticals, especially those known to affect coagulation. It is recommended that use of these products be discontinued 14 days before dental or surgical procedures. The requesting health care practitioner and laboratory should be advised if the patient regularly uses these products so that their effects can be taken into consideration when reviewing results.

▶ Review the procedure with the patient. Inform the patient that specimen collection takes approximately 5 to 10 minutes. Address concerns about pain related to the procedure. Explain to the patient that there may be some discomfort during the venipuncture.

▶ *Sensitivity to social and cultural issues,* as well as concern for modesty, is important in providing psychological support before, during, and after the procedure.

▶ There are no food, fluid, or medication restrictions, unless by medical direction.

Intratest:

▶ If the patient has a history of severe allergic reaction to latex, care should be taken to avoid the use of equipment containing latex.

▶ Instruct the patient to cooperate fully and to follow directions. Direct the patient to breathe normally and to avoid unnecessary movement.

▶ Observe standard precautions, and follow the general guidelines in Appendix A. Positively identify the patient, and label the appropriate tubes with the corresponding patient demographics, date, and time of collection. Perform a venipuncture; collect the specimen in a special blue-top tube.

▶ Remove the needle, and apply a pressure dressing over the puncture site.

▶ Promptly transport the specimen to

the laboratory for processing and analysis.

➤ The results are recorded manually or in a computerized system for recall and postprocedure interpretation by the appropriate health care practitioner.

Post-test:

➤ Observe venipuncture site for bleeding or hematoma formation. Apply paper tape or other adhesive to hold pressure bandage in place, or replace with a plastic bandage.

➤ Instruct the patient to report bleeding from skin or mucous membranes, ecchymosis, petechiae, hematuria and occult blood.

➤ Inform the patient with increased levels of fibrin degradation products of the importance of taking precautions against bruising and bleeding, including the use of a soft bristle toothbrush, use of an electric razor, avoidance of constipation, avoidance of acetylsalicylic acid and similar products, and avoidance of intramuscular injections.

➤ A written report of the examination will be sent to the requesting health care practitioner, who will discuss the results with the patient.

➤ Reinforce information given by the patient's health care provider regarding further testing, treatment, or referral to another health care provider. Answer any questions or address any concerns voiced by the patient or family.

➤ Depending on the results of this procedure, additional testing may be performed to evaluate or monitor progression of the disease process and determine the need for a change in therapy. Evaluate test results in relation to the patient's symptoms and other tests performed.

Related laboratory tests:

➤ Related laboratory tests include activated partial thromboplastin time, aspartate alanino aminotransbilirubin, BUN creatinine, complete blood count, D-dimer, fibrinogen, plasminogen, and platelet count.

FIBRINOGEN

SYNONYM/**A**CRONYM: Factor I.

SPECIMEN: Plasma (1 mL) collected in blue-top (sodium citrate) tube.

REFERENCE **VALUE:** (Method: Photo-optical clot detection)

Age	Conventional Units	SI Units (Conventional Units × 0.01)
Newborn	125–300 mg/dL	1.25–3.00 g/L
Adult	200–400 mg/dL	2.00–4.00 g/L

DESCRIPTION & RATIONALE: Fibrinogen (factor I) is synthesized in the liver. In the common final pathway of the coagulation sequence, thrombin converts fibrinogen to fibrin, which then clots blood as it combines with platelets. In normal, healthy individuals, the serum should contain no residual fibrinogen after clotting has occurred. ∎

INDICATIONS:
- Assist in the diagnosis of suspected disseminated intravascular coagulation (DIC), as indicated by decreased fibrinogen levels

- Evaluate congenital or acquired dysfibrinogenemias

- Monitor hemostasis in disorders associated with low fibrinogen levels or elevated levels that can predispose patients to excessive thrombosis

RESULT

Increased in:
- Acute myocardial infarction
- Cancer
- Eclampsia
- Hodgkin's disease
- Inflammation
- Multiple myeloma
- Nephrotic syndrome
- Pregnancy
- Tissue necrosis

Decreased in:
- Congenital fibrinogen deficiency (rare)
- DIC
- Dysfibrinogenemia
- Liver disease (severe)
- Primary fibrinolysis

CRITICAL VALUE:
Less than 80 mg/dL.

Note and immediately report to the health care practitioner any critically decreased values and related symptoms. Signs and symptoms of microvascular thrombosis include cyanosis, ischemic tissue necrosis, hemorrhagic necrosis, tachypnea, dyspnea, pulmonary emboli, venous distention, abdominal pain, and oliguria. Possible interventions include identification and treatment of the underlying cause, support through administration of required blood products (platelets, cryoprecipitate, or fresh frozen plasma), and administration of heparin.

INTERFERING FACTORS:
- Drugs that may increase fibrinogen levels include acetylsalicylic acid, norethandrolone, oral contraceptives, oxandrolone, and oxymetholone.

- Drugs that may decrease fibrinogen levels include anabolic steroids, asparaginase, bezafibrate, danazol, dextran, fenofibrate, fish oils, gemfibrozil, lovastatin, pentoxifylline, phosphorus, and ticlopidine.

- Transfusions of whole blood, plasma, or fractions within 4 weeks of the test invalidate results.

- Placement of tourniquet for longer than 1 minute can result in venous stasis and changes in the concentration of plasma proteins to be measured. Platelet activation may also occur under these conditions, causing erroneous results.

- Vascular injury during phlebotomy can activate platelets and coagulation factors, causing erroneous results.

- Hemolyzed specimens must be rejected because hemolysis is an indication of platelet and coagulation factor activation.

- Incompletely filled tubes contaminated with heparin or clotted specimens must be rejected.

- Icteric or lipemic specimens interfere with optical testing methods, producing erroneous results.

- Traumatic venipuncture and excessive agitation of the sample can alter test results.

Nursing Implications and Procedure • • • • • • • • • • •

Pretest:

➤ Inform the patient that the test is used to evaluate fibrinolytic activity as well as identify congenital deficiency and DIC.

➤ Obtain a history of the patient's complaints, including a list of known allergens (especially allergies or sensitivities to latex), and inform the appropriate health care practitioner accordingly.

➤ Obtain a history of the patient's hematopoietic and hepatobiliary systems, as well as results of previously performed laboratory tests, surgical procedures, and other diagnostic procedures. For related laboratory tests, refer to the Hematopoietic and Hepatobiliary System tables.

➤ Note any recent procedures that can interfere with test results.

➤ Obtain a list of medications the patient is taking, including herbs, nutritional supplements, and nutraceuticals. The requesting health care practitioner and laboratory should be advised if the patient regularly takes these products so that their effects can be taken into consideration when reviewing results.

➤ Review the procedure with the patient. Inform the patient that specimen collection takes approximately 5 to 10 minutes. Address concerns about pain related to the procedure. Explain to the patient that there may be some discomfort during the venipuncture.

➤ There are no food, fluid, or medication restrictions, unless by medical direction.

Intratest:

➤ If the patient has a history of severe allergic reaction to latex, care should be taken to avoid the use of equipment containing latex.

➤ Instruct the patient to cooperate fully and to follow directions. Direct the patient to breathe normally and to avoid unnecessary movement.

➤ Observe standard precautions, and follow the general guidelines in Appendix A. Positively identify the patient, and label the appropriate tubes with the corresponding patient demographics, date, and time of collection. Perform a venipuncture; collect the specimen in a 5-mL blue-top tube. Fill the tube completely. *Important note:* Two different concentrations of sodium citrate preservative are currently added to blue-top tubes for coagulation studies: 3.2% and 3.8%. The Clinical and Laboratory Standards Institute/CLSI (formerly the National Committee for Clinical Laboratory Standards/NCCLS) guideline for sodium citrate is 3.2%. Laboratories establish reference ranges for coagulation testing based on numerous factors, including sodium citrate concentration, test equipment, and test reagents. It is important to inquire from the laboratory which concentration it recommends, because each concentration will have its own specific reference range.

➤ When multiple specimens are drawn, the blue-top tube should be collected after sterile (i.e., blood culture) and nonadditive red-top tubes. When coagulation testing is the only work to be done, an extra red-top tube should be collected before the blue-top tube to avoid contaminating the specimen with tissue thromboplastin, which can falsely decrease values.

➤ Remove the needle, and apply a pressure dressing over the puncture site.

➤ Promptly transport the specimen to the laboratory for processing and analysis. The CLSI recommendation for processed and unprocessed specimens stored in unopened tubes is that testing should be completed within 1 to 4 hours of collection.

➤ The results are recorded manually or in a computerized system for recall and postprocedure interpretation by the appropriate health care practitioner.

Post-test:

➤ Observe venipuncture site for bleeding or hematoma formation. Apply paper tape or other adhesive to hold pressure bandage in place, or replace with a plastic bandage.

➤ Instruct the patient to report bruising, petechiae, and bleeding from mucous membranes, hematuria and occult blood.

➤ Inform the patient with a decreased fibrinogen level of the importance of taking precautions against bruising and bleeding, including the use of a soft bristle toothbrush, use of an electric razor, avoidance of constipation, avoidance of acetylsalicylic acid and similar products, and avoidance of intramuscular injections.

➤ A written report of the examination will be sent to the requesting health care practitioner, who will discuss the results with the patient.

➤ Reinforce information given by the patient's health care provider regarding further testing, treatment, or referral to another health care provider. Answer any questions or address any concerns voiced by the patient or family.

➤ Depending on the results of this procedure, additional testing may be performed to evaluate or monitor progression of the disease process and determine the need for a change in therapy. Evaluate test results in relation to the patient's symptoms and other tests performed.

Related laboratory tests:

➤ Related laboratory tests include activated partial thromboplastin time, alanine aminotransferase, albumin, alkaline phosphatase, aspartate aminotransferase, bilirubin, clot retraction, D-dimer, erythrocyte sedimentation rate, fibrin degradation products, γ-glutamyl transpeptidase, liver biopsy, plasminogen, and prothrombin time.

FLUORESCEIN ANGIOGRAPHY

• •

SYNONYM/ACRONYM: FA.

AREA OF APPLICATION: Eyes.

CONTRAST: Fluorescein dye.

DESCRIPTION & RATIONALE: This test involves the color radiographic examination of the retinal vasculature following a rapid injection of a contrast medium known as sodium fluoroscein. A special fundus camera is used that allows for images to be taken in sequence and manipulated by a computer to provide views of abnormalities of the retinal vessels during filling and emptying of the dye. The camera allows only light waves at 490 nm in the blue range to strike the fundus of the eye. When the fluorescein dye is injected into the eye, the blue light excites the dye molecules to a higher state of activity and causes them to emit a greenish-yellow fluoresence that is recorded. ∎

INDICATIONS:
- Detect arterial or venous occlusion evidenced by the reduced, delayed, or absent flow of the contrast medium through the vessels or possible vessel leakage of the medium
- Detect possible vascular disorders affecting visual acuity
- Detect presence of microaneurysms caused by hypertensive retinopathy
- Detect the presence of tumors, retinal edema, or inflammation, as evidenced by abnormal patterns of degree of fluorescence
- Diagnose diabetic retinopathy
- Diagnose past reduced flow or patency of the vascular circulation of the retina, as evidenced by neovascularization
- Diagnose presence of macular degeneration and any other degeneration and any associated hemorrhaging
- Observe ocular effects resulting from the long-term use of high-risk medications

RESULT

Normal Findings:
- No leakage of dye from retinal blood vessels
- Normal retina and retinal and choroidal vessels
- No evidence of vascular abnormalities, such as hemorrhage, retinopathy, aneurysms, or obstructions caused by stenosis and resulting in collateral circulation

Abnormal Findings:
- Aneurysm
- Arteriovenous shunts
- Diabetic retinopathy
- Macular degeneration
- Neovascularization
- Obstructive disorders of the arteries or veins that lead to collateral circulation

CRITICAL VALUES: N/A

INTERFERING FACTORS:

This procedure is contraindicated for:
- Patients with a past history of hypersensitivity to radiographic dyes
- Patients with narrow-angle glaucoma if pupil dilation is performed as dilation can initiate a severe and sight-threatening open-angle attack
- Patients with allergies to mydriatics if pupil dilation using mydriatics is performed

Factors that may impair the results of the examination:
- Inability of the patient to cooperate or remain still during the test because of age, significant pain, or mental status may interfere with the test results.
- Presence of cataracts may interfere with fundal view.
- Ineffective dilation of the pupils may impair clear imaging.
- Allergic reaction to radiographic dye, including nausea and vomiting.
- Failure to follow medication restrictions before the procedure may cause the procedure to be canceled or repeated.

Nursing Implications and Procedure • • • • • • • • • • •

➤ Inform the patient that the test detects possible vascular disorders of the eye.

➤ Obtain a history of the patient's complaints, including a list of known allergens, especially allergies or sensitivities to radiographic dyes, shellfish, and bee venom.

➤ Obtain a history of the patient's known or suspected vision loss, changes in visual acuity, including type and cause; use of glasses or contact lenses; eye conditions with treatment regimens; eye surgery; and other tests and procedures to assess and diagnose visual deficit.

➤ Obtain a history of results of previously performed laboratory tests, surgical procedures, and other diagnostic procedures.

➤ Obtain a list of the medications the patient is taking, including herbs, nutritional supplements, and nutraceuticals. The requesting health care practitioner should be advised if the patient regularly uses these products so that their effects can be taken into consideration when reviewing results.

➤ Instruct the patient to remove contact lenses or glasses, as appropriate. Instruct the patient regarding the importance of keeping the eyes open for the test.

➤ Review the procedure with the patient. Explain that the patient will be requested to fixate the eyes during the procedure. Address concerns about pain related to the procedure. Explain to the patient that mydriatics, if used, may cause blurred vision and sensitivity to light. There may also be a brief stinging sensation when the drop is put in the eye. Explain to the patient that some discomfort may be experienced during the insertion of the intermittent infusion device. Inform the patient that, when fluoresecein dye is injected, it may

cause facial flushing or nausea and vomiting. Inform the patient that a technician, optometrist, or health care practitioner performs the test, in a quiet, darkened room, and that to dilate and evaluate both eyes, the test can take up 60 minutes.

➤ Explain that an intravenous (IV) line may be inserted to allow infusion of dye.

➤ There are no food or fluid restrictions, unless by medical direction.

➤ The patient should avoid eye medications (particularly mydriatic eye drops if the patient has glaucoma) for at least 1 day prior to the test.

➤ Ensure that the patient understands that he or she must refrain from driving until the pupils return to normal (about 4 hours) after the test and has made arrangements to have someone else be responsible for transportation after the test.

➤ *Make sure a written and informed consent has been signed prior to the procedure and before administering any medications.*

➤ Ensure that the patient has complied with medication restrictions; assure that eye medications, especially mydriatics, have been withheld for at least 1 day prior to the test.

➤ Have emergency equipment readily available.

➤ Instruct the patient to cooperate fully and to follow directions. Ask the patient to remain still during the procedure because movement produces unreliable results.

➤ Seat the patient in a chair that faces the camera. Instruct the patient to look at directed target while the eyes are examined.

➤ If dilation is to be performed, administer the ordered mydriatic to each eye and repeat in 5 to 15 minutes. Drops are placed in the eye with the patient looking up and the solution directed at the six o'clock position of the sclera (white of the eye) near the limbus (grey, semitransparent area of the eyeball where the cornea and sclera meet). The dropper bottle should not touch the eyelashes.

➤ Insert an intermittent infusion device, as ordered, for subsequent injection of the contrast media or emergency medications.

➤ After the eyedrops are administered but before the dye is injected, color photographs are taken.

➤ Ask the patient to place the chin in the chin rest and gently press the forehead against the support bar. Ask the patient to open his or her eyes wide and look at the desired target.

➤ Fluorescein dye is then injected into the brachial vein using the intermittent infusion device, and a rapid sequence of photographs are taken and repeated after the dye has reached the retinal vascular system. Follow-up photographs are taken in 20 to 30 minutes.

➤ At the conclusion of the procedure, the IV needle is removed, and an adhesive strip is applied to the site.

➤ Observe for hypersensitive reaction to the dye. The patient may become nauseous and vomit.

➤ The results are recorded on developed color film or electronically on computerized equipment for recall and postprocedure interpretation by the appropriate health care practitioner.

Post-test:

➤ Instruct the patient to resume usual medications, as directed by the health care practitioner.

➤ A written report of the examination will be completed by a health care practitioner specializing in this branch of medicine. The report will be sent to the requesting health care practitioner, who will discuss the results with the patient.

➤ Recognize anxiety related to test results, and be supportive of impaired activity related to vision loss or perceived loss of driving privileges. Discuss the implications of abnormal test results on the patient's lifestyle. Provide teaching and information regarding the clinical implications of the test results, as appropriate.

➤ Reinforce information given by the patient's health care provider regarding further testing, treatment, or referral to another health care provider. Inform the patient that visual acuity and resposnses to light may change. Suggest that the patient wear dark glasses after the test until the pupils return to normal size. Inform the patient that yellow discoloration of the skin and urine from the radiographic dye is normally present for up to 2 days. Answer any questions or address any concerns voiced by the patient or family.

➤ Depending on the results of this procedure, additional testing may be performed to evaluate or monitor progression of the disease process and determine the need for a change in therapy. Evaluate test results in relation to the patient's symptoms and other tests performed.

Related diagnostic tests:

➤ Related diagnostic tests include fundus photography, gonioscopy, and visual field testing.

FOLATE

SYNONYM/ACRONYM: Folic acid.

SPECIMEN: Serum (1 mL) collected in a red- or tiger-top tube.

REFERENCE VALUE: (Method: Radioimmunoassay)

Age	Conventional Units	SI Units (Conventional Units × 2.265)
Newborn–1 y	5–21 ng/mL	11–48 nmol/L
Adult	Greater than 2.5 ng/mL	Greater than 5.7 nmol/L

DESCRIPTION & RATIONALE: Folate, a water-soluble vitamin, is produced by bacteria in the intestines and stored in small amounts in the liver. Dietary folate is absorbed through the intestinal mucosa and stored in the liver. Folate is necessary for normal red blood cell and white blood cell function, DNA replication, and cell division. Folate levels are often measured in association with serum vitamin B_{12} determinations. Hyperhomocystinemia resulting from folate deficiency in pregnant women is believed to increase the risk of neural tube defects. Elevated levels of homocysteine are thought to cause chemical damage to the exposed neural tissue of the developing fetus. ■

INDICATIONS:
- Assist in the diagnosis of megaloblastic anemia resulting from deficient folate intake or increased folate requirements, such as in pregnancy and hemolytic anemia
- Monitor the effects of prolonged parenteral nutrition
- Monitor response to disorders that may lead to folate deficiency or decreased absorption and storage

RESULT

Increased in:
- Blind loop syndrome
- Distal small bowel disease
- Excessive dietary intake of folate or folate supplements
- Pernicious anemia
- Vitamin B_{12} deficiency

Decreased in:
- Chronic alcoholism
- Crohn's disease
- Exfoliative dermatitis
- Hemolytic anemias
- Infantile hyperthyroidism
- Liver disease

- Malnutrition
- Megaloblastic anemia
- Myelofibrosis
- Neoplasms
- Pregnancy
- Regional enteritis
- Scurvy
- Sideroblastic anemias
- Sprue
- Ulcerative colitis
- Whipple's disease

CRITICAL VALUES: N/A

INTERFERING FACTORS:

- Drugs that may decrease folate levels include aminopterin, ampicillin, antacids, anticonvulsants, barbiturates, chloramphenicol, chloroguanide, erythromycin, ethanol, glutethimide, lincomycin, metformin, methotrexate, nitrofurans, oral contraceptives, penicillin, pentamidine, phenytoin, pyrimethamine, tetracycline, and triamterene.

- Recent radioactive scans or radiation within 1 week before the test can interfere with test results when radioimmunoassay is the test method.

Nursing Implications and Procedure • • • • • • • • • • • •

Pretest:

➤ Inform the patient that the test is used to detect folate deficiency and to monitor folate therapy.

➤ Obtain a history of the patient's complaints, including a list of known allergens (especially allergies or sensitivities to latex), and inform the appropriate health care practitioner accordingly.

➤ Obtain a history of the patient's gastrointestinal and hematopoietic systems, as well as results of previously performed laboratory tests, surgical procedures, and other diagnostic procedures. For related laboratory tests, refer to the Gastrointestinal and Hematopoietic System tables.

➤ Note any recent procedures that can interfere with test results.

➤ Obtain a list of medications the patient is taking, including herbs, nutritional supplements, and nutraceuticals. The requesting health care practitioner and laboratory should be advised if the patient regularly uses these products so that their effects can be taken into consideration when reviewing results.

➤ Review the procedure with the patient. Inform the patient that specimen collection takes approximately 5 to 10 minutes. Address concerns about pain related to the procedure. Explain to the patient that there may be some discomfort during the venipuncture.

➤ There are no food, fluid, or medication restrictions, unless by medical direction.

Intratest:

➤ If the patient has a history of severe allergic reaction to latex, care should be taken to avoid the use of equipment containing latex.

➤ Instruct the patient to cooperate fully and to follow directions. Direct the patient to breathe normally and to avoid unnecessary movement.

➤ Observe standard precautions, and follow the general guidelines in Appendix A. Positively identify the patient, and label the appropriate tubes with the corresponding patient demographics, date, and time of collection. Perform a venipuncture; collect the specimen in a 5-mL red- or tiger-top tube. Protect the specimen from light.

➤ Remove the needle, and apply a pressure dressing over the puncture site.

➤ Promptly transport the specimen to

the laboratory for processing and analysis.

➤ The results are recorded manually or in a computerized system for recall and postprocedure interpretation by the appropriate health care practitioner.

Post-test:

➤ Observe venipuncture site for bleeding or hematoma formation. Apply paper tape or other adhesive to hold pressure bandage in place, or replace with a plastic bandage.

➤ *Nutritional considerations:* Instruct the folate-deficient patient (especially pregnant women), as appropriate, to eat foods rich in folate, such as liver, salmon, eggs, asparagus, green leafy vegetables, broccoli, sweet potatoes, beans, and whole wheat.

➤ A written report of the examination will be sent to the requesting health care practitioner, who will discuss the results with the patient.

➤ Reinforce information given by the patient's health care provider regarding further testing, treatment, or referral to another health care provider. Answer any questions or address any concerns voiced by the patient or family.

➤ Depending on the results of this procedure, additional testing may be performed to evaluate or monitor progression of the disease process and determine the need for a change in therapy. Evaluate test results in relation to the patient's symptoms and other tests performed.

Related laboratory tests:

➤ Related laboratory tests include complete blood count, homocysteine, and vitamin B_{12}.

FOLLICLE-STIMULATING HORMONE

SYNONYM/ACRONYM: Follitropin, FSH.

SPECIMEN: Serum (1 mL) collected in a red- or tiger-top tube.

REFERENCE VALUE: (Method: Immunoassay)

Status	Conventional Units	SI Units (Conventional Units × 1)
Prepuberty	Less than 10 mIU/mL	Less than 10 IU/L
Men	1.4–15.5 mIU/mL	1.4–15.5 IU/L
Women		
Follicular phase	1.4–9.9 mIU/mL	1.4–9.9 IU/L
Ovulatory peak	6.2–17.2 mIU/mL	6.2–17.2 IU/L
Luteal phase	1.1–9.2 mIU/mL	1.1–9.2 IU/L
Postmenopause	19–100 mIU/mL	19–100 IU/L

DESCRIPTION & RATIONALE: Follicle-stimulating hormone (FSH) is produced and stored in the anterior portion of the pituitary gland. In women, FSH promotes maturation of the graafian (germinal) follicle, causing estrogen secretion and allowing the ovum to mature. In men, FSH partially controls spermatogenesis, but the presence of testosterone is also necessary. Gonadotropin-releasing hormone secretion is stimulated by a decrease in estrogen and testosterone levels. Gonadotropin-releasing hormone secretion stimulates FSH secretion. FSH production is inhibited by an increase in estrogen and testosterone levels. FSH production is pulsatile, episodic, and cyclic, and is subject to diurnal variation. Serial measurement is often required. ■

INDICATIONS:
- Assist in distinguishing between primary and secondary (pituitary or hypothalamic) gonadal failure
- Define menstrual cycle phases as a part of infertility testing
- Evaluate ambiguous sexual differentiation in infants
- Evaluate early sexual development in girls younger than age 9 or boys younger than age 10 (precocious puberty associated with elevated levels)
- Evaluate failure of sexual maturation in adolescence
- Evaluate testicular dysfunction
- Investigate impotence, gynecomastia, and menstrual disturbances

RESULT

Increased in:
- Alcoholism
- Castration
- Gonadal failure
- Gonadotropin-secreting pituitary tumors
- Klinefelter's syndrome
- Menopause
- Orchitis
- Precocious puberty in children
- Primary hypogonadism
- Reifenstein's syndrome
- Turner's syndrome

Decreased in:
- Anorexia nervosa
- Anterior pituitary hypofunction
- Hemochromatosis
- Hyperprolactinemia
- Hypothalamic disorders
- Polycystic ovary disease
- Pregnancy
- Sickle cell anemia

CRITICAL VALUES: N/A

INTERFERING FACTORS:
- Drugs that may increase FSH levels include cimetidine, clomiphene, digitalis, gonadotropin-releasing hormone, ketoconazole, levodopa, nafarelin, naloxone, nilutamide, oxcarbazepine, and pravastatin.
- Drugs that may decrease FSH levels include anabolic steroids, anticonvulsants, buserelin, estrogens, corticotropin-releasing hormone, goserelin, megestrol, mestranol, oral contraceptives, phenothiazine, pimozide, pravastatin, progesterone, stanozolol, tamoxifen, toremifene, and valproic acid.
- In menstruating women, values vary in relation to the phase of the menstrual cycle. Values are higher in postmenopausal women.

Nursing Implications and Procedure • • • • • • • • • • •

➤ Inform the patient that the test is used to distinguish primary causes of gonadal failure from secondary causes, evaluate menstrual disturbances, and assist in infertility evaluations.

➤ Obtain a history of the patient's complaints, including a list of known allergens (especially allergies or sensitivities to latex), and inform the appropriate health care practitioner accordingly.

➤ Obtain a history of the patient's endocrine and reproductive systems, as well as phase of menstrual cycle and results of previously performed laboratory tests, surgical procedures, and other diagnostic procedures. For related laboratory tests, refer to the Endocrine and Reproductive System tables.

➤ Obtain a list of medications the patient is taking, including herbs, nutritional supplements, and nutraceuticals. The requesting health care practitioner and laboratory should be advised if the patient regularly uses these products so that their effects can be taken into consideration when reviewing results.

➤ Review the procedure with the patient. Inform the patient that specimen collection takes approximately 5 to 10 minutes. Address concerns about pain related to the procedure. Explain to the patient that there may be some discomfort during the venipuncture.

➤ There are no food, fluid, or medication restrictions, unless by medical direction.

➤ If the patient has a history of severe allergic reaction to latex, care should be taken to avoid the use of equipment containing latex.

➤ Instruct the patient to cooperate fully and to follow directions. Direct the patient to breathe normally and to avoid unnecessary movement.

➤ Observe standard precautions, and follow the general guidelines in Appendix A. Positively identify the patient, and label the appropriate tubes with the corresponding patient demographics, date, and time of collection. Perform a venipuncture; collect the specimen in a 5-mL red- or tigertop tube.

➤ Remove the needle, and apply a pressure dressing over the puncture site.

➤ Promptly transport the specimen to the laboratory for processing and analysis.

➤ The results are recorded manually or in a computerized system for recall and postprocedure interpretation by the appropriate health care practitioner.

➤ Observe venipuncture site for bleeding or hematoma formation. Apply paper tape or other adhesive to hold pressure bandage in place, or replace with a plastic bandage.

➤ A written report of the examination will be sent to the requesting health care practitioner, who will discuss the results with the patient.

➤ *Social and cultural considerations:* Recognize anxiety related to test results and provide a supportive, nonjudgmental environment when assisting a patient through the process of fertility testing. Discuss the implications of abnormal test results on the patient's lifestyle. Provide teaching and information regarding the clinical implications of the test results, as appropriate. Educate the patient and partner regarding access to counseling services, as appropriate.

➤ Reinforce information given by the patient's health care provider regarding further testing, treatment, or referral to another health care provider. Inform the patient that multiple specimens may be required. Answer any questions or address any concerns voiced by the patient or family.

➤ Depending on the results of this procedure, additional testing may be performed to evaluate or monitor progression of the disease process and determine the need for a change in therapy. Evaluate test results in relation to the patient's symptoms and other tests performed.

Related laboratory tests:

➤ Related laboratory tests include estradiol, luteinizing hormone, prolactin, and testosterone.

FRUCTOSAMINE

SYNONYM/ACRONYM: Glycated albumin.

SPECIMEN: Serum (1 mL) collected in a red- or tiger-top tube.

REFERENCE VALUE: (Method: Spectrophotometry)

Status	Conventional Units	SI Units (Conventional Units × 0.01)
Normal	174–286 μmol/L	1.74–2.86 mmol/L
Diabetic		
Controlled	210–421 μmol/L	2.10–4.21 mmol/L
Uncontrolled	268–870 μmol/L	2.68–8.70 mmol/L

DESCRIPTION & RATIONALE: Fructosamine is the result of a covalent linkage between glucose and albumin or other proteins. Similar to glycated hemoglobin, fructosamine can be used to monitor long-term control of glucose in diabetics. It has a shorter half-life than glycated hemoglobin and is thought to be more sensitive to short-term fluctuations in glucose concentrations. Some glycated hemoglobin methods are affected by hemoglobin variants. Fructosamine is not subject to this interference. ∎

INDICATIONS: Evaluate diabetic control

RESULT

Increased in: Diabetic patients with poor glucose control

Decreased in: Severe hypoproteinemia

CRITICAL VALUES: N/A

INTERFERING FACTORS:
• Drugs that may increase fructosamine levels include bendroflumethiazide and captopril.

- Drugs that may decrease fructosamine levels include ascorbic acid, pyridoxine, and terazosin.

- Decreased albumin levels may result in falsely decreased fructosamine levels.

Nursing Implications and Procedure . . . .

Pretest:

➤ Inform the patient that the test is used to evaluate diabetic control.

➤ Obtain a history of the patient's complaints, especially related to diabetic control. Obtain a list of known allergens, especially allergies or sensitivities to latex, and inform the appropriate health care practitioner accordingly.

➤ Obtain a history of the patient's endocrine and gastrointestinal systems, as well as results of previously performed laboratory tests, surgical procedures, and other diagnostic procedures. For related laboratory tests, refer to the Endocrine and Gastrointestinal System tables.

➤ Obtain a list of medications the patient is taking, including herbs, nutritional supplements, and nutraceuticals. The requesting health care practitioner and laboratory should be advised if the patient regularly uses these products so that their effects can be taken into consideration when reviewing results.

➤ Review the procedure with the patient. Inform the patient that specimen collection takes approximately 5 to 10 minutes. Address concerns about pain related to the procedure. Explain to the patient that there may be some discomfort during the venipuncture.

➤ There are no food, fluid, or medication restrictions, unless by medical direction.

Intratest:

➤ If the patient has a history of severe allergic reaction to latex, care should be taken to avoid the use of equipment containing latex.

➤ Instruct the patient to cooperate fully and to follow directions. Direct the patient to breathe normally and to avoid unnecessary movement.

➤ Observe standard precautions, and follow the general guidelines in Appendix A. Positively identify the patient, and label the appropriate tubes with the corresponding patient demographics, date, and time of collection. Perform a venipuncture; collect the specimen in a 5-mL red- or tiger-top tube.

➤ Remove the needle, and apply a pressure dressing over the puncture site.

➤ Promptly transport the specimen to the laboratory for processing and analysis.

➤ The results are recorded manually or in a computerized system for recall and postprocedure interpretation by the appropriate health care practitioner.

Post-test:

➤ Observe venipuncture site for bleeding or hematoma formation. Apply paper tape or other adhesive to hold pressure bandage in place, or replace with a plastic bandage.

➤ *Nutritional considerations:* Abnormal fructosamine levels may be associated with conditions resulting from poor glucose control. Instruct the diabetic patient, as appropriate, in nutritional management of the disease. Patients who adhere to dietary recommendations report a better general feeling of health, better weight management, greater control of glucose and lipid values, and improved use of insulin. There is no "diabetic diet"; however, many meal-planning approaches with nutritional goals are endorsed by the American Dietetic Association. The nutritional needs of each diabetic patient must be determined individually with the appropriate health care professionals, particularly professionals trained in nutrition.

➤ Instruct the patient and caregiver to report signs and symptoms of hypoglycemia (weakness, confusion, diaphoresis, rapid pulse) or hyperglycemia (thirst, polyuria, hunger, lethargy).

➤ A written report of the examination will be sent to the requesting health care practitioner, who will discuss the results with the patient.

➤ Recognize anxiety related to test results, and be supportive of impaired activity related to perceived loss of independence and fear of shortened life expectancy. Discuss the implications of abnormal test results on the patient's lifestyle. Provide teaching and information regarding the clinical implications of the test results, as appropriate. Emphasize, as appropriate, that good control of glucose levels delays the onset and slows the progression of diabetic retinopathy, nephropathy, and neuropathy. Educate the patient regarding access to counseling services. Provide contact information, if desired, for the American Diabetes Association *(http://www.diabetes.org)*.

➤ Reinforce information given by the patient's health care provider regarding further testing, treatment, or referral to another health care provider. Answer any questions or address any concerns voiced by the patient or family.

➤ Depending on the results of this procedure, additional testing may be performed to evaluate or monitor progression of the disease process and determine the need for a change in therapy. Evaluate test results in relation to the patient's symptoms and other tests performed.

Related laboratory tests:

➤ Related laboratory tests include cortisol, C-peptide, glucose, glucose tolerance test, glycated hemoglobin A_{1C}, insulin, insulin antibodies, ketones, and microalbumin.

FUNDUS PHOTOGRAPHY

. . . .

SYNONYMS/ACRONYMS: N/A.

AREA OF APPLICATION: Eyes.

CONTRAST: N/A.

DESCRIPTION & RATIONALE: This test involves the photographic examination of the structures of the eye to document the condition of the eye, detect abnormalities, and assist in following the progress of treatment. ■

INDICATIONS:

• Detect the presence of choroidal nevus

• Detect various types and stages of glaucoma

• Document the presence of diabetic retinopathy

- Document the presence of macular degeneration and any other degeneration and any associated hemorrhaging

- Observe ocular effects resulting from the long-term use of high-risk medications

RESULT

Normal Findings:
- Normal optic nerve and vessels
- No evidence of other ocular abnormalities

Abnormal Findings:
- Aneurysm
- Choroidal nevus
- Diabetic retinopathy
- Macular degeneration
- Obstructive disorders of the arteries or veins that lead to collateral circulation

CRITICAL VALUES: N/A

INTERFERING FACTORS:

This procedure is contraindicated for:
- Patients with narrow-angle glaucoma if pupil dilation is performed as dilation can initiate a severe and sight-threatening open-angle attack
- Patients with allergies to mydriatics if pupil dilation using mydriatics is performed

Factors that may impair the results of the examination:
- Inability of the patient to cooperate or remain still during the test because of age, significant pain, or mental status may interfere with the test results.
- Presence of cataracts may interfere with fundal view.
- Ineffective dilation of the pupils may impair clear imaging.
- Rubbing or squeezing the eyes may affect results.

- Failure to follow medication restrictions before the procedure may cause the procedure to be canceled or repeated.

Nursing Implications and Procedure ● ● ● ● ● ● ● ● ● ● ●

Pretest:

➤ Inform the patient that the procedure detects possible vascular or other structural abnormalities of the eye.

➤ Obtain a history of the patient's complaints, including a list of known allergens, especially mydriatics if dilation is to be performed.

➤ Obtain a history of the patient's known or suspected vision loss, changes in visual acuity, including type and cause; use of glasses or contact lenses; eye conditions with treatment regimens; eye surgery; and other tests and procedures to assess and diagnose visual deficit.

➤ Obtain a history of results of previously performed laboratory tests, surgical procedures, and other diagnostic procedures. For related diagnostic tests, refer to the table of tests associated with the Ocular System.

➤ Obtain a list of the medications the patient is taking, including herbs, nutritional supplements, and nutraceuticals. The requesting health care practitioner should be advised if the patient regularly uses these products so that their effects can be taken into consideration when reviewing results.

➤ Instruct the patient to remove contact lenses or glasses, as appropriate. Instruct the patient regarding the importance of keeping the eyes open for the test.

➤ Review the procedure with the patient. Explain that the patient will be requested to fixate the eyes during the procedure. Address concerns about pain related to the procedure. Explain to the patient that mydriatics, if used, may cause blurred vision and sensitivity to light. There may also be a brief stinging sensation when the drop is put in the eye but that no discomfort will be experienced during the examination. Inform the patient that a technician, optometrist, or health care practitioner performs the test, in a quiet, darkened room, and that to dilate and evaluate both eyes, the test can take up 60 minutes.

➤ There are no food or fluid restrictions, unless by medical direction.

➤ The patient should avoid eye medications (particularly mydriatic eye drops if the patient has glaucoma) for at least 1 day prior to the test.

➤ Ensure that the patient understands that he or she must refrain from driving until the pupils return to normal (about 4 hours) after the test and has made arrangements to have someone else be responsible for transportation after the test.

Intratest:

➤ Ensure that the patient has complied with medication restrictions; assure that eye medications, especially mydriatics, have been restricted for at least 1 day prior to the test.

➤ Instruct the patient to cooperate fully and to follow directions. Ask the patient to remain still during the procedure because movement produces unreliable results.

➤ Seat the patient in a chair that faces the camera. Instruct the patient to look at directed target while the eyes are examined.

➤ If dilation is to be performed, administer the ordered mydriatic to each eye and repeat in 5 to 15 minutes. Drops are placed in the eye with the patient looking up and the solution directed at the six o'clock position of the sclera (white of the eye) near the limbus (grey, semitransparent area of the eyeball where the cornea and sclera meet). The dropper bottle should not touch the eyelashes.

➤ Ask the patient to place the chin in the chin rest and gently press the forehead against the support bar. Ask the patient to open his or her eyes wide and look at desired target while a sequence of photographs are taken.

➤ The results are recorded on developed photographic film or electronically on computerized equipment for recall and postprocedure interpretation by the appropriate health care practitioner.

Post-test:

➤ Instruct the patient to resume usual medications, as directed by the health care practitioner.

➤ A written report of the examination will be completed by a health care practitioner specializing in this branch of medicine. The report will be sent to the requesting health care practitioner, who will discuss the results with the patient.

➤ Recognize anxiety related to test results, and be supportive of impaired activity related to vision loss or perceived loss of driving privileges Discuss the implications of abnormal test results on the patient's lifestyle. Provide teaching and information regarding the clinical implications of the test results, as appropriate.

➤ Reinforce information given by the patient's health care provider regarding further testing, treatment, or referral to another health care provider. Inform the patient that visual acuity and responses to light may change. Suggest that the patient wear dark glasses after the test until the pupils return to normal size. Answer any questions or address any concerns voiced by the patient or family.

➤ Depending on the results of this procedure, additional testing may be performed to evaluate or monitor progression of the disease process and determine the need for a change in therapy. Evaluate test results in relation to the patient's symptoms and other tests performed.

Related diagnostic tests:

➤ Related diagnostic tests include fluorescein angiography, gonioscopy, intraocular pressure, refraction, slit-lamp biomicroscopy, and visual field testing.

GALLIUM SCAN

SYNONYMS/ACRONYM: Gallium scan, tumor; gallium scan, abscess; gallium scan, fever of undetermined origin.

AREA OF APPLICATION: Whole body.

CONTRAST: Intravenous radioactive gallium-67 citrate.

DESCRIPTION & RATIONALE: Gallium imaging is a nuclear medicine study that assists in diagnosing neoplasm and inflammation activity. Gallium, which has 90% sensitivity for inflammatory disease, is readily distributed throughout plasma and body tissues. Gallium imaging is sensitive in detecting abscesses, pneumonia, pyelonephritis, active sarcoidosis, and active tuberculosis. In immunocompromised patients, such as patients with acquired immunodeficiency syndrome, gallium imaging can detect complications such as *Pneumocystis jiroveci* (formerly *carinii*) pneumonitis. Gallium imaging is useful but less commonly performed in the diagnosis and staging of some neoplasms, including Hodgkin's disease, lymphoma, melanoma, and leukemia. Imaging can be performed 6 to 72 hours after gallium injection. A gamma camera detects the radiation emitted from the injected radioactive material, and a representative image of the distribution of the radioactive material is obtained. The nonspecificity of gallium imaging requires correlation with other diagnostic studies, such as computed tomography, magnetic resonance imaging, and ultrasonography. ■

INDICATIONS:
- Aid in the diagnosis of infectious or inflammatory diseases
- Evaluate lymphomas
- Evaluate recurrent lymphomas or tumors after radiation therapy or chemotherapy
- Perform as a screening examination for fever of undetermined origin

RESULT

Normal Findings:
- Normal distribution of gallium. Some localization of the radionuclide within the liver, spleen, bone, nasopharynx, lacrimal glands, breast, and bowel is expected.

Abnormal Findings:
- Abscess
- Infection
- Inflammation
- Lymphoma
- Tumor

CRITICAL VALUES: N/A

INTERFERING FACTORS:

This procedure is contraindicated for:

- Patients who are pregnant or suspected of being pregnant, unless the potential benefits of the procedure far outweigh the risks to the fetus and mother

Factors that may impair clear imaging:

- Inability of the patient to cooperate or remain still during the procedure because of age, significant pain, or mental status

- Improper adjustment of the radiographic equipment to accommodate obese or thin patients, which can cause overexposure or underexposure and a poor-quality study

- Metallic objects within the examination field (e.g., jewelry, body rings), which may inhibit organ visualization and can produce unclear images

- Patients who are very obese, who may exceed the weight limit for the equipment

- Incorrect positioning of the patient, which may produce poor visualization of the area to be examined

- Performance of other nuclear scans within the preceding 24 to 48 hours

- Administration of certain medications (e.g., gastrin, cholecystokinin), which may interfere with gastric emptying

Other considerations:

- Improper injection of the radionuclide may allow the tracer to seep deep into the muscle tissue, producing erroneous hot spots.

- Consultation with a health care practitioner should occur before the procedure for radiation safety concerns regarding younger patients or patients who are lactating.

- Risks associated with radiologic overexposure can result from frequent x-ray procedures. Personnel in the room with the patient should wear a protective lead apron, stand behind a shield, or leave the area while the examination is being done. Badges that reveal the level of exposure to radiation should be worn by persons working in the area where the examination is being done.

Nursing Implications and Procedure . . . .

Pretest:

➤ Inform the patient that the test detects inflammation, infection, or tumor.

➤ Obtain a history of the patient's complaints and symptoms, including a list of known allergens.

➤ Obtain a history of results of previously performed diagnostic procedures, surgical procedures, and laboratory tests For related diagnostic tests, refer to the Musculoskeletal, Respiratory, and Immune System tables.

➤ Record the date of the last menstrual period and determine the possibility of pregnancy in perimenopausal women.

➤ Obtain a list of the patient's current medications.

➤ Review the procedure with the patient. Explain to the patient that some pain may be experienced during the test, and there may be moments of discomfort. Explain the purpose of the test and how the procedure is performed. Inform the patient that the procedure is performed in a nuclear medicine department, usually by a technologist and support staff, and takes approximately 30 to 60 minutes. Delayed images are needed 72 hours after the initial injection. Inform the patient that the technologist will inject gallium in an arm vein and ask the patient to return later for the imaging procedure, at which time the patient will be placed in a supine position on a flat table.

➤ *Sensitivity to cultural and social issues,* as well as concern for modesty, is important in providing psychological support before, during, and after the procedure.

➤ There are no food, fluid, or medication restrictions, unless by medical direction.

➤ Instruct the patient to remove dentures, jewelry (including watches), hairpins, credit cards, and other metallic objects.

➤ *Make sure a written and informed consent has been signed prior to the procedure and before administering any medications.*

Intratest:

➤ Ensure that the patient has removed jewelry, dentures, all external metallic objects, and the like prior to the procedure.

➤ Patients are given a gown, robe, and foot coverings to wear and instructed to void prior to the procedure.

➤ Instruct the patient to cooperate fully and to follow directions. Instruct the patient to lie still during the procedure because movement produces unclear images.

➤ Observe standard precautions, and follow the general guidelines in Appendix A.

➤ Administer sedative to a child or to an uncooperative adult, as ordered.

➤ The radionuclide is administered intravenously. Delayed views may be taken at 6, 24, 48, and 72 hours after the injection.

➤ If an abdominal abscess or infection is suspected, laxatives or enemas may be ordered before delayed imaging at 48 or 72 hours after the injection.

➤ The results are recorded on film or in a computerized system for recall and postprocedure interpretation by the appropriate health care practitioner.

Post-test:

➤ Instruct the patient to resume usual diet, medication, and activity, after imaging is complete, as directed by the health care practitioner.

➤ Advise the patient to drink increased amounts of fluids for several days to eliminate the radionuclide from the body, unless contraindicated. Tell the patient the radionuclide is eliminated from the body within 48 to 72 hours.

➤ Inform the patient to flush the toilet immediately after each voiding following the procedure, and to wash hands meticulously with soap and water after each voiding for 72 hours after the procedure.

➤ Tell all caregivers to wear gloves when discarding urine for 48 hours after the procedure. Wash gloved hands with soap and water before removing gloves. Then wash ungloved hands after removing the gloves.

➤ Instruct the patient in the care and assessment of the injection site. Observe the site for bleeding, hematoma formation, and inflammation.

➤ A written report of the examination will be completed by a health care practitioner specializing in this branch of medicine. The report will be sent to the requesting health care practitioner, who will discuss the results with the patient.

➤ Reinforce information given by the patient's health care provider regarding further testing, treatment, or referral to another health care provider. Answer any questions or address any concerns voiced by the patient or family.

➤ Depending on the results of this procedure, additional testing may be needed to evaluate or monitor progression of the disease process and determine the need for a change in therapy. Evaluate test results in relation to the patient's symptoms and other tests performed.

Related diagnostic tests:

➤ Related diagnostic tests include chest x-ray; computed tomography of the thorax, abdomen, and pelvis; and magnetic resonance imaging of the chest and abdomen.

GASTRIC ACID STIMULATION TEST

SYNONYM/ACRONYM: N/A.

SPECIMEN: Gastric fluid collected in eight plastic tubes at 15-minute intervals.

REFERENCE VALUE: (Method: Volume measurement and pH by ion-selective electrode)

Basal acid output (BAO)	*Male:* 0–10.5 mmol/h
	Female: 0–5.6 mmol/h
Peak acid output (PAO)	*Male:* 12–60 mmol/h
	Female: 8–40 mmol/h
Peak response time	*Pentagastrin, intramuscular:* 15–45 min
	Pentagastrin, subcutaneous: 10–30 min
BAO/PAO ratio	Less than 0.20

DESCRIPTION & RATIONALE: The gastric acid stimulation test is performed to determine the response to substances administered to induce increased gastric acid production. Pentagastrin is the usual drug of choice to induce gastric secretion because it has no major side effects. The samples obtained from gastric acid stimulation tests are examined for volume, pH, and amount of acid secreted. First, basal acid output (BAO) is determined by averaging the results of gastric samples collected before the administration of a gastric stimulant. Then a gastric stimulant is administered and peak acid output (PAO) is determined by adding together the gastric acid output of the highest two consecutive 15-minute stimulation samples. Finally, BAO and PAO are compared as a ratio, which is normally less than 0.20. ∎

INDICATIONS:
• Detect duodenal ulcer

• Detect gastric carcinoma

• Detect pernicious anemia

• Detect Zollinger-Ellison syndrome

• Evaluate effectiveness of vagotomy in the treatment of peptic ulcer disease

RESULT

Increased:
• BAO
  Basophilic leukemia
  Duodenal ulcer
  G-cell hyperplasia
  Recurring peptic ulcer
  Retained antrum syndrome

Systemic mastocytosis
Vagal hyperfunction
Zollinger-Ellison syndrome

- PAO
Duodenal ulcer
Zollinger-Ellison syndrome

Decreased:
- BAO
Gastric ulcer

- PAO
Chronic gastritis
Gastric cancers
Gastric polyps
Gastric ulcer
Myxedema
Pernicious anemia

CRITICAL VALUES: N/A

INTERFERING FACTORS:
- Drugs that may increase gastric volume include atropine, diazepam, ganglionic blocking agents, and insulin.

- Drugs and substances that may increase gastric pH include caffeine, calcium salts, corticotropin, ethanol, rauwolfia, reserpine, and tolazoline.

- Drugs and substances that may decrease gastric pH include atropine, cimetidine, diazepam, famotidine, ganglionic blocking agents, glucagon, nizatidine, omeprazole, oxmetidine, propranolol, prostaglandin F_{2a}, ranitidine, and secretin.

- Gastric intubation is contraindicated in patients with esophageal varices, diverticula, stenosis, malignant neoplasm of the esophagus, aortic aneurysm, severe gastric hemorrhage, and congenital heart failure.

- The use of histamine diphosphate is contraindicated in patients with a history of asthma, paroxysmal hypertension, urticaria, or other allergic conditions.

- Failure to follow dietary restrictions may result in stimulation of gastric secretions.

- Failure to follow dietary restrictions before the procedure may cause the procedure to be canceled or repeated.

- Exposure to the sight, smell, or thought of food immediately before and during the test may result in stimulation of gastric secretions.

Nursing Implications and Procedure ● ● ● ● ● ● ● ● ● ● ●

Pretest:

➤ Inform the patient that the test is used to asist in the differential diagnosis of gastrointestinal disorders.

➤ Obtain a history of the patient's complaints, including a list of known allergens (especially allergies or sensitivities to latex), and inform the appropriate health care practitioner accordingly.

➤ Obtain a history of the patient's gastrointestinal system, as well as results of previously performed laboratory tests, surgical procedures, and other diagnostic procedures. For related laboratory tests, refer to the Gastrointestinal System table.

➤ Obtain a list of the medications the patient is taking, including herbs, nutritional supplements, and nutraceuticals. The requesting health care practitioner and laboratory should be advised if the patient regularly uses these products so that their effects can be taken into consideration when reviewing results.

➤ Review the procedure with the patient. Inform the patient that specimen collection takes approximately 60 to 120 minutes. Address concerns about pain related to the procedure. Explain that some discomfort is experienced from insertion of the nasogastric tube.

➤ *Sensitivity to social and cultural issues,* as well as concern for modesty, is important in providing psychological support before, during, and after the procedure.

➤ Drugs and substances that may alter gastric secretions (e.g., alcohol, histamine, nicotine, adrenocorticotropic steroids, insulin, para-sympathetic agents, belladonna alkaloids, anticholinergic drugs, histamine receptor antagonists) should be restricted by medical direction for 72 hours before the test.

➤ Instruct the patient to fast from food after the evening meal the night before the test, and not to drink water for 1 hour before the test. The patient should be instructed to refrain from chewing gum or smoking for at least 12 hours before the test.

➤ *Make sure a written and informed consent has been signed prior to the procedure and before administering any medications.*

Intratest:

➤ Ensure that the patient has complied with dietary restrictions and other pretesting preparations; assure that food has been restricted for at least 12 hours prior to the procedure.

➤ If the patient has a history of severe allergic reaction to latex, care should be taken to avoid the use of equipment containing latex.

➤ Ensure that the patient does not have a history of asthma, paroxysmal hypertension, urticaria, or other allergic conditions if histamine diphosphate is being considered for use in the test.

➤ Record baseline vital signs.

➤ If the patient is wearing dentures, remove them.

➤ Have the patient sit, or help the patient recline on the left side.

➤ Instruct the patient to cooperate fully and to follow directions. Direct the patient to breathe normally and to avoid unnecessary movement.

➤ Observe standard precautions, and follow the general guidelines in Appendix A. Positively identify the patient, and label the appropriate collection containers with the corresponding patient demographics, date, and time of collection.

➤ A cold lubricated gastric (Levine) tube is inserted orally. Alternatively, if the patient has a hyperactive gag reflex, the tube can be inserted nasally. The tube must have a radiopaque tip.

➤ Fluoroscopy or x-ray is used to confirm proper position of the tube before the start of the test.

➤ Using a constant but gentle suction, gastric contents are collected. Do not use specimens obtained from the first 15 to 30 minutes of suctioning.

➤ The gastric stimulant is administered, and the peak basal specimens are collected over a 60-minute period as four 15-minute specimens. Number the specimen tubes in the order in which they were collected.

➤ Promptly transport the specimen to the laboratory for processing and analysis.

➤ The results are recorded manually or in a computerized system for recall and postprocedure interpretation by the appropriate health care practitioner.

Post-test:

➤ Instruct the patient to resume usual diet and medication, as directed by the health care practitioner.

➤ Monitor vital signs and neurologic status every 15 minutes for 1 hour, then every 2 hours for 4 hours, and then as ordered by the health care practitioner for evaluation. Protocols may vary from facility to facility.

➤ Instruct the patient to report any chest pain, upper abdominal pain, pain on swallowing, difficulty breathing, or expectoration of blood. Report these to the health care practitioner immediately.

➤ Monitor for side effects of drugs administered to induce gastric secretion (e.g., flushing, headache, nasal stuffiness, dizziness, faintness, nausea).

➤ A written report of the examination will be sent to the requesting health care practitioner, who will discuss the results with the patient.

➤ Recognize anxiety related to test results. Discuss the implications of abnormal test results on the patient's lifestyle. Provide teaching and information regarding the clinical implications of the test results, as appropriate.

➤ Reinforce information given by the patient's health care provider regarding further testing, treatment, or referral to another health care provider. Answer any questions or address any concerns voiced by the patient or family.

➤ Instruct the patient in the use of any ordered medications. Explain the importance of adhering to the therapy regimen. As appropriate, instruct the patient in significant side effects and systemic reactions associated with the prescribed medication. Encourage him or her to review corresponding literature provided by a pharmacist.

➤ Depending on the results of this procedure, additional testing may be performed to evaluate or monitor progression of the disease process and determine the need for a change in therapy. Evaluate test results in relation to the patient's symptoms and other tests performed.

Related laboratory tests:

➤ Related laboratory tests include complete blood count, folate, gastrin, *Helicobacter pylori* antibody, intrinsic factor antibodies, and vitamin B_{12}.

GASTRIC EMPTYING SCAN

• •

SYNONYMS/ACRONYM: Gastric emptying quantitation, gastric emptying scintigraphy.

AREA OF APPLICATION: Esophagus, stomach, small bowel.

CONTRAST: Oral radioactive technetium-99m sulfur colloid.

DESCRIPTION & RATIONALE: A gastric emptying scan quantifies gastric emptying physiology. The procedure is indicated for patients with gastric motility symptoms, including diabetic gastroparesis, anorexia nervosa, gastric outlet obstruction syndromes, postvagotomy and postgastrectomy syndromes, and assessment of medical and surgical treatments for diseases known to affect gastric motility. A radionuclide is administered, and the clearance of solids and liquids may be evaluated. The images are recorded electronically, showing the gastric emptying function over time. ∎

INDICATIONS:

- Investigate the cause of rapid or slow rate of gastric emptying
- Measure gastric emptying rate

RESULT

Normal Findings:

- Mean time emptying of liquid phase: 30 minutes (range, 11 to 49 minutes)
- Mean time emptying of solid phase: 40 minutes (range, 28 to 80 minutes)
- No delay in gastric emptying rate

Abnormal Findings:

- Decreased rate:
  Dumping syndrome
  Duodenal ulcer
  Malabsorption syndromes
  Zollinger-Ellison syndrome

- Increased rate:
  Amyloidosis
  Anorexia nervosa
  Diabetes
  Gastric outlet obstruction
  Gastric ulcer
  Gastroenteritis
  Gastroesophageal reflux
  Hypokalemia, hypomagnesemia
  Post–gastric surgery period
  Postoperative ileus
  Post–radiation therapy period
  Scleroderma

CRITICAL VALUES: N/A

INTERFERING FACTORS:

This procedure is contraindicated for:

- Patients who are pregnant or suspected of being pregnant, unless the potential benefits of the procedure far outweigh the risks to the fetus and mother
- Patients with esophageal motor disorders or swallowing difficulties

Factors that may impair clear imaging:

- Inability of the patient to cooperate or remain still during the procedure because of age, significant pain, or mental status
- Improper adjustment of the radiographic equipment to accommodate obese or thin patients, which can cause a poor-quality study
- Metallic objects within the examination field (e.g., jewelry, body rings), which may inhibit organ visualization and can produce unclear images
- Retained barium from a previous radiologic procedure
- Patients who are very obese, who may exceed the weight limit for the equipment
- Incorrect positioning of the patient, which may produce poor visualization of the area to be examined
- Performance of other nuclear scans within the preceding 24 to 48 hours
- Administration of certain medications (e.g., gastrin, cholecystokinin), which may interfere with gastric emptying

Other considerations:

- Failure to follow dietary restrictions before the procedure may cause the procedure to be canceled or repeated.
- Consultation with a health care practitioner should occur before the procedure for radiation safety concerns regarding younger patients or patients who are lactating.
- Risks associated with radiologic overexposure can result from frequent x-ray procedures. Personnel in the room with the patient should wear a protective lead apron, stand behind a shield, or leave the area while the examination is being done. Badges that reveal the level of exposure to radiation should be worn by persons working in the area where the examination is being done.

Nursing Implications and Procedure • • • • • • • • • • •

Pretest:

➤ Inform the patient that the procedure assesses gastric emptying.

➤ Obtain a history of the patient's complaints and symptoms, including a list of known allergens, especially to eggs.

➤ Obtain a history of the patient's gastrointestinal system, as well as results of previously performed diagnostic procedures, surgical procedures, and laboratory tests. For related diagnostic tests, refer to the Gastrointestinal System table.

➤ Record the date of the last menstrual period and determine the possibility of pregnancy in perimenopausal women.

➤ Obtain a list of the patient's current medications.

➤ Review the procedure with the patient. Address concerns about pain related to the procedure. Explain to the patient that some pain may be experienced during the test, and there may be moments of discomfort. Explain the purpose of the test and how the procedure is performed. Reassure the patient that the radionuclide poses no radioactive hazard and rarely produces side effects. Inform the patient that the procedure is performed in a nuclear medicine department, usually by a technologist and support staff, and takes approximately 30 to 120 minutes. Inform the patient that the technologist will place him or her in an upright position in front of the gamma camera (scanner).

➤ *Sensitivity to cultural and social issues,* as well as concern for modesty, is important in providing psychological support before, during and after the procedure.

➤ Restrict food and fluids for 6 to 8 hours before the scan.

➤ Instruct the patient to remove dentures, jewelry (including watches), hairpins, credit cards, and other metallic objects.

Intratest:

➤ Ensure that the patient has complied with dietary and fluids restrictions and pretesting preparations. Ensure that the patient has removed all external metallic objects (jewelry, dentures, etc.) prior to the procedure.

➤ Patients are given a gown, robe, and foot coverings to wear and instructed to void prior to the procedure.

➤ Obtain and record baseline vital signs.

➤ Instruct the patient to cooperate fully and to follow directions. Instruct the patient to lie still during the procedure because movement produces unclear images.

➤ Observe standard precautions, and follow the general guidelines in Appendix A.

➤ Administer sedative to a child or to an uncooperative adult, as ordered.

➤ Place the patient in an upright position in front of the gamma camera.

➤ Ask the patient to take the radionuclide orally, combined with eggs or as a liquid.

➤ Images are recorded over a period of time (30 to 60 minutes) and evaluated with regard to the amount of time the stomach takes to empty its contents.

➤ The results are recorded on film or in a computerized system for recall and postprocedure interpretation by the appropriate health care practitioner.

Post-test:

➤ Instruct the patient to resume usual diet, medication, and activity, as directed by the health care practitioner.

➤ Monitor vital signs every 15 minutes for 1 hour, then every 2 hours for 4 hours, and then as ordered by the health care practitioner. Compare with baseline values. Protocols may vary from facility to facility.

➤ Advise the patient to drink increased

amounts of fluids for 24 to 48 hours to eliminate the radionuclide from the body, unless contraindicated. Tell the patient that radionuclide is eliminated from the body within 6 to 24 hours.

➤ Inform the patient to flush the toilet immediately after each voiding following the procedure, and to wash hands meticulously with soap and water after each voiding for 24 hours after the procedure.

➤ Tell all caregivers to wear gloves when discarding urine for 24 hours after the procedure. Wash gloved hands with soap and water before removing gloves. Then wash hands after removing the gloves.

➤ A written report of the examination will be completed by a health care practitioner specializing in this branch of medicine. The report will be sent to the requesting health care practitioner, who will discuss the results with the patient.

➤ Reinforce information given by the patient's health care provider regarding further testing, treatment, or referral to another health care provider. Answer any questions or address any concerns voiced by the patient or family.

➤ Depending on the results of this procedure, additional testing may be needed to evaluate or monitor progression of the disease process and determine the need for a change in therapy. Evaluate test results in relation to the patient's symptoms and other tests performed.

Related diagnostic tests:

➤ Related diagnostic tests include computed tomography of the abdomen, and upper gastrointestinal and small bowel series.

GASTRIN AND GASTRIN STIMULATION TEST

• •

SYNONYM/ACRONYM: N/A.

SPECIMEN: Serum (1 mL) collected in a red- or tiger-top tube.

REFERENCE VALUE: (Method: Radioimmunoassay)

Age	Conventional Units	SI Units (Conventional Units × 1)
Infant	120–183 pg/mL	120–183 ng/L
Child	Less than 10–125 pg/mL	Less than 10–125 ng/L
Adult		
Up to 60 y	25–90 pg/mL	25–90 ng/L
60 y and older	Less than 100 pg/mL	Less than 100 ng/L

Stimulation Tests

Gastrin stimulation test with calcium or secretin	No response or slight increase over baseline

DESCRIPTION & RATIONALE: Gastrin is a hormone secreted by the stomach and duodenum in response to vagal stimulation; the presence of food, alcohol, or calcium in the stomach; and the alkalinity of gastric secretions. After its absorption into the circulation, gastrin returns to the stomach and acts as a stimulant for acid, insulin, pepsin, and intrinsic factor secretion. Gastrin stimulation tests can be performed after a test meal or intravenous infusion of calcium or secretin. ■

INDICATIONS:
• Assist in the diagnosis of gastric carcinoma, pernicious anemia, or G-cell hyperplasia

• Assist in the diagnosis of Zollinger-Ellison syndrome

• Assist in the differential diagnosis of ulcers from other gastrointestinal peptic disorders

RESULT

Increased in:
• Chronic gastritis

• Chronic renal failure

• Gastric and duodenal ulcers

• Gastric carcinoma

• G-cell hyperplasia

• Hyperparathyroidism

• Pernicious anemia

• Pyloric obstruction

• Retained antrum

• Zollinger-Ellison syndrome

Decreased in:
• Hypothyroidism

• Vagotomy

CRITICAL VALUES: N/A

INTERFERING FACTORS:
• Drugs and substances that may increase gastrin levels include amino acids, catecholamines, cimetidine, insulin, morphine, omeprazole, pantoprazole, sufotidine, terbutaline, calcium products, and coffee.

• Drugs that may decrease gastrin levels include atropine, enprostil, glucagon, secretin, streptozocin, and tolbutamide.

• In some cases, protein ingestion elevates serum gastrin levels.

• Recent radioactive scans or radiation within 1 week before the test can interfere with test results when radioimmunoassay is the test method.

• Failure to follow dietary and medication restrictions before the procedure may cause the procedure to be canceled or repeated.

Nursing Implications and Procedure • • • • • • • • • • •

Pretest:

➤ Inform the patient that the test is used to assist in the diagnosis of Zollinger-Ellison syndrome and gastrinoma.

➤ Obtain a history of the patient's complaints, including a list of known allergens (especially allergies or sensitivities to latex), and inform the appropriate health care practitioner accordingly.

➤ Obtain a history of the patient's endocrine and gastrointestinal systems, as well as results of previously performed laboratory tests, surgical procedures, and other diagnostic procedures. For related laboratory tests, refer to the Endocrine and Gastrointestinal System tables.

➤ Note any recent procedures that can interfere with test results.

➤ Obtain a list of medications the patient is taking, including herbs, nutritional supplements, and nutraceuticals. The requesting health care practitioner and laboratory should be advised if the patient regularly uses these products so that their effects can be taken into consideration when reviewing results.

➤ Review the procedure with the patient. Inform the patient that specimen collection takes approximately 5 to 10 minutes. Address concerns about pain related to the procedure. Explain to the patient that there may be some discomfort during the venipuncture.

➤ Instruct the patient to fast for 12 hours before the test.

➤ Instruct the patient to withhold medications and alcohol for 12 to 24 hours, as ordered by the health care practitioner.

➤ There are no fluid restrictions, unless by medical direction.

Intratest:

➤ Ensure that the patient has complied with dietary and medication restrictions and other pretesting preparations; assure that food and medications have been withheld for at least 12 hours prior to the procedure.

➤ If the patient has a history of severe allergic reaction to latex, care should be taken to avoid the use of equipment containing latex.

➤ Instruct the patient to cooperate fully and to follow directions. Direct the patient to breathe normally and to avoid unnecessary movement.

➤ Administer gastrin stimulators as appropriate.

➤ Observe standard precautions, and follow the general guidelines in Appendix A. Positively identify the patient, and label the appropriate tubes with the corresponding patient demographics, date, and time of collection. Perform a venipuncture; collect the specimen in a 5-mL red- or tiger-top tube.

➤ Remove the needle, and apply a pressure dressing over the puncture site.

➤ Promptly transport the specimen to the laboratory for processing and analysis.

➤ The results are recorded manually or in a computerized system for recall and postprocedure interpretation by the appropriate health care practitioner.

Post-test:

➤ Observe venipuncture site for bleeding or hematoma formation. Apply paper tape or other adhesive to hold pressure bandage in place, or replace with a plastic bandage.

➤ Instruct the patient to resume usual diet and medications, as directed by the health care practitioner.

➤ *Nutritional considerations:* Nutritional support with calcium, iron, and vitamin B_{12} supplementation may be ordered, as appropriate.

➤ A written report of the examination will be sent to the requesting health care practitioner, who will discuss the results with the patient.

➤ Reinforce information given by the patient's health care provider regarding further testing, treatment, or referral to another health care provider. Answer any questions or address any concerns voiced by the patient or family.

➤ Depending on the results of this procedure, additional testing may be performed to evaluate or monitor progression of the disease process and determine the need for a change

in therapy. Evaluate test results in relation to the patient's symptoms and other tests performed.

Related laboratory tests:

➤ Related laboratory tests include complete blood count, folate, gastric acid stimulation, glucose, *Helicobacter pylori* antibody, and vitamin B_{12}.

GASTROESOPHAGEAL REFLUX SCAN

SYNONYMS/ACRONYM: Aspiration scan, GER scan, GERD scan.

AREA OF APPLICATION: Esophagus and stomach.

CONTRAST: Oral radioactive technetium-99m sulfur colloid.

DESCRIPTION & RATIONALE: The gastroesophageal reflux (GER) scan assesses gastric reflux across the esophageal sphincter. Symptoms of GER include heartburn, regurgitation, vomiting, dysphagia, and a bitter taste in the mouth. This procedure may be used to evaluate the medical or surgical treatment of patients with GER and to detect aspiration of gastric contents into the lungs. A radionuclide such as technetium-99m sulfur colloid is ingested orally in orange juice. Scanning studies are done immediately to assess the amount of liquid that has reached the stomach. An abdominal binder is applied and then tightened gradually to obtain images at increasing degrees of abdominal pressure: 0, 20, 40, 60, 80, and 100 mm Hg.

Computer calculation determines the amount of reflux into the esophagus at each of these abdominal pressures as recorded on the images. For aspiration scans, images are taken over the lungs to detect tracheoesophageal aspiration of the radionuclide.

In infants, the study distinguishes between vomiting and reflux. Reflux occurs predominantly in infants younger than age 2, who are mainly on a milk diet. This procedure is indicated when an infant has symptoms such as failure to thrive, feeding problems, and episodes of wheezing with chest infection. The radionuclide is added to the infant's milk, images are obtained of the gastric and esophageal area, and the images are evaluated visually and by computer. ∎

INDICATIONS:
- Aid in the diagnosis of GER in patients with unexplained nausea and vomiting
- Distinguish between vomiting and reflux in infants with failure to thrive, feeding problems, and wheezing combined with chest infection

RESULT

Normal Findings:
- Reflux less than or equal to 4% across the esophageal sphincter

Abnormal Findings:
- Reflux of greater than 4% at any pressure level
- Pulmonary aspiration

CRITICAL VALUES: N/A

INTERFERING FACTORS:

This procedure is contraindicated for:
- Patients who are pregnant or suspected of being pregnant, unless the potential benefits of the procedure far outweigh the risks to the fetus and mother
- Patients with hiatal hernia, esophageal motor disorders, or swallowing difficulties

Factors that may impair clear imaging:
- Inability of the patient to cooperate or remain still during the procedure because of age, significant pain, or mental status
- Improper adjustment of the radiographic equipment to accommodate obese or thin patients, which can cause overexposure or underexposure and a poor-quality study
- Patients who are very obese, who may exceed the weight limit for the equipment

- Incorrect positioning of the patient, which may produce poor visualization of the area to be examined
- Retained barium from a previous radiologic procedure
- Other nuclear scans done within the previous 24 to 48 hours
- Metallic objects within the examination field (e.g., jewelry, body rings), which may inhibit organ visualization and can produce unclear images

Other considerations:
- Consultation with a health care practitioner should occur before the procedure for radiation safety concerns regarding younger patients or patients who are lactating.
- Risks associated with radiologic overexposure can result from frequent x-ray procedures. Personnel in the room with the patient should wear a protective lead apron, stand behind a shield, or leave the area while the examination is being done. Badges that reveal the level of exposure to radiation should be worn by persons working in the area where the examination is being done.

Nursing Implications and Procedure ․․․․․․․․․․

Pretest:

➤ Inform the patient that the procedure evaluates gastric reflux.

➤ Obtain a history of the patient's complaints and symptoms, including a list of known allergens.

➤ Obtain a history of the patient's gastrointestinal system, signs and symptoms of gastroesophageal reflux, and results of previously performed diagnostic procedures, surgical procedures, and laboratory tests. For related diagnostic tests, refer to the Gastrointestinal and Musculoskeletal System tables.

- Record the date of the last menstrual period and determine the possibility of pregnancy in perimenopausal women.

- Note any recent procedures that can interfere with test results; including examinations using iodine-based contrast medium or barium.

- Obtain a list of the medications the patient is taking, including anticoagulant therapy, acetylsalicylic acid, herbs, nutritional supplements, and nutraceuticals, especially those known to affect coagulation (see Appendix F). It is recommended that use be discontinued 14 days before surgical procedures. The requesting health care practitioner and laboratory should be advised if the patient regularly uses these products so that their effects can be taken into consideration when reviewing results.

- Review the procedure with the patient. Address concerns about pain related to the procedure. Explain to the patient that some pain may be experienced during the test, or there may be moments of discomfort. Explain that the radioactive colloid is ingested orally in either orange juice or milk. Reassure the patient that the radionuclide poses no radioactive hazard and rarely produces side effects. Inform the patient that the procedure is performed in a special department, usually in a radiology department, by a healthcare practitioner and support staff and takes approximately 30 to 60 minutes.

- *Sensitivity to social and cultural issues,* as well as concern for modesty, is important in providing psychological support before, during and after the procedure.

- Fasting before the scan is not required; the patient may be encouraged to eat a full meal before the procedure.

- Instruct the patient to remove dentures, jewelry (including watches), hairpins, credit cards, and other metallic objects in the area to be examined.

Intratest:

- Ensure the patient has removed all external metallic objects (jewelry, dentures, etc.) prior to the procedure.

- Have emergency equipment readily available.

- If the patient has a history of severe allergic reactions to any substance or drug, administer ordered prophylactic steroids or antihistamines before the procedure. Use nonionic contrast medium for the procedure.

- Patients are given a gown, robe, and foot coverings to wear and instructed to void prior to the procedure.

- Record baseline vital signs and assess neurologic status. Protocols may vary from facility to facility.

- Instruct the patient to cooperate fully and to follow directions. Instruct the patient to remain still throughout the procedure because movement produces unreliable results.

- Observe standard precautions, and follow the general guidelines in Appendix A.

- Establish an intravenous fluid line for the injection of emergency drugs and of sedatives.

- Administer an antianxiety agent, as ordered, if the patient has claustrophobia. Administer a sedative to a child or to an uncooperative adult, as ordered.

- Place the patient in a supine position on a flat table with foam wedges, which help maintain position and immobilization. Images are recorded to confirm swallowing of the liquid and emptying into the stomach.

- The abdominal binder is applied, and scans are taken as the binder is tightened at various pressures, as described previously.

- If reflux occurs at lower pressures, an additional 30 mL of water may be given to clear the esophagus.

- Wear gloves during the radionuclide administration and while handling the patient's urine.

➤ Instruct the patient to take slow, deep breaths if nausea occurs during the procedure. Monitor and administer an antiemetic agent if ordered. Ready an emesis basin for use.

➤ Monitor the patient for complications related to the procedure (e.g., allergic reaction, anaphylaxis, bronchospasm).

➤ The results are recorded on film or in a computerized system for recall and postprocedure interpretation by the appropriate health care practitioner.

Post-test:

➤ Monitor vital signs and neurologic status every 15 minutes for 1 hour, then every 2 hours for 4 hours, and then as ordered by the health care practitioner. Compare with baseline values. Protocols may vary from facility to facility.

➤ Observe for delayed allergic reactions, such as rash, urticaria, tachycardia, hyperpnea, hypertension, palpitations, nausea, or vomiting.

➤ Instruct the patient to immediately report symptoms such as fast heart rate, difficulty breathing, skin rash, itching, or decreased urinary output.

➤ Instruct the patient to drink increased amounts of fluids for 24 to 48 hours to eliminate the radionuclide from the body, unless contraindicated. Tell the patient that radionuclide is eliminated from the body within 6 to 24 hours.

➤ Instruct the patient to flush the toilet immediately after each voiding following the procedure, and to wash hands meticulously with soap and water after each voiding for 24 hours after the procedure.

➤ Instruct all caregivers to wear gloves when discarding urine for 24 hours after the procedure. Wash gloved hands with soap and water before removing gloves. Then wash hands after the gloves are removed.

➤ If a woman who is breast-feeding must have a nuclear scan, she should not breast-feed the infant until the radionuclide has been eliminated. This could take as long as 3 days. She should be instructed to express the milk and discard it during the 3-day period to prevent cessation of milk production.

➤ *Nutritional considerations:* A low-fat, low-cholesterol, and low-sodium diet should be consumed to reduce current disease processes. High fat consumption increases the amount of bile acids in the colon and should be avoided.

➤ No other radionuclide tests should be scheduled for 24 to 48 hours after this procedure.

➤ A written report of the examination will be completed by a health care practitioner specializing in this branch of medicine. The report will be sent to the requesting health care practitioner, who will discuss the results with the patient.

➤ Recognize anxiety related to test results, and be supportive of perceived loss of independent function. Discuss the implications of abnormal test results on the patient's lifestyle. Provide teaching and information regarding the clinical implications of the test results, as appropriate.

➤ Reinforce information given by the patient's health care provider regarding further testing, treatment, or referral to another health care provider. Answer any questions or address any concerns voiced by the patient or family.

➤ Instruct the patient in the use of any ordered medications. Explain the importance of adhering to the therapy regimen. As appropriate, instruct the patient in significant side effects and systemic reactions associated with the prescribed medication. Encourage him or her to review corresponding literature provided by a pharmacist.

➤ Depending on the results of this procedure, additional testing may be

needed to evaluate or monitor progression of the disease process and determine the need for a change in therapy. Evaluate test results in relation to the patient's symptoms and other tests performed.

Related diagnostic tests:

➤ Related diagnostic tests include computed tomography of the abdomen, gastric emptying scan, and upper gastrointestinal and small bowel series.

GASTROINTESTINAL BLOOD LOSS SCAN

SYNONYMS/ACRONYM: Gastrointestinal bleed localization study, GI bleed scintigraphy, lower GI blood loss scan, GI scintigram.

AREA OF APPLICATION: Abdomen.

CONTRAST: Intravenous radioactive technetium-99m–labeled red blood cells.

DESCRIPTION & RATIONALE: Gastrointestinal (GI) blood loss scan is a nuclear medicine study that assists in detecting and localizing active GI tract bleeding (2 or 3 mL/min) for the purpose of better directing endoscopic or angiographic studies. This procedure can detect bleeding if the rate is greater than 0.5 mL/min, but it is not specific for site localization or cause of bleeding. Endoscopy is the procedure of choice for diagnosing upper GI bleeding. After injection of technetium-99m–labeled red blood cells, immediate and delayed images of various views of the abdomen are obtained. The radionuclide remains in the circulation long enough to extravasate and accumulate within the bowel lumen at the site of active bleeding. This procedure is valuable for the detection and localization of recent non-GI intra-abdominal hemorrhage. Images may be taken over an extended period to show intermittent bleeding. ■

INDICATIONS: Diagnose unexplained abdominal pain and GI bleeding

RESULT

Normal Findings:
• Normal distribution of radionuclide in the large vessels with no extravascular activity

Abnormal Findings:
• Angiodysplasia
• Aortoduodenal fistula

- Diverticulosis
- GI bleeding
- Inflammatory bowel disease
- Polyps
- Tumor
- Ulcer

CRITICAL VALUES: N/A

INTERFERING FACTORS:

This procedure is contraindicated for:
- Patients who are pregnant or suspected of being pregnant, unless the potential benefits of the procedure far outweigh the risks to the fetus and mother

Factors that may impair clear imaging:
- Inability of the patient to cooperate or remain still during the procedure because of age, significant pain, or mental status
- Retained barium from a previous radiologic procedure
- Metallic objects within the examination field (e.g., jewelry, body rings), which may inhibit organ visualization and can produce unclear images
- Improper adjustment of the radiographic equipment to accommodate obese or thin patients, which can cause overexposure or underexposure and a poor-quality study
- Patients who are very obese, who may exceed the weight limit for the equipment
- Incorrect positioning of the patient, which may produce poor visualization of the area to be examined
- Other nuclear scans done within the previous 24 to 48 hours
- Inaccurate timing of imaging after the radionuclide injection

Other considerations:
- The examination detects only active or intermittent bleeding.
- The procedure is of little value in patients with chronic anemia or slowly decreasing hematocrit.
- The scan is less accurate for localization of bleeding sites in the upper GI tract.
- Improper injection of the radionuclide allows the tracer to seep deep into the muscle tissue, producing erroneous hot spots.
- The test is not specific and does not indicate the exact pathologic condition causing the bleeding, and may miss small sites of bleeding (less than 0.5 mL/min) caused by diverticular disease or angiodysplasia.
- Physiologically unstable patients may be unable to be scanned over long periods or may need to go to surgery before the procedure is complete.
- Consultation with a health care practitioner should occur before the procedure for radiation safety concerns regarding younger patients or patients who are lactating.
- Risks associated with radiographic overexposure can result from frequent x-ray procedures. Personnel in the room with the patient should wear a protective lead apron, stand behind a shield, or leave the area while the examination is being done. Personnel working in the area where the examination is being done should wear badges that reveal their level of exposure to radiation.

Nursing Implications and Procedure

Pretest:

➤ Inform the patient that the procedure evaluates GI bleeding.

➤ Obtain a history of the patient's complaints and symptoms, including a list of known allergens.

> Obtain a history of the patient's gastrointestinal system, including signs and symptoms of GI bleeding, pain, intussusception, volvulus, or diverticulitis, as well as results of previously performed diagnostic procedures, surgical procedures, and laboratory tests. For related diagnostic tests, refer to the Gastrointestinal and Hematopoietic System tables.

> Note any recent procedures that can interfere with test results; including examinations using iodine-based contrast medium or barium.

> Record the date of the last menstrual period and determine the possibility of pregnancy in perimenopausal women.

> Obtain a list of the medications the patient is taking, including anticoagulant therapy, acetylsalicylic acid, herbs, nutritional supplements, and nutraceuticals, especially those known to affect coagulation (see Appendix F). It is recommended that use be discontinued 14 days before surgical procedures. The requesting health care practitioner and laboratory should be advised if the patient regularly uses these products so that their effects can be taken into consideration when reviewing results.

> Review the procedure with the patient. Address concerns about pain related to the procedure. Explain to the patient that some pain may be experienced during the test, or there may be moments of discomfort. Reassure the patient that the radionuclide poses no radioactive hazard and rarely produces side effects. Inform the patient that the procedure is performed in a special department, usually in a radiology department, by a health care practitioner and support staff, and takes approximately 60 minutes to complete, with additional images taken periodically over 24 hours.

> Explain that an intravenous (IV) line may be inserted to allow infusion of IV fluids, contrast medium, dye, or sedatives. Usually normal saline is infused.

> *Sensitivity to social and cultural issues,* as well as concern for modesty, is important in providing psychological support before, during and after the procedure.

> Fasting before the scan is not needed, unless otherwise indicated.

> Instruct the patient to remove dentures, jewelry, including watches, hairpins, credit cards, and other metallic objects in the area to be examined.

> *Make sure a written and informed consent has been signed prior to the procedure and before administering any medications.*

Intratest:

> Ensure that the patient has removed all external metallic objects (jewelry, dentures, etc.) prior to the procedure.

> Have emergency equipment readily available.

> If the patient has a history of severe allergic reactions to any substance or drug, administer ordered prophylactic steroids or antihistamines before the procedure. Use nonionic contrast medium for the procedure.

> Patients are given a gown, robe, and foot coverings to wear and instructed to void prior to the procedure.

> Record baseline vital signs and assess neurologic status. Protocols may vary from facility to facility.

> Instruct the patient to cooperate fully and to follow directions. Instruct the patient to remain still throughout the procedure because movement produces unreliable results.

> Observe standard precautions, and follow the general guidelines in Appendix A.

> Establish IV fluid line for the injection of emergency drugs, radionuclide, and sedatives.

> Administer an antianxiety agent, as ordered, if the patient has claustrophobia. Administer a sedative to a child or to an uncooperative adult, as ordered.

> Place the patient in a supine position

on a flat table with foam wedges to help maintain position and immobilization. The radionuclide is administered intravenously, and the abdomen is scanned immediately for 1 minute to screen for vascular lesions that cause bleeding. Images are taken every 5 minutes for the next 60 minutes in the anterior, oblique, and lateral views, and a postvoid anterior view is taken.

➤ Wear gloves during the radionuclide injection and while handling the patient's urine.

➤ Instruct the patient to take slow, deep breaths if nausea occurs during the procedure. Monitor and administer an antiemetic agent if ordered. Ready an emesis basin for use.

➤ Monitor the patient for complications related to the procedure (e.g., allergic reaction, anaphylaxis, bronchospasm).

➤ The needle or catheter is removed, and a pressure dressing is applied over the puncture site.

➤ The results are recorded on film or in a computerized system for recall and postprocedure interpretation by the appropriate health care practitioner.

Post-test:

➤ Monitor vital signs and neurologic status every 15 minutes for 1 hour, then every 2 hours for 4 hours, and then as ordered by the health care practitioner. Compare with baseline values. Protocols may vary from facility to facility.

➤ Observe for delayed allergic reactions, such as rash, urticaria, tachycardia, hyperpnea, hypertension, palpitations, nausea, or vomiting.

➤ Advise the patient to immediately report symptoms such as fast heart rate, difficulty breathing, skin rash, itching, or decreased urinary output.

➤ Observe the needle/catheter insertion site for bleeding, inflammation, or hematoma formation.

➤ Instruct the patient to apply cold compresses to the puncture site, as needed, to reduce discomfort or edema.

➤ Instruct the patient to drink increased amounts of fluids for 24 to 48 hours to eliminate the radionuclide from the body, unless contraindicated. Tell the patient that radionuclide is eliminated from the body within 6 to 24 hours.

➤ Instruct the patient to flush the toilet immediately after each voiding following the procedure, and to wash hands meticulously with soap and water after each voiding for 24 hours after the procedure.

➤ Instruct all caregivers to wear gloves when discarding urine for 24 hours after the procedure. Wash gloved hands with soap and water before removing gloves. Then wash hands after the gloves are removed.

➤ If a woman who is breast-feeding must have a nuclear scan, she should not breast-feed the infant until the radionuclide has been eliminated. This could take as long as 3 days. She should be instructed to express the milk and discard it during the 3-day period to prevent cessation of milk production.

➤ *Nutritional considerations:* A low-fat, low-cholesterol, and low-sodium diet should be consumed to reduce current disease processes. High fat consumption increases the amount of bile acids in the colon and should be avoided.

➤ No other radionuclide tests should be scheduled for 24 to 48 hours after this procedure.

➤ A written report of the examination will be completed by a health care practitioner specializing in this branch of medicine. The report will be sent to the requesting health care practitioner, who will discuss the results with the patient.

➤ Recognize anxiety related to test results, and be supportive of perceived loss of independent function. Discuss the implications of abnormal test results on the patient's lifestyle. Provide teaching and information

regarding the clinical implications of the test results, as appropriate.

➤ Reinforce information given by the patient's health care provider regarding further testing, treatment, or referral to another health care provider. Answer any questions or address any concerns voiced by the patient or family.

➤ Instruct the patient in the use of any ordered medications. Explain the importance of adhering to the therapy regimen. As appropriate, instruct the patient in significant side effects and systemic reactions associated with the prescribed medication. Encourage him or her to review corresponding literature provided by a pharmacist.

➤ Depending on the results of this procedure, additional testing may be needed to evaluate or monitor progression of the disease process and determine the need for a change in therapy. Evaluate test results in relation to the patient's symptoms and other tests performed.

Related diagnostic tests:

➤ Related diagnostic tests include angiography of the abdomen, computed tomography of the abdomen, and magnetic resonance imaging of the abdomen.

GLUCAGON

. . . .

SYNONYM/ACRONYM: N/A.

SPECIMEN: Plasma (1 mL) collected in chilled, lavender-top (EDTA) tube. Specimen should be transported tightly capped and in an ice slurry.

REFERENCE VALUE: (Method: Radioimmunoassay)

Age	Conventional Units	SI Units (Conventional Units ×1)
Cord blood	0–215 pg/mL	0–215 ng/L
1–3 d	0–1750 pg/mL	0–1750 ng/L
4–14 y	0–148 pg/mL	0–148 ng/L
Adult	20–100 pg/mL	20–100 ng/L

DESCRIPTION & RATIONALE: Glucagon is a hormone secreted by the alpha cells of the islets of Langerhans in the pancreas in response to hypoglycemia. This hormone acts primarily on the liver to promote glucose production and to control glucose storage. The coordinated release of insulin, glucagon, and somatostatin ensures an adequate fuel supply while maintaining stable blood glucose. Patients with glucagonoma have values greater than 500 ng/L. Values greater than 1000 ng/L are diagnostic for this condition. Glucagonoma causes three different syndromes:

1. *Syndrome 1:* A characteristic skin rash, diabetes or impaired glucose tolerance, weight loss, anemia, and venous thrombosis
2. *Syndrome 2:* Severe diabetes
3. *Syndrome 3:* Multiple endocrine neoplasia

A dramatic increase in glucagon occurring soon after renal transplant may indicate organ rejection. In the case of kidney transplant rejection, glucagon levels increase several days before an increase in creatinine levels.

Glucagon deficiency can be confirmed by measuring glucagon levels before and after intravenous infusion of 0.5 g arginine/kg. Glucagon deficiency is confirmed when levels fail to rise 30 to 60 minutes after infusion. Newborn infants of diabetic mothers have impaired glucagon secretion, which may play a role in their hypoglycemia. ■

INDICATIONS:

• Assist in confirming glucagon deficiency

• Assist in the diagnosis of suspected glucagonoma (alpha islet-cell neoplastic tumor)

• Assist in the diagnosis of suspected renal failure or renal transplant rejection

RESULT

Increased in:
• Acromegaly
• Acute pancreatitis
• Burns
• Cirrhosis
• Cushing's syndrome
• Diabetes (uncontrolled)
• Glucagonoma
• Hyperlipoproteinemia types III and IV
• Hypoglycemia
• Infections
• Kidney transplant rejection
• Renal failure
• Stress
• Trauma

Decreased in:
• Chronic pancreatitis
• Cystic fibrosis
• Postpancreatectomy period

CRITICAL VALUES: N/A

INTERFERING FACTORS:

• Drugs that may increase glucagon levels include amino acids (e.g., arginine), cholecystokinin, danazol, gastrin, glucocorticoids, insulin, and nifedipine.

• Drugs that may decrease glucagon levels include atenolol, pindolol, propranolol, secretin, and verapamil.

• Recent radioactive scans or radiation within 1 week before the test can interfere with test results when radioimmunoassay is the test method.

• Failure to follow dietary restrictions before the procedure may cause the procedure to be canceled or repeated.

Nursing Implications and Procedure • • • • • • • • • • •

➤ Inform the patient that the test is used to assist in the diagnosis of glucagonoma.

➤ Obtain a history of the patient's complaints, including a list of known allergens (especially allergies or sensitivities to latex), and inform the appropriate health care practitioner accordingly.

➤ Obtain a history of the patient's endocrine system as well as results of previously performed laboratory tests, surgical procedures, and other diagnostic procedures. For related laboratory tests, refer to the Endocrine System table.

➤ Note any recent procedures that can interfere with test results.

➤ Obtain a list of medications the patient is taking, including herbs, nutritional supplements, and nutraceuticals. The requesting health care practitioner and laboratory should be advised if the patient regularly uses these products so that their effects can be taken into consideration when reviewing results.

➤ Review the procedure with the patient. Inform the patient that specimen collection takes approximately 5 to 10 minutes. Address concerns about pain related to the procedure. Explain to the patient that there may be some discomfort during the venipuncture.

➤ Instruct the patient to fast for at least 12 hours before specimen collection for baseline values. Diabetic patients should be in good glycemic control before testing.

➤ There are no fluid or medication restrictions unless by medical direction.

➤ Prepare an ice slurry in a cup or plastic bag to have ready for immediate transport of the specimen to the laboratory. Prechill the lavender-top tube in the ice slurry.

➤ Ensure that the patient has complied with dietary restrictions; assure that food has been restricted for at least 12 hours prior to the procedure.

➤ If the patient has a history of severe allergic reaction to latex, care should be taken to avoid the use of equipment containing latex.

➤ Instruct the patient to cooperate fully and to follow directions. Direct the patient to breathe normally and to avoid unnecessary movement.

➤ Observe standard precautions, and follow the general guidelines in Appendix A. Positively identify the patient, and label the appropriate tubes with the corresponding patient demographics, date, and time of collection. Perform a venipuncture; collect the specimen in a chilled 5-mL lavender-top tube. The sample should be placed in an ice slurry immediately after collection. Information on the specimen label can be protected from water in the ice slurry if the specimen is first placed in a protective plastic bag.

➤ Remove the needle, and apply a pressure dressing over the puncture site.

➤ Promptly transport the specimen to the laboratory for processing and analysis.

➤ The results are recorded manually or in a computerized system for recall and postprocedure interpretation by the appropriate health care practitioner.

➤ Observe venipuncture site for bleeding or hematoma formation. Apply paper tape or other adhesive to hold pressure bandage in place, or replace with a plastic bandage.

➤ Instruct the patient to resume usual diet, as directed by the health care practitioner.

➤ *Nutritional considerations:* Instruct the diabetic patient, as appropriate, in nutritional management of the disease. Patients who adhere to dietary recommendations report a better general feeling of health, better weight management, greater control of glucose and lipid values, and improved use of insulin. There is no "diabetic diet"; however, many meal-planning approaches with nutritional goals are endorsed by the American Dietetic Association. The nutritional needs of each diabetic patient must be determined individually with the appropriate health care professionals, particularly professionals trained in nutrition.

➤ Increased glucagon levels may be associated with diabetes. Instruct the patient and caregiver to report signs and symptoms of hypoglycemia (weakness, confusion, diaphoresis, rapid pulse) or hyperglycemia (thirst, polyuria, hunger, lethargy).

➤ A written report of the examination will be sent to the requesting health care practitioner, who will discuss the results with the patient.

➤ Recognize anxiety related to test results, and be supportive of perceived loss of independence and fear of shortened life expectancy. Discuss the implications of abnormal test results on the patient's lifestyle. Provide teaching and information regarding the clinical implications of the test results, as appropriate. Emphasize, as appropriate, that good glycemic control delays the onset and slows the progression of diabetic retinopathy, nephropathy, and neuropathy. Educate the patient regarding access to counseling services. Provide contact information, if desired, for the American Diabetes Association *(http://www.diabetes.org)*.

➤ Reinforce information given by the patient's health care provider regarding further testing, treatment, or referral to another health care provider. Answer any questions or address any concerns voiced by the patient or family.

➤ Depending on the results of this procedure, additional testing may be performed to evaluate or monitor progression of the disease process and determine the need for a change in therapy. Evaluate test results in relation to the patient's symptoms and other tests performed.

Related laboratory tests:

➤ Related laboratory tests include glucose, glucose tolerance tests, glycated hemoglobin A_{1C}, insulin, insulin antibodies, and microalbumin.

GLUCOSE

. . . .

SYNONYMS/ACRONYMS: Blood sugar, fasting blood sugar (FBS), postprandial glucose, 2-hour PC.

SPECIMEN: Serum (1 mL) collected in a red- or tiger-top tube. Plasma (1 mL) collected in gray-top (sodium fluoride) or green-top (heparin) tube is also acceptable.

REFERENCE VALUE: (Method: Spectrophotometry)

Age	Conventional Units	SI Units (Conventional Units ×0.0555)
Fasting		
Cord blood	45–96 mg/dL	2.5–5.3 mmol/L
Premature infant	20–60 mg/dL	1.1–3.3 mmol/L
Neonate	30–60 mg/dL	1.7–3.3 mmol/L
Newborn 1 d	40–60 mg/dL	2.2–3.3 mmol/L
Newborn 2 d–2 y	50–80 mg/dL	2.8–4.4 mmol/L
Child	60–100 mg/dL	3.3–5.6 mmol/L
Adult	65–99 mg/dL	3.6–5.5 mmol/L
Prediabetes or Impaired Fasting Glucose	100–125 mg/dL	5.6–6.9 mmol/L
2-Hour Postprandial		
2-h Postprandial	Less than 105 mg/dL	Less than 5.8 mmol/L

DESCRIPTION & RATIONALE: Glucose, a simple six-carbon sugar (monosaccharide), enters the diet as part of the sugars sucrose, lactose, and maltose and as the major constituent of the complex polysaccharide called dietary starch. The body acquires most of its energy from the oxidative metabolism of glucose. Excess glucose is stored in the liver or in muscle tissue as glycogen.

Diabetes is a group of diseases characterized by hyperglycemia or elevated glucose levels. Hyperglycemia results from a defect in insulin secretion (type 1 diabetes), a defect in insulin action, or a combination of defects in secretion and action (type 2 diabetes). The chronic hyperglycemia of diabetes may result over time in damage, dysfunction, and eventually failure of the eyes, kidneys, nerves, heart, and blood vessels. The American Diabetes Association's criteria for diagnosing diabetes include any combination of the following findings or confirmation of any of the individual findings by repetition on a subsequent day:

- Symptoms of diabetes (e.g., polyuria, polydipsia, unexplained weight loss) in addition to a random glucose level greater than 200 mg/dL
- Fasting blood glucose greater than 126 mg/dL, after a minimum of an 8-hour fast
- Glucose level greater than 200 mg/dL 2 hours after glucose challenge with standardized 75-mg load ■

INDICATIONS:
- Assist in the diagnosis of insulinoma
- Determine insulin requirements
- Evaluate disorders of carbohydrate metabolism
- Identify hypoglycemia
- Screen for diabetes

RESULT

Increased in:
- Acromegaly, gigantism
- Acute stress reaction
- Cerebrovascular accident
- Cushing's syndrome

- Diabetes
- Glucagonoma
- Hemochromatosis
- Liver disease (severe)
- Myocardial infarction
- Pancreatic adenoma
- Pancreatitis (acute and chronic)
- Pancreatitis due to mumps
- Pheochromocytoma
- Renal disease (severe)
- Shock, trauma
- Somatostatinoma
- Strenuous exercise
- Syndrome X (metabolic syndrome)
- Thyrotoxicosis
- Vitamin B_1 deficiency

Decreased in:
- Acute alcohol ingestion
- Addison's disease
- Ectopic insulin production from tumors (adrenal carcinoma, carcinoma of the stomach, fibrosarcoma)
- Excess insulin by injection
- Galactosemia
- Glucagon deficiency
- Glycogen storage diseases
- Hereditary fructose intolerance
- Hypopituitarism
- Hypothyroidism
- Insulinoma
- Malabsorption syndromes
- Maple syrup urine disease
- Poisoning resulting in severe liver disease
- Postgastrectomy
- Starvation
- von Gierke disease

CRITICAL VALUES:
Less than 40 mg/dL
Greater than 400 mg/dL
Note and immediately report to the health care practitioner any critically increased or decreased values and related symptoms.

Symptoms of decreased glucose levels include headache, confusion, hunger, irritability, nervousness, restlessness, sweating, and weakness. Possible interventions include oral or intravenous (IV) administration of glucose, IV or intramuscular injection of glucagon, and continuous glucose monitoring.

Symptoms of elevated glucose levels include abdominal pain, fatigue, muscle cramps, nausea, vomiting, polyuria, and thirst. Possible interventions include subcutaneous or IV injection of insulin with continuous glucose monitoring.

INTERFERING FACTORS:
- Drugs that may increase glucose levels include acetazolamide, alanine, albuterol, anesthetic agents, antipyrine, atenolol, betamethasone, cefotaxime, chlorpromazine, chlorprothixene, clonidine, clorexolone, corticotropin, cortisone, cyclic AMP, cyclopropane, dexamethasone, dextroamphetamine, diapamide, epinephrine, enflurane, ethacrynic acid, ether, fludrocortisone, fluoxymesterone, furosemide, glucagon, glucocorticoids, homoharringtonine, hydrochlorothiazide, hydroxydione, isoniazid, maltose, meperidine, meprednisone, methyclothiazide, metolazone, niacin, nifedipine, nortriptyline, octreotide, oral contraceptives, oxyphenbutazone, pancreozymin, phenelzine, phenylbutazone, piperacetazine, polythiazide, prednisone, quinethazone, reserpine, rifampin, ritodrine, salbutamol, secretin, somatostatin, thiazides, thyroid hormone, and triamcinolone.

- Drugs that may decrease glucose levels include acarbose, acetylsalicylic acid, acipimox, alanine, allopurinol, antimony compounds, arsenicals, ascorbic acid, benzene, buformin, cannabis, captopril, carbutamide, chloroform, clofibrate, dexfenfluramine, enalapril, enprostil, erythromycin, fenfluramine, gemfibrozil, glibornuride, glyburide, guanethidine, niceritrol, nitrazepam, oral contraceptives, oxandrolone, oxymetholone, phentolamine, phosphorus, promethazine, ramipril, rotenone, sulfonylureas, thioclaride, tolbutamide, tromethamine, and verapamil.

- Elevated urea levels and uremia can lead to falsely elevated glucose levels.

- Extremely elevated white blood cell counts can lead to falsely decreased glucose values.

- Failure to follow dietary restrictions before the fasting test can lead to falsely elevated glucose values.

- Administration of insulin or oral hypoglycemic agents within 8 hours of a fasting blood glucose can lead to falsely decreased values.

- Specimens should never be collected above an intravenous (IV) line because of the potential for dilution when the specimen and the IV solution combine in the collection container, falsely decreasing the result. There is also the potential of contaminating the sample with the substance of interest, if it is present in the IV solution, falsely increasing the result.

- Failure to follow dietary restrictions before the procedure may cause the procedure to be canceled or repeated.

Nursing Implications and Procedure • • • • • • • • • • •

Pretest:

> Inform the patient that the test is used to to assist in the diagnosis of diabetes and to evaluate disorders of carbohydrate metabolism.

> Obtain a history of the patient's complaints, including a list of known allergens (especially allergies or sensitivities to latex), and inform the appropriate health care practitioner accordingly.

> Obtain a history of the patient's endocrine system as well as results of previously performed laboratory tests, surgical procedures, and other diagnostic procedures. For related laboratory tests, refer to the Endocrine System table.

> Obtain a list of medications the patient is taking, including herbs, nutritional supplements, nutraceuticals, insulin, and any other substances used to regulate glucose levels. The requesting health care practitioner and laboratory should be advised if the patient regularly uses these products so that their effects can be taken into consideration when reviewing results.

> Review the procedure with the patient. Inform the patient that specimen collection takes approximately 5 to 10 minutes. Address concerns about pain related to the procedure. Explain to the patient that there may be some discomfort during the venipuncture.

> For the fasting glucose test, the patient should fast for at least 12 hours before specimen collection.

> There are no fluid or medication restrictions, unless by medical direction.

> The patient should follow the instructions given for 2-hour postprandial glucose test. Some health care practitioners may order administration of a standard glucose solution, whereas others may instruct the patient to eat a meal with a known carbohydrate composition.

Intratest:

> Ensure that the patient has complied with dietary restrictions and other pretesting preparations; assure that food has been restricted for at least 12 hours prior to the fasting procedure.

> If the patient has a history of severe allergic reaction to latex, care should

be taken to avoid the use of equipment containing latex.

➤ Instruct the patient to cooperate fully and to follow directions. Direct the patient to breathe normally and to avoid unnecessary movement.

➤ Observe standard precautions, and follow the general guidelines in Appendix A. Positively identify the patient, and label the appropriate tubes with the corresponding patient demographics, date, and time of collection. Perform a venipuncture; collect the specimen in a 5-mL gray-top tube.

➤ Remove the needle, and apply a pressure dressing over the puncture site.

➤ Promptly transport the specimen to the laboratory for processing and analysis.

➤ The results are recorded manually or in a computerized system for recall and postprocedure interpretation by the appropriate health care practitioner.

Post-test:

➤ Observe venipuncture site for bleeding or hematoma formation. Apply paper tape or other adhesive to hold pressure bandage in place, or replace with a plastic bandage.

➤ Instruct the patient to resume usual diet, as directed by the health care practitioner.

➤ *Nutritional considerations:* Increased glucose levels may be associated with diabetes. Instruct the diabetic patient, as appropriate, in nutritional management of the disease. Patients who adhere to dietary recommendations report a better general feeling of health, better weight management, greater control of glucose and lipid values, and improved use of insulin. There is no "diabetic diet"; however, many meal-planning approaches with nutritional goals are endorsed by the American Dietetic Association. The nutritional needs of each diabetic patient must be determined individually with the appropriate health care professionals,

particularly professionals trained in nutrition.

➤ Instruct the patient and caregiver to report signs and symptoms of hypoglycemia (weakness, confusion, diaphoresis, rapid pulse) or hyperglycemia (thirst, polyuria, hunger, lethargy).

➤ A written report of the examination will be sent to the requesting health care practitioner, who will discuss the results with the patient.

➤ Recognize anxiety related to test results, and be supportive of perceived loss of independence and fear of shortened life expectancy. Discuss the implications of abnormal test results on the patient's lifestyle. Provide teaching and information regarding the clinical implications of the test results, as appropriate. Emphasize, as appropriate, that good glycemic control delays the onset of and slows the progression of diabetic retinopathy, nephropathy, and neuropathy. Educate the patient regarding access to counseling services. Provide contact information, if desired, for the American Diabetes Association *(http://www.diabetes. org).*

➤ Reinforce information given by the patient's health care provider regarding further testing, treatment, or referral to another health care provider. Answer any questions or address any concerns voiced by the patient or family.

➤ Depending on the results of this procedure, additional testing may be performed to evaluate or monitor progression of the disease process and determine the need for a change in therapy. Evaluate test results in relation to the patient's symptoms and other tests performed.

Related laboratory tests:

➤ Related laboratory tests include blood urea nitrogen, C-peptide, creatinine, fructosamine, glucose tolerance tests, glycated hemoglobin A_{1C}, insulin, insulin antibodies, ketones, and microalbumin.

GLUCOSE-6-PHOSPHATE DEHYDROGENASE

SYNONYM/ACRONYM: G6PD.

SPECIMEN: Whole blood (1 mL) collected in a lavender-top (ethylenediaminetetra-acetic acid [EDTA]) tube.

REFERENCE VALUE: (Method: Fluorescent) Qualitative assay—enzyme activity detected; quantitative assay—the following table reflects enzyme activity in units per gram of hemoglobin and in units per milliliter of erythrocytes:

Age	Conventional Units	SI Units
		(Conventional Units ×0.0645)
Newborn	7.8–14.4 U/g hemoglobin	0.5–0.93 MU/mol hemoglobin
Adult	5.5–9.3 U/g hemoglobin	0.35–0.60 MU/mol hemoglobin
		(Conventional Units ×1)
Newborn	2.65–4.90 U/mL erythrocytes	2.65–4.90 kU/L erythrocytes
Adult	1.87–3.16 U/mL erythrocytes	1.87–3.16 kU/L erythrocytes

DESCRIPTION & RATIONALE: Glucose-6-phosphate dehydrogenase (G6PD) is a red blood cell enzyme. It is involved in the hexose monophosphate shunt, and its function is to protect hemoglobin from oxidation. G6PD deficiency is an inherited X-linked abnormality; approximately 20% of female carriers are heterozygous. This deficiency results in hemolysis of varying degrees and acuity depending on the severity of the abnormality. There are three G6PD variants of high frequency in different ethnic groups. G6PD A⁻ is more common in African-Americans (10% of males). G6PD Mediterranean is especially common in Iraqis, Kurds, Sephardic Jews, and Lebanese and less

common in Greeks, Italians, Turks, North Africans, Spaniards, Portuguese, and Ashkenazic Jews. G6PD Mahidol is common in Southeast Asians (22% of males). ■

INDICATIONS:
- Assist in identifying the cause of hemolytic anemia resulting from drug sensitivity, metabolic disorder, or infection
- Assist in identifying the cause of hemolytic anemia resulting from enzyme deficiency

RESULT

Increased in:
- Hepatic coma
- Hyperthyroidism

- Idiopathic thrombocytopenic purpura
- Myocardial infarction
- Pernicious anemia
- Viral hepatitis

Decreased in:
- Congenital nonspherocytic anemia
- G6PD deficiency
- Nonimmunologic hemolytic disease of the newborn

CRITICAL VALUES: N/A

INTERFERING FACTORS:
- Sulfates may decrease G6PD levels.
- G6PD levels are increased in reticulocytes; the test results may be falsely positive when a patient is in a period of acute hemolysis. G6PD levels can also be affected by the presence of large numbers of platelets and white blood cells, which also contain significant amounts of the enzyme.

Nursing Implications and Procedure • • • • • • • • • • •

Pretest:

➤ Inform the patient that the test is used to identify an enzyme deficiency that can result in red blood cell hemolysis.

➤ Obtain a history of the patient's complaints, including a list of known allergens (especially allergies or sensitivities to latex), and inform the appropriate health care practitioner accordingly.

➤ Obtain a history of the patient's hematopoietic system as well as results of previously performed laboratory tests, surgical procedures, and other diagnostic procedures. For related laboratory tests, refer to the Hematopoietic System table.

➤ Obtain a list of medications the patient is taking, including herbs, nutritional supplements, and nutraceuticals. The requesting health care practitioner and laboratory should be advised if the patient regularly uses these products so that their effects can be taken into consideration when reviewing results.

➤ Review the procedure with the patient. Inform the patient that specimen collection takes approximately 5 to 10 minutes. Address concerns about pain related to the procedure. Explain to the patient that there may be some discomfort during the venipuncture.

➤ There are no food, fluid, or medication restrictions, unless by medical direction.

Intratest:

➤ If the patient has a history of severe allergic reaction to latex, care should be taken to avoid the use of equipment containing latex.

➤ Instruct the patient to cooperate fully and to follow directions. Direct the patient to breathe normally and to avoid unnecessary movement.

➤ Observe standard precautions, and follow the general guidelines in Appendix A. Positively identify the patient, and label the appropriate tubes with the corresponding patient demographics, date, and time of collection. Perform a venipuncture; collect the specimen in a 5-mL lavender-top tube.

➤ Remove the needle, and apply a pressure dressing over the puncture site.

➤ Promptly transport the specimen to the laboratory for processing and analysis.

➤ The results are recorded manually or in a computerized system for recall and postprocedure interpretation by the appropriate health care practitioner.

Post-test:

➤ Observe venipuncture site for bleeding or hematoma formation. Apply paper tape or other adhesive to hold pressure bandage in place, or replace with a plastic bandage.

➤ *Nutritional considerations:* Educate the patient with G6PD deficiency, as appropriate, to avoid certain foods, vitamins, and drugs that may precipitate an acute episode of intravascular hemolysis, including fava beans, ascorbic acid (large doses), acetanilid, antimalarials, furazolidone, isobutyl nitrate, methylene blue, nalidixic acid, naphthalene, niridazole, nitrofurantoin, phenazopyridine, phenylhydrazine, primaquine, sulfacetamide, sulfamethoxazole, sulfanilamide, sulfapyridine, thiazolesulfone, toluidine blue, trinitrotoluene, and urate oxidase.

➤ A written report of the examination will be sent to the requesting health care practitioner, who will discuss the results with the patient.

➤ Reinforce information given by the patient's health care provider regarding further testing, treatment, or referral to another health care provider. Answer any questions or address any concerns voiced by the patient or family.

➤ Depending on the results of this procedure, additional testing may be performed to evaluate or monitor progression of the disease process and determine the need for a change in therapy. Evaluate test results in relation to the patient's symptoms and other tests performed.

Related laboratory tests:

➤ Related laboratory tests include bilirubin, complete blood count (including examination of peripheral smear for red blood cell abnormalities and the presence of Heinz bodies), Ham's test, haptoglobin, hemosiderin, osmotic fragility, reticulocyte count, urinalysis (for hemoglobin and urobilinogen), and vitamin B_{12}.

GLUCOSE TOLERANCE TESTS

. . . .

SYNONYMS/ACRONYM: Standard oral tolerance test, standard gestational screen, standard gestational tolerance test, GTT.

SPECIMEN: Plasma (1 mL) collected in gray-top (sodium fluoride) tube. Serum (1 mL) collected in a red- or tiger-top tube or plasma collected in a green-top (heparin) tube is also acceptable. It is important to use the same type of collection container throughout the entire test.

REFERENCE VALUE: (Method: Spectrophotometry)

	Conventional Units	SI Units (Conventional Units × 0.0555)
Standard Oral Tolerance		
Fasting sample	Less than 126 mg/dL	Less than 7.0 mmol/L
2-h sample	Less than 200 mg/dL	Less than 11.1 mmol/L
Prediabetes or Impaired Glucose Tolerance	140–199 mg/dL	7.8–11.0 mmol/L
Standard Gestational Screen	Less than 141 mg/dL	Less than 7.8 mmol/L

(Continued on the following page)

	Conventional Units	SI Units (Conventional Units × 0.0555)
Standard Gestational Tolerance		
Fasting sample	75–104 mg/dL	4.2–5.8 mmol/L
1-h sample	75–180 mg/dL	4.2–10.0 mmol/L
2-h sample	75–164 mg/dL	4.2–9.1 mmol/L
3-h sample	75–144 mg/dL	4.2–8.0 mmol/L

Plasma glucose values are reported to be 10%–20% higher than serum values.

DESCRIPTION & RATIONALE: The glucose tolerance test (GTT) measures glucose levels after administration of an oral or intravenous carbohydrate challenge. Patients with diabetes are unable to metabolize glucose at a normal rate. The oral GTT is used for individuals who are able to eat and who are not known to have problems with gastrointestinal malabsorption. The intravenous GTT is used for individuals who are unable to tolerate oral glucose.

Diabetes is a group of diseases characterized by hyperglycemia or elevated glucose levels. Hyperglycemia results from a defect in insulin secretion (type 1 diabetes), a defect in insulin action, or a combination of dysfunction secretion and action (type 2 diabetes). The chronic hyperglycemia of diabetes over time results in damage, dysfunction, and eventually failure of the eyes, kidneys, nerves, heart, and blood vessels. The American Diabetes Association's criteria for diagnosing diabetes include any combination of the following findings or confirmation of any of the individual findings by repetition on a subsequent day:

- Symptoms of diabetes (e.g., polyuria, polydipsia, and unexplained weight loss) in addition to a random glucose level greater than 200 mg/dL

- Fasting blood glucose greater than 126 mg/dL, after a minimum of an 8-hour fast
- Glucose level greater than 200 mg/dL 2 hours after glucose challenge with standardized 75-mg load ■

INDICATIONS:
- Evaluate abnormal fasting or postprandial blood glucose levels that do not clearly indicate diabetes
- Evaluate glucose metabolism in women of childbearing age, especially women who are pregnant and have (1) a history of previous fetal loss or birth of infants weighing 9 pounds or more, and/or (2) a family history of diabetes
- Identify abnormal renal tubular function if glycosuria occurs without hyperglycemia
- Identify impaired glucose metabolism without overt diabetes
- Support the diagnosis of hyperthyroidism and alcoholic liver disease, which are characterized by a sharp rise in blood glucose followed by a decline to subnormal levels

RESULT

Tolerance increased in:
- Decreased absorption of glucose:
  Adrenal insufficiency (Addison's disease, hypopituitarism)
  Hypothyroidism

Intestinal diseases, such as celiac disease and tropical sprue
Whipple's disease

- Increased insulin secretion:
Pancreatic islet cell tumor

Tolerance impaired in:
- Increased absorption of glucose:
Excessive intake of glucose
Gastrectomy
Gastroenterostomy
Hyperthyroidism
Vagotomy

- Decreased usage of glucose:
Central nervous system lesions
Cushing's syndrome
Diabetes
Hemochromatosis
Hyperlipidemia

- Decreased glycogenesis:
Hyperthyroidism
Infections
Liver disease (severe)
Pheochromocytoma
Pregnancy
Stress
von Gierke disease

CRITICAL VALUES:
Less than 40 mg/dL
Greater than 400 mg/dL
Note and immediately report to the health care practitioner any critically increased or decreased values and related symptoms.

Symptoms of decreased glucose levels include headache, confusion, hunger, irritability, nervousness, restlessness, sweating, and weakness. Possible interventions include oral or intravenous (IV) administration of glucose, IV or intramuscular injection of glucagon, and continuous glucose monitoring.

Symptoms of elevated glucose levels include abdominal pain, fatigue, muscle cramps, nausea, vomiting, polyuria, and thirst. Possible interventions include sub- cutaneous or IV injection of insulin with continuous glucose monitoring.

INTERFERING FACTORS:
- Drugs and substances that may increase GTT values include acetylsalicylic acid, atenolol, bendroflumethiazide, clofibrate, fenfluramine, fluoxymesterone, glyburide, guanethidine, lisinopril, methandrostenolone, metoprolol, nandrolone, niceritrol, nifedipine, nitrendipine, norethisterone, phenformin, phenobarbital, prazosin, terazosin, and caffeine.

- Drugs and substances that may decrease GTT values include acebutolol, beclomethasone, bendroflumethiazide, betamethasone, calcitonin, catecholamines, chlorothiazide, chlorpromazine, chlorthalidone, cimetidine, corticotropin, cortisone, danazol, deflazacort, dexamethasone, diapamide, diethylstilbestrol, ethacrynic acid, fludrocortisone, furosemide, glucagon, glucocorticosteroids, heroin, hydrochlorothiazide, mephenytoin, mestranol, methadone, methandrostenolone, methylprednisolone, muzolimine, niacin, nifedipine, norethindrone, norethy nodrel, oral contraceptives, paramethasone, perphenazine, phenolphthalein, phenothiazine, phenytoin, pindolol, prednisolone, prednisone, propranolol, quinethazone, thiazides, triamcinolone, triamterene, and verapamil.

- The test should be performed on ambulatory patients. Impaired physical activity can lead to falsely increased values.

- Excessive physical activity before or during the test can lead to falsely decreased values.

- Failure of the patient to ingest a diet with sufficient carbohydrate content (e.g., 150 g/day) for at least 3 days before the test can result in falsely decreased values.

- Smoking before or during the test can lead to falsely increased values.

- The patient should not be under recent or current physiologic stress during the test. If the patient has had recent surgery (less than 2 weeks previously), an infectious disease, or a major illness (e.g., myocardial infarction), the test should be delayed or rescheduled.

- Failure to follow dietary restrictions before the procedure may cause the procedure to be canceled or repeated.

Nursing Implications and Procedure • • • • • • • • • • • •

Pretest:

➤ Inform the patient that the test is used to assist in the diagnosis of diabetes.

➤ Obtain a history of the patient's complaints, including a list of known allergens (especially allergies or sensitivities to latex), and inform the appropriate health care practitioner accordingly.

➤ Obtain a history of the patient's endocrine system as well as results of previously performed laboratory tests, surgical procedures, and other diagnostic procedures. For related laboratory tests, refer to the Endocrine System table.

➤ Obtain a list of medications the patient is taking, including herbs, nutritional supplements, and nutraceuticals. The requesting health care practitioner and laboratory should be advised if the patient regularly uses these products so that their effects can be taken into consideration when reviewing results.

➤ Review the procedure with the patient. Inform the patient that specimen collection takes approximately 5 to 10 minutes. Inform the patient that multiple specimens may be required. Address concerns about pain related to the procedure. Explain to the patient that there may be some discomfort during the venipuncture.

➤ The patient should fast for at least 8

to 12 hours before the standard oral and standard gestational GTTs.

➤ There are no fluid or medication restrictions, unless by medical direction.

Intratest:

➤ Ensure that the patient has complied with dietary and activity restrictions as well as other pretesting preparations; assure that food has been restricted for at least 8 to 12 hours prior to the procedure.

➤ If the patient has a history of severe allergic reaction to latex, care should be taken to avoid the use of equipment containing latex.

➤ Instruct the patient to cooperate fully and to follow directions. Direct the patient to breathe normally and to avoid unnecessary movement.

➤ Observe standard precautions, and follow the general guidelines in Appendix A. Positively identify the patient, and label the appropriate tubes with the corresponding patient demographics, date, and time of collection. Perform a venipuncture; collect the specimen in a 5-mL gray-top tube.

➤ Remove the needle, and apply a pressure dressing over the puncture site.

➤ Promptly transport the specimen to the laboratory for processing and analysis. Do not wait until all specimens have been collected to transport.

➤ The results are recorded manually or in a computerized system for recall and postprocedure interpretation by the appropriate health care practitioner.

Standard oral GTT:

➤ The standard oral GTT takes 2 hours. A fasting blood glucose is determined before administration of an oral glucose load. If the fasting blood glucose is less than 126 mg/dL, the patient is given an oral glucose load.

➤ An oral glucose load should not be administered *before* the value of the fasting specimen has been received. *If the fasting blood glucose is greater than 126 mg/dL, the standard glucose load is not administered and the test is canceled.* The laboratory will follow its protocol as far as notifying the patient of his or her glucose level and the reason why the test was canceled. The requesting health care practitioner will then be issued a report indicating the glucose level and the cancellation of the test. A fasting glucose greater than 126 mg/dL indicates diabetes; therefore, the glucola would never be administered before allowing the requesting health care practitioner to evaluate the clinical situation.

➤ Adults receive 75 g and children receive 1.75 g/kg ideal weight, not to exceed 75 g. The glucose load should be consumed within 5 minutes, and time 0 begins as soon as the patient begins to ingest the glucose load. A second specimen is collected at 2 hours, concluding the test. The test is discontinued if the patient vomits before the second specimen has been collected.

Standard gestational screen:

➤ The standard gestational screen is performed on pregnant women. If results from the screen are abnormal, a full gestational GTT is performed. The gestational screen does not require a fast. The patient is given a 50-g oral glucose load. The glucose load should be consumed within 5 minutes, and time 0 begins as soon as the patient begins to ingest the glucose load. One hour after ingestion, a specimen is collected. The test is discontinued if the patient vomits before the 1-hour specimen has been collected.

Standard gestational GTT:

➤ The standard gestational GTT takes 3 hours. A fasting blood glucose is determined before administration of a 100-g oral glucose load. If the fasting blood glucose is less than 126 mg/dL, the patient is given an oral glucose load.

➤ An oral glucose load should not be administered *before* the value of the fasting specimen has been received. *If the fasting blood glucose is greater than 126 mg/dL, the glucola is not administered and the test is canceled* (see previous explanation).

➤ The glucose load should be consumed within 5 minutes, and time 0 begins as soon as the patient begins to ingest the glucose load. Subsequent specimens are collected at 1, 2, and 3 hours, concluding the test. The test is discontinued if the patient vomits before all specimens have been collected.

Post-test:

➤ Observe venipuncture site for bleeding or hematoma formation. Apply paper tape or other adhesive to hold pressure bandage in place, or replace with a plastic bandage.

➤ Instruct the patient to resume usual diet and activity, as directed by the health care practitioner.

➤ *Nutritional considerations:* Increased glucose levels may be associated with diabetes. Instruct the diabetic patient, as appropriate, in nutritional management of the disease. Patients who adhere to dietary recommendations report a better general feeling of health, better weight management, greater control of glucose and lipid values, and improved use of insulin. There is no "diabetic diet"; however, many meal-planning approaches with nutritional goals are endorsed by the American Dietetic Association. The nutritional needs of each diabetic patient need to be determined individually with the appropriate health care professionals, particularly professionals trained in nutrition.

➤ Impaired glucose tolerance may be associated with diabetes. Instruct the patient and caregiver to report signs and symptoms of hypoglycemia (weakness, confusion, diaphoresis, rapid pulse) or hyperglycemia (thirst, polyuria, hunger, lethargy).

➤ A written report of the examination

will be sent to the requesting health care practitioner, who will discuss the results with the patient.

➤ Recognize anxiety related to test results, and be supportive of perceived loss of independence and fear of shortened life expectancy. Discuss the implications of abnormal test results on the patient's lifestyle. Provide teaching and information regarding the clinical implications of the test results, as appropriate. Emphasize, as appropriate, that good glycemic control delays the onset of and slows the progression of diabetic retinopathy, nephropathy, and neuropathy. Educate the patient regarding access to counseling services. Provide contact information, if desired, for the American Diabetes Association *(http://www.diabetes. org)*.

➤ Reinforce information given by the patient's health care provider regarding further testing, treatment, or referral to another health care provider. Answer any questions or address any concerns voiced by the patient or family.

➤ Depending on the results of this procedure, additional testing may be performed to evaluate or monitor progression of the disease process and determine the need for a change in therapy. Evaluate test results in relation to the patient's symptoms and other tests performed.

Related laboratory tests:

➤ Related laboratory tests include blood urea nitrogen, C-peptide, cholesterol (total and HDL), creatinine, fructosamine, glucose, glycated hemoglobin A_{1c}, insulin, insulin antibodies, ketones, microalbumin, and triglycerides.

γ-GLUTAMYLTRANSFERASE

SYNONYMS/ACRONYMS: Serum γ-glutamyltransferase, γ-glutamyl transpeptidase, GGT, SGGT.

SPECIMEN: Serum (1 mL) collected in a red- or tiger-top tube. Plasma (1 mL) collected in green-top (heparin) tube is also acceptable.

REFERENCE VALUE: (Method: Spectrophotometry)

Sex	Conventional & SI Units
Male	1–94 U/L
Female	1–70 U/L

DESCRIPTION & RATIONALE: γ-Glutamyltransferase (GGT) assists with the reabsorption of amino acids and peptides from the glomerular filtrate and intestinal lumen. Hepatobiliary, renal tubular, and pancreatic tissues contain large amounts of GGT. Other sources include the prostate gland, brain, and heart. GGT is elevated in all types of liver disease and is more responsive to biliary obstruction, cholangitis, or cholecystitis than any of the other enzymes used as markers for liver disease. ■

INDICATIONS:

- Assist in the diagnosis of obstructive jaundice in neonates
- Detect the presence of liver disease
- Evaluate and monitor patients with known or suspected alcohol abuse (levels rise after ingestion of small amounts of alcohol)

RESULT

Increased in:
- Cirrhosis
- Diabetes with hypertension
- Hepatitis
- Hepatobiliary tract disorders
- Hepatocellular carcinoma
- Hyperthyroidism
- Obstructive liver disease
- Pancreatitis
- Renal transplantation
- Significant alcohol ingestion

Decreased in:
- Hypothyroidism

CRITICAL VALUES: N/A

INTERFERING FACTORS:
- Drugs that may increase GGT levels include acetaminophen, aminoglutethimide, anticonvulsants, barbiturates, captopril, clotiazepam, disulfiram, methyldopa, oral contraceptives, phenothiazines, rifampin, and streptokinase.
- Drugs that may decrease GGT levels include bezafibrate, cefotaxime, clofibrate, fenofibrate, and ursodiol.

Nursing Implications and Procedure • • • • • • • • • • •

Pretest:

➤ Inform the patient that the test is used to assess liver function.

➤ Obtain a history of the patient's complaints, including a list of known allergens (especially allergies or sensitivities to latex), and inform the appropriate health care practitioner accordingly.

➤ Obtain a history of the patient's hepatobiliary system as well as results of previously performed laboratory tests, surgical procedures, and other diagnostic procedures. For related laboratory tests, refer to the Hepatobiliary System table.

➤ Obtain a history of intravenous drug use, alcohol use, high-risk sexual activity, and occupational exposure.

➤ Obtain a list of the medications the patient is taking, including herbs, nutritional supplements, and nutraceuticals. The requesting health care practitioner and laboratory should be advised if the patient regularly uses these products so that their effects can be taken into consideration when reviewing results.

➤ Review the procedure with the patient. Inform the patient that specimen collection takes approximately 5 to 10 minutes. Address concerns about pain related to the procedure. Explain to the patient that there may be some discomfort during the venipuncture.

➤ *Sensitivity to social and cultural issues,* as well as concern for modesty, is important in providing psychological support before, during, and after the procedure.

➤ There are no food, fluid, or medication restrictions, unless by medical direction.

Intratest:

➤ If the patient has a history of severe allergic reaction to latex, care should be taken to avoid the use of equipment containing latex.

➤ Instruct the patient to cooperate fully and to follow directions. Direct the patient to breathe normally and to avoid unnecessary movement.

➤ Observe standard precautions, and follow the general guidelines in Appendix A. Positively identify the patient, and label the appropriate tubes with the corresponding patient demographics, date, and time of collection. Perform a venipuncture; collect the specimen in a 5-mL red- or tiger-top tube.

➤ Remove the needle, and apply a pressure dressing over the puncture site.

➤ Promptly transport the specimen to the laboratory for processing and analysis.

➤ The results are recorded manually or in a computerized system for recall and postprocedure interpretation by the appropriate health care practitioner.

Post-test:

➤ Observe venipuncture site for bleeding or hematoma formation. Apply paper tape or other adhesive to hold pressure bandage in place, or replace with a plastic bandage.

➤ *Nutritional considerations:* Increased GGT levels may be associated with liver disease. Dietary recommendations may be indicated and vary depending on the condition and its severity. Currently, there are no specific medications that can be given to cure hepatitis, but elimination of alcohol ingestion and a diet optimized for convalescence are commonly included in the treatment plan. A high-calorie, high-protein, moderate-fat diet with a high fluid intake is often recommended for patients with hepatitis. Treatment of cirrhosis is different because a low-protein diet may be in order if the patient's liver has lost the ability to process the end products of protein metabolism. A diet of soft foods also may be required if esophageal varices have developed. Ammonia levels may be used to determine whether protein should be added to or reduced from the diet. The patient should be encouraged to eat simple carbohydrates and emulsified fats (as in homogenized milk or eggs), as opposed to complex carbohydrates (e.g., starch, fiber, and glycogen [animal carbohydrates]) and complex fats, which would require additional bile to emulsify them so that they can be used. The cirrhotic patient should also be carefully observed for the development of ascites, in which case fluid and electrolyte balance requires strict attention. The alcoholic patient should be encouraged to avoid alcohol and to seek appropriate counseling for substance abuse.

➤ A written report of the examination will be sent to the requesting health care practitioner, who will discuss the results with the patient.

➤ Recognize anxiety related to test results, and be supportive of impaired activity related to lack of neuromuscular control, perceived loss of independence, and fear of shortened life expectancy. Discuss the implications of abnormal test results on the patient's lifestyle. Provide teaching and information regarding the clinical implications of the test results, as appropriate. Educate the patient regarding access to counseling services.

➤ Reinforce information given by the patient's health care provider regarding further testing, treatment, or referral to another health care provider. Answer any questions or address any concerns voiced by the patient or family.

Depending on the results of this procedure, additional testing may be performed to evaluate or monitor progression of the disease process and determine the need for a change in therapy. Evaluate test results in relation to the patient's symptoms and other tests performed.

Related laboratory tests:

Related laboratory tests include alanine aminotransferase, alkaline phosphatase and isoenzymes, ammonia, aspartate aminotransferase, bilirubin, electrolytes, hepatitis A antibody, hepatitis B antigen and antibody, and hepatitis C antibody.

GLYCATED HEMOGLOBIN A$_{1C}$

Synonyms/Acronym: Hemoglobin A$_{1C}$, A$_{1C}$.

Specimen: Whole blood (1 mL) collected in a lavender-top (ethylenediaminetetra-acetic acid [EDTA]) tube.

Reference Value: (Method: Chromatography)

Total A$_1$	4.0–7.0%
A$_{1C}$	4.0–5.5%

Values vary widely by method.

Description & Rationale: *Glycosylated* or *glycated hemoglobin* is a term used to describe the combination of glucose and hemoglobin into a ketamine; the rate at which this occurs is proportional to glucose concentration. The average life span of a red blood cell is approximately 120 days; measurement of glycated hemoglobin is a way to monitor long-term diabetic management.

Diabetes is a group of diseases characterized by hyperglycemia or elevated glucose levels. Hyperglycemia results from a defect in insulin secretion (type 1 diabetes), a defect in insulin action, or a combination of dysfunction secretion and action (type 2 diabetes). The chronic hyperglycemia of diabetes over time results in damage, dysfunction, and eventually failure of the eyes, kidneys, nerves, heart, and blood vessels. Hemoglobin A$_{1C}$ levels are not age dependent and are not affected by exercise, diabetic medications, or nonfasting state before specimen collection. ∎

Indications: Assess long-term glucose control in diabetics

Result

Increased in:
- Diabetes (poorly controlled or uncontrolled)

Decreased in:

• Chronic blood loss

• Chronic renal failure

• Conditions that decrease red blood cell life span

• Hemolytic anemia

• Pregnancy

CRITICAL VALUES: N/A

INTERFERING FACTORS:

• Drugs that may increase glycated hemoglobin A_{1C} values include hydrochlorothiazide, indapamide, insulin, morphine, propranolol, and sulfonylureas.

• Drugs that may decrease glycated hemoglobin A_{1C} values include carbamate, galactose, and metformin.

• Conditions involving abnormal hemoglobins (hemoglobinopathies) affect the reliability of glycated hemoglobin A_{1C} values, causing (1) falsely increased values, (2) falsely decreased values, or (3) discrepancies in either direction depending on the method.

Nursing Implications and Procedure • • • • • • • • • • •

Pretest:

➤ Inform the patient that the test is used to assess long-term glycemic control (past 3 months).

➤ Obtain a history of the patient's complaints, including a list of known allergens (especially allergies or sensitivities to latex), and inform the appropriate health care practitioner accordingly.

➤ Obtain a history of the patient's endocrine system as well as results of previously performed laboratory tests, surgical procedures, and other diagnostic procedures. For related laboratory tests, refer to the Endocrine System table.

➤ Obtain a list of the medications the patient is taking, including herbs, nutritional supplements, and nutraceuticals. The requesting health care practitioner and laboratory should be advised if the patient regularly uses these products so that their effects can be taken into consideration when reviewing results.

➤ Review the procedure with the patient. Inform the patient that specimen collection takes approximately 5 to 10 minutes. Address concerns about pain related to the procedure. Explain to the patient that there may be some discomfort during the venipuncture.

➤ There are no food, fluid, or medication restrictions, unless by medical direction.

Intratest:

➤ If the patient has a history of severe allergic reaction to latex, care should be taken to avoid the use of equipment containing latex.

➤ Instruct the patient to cooperate fully and to follow directions. Direct the patient to breathe normally and to avoid unnecessary movement.

➤ Observe standard precautions, and follow the general guidelines in Appendix A. Positively identify the patient, and label the appropriate tubes with the corresponding patient demographics, date, and time of collection. Perform a venipuncture; collect the specimen in a 5-mL lavender top tube.

➤ Remove the needle, and apply a pressure dressing over the puncture site.

➤ Promptly transport the specimen to the laboratory for processing and analysis.

➤ The results are recorded manually or in a computerized system for recall and postprocedure interpretation by the appropriate health care practitioner.

Post-test:

➤ Observe venipuncture site for bleeding or hematoma formation. Apply

paper tape or other adhesive to hold pressure bandage in place, or replace with a plastic bandage.

➤ *Nutritional considerations:* Increased glycated hemoglobin A_{1C} levels may be associated with diabetes. Instruct the diabetic patient, as appropriate, in nutritional management of the disease. Patients who adhere to dietary recommendations report a better general feeling of health, better weight management, greater control of glucose and lipid values, and improved use of insulin. There is no "diabetic diet"; however, many meal-planning approaches with nutritional goals are endorsed by the American Dietetic Association. The nutritional needs of each diabetic patient must be determined individually with the appropriate health care professionals, particularly professionals trained in nutrition.

➤ Instruct the patient and caregiver to report signs and symptoms of hypoglycemia (weakness, confusion, diaphoresis, rapid pulse) or hyperglycemia (thirst, polyuria, hunger, lethargy).

➤ A written report of the examination will be sent to the requesting health care practitioner, who will discuss the results with the patient.

➤ Recognize anxiety related to test results, and be supportive of perceived loss of independence and fear of shortened life expectancy.

➤ Discuss the implications of abnormal test results on the patient's lifestyle. Provide teaching and information regarding the clinical implications of the test results, as appropriate. Emphasize, as appropriate, that good glycemic control delays the onset of and slows the progression of diabetic retinopathy, nephropathy, and neuropathy. Educate the patient regarding access to counseling services. Provide contact information, if desired, for the American Diabetes Association *(http://www.diabetes.org)*.

➤ Reinforce information given by the patient's health care provider regarding further testing, treatment, or referral to another health care provider. Answer any questions or address any concerns voiced by the patient or family.

➤ Depending on the results of this procedure, additional testing may be performed to evaluate or monitor progression of the disease process and determine the need for a change in therapy. Evaluate test results in relation to the patient's symptoms and other tests performed.

Related laboratory tests:

➤ Related laboratory tests include C-peptide, cholesterol (total and HDL), fructosamine, glucose, glucose tolerance tests, insulin, insulin antibodies, ketones, microalbumin, and triglycerides.

GONIOSCOPY

SYNONYMS/ACRONYMS: N/A.

AREA OF APPLICATION: Eyes.

CONTRAST: N/A.

DESCRIPTION & RATIONALE:

Gonioscopy is a technique that is used for examination of the anterior chamber structures of the eye; the trabecular meshwork and the anatomic relationship of the trabecular meshwork to the iris. The trabecular meshwork is the drainage system of the eye, and gonioscopy is performed to determine if it is suspected that the drainage angle may be damaged, blocked, or clogged. Gonioscopy in combination with biomicroscopy is considered to be the most thorough basis to confirm a diagnosis of glaucoma and to differentiate between open-angle and angle-closure glaucoma. The angle structures of the anterior chamber are normally not visible because light entering the eye through the cornea is reflected back into the anterior chamber. Placement of a special contact lens (goniolens) over the cornea allows reflected light to pass back through the cornea and onto a reflective mirror in the contact lens. It is in this way that the angle structures can be visualized. There are two types of gonioscopy; indirect and direct. The more commonly used indirect technique employs a mirrored goniolens and biomicroscope. Direct gonioscopy is performed with a gonioscope containing a dome-shaped contact lens known as a gonioprism. The gonioprism eliminates internally reflected light, allowing direct visualization of the angle. Interpretation of visual examination is usually documented in a color hand-drawn diagram. Scheie's classification is used to standardize definition of angles based on appearance by gonioscopy. Shaffer's classification is based on the angular width of the angle recess. ∎

INDICATIONS:

- Assessment of peripheral anterior synechiae (PAS)

- Conditions affecting the ciliary body

- Degenerative conditions of the anterior chamber

- Evaluation of glaucoma (confirmation of normal structures and estimation of angle width)

- Growth or tumor in the angle

- Hyperpigmentation

- Post-trauma evaluation for angle recession

- Suspected neovascularization of the angle

- Uveitis

RESULT

Scheie's Classification Based on Visible Angle Structures	
Classification	*Appearance*
Wide Open	All angle structures seen
Grade I Narrow	Difficult to see over the iris root
Grade II Narrow	Ciliary band obscured
Grade III Narrow	Posterior trabeculum hazy
Grade IV Narrow	Only Schwalbe's line visible

Shaffer's Classification Based on Angle Width	
Classification	Appearance
Wide Open (20°–45°)	Closure improbable
Moderately Narrow (10°–20°)	Closure possible
Extremely Narrow (less than 10°)	Closure possible
Partially/Totally Closed	Closure present

Normal Findings:

- Normal appearance of anterior chamber structures and wide, unblocked, normal angle

Abnormal Findings:

- Corneal endothelial disorders (Fuchs endothelial dystrophy, iridocorneal endothelial syndrome)

- Glaucoma

- Lens disorders (cataract, displaced lens)

- Malignant ocular neoplasm in angle

- Neovascularization in angle

- Ocular hemorrhage

- PAS

- Schwartz syndrome

- Trauma

- Tumors

- Uveitis

CRITICAL VALUES: N/A

INTERFERING FACTORS:

- Inability of the patient to cooperate or remain still during the test because of age, significant pain, or mental status may interfere with the test results.

Nursing Implications and Procedure • • • • • • • • • • •

Pretest:

➤ Inform the patient that the procedure detects abnormailities in the structures of the anterior chamber of the eye.

➤ Obtain a history of the patient's complaints, including a list of known allergens.

➤ Obtain a history of the patient's known or suspected vision loss, changes in visual acuity, including type and cause; use of glasses or contact lenses; eye conditions with treatment regimens; eye surgery; and other tests and procedures to assess and diagnose visual deficit.

➤ Obtain a history of results of previously performed laboratory tests, surgical procedures, and other diagnostic procedures. For related diagnostic tests, refer to the table of tests associated with the Ocular System.

➤ Obtain a list of the medications the patient is taking, including herbs, nutritional supplements, and nutraceuticals. The requesting health care practitioner should be advised if the patient regularly uses these products so that their effects can be taken into consideration when reviewing results.

➤ Instruct the patient to remove contact lenses or glasses, as appropriate. Instruct the patient regarding the importance of keeping the eyes open for the test.

➤ Review the procedure with the patient. Explain that the patient will be requested to fixate the eyes during the procedure. Address concerns about pain related to the procedure. Explain to the patient that no pain will be experienced during the test, but there may be moments of discomfort. Explain to the patient that some discomfort may be experienced after the test when the numbness wears off from anesthetic drops adminstered prior to the test. Tell the patient that the test is performed by a health care practitioner or optometrist and takes about 5 minutes to complete.

➤ There are no food, fluid, or medication restrictions, unless by medical direction.

Intratest:

➤ Instruct the patient to cooperate fully and to follow directions. Ask the patient to remain still during the procedure because movement produces unreliable results.

➤ Seat the patient comfortably. Instill ordered topical anesthetic in each eye, as ordered, and allow time for it to work. Topical anesthetic drops are placed in the eye with the patient looking up and the solution directed at the six o'clock position of the sclera (white of the eye) near the limbus (grey, semitransparent area of the eyeball where the cornea and sclera meet). The dropper bottle should not touch the eyelashes.

➤ Ask the patient to place the chin in the chin rest and gently press the forehead against the support bar. Ask the patient to open his or her eyes wide and look at desired target. Explain that the health care practitioner or optometrist will place a lens on the eye while a narrow beam of light is focused on the eye.

➤ The results are recorded manually for recall and postprocedure interpretation by the appropriate health care practitioner.

Post-test:

➤ A written report of the examination will be completed by a health care practitioner specializing in this branch of medicine. The report will be sent to the requesting health care practitioner, who will discuss the results with the patient.

➤ Recognize anxiety related to test results, and be supportive of impaired activity related to vision loss or perceived loss of driving privileges. Discuss the implications of abnormal test results on the patient's lifestyle. Provide teaching and information regarding the clinical implications of the test results, as appropriate.

➤ Reinforce information given by the patient's health care provider regarding further testing, treatment, or referral to another health care provider. Answer any questions or address any concerns voiced by the patient or family.

➤ Depending on the results of this procedure, additional testing may be performed to evaluate or monitor progression of the disease process and determine the need for a change in therapy. Evaluate test results in relation to the patient's symptoms and other tests performed.

Related diagnostic tests:

➤ Related diagnostic tests include fundus photography, pachymetry, slit-lamp biomicroscopy, and visual field testing.

GRAM STAIN

SYNONYM/ACRONYM: N/A.

SPECIMEN: Blood, biopsy specimen, or body fluid as collected for culture.

REFERENCE VALUE: N/A.

DESCRIPTION & RATIONALE: Gram stain is a technique commonly used to identify bacterial organisms based on their specific staining characteristics. The method involves smearing a small amount of specimen on a slide, and then exposing it to gentian or crystal violet, iodine, alcohol, and safranin O. Gram-positive bacteria retain the gentian or crystal violet and iodine stain complex after a decolorization step and appear purple-blue in color. Gram-negative bacteria do not retain the stain after decolorization but can pick up the pink color of the safranin O counterstain. Gram stain results should be correlated with culture results to interpret the significance of isolated organisms. A sputum Gram stain showing greater than 25 squamous epithelial cells per low-power field, regardless of the number of polymorphonuclear white blood cells, indicates contamination of the specimen with saliva, and the specimen should be rejected for subsequent culture. The occasional presence of bacteria in an unspun urine Gram stain suggests a correlating colony count of 10,000 bacteria/mL. The presence of bacteria in most fields is clinically significant and suggests greater than 100,000 bacteria/mL of urine. ■

INDICATIONS:
- Provide a rapid determination of the acceptability of the specimen for further analysis
- Provide rapid, presumptive information about the type of potential pathogen present in the specimen (i.e., gram-positive bacteria, gram-negative bacteria, or yeast)

RESULT

Gram Positive	Gram Negative			Acid Fast or Partial Acid Fast
Actinomadura	Acinetobacter	Helicobacter	Xanthomonas	Nocardia
Actinomyces	Aeromonas	Klebsiella	Yersinia	Mycobacterium
Bacillus	Alcaligenes	Legionella		
Clostridium	Bacteroides	Leptospira		
Corynebacterium	Bordetella	Moraxella		
Enterococcus	Borrelia	Neisseria		
Erysipelothrix	Brucella	Pasteurella		
Lactobacillus	Campylobacter	Plesiomonas		
Listeria	Citrobacter	Porphyromonas		
Micrococcus	Chlamydia	Prevotella		
Mycobacterium (gram variable)	Enterobacter	Proteus		
Peptostreptococcus	Escherichia	Pseudomonas		

(Continued on the following page)

Gram Positive		Gram Negative		Acid Fast or Partial Acid Fast
Propionibacterium	Flavobacter	Rickettsia		
Rhodococcus	Francisella	Salmonella		
Staphylococcus	Fusobacterium	Serratia		
Streptococcus	Gardnerella	Shigella		
	Haemophilus	Vibrio		

Note: *Treponema* species are classified as gram-negative spirochetes, but they are most often visualized using dark-field or silver staining techniques.

CRITICAL VALUES:
Note and immediately report to the health care practitioner any positive results in blood, cerebrospinal fluid, or any body cavity fluid, along with related symptoms.

INTERFERING FACTORS: Very young, very old, or dead cultures may react atypically to the Gram stain technique.

Nursing Implications and Procedure • • • • • • • • • • •

Pretest:

➤ Inform the patient that the test is used to assist in identifying the presence of pathogenic organisms.

➤ Obtain a history of the patient's complaints, including a list of known allergens (especially allergies or sensitivities to latex), and inform the appropriate health care practitioner accordingly.

➤ Obtain a history of the patient's gastrointestinal, genitourinary, immune, reproductive, and respiratory systems, as well as results of previously performed laboratory tests, surgical procedures, and other diagnostic procedures. For related laboratory tests, refer to the Gastrointestinal, Genitourinary, Immune, Reproductive, and Respiratory System tables.

➤ Obtain a list of medications the patient is taking, including herbs, nutritional supplements, and nutra-

ceuticals. The requesting health care practitioner and laboratory should be advised if the patient regularly uses these products so that their effects can be taken into consideration when reviewing results.

➤ Review the procedure with the patient. Inform the patient that the time it takes to collect a proper specimen varies according to the patient's level of cooperation as well as the specimen collection site. Address concerns about pain related to the procedure. Explain to the patient that there may be some discomfort during the procedure.

➤ *Sensitivity to social and cultural issues,* as well as concern for modesty, is important in providing psychological support before, during, and after the procedure.

➤ There are no food, fluid, or medication restrictions, unless by medical direction.

Intratest:

➤ Instruct the patient to cooperate fully and to follow directions.

➤ Observe standard precautions, and follow the general guidelines in Appendix A. Positively identify the patient, and label the appropriate collection container with the corresponding patient demographics, date, and time of collection.

➤ Specific collection instructions are found in the associated culture monographs.

➤ Promptly transport the specimen to

the laboratory for processing and analysis.

➤ The results are recorded manually or in a computerized system for recall and postprocedure interpretation by the appropriate health care practitioner.

Post-test:

➤ Administer antibiotics as ordered, and instruct the patient in the importance of completing the entire course of antibiotic therapy even if no symptoms are present.

➤ A written report of the examination will be sent to the requesting health care practitioner, who will discuss the results with the patient.

➤ Recognize anxiety related to test results. Discuss the implications of abnormal test results on the patient's lifestyle. Provide teaching and information regarding the clinical implications of the test results, as appropriate.

➤ Reinforce information given by the patient's health care provider regarding further testing, treatment, or referral to another health care provider. Answer any questions or address any concerns voiced by the patient or family.

➤ Depending on the results of this procedure, additional testing may be performed to evaluate or monitor progression of the disease process and determine the need for a change in therapy. Evaluate test results in relation to the patient's symptoms and other tests performed.

Related laboratory tests:

➤ Related laboratory tests include bacterial and viral cultures, cerebrospinal fluid analysis, complete blood count, and urinalysis.

GROUP A STREPTOCOCCAL SCREEN

· ·

SYNONYMS/ACRONYM: Strep screen, rapid strep screen, direct strep screen.

SPECIMEN: Throat swab (two swabs should be submitted so that a culture can be performed if the screen is negative).

REFERENCE VALUE: (Method: Enzyme immunoassay or latex agglutination) Negative.

DESCRIPTION & RATIONALE: Rheumatic fever is a possible sequela to an untreated streptococcal infection. Early diagnosis and treatment appear to lessen the seriousness of symptoms during the acute phase and overall duration of the infection and sequelae. The onset of strep throat is sudden and includes symptoms such as chills, headache, sore throat, malaise, and exudative gray-white patches on the tonsils or pharynx. The group

A streptococcal screen should not be ordered unless the results would be available within 1 to 2 hours of specimen collection to make rapid, effective therapeutic decisions. A positive result can be a reliable basis for the initiation of therapy. A negative result is presumptive for infection and should be backed up by culture results. In general, specimens showing growth of less than 10 colonies on culture yield negative results by the rapid screening method. Evidence of group A streptococci disappears rapidly after the initiation of antibiotic therapy. A nucleic acid probe method has also been developed for rapid detection of group A streptococci. ■

INDICATIONS: Assist in the rapid determination of the presence of group A streptococci

RESULT

Positive findings in:
• Rheumatic fever

• Scarlet fever

• Strep throat

• Streptococcal glomerulonephritis

• Tonsillitis

CRITICAL VALUES: N/A

INTERFERING FACTORS:
• Polyester swabs are favored over cotton for best chance of detection.

• Sensitivity of the method varies from manufacturer to manufacturer.

• Adequate specimen collection in children may be difficult to achieve, which explains the higher percentage of false-negative results in this age group.

Nursing Implications and Procedure • • • • • • • • • • •

Pretest:

➤ Inform the patient that the test is used to detect group A streptococcal infection.

➤ Obtain a history of the patient's complaints, including a list of known allergens (especially allergies or sensitivities to latex), and inform the appropriate health care practitioner accordingly.

➤ Obtain a history of the patient's immune and respiratory systems, as well as results of previously performed laboratory tests, surgical procedures, and other diagnostic procedures. For related laboratory tests, refer to the Immune and Respiratory System tables.

➤ Obtain a history of prior antibiotic therapy.

➤ Obtain a list of medications the patient is taking, including herbs, nutritional supplements, and nutraceuticals. The requesting health care practitioner and laboratory should be advised if the patient regularly uses these products so that their effects can be taken into consideration when reviewing results.

➤ Before specimen collection, verify with the laboratory whether wet or dry swabs are preferred for collection.

➤ Review the procedure with the patient. Inform the patient that specimen collection takes approximately 5 to 10 minutes. Address concerns about pain related to the procedure. Explain to the patient that there may be some discomfort during the swabbing procedure.

➤ There are no food, fluid, or medication restrictions, unless by medical direction.

Intratest:

➤ Instruct the patient to cooperate fully and to follow directions. Direct the

patient to breathe normally and to avoid unnecessary movement.

➤ Observe standard precautions, and follow the general guidelines in Appendix A. Positively identify the patient, and label the appropriate specimen container with the corresponding patient demographics, date, and time of collection. Vigorous swabbing of both tonsillar pillars and the posterior throat enhances the probability of streptococcal antigen detection.

➤ Promptly transport the specimen to the laboratory for processing and analysis.

➤ The results are recorded manually or in a computerized system for recall and postprocedure interpretation by the appropriate health care practitioner.

course of antibiotic therapy even if no symptoms are present.

➤ A written report of the examination will be sent to the requesting health care practitioner, who will discuss the results with the patient.

➤ Reinforce information given by the patient's health care provider regarding further testing, treatment, or referral to another health care provider. Answer any questions or address any concerns voiced by the patient or family.

➤ Depending on the results of this procedure, additional testing may be performed to evaluate or monitor progression of the disease process and determine the need for a change in therapy. Evaluate test results in relation to the patient's symptoms and other tests performed.

Post-test:

➤ Administer antibiotics as ordered, and emphasize to the patient the importance of completing the entire

Related laboratory tests:

➤ Related laboratory tests include complete blood count, Gram stain, and relevant cultures.

GROWTH HORMONE, STIMULATION AND SUPPRESSION TESTS

· ·

SYNONYMS/ACRONYMS: Somatotropic hormone, somatotropin, GH, hGH.

SPECIMEN: Serum (1 mL) collected in a red- or tiger-top tube.

REFERENCE VALUE: (Method: Radioimmunoassay)

Growth Hormone

Age	Conventional Units	SI Units (Conventional Units × 1)
Cord blood	8–40 ng/mL	8–40 μg/L
1 d	5–50 ng/mL	5–50 μg/L
1 wk	5–25 ng/mL	5–25 μg/L
Child	2–10 ng/mL	2–10 μg/L
Adult		
Male	0–5 ng/mL	0–5 μg/L
Female	0–10 ng/mL	0–10 μg/L
Male older than 60 y	0–10 ng/mL	0–10 μg/L
Female older than 60 y	0–14 ng/mL	0–14 μg/L
Stimulation Tests		
Rise above baseline	Greater than 5 ng/mL	Greater than 5 μg/L
Peak response	Greater than 10 ng/mL	Greater than 10 μg/L
Suppression Tests		
	0–2 ng/mL	0–2 μg/L

DESCRIPTION & RATIONALE: Human growth hormone (GH) is secreted in episodic bursts by the anterior pituitary gland; the highest level is usually secreted during deep sleep. GH plays an integral role in growth from birth to puberty. GH promotes skeletal growth by stimulating hepatic production of proteins; it also affects lipid and glucose metabolism. Random levels are rarely useful because secretion of GH is episodic and pulsatile. Stimulation tests with arginine, glucagon, insulin, or L-dopa, as well as suppression tests with glucose, provide useful information. ■

INDICATIONS:

- Assist in the diagnosis of acromegaly in adults
- Assist in establishing a diagnosis of dwarfism or growth retardation in children with decreased GH levels, indicative of a pituitary cause
- Assist in establishing a diagnosis of gigantism in children with GH increased levels, indicative of a pituitary cause
- Detect suspected disorder associated with decreased GH
- Monitor response to treatment of growth retardation

RESULT

Increased in:
- Acromegaly
- Anorexia nervosa
- Cirrhosis
- Diabetes (uncontrolled)
- Ectopic GH secretion (neoplasms of stomach, lung)
- Exercise
- Gigantism (pituitary)
- Hyperpituitarism

- Laron dwarfism
- Malnutrition
- Renal failure
- Stress

Decreased in:
- Adrenocortical hyperfunction
- Dwarfism (pituitary)
- Hypopituitarism

CRITICAL VALUES: N/A

INTERFERING FACTORS:
- Drugs that may increase GH levels include alanine, anabolic steroids, angiotensin II, apomorphine, arginine, clonidine, corticotropin, cyclic AMP, desipramine, dexamethasone, dopamine, fenfluramine, galanin, glucagon, GH-releasing hormone, hydrazine, levodopa, methamphetamine, methyldopa, metoclopramide, midazolam, niacin, oral contraceptives, phenytoin, propranolol, and vasopressin.
- Drugs that may decrease GH levels include corticosteroids, corticotropin, hydrocortisone, octreotide, and pirenzepine.
- Recent radioactive scans or radiation within 1 week before the test can interfere with test results when radioimmunoassay is the test method.
- Failure to follow dietary and activity restrictions before the procedure may cause the procedure to be canceled or repeated.

Nursing Implications and Procedure · · · · · · · · · · ·

Pretest:

➤ Inform the patient that the test is used to assess pituitary function.

➤ Obtain a history of the patient's complaints, including a list of known allergens (especially allergies or sensitivities to latex), and inform the appropriate health care practitioner accordingly.

➤ Obtain a history of the patient's endocrine system as well as results of previously performed laboratory tests, surgical procedures, and other diagnostic procedures. For related laboratory tests, refer to the Endocrine System table.

➤ Record pertinent information related to diet, sleep pattern, and activity at the time of the test.

➤ Note any recent procedures that can interfere with test results.

➤ Obtain a list of medications the patient is taking, including herbs, nutritional supplements, and nutraceuticals. The requesting health care practitioner and laboratory should be advised if the patient regularly uses these products that so their effects can be taken into consideration when reviewing results.

➤ Review the procedure with the patient. The patient should have bed rest for 1 hour before each sample is obtained. Inform the patient that multiple specimens may be required. Inform the patient that specimen collection takes approximately 5 to 10 minutes. Address concerns about pain related to the procedure. Explain to the patient that there may be some discomfort during the venipuncture.

➤ The patient should fast and avoid strenuous exercise for 12 hours before specimen collection.

➤ There are no fluid or medication restrictions, unless by medical direction.

Intratest:

➤ Ensure that the patient has complied with dietary and activity restrictions; assure that food and strenuous activity have been restricted for at least 12 hours prior to the procedure.

➤ If the patient has a history of severe allergic reaction to latex, care should be taken to avoid the use of equipment containing latex.

➤ Instruct the patient to cooperate fully

and to follow directions. Direct the patient to breathe normally and to avoid unnecessary movement.

➤ Observe standard precautions, and follow the general guidelines in Appendix A. Positively identify the patient, and label the appropriate tubes with the corresponding patient demographics, date, and time of collection. Perform a venipuncture; collect the specimen in a 5-mL red- or tiger-top tube. Test samples may be requested at baseline and 10-, 20-, 30-, 45-, and 60-minute intervals after stimulation and at baseline and 30-, 60-, 90-, and 120-minute intervals after suppression.

➤ Remove the needle, and apply a pressure dressing over the puncture site.

➤ Promptly transport the specimen to the laboratory for processing and analysis.

➤ The results are recorded manually or in a computerized system for recall and postprocedure interpretation by the appropriate health care practitioner.

paper tape or other adhesive to hold pressure bandage in place, or replace with a plastic bandage.

➤ Instruct the patient to resume usual diet, fluids, medications, or activity, as directed by the health care practitioner.

➤ A written report of the examination will be sent to the requesting health care practitioner, who will discuss the results with the patient.

➤ Reinforce information given by the patient's health care provider regarding further testing, treatment, or referral to another health care provider. Answer any questions or address any concerns voiced by the patient or family.

➤ Depending on the results of this procedure, additional testing may be performed to evaluate or monitor progression of the disease process and determine the need for a change in therapy. Evaluate test results in relation to the patient's symptoms and other tests performed.

Post-test:

Observe venipuncture site for bleeding or hematoma formation. Apply

Related laboratory tests:

➤ A related laboratory test is adrenocorticotropic hormone.

HAM'S TEST FOR PAROXYSMAL NOCTURNAL HEMOGLOBINURIA

· ·

SYNONYM/ACRONYM: Acid hemolysis test for PNH.

SPECIMEN: Whole blood (5 mL) collected in lavender-top (EDTA) top tube and serum (3 mL) collected in red-top tube.

REFERENCE VALUE: (Method: Acidified hemolysis) No hemolysis seen.

DESCRIPTION & RATIONALE: Paroxysmal nocturnal hemoglobinuria (PNH) is a condition in which the patient experiences nocturnal hemoglobinuria, chronic hemolytic anemia, diminished or absent generation of new red blood cells (RBCs), and a tendency to thrombose. It is caused by an acquired defect in hematopoietic stem cells. In patients with PNH, erythrocytes have an increased sensitivity to complement and will lyse when mixed with acidified serum containing complement. The patient's RBCs are also mixed with fresh normal serum that is ABO compatible with the patient's cells. Some of the control serum is acidified, and some is heated to inactivate the complement. The result is positive if 10% to 50% cell lysis occurs in the samples mixed with patient and control acidified serum. No hemolysis should occur in the heated control serum. The sugar water test can also be performed to investigate the presence of PNH. Platelet and granulocyte membranes are affected as well, but RBC hemolysis in a positive test is clear evidence of PNH. ∎

INDICATIONS:

• Evaluate hemolytic anemia, especially with hemosiderinuria

• Evaluate suspected congenital dyserythropoietic anemia, type II (also known as HEMPAS [*h*ereditary *e*rythroblastic *m*ultinuclearity with *p*ositive *a*cidified *s*erum test])

• Evaluate suspected PNH

RESULT

Increased in:

• Congenital dyserythropoietic anemia, type II

• Paroxysmal nocturnal hemoglobinuria

Decreased in: N/A

CRITICAL VALUES: N/A

INTERFERING FACTORS:

• False-positives may occur in the presence of other disorders, such as aplastic anemia, HEMPAS, hereditary or acquired spherocytosis, leukemia, and myeloproliferative syndromes. False-positives may also occur with aged RBCs. The sugar water test is negative in HEMPAS.

• False-negatives can occur if the patient's serum sample contains a low level of complement.

Nursing Implications and Procedure • • • • • • • • • •

Pretest:

▶ Inform the patient that the test is used to assist in the diagnosis of PNH.

▶ Obtain a history of the patient's complaints, including a list of known allergens (especially allergies or sensitivities to latex), and inform the appropriate health care practitioner accordingly.

▶ Obtain a history of the patient's hematopoietic system, as well as results of previously performed laboratory tests, surgical procedures, and other diagnostic procedures. For related laboratory tests, refer to the Hematopoietic System table.

▶ Obtain a list of the medications the patient is taking, including herbs, nutritional supplements, and nutraceuticals. The requesting health care practitioner and laboratory should be advised if the patient regularly uses these products so that their effects can be taken into consideration when reviewing results.

▶ Review the procedure with the patient. Inform the patient that specimen collection takes approximately

5 to 10 minutes. Address concerns about pain related to the procedure. Explain to the patient that there may be some discomfort during the venipuncture.

➤ There are no food, fluid, or medication restrictions, unless by medical direction.

Intratest:

➤ If the patient has a history of severe allergic reaction to latex, care should be taken to avoid the use of equipment containing latex.

➤ Instruct the patient to cooperate fully and to follow directions. Direct the patient to breathe normally and to avoid unnecessary movement.

➤ Observe standard precautions, and follow the general guidelines in Appendix A. Positively identify the patient, and label the appropriate tubes with the corresponding patient demographics, date, and time of collection. Perform a venipuncture; collect the specimen in a 5-mL lavender and a 5-mL red-top tube.

➤ Remove the needle, and apply a pressure dressing over the puncture site.

➤ Promptly transport the specimen to the laboratory for processing and analysis.

➤ The results are recorded manually or in a computerized system for recall and postprocedure interpretation by the appropriate health care practitioner.

Post-test:

➤ Observe venipuncture site for bleeding or hematoma formation. Apply paper tape or other adhesive to hold pressure bandage in place, or replace with a plastic bandage.

➤ A written report of the examination will be sent to the requesting health care practitioner, who will discuss the results with the patient.

➤ Reinforce information given by the patient's health care provider regarding further testing, treatment, or referral to another health care provider. Answer any questions or address any concerns voiced by the patient or family.

➤ Depending on the results of this procedure, additional testing may be performed to evaluate or monitor progression of the disease process and determine the need for a change in therapy. Evaluate test results in relation to the patient's symptoms and other tests performed.

Related laboratory tests:

➤ Related laboratory tests include bone marrow biopsy, complete blood count, direct Coombs' test, glucose-6-phosphate dehydrogenase, haptoglobin, hematocrit, hemoglobin, hemosiderin, leukocyte alkaline phosphatase, and osmotic fragility.

HAPTOGLOBIN

· ·

SYNONYMS/ACRONYMS: Hapto, HP, Hp.

SPECIMEN: Serum (1 mL) collected in a red- or tiger-top tube.

REFERENCE VALUE: (Method: Nephelometry)

Age	Conventional Units	SI Units (Conventional Units × 0.01)
Newborn	5–48 mg/dL	0.05–0.48 g/L
6 mo–16 y	25–138 mg/dL	0.25–1.38 g/L
Adult	15–200 mg/dL	0.15–2.00 g/L

DESCRIPTION & RATIONALE: Haptoglobin is an α_2-globulin produced in the liver. It binds with the free hemoglobin released when red blood cells (RBCs) are lysed. If left unchecked, free hemoglobin in the plasma can cause renal damage; haptoglobin prevents it from accumulating. In conditions such as hemolytic anemia, so many hemolyzed RBCs are available for binding that the liver cannot compensate by producing additional haptoglobin fast enough, resulting in low serum levels. ∎

INDICATIONS:
- Assist in the investigation of suspected transfusion reaction

- Evaluate known or suspected chronic liver disease, as indicated by decreased levels

- Evaluate known or suspected disorders characterized by excessive RBC hemolysis, as indicated by decreased levels

- Evaluate known or suspected disorders involving a diffuse inflammatory process or tissue destruction, as indicated by elevated levels

RESULT

Increased in:
- Biliary obstruction

- Disorders involving tissue destruction, such as cancers, burns, and acute myocardial infarction

- Infection or inflammatory diseases, such as ulcerative colitis, arthritis, and pyelonephritis

- Neoplasms

- Steroid therapy

Decreased in:
- Autoimmune hemolysis

- Hemolysis due to drug reaction

- Hemolysis due to mechanical destruction (e.g., artificial heart valves, contact sports, subacute bacterial endocarditis)

- Hemolysis due to RBC membrane or metabolic defects

- Hemolysis due to transfusion reaction

- Hypersplenism

- Ineffective hematopoiesis due to conditions such as folate deficiency or hemoglobinopathies

- Liver disease

CRITICAL VALUES: N/A

INTERFERING FACTORS:
- Drugs that may increase haptoglobin levels include anabolic steroids, danazol, ethylestrenol, fluoxymesterone, methandrostenolone, norethandrolone, oxandrolone, oxymetholone, and stanozolol.

- Drugs that may decrease haptoglobin levels include acetanilid, aminosalicylic acid, chlorpromazine, dapsone, dextran, diphenhydramine, furadaltone, furazolidone, isoniazid, nitrofurantoin, norethindrone, oral contraceptives, quinidine, resorcinol, stibophen, tamoxifen, thiazolsulfone, and tripelennamine.

Nursing Implications and Procedure • • • • • • • • • • •

Pretest:

➤ Inform the patient that the test is primarily used to investigate hemolytic states.

➤ Obtain a history of the patient's complaints, including a list of known allergens (especially allergies or sensitivities to latex), and inform the appropriate health care practitioner accordingly.

➤ Obtain a history of the patient's hematopoietic, hepatobiliary, and immune systems, as well as results of previously performed laboratory tests, surgical procedures, and other diagnostic procedures. For related laboratory tests, refer to the Hematopoietic, Hepatobiliary, and Immune System tables.

➤ Obtain a list of the medications the patient is taking, including herbs, nutritional supplements, and nutraceuticals. The requesting health care practitioner and laboratory should be advised if the patient regularly uses these products so that their effects can be taken into consideration when reviewing results.

➤ Review the procedure with the patient. Inform the patient that specimen collection takes approximately 5 to 10 minutes. Address concerns about pain related to the procedure. Explain to the patient that there may be some discomfort during the venipuncture.

➤ There are no food, fluid, or medication restrictions, unless by medical direction.

Intratest:

➤ If the patient has a history of severe allergic reaction to latex, care should be taken to avoid the use of equipment containing latex.

➤ Instruct the patient to cooperate fully and to follow directions. Direct the patient to breathe normally and to avoid unnecessary movement.

➤ Observe standard precautions, and follow the general guidelines in Appendix A. Positively identify the patient, and label the appropriate tubes with the corresponding patient demographics, date, and time of collection. Perform a venipuncture; collect the specimen in a 5-mL red-top tube.

➤ Remove the needle, and apply a pressure dressing over the puncture site.

➤ Promptly transport the specimen to the laboratory for processing and analysis.

➤ The results are recorded manually or in a computerized system for recall and postprocedure interpretation by the appropriate health care practitioner.

Post-test:

➤ Observe venipuncture site for bleeding or hematoma formation. Apply paper tape or other adhesive to hold pressure bandage in place, or replace with a plastic bandage.

➤ Instruct the patient to immediately report symptoms of hemolysis, including chills, fever, flushing, back pain, and fast heartbeat, to the health care practitioner.

➤ A written report of the examination will be sent to the requesting health care practitioner, who will discuss the results with the patient.

➤ Reinforce information given by the patient's health care provider regarding further testing, treatment, or referral to another health care provider. Answer any questions or address any concerns voiced by the patient or family.

➤ Depending on the results of this procedure, additional testing may be

performed to evaluate or monitor progression of the disease process and determine the need for a change in therapy. Evaluate test results in relation to the patient's symptoms and other tests performed.

HELICOBACTER PYLORI ANTIBODY

SYNONYM/ACRONYM: *H. pylori.*

SPECIMEN: Serum (1 mL) collected in a plain red-top tube.

REFERENCE VALUE: (Method: Enzyme-linked immunosorbent assay [ELISA]) Negative.

DESCRIPTION & RATIONALE: There is a strong association between *Helicobacter pylori* infection and gastric cancer, duodenal and gastric ulcer, and chronic gastritis. Immunoglobulin G (IgG) antibodies can be detected for up to 1 year after treatment. The presence of *H. pylori* can also be demonstrated by a positive urea breath test, positive stool culture, or positive endoscopic biopsy. Patients with symptoms and evidence of *H. pylori* infection are considered to be *infected* with the organism; patients who demonstrate evidence of *H. pylori* but are without symptoms are said to be *colonized.* ∎

INDICATIONS:
• Assist in differentiating between *H. pylori* infection and nonsteroidal anti-inflammatory drug use as the cause of gastritis or peptic or duodenal ulcer

• Assist in establishing a diagnosis of gastritis, gastric carcinoma, or peptic or duodenal ulcer

RESULT

Positive findings in:
• *H. pylori* infection
• *H. pylori* colonization

Negative findings in: N/A

CRITICAL VALUES: N/A

INTERFERING FACTORS: N/A

Nursing Implications and Procedure • • • • • • • • • •

Pretest:

➤ Inform the patient that the test is used to assist in the diagnosis of *H.*

pylori infection in patients with duodenal and gastric disease.

▶ Obtain a history of the patient's complaints, including a list of known allergens (especially allergies or sensitivities to latex), and inform the appropriate health care practitioner accordingly.

▶ Obtain a history of the patient's gastrointestinal and immune systems, as well as results of previously performed laboratory tests, surgical procedures, and other diagnostic procedures. For related laboratory tests, refer to the Gastrointestinal and Immune System tables.

▶ Obtain a list of the medications the patient is taking, including herbs, nutritional supplements, and nutraceuticals. The requesting health care practitioner and laboratory should be advised if the patient regularly uses these products so that their effects can be taken into consideration when reviewing results.

▶ Review the procedure with the patient. Inform the patient that specimen collection takes approximately 5 to 10 minutes. Address concerns about pain related to the procedure. Explain to the patient that there may be some discomfort during the venipuncture.

▶ There are no food, fluid, or medication restrictions, unless by medical direction.

Intratest:

▶ If the patient has a history of severe allergic reaction to latex, care should be taken to avoid the use of equipment containing latex.

▶ Instruct the patient to cooperate fully and to follow directions. Direct the patient to breathe normally and to avoid unnecessary movement.

▶ Observe standard precautions, and follow the general guidelines in Appendix A. Positively identify the patient, and label the appropriate tubes with the corresponding patient demographics, date, and time of collection. Perform a venipuncture; collect the specimen in a 5-mL redtop tube.

▶ Remove the needle, and apply a pressure dressing over the puncture site.

▶ Promptly transport the specimen to the laboratory for processing and analysis.

▶ The results are recorded manually or in a computerized system for recall and postprocedure interpretation by the appropriate health care practitioner.

Post-test:

▶ Observe venipuncture site for bleeding or hematoma formation. Apply paper tape or other adhesive to hold pressure bandage in place, or replace with a plastic bandage.

▶ A written report of the examination will be sent to the requesting health care practitioner, who will discuss the results with the patient.

▶ Reinforce information given by the patient's health care provider regarding further testing, treatment, or referral to another health care provider. Inform the patient that a positive test result constitutes an independent risk factor for gastric cancer. Answer any questions or address any concerns voiced by the patient or family.

▶ Depending on the results of this procedure, additional testing may be performed to evaluate or monitor progression of the disease process and determine the need for a change in therapy. Evaluate test results in relation to the patient's symptoms and other tests performed.

Related laboratory tests:

▶ Related laboratory tests include gastric acid stimulation and gastrin.

HEMATOCRIT

. . . .

SYNONYMS/ACRONYMS: Packed cell volume (PCV), Hct.

SPECIMEN: Whole blood from one full lavender-top (EDTA) tube, Microtainer, or capillary. Whole blood from a green-top (lithium or sodium heparin) tube may also be submitted.

REFERENCE VALUE: (Method: Automated, computerized, multichannel analyzers)

Age	Conventional Units (%)	SI Unit (Volume Fraction, Conventional Units × 0.01)
Cord blood	47–57	0.47–0.57
1 d	51–65	0.51–0.65
2 wk	47–57	0.47–0.57
1 mo	38–52	0.38–0.52
6 mo	35–41	0.35–0.41
1 y	37–41	0.37–0.41
10 y	36–42	0.36–0.42
Adult		
Male	43–49	0.43–0.49
Female	38–44	0.38–0.44

DESCRIPTION & RATIONALE: Blood consists of a fluid portion (plasma) and a solid portion that includes red blood cells (RBCs), white blood cells, and platelets. The hematocrit, or packed cell volume, is the percentage of RBCs in a volume of whole blood. For example, a hematocrit (Hct) of 45% means that a 100-mL sample of blood contains 45 mL of packed RBCs. Although the Hct depends primarily on the number of RBCs, the average size of the RBCs plays a role. Conditions that cause the RBCs to swell, such as when the serum sodium concentration is elevated, may increase the Hct level.

Hct level is included in the complete blood count (CBC) and is generally tested together with hemoglobin (Hgb). These levels parallel each other and are the best determinant of the degree of anemia or polycythemia. *Polycythemia* is a term used in conjunction with conditions resulting from an abnormal increase in Hgb, Hct, and RBC count. *Anemia* is a term associated with conditions resulting from an abnormal decrease in Hgb, Hct, and RBC count. Results of the Hgb, Hct, and RBC count should be evaluated simultaneously because the same underlying conditions affect this triad of tests similarly. The RBC count multiplied by 3 should approximate the Hgb concentration. The Hct should be within three times the Hgb if the RBC population is normal in size and shape. The Hct plus 6 should approximate the first two figures of the RBC count within 3 (e.g., Hct is 40%; therefore 40 + 6 = 46, and the RBC count should be 4.3 to 4.9). There are some cultural variations in Hgb and Hct (H&H) values. After the first decade of life, the mean Hgb in African Americans is 0.5 to 1.0 g lower than in whites. Mexican Americans and Asian Americans have higher H&H values than whites. ▪

INDICATIONS:

• Detect hematologic disorder, neoplasm, or immunologic abnormality

• Determine the presence of hereditary hematologic abnormality

• Evaluate known or suspected anemia and related treatment, in combination with Hgb

• Monitor blood loss and response to blood replacement, in combination with Hgb

• Monitor the effects of physical or emotional stress on the patient

• Monitor fluid imbalances or their treatment

• Monitor hematologic status during pregnancy, in combination with Hgb

• Monitor the progression of nonhematologic disorders such as chronic obstructive pulmonary disease, malabsorption syndromes, cancer, and renal disease

• Monitor response to drugs or chemotherapy, and evaluate undesired reactions to drugs that may cause blood dyscrasias

• Provide screening as part of a CBC count in a general physical examination, especially upon admission to a health care facility or before surgery

RESULT

Increased in:
• Burns

• Congestive heart failure

• COPD

• Dehydration

• Erythrocytosis

• Hemoconcentration

• High altitudes

• Polycythemia

• Shock

Decreased in:
• Anemia

• Blood loss (acute and chronic)

• Bone marrow hyperplasia

• Chronic disease

• Hemolytic disorders

• Hemorrhage (acute and chronic)

• Fluid retention

• Nutritional deficit

• Pregnancy

• Splenomegaly

CRITICAL VALUES:

Less than 18%

Greater than 54%

Note and immediately report to the health care practitioner any critically increased or decreased values and related symptoms.

• Low Hct leads to anemia. Anemia can be caused by blood loss, decreased blood cell production, increased blood cell destruction, and hemodilution. Causes of blood loss include menstrual excess or frequency, gastrointestinal bleeding, inflammatory bowel disease, and hematuria. Decreased blood cell production can be caused by folic acid deficiency, vitamin B_{12} deficiency, iron deficiency, and chronic disease. Increased blood cell destruction can be caused by a hemolytic reaction, chemical reaction, medication reaction, and sickle cell disease. Hemodilution can be caused by congestive heart failure, renal failure, polydipsia, and overhydration. Symptoms of anemia (due to these causes) include anxiety, dyspnea, edema, hypertension, hypotension, hypoxia, jugular venous distention, fatigue, pallor, rales, restlessness, and weakness. Treatment of anemia depends on the cause.

• High Hct leads to polycythemia. Polycythemia can be caused by dehydration, decreased oxygen levels in the body, and an overproduction of RBCs by the bone marrow. Dehydration from diuretic use, vomiting, diarrhea, excessive sweating, severe burns, or decreased fluid intake decreases the plasma component of whole blood, thereby increasing the ratio of RBCs to plasma, and leads to a higher than normal Hct. Causes of decreased oxygen include smoking, exposure to carbon monoxide, high altitude, and chronic lung disease, which leads to a mild hemoconcentration of blood in the body to carry more oxygen to the body's tissues. An overproduction of RBCs by the bone marrow leads to polycythemia vera, which is a rare chronic myeloproliferative disorder that leads to a severe hemoconcentration of blood. Severe hemoconcentration can lead to thrombosis (spontaneous blood clotting). Symptoms of hemoconcentration include

decreased pulse pressure and volume, loss of skin turgor, dry mucous membranes, headaches, hepatomegaly, low central venous pressure, orthostatic hypotension, pruritis (especially after a hot bath), splenomegaly, tachycardia, thirst, tinnitus, vertigo, and weakness. Treatment of polycythemia depends on the cause. Possible interventions for hemoconcentration due to dehydration include intravenous fluids and discontinuance of diuretics if they are believed to be contributing to critically elevated Hct. Polycythemia due to decreased oxygen states can be treated by removal of the offending substance, such as smoke or carbon monoxide. Treatment includes oxygen therapy in cases of smoke inhalation, carbon monoxide poisioning, and desaturating chronic lung disease. Symptoms of polycythemic overload crisis include signs of thrombosis, pain and redness in the extremities, facial flushing, and irritability. Possible interventions for hemoconcentration due to polycythemia include therapeutic phlebotomy and intravenous fluids.

INTERFERING FACTORS:

• Drugs and substances that may cause a decrease in Hct include those that induce hemolysis due to drug sensitivity or enzyme deficiency, such as acetaminophen, aminopyrine, aminosalicylic acid, amphetamine, anticonvulsants, antimalarials, antipyretics, antipyrine, arsenicals, benzene, busulfan, carbenicillin, cephalothin, chemotherapy drugs, chlorate, chloroquine, chlorothiazide, chlorpromazine, colchicine, corticosteroids, dapsone, dimercaprol, diphenhydramine, dipyrone, glucosulfone, glycerin, gold, hydroflumethiazide, indomethacin, mephytoin, methyldopa, nalidixic acid, neomycin, niridazole, nitrobenzene, nitrofurantoin, novobiocin, penicillin, phenacemide, phenazopyridine, phenothiazines, and pipobroman (intended effect for polycythemia); and those that result in anemia, such as miconazole, penicillamine, phenylhydrazine, primaquine, probenecid, pyrazolones, pyrimethamine, quinines, streptomycin, sulfamethizole, sulfamethoxypyridazine, sulfisoxazole, suramin, thioridazine, tolbutamide, trimethadione, and tripelennamine.

- Some drugs may also affect Hct values by increasing or decreasing the RBC count (see monograph titled "Red Blood Cell Count").

- The results of RBC counts may vary depending on the patient's position: Hct can decrease when the patient is recumbent as a result of hemodilution and can increase when the patient rises as a result of hemoconcentration.

- Leaving the tourniquet in place for longer than 60 seconds can falsely increase Hct levels by 2% to 5%.

- Traumatic venipuncture and hemolysis may result in falsely decreased Hct values.

- Failure to fill the tube sufficiently (i.e., tube less than three-quarters full) may yield inadequate sample volume for automated analyzers and may be a reason for specimen rejection.

- Clotted or hemolized specimens must be rejected for analysis.

- Care should be taken in evaluating the Hct during the first few hours after transfusion or acute blood loss because the value may appear to be normal and may not be a reliable indicator of anemia.

- Abnormalities in the RBC size (macrocytes, microcytes) or shape (spherocytes, sickle cells) may alter Hct values, as in diseases and conditions including sickle cell anemia, hereditary spherocytosis, and iron deficiency.

- Elevated blood glucose or serum sodium levels may produce elevated

Hct levels because of swelling of the erythrocytes.

Nursing Implications and Procedure

Pretest:

➤ Inform the patient that the test is used to evaluate anemia, polycythemia, and hydration status and to monitor therapy.

➤ Obtain a history of the patient's complaints, including a list of known allergens (especially allergies or sensitivities to latex), and inform the appropriate health care practitioner accordingly.

➤ Obtain a history of the patient's cardiovascular, gastrointestinal, hematopoietic, hepatobiliary, immune, musculoskeletal, and respiratory systems, as well as results of previously performed laboratory tests, surgical procedures, and other diagnostic procedures. For related laboratory tests, refer to the Cardiovascular, Gastrointestinal, Hematopoietic, Hepatobiliary, Immune, Musculoskeletal, and Respiratory System tables.

➤ Note any recent procedures that can interfere with test results.

➤ Obtain a list of the medications the patient is taking, including herbs, nutritional supplements, and nutraceuticals. The requesting health care practitioner and laboratory should be advised if the patient regularly uses these products so their that effects can be taken into consideration when reviewing results.

➤ Review the procedure with the patient. Inform the patient that specimen collection takes approximately 5 to 10 minutes. Address concerns about pain related to the procedure. Explain to the patient that there may be some discomfort during the venipuncture.

➤ *Sensitivity to social and cultural issues,* as well as concern for mod-

esty, is important in providing psychological support before, during, and after the procedure.

➤ There are no food, fluid, or medication restrictions, unless by medical direction.

Intratest:

➤ If the patient has a history of severe allergic reaction to latex, care should be taken to avoid the use of equipment containing latex.

➤ Instruct the patient to cooperate fully and to follow directions. Direct the patient to breathe normally and to avoid unnecessary movement.

➤ Observe standard precautions, and follow the general guidelines in Appendix A. Positively identify the patient, and label the appropriate tubes with the corresponding patient demographics, date, and time of collection. Perform a venipuncture; collect the specimen in a 5-mL lavender-top (EDTA) tube. An EDTA Microtainer sample may be obtained from infants, children, and adults for whom venipuncture may not be feasible. The specimen should be mixed gently by inverting the tube 10 times. The specimen should be analyzed within 6 hours when stored at room temperature or within 24 hours if stored at refrigerated temperature. If it is anticipated the specimen will not be analyzed within 4 to 6 hours, two blood smears should be made immediately after the venipuncture and submitted with the blood sample. Smears made from specimens older than 6 hours will contain an unacceptable number of misleading artifactual abnormalities of the RBCs, such as echinocytes and spherocytes, as well as necrobiotic white blood cells.

➤ Remove the needle, and apply a pressure dressing over the puncture site.

➤ Promptly transport the specimen to the laboratory for processing and analysis.

➤ The results are recorded manually or in a computerized system for recall and postprocedure interpretation by the appropriate health care practitioner.

Post-test:

➤ Observe venipuncture site for bleeding or hematoma formation. Apply paper tape or other adhesive to hold pressure bandage in place, or replace with a plastic bandage.

➤ *Nutritional considerations:* Nutritional therapy may be indicated for patients with decreased Hct. Iron deficiency is the most common nutrient deficiency in the United States. Patients at risk (e.g., children, pregnant women and women of childbearing age, low-income populations) should be instructed to include foods that are high in iron in their diet, such as meats (especially liver), eggs, grains, green leafy vegetables, and multivitamins with iron. Iron absorption is affected by numerous factors (see monograph titled "Iron").

➤ A written report of the examination will be sent to the requesting health care practitioner, who will discuss the results with the patient.

➤ Reinforce information given by the patient's health care provider regarding further testing, treatment, or referral to another health care provider. Answer any questions or address any concerns voiced by the patient or family.

➤ Depending on the results of this procedure, additional testing may be performed to evaluate or monitor progression of the disease process and determine the need for a change in therapy. Evaluate test results in relation to the patient's symptoms and other tests performed.

Related laboratory tests:

➤ Related laboratory tests include CBC, erythropoietin, ferritin, iron/total iron-binding capacity, peripheral blood smear, and reticulocyte count.

HEMOGLOBIN

SYNONYM/ACRONYM: Hgb.

SPECIMEN: Whole blood from one full lavender-top (EDTA) tube, Microtainer, or capillary. Whole blood from a green-top (lithium or sodium heparin) tube may also be submitted.

REFERENCE VALUE: (Method: Spectrophotometry)

Age	Conventional Units	SI Units (Conventional Units × 10)
Cord blood	13.5–20.5 g/dL	135–205 mmol/L
2 wk	13.4–19.8 g/dL	134–198 mmol/L
1 mo	10.7–17.1 g/dL	107–171 mmol/L
6 mo	11.1–14.4 g/dL	111–144 mmol/L
1 y	11.3–14.1 g/dL	113–141 mmol/L
9–14 y	12.0–14.4 g/dL	120–144 mmol/L
Adult		
Male	13.2–17.3 g/dL	132–173 mmol/L
Female	11.7–15.5 g/dL	117–155 mmol/L
Older adult (65–74 y)		
Male	12.6–17.4 g/dL	126–174 mmol/L
Female	11.7–16.1 g/dL	117–161 mmol/L

DESCRIPTION & RATIONALE: Hemoglobin (Hgb) is the main intracellular protein of erythrocytes. It carries oxygen (O_2) to and removes carbon dioxide (CO_2) from red blood cells (RBCs). It also serves as a buffer to maintain acid-base balance in the extracellular fluid. Each Hgb molecule consists of heme and globulin. Copper is a cofactor necessary for the enzymatic incorporation of iron molecules into heme. Heme contains iron and porphyrin molecules that have a high affinity for O_2. The affinity of Hgb molecules for O_2 is influenced by 2,3-diphosphoglycerate (2,3-DPG), a substance produced by anaerobic glycolysis to generate energy for the RBCs. When Hgb binds with 2,3-DPG, O_2 affinity decreases. The ability of Hgb to bind and release O_2 can be graphically represented by an oxyhemoglobin dissociation curve. The term *shift to the left* is used to describe an increase in the affinity of Hgb for O_2. Conditions that can cause this leftward shift include decreased body temperature, decreased 2,3-DPG, decreased CO_2 concentration, and increased pH. Conversely, a *shift to the right* represents a decrease in the affinity of Hgb for O_2. Conditions that can cause a rightward shift include increased body temperature, increased 2,3-DPG levels, increased CO_2 concentration, and decreased pH.

Hgb levels are a direct reflection of the O_2-combining capacity of the blood. It is the combination of heme and O_2 that gives blood its characteristic red color. RBC counts parallel the O_2-combining capacity of Hgb, but because some RBCs contain more Hgb than other cells, the relationship is not directly proportional. As CO_2 diffuses into RBCs, an enzyme called carbonic anhydrase converts the CO_2 into bicarbonate and hydrogen ions. Hgb that is not bound to O_2 combines with the free hydrogen ions, increasing pH. As this binding is occurring, bicarbonate is leaving the RBC in exchange for chloride ions. (For additional information about the relationship between the respiratory and renal components of this buffer system, see monograph titled "Blood Gases.")

Hgb is included in the complete blood count (CBC) and generally performed with a hematocrit (Hct). These levels parallel each other and are frequently used to evaluate anemia. *Polycythemia* is a term used in conjunction with conditions resulting from an abnormal increase in Hgb, Hct, and RBC count. *Anemia* is a term associated with conditions resulting from an abnormal decrease in Hgb, Hct, and RBC count. Results of the Hgb, Hct, and RBC count should be evaluated simultaneously because the same underlying condi-

tions affect this triad of tests similarly. The RBC count multiplied by 3 should approximate the Hgb concentration. The Hct should be within three times the Hgb if the RBC population is normal in size and shape. The Hct plus 6 should approximate the first two figures of the RBC count within 3 (e.g., Hct is 40%; therefore 40 + 6 = 46, and the RBC count should be 4.6 or in the range of 4.3 to 4.9). There are some cultural variations in Hgb and Hct (H&H) values. After the first decade of life, the mean Hgb in African Americans is 0.5 to 1.0 g lower than in whites. Mexican Americans and Asian Americans have higher Hgb and H&H values than whites. ■

INDICATIONS:

- Detect hematologic disorder, neoplasm, or immunologic abnormality

- Determine the presence of hereditary hematologic abnormality

- Evaluate known or suspected anemia and related treatment, in combination with Hct

- Monitor blood loss and response to blood replacement, in combination with Hct

- Monitor the effects of physical or emotional stress on the patient

- Monitor fluid imbalances or their treatment

- Monitor hematologic status during pregnancy, in combination with Hct

- Monitor the progression of nonhematologic disorders, such as chronic obstructive pulmonary disease (COPD), malabsorption syndromes, cancer, and renal disease

- Monitor response to drugs or chemotherapy, and evaluate undesired reactions to drugs that may cause blood dyscrasias

• Provide screening as part of a CBC in a general physical examination, especially upon admission to a health care facility or before surgery

RESULT

Increased in:

• Burns

• Congestive heart failure

• COPD

• Dehydration

• Erythrocytosis

• Hemoconcentration

• High altitudes

• Polycythemia vera

Decreased in:

• Anemias

• Carcinoma

• Fluid retention

• Hemoglobinopathies

• Hemolytic disorders

• Hemorrhage (acute and chronic)

• Hodgkin's disease

• Incompatible blood transfusion

• Intravenous overload

• Leukemia

• Lymphomas

• Nutritional deficit

• Pregnancy

• Splenomegaly

CRITICAL VALUES:
Less than 6.0 g/dL
Greater than 18.0 g/dL
Note and immediately report to the health care practitioner any critically

increased or decreased values and related symptoms.

• Low Hgb leads to anemia. Anemia can be caused by blood loss, decreased blood cell production, increased blood cell destruction, and hemodilution. Causes of blood loss include menstrual excess or frequency, gastrointestinal bleeding, inflammatory bowel disease, and hematuria. Decreased blood cell production can be caused by folic acid deficiency, vitamin B_{12} deficiency, iron deficiency, and chronic disease. Increased blood cell destruction can be caused by a hemolytic reaction, chemical reaction, medication reaction, and sickle cell disease. Hemodilution can be caused by congestive heart failure, renal failure, polydipsia, and overhydration. Symptoms of anemia (due to these causes) include anxiety, dyspnea, edema, hypertension, hypotension, hypoxia, jugular venous distention, fatigue, pallor, rales, restlessness, and weakness. Treatment of anemia depends on the cause.

• High Hgb leads to polycythemia. Polycythemia can be caused by dehydration, decreased oxygen levels in the body, and an overproduction of RBCs by the bone marrow. Dehydration from diuretic use, vomiting, diarrhea, excessive sweating, severe burns, or decreased fluid intake decreases the plasma component of whole blood, thereby increasing the ratio of RBCs to plasma and leads to a higher than normal Hgb. Causes of decreased oxygen include smoking, exposure to carbon monoxide, high altitude, and chronic lung disease, which leads to a mild hemoconcentration of blood in the body to carry more oxygen to the body's tissues. An overproduction of RBCs by the bone marrow leads to polycythemia vera, which is a rare chronic myeloproliferative disorder that leads to a severe hemoconcentration of blood. Severe hemoconcentration can lead to thrombosis (spontaneous blood clotting).

Symptoms of hemoconcentration include decreased pulse pressure and volume, loss of skin turgor, dry mucous membranes, headaches, hepatomegaly, low central venous pressure, orthostatic hypotension, pruritis (especially after a hot bath), splenomegaly, tachycardia, thirst, tinnitus, vertigo, and weakness. Treatment of polycythemia depends on the cause. Possible interventions for hemoconcentration due to dehydration include intravenous fluids and discontinuance of diuretics if they are believed to be contributing to critically elevated Hgb. Polycythemia due to decreased oxygen states can be treated by removal of the offending substance, such as smoke or carbon monoxide. Treatment includes oxygen therapy in cases of smoke inhalation, carbon monoxide poisioning, and desaturating chronic lung disease. Symptoms of polycythemic overload crisis include signs of thrombosis, pain and redness in extremities, facial flushing, and irritability. Possible interventions for hemoconcentration due to polycythemia include therapeutic phlebotomy and intravenous fluids.

INTERFERING FACTORS:

- Drugs and substances that may cause a decrease in Hgb levels include those that induce hemolysis due to drug sensitivity or enzyme deficiency, such as acetaminophen, aminopyrine, aminosalicylic acid, amphetamine, anticonvulsants, antimalarials, antipyretics, antipyrine, arsenicals, benzene, busulfan, carbenicillin, cephalothin, chemotherapy drugs, chlorate, chloroquine, chlorothiazide, chlorpromazine, colchicine, corticosteroids, dapsone, dimercaprol, diphenhydramine, dipyrone, glucosulfone, glycerin, gold, hydroflumethiazide, indomethacin, mepheytoin, methyldopa, nalidixic acid, neomycin, niridazole, nitrobenzene, nitrofurantoin, novobiocin, penicillin, phenacemide, phenazopyridine, and phenothiazines; and those that result in

anemia, such as miconazole, penicillamine, phenylhydrazine, primaquine, probenecid, pyrazolones, pyrimethamine, quinines, streptomycin, sulfamethizole, sulfamethoxypyridazine, sulfisoxazole, suramin, thioridazine, tolbutamide, trimethadione, and tripelennamine.

- Some drugs may also affect Hgb values by increasing or decreasing the RBC count (see monograph titled "Red Blood Cell Count").

- The results of RBC counts may vary depending on the patient's position: Hgb can decrease when the patient is recumbent as a result of hemodilution and can increase when the patient rises as a result of hemoconcentration.

- Use of the neutraceutical liver extract is strongly contraindicated in iron-storage disorders, such as hemochromatosis, because it is rich in heme (the iron-containing pigment in Hgb).

- A severe copper deficiency may result in decreased Hgb levels.

- Cold agglutinins may falsely increase the mean corpuscular Hgb concentration (MCHC) and decrease the RBC count, affecting Hgb values. This can be corrected by warming the blood or replacing the plasma with warmed saline and repeating the analysis.

- Leaving the tourniquet in place for longer than 60 seconds can falsely increase Hgb levels by 2% to 5%.

- Failure to fill the tube sufficiently (i.e., tube less than three-quarters full) may yield inadequate sample volume for automated analyzers and may be a reason for specimen rejection.

- Clotted or hemolyzed specimens must be rejected for analysis.

- Care should be taken in evaluating the Hgb during the first few hours after transfusion or acute blood loss because the value may appear to be normal.

- Abnormalities in the RBC size (macrocytes, microcytes) or shape (spherocytes, sickle cells) may alter Hgb values, as in diseases and conditions including sickle cell anemia, hereditary spherocytosis, and iron deficiency.

- Lipemia will falsely increase the Hgb measurement, also affecting the mean corpuscular volume (MCV) and MCHC. This can be corrected by replacing the plasma with saline, repeating the measurement, and manually correcting the Hgb, MCH, and MCHC using specific mathematical formulas.

Nursing Implications and Procedure • • • • • • • • • • •

Pretest:

➤ Inform the patient that the test is used to evaluate anemia, polycythemia, and hydration status and to monitor therapy.

➤ Obtain a history of the patient's complaints, including a list of known allergens (especially allergies or sensitivities to latex), and inform the appropriate health care practitioner accordingly.

➤ Obtain a history of the patient's cardiovascular, gastrointestinal, hematopoietic, hepatobiliary, immune, musculoskeletal, and respiratory systems, as well as results of previously performed laboratory tests, surgical procedures, and other diagnostic procedures. For related laboratory tests, refer to the Cardiovascular, Gastrointestinal, Hematopoietic, Hepatobiliary, Immune, Musculoskeletal, and Respiratory System tables.

➤ Note any recent procedures that can interfere with test results.

➤ Obtain a list of the medications the patient is taking, including herbs, nutritional supplements, and nutraceuticals. The requesting health care practitioner and laboratory should be

advised if the patient regularly uses these products so that their effects can be taken into consideration when reviewing results.

➤ Review the procedure with the patient. Inform the patient that specimen collection takes approximately 5 to 10 minutes. Address concerns about pain related to the procedure. Explain to the patient that there may be some discomfort during the venipuncture.

➤ *Sensitivity to social and cultural issues,* as well as concern for modesty, is important in providing psychological support before, during, and after the procedure.

➤ There are no food, fluid, or medication restrictions, unless by medical direction.

Intratest:

➤ If the patient has a history of severe allergic reaction to latex, care should be taken to avoid the use of equipment containing latex.

➤ Instruct the patient to cooperate fully and to follow directions. Direct the patient to breathe normally and to avoid unnecessary movement.

➤ Observe standard precautions, and follow the general guidelines in Appendix A. Positively identify the patient, and label the appropriate tubes with the corresponding patient demographics, date, and time of collection. Perform a venipuncture; collect the specimen in a 5-mL lavender-top (EDTA) tube. An EDTA Microtainer sample may be obtained from infants, children, and adults for whom venipuncture may not be feasible. The specimen should be mixed gently by inverting the tube 10 times. The specimen should be analyzed within 6 hours when stored at room temperature or within 24 hours if stored at refrigerated temperature. If it is anticipated the specimen will not be analyzed within 4 to 6 hours, two blood smears should be made immediately after the venipuncture and submitted with the blood sample. Smears made from specimens older than 6 hours will contain an unacceptable number of misleading artifactual abnormalities of the RBCs, such as echinocytes and spherocytes, as well as necrobiotic white blood cells.

➤ Remove the needle, and apply a pressure dressing over the puncture site.

➤ Promptly transport the specimen to the laboratory for processing and analysis.

➤ The results are recorded manually or in a computerized system for recall and postprocedure interpretation by the appropriate health care practitioner.

Post-test:

➤ Observe venipuncture site for bleeding or hematoma formation. Apply paper tape or other adhesive to hold pressure bandage in place, or replace with a plastic bandage.

➤ *Nutritional considerations:* Nutritional therapy may be indicated for patients with decreased Hgb. Iron deficiency is the most common nutrient deficiency in the United States. Patients at risk (e.g., children, pregnant women and women of childbearing age, low-income populations) should be instructed to include foods that are high in iron in their diet, such as meats (especially liver), eggs, grains, green leafy vegetables, and multivitamins with iron. Iron absorption is affected by numerous factors (see monograph titled "Iron").

➤ A written report of the examination will be sent to the requesting health care practitioner, who will discuss the results with the patient.

➤ Reinforce information given by the patient's health care provider regarding further testing, treatment, or referral to another health care provider. Answer any questions or address any concerns voiced by the patient or family.

➤ Depending on the results of this procedure, additional testing may be performed to evaluate or monitor progression of the disease process and determine the need for a change in therapy. Evaluate test results in relation to the patient's symptoms and other tests performed.

Related laboratory tests:

➤ Related laboratory tests include CBC, erythropoietin, ferritin, iron/total iron-binding capacity, peripheral blood smear, and reticulocyte count.

HEMOGLOBIN ELECTROPHORESIS

SYNONYM/ACRONYM: N/A.

SPECIMEN: Whole blood (1 mL) collected in a lavender-top (EDTA) tube.

REFERENCE VALUE: (Method: Electrophoresis)

Hgb A	
Adult	Greater than 95%
Hgb A₂	
Adult	1.5–3.7%
Hgb F	
Newborns and infants	
1 d–3 wk	70–77%
6–9 wk	42–64%
3–4 mo	7–39%
6 mo	3–7%
8–11 mo	0.6–2.6%
Adult	Less than 2%

DESCRIPTION & RATIONALE: Hemoglobin (Hgb) electrophoresis is a separation process used to identify normal and abnormal forms of Hgb. Hgb A is the main form of Hgb in the normal adult. Hgb F is the main form of Hgb in the fetus, the remainder being composed of Hgb A_1 and A_2. Small amounts of Hgb F are normal in the adult. Hgb D, E, H, S, and C result from abnormal amino acid substitutions during the formation of Hgb and are inherited hemoglobinopathies. ■

INDICATIONS:

• Assist in the diagnosis of Hgb C disease

• Assist in the diagnosis of thalassemia, especially in patients with a family history positive for the disorder

• Differentiate among thalassemia types

• Evaluate hemolytic anemia of unknown cause

• Evaluate a positive sickle cell screening test to differentiate sickle cell trait from sickle cell disease

RESULT

Increased:

• Hgb A_2:

Megaloblastic anemia
Thalassemias

• Hgb F:
Acquired aplastic anemia
Hereditary persistence of fetal Hgb
Hyperthyroidism
Leakage of fetal blood into
   maternal circulation
Leukemia (acute or chronic)
Myeloproliferative disorders
Sickle cell disease
Thalassemias

• β-Chain substitutions:
Hgb C (second most common
   variant in the United States, it
   has a higher prevalence among
   African Americans):

• Hgb C disease
Hgb D (rare hemoglobinopathy that
   may also be found in
   combination with Hgb S or
   thalassemia):

• Splenomegaly without other significant clinical implications
Hgb E (second most common
   hemoglobinopathy in the world,
   occurs with the highest
   frequency in Southeast Asians
   and African-Americans):

• Thalassemia-like condition

Hgb S (most common variant in the United States, occurs with a frequency of about 8% among African Americans):

- Sickle cell trait or disease

- α-Chain substitutions: Hgb H:

- α-Thalassemias Bart's Hgb:

- α-Thalassemias

- Hgb Bart's hydrops fetalis syndrome

Decreased:
- Hgb A_2: Erythroleukemia:

- Hgb H disease

- Iron-deficiency anemia (untreated)

- Sideroblastic anemia

CRITICAL VALUES: N/A

INTERFERING FACTORS:
- High altitude and dehydration may increase values.

- Iron deficiency may decrease Hgb A_2, C, and S.

- In patients less than 3 months of age, false-negative results for Hgb S occur in coincidental polycythemia.

- Red blood cell transfusion within 4 months of test can mask abnormal Hgb levels.

Nursing Implications and Procedure

Pretest:

➤ Inform the patient that the test is used to identify hemoglobin variants and diagnose thalassemias.

➤ Obtain a history of the patient's complaints, including a list of known allergens (especially allergies or sen-

sitivities to latex), and inform the appropriate health care practitioner accordingly.

➤ Obtain a history of the patient's hematopoietic system, as well as results of previously performed laboratory tests, surgical procedures, and other diagnostic procedures. For related laboratory tests, refer to the Hematopoietic System table.

➤ Note any recent procedures that can interfere with test results.

➤ Obtain a list of the medications the patient is taking, including herbs, nutritional supplements, and nutraceuticals. The requesting health care practitioner and laboratory should be advised if the patient is regularly using these products so that their effects can be taken into consideration when reviewing results.

➤ Review the procedure with the patient. Inform the patient that specimen collection takes approximately 5 to 10 minutes. Address concerns about pain related to the procedure. Explain to the patient that there may be some discomfort during the venipuncture.

➤ *Sensitivity to social and cultural issues,* as well as concern for modesty, is important in providing psychological support before, during, and after the procedure.

➤ There are no food, fluid, or medication restrictions, unless by medical direction.

Intratest:

➤ If the patient has a history of severe allergic reaction to latex, care should be taken to avoid the use of equipment containing latex.

➤ Instruct the patient to cooperate fully and to follow directions. Direct the patient to breathe normally and to avoid unnecessary movement.

➤ Observe standard precautions, and follow the general guidelines in Appendix A. Positively identify the patient, and label the appropriate tubes with the corresponding patient

demographics, date, and time of collection. Perform a venipuncture; collect the specimen in a 5-mL lavender-top tube.

➤ Remove the needle, and apply a pressure dressing over the puncture site.

➤ Promptly transport the specimen to the laboratory for processing and analysis.

➤ The results are recorded manually or in a computerized system for recall and postprocedure interpretation by the appropriate health care practitioner.

Post-test:

➤ Observe venipuncture site for bleeding or hematoma formation. Apply paper tape or other adhesive to hold pressure bandage in place, or replace with a plastic bandage.

➤ A written report of the examination will be sent to the requesting health care practitioner, who will discuss the results with the patient.

➤ Reinforce information given by the patient's health care provider regarding further testing, treatment, or referral to another health care provider. Answer any questions or address any concerns voiced by the patient or family.

➤ Depending on the results of this procedure, additional testing may be performed to evaluate or monitor progression of the disease process and determine the need for a change in therapy. Evaluate test results in relation to the patient's symptoms and other tests performed.

Related laboratory tests:

➤ Related laboratory tests include blood gases, complete blood count (including evaluation of blood smear for RBC morphology), methemoglobin, and sickle cell screen.

HEMOSIDERIN

SYNONYMS/ACRONYM: Hemosiderin stain, Pappenheimer body stain, iron stain.

SPECIMEN: Urine (5 mL) from a random first morning sample, collected in a clean plastic collection container.

REFERENCE VALUE: (Method: Microscopic examination of Prussian blue–stained specimen) None seen.

DESCRIPTION & RATIONALE: Hemosiderin stain is used to indicate the presence of iron storage granules called *hemosiderin* by microscopic examination of urine sediment. Granules of hemosiderin stain blue when potassium ferrocyanide is added to the sample. Hemosiderin is normally found in the liver, spleen, and bone marrow, but not in the urine. Under normal conditions, hemosiderin is absorbed by the renal tubules; however, in extensive hemolysis, renal tubule damage, or an iron metabolism disorder, hemosiderin filters its way into the urine. The Prussian blue stain may also be used to identify siderocytes (iron-containing red blood cells [RBCs]) in peripheral blood. The presence of siderocytes in circulating RBCs is abnormal. ▪

INDICATIONS:

• Assist in the diagnosis of hemochromatosis (tissue damage caused by iron toxicity)

• Detect excessive RBC hemolysis within the systemic circulation

• Evaluate renal tubule dysfunction

RESULT

Increased in:

• Burns

• Cold hemagglutinin disease

• Hemochromatosis

• Hemolytic transfusion reactions

• Mechanical trauma to RBCs

• Megaloblastic anemia

• Microangiopathic hemolytic anemia

• Paroxysmal nocturnal hemoglobinuria

• Pernicious anemia

• Sickle cell anemia

• Thalassemia major

Decreased in: N/A

CRITICAL VALUES: N/A

INTERFERING FACTORS: N/A

Nursing Implications and Procedure • • • • • • • • • • • •

Pretest:

➤ Inform the patient that the test is used to indicate recent intravascular hemolysis and to assist in the diagnosis of unexplained anemia.

➤ Obtain a history of the patient's complaints, including a list of known allergens, and inform the appropriate health care practitioner accordingly.

➤ Obtain a history of the patient's hematopoietic and genitourinary systems, especially a history of hemolytic anemia, as well as results of previously performed laboratory tests, surgical procedures, and other diagnostic procedures. For related laboratory tests, refer to the Hematopoietic and Genitourinary System tables.

➤ Obtain a list of the medications the patient is taking, including herbs, nutritional supplements, and nutraceuticals. The requesting health care practitioner and laboratory should be advised if the patient regularly uses these products so that their effects can be taken into consideration when reviewing results.

➤ Review the procedure with the patient. Inform the patient that specimen collection takes approximately 5 to 10 minutes. Address concerns about pain related to the procedure. Explain to the patient that there should be no discomfort during the procedure.

➤ *Sensitivity to social and cultural issues,* as well as concern for modesty, is important in providing psychological support before, during, and after the procedure.

➤ There are no food, fluid, or medication restrictions, unless by medical direction.

Intratest:

➤ If the patient has a history of severe allergic reaction to latex, care should

be taken to avoid the use of equipment containing latex.

➤ Instruct the patient to cooperate fully and to follow directions.

➤ Observe standard precautions, and follow the general guidelines in Appendix A. Positively identify the patient, and label the appropriate collection container with the corresponding patient demographics, date, and time of collection.

Clean-catch specimen:

➤ Instruct the male patient to (1) thoroughly wash his hands, (2) cleanse the meatus, (3) void a small amount into the toilet, and (4) void directly into the specimen container.

➤ Instruct the female patient to (1) thoroughly wash her hands; (2) cleanse the labia from front to back; (3) while keeping the labia separated, void a small amount into the toilet; and (4) without interrupting the urine stream, void directly into the specimen container.

Indwelling catheter:

➤ Put on gloves. Empty drainage tube of urine. It may be necessary to clamp off the catheter for 15 to 30 minutes before specimen collection. Cleanse specimen port with antiseptic swab, and then aspirate 5 mL of urine with a 21- to 25-gauge needle and syringe. Transfer urine to a collection container.

General:

➤ Promptly transport the specimen to the laboratory for processing and analysis.

➤ The results are recorded manually or in a computerized system for recall and postprocedure interpretation by the appropriate health care practitioner.

Post-test:

➤ A written report of the examination will be sent to the requesting health care practitioner, who will discuss the results with the patient.

➤ Recognize anxiety related to test results. Discuss the implications of abnormal test results on the patient's lifestyle. Provide teaching and information regarding the clinical implications of the test results, as appropriate.

➤ Reinforce information given by the patient's health care provider regarding further testing, treatment, or referral to another health care provider. Answer any questions or address any concerns voiced by the patient or family.

➤ Depending on the results of this procedure, additional testing may be performed to evaluate or monitor progression of the disease process and determine the need for a change in therapy. Evaluate test results in relation to the patient's symptoms and other tests performed.

Related laboratory tests:

➤ Related laboratory tests include bone marrow studies, complete blood count, ferritin, iron/total iron-binding capacity, kidney biopsy, lead, and RBC morphology.

HEPATITIS A ANTIBODY

SYNONYM/ACRONYM: HAV serology.

SPECIMEN: Serum (1 mL) collected in a red- or tiger-top tube.

REFERENCE VALUE: (Method: Enzyme immunoassay) Negative.

DESCRIPTION & RATIONALE: The hepatitis A virus is classified as a picornavirus. Its primary mode of transmission is by the fecal-oral route under conditions of poor personal hygiene or inadequate sanitation. The incubation period is about 28 days, with a range of 15 to 50 days. Onset is usually abrupt, with the acute disease lasting about 1 week. Therapy is supportive, and there is no development of chronic or carrier states. Assays for total (immunoglobulin G and immunoglobulin M [IgM]) hepatitis A antibody and IgM-specific hepatitis A antibody assist in differentiating recent infection from prior exposure. If results from the IgM-specific or from both assays are positive, recent infection is suspected. If the IgM-specific test results are negative and the total antibody test results are positive, past infection is indicated. The clinically significant assay—IgM-specific antibody—is often the only test requested. Jaundice occurs in 70% to 80% of adult cases of HAV infection and in 70% of pediatric cases. ■

INDICATIONS:
• Screen individuals at high risk of exposure, such as those in long-term residential facilities or correctional facilities

• Screen individuals with suspected HAV infection

RESULT

Positive findings in:
• Individuals with current hepatitis A infection

• Individuals with past hepatitis A infection

CRITICAL VALUES: N/A

INTERFERING FACTORS: N/A

Nursing Implications and Procedure

Pretest:

➤ Inform the patient that the test is used to test blood for the presence of antibodies that would indicate past or current hepatitis A infection.

➤ Obtain a history of the patient's complaints, including a list of known allergens (especially allergies or sensitivities to latex), and inform the appropriate health care practitioner accordingly.

➤ Obtain a history of the patient's hepatobiliary and immune systems and results of previously performed laboratory tests, surgical procedures, and other diagnostic procedures. For related laboratory tests, refer to the Hepatobiliary and Immune System tables.

➤ Obtain a list of the medications the patient is taking, including herbs, nutritional supplements, and nutraceuticals. The requesting health care practitioner and laboratory should be advised if the patient regularly uses these products so that their effects can be taken into consideration when reviewing results.

➤ Review the procedure with the patient. Inform the patient that specimen collection takes approximately 5 to 10 minutes. Address concerns about pain related to the procedure. Explain to the patient that there may be some discomfort during the venipuncture.

➤ There are no food, fluid, or medication restrictions, unless by medical direction.

Intratest:

➤ If the patient has a history of severe allergic reaction to latex, care should be taken to avoid the use of equipment containing latex.

➤ Instruct the patient to cooperate fully and to follow directions. Direct the patient to breathe normally and to avoid unnecessary movement.

➤ Observe standard precautions, and follow the general guidelines in Appendix A. Positively identify the patient, and label the appropriate tubes with the corresponding patient demographics, date, and time of collection. Perform a venipuncture; collect the specimen in a 5-mL red- or tiger-top tube.

➤ Remove the needle, and apply a pressure dressing over the puncture site.

➤ Promptly transport the specimen to the laboratory for processing and analysis.

➤ The results are recorded manually or in a computerized system for recall and postprocedure interpretation by the appropriate health care practitioner.

Post-test:

➤ Observe venipuncture site for bleeding or hematoma formation. Apply paper tape or other adhesive to hold pressure bandage in place, or replace with a plastic bandage.

➤ *Nutritional considerations:* Dietary recommendations may be indicated and will vary depending on the type and severity of the condition. Elimination of alcohol ingestion and a diet optimized for convalescence are commonly included in the treatment plan.

➤ A written report of the examination will be sent to the requesting health care practitioner, who will discuss the results with the patient.

➤ *Social and cultural considerations:* Recognize anxiety related to test results, and offer support. Discuss the implications of abnormal test results on the patient's lifestyle. Provide teaching and information regarding the clinical implications of the test results, as appropriate. Counsel the patient, as appropriate, regarding risk of transmission and proper prophylaxis. Immune globulin can be given before exposure (in the case of individuals who may be traveling to a location where the disease is endemic) or after exposure, during the incubation period. Prophylaxis is most effective when administered 2 weeks after exposure.

➤ Reinforce information given by the patient's health care provider regarding further testing, treatment, or referral to another health care provider. Answer any questions or address any concerns voiced by the patient or family.

Depending on the results of this procedure, additional testing may be performed to evaluate or monitor progression of the disease process and determine the need for a change in therapy. Evaluate test results in relation to the patient's symptoms and other tests performed.

Related laboratory tests include alanine aminotransferase, alkaline phosphatase, aspartate aminotransferase, bilirubin, γ-glutamyltranspeptidase, and hepatitis B and C antigens and antibodies.

HEPATITIS B ANTIGEN AND ANTIBODY

SYNONYMS/ACRONYMS: HBeAg, HBeAb, HBcAb, HBsAb, HBsAg.

SPECIMEN: Serum (1 mL) collected in a red- or tiger-top tube.

REFERENCE VALUE: (Method: Enzyme immunoassay) Negative.

DESCRIPTION & RATIONALE: The hepatitis B virus (HBV) is classified as a double-stranded DNA retrovirus of the Hepadnaviridae family. Its primary modes of transmission are parenteral, perinatal, and sexual contact. Serologic profiles vary with different scenarios (i.e., asymptomatic infection, acute/resolved infection, coinfection, and chronic carrier state). The formation and detectability of markers is also dose dependent. The following description refers to HBV infection that becomes resolved. The incubation period is generally 6 to 16 weeks. The hepatitis B surface antigen (HBsAg) is the first marker to appear after infection. It is detectable 8 to 12 weeks after exposure and often precedes symptoms. At about the time liver enzymes fall back to normal levels, the HBsAg titer has fallen to nondetectable levels. If the HBsAg remains detectable after 6 months, the patient will likely become a chronic carrier who can transmit the virus. Hepatitis Be antigen (HBeAg) appears in the serum 10 to 12 weeks after exposure. HBeAg can be found in the serum of patients with acute or chronic HBV infection and is a sign of active viral replication and infectivity. Levels of hepatitis Be antibody (HBeAb) appear about 14 weeks after exposure, suggesting resolution of the infection and reduction of the patient's ability to transmit the disease. The more quickly HBeAg disappears, the shorter the acute phase of the infection. Immunoglobulin M–specific hepatitis B core antibody (HBcAb) appears 6 to 14 weeks after exposure to HBsAg and continues to be detectable either until the infection is resolved or over the life span in patients who are in a chronic carrier state. In some cases, HBcAb may be the only detectable marker; hence its lone appearance has sometimes been referred to as the *core window*. HBcAb is not an indicator of recovery or immunity; however, it does indicate current or previous infection. Hepatitis B surface antibody (HBsAb) appears 2 to 16 weeks after HBsAg disappears. Appearance of HBsAb represents clinical recovery and immunity to the virus.

Onset of HBV infection is usually insidious. Most children and half of infected adults are asymptomatic. During the acute phase of infection, symptoms range from mild to severe. Chronicity decreases with age. HBsAg and HBcAb tests are used to screen donated blood before transfusion. HBsAg testing is often part of the routine prenatal screen. ▪

INDICATIONS:
• Detect exposure to HBV
• Detect possible carrier status
• Screen donated blood before transfusion
• Screen for individuals at high risk of exposure, such as hemodialysis patients, persons with multiple sex partners, persons with a history of other sexually transmitted diseases, intravenous drug abusers, infants born to infected mothers, individuals residing in long-term residential facilities or correctional facilities, recipients of blood- or plasma-derived products, allied health care workers, and public service employees who come in contact with blood and blood products.

RESULT

Positive findings in:
• Patients currently infected with HBV
• Patients with a past HBV infection

CRITICAL VALUES: N/A

INTERFERING FACTORS: Drugs that may decrease HBeAb and HBsAb include interferon.

Nursing Implications and Procedure ・・・・・・・・・・・

Pretest:

➤ Inform the patient that the test is used to identify and confirm hepatitis B infection.

➤ Obtain a history of the patient's complaints, including a list of known allergens (especially allergies or sensitivities to latex), and inform the appropriate health care practitioner accordingly.

➤ Obtain a history of the patient's hepatobiliary and immune systems, as well as results of previously performed laboratory tests, surgical procedures, and other diagnostic procedures. For related laboratory tests, refer to the Hepatobiliary and Immune System tables.

➤ Obtain a history of intravenous drug use, high-risk sexual activity, or occupational exposure.

➤ Obtain a list of the medications the patient is taking, including herbs, nutritional supplements, and nutraceuticals. The requesting health care practitioner and laboratory should be advised if the patient is regularly using these products so that their effects can be taken into consideration when reviewing results.

➤ Review the procedure with the patient. Inform the patient that specimen collection takes approximately 5 to 10 minutes. Address concerns about pain related to the procedure. Explain to the patient that there may be some discomfort during the venipuncture.

➤ *Sensitivity to social and cultural issues,* as well as concern for modesty, is important in providing psychological support before, during, and after the procedure.

➤ There are no food, fluid, or medication restrictions, unless by medical direction.

Intratest:

➤ If the patient has a history of severe allergic reaction to latex, care should be taken to avoid the use of equipment containing latex.

➤ Instruct the patient to cooperate fully and to follow directions. Direct the patient to breathe normally and to avoid unnecessary movement.

➤ Observe standard precautions, and follow the general guidelines in Appendix A. Positively identify the patient, and label the appropriate tubes with the corresponding patient demographics, date, and time of collection. Perform a venipuncture; collect the specimen in a 5-mL red- or tiger-top tube.

➤ Remove the needle, and apply a pressure dressing over the puncture site.

➤ Promptly transport the specimen to the laboratory for processing and analysis.

➤ The results are recorded manually or in a computerized system for recall and postprocedure interpretation by the appropriate health care practitioner.

Post-test:

➤ Observe venipuncture site for bleeding or hematoma formation. Apply paper tape or other adhesive to hold pressure bandage in place, or replace with a plastic bandage.

➤ *Nutritional considerations:* Dietary recommendations may be indicated and will vary depending on the type and severity of the condition. Elimination of alcohol ingestion, and a diet optimized for convalescence are commonly included in the treatment plan. A high-calorie, high-protein, moderate-fat diet with a high fluid intake is often recommended for patients with hepatitis.

➤ A written report of the examination will be sent to the requesting health care practitioner, who will discuss the results with the patient.

➤ *Cultural and social considerations:* Recognize anxiety related to test results, and be supportive of impaired activity related to lack of neuromuscular control, perceived loss of independence, and fear of shortened life expectancy. Discuss the implications of abnormal test results on the patient's lifestyle. Provide teaching and information regarding the clinical implications of the test results, as appropriate. Educate the patient regarding access to counseling services. Counsel the patient, as appropriate, regarding risk of transmission and proper prophylaxis. Hepatitis B immune globulin (HBIG) vaccination should be given immediately after situations in which there is a potential for HBV exposure (e.g., accidental needle stick, perinatal period, sexual contact) for temporary, passive protection. Some studies have indicated that interferon alfa may be useful in the treatment of chronic hepatitis B.

➤ Counsel the patient and significant contacts, as appropriate, that HBIG immunization is available and has in fact become a requirement in many places as part of childhood immunization and employee health programs. Parents may choose to sign a waiver preventing their newborns from receiving the vaccine; they may choose not to vaccinate on the basis of philosophical, religious, or medical reasons. Vaccination regulations vary from state to state.

➤ Inform the patient that positive findings must be reported to local health department officials, who will question him or her regarding sexual partners.

➤ Offer support, as appropriate, to patients who may be the victims of rape or other forms of sexual assault, including children and elderly individuals. Educate the patient regarding access to counseling services. Provide a nonjudgmental, nonthreatening atmosphere for a discussion during which the risks of sexually transmitted diseases are explained. It is also important to discuss the problems that the patient may experience (e.g., guilt, depression, anger).

➤ Reinforce information given by the patient's health care provider regarding further testing, treatment, or referral to another health care provider. Answer any questions or address any concerns voiced by the patient or family.

➤ Depending on the results of this procedure, additional testing may be performed to evaluate or monitor progression of the disease process and determine the need for a change in therapy. Evaluate test results in relation to the patient's symptoms and other tests performed.

Related laboratory tests:

➤ Related laboratory tests include alanine aminotransferase, alkaline phosphatase, aspartate aminotransferase, bilirubin, culture anal and chlamydia group antibody, γ-glutamyltranspeptidase, hepatitis C serology, human immunodeficiency virus serology, liver biopsy, and syphilis serology.

HEPATITIS C ANTIBODY

SYNONYMS/ACRONYMS: HCV serology, hepatitis non-A/non-B.

SPECIMEN: Serum (1 mL) collected in a red- or tiger-top tube.

REFERENCE VALUE: (Method: Enzyme immunoassay, branched chain DNA [bDNA], polymerase chain reaction [PCR], recombinant immunoblot assay [RIBA]) Negative.

DESCRIPTION & RATIONALE: The hepatitis C virus (HCV) causes the majority of blood-borne non-A, non-B hepatitis cases. Its primary modes of transmission are parenteral, perinatal, and sexual contact. The virus is thought to be a flavivirus and contains a single-stranded RNA core. The incubation period varies widely, from 2 to 52 weeks. Onset is insidious, and the risk of chronic liver disease after infection is high. On average, antibodies to hepatitis C are detectable in approximately 45% of infected individuals within 6 weeks of infection. The remaining 55% produce antibodies within the next 6 to 12 months. Once infected with HCV, 50% of patients will become chronic carriers. Infected individuals and carriers have a high frequency of chronic liver diseases such as cirrhosis and chronic active hepatitis, and they have a higher risk of developing hepatocellular cancer. The transmission of hepatitis C by blood transfusion has decreased dramatically since it became part of the routine screening panel for blood donors. The possibility of prenatal transmission exists, especially in the presence of human immunodeficiency virus (HIV) coinfection. Therefore, this test is often included in prenatal testing packages. ■

INDICATIONS:

• Assist in the diagnosis of non-A, non-B viral hepatitis infection

• Monitor patients suspected of HCV infection but who have not yet produced antibody

• Screen donated blood before transfusion

RESULT

Positive findings in:
• Patients currently infected with HCV

• Patients with a past HCV infection

Negative findings in: N/A

CRITICAL VALUES: N/A

INTERFERING FACTORS: Drugs that may decrease hepatitis C antibody levels include interferon.

Nursing Implications and Procedure • • • • • • • • • • •

Pretest: ■

➤ Inform the patient that the test is used to identify and confirm hepatitis C infection.

➤ Obtain a history of the patient's complaints, including a list of known allergens (especially allergies or sensitivities to latex), and inform the appropriate health care practitioner accordingly.

➤ Obtain a history of the patient's hepatobiliary and immune systems, as well as results of previously performed laboratory tests, surgical procedures, and other diagnostic procedures. For related laboratory tests, refer to the Hepatobiliary and Immune System tables.

➤ Obtain a history of intravenous drug use, high-risk sexual activity, or occupational exposure.

➤ Obtain a list of the medications the patient is taking, including herbs, nutritional supplements, and nutraceuticals. The requesting health care practitioner and laboratory should be advised if the patient is regularly using these products so that their effects can be taken into consideration when reviewing results.

➤ Review the procedure with the patient. Inform the patient that specimen collection takes approximately 5 to 10 minutes. Address concerns about pain related to the procedure. Explain to the patient that there may be some discomfort during the venipuncture.

➤ *Sensitivity to social and cultural issues,* as well as concern for modesty, is important in providing psychological support before, during, and after the procedure.

➤ There are no food, fluid, or medication restrictions, unless by medical direction.

Intratest:

➤ If the patient has a history of severe allergic reaction to latex, care should be taken to avoid the use of equipment containing latex.

➤ Instruct the patient to cooperate fully and to follow directions. Direct the patient to breathe normally and to avoid unnecessary movement.

➤ Observe standard precautions, and follow the general guidelines in Appendix A. Positively identify the patient, and label the appropriate tubes with the corresponding patient demographics, date, and time of collection. Perform a venipuncture; collect the specimen in a 5-mL red- or tiger-top tube.

➤ Remove the needle, and apply a pressure dressing over the punc-ture site.

➤ Promptly transport the specimen to the laboratory for processing and analysis.

➤ The results are recorded manually or in a computerized system for recall and postprocedure interpretation by the appropriate health care practitioner.

Post-test:

➤ Observe venipuncture site for bleeding or hematoma formation. Apply paper tape or other adhesive to hold pressure bandage in place, or replace with a plastic bandage.

➤ *Nutritional considerations:* Dietary recommendations may be indicated and will vary depending on the type and severity of the condition. Currently, for example, there are no specific medications that can be given to cure hepatitis; however, bed rest, elimination of alcohol ingestion, and a diet optimized for convalescence are commonly included in the treatment plan. A high-calorie, high-protein, moderate-fat diet with a high fluid intake is often recommended for patients with hepatitis.

➤ A written report of the examination will be sent to the requesting health care practitioner, who will discuss the results with the patient.

➤ *Cultural and social considerations:* Recognize anxiety related to test results, and be supportive of impaired activity related to lack of neuromuscular control, perceived loss of independence, and fear of shortened life expectancy. Discuss the implications of abnormal test results on the patient's lifestyle. Provide teaching and information regarding the clinical implications of the test results, as appropriate. Educate the patient regarding access to counseling services. Counsel the patient, as appropriate, regarding the risk of transmission and proper prophylaxis. Interferon alfa was approved in 1991 by the U.S. Food and Drug Administration for use as a therapeutic agent in the treatment of chronic HCV infection.

➤ Inform the patient that positive findings must be reported to local health department officials, who will question him or her regarding sexual partners.

➤ Offer support, as appropriate, to patients who may be the victims of rape or other forms of sexual assault, including children and elderly individuals. Educate the patient regarding access to counseling services. Provide a nonjudgmental, nonthreatening atmosphere for a discussion during which the risks of sexually transmitted diseases are explained. It is also important to discuss the problems that the patient may experience (e.g., guilt, depression, anger).

➤ Reinforce information given by the patient's health care provider regarding further testing, treatment, or referral to another health care provider. Answer any questions or

address any concerns voiced by the patient or family.

➤ Depending on the results of this procedure, additional testing may be performed to evaluate or monitor progression of the disease process and determine the need for a change in therapy. Evaluate test results in relation to the patient's symptoms and other tests performed.

➤ Related laboratory tests include alanine aminotransferase, alkaline phosphatase, aspartate aminotransferase, bilirubin, culture anal and chlamydia group antibody, γ-glutamyltranspeptidase, hepatitis B serology, HIV serology, liver biopsy, and syphilis serology.

HEPATITIS D ANTIBODY

SYNONYM/ACRONYM: Delta hepatitis.

SPECIMEN: Serum (1 mL) collected in a red- or tiger-top tube.

REFERENCE VALUE: (Method: Enzyme immunoassay, EIA) Negative.

DESCRIPTION & RATIONALE: Symptoms of hepatitis D virus (HDV) infection are similar but often more severe than those of hepatitis B virus (HBV) infection. As with HBV, the primary modes of HDV transmission are parenteral, perinatal, and sexual contact. The virus contains a single-stranded RNA core. In order to replicate, it requires the presence of the hepatitis B outer coat. Therefore, HDV infection can only occur with hepatitis B coinfection or superinfection. Onset is abrupt, after an incubation period of 3 to 13 weeks. Because of its dependence on HBV, prevention can be accomplished by using the same pre-exposure and postexposure protective measures used for HBV

(see monograph titled "Hepatitis B Antigen and Antibody.") ■

INDICATIONS: Establish the presence of coinfection or superinfection in patients with HBV (clinical course of superinfection is more severe)

RESULT

Positive findings in:
• Individuals currently infected with HDV
• Individuals with a past HDV infection

CRITICAL VALUES: N/A

INTERFERING FACTORS: Drugs that may decrease hepatitis D antibody levels include interferon.

Nursing Implications and Procedure • • • • • • • • • • •

➤ Inform the patient that the test is used to test blood for the presence of antibodies that would indicate past or current hepatitis D infection.

➤ Obtain a history of the patient's complaints, including a list of known allergens (especially allergies or sensitivities to latex), and inform the appropriate health care practitioner accordingly.

➤ Obtain a history of the patient's hepatobiliary and immune systems and results of previously performed laboratory tests, surgical procedures, and other diagnostic procedures. For related laboratory tests, refer to the Hepatobiliary and Immune System tables.

➤ Obtain a history of intravenous drug use, high-risk sexual activity, or occupational exposure.

➤ Obtain a list of the medications the patient is taking, including herbs, nutritional supplements, and nutraceuticals. The requesting health care practitioner and laboratory should be advised if the patient is regularly using these products so that their effects can be taken into consideration when reviewing results.

➤ Review the procedure with the patient. Inform the patient that specimen collection takes approximately 5 to 10 minutes. Address concerns about pain related to the procedure. Explain to the patient that there may be some discomfort during the venipuncture.

➤ *Sensitivity to social and cultural issues*, as well as concern for modesty, is important in providing psychological support before, during, and after the procedure.

➤ There are no food, fluid, or medication restrictions, unless by medical direction.

➤ If the patient has a history of severe allergic reaction to latex, care should be taken to avoid the use of equipment containing latex.

➤ Instruct the patient to cooperate fully and to follow directions. Direct the patient to breathe normally and to avoid unnecessary movement.

➤ Observe standard precautions, and follow the general guidelines in Appendix A. Positively identify the patient, and label the appropriate tubes with the corresponding patient demographics, date, and time of collection. Perform a venipuncture; collect the specimen in a 5-mL red- or tiger-top tube.

➤ Remove the needle, and apply a pressure dressing over the puncture site.

➤ Promptly transport the specimen to the laboratory for processing and analysis.

➤ The results are recorded manually or in a computerized system for recall and postprocedure interpretation by the appropriate health care practitioner.

➤ Observe venipuncture site for bleeding or hematoma formation. Apply paper tape or other adhesive to hold pressure bandage in place, or replace with a plastic bandage.

➤ *Nutritional considerations:* Dietary recommendations may be indicated and will vary depending on the type and severity of the condition. Elimination of alcohol ingestion, and a diet optimized for convalescence are commonly included in the treatment plan. A high-calorie, high-protein, moderate-fat diet with a high fluid intake is often recommended for patients with hepatitis.

➤ A written report of the examination will be sent to the requesting health care practitioner, who will discuss the results with the patient.

➤ *Cultural and social considerations:*

Recognize anxiety related to test results, and and be supportive of impaired activity related to lack of neuromuscular control, perceived loss of independence, and fear of shortened life expectancy. Discuss the implications of abnormal test results on the patient's lifestyle. Provide teaching and information regarding the clinical implications of the test results, as appropriate. Educate the patient regarding access to counseling services. Counsel the patient, as appropriate, regarding the risk of transmission and proper prophylaxis. Hepatitis B immune globulin (HBIG) vaccination should be given immediately after situations in which there is a potential for HBV exposure (e.g., accidental needle stick, perinatal period, sexual contact) for temporary, passive protection.

➤ Counsel the patient and significant contacts, as appropriate, that HBIG immunization is available and has in fact become a requirement in many places as part of childhood immunization and employee health programs. Parents may choose to sign a waiver preventing their newborns from receiving the vaccine; they may choose not to vaccinate on the basis of philosophical, religious, or medical reasons. Vaccination regulations vary from state to state.

➤ Reinforce information given by the patient's health care provider regarding further testing, treatment, or referral to another health care provider. Answer any questions or address any concerns voiced by the patient or family.

➤ Depending on the results of this procedure, additional testing may be performed to evaluate or monitor progression of the disease process and determine the need for a change in therapy. Evaluate test results in relation to the patient's symptoms and other tests performed.

Related laboratory tests:

➤ Related laboratory tests include alanine aminotransferase, alkaline phosphatase, aspartate aminotransferase, bilirubin, culture anal and chlamydia group antibody, γ-glutamyltranspeptidase, hepatitis B and C antibodies/antigens human immunodeficiency virus serology, liver biopsy, and syphilis serology.

HEPATOBILIARY SCAN

SYNONYM/ACRONYM: Hepatobiliary imaging, biliary tract radionuclide scan, hepatobiliary scintigraphy, gallbladder scan, cholescintigraphy, HIDA (a technetium-99m disopropyl analogue) scan.

AREA OF APPLICATION: Bile ducts.

CONTRAST: Intravenous contrast medium (aminodiacetic acid compounds), usually combined with technetium-99m.

DESCRIPTION & RATIONALE: The hepatobiliary scan is a nuclear medicine study of the hepatobiliary excretion system. It is primarily used to determine the patency of the cystic and common bile ducts, but it can also be used to determine overall hepatic function, gallbladder function, presence of gallstones (indirectly), and sphincter of Oddi dysfunction. Technetium (Tc-99m) HIDA (tribromoethyl, an aminodiacetic acid) is injected intravenously (IV) and excreted into the bile duct system. A gamma camera detects the radiation emitted from the injected contrast medium, and a representative image of the duct system is obtained. The results are correlated with other diagnostic studies, such as IV cholangiography, computed tomography (CT) scan of the gallbladder, and ultrasonography. Gallbladder emptying or ejection fraction can be determined by administering a fatty meal or cholecystokinin to the patient. This procedure can be used before and after surgery to determine the extent of bile reflux. ■

INDICATIONS:
- Aid in the diagnosis of acute and chronic cholecystitis
- Aid in the diagnosis of suspected gallbladder disorders, such as inflammation, perforation, or calculi
- Assess enterogastric reflux
- Assess obstructive jaundice when done in combination with radiography or ultrasonography
- Determine common duct obstruction caused by tumors or choledocholithiasis
- Evaluate biliary enteric bypass patency

- Postoperatively evaluate gastric surgical procedures and abdominal trauma

RESULT

Normal Findings:
- Normal shape, size, and function of the gallbladder with patent cystic and common bile ducts

Abnormal Findings:
- Acalculous cholecystitis
- Acute cholecystitis
- Chronic cholecystitis
- Common bile duct obstruction secondary to gallstones, tumor, or stricture
- Congenital biliary atresia or choledochal cyst
- Postoperative biliary leak, fistula, or obstruction
- Trauma-induced bile leak or cyst

CRITICAL VALUES: N/A

INTERFERING FACTORS:

This procedure is contraindicated for:
- Patients who are pregnant or suspected of being pregnant, unless the potential benefits of the procedure far outweigh the risks to the fetus and mother

Factors that may impair clear imaging:
- Inability of the patient to cooperate or remain still during the procedure because of age, significant pain, or mental status
- Improper adjustment of the radiographic equipment to accommodate obese or thin patients, which can cause overexposure or underexposure and poor-quality study
- Patients who are very obese, who may exceed the weight limit for the equipment

- Incorrect positioning of the patient, which may produce poor visualization of the area to be examined

- Retained barium from a previous radiologic procedure

- Metallic objects within the examination field (e.g., jewelry, body rings), which may inhibit organ visualization and can produce unclear images

- Bilirubin levels greater than or equal to 30 mg/dL, depending on the radionuclide used, which may decrease hepatic uptake

- Other nuclear scans done within the previous 24 to 48 hours

- Fasting for more than 24 hours before the procedure, total parenteral nutrition, and alcoholism

- Ingestion of food or liquids within 2 to 4 hours before the scan

Other considerations:

- Failure to follow dietary restrictions before the procedure may cause the procedure to be canceled or repeated.

- Improper injection of the radionuclide that allows the tracer to seep deep into the muscle tissue can produce erroneous hot spots.

- Inaccurate timing of imaging after the radionuclide injection can affect the results.

- Consultation with a health care practitioner should occur before the procedure for radiation safety concerns regarding younger patients or patients who are lactating.

- Risks associated with radiologic overexposure can result from frequent x-ray procedures. Personnel in the room with the patient should wear a protective lead apron, stand behind a shield, or leave the area while the examination is being done. Personnel working in the area where the examination is being done should wear badges that reveal their level of exposure to radiation.

Nursing Implications and Procedure

Pretest:

➤ Inform the patient that the procedure detects inflammation or obstruction of the gallbladder or bile duct system.

➤ Obtain a history of the patient's complaints and symptoms, including a list of known allergens.

➤ Obtain a history of results of previously performed diagnostic procedures, surgical procedures, and laboratory tests. For related diagnostic tests, refer to the Hepatobiliary System table.

➤ Record the date of the last menstrual period and determine the possibility of pregnancy in perimenopausal women.

➤ Obtain a list of the patient's current medications.

➤ Review the procedure with the patient. Address concerns about pain related to the procedure. Explain to the patient that some pain may be experienced during the test, and there may be moments of discomfort. Explain the purpose of the test and how the procedure is performed. Inform the patient that the procedure is performed in a nuclear medicine department, usually by a technologist and support staff, and usually takes approximately 60 to 90 minutes. Inform the patient that the technologist will place him or her in a supine position on a flat table for the injection of contrast medium. Delayed images are needed up to 24 hours after the initial injection. The patient may leave the department and return later to undergo delayed imaging.

➤ *Sensitivity to cultural and social issues,* as well as concern for modesty, is important in providing psychological support before, during, and after the procedure.

➤ Restrict food and fluids for 4 to 6 hours before the scan.

➤ Instruct the patient to remove dentures, jewelry (including watches), hairpins, credit cards, and other metallic objects.

➤ *Make sure a written and informed consent has been signed prior to the procedure and before administering any medications.*

Intratest:

➤ Ensure that the patient fasted for 4 to 6 hours before the scan, unless otherwise indicated.

➤ Ask patient to remove jewelry, including watches, and any other metallic objects.

➤ Patients are given a gown, robe, and foot coverings to wear and instructed to void prior to the procedure.

➤ Instruct the patient to cooperate fully and to follow directions. Instruct the patient to lie still during the procedure because movement produces unclear images.

➤ Observe standard precautions, and follow the general guidelines in Appendix A.

➤ Administer sedative to a child or to an uncooperative adult, as ordered.

➤ Place the patient in a supine position on a flat table with foam wedges to help maintain position and immobilization.

➤ IV radionuclide is administered, and the upper-right quadrant of the abdomen is scanned immediately, with images then taken every 5 minutes for the first 30 minutes and every 10 minutes for the next 30 minutes. Delayed views are taken in 2, 4, and 24 hours if the gallbladder cannot be visualized, in order to differentiate acute from chronic cholecystitis or to detect the degree of obstruction.

➤ IV morphine may be administered during the study to initiate spasms of the sphincter of Oddi, forcing the radionuclide into the gallbladder, if the organ is not visualized within 1 hour of injection of the radionuclide. Imaging is then done 20 to 50 minutes later to determine delayed visualization or nonvisualization of the gallbladder.

➤ If gallbladder function or bile reflux is being assessed, the patient will be given a fatty meal or cholecystokinin 60 minutes after the injection.

➤ Wear gloves during the radionuclide administration and while handling the patient's urine.

➤ The results are recorded on film or in a computerized system for recall and postprocedure interpretation by the appropriate health care practitioner.

Post-test:

➤ Instruct the patient to resume usual diet, medications, and activity, after imaging is complete, as directed by the health care practitioner.

➤ Advise patient to drink increased amounts of fluids for 24 to 48 hours to eliminate the radionuclide from the body, unless contraindicated. Tell the patient that radionuclide is eliminated from the body within 6 to 24 hours.

➤ Inform the patient to immediately flush the toilet after each voiding after the procedure, and to meticulously wash hands with soap and water after each voiding for 24 hours after the procedure.

➤ Tell all caregivers to wear gloves when discarding urine for 24 hours after the procedure. Wash gloved hands with soap and water before removing gloves. Then wash ungloved hands after the gloves are removed.

➤ Instruct the patient in the care and assessment of the injection site. Observe for bleeding, hematoma formation, and inflammation.

➤ A written report of the examination will be completed by a health care practitioner specializing in this branch of medicine. The report will be sent to the requesting health care practitioner, who will discuss the results with the patient.

➤ Reinforce information given by the patient's health care provider regarding further testing, treatment, or referral to another health care provider. Answer any questions or address any concerns voiced by the patient or family.

➤ Depending on the results of this procedure, additional testing may be needed to evaluate or monitor progression of the disease process and determine the need for a change in therapy. Evaluate test results in relation to the patient's symptoms and other tests performed.

Related diagnostic tests:

➤ Related diagnostic tests include computed tomography of the abdomen, magnetic resonance imaging of the abdomen, and ultrasound of the liver and bile ducts.

HER-2/NEU ONCOPROTEIN

SYNONYM/ACRONYM: c-erb-B2.

SPECIMEN: Breast tissue or cells.

REFERENCE VALUE: (Method: Immunocytochemical) Negative.

DESCRIPTION & RATIONALE: Breast cancer is the most common newly diagnosed cancer in American women. It is the second leading cause of cancer-related death. The presence of abnormal amounts of a protein called human epidermal growth factor receptor 2 (HER-2/neu oncoprotein) is helpful in establishing histologic evidence of metastatic breast cancer. Overexpression of this protein results from an acquired genetic mutation and occurs in 25% to 30% of patients with metastatic breast cancer. Metastatic breast cancer patients with high levels of HER-2/neu oncoprotein have a poor prognosis: They have rapid tumor progression, increased rate of recurrence, poor response to standard therapies, and a lower survival rate.

The specimen is collected by fine-needle or open biopsy. The tissue sample is treated with a material that binds to HER-2/neu oncoprotein. A dye is added to the tissue sample; areas of tissue that have large amounts of HER-2/neu oncoprotein are indicated by high-intensity color on the tissue sample. ■

INDICATIONS: Evidence of breast lesion by palpation, mammography, or ultrasound

RESULT

Positive findings in: Breast cancer

CRITICAL VALUES: N/A

INTERFERING FACTORS: N/A

Nursing Implications and Procedure . . . .

Pretest:

➤ Inform the patient that the test is primarily used to assist in the prognosis and in the management of response to therapy for breast cancer.

➤ Obtain a history of the patient's complaints, including a list of known allergens (especially allergies or sensitivities to latex), and inform the appropriate health care practitioner accordingly.

➤ Obtain a history of the patient's immune and reproductive systems and results of previously performed laboratory tests, surgical procedures, and other diagnostic procedures. For related laboratory tests, refer to the Immune and Reproductive System tables.

➤ Record the date of the last menstrual period and determine the possibility of pregnancy in perimenopausal women.

➤ Obtain a list of the medications the patient is taking, including anticoagulant therapy, acetylsalicylic acid, herbs, nutritional supplements, and nutraceuticals, especially those known to affect coagulation. It is recommended that use be discontinued 14 days before dental or surgical procedures. The requesting health care practitioner and laboratory should be advised if the patient regularly uses these products so that their effects can be taken into consideration when reviewing results.

➤ Review the procedure with the patient. Inform the patient that it may be necessary to shave the site before the procedure. Instruct that prophylactic antibiotics may be administered prior to the procedure. Address concerns about pain related to the procedure. Explain that a sedative and/or analgesia will be administered to promote relaxation and reduce discomfort prior to the percutaneous biopsy; a general anesthesia will be administered prior to the open biopsy. Explain to the patient that no pain will be experienced during the test when general anesthesia is used, but that any discomfort with a needle biopsy will be minimized with local anesthetics and systemic analgesics. Inform the patient that the biopsy is performed under sterile conditions by a health care practitioner specializing in this procedure. The surgical procedure usually takes about 20 to 30 minutes to complete, and that sutures may be necessary to close the site. A needle biopsy usually takes about 15 minutes to complete.

➤ *Sensitivity to cultural and social issues,* as well as concern for modesty, is important in providing psychological support before, during and after the procedure.

➤ Explain that an intravenous (IV) line will be inserted to allow infusion of IV fluids, antibiotics, anesthetics, and analgesics.

➤ Ensure that anticoagulant therapy has been withheld for the appropriate amount of days prior to the procedure. Amount of days to withhold medication is dependant on the type of anticoagulant. Notify health care practitioner if patient anticoagulant therapy has not been withheld.

Open biopsy:

➤ Instruct the patient that nothing should be taken by mouth for 6 to 8 hours prior to a general anesthetic.

Needle biopsy:

➤ Instruct the patient that nothing should be taken by mouth for at least 4 hours prior to the procedure to reduce the risk of nausea and vomiting.

General:

➤ *Make sure a written and informed consent has been signed prior to the procedure and before administering any medications.*

Intratest:

➤ Ensure that the patient has complied with dietary restrictions; assure that food has been restricted for at least 4 to 8 hours prior to the procedure, depending on the anesthetic chosen for the procedure.

➤ Have emergency equipment readily available.

➤ Have the patient void before the procedure.

➤ Observe standard precautions, and follow the general guidelines in Appendix A. Positively identify the patient, and label the appropriate collection containers with the corresponding patient demographics, date and time of collection, and site location, especially left or right breast.

➤ Assist the patient to the desired position depending on the test site to be used, and direct the patient to breath normally during the beginning of the general anesthesia. Instruct the patient to cooperate fully and to follow directions. Direct the patient to breathe normally and to avoid unnecessary movement during the local anesthetic and the procedure.

➤ Record baseline vital signs and continue to monitor throughout the procedure. Protocols may vary from facility to facility.

➤ After the administration of general or local anesthesia, cleanse the site with an antiseptic solution, and drape the area with sterile towels.

Open biopsy:

➤ After administration of general anesthesia and surgical prep is completed, an incision is made, suspi-

cious area(s) are located, and tissue samples are collected.

Needle biopsy:

➤ Direct the patient to take slow deep breaths when the local anesthetic is injected. Protect the site with sterile drapes. Instruct the patient to take a deep breath, exhale forcefully, and hold the breath while the biopsy needle is inserted and rotated to obtain a core of breast tissue. Once the needle is removed, the patient may breathe. Pressure is applied to the site for 3 to 5 minutes, then a sterile pressure dressing is applied.

General:

➤ Monitor the patient for complications related to the procedure (e.g., allergic reaction, anaphylaxis).

➤ Apply a sterile dressing to the site.

➤ Place tissue samples in properly labeled specimen container containing formalin solution, and promptly transport the specimen to the laboratory for processing and analysis.

➤ The results are recorded manually or in a computerized system for recall and postprocedure interpretation by the appropriate health care practitioner.

Post-test:

➤ Instruct the patient to resume preoperative diet, as directed by the health care practitioner.

➤ Monitor vital signs every 15 minutes for 1 hour, and then every 2 hours for 4 hours, and then as ordered by the health care practitioner. Monitor temperature every 4 hours for 24 hours. Compare with baseline values. Notify the health care practitioner if temperature is elevated. Protocols may vary from facility to facility.

➤ Observe for delayed allergic reactions, such as rash, urticaria, tachycardia, hyperpnea, hypertension, palpitations, nausea, or vomiting.

➤ Observe the biopsy site for bleeding, inflammation, or hematoma formation.

➤ Instruct the patient in the care and assessment of the site. Instruct the patient to report any redness, edema, bleeding, or pain at the biopsy site. Instruct the patient to immediately report chills or fever. Instruct the patient to keep the site clean and change the dressing as needed.

➤ Assess for nausea and pain. Administer antiemetic and analgesic medications as needed and as directed by the health care practitioner.

➤ Administer antibiotic therapy if ordered. Remind the patient of the importance of completing the entire course of antibiotic therapy, even if signs and symptoms disappear before completion of therapy.

➤ A written report of the examination will be completed by a health care practitioner specializing in this branch of medicine. The report will be sent to the requesting health care practitioner, who will discuss the results with the patient.

➤ Recognize anxiety related to test results, and offer support. Discuss the implications of abnormal test results on the patient's lifestyle Provide teaching and information regarding the clinical implications of the test results, as appropriate. Inform the patient about hormone therapy, as appropriate based on test results. Educate the patient regarding access to counseling services.

➤ Reinforce information given by the patient's health care provider regarding further testing, treatment, or referral to another health care provider. Inform the patient of a follow-up appointment for removal of sutures, if indicated. Instruct and educate the patient on how to perform monthly breast self-examination and emphasize, as appropriate, the importance of having a mammogram performed annually. Answer any questions or address any concerns voiced by the patient or family.

➤ Instruct the patient in the use of any ordered medications. Explain the importance of adhering to the therapy regimen. As appropriate, instruct the patient in significant side effects and systemic reactions associated with the prescribed medication. Encourage him or her to review corresponding literature provided by a pharmacist.

➤ Depending on the results of this procedure, additional testing may be performed to evaluate or monitor progression of the disease process and determine the need for a change in therapy. Evaluate test results in relation to the patient's symptoms and other tests performed.

Related laboratory tests:

➤ Related laboratory tests include breast biopsy, CA 15-3, carcinoembryonic antigen, and estrogen and progesterone receptors.

HEXOSAMINIDASE A AND B

SYNONYM/ACRONYM: N/A.

SPECIMEN: Serum (3 mL) collected in a red-top tube. After the specimen is collected, it *must* be brought immediately to the laboratory. The specimen must be allowed to clot for 1 to 1.5 hours in the refrigerator. The serum should be removed and frozen immediately.

REFERENCE VALUE: (Method: Fluorometry)

Total Hexosaminidase	Conventional Units	SI Units (Conventional Units × 0.0167)
Noncarrier	589–955 nmol/h/mL	9.83–15.95 U/L
Heterozygote	465–675 nmol/h/mL	3.30–5.39 U/L
Tay-Sachs homozygote	Greater than 1027 nmol/h/mL	Greater than 17.15 U/L

Hexosaminidase A	Conventional Units	SI Units (Conventional Units × 0.0167)
Noncarrier	456–592 nmol/h/mL	7.2–9.88 U/L
Heterozygote	197–323 nmol/h/mL	3.3–5.39 U/L
Tay-Sachs homozygote	0 nmol/h/mL	0 U/L

Hexosaminidase B	Conventional Units	SI Units (Conventional Units × 0.0167)
Noncarrier	12–32 nmol/h/mL	0.2–0.54 U/L
Heterozygote	21–81 nmol/h/mL	0.35–1.35 U/L
Tay-Sachs homozygote	Greater than 305 nmol/h/mL	Greater than 5.09 U/L

DESCRIPTION & RATIONALE: Hexosaminidase is a lysosomal enzyme. There are three predominant isoenzymes: hexosaminidase A, B, and S. Deficiency results in the accumulation of complex sphingolipids and gangliosides in the brain. There are more than 70 lysozymal enzyme disorders. Testing for hexosaminidase A is done to determine the presence of Tay-Sachs disease, a genetic autosomal recessive condition characterized by early and progressive retardation of physical and mental development.

This enzyme deficiency is most common among Ashkenazic Jews. Patients who are homozygous for this trait have no hexosaminidase A and have greatly elevated levels of hexosaminidase B; signs and symptoms include red spot in the retina, blindness, and muscular weakness. Tay-Sachs disease results in early death, usually by age 3 or 4 years. ∎

INDICATIONS:
- Assist in the diagnosis of Tay-Sachs disease

• Identify carriers with hexosaminidase deficiency

RESULT

Increased in:
• Total
  Gastric cancer
  Hepatic disease
  Myeloma
  Myocardial infarction
  Pregnancy
  Symptomatic porphyria
  Vascular complications of diabetes

• Hexosaminidase A
  Diabetes
  Pregnancy

• Hexosaminidase B
  Tay-Sachs disease

Decreased in:
• Total
  Sandhoff's disease

• Hexosaminidase A
  Tay-Sachs disease

• Hexosaminidase B
  Sandhoff's disease

CRITICAL VALUES: N/A

INTERFERING FACTORS: Drugs that may increase hexosaminidase levels include ethanol, isoniazid, oral contraceptives, and rifampin.

Nursing Implications and Procedure

Pretest:

➤ Inform the patient that the test is used to identify carrier status for Tay-Sachs disease.

➤ Obtain a history of the patient's complaints, including a list of known allergens (especially allergies or sensitivities to latex), and inform the

appropriate health care practitioner accordingly.

➤ Obtain a history of the patient's reproductive system and results of previously performed laboratory tests, surgical procedures, and other diagnostic procedures. For related laboratory tests, refer to the Reproductive System table.

➤ Obtain a list of the medications the patient is taking, including herbs, nutritional supplements, and nutraceuticals. The requesting health care practitioner and laboratory should be advised if the patient regularly uses these products so that their effects can be taken into consideration when reviewing results.

➤ Review the procedure with the patient. Inform the patient that specimen collection takes approximately 5 to 10 minutes. Address concerns about pain related to the procedure. Explain to the patient that there may be some discomfort during the venipuncture.

➤ *Sensitivity to social and cultural issues,* as well as concern for modesty, is important in providing psychological support before, during, and after the procedure.

➤ There are no food, fluid, or medication restrictions, unless by medical direction.

Intratest:

➤ If the patient has a history of severe allergic reaction to latex, care should be taken to avoid the use of equipment containing latex.

➤ Instruct the patient to cooperate fully and to follow directions. Direct the patient to breathe normally and to avoid unnecessary movement.

➤ Observe standard precautions, and follow the general guidelines in Appendix A. Positively identify the patient, and label the appropriate tubes with the corresponding patient demographics, date, and time of collection. Perform a venipuncture; collect the specimen in a 5-mL red-top tube.

➤ Remove the needle, and apply a pressure dressing over the puncture site.

➤ Promptly transport the specimen to the laboratory for processing and analysis.

➤ The results are recorded manually or in a computerized system for recall and postprocedure interpretation by the appropriate health care practitioner.

Post-test:

➤ Observe venipuncture site for bleeding or hematoma formation. Apply paper tape or other adhesive to hold pressure bandage in place, or replace with a plastic bandage.

➤ A written report of the examination will be sent to the requesting health care practitioner, who will discuss the results with the patient.

➤ Recognize anxiety related to test results, and be supportive fear of shortened life expectancy. Discuss the implications of abnormal test results on the patient's lifestyle. Provide teaching and information regarding the clinical implications of the test results, as appropriate.

Encourage the family to seek genetic counseling if results are abnormal. It is also important to discuss feelings the mother and father may experience (e.g., guilt, depression, anger) if abnormalities are detected. Educate the patient regarding access to counseling services. Provide contact information, if desired, for the National Tay Sachs and Allied Diseases Association (http://www.ntsad.org).

➤ Reinforce information given by the patient's health care provider regarding further testing, treatment, or referral to another health care provider. Answer any questions or address any concerns voiced by the patient or family.

➤ Depending on the results of this procedure, additional testing may be performed to evaluate or monitor progression of the disease process and determine the need for a change in therapy. Evaluate test results in relation to the patient's symptoms and other tests performed.

Related laboratory tests:

➤ A related laboratory test is chromosome analysis.

HOLTER MONITOR

SYNONYMS/ACRONYM: Holter electrocardiography, ambulatory monitoring, ambulatory electrocardiography, event recorder.

AREA OF APPLICATION: Heart.

CONTRAST: None.

DESCRIPTION & RATIONALE: The Holter monitor records electrical cardiac activity on a continuous basis for 24 to 48 hours. This noninvasive study includes the use of a portable device worn around the waist or over the shoulder that records cardiac electrical impulses on a magnetic tape.

The recorder has a clock that allows accurate time markings on the tape. The patient is asked to keep a log or diary of daily activities and to record any occurrence of cardiac symptoms. When the client pushes a button indicating that symptoms (e.g., pain, palpitations, dyspnea, syncope) have occurred, an event marker is placed on the tape for later comparison with the cardiac activity recordings and the daily activity log. Some recorders allow the data to be transferred to the physician's office by telephone, where the tape is interpreted by a computer to detect any significantly abnormal variations in the recorded waveform patterns. ■

INDICATIONS:
- Detect arrhythmias that occur during normal daily activities, and correlate them with symptoms experienced by the patient
- Evaluate activity intolerance related to oxygen supply and demand imbalance
- Evaluate chest pain, dizziness, syncope, and palpitations
- Evaluate the effectiveness of antiarrhythmic medications for dosage adjustment, if needed
- Evaluate pacemaker function
- Monitor for ischemia and arrhythmias after myocardial infarction or cardiac surgery before changing rehabilitation and other therapy regimens

RESULT

Normal Findings:
- Normal sinus rhythm

Abnormal Findings:
- Arrhythmias such as premature ventricular contractions, bradyarrhythmias,

tachyarrhythmias, conduction defects, and bradycardia
- Cardiomyopathy
- Hypoxic or ischemic changes
- Mitral valve abnormality
- Palpitations

CRITICAL VALUES: N/A

INTERFERING FACTORS:

Factors that may impair the results of the examination:
- Improper placement of the electrodes or movement of the electrodes
- Failure of the patient to maintain a daily log of symptoms or to push the button to produce a mark on the strip when experiencing a symptom

---

Nursing Implications and Procedure

Pretest:

➤ Inform the patient that the procedure evaluates how the heart responds to normal activity or to a medication regimen.

➤ Obtain a history of the patient's cardiovascular system, cardiac disease, and present cardiovascular status, as well as results of previously performed laboratory tests, surgical procedures, and other diagnostic procedures. For related diagnostic tests, refer to the Cardiovascular System table.

➤ Obtain a list of the medications the patient is taking, including herbs, nutritional supplements, and nutraceuticals. The requesting health care practitioner and laboratory should be advised if the patient regularly uses these products so that their effects can be taken into consideration when reviewing results.

➤ Review the procedure with the patient. Address concerns about pain related to the procedure. Explain that no electricity is delivered to the body during this procedure and that no discomfort is experienced during monitoring. Inform the patient that the electrocardiography (ECG) recorder is worn for 24 to 48 hours, at which time the patient is to return to the laboratory with an activity log to have the monitor and strip removed for interpretation.

➤ Advise the patient to avoid contact with electrical devices that can affect the strip tracings (e.g., shavers, toothbrush, massager, blanket) and to avoid showers and tub bathing.

➤ Instruct the patient to perform normal activities, such as walking, sleeping, climbing stairs, sexual activity, bowel or urinary elimination, cigarette smoking, emotional upsets, and medications, and to record them in an activity log.

➤ Instruct the patient to wear loose-fitting clothing over the electrodes and not to disturb or disconnect the electrodes or wires.

➤ Instruct the patient regarding recording and pressing the button upon experiencing pain or discomfort.

➤ Advise the patient to report a light signal on the monitor, which indicates equipment malfunction or that an electrode has come off.

➤ *Sensitivity to cultural and social issues,* as well as concern for modesty, is important in providing psychological support before, during and after the procedure.

Intratest:

➤ Patients are given a gown, robe, and foot coverings to wear and instructed to void prior to the procedure.

➤ Instruct the patient to cooperate fully and to follow directions.

➤ Observe standard precautions, and follow the general guidelines in Appendix A.

➤ Place the patient in a supine position.

➤ Expose the chest. Shave excessive hair at the skin sites; cleanse thoroughly with alcohol and rub until red in color.

➤ Apply electropaste to the skin sites to provide conduction between the skin and electrodes, or apply disk electrodes that are prelubricated and disposable.

➤ Apply two electrodes on the manubrium (negative electrodes), one in the V_1 position (fourth intercostal space at the border of the right sternum), and one at the V_5 position (level of the fifth intercostal space at the midclavicular line, horizontally and at the left axillary line). A ground electrode is also placed and secured to the skin of the chest or abdomen.

➤ After checking to ensure that the electrodes are secure, attach the electrode cable to the monitor and the lead wires to the electrodes.

➤ Check the monitor for paper supply and battery, insert the tape, and turn on the recorder. Tape all wires to the chest, and place the belt or shoulder strap in the proper position.

Post-test:

➤ Gently remove the tape and other items securing the electrodes to the patient.

➤ Advise the patient to immediately report symptoms such as fast heart rate or difficulty breathing.

➤ Compare the activity log and tape recordings for changes during the monitoring period.

➤ A written report of the examination will be completed by a health care practitioner specializing in this branch of medicine. The report will be sent to the requesting health care practitioner, who will discuss the results with the patient.

➤ Recognize anxiety related to test results, and be supportive of perceived loss of independence and fear of shortened life expectancy. Discuss the implications of abnormal test results on the patient's lifestyle. Provide teaching and information regarding the clinical implications of the test results, as appropriate. Educate the patient regarding access to counseling services.

➤ Depending on the results of this procedure, additional testing may be needed to evaluate or monitor progression of the disease process and determine the need for a change in therapy. Evaluate test results in relation to the patient's symptoms and other tests performed.

Related diagnostic tests:

➤ Related diagnostic tests include echocardiography and electrocardiogram.

HOMOCYSTEINE AND METHYLMALONIC ACID

· ·

SYNONYM/ACRONYM: N/A.

SPECIMEN: Serum (4 mL) collected in a red- or tiger-top tube if methylmalonic acid and homocysteine are to be measured together. Alternatively, plasma collected in a lavender-top (EDTA) tube may be acceptable for the homocysteine measurement. The laboratory should be consulted before specimen collection because specimen type may be method dependent. Care must be taken to use the same type of collection container if serial measurements are to be taken.

REFERENCE VALUE: (Method: Chromatography) Homocysteine: 8 to 20 μmol/L; methylmalonic acid: 80 to 560 μmol/L.

DESCRIPTION & RATIONALE: Homocysteine is an amino acid formed from methionine. Normally homocysteine is rapidly remetabolized in a biochemical pathway that requires vitamin B_{12} and folate, preventing the buildup of homocysteine in the blood. Excess levels damage the endothelial lining of blood vessels; change coagulation factor levels, increasing the risk of blood clot formation; prevent smaller arter-

ies from dilating, increasing the risk of plaque formation; cause platelet aggregation; and cause smooth muscle cells lining the arterial wall to multiply, promoting atherosclerosis.

Approximately one-third of patients with hyperhomocystinuria have normal fasting levels. Patients with a heterozygous biochemical enzyme defect in cystathionine B synthase or with a nutritional deficiency in vitamin B_6

can be identified through the administration of a methionine challenge or loading test. Specimens are collected while fasting and 2 hours later. An increase in homocysteine after 2 hours is indicative of hyperhomocystinuria. In patients with vitamin B_{12} deficiency, elevated levels of methylmalonic acid and homocysteine develop fairly early in the course of the disease. Unlike vitamin B_{12} levels, homocysteine levels will remain elevated for at least 24 hours after the start of vitamin therapy. This may be useful if vitamin therapy is inadvertently begun before specimen collection. Patients with folate deficiency, for the most part, will only develop elevated homocysteine levels. Hyperhomocystinemia due to folate deficiency in pregnant women is believed to increase the risk of neural tube defects. Elevated levels of homocysteine are thought to chemically damage the exposed neural tissue of the developing fetus. ■

INDICATIONS:
• Evaluate inherited enzyme deficiencies that result in homocystinuria

• Evaluate the risk for cardiovascular disease

• Evaluate the risk for venous thrombosis

RESULT

Increased in:
• Chronic renal failure

• Coronary artery disease

• Folic acid deficiency

• Homocystinuria

• Vitamin B_{12} deficiency

Decreased in: N/A

CRITICAL VALUES: N/A

INTERFERING FACTORS:
• Drugs that may increase plasma homocysteine levels include anticonvulsants, cycloserine, hydralazine, isoniazid, methotrexate, penicillamine, phenelzine, and theophylline.

• Specimens should be kept at a refrigerated temperature and delivered immediately to the laboratory for processing.

Nursing Implications and Procedure ●●●●●●●●●●●●

Pretest:

➤ Inform the patient that the test is used to screen for risk of cardiovascular disease and stroke.

➤ Obtain a history of the patient's complaints, including a list of known allergens (especially allergies or sensitivities to latex), and inform the appropriate health care practitioner accordingly.

➤ Obtain a history of the patient's cardiovascular and hematopoietic systems, as well as results of previously performed laboratory tests, surgical procedures, and other diagnostic procedures. For related laboratory tests, refer to the Cardiovascular and Hematopoietic System tables.

➤ Obtain a list of the medications the patient is taking, including herbs, nutritional supplements, and nutraceuticals. The requesting health care practitioner and laboratory should be advised if the patient regularly uses these products so that their effects can be taken into consideration when reviewing results.

➤ Review the procedure with the patient. Inform the patient that specimen collection takes approximately 5 to 10 minutes. Address concerns about pain related to the procedure. Explain to the patient that there may be some discomfort during the venipuncture.

➤ There are no food, fluid, or medication restrictions, unless by medical direction.

Intratest:

➤ If the patient has a history of severe allergic reaction to latex, care should be taken to avoid the use of equipment containing latex.

➤ Instruct the patient to cooperate fully and to follow directions. Direct the patient to breathe normally and to avoid unnecessary movement.

➤ Observe standard precautions, and follow the general guidelines in Appendix A. Positively identify the patient, and label the appropriate tubes with the corresponding patient demographics, date, and time of collection. Perform a venipuncture; collect the specimen for combined methylmalonic acid and homocysteine studies in two 5-mL red- or tiger-top tubes. If only homocysteine is to be measured, a 5-mL lavender-top tube is acceptable.

➤ Remove the needle, and apply a pressure dressing over the puncture site.

➤ Promptly transport the specimen to the laboratory for processing and analysis.

➤ The results are recorded manually or in a computerized system for recall and postprocedure interpretation by the appropriate health care practitioner.

Post-test:

➤ Observe venipuncture site for bleeding or hematoma formation. Apply paper tape or other adhesive to hold pressure bandage in place, or replace with a plastic bandage.

➤ *Nutritional considerations:* Increased homocysteine levels may be associated with atherosclerosis and coronary artery disease. Nutritional therapy is recommended for individuals identified to be at high risk for developing coronary artery disease. If overweight, these patients should be encouraged to achieve a normal weight. The American Heart Association has Step 1 and Step 2 diets that may be helpful in achieving a goal of lowering total cholesterol and triglyceride levels. The Step 1 diet emphasizes a reduction in foods high in saturated fats and cholesterol. Red meats, eggs, and dairy products are the major sources of saturated fats and cholesterol. If triglycerides are also elevated, patients should be advised to eliminate or reduce alcohol and simple carbohydrates from their diet. The Step 2 diet recommends stricter reductions.

➤ *Nutritional considerations:* Diets rich in fruits, grains, and cereals, in addition to a multivitamin containing B_{12} and folate, may be recommended for patients with elevated homocysteine levels. Processed and refined foods should be kept to a minimum.

➤ A written report of the examination will be sent to the requesting health care practitioner, who will discuss the results with the patient.

➤ Recognize anxiety related to test results, and be supportive of fear of shortened life expectancy. Discuss the implications of abnormal test results on the patient's lifestyle. Provide teaching and information regarding the clinical implications of the test results, as appropriate. Educate the patient regarding access to counseling services. Provide contact information, if desired, for the American Heart Association (*http://www.americanheart.org*).

➤ Reinforce information given by the patient's health care provider regarding further testing, treatment, or referral to another health care provider. Answer any questions or address any concerns voiced by the patient or family.

➤ Depending on the results of this procedure, additional testing may be performed to evaluate or monitor progression of the disease process and determine the need for a change in therapy. Evaluate test results in relation to the patient's symptoms and other tests performed.

HOMOVANILLIC ACID

SYNONYM/ACRONYM: HVA.

SPECIMEN: Urine (10 mL) from a timed specimen collected in a clean plastic collection container with 6N HCl as a preservative.

REFERENCE VALUE: (Method: Chromatography)

Age	Conventional Units	SI Units
Homovanillic acid		
		(Conventional Units × 5.49)
3–6 y	1.4–4.3 mg/24 h	8–24 μmol/24 h
7–10 y	2.1–4.7 mg/24 h	12–26 μmol/24 h
11–16 y	2.4–8.7 mg/24 h	13–48 μmol/24 h
Adult	1.4–8.8 mg/24 h	8–48 μmol/24 h
Vanillylmandelic Acid		
		(Conventional Units × 5.05)
3–6 y	1.0–2.6 mg/24 h	5–13 μmol/24 h
7–10 y	2.0–3.2 mg/24 h	10–16 μmol/24 h
11–16 y	2.3–5.2 mg/24 h	12–26 μmol/24 h
Adult	1.4–6.5 mg/24 h	7–33 μmol/24 h

DESCRIPTION & RATIONALE: Homovanillic acid (HVA) is the main terminal metabolite of dopamine. Vanillylmandelic acid is a major metabolite of epinephrine and norepinephrine. Both of these tests should be evaluated together for the diagnosis of neuroblastoma. Excretion may be intermittent; therefore, a 24-hour specimen is preferred. Creatinine is usually measured simultaneously to ensure adequate collection and to calculate an excretion ratio of metabolite to creatinine. ■

INDICATIONS:
* Assist in the diagnosis of pheochromocytoma, neuroblastoma, and ganglioblastoma
* Monitor the course of therapy

RESULT

Increased in:
* Ganglioblastoma
* Neuroblastoma
* Pheochromocytoma
* Riley-Day syndrome

Decreased in:
* Schizotypal personality disorders

CRITICAL VALUES: N/A

INTERFERING FACTORS:
* Drugs that may increase HVA levels include acetylsalicylic acid, disulfiram, levodopa, pyridoxine, and reserpine.
* Drugs that may decrease HVA levels include moclobemide.
* All urine voided for the timed collection period must be included in the collection or else falsely decreased values may be obtained. Compare output records with volume collected to verify that all voids were included in the collection.

Nursing Implications and Procedure • • • • • • • • • •

Pretest:

➤ Inform the patient that the test is used to diagnose neuroblas-

toma, pheochromocytoma, and ganglioblastoma and to monitor therapy.

➤ Obtain a history of the patient's complaints, including a list of known allergens (especially allergies or sensitivities to latex), and inform the appropriate health care practitioner accordingly.

➤ Obtain a history of the patient's endocrine system, as well as results of previously performed laboratory tests, surgical procedures, and other diagnostic procedures. For related laboratory tests, refer to the Endocrine System table.

➤ Obtain a list of the medications the patient is taking, including herbs, nutritional supplements, and nutraceuticals. The requesting health care practitioner and laboratory should be advised if the patient regularly uses these products so that their effects can be taken into consideration when reviewing results.

➤ Review the procedure with the patient. Provide a nonmetallic urinal, bedpan, or toilet-mounted collection device. Address concerns about pain related to the procedure. Explain to the patient that there should be no discomfort during the procedure.

➤ Usually a 24-hour time frame for urine collection is ordered. Inform the patient that all urine must be saved during that 24-hour period. Instruct the patient not to void directly into the laboratory collection container. Instruct the patient to avoid defecating in the collection device and to keep toilet tissue out of the collection device to prevent contamination of the specimen. Place a sign in the bathroom to remind the patient to save all urine.

➤ Instruct the patient to void all urine into the collection device and then to pour the urine into the laboratory collection container. Alternatively, the specimen can be left in the collection device for a health care staff member to add to the laboratory collection container.

➤ *Sensitivity to social and cultural issues*, as well as concern for modesty, is important in providing psychological support before, during, and after the procedure.

➤ If possible, and with medical direction, patients should withhold acetylsalicylic acid, disulfiram, pyridoxine, and reserpine for 2 days before specimen collection. Levodopa should be withheld for 2 weeks before specimen collection.

➤ There are no food or fluid restrictions, unless by medical direction.

Intratest:

➤ Ensure that the patient has complied with medication restrictions; assure that specified medications, with medical direction, have been restricted for at least 2 days prior to the procedure.

➤ If the patient has a history of severe allergic reaction to latex, care should be taken to avoid the use of equipment containing latex.

➤ Instruct the patient to cooperate fully and to follow directions.

➤ Observe standard precautions, and follow the general guidelines in Appendix A. Positively identify the patient, and label the appropriate tubes with the corresponding patient demographics, date, and time of collection.

Timed specimen:

➤ Obtain a clean 3-L urine specimen container, toilet-mounted collection device, and plastic bag (for transport of the specimen container). The specimen must be refrigerated or kept on ice throughout the entire collection period. If an indwelling urinary catheter is in place, the drainage bag must be kept on ice.

➤ Begin the test between 6 a.m. and 8 a.m., if possible. Collect first voiding and discard. Record the time the specimen was discarded as the beginning of the timed collection period. The next morning, ask the patient to void at the same time the collection was started and add this last voiding to the container.

➤ If an indwelling catheter is in place,

replace the tubing and container system at the start of the collection time. Keep the container system on ice during the collection period, or empty the urine into a larger container periodically during the collection period; monitor to ensure continued drainage, and conclude the test the next morning at the same hour the collection was begun.

➤ At the conclusion of the test, compare the quantity of urine with the urinary output record for the collection; if the specimen contains less than what was recorded as output, some urine may have been discarded, invalidating the test.

➤ Include on the collection container's label the amount of urine, test start and stop times, and ingestion of any foods or medications that can affect test results.

➤ Promptly transport the specimen to the laboratory for processing and analysis.

➤ The results are recorded manually or in a computerized system for recall and postprocedure interpretation by the appropriate health care practitioner.

Post-test:

➤ Instruct the patient to resume usual medications, as directed by the health care practitioner.

➤ A written report of the examination will be sent to the requesting health care practitioner, who will discuss the results with the patient.

➤ Recognize anxiety related to test results. Discuss the implications of abnormal test results on the patient's lifestyle. Provide teaching and information regarding the clinical implications of the test results, as appropriate. Educate the patient regarding access to counseling services.

➤ Reinforce information given by the patient's health care provider regarding further testing, treatment, or referral to another health care provider. Answer any questions or

address any concerns voiced by the patient or family.

➤ Depending on the results of this procedure, additional testing may be performed to evaluate or monitor progression of the disease process and determine the need for a change in therapy. Evaluate test results in relation to the patient's symptoms and other tests performed.

Related laboratory tests:

➤ Related laboratory tests include carcinoembryonic antigen, catecholamines (blood and urine), metanephrines, and vanillylmandelic acid.

HUMAN CHORIONIC GONADOTROPIN

SYNONYMS/ACRONYMS: Chorionic gonadotropin, pregnancy test, HCG, hCG, β-HCG, β-subunit HCG.

SPECIMEN: Serum (1 mL) collected in a red- or tiger-top tube. Plasma (1 mL) collected in green-top (heparin) tube is also acceptable.

REFERENCE VALUE: (Method: Immunoassay)

	Conventional Units	SI Units (Conventional Units × 1)
Males and nonpregnant females	Less than 5 mIU/mL	Less than 5 IU/L
Pregnant females by week of gestation:		
Less than 1 wk	5–50 mIU/mL	5–50 IU/L
2 wk	50–500 mIU/mL	50–500 IU/L
3 wk	100–10,000 mIU/mL	100–10,000 IU/L
4 wk	1,000–30,000 mIU/mL	1,000–30,000 IU/L
5 wk	3,500–115,000 mIU/mL	3,500–115,000 IU/L
6–8 wk	12,000–270,000 mIU/mL	12,000–270,000 IU/L
12 wk	15,000–220,000 mIU/mL	15,000–220,000 IU/L

DESCRIPTION & RATIONALE: Human chorionic gonadotropin (HCG) is a hormone secreted by the placenta beginning 8 to 10 days after conception, which coincides with implantation of the fertilized ovum. It stimulates secretion of progesterone by the corpus luteum. HCG levels peak at 8 to 12 weeks of gestation and then fall to less than 10% of first trimester levels by the end of pregnancy. By postpartum week 2, levels are undetectable. HCG levels increase at a slower rate in ectopic pregnancy and spontaneous abortion than in normal pregnancy; a low rate of change between serial specimens is predictive of a nonviable fetus. As assays improve in sensitivity over time, ectopic pregnancies are increasingly being identified before rupture. HCG is used along with estriol and α_1-fetoprotein in prenatal screening for neural tube defects. These prenatal measurements are also known as *triple markers.* Serial measurements are needed for an accurate estimate of gestational stage and determination of fetal viability. Triple marker testing has also been used to screen for trisomy 21 (Down syndrome). (To compare HCG to other tests in the triple marker screening procedure, see monograph titled "α_1-Fetoprotein.") HCG is also produced by some germ cell tumors. Most assays measure both the intact and free β-HCG subunit, but if HCG is to be used as a tumor marker, the assay must be capable of detecting both intact and free β-HCG. ▪

INDICATIONS:

• Assist in the diagnosis of suspected HCG-producing tumors, such as choriocarcinoma, germ cell tumors of the ovary and testes, or hydatidiform moles

• Confirm pregnancy, assist in the diagnosis of suspected ectopic pregnancy, or determine threatened or incomplete abortion

• Determine adequacy of hormonal levels to maintain pregnancy

• Monitor effects of surgery or chemotherapy

• Monitor ovulation induction treatment

• Prenatally detect neural tube defects and trisomy 21 (Down syndrome)

RESULT

Increased in:
• Choriocarcinoma

• Ectopic HCG-producing tumors (stomach, lung, colon, pancreas, liver, breast)

• Erythroblastosis fetalis

• Germ cell tumors (ovary and testes)

• Hydatidiform mole

• Islet cell tumors

• Multiple gestation pregnancy

• Pregnancy

Decreased in:
• Ectopic pregnancy

• Incomplete abortion

• Intrauterine fetal demise

• Spontaneous abortion

• Threatened abortion

CRITICAL VALUES: N/A

INTERFERING FACTORS:
• Drugs that may decrease HCG levels include epostane and mifepristone.

• Results may vary widely depending on the sensitivity and specificity of the assay. Performance of the test too early in pregnancy may cause false-negative results. HCG is composed of an α and a β subunit. The structure of the α subunit is essentially identical to the α subunit of follicle-stimulating hormone, luteinizing hormone, and thyroid-stimulating hormone. The structure of the β subunit differentiates HCG from the other hormones. False-positive results can therefore be obtained if the HCG assay does not detect β subunit.

Nursing Implications and Procedure • • • • • • • • • • •

Pretest:

➤ Inform the patient, as appropriate, that the test is used to verify pregnancy, screen for neural tube defects, or detect HCG-secreting tumors.

➤ Obtain a history of the patient's complaints, including a list of known allergens (especially allergies or sensitivities to latex), and inform the appropriate health care practitioner accordingly.

➤ Obtain a history of the patient's endocrine, immune, and reproductive systems and results of previously performed laboratory tests, surgical procedures, and other diagnostic procedures. For related laboratory tests, refer to the Endocrine, Immune, and Reproductive System tables.

➤ Record the date of the last menstrual period and determine the possibility of pregnancy in perimenopausal women.

➤ Obtain a list of the medications the patient is taking, including herbs, nutritional supplements, and nutraceuticals. The requesting health care practitioner and laboratory should be advised if the patient regularly uses these products so that their effects can be taken into consideration when reviewing results.

➤ Review the procedure with the patient. Inform the patient that specimen collection takes approximately 5 to 10 minutes. Address concerns about pain related to the procedure. Explain to the patient that there may be some discomfort during the venipuncture.

➤ There are no food, fluid, or medication restrictions, unless by medical direction.

Intratest:

➤ If the patient has a history of severe allergic reaction to latex, care should be taken to avoid the use of equipment containing latex.

➤ Instruct the patient to cooperate fully and to follow directions. Direct the patient to breathe normally and to avoid unnecessary movement.

➤ Observe standard precautions, and follow the general guidelines in Appendix A. Positively identify the patient, and label the appropriate tubes with the corresponding patient demographics, date, and time of collection. Perform a venipuncture; collect the specimen in a 5-mL red- or tiger-top tube.

➤ Remove the needle, and apply a pressure dressing over the puncture site.

➤ Promptly transport the specimen to the laboratory for processing and analysis.

➤ The results are recorded manually or in a computerized system for recall and postprocedure interpretation by the appropriate health care practitioner.

Post-test:

➤ Observe venipuncture site for bleeding or hematoma formation. Apply paper tape or other adhesive to hold pressure bandage in place, or replace with a plastic bandage.

➤ A written report of the examination will be sent to the requesting health care practitioner, who will discuss the results with the patient.

➤ *Social and cultural considerations:* Recognize anxiety related to abnormal test results, and encourage the family to seek counseling if concerned with pregnancy termination or to seek genetic counseling if a chromosomal abnormality is determined. Provide teaching and information regarding the clinical implications of the test results, as appropriate. Decisions regarding elective abortion should take place in the presence of both parents. Provide a nonjudgmental, nonthreatening atmosphere for discussing the risks and difficulties of delivering and raising a developmentally challenged infant, as well as exploring other options (termination of pregnancy or adoption). It is also important to discuss feelings the mother and father may experience (e.g., guilt, depression, anger) if fetal abnormalities are detected.

➤ *Social and cultural considerations:* Offer support, as appropriate, to patients who may be the victims of rape or sexual assault. Educate the patient regarding access to counseling services. Provide a nonjudgmental, nonthreatening atmosphere for a discussion during which risks of sexually transmitted diseases are explained. It is also important to discuss problems the victim of sexual assault may experience (e.g., guilt, depression, anger) if there is possibility of pregnancy related to the assault.

➤ *Social and cultural considerations:* In patients with carcinoma, recognize anxiety related to test results and offer support. Provide teaching and information regarding the clinical implications of abnormal test results, as appropriate. Educate the patient

regarding access to counseling services, as appropriate.

➤ Reinforce information given by the patient's health care provider regarding further testing, treatment, or referral to another health care provider. Answer any questions or address any concerns voiced by the patient or family.

➤ Depending on the results of this procedure, additional testing may be performed to evaluate or monitor the patient's condition and determine the need for a change in therapy. Evaluate test results in relation to the patient's symptoms and other tests performed.

Related laboratory tests:

➤ Related laboratory tests include *Chlamydia* group antibody, chorionic villus biopsy, chromosome analysis, cytomegalovirus antibody, estradiol, fetal fibronectin, α_1-fetoprotein, hemwatocrit, hemoglobin, progesterone, rubella antibody, rubeola antibody, syphilis serology, toxoplasma antibody, and white blood cell count.

HUMAN IMMUNODEFICIENCY VIRUS TYPE 1 AND TYPE 2 ANTIBODIES

· ·

SYNONYM/ACRONYM: HIV-1/HIV-2.

SPECIMEN: Serum (1 mL) collected in a red-top tube.

REFERENCE VALUE: (Method: Enzyme immunoassay) Negative.

DESCRIPTION & RATIONALE: Human immunodeficiency virus (HIV) is the etiologic agent of acquired immunodeficiency syndrome (AIDS) and is transmitted through bodily secretions, especially by blood or sexual contact. The virus preferentially binds to the T4 helper lymphocytes and replicates within the cells. Current assays detect several viral proteins. Positive results should be confirmed by Western blot assay. This test is routinely recommended as part of a prenatal workup and is required for evaluating donated blood units before release for transfusion. ■

INDICATIONS:

• Evaluate donated blood units before transfusion

• Perform as part of prenatal screening

• Screen organ transplant donors

• Test individuals who have documented and significant exposure to other infected individuals

• Test exposed high-risk individuals for detection of antibody (e.g., persons with multiple sex partners, persons with a history of other sexually transmitted diseases, intravenous drug users, infants born to infected mothers, allied health care workers, public service employees who have contact with blood and blood products)

RESULT

Positive findings in: HIV-1 or HIV-2 infection

CRITICAL VALUES: N/A

INTERFERING FACTORS:

• Drugs that may decrease HIV antibody levels include didanosine, dideoxycytidine, zalcitabine, and zidovudine.

• Nonreactive HIV test results occur during the acute stage of the disease, when the virus is present but antibodies have not sufficiently developed to be detected. It may take up to 6 months for the test to become positive. During this stage, the test for HIV antigen may not confirm an HIV infection.

• Test kits for HIV are very sensitive. As a result, nonspecific reactions may occur, leading to a false-positive result.

Nursing Implications and Procedure • • • • • • • • • • •

Pretest:

➤ Inform the patient that the test is used to test blood for the presence of antibodies to human inmmunodeficiency virus.

➤ Obtain a history of the patient's complaints, including a list of known allergens (especially allergies or sensitivities to latex), and inform the appropriate health care practitioner accordingly.

➤ Obtain a history of the patient's immune and reproductive systems, a history of high-risk behaviors, and results of previously performed laboratory tests, surgical procedures, and other diagnostic procedures. For related laboratory tests, refer to the Immune and Reproductive System tables.

➤ Obtain a list of the medications the patient is taking, including herbs, nutritional supplements, and nutraceuticals. The requesting health care practitioner and laboratory should be advised if the patient regularly uses these products so that their effects can be taken into consideration when reviewing results.

➤ Review the procedure with the patient. Inform the patient that specimen collection takes approximately 5 to 10 minutes. Address concerns about pain related to the procedure. Explain to the patient that there may be some discomfort during the venipuncture.

➤ There are no food, fluid, or medication restrictions, unless by medical direction.

➤ *Make sure a written and informed consent has been signed prior to the procedure and before administering any medications.*

Intratest:

➤ If the patient has a history of severe allergic reaction to latex, care should be taken to avoid the use of equipment containing latex.

➤ Instruct the patient to cooperate fully and to follow directions. Direct the patient to breathe normally and to avoid unnecessary movement.

➤ Observe standard precautions, and follow the general guidelines in Appendix A. Positively identify the patient, and label the appropriate tubes with the corresponding patient demographics, date, and time of collection. Perform a venipuncture; collect the specimen in a 5-mL red-top tube.

➤ Remove the needle, and apply a pressure dressing over the puncture site.

➤ Promptly transport the specimen to the laboratory for processing and analysis.

➤ The results are recorded manually or in a computerized system for recall and postprocedure interpretation by the appropriate health care practitioner.

Post-test:

➤ Observe venipuncture site for bleeding or hematoma formation. Apply paper tape or other adhesive to hold pressure bandage in place, or replace with a plastic bandage.

➤ A written report of the examination will be sent to the requesting health care practitioner, who will discuss the results with the patient.

➤ Warn the patient that false-positive results occur and that the absence of antibody does not guarantee absence of infection, because the virus may be latent or may not have produced detectable antibody at the time of testing.

➤ *Social and cultural considerations:* Recognize anxiety related to test results, and be supportive of impaired activity related to weakness, perceived loss of independence, and fear of shortened life expectancy. Discuss the implications of abnormal test results on the patient's lifestyle. Provide teaching and information regarding the clinical implications of the test results, as appropriate. Educate the patient regarding access to counseling services. Provide contact information, if desired, for AIDS information provided by the National Institutes of Health *(http://www.aidsinfo.nih.gov).*

➤ *Social and cultural considerations:* Counsel the patient, as appropriate, regarding risk of transmission and proper prophylaxis, and reinforce the importance of strict adherence to the treatment regimen.

➤ *Social and cultural considerations:* Inform patients that positive findings must be reported to local health department officials, who will question him or her regarding sexual partners.

➤ *Social and cultural considerations:* Offer support, as appropriate, to patients who may be the victims of rape or sexual assault. Educate the patient regarding access to counseling services. Provide a nonjudgmental, nonthreatening atmosphere for a discussion during which risks of sexually transmitted diseases are explained. It is also important to discuss problems the patient may experience (e.g., guilt, depression, anger).

➤ Inform the patient that retesting may be necessary.

➤ Reinforce information given by the patient's health care provider regarding further testing, treatment, or referral to another health care provider. Answer any questions or

address any concerns voiced by the patient or family.

➤ Depending on the results of this procedure, additional testing may be performed to evaluate or monitor progression of the disease process and determine the need for a change in therapy. Evaluate test results in relation to the patient's symptoms and other tests performed.

Related laboratory tests:

➤ Related laboratory tests include CD4/CD8 enumeration, *Chlamydia* group antibody, complete blood count, cytomegalovirus, hepatitis B antibody and antigen, hepatitis C antibody, human T-cell lymphotropic virus types I and II, β_2-microglobulin, skin culture, and syphilis serology.

HUMAN LEUKOCYTE ANTIGEN B27

SYNONYM/ACRONYM: HLA-B27.

SPECIMEN: Whole blood (5 mL) collected in green-top (heparin) or yellow-top (acid-citrate-dextrose [ACD]) tube.

REFERENCE VALUE: (Method: Flow cytometry) Negative (indicating absence of the antigen).

DESCRIPTION & RATIONALE: The human leukocyte antigens (HLAs) are gene products of the major histocompatibility complex, derived from their respective loci on the short arm of chromosome 6. There are more than 27 identified HLAs. HLA-B27 is an allele (one of two or more genes for an inheritable trait that occupy the same location on each chromosome, paternal and maternal) of the HLA-B locus. The presence of HLA-B27 is associated with several specific conditions, as listed later, but HLA-B27 should not be used as a screening test for these conditions. ∎

INDICATIONS: Assist in diagnosing ankylosing spondylitis and Reiter's syndrome

RESULT

Positive findings in:

• Ankylosing spondylitis

• Juvenile rheumatoid arthritis

• Psoriatic arthritis

• Reiter's syndrome

CRITICAL VALUES: N/A

INTERFERING FACTORS:

• The specimen should be stored at room temperature and should be received by the laboratory performing the assay within 24 hours of collection. It is highly recommended that the laboratory be contacted before specimen collection to avoid specimen rejection.

Nursing Implications and Procedure • • • • • • • • • •

Pretest: ■

➤ Inform the patient that the test is used to evaluate ankylosing spondylitis and other disorders associated with HLA-B27.

➤ Obtain a history of the patient's complaints, including a list of known allergens (especially allergies or sensitivities to latex), and inform the appropriate health care practitioner accordingly.

➤ Obtain a history of the patient's immune and musculoskeletal systems as well as results of previously performed laboratory tests, surgical procedures, and other diagnostic procedures. For related laboratory tests, refer to the Immune and Musculoskeletal System tables.

➤ Obtain a list of the medications the patient is taking, including herbs, nutritional supplements, and nutraceuticals. The requesting health care practitioner and laboratory should be advised if the patient regularly uses these products so that their effects can be taken into consideration when reviewing results.

➤ Review the procedure with the patient. Inform the patient that specimen collection takes approximately 5 to 10 minutes. Address concerns about pain related to the procedure. Explain to the patient that there may be some discomfort during the venipuncture.

➤ *Sensitivity to social and cultural issues,* as well as concern for modesty, is important in providing psychological support before, during, and after the procedure.

➤ There are no food, fluid, or medication restrictions, unless by medical direction.

Intratest: ■

➤ If the patient has a history of severe allergic reaction to latex, care should be taken to avoid the use of equipment containing latex.

➤ Instruct the patient to cooperate fully and to follow directions. Direct the patient to breathe normally and to avoid unnecessary movement.

➤ Observe standard precautions, and follow the general guidelines in Appendix A. Positively identify the patient, and label the appropriate tubes with the corresponding patient demographics, date, and time of collection. Perform a venipuncture; collect the specimen in a 5-mL green- or yellow-top tube.

➤ Remove the needle, and apply a pressure dressing over the puncture site.

➤ Promptly transport the specimen to the laboratory for processing and analysis.

➤ The results are recorded manually or in a computerized system for recall and postprocedure interpretation by the appropriate health care practitioner.

Post-test: ■

➤ Observe venipuncture site for bleeding or hematoma formation. Apply paper tape or other adhesive to hold pressure bandage in place, or replace with a plastic bandage.

➤ A written report of the examination will be sent to the requesting health care practitioner, who will discuss the results with the patient.

➤ Recognize anxiety related to test results, and be supportive of perceived loss of independence and and fear of shortened life expectancy. These diseases can be moderately to severely debilitating, resulting in significant lifestyle changes. Discuss the implications of abnormal test results on the patient's lifestyle. Provide teaching and information regarding the clinical implications of the test results, as appropriate. Educate the patient regarding access to counseling services.

➤ Reinforce information given by the patient's health care provider regarding further testing, treatment, or referral to another health care provider. Inform the patient that false-positive test results occur and that retesting may be required. Answer any questions or address any concerns voiced by the patient or family.

➤ Depending on the results of this procedure, additional testing may be performed to evaluate or monitor progression of the disease process and determine the need for a change

in therapy. Evaluate test results in relation to the patient's symptoms and other tests performed.

Related laboratory tests:

➤ A related laboratory test is rheumatoid factor.

HUMAN T-LYMPHOTROPIC VIRUS TYPE I AND TYPE II ANTIBODIES

SYNONYM/ACRONYM: HTLV-I/HTLV-II.

SPECIMEN: Serum (1 mL) collected in a red-top tube.

REFERENCE VALUE: (Method: Enzyme immunoassay) Negative.

DESCRIPTION & RATIONALE: Human T-lymphotropic virus type I (HTLV-I) and type II (HTLV-II) are two closely related retroviruses known to remain latent for extended periods before becoming reactive. The viruses are transmitted by sexual contact, contact with blood, placental transfer from mother to fetus, or ingestion of breast milk. As with human immunodeficiency virus type 1 (HIV-1) and type 2 (HIV-2), HTLV targets the T4 lymphocytes. The disease is uncommon in the United States, but retrospective studies conducted by the American Red Cross demonstrated that a small percentage of transfusion recipients became infected by HTLV-positive blood. The results of this study led to a requirement that all donated blood

units be tested for HTLV-I/HTLV-II before release for transfusion. ∎

INDICATIONS:

• Distinguish HTLV-I/HTLV-II infection from spastic myelopathy

• Establish HTLV-I as the causative agent in adult lymphoblastic (T-cell) leukemia

• Evaluate donated blood units before transfusion

• Evaluate HTLV-II as a contributing cause of chronic neuromuscular disease

RESULT

Positive findings in: HTLV-I/HTLV-II infection

CRITICAL VALUES: N/A

INTERFERING FACTORS: N/A

Nursing Implications and Procedure • • • • • • • • • • •

Pretest:

➤ Inform the patient that the test is used to test blood for the presence of antibodies that would indicate past or current HTLV infection.

➤ Obtain a history of the patient's complaints, including a list of known allergens (especially allergies or sensitivities to latex), and inform the appropriate health care practitioner accordingly.

➤ Obtain a history of the patient's immune system, a history of high-risk behaviors, and results of previously performed laboratory tests, surgical procedures, and other diagnostic procedures. For related laboratory tests, refer to the Immune System table.

➤ Obtain a list of the medications the patient is taking, including herbs, nutritional supplements, and nutraceuticals. The requesting health care practitioner and laboratory should be advised if the patient regularly uses these products so that their effects can be taken into consideration when reviewing results.

➤ Review the procedure with the patient. Inform the patient that specimen collection takes approximately 5 to 10 minutes. Address concerns about pain related to the procedure. Explain to the patient that there may be some discomfort during the venipuncture.

➤ There are no food, fluid, or medication restrictions, unless by medical direction.

Intratest:

➤ If the patient has a history of severe allergic reaction to latex, care should be taken to avoid the use of equipment containing latex.

➤ Instruct the patient to cooperate fully and to follow directions. Direct the patient to breathe normally and to avoid unnecessary movement.

➤ Observe standard precautions, and follow the general guidelines in Appendix A. Positively identify the patient, and label the appropriate tubes with the corresponding patient demographics, date, and time of collection. Perform a venipuncture; collect the specimen in a 5-mL red-top tube.

➤ Remove the needle, and apply a pressure dressing over the puncture site.

➤ Promptly transport the specimen to the laboratory for processing and analysis.

➤ The results are recorded manually or in a computerized system for recall and postprocedure interpretation by the appropriate health care practitioner.

Post-test:

➤ Observe venipuncture site for bleeding or hematoma formation. Apply paper tape or other adhesive to hold pressure bandage in place, or replace with a plastic bandage.

➤ A written report of the examination will be sent to the requesting health care practitioner, who will discuss the results with the patient.

➤ Warn the patient that false-positive results occur and that the absence of antibody does not guarantee absence of infection, because the virus may be latent or not have produced detectable antibody at the time of testing.

➤ *Social and cultural considerations:* Recognize anxiety related to test results, and be supportive of impaired activity related to weakness, perceived loss of independence, and fear of shortened life expectancy. Discuss the implications of positive test results on the patient's lifestyle. Provide teaching and information regarding the clinical implications of the test results, as appropriate. Educate the patient regarding access to counseling services.

➤ *Social and cultural considerations:* Counsel the patient, as appropriate, regarding risk of transmission and proper prophylaxis, and reinforce the importance of strict adherence to the treatment regimen.

➤ Inform the patient that the presence of HTLV-I/HTLV-II antibodies precludes blood donation, but it does not mean that leukemia or a neurologic disorder is present or will develop.

➤ Inform the patient that subsequent retesting may be necessary.

➤ Reinforce information given by the patient's health care provider regarding further testing, treatment, or referral to another health care provider. Answer any questions or address any concerns voiced by the patient or family.

➤ Depending on the results of this procedure, additional testing may be performed to evaluate or monitor progression of the disease process and determine the need for a change in therapy. Evaluate test results in relation to the patient's symptoms and other tests performed.

Related laboratory tests:

➤ Related laboratory tests include complete blood count, hepatitis B, C, and D antigens and antibodies, and HIV-1/HIV-2.

5-HYDROXYINDOLEACETIC ACID

SYNONYM/ACRONYM: 5-HIAA.

SPECIMEN: Urine (10 mL) from a timed specimen collected in a clean plastic collection container with boric acid as a preservative.

REFERENCE VALUE: (Method: High-pressure liquid chromatography)

Conventional Units	SI Units (Conventional Units × 5.23)
2–7 mg/24 h	10.5–36.6 μmol/24 h

DESCRIPTION & RATIONALE: Because 5-hydroxyindoleacetic acid (5-HIAA) is a metabolite of serotonin, 5-HIAA levels reflect plasma serotonin concentrations. 5-HIAA is excreted in the urine. Increased urinary excretion occurs in the presence of carcinoid tumors. This test, which replaces serotonin measurement, is most accurate when obtained from a 24-hour urine specimen. ■

INDICATIONS: Detect early, small, or intermittently secreting carcinoid tumors

RESULT

Increased in:
- Celiac and tropical sprue
- Cystic fibrosis
- Foregut and midgut carcinoid tumors
- Oat cell carcinoma of the bronchus
- Ovarian carcinoid tumors
- Whipple's disease

Decreased in:
- Depressive illnesses
- Hartnup disease
- Mastocytosis
- Phenylketonuria
- Renal disease
- Small intestine resection

CRITICAL VALUES: N/A

INTERFERING FACTORS:
- Drugs that may increase 5-HIAA levels include acetaminophen, cisplatin, ephedrine, fluorouracil, cough syrups containing glyceryl guaiacolate, melphalan, mephenesin, methocarbamol, naproxen, phenacetin, pindolol, and rauwolfia alkaloids.
- Drugs that may decrease 5-HIAA levels include corticotropin, ethanol, imipramine, isoniazid, levodopa, methenamine, methyldopa, monoamine oxidase inhibitors, and phenothiazines.
- Foods containing serotonin, such as avocados, bananas, chocolate, eggplant, pineapples, plantain, red plums, tomatoes, and walnuts, can falsely elevate levels if ingested within 4 days of specimen collection.
- Severe gastrointestinal disturbance or diarrhea can interfere with test results.
- Failure to collect all the urine and store the specimen properly during the 24-hour test period invalidates the results.
- Failure to follow dietary restrictions before the procedure may cause the procedure to be canceled or repeated.

Nursing Implications and Procedure

Pretest:

➤ Inform the patient that the test is used to diagnose carcinoid tumors.

➤ Obtain a history of the patient's complaints, including a list of known allergens (especially allergies or sensitivities to latex), and inform the appropriate health care practitioner accordingly.

➤ Obtain a history of the patient's endocrine, gastrointestinal, and immune system and results of previously performed laboratory tests, surgical procedures, and other diagnostic procedures. For related laboratory tests, refer to the Endocrine, Gastrointestinal, and Immune System tables.

➤ Obtain a list of the medications the patient is taking, including herbs, nutritional supplements, and nutraceuticals. The requesting health care practitioner and laboratory should be advised if the patient regularly uses these products so that their effects can be taken into consideration when reviewing results.

➤ Review the procedure with the patient. Provide a nonmetallic urinal, bedpan, or toilet-mounted collection device. Address concerns about pain related to the procedure. Explain to the patient that there should be no discomfort during the procedure.

➤ Inform the patient that all urine collected over a 24-hour period must be saved; if a preservative has been added to the container, instruct the patient not to discard the preservative. Instruct the patient not to void directly into the container. Instruct the patient to avoid defecating in the collection device and to keep toilet tissue out of the collection device to prevent contamination of the specimen. Place a sign in the bathroom as a reminder to save all urine.

➤ Instruct the patient to void all urine into the collection device, then pour the urine into the laboratory collection container. Alternatively, the specimen can be left in the collection device for a health care staff member to add to the laboratory collection container.

➤ *Sensitivity to social and cultural issues,* as well as concern for modesty, is important in providing psychological support before, during, and after the procedure.

➤ There are no fluid restrictions unless by medical direction.

➤ Inform the patient that foods and medications (herbs, nutritional supplements, and nutraceuticals) listed under "Interfering Factors" should be restricted by medical direction for at least 4 days before specimen collection.

Intratest:

➤ Ensure that the patient has complied with dietary and medication restrictions; assure foods and medications listed under "Interfering Factors" have been restricted for at least 4 days prior to the procedure.

➤ If the patient has a history of severe allergic reaction to latex, care should be taken to avoid the use of equipment containing latex.

➤ Instruct the patient to cooperate fully and to follow directions.

➤ Observe standard precautions, and follow the general guidelines in Appendix A. Positively identify the patient, and label the appropriate collection container with the corresponding patient demographics, date, and time of collection.

Timed specimen:

➤ Obtain a clean 3-L urine specimen container, toilet-mounted collection device, and plastic bag (for transport of the specimen container). The specimen must be refrigerated or kept on ice throughout the entire collection period. If an indwelling urinary catheter is in place, the drainage bag must be kept on ice.

➤ Begin the test between 6 and 8 a.m., if possible. Collect first voiding and discard. Record the time the specimen was discarded as the beginning of the timed collection period. The next morning, ask the patient to void at the same time the collection was started, and add this last voiding to the container.

➤ If an indwelling catheter is in place, replace the tubing and container system at the start of the collection time. Keep the container system on ice during the collection period, or empty the urine into a larger container periodically during the collection period; monitor to ensure continued drainage. Conclude the test the next morning at the same hour the collection was begun.

➤ At the conclusion of the test, compare the quantity of urine with the urinary output record for the collection; if the specimen contains less than what was recorded as output, some urine may have been discarded, invalidating the test.

➤ Include on the specimen collection container's label the amount of urine, test start and stop times, and ingestion of any foods or medications that can affect test results. Promptly transport the specimen to the laboratory for processing and analysis.

➤ The results are recorded manually or in a computerized system for recall and postprocedure interpretation by the appropriate health care practitioner.

Post-test:

➤ Instruct the patient to resume usual diet, as directed by the health care practitioner. Consideration may be given to niacin supplementation and increased protein, if appropriate, for patients with abnormal findings. In some cases, the tumor may divert dietary tryptophan to serotonin, resulting in pellagra.

➤ A written report of the examination will be sent to the requesting health care practitioner, who will discuss the results with the patient.

➤ Recognize anxiety related to test results. Discuss the implications of abnormal test results on the patient's lifestyle. Provide teaching and information regarding the clinical implications of the test results, as appropriate.

➤ Reinforce information given by the patient's health care provider regard-

ing further testing, treatment, or referral to another health care provider. Answer any questions or address any concerns voiced by the patient or family.

➤ Depending on the results of this procedure, additional testing may be performed to evaluate or monitor progression of the disease process and determine the need for a change in therapy. Evaluate test results in relation to the patient's symptoms and other tests performed.

Related laboratory tests:

➤ A related laboratory test is biopsy of the affected tissue.

HYPERSENSITIVITY PNEUMONITIS SEROLOGY

• •

Synonym/Acronym: Farmer's lung disease serology, extrinsic allergic alveolitis.

Specimen: Serum (2 mL) collected in a red-top tube.

Reference value: (Method: Immunodiffusion) Negative.

Description & Rationale: Hypersensitivity pneumonitis is a respiratory disease caused by the inhalation of organisms from an organic source. Affected and symptomatic individuals will demonstrate acute bronchospastic reaction 4 to 6 hours after exposure to the offending antigen. Inhalation of the antigen stimulates the production of immunoglobulin (Ig) G antibodies. The combination of immunecom-

plexing and cell-mediated immunopathogenesis results in a chronic granulomatous pneumonitis of the interstitial space of the lung. Hypersensitivity pneumonitis serology includes detection of antibodies to *Aspergillus fumigatus, Micropolyspora faeni, Thermoactinomyces vulgaris,* and *T. candidus.* A negative test result does not rule out hypersensitivity pneumonitis as a possible diagnosis, nor does a positive test result confirm the diagnosis. Also, individuals with a positive test result may not exhibit the typical symptoms, and patients with severe symptoms may not have detectable levels of antibody while their disease is inactive. To confirm the diagnosis, it is necessary to obtain a sputum culture and chest x-rays. ▪

INDICATIONS: Assist in establishing a diagnosis of hypersensitivity pneumonitis in patients experiencing fever, chills, and dyspnea after repeated exposure to moist organic sources

RESULT

> ***Increased in:*** Hypersensitivity pneumonitis

CRITICAL VALUES: N/A

INTERFERING FACTORS: N/A

Nursing Implications and Procedure • • • • • • • • • • •

Pretest:

➤ Inform the patient that the test is used to establish a diagnosis of hypersensitivity pneumonitis.

➤ Obtain a history of the patient's complaints, including a list of known allergens (especially allergies or sensitivities to latex), and inform the appropriate health care practitioner accordingly.

➤ Obtain a history of the patient's immune and respiratory systems, as well as results of previously performed laboratory tests, surgical procedures, and other diagnostic procedures. For related laboratory tests, refer to the Immune and Respiratory System tables.

➤ Obtain a list of the medications the patient is taking, including herbs, nutritional supplements, and nutra-

ceuticals. The requesting health care practitioner and laboratory should be advised if the patient regularly uses these products so that their effects can be taken into consideration when reviewing results.

➤ Review the procedure with the patient. Inform the patient that specimen collection takes approximately 5 to 10 minutes. Address concerns about pain related to the procedure. Explain to the patient that there may be some discomfort during the venipuncture.

➤ There are no food, fluid, or medication restrictions, unless by medical direction.

Intratest:

➤ If the patient has a history of severe allergic reaction to latex, care should be taken to avoid the use of equipment containing latex.

➤ Instruct the patient to cooperate fully and to follow directions. Direct the patient to breathe normally and to avoid unnecessary movement.

➤ Observe standard precautions, and follow the general guidelines in Appendix A. Positively identify the patient, and label the appropriate tubes with the corresponding patient demographics, date, and time of collection. Perform a venipuncture; collect the specimen in a 5-mL red-top tube.

➤ Remove the needle, and apply a pressure dressing over the puncture site.

➤ Promptly transport the specimen to the laboratory for processing and analysis.

➤ The results are recorded manually or in a computerized system for recall and postprocedure interpretation by the appropriate health care practitioner.

Post-test:

➤ Observe venipuncture site for bleeding or hematoma formation. Apply paper tape or other adhesive to hold pressure bandage in place, or replace with a plastic bandage.

➤ *Nutritional considerations:* Positive test results may be associated with respiratory disease. Malnutrition is commonly seen in patients with severe respiratory disease for reasons including fatigue and lack of appetite. The importance of following the prescribed diet should be stressed to the patient and/or caregiver.

➤ Instruct the patient in preventive measures for protecting his or her lungs (e.g., avoid contact with persons who have respiratory or other infections, avoid use of tobacco, avoid highly polluted areas as well as work environments with hazards such as fumes, dust, and other respiratory pollutants).

➤ Instruct the patient in deep breathing and pursed-lip breathing to enhance breathing patterns, as appropriate.

➤ Inform the patient of smoking cessation programs, as appropriate.

➤ A written report of the examination will be sent to the requesting health care practitioner, who will discuss the results with the patient.

➤ Recognize anxiety related to test results, and be supportive of impaired activity related to lack of respiratory function, perceived loss of independence, and fear of short-ened life expectancy. Discuss the implications of abnormal test results on the patient's lifestyle. Provide teaching and information regarding the clinical implications of the test results, as appropriate. Educate the patient regarding access to counseling services. Provide contact information, if desired, for the American Lung Association *(http://www.lungusa.org).*

➤ Reinforce information given by the patient's health care provider regarding further testing, treatment, or referral to another health care provider. Answer any questions or address any concerns voiced by the patient or family.

➤ Depending on the results of this procedure, additional testing may be performed to evaluate or monitor progression of the disease process and determine the need for a change in therapy. Evaluate test results in relation to the patient's symptoms and other tests performed.

Related laboratory tests:

➤ Related tests include allergen-specific IgE, arterial/alveolar oxygen ratio, chest x-ray, complete blood count, eosinophil count, lung biopsy, and sputum culture.

HYSTEROSALPINGOGRAPHY

S<small>YNONYMS/</small>A<small>CRONYM:</small> Uterography, uterosalpingography, hysterogram.

A<small>REA OF</small> A<small>PPLICATION:</small> Uterus and fallopian tubes.

C<small>ONTRAST:</small> Iodinated contrast medium.

DESCRIPTION & RATIONALE: Hysterosalpingography is generally performed as part of an infertility study to identify anatomic abnormalities of the uterus or occlusion of the fallopian tubes. The procedure allows visualization of the uterine cavity, fallopian tubes, and peritubal area after the injection of contrast medium into the cervix. The contrast medium should flow through the uterine cavity, through the fallopian tubes, and into the peritoneal cavity, where it can be absorbed if no obstruction exists. Passage of the contrast medium through the tubes may clear mucous plugs, straighten kinked tubes, or break up adhesions, thus restoring fertility. This procedure is also used to evaluate the fallopian tubes after tubal ligation and to evaluate the results of reconstructive surgery. Risks include uterine perforation, exposure to radiation, infection, allergic reaction to contrast medium, bleeding, and pulmonary embolism. ∎

INDICATIONS:
• Confirm the presence of fistulas or adhesions

• Confirm tubal abnormalities such as adhesions and occlusions

• Confirm uterine abnormalities such as congenital malformation, traumatic injuries, or the presence of foreign bodies

• Detect bicornate uterus

• Evaluate adequacy of surgical tubal ligation and reconstructive surgery

RESULT

Normal Findings:
• Contrast medium flowing freely into the fallopian tubes and not leaking from the uterus

• Normal position, shape, and size of the uterine cavity

Abnormal Findings:
• Bicornate uterus

• Developmental abnormalities

• Extrauterine pregnancy

• Internal scarring

• Kinking of the fallopian tubes due to adhesions

• Partial or complete blockage of fallopian tube(s)

• Tumors

• Uterine cavity anomalies

• Uterine fistulas

• Uterine masses or foreign body

• Uterine fibroid tumors (leiomyomas)

INTERFERING FACTORS:

This procedure is contraindicated for:
• ⚠ Patients with allergies to shellfish or iodinated dye. The contrast medium used may cause a life-threatening allergic reaction. Patients with a known hypersensitivity to the contrast medium may benefit from premedication with corticosteroids or the use of nonionic contrast medium.

• Patients with bleeding disorders.

• Patients who are pregnant or suspected of being pregnant, unless the potential benefits of the procedure far outweigh the risks to the fetus and mother.

• ⚠ Elderly and other patients who are chronically dehydrated before the test, because of their risk of contrast-induced renal failure.

• ⚠ Patients who are in renal failure.

• Patients with menses, undiagnosed vaginal bleeding, or pelvic inflammatory disease.

- Young patients (17 years and younger), unless the benefits of the x-ray diagnosis outweigh the risks of exposure to high levels of radiation.

***Factors that may
impair clear imaging:***

- Gas or feces in the gastrointestinal tract resulting from inadequate cleansing or failure to restrict food intake before the study

- Retained barium from a previous radiologic procedure

- Metallic objects within the examination field (e.g., jewelry, body rings), which may inhibit organ visualization and can produce unclear images

- Improper adjustment of the radiographic equipment to accommodate obese or thin patients, which can cause overexposure or underexposure and a poor-quality study

- Patients who are very obese, who may exceed the weight limit for the equipment

- Incorrect positioning of the patient, which may produce poor visualization of the area to be examined

- Inability of the patient to cooperate or remain still during the procedure because of age, significant pain, or mental status

- Insufficient injection of contrast medium

- Excessive traction during the test or tubal spasm, which may cause the appearance of a stricture in an otherwise normal fallopian tube

Other considerations:

- Excessive traction during the test may displace adhesions, making the fallopian tubes appear normal.

- The procedure may be terminated if chest pain or severe cardiac arrhythmias occur.

- Failure to follow dietary restrictions and other pretesting preparations may cause the procedure to be canceled or repeated.

- Consultation with a health care practitioner should occur before the procedure for radiation safety concerns regarding younger patients or patients who are lactating.

- Risks associated with radiographic overexposure can result from frequent x-ray procedures. Personnel in the room with the patient should wear a protective lead apron, stand behind a shield, or leave the area while the examination is being done. Personnel working in the area where the examination is being done should wear badges that reveal their level of exposure to radiation.

Nursing Implications and Procedure • • • • • • • • • • •

Pretest:

▶ Inform the patient that the procedure assesses the uterus and fallopian tubes.

▶ Obtain a history of the patient's complaints, including a list of known allergens, especially allergies or sensitivities to latex, iodine, seafood, contrast medium, and dyes.

▶ Obtain a history of the patient's reproductive and genitourinary systems, and results of previously performed diagnostic procedures, surgical procedures, and laboratory tests. For related diagnostic tests, refer to the Reproductive and Genitourinary System tables.

▶ Ensure that this procedure is performed before an upper gastrointestinal study or barium swallow.

▶ Record the date of the last menstrual period and determine the possibility of pregnancy in perimenopausal women.

▶ Obtain a list of the medications the patient is taking.

▶ Review the procedure with the patient. Address concerns about pain related to the procedure. Explain to the patient that some pain may be experienced during the test, and there may be moments of discomfort. Explain to the patient that she may feel temporary sensations of nausea, dizziness, slow heartbeat, and menstrual-like cramping during the procedure and shoulder pain from subphrenic irritation from the contrast medium as it spills into the peritoneal cavity. Explain the purpose of the test and how the procedure is performed. Inform the patient that the procedure is performed in a radiology department, usually by a health care practitioner and support staff, and takes approximately 30 to 60 minutes.

➤ *Sensitivity to cultural and social issues,* as well as concern for modesty, is important in providing psychological support before, during and after the procedure.

➤ Instruct the patient to fast and restrict fluids for 8 hours prior to the procedure.

➤ Patients receiving metformin (Glucophage) for non–insulin-dependent (type 2) diabetes should discontinue the drug on the day of the test and continue to withhold it for 48 hours after the test. Failure to do so may result in lactic acidosis.

➤ Instruct the patient to take a laxative or a cathartic, as ordered, on the evening before the examination.

➤ Instruct the patient to remove jewelry (including watches), credit cards, and other metallic objects.

➤ *Make sure a written and informed consent has been signed prior to the procedure and before administering any medications.*

Intratest:

➤ Ensure that the patient has complied with dietary and medication restrictions and pretesting preparations for at least 6 hours prior to the procedure. Ensure the patient has removed all external metallic objects prior to the procedure.

➤ Assess for completion of bowel preparation according to the institu-

tion's procedure. Administer enemas or suppositories on the morning of the test, as ordered.

➤ Have emergency equipment readily available.

➤ Patients are given a gown and robe to wear and instructed to void prior to the procedure.

➤ Instruct the patient to cooperate fully and to follow directions. Instruct the patient to remain still throughout the procedure because movement produces unreliable results.

➤ Observe standard precautions, and follow the general guidelines in Appendix A.

➤ Remove any wires connected to electrodes, if allowed.

➤ Place the patient in a lithotomy position on the fluoroscopy table.

➤ A kidney, ureter, and bladder (KUB) film is taken to ensure that no stool, gas, or barium will obscure visualization of the uterus and fallopian tubes.

➤ A speculum is inserted into the vagina, and contrast medium is introduced into the uterus through the cervix via a cannula, after which both fluoroscopic and radiographic films are taken.

➤ To take oblique views, the table may be tilted or the patient may be asked to change position during the procedure.

➤ The results are recorded manually, on film, or by automated equipment in a computerized system for recall and postprocedure interpretation by the appropriate health care practitioner.

Post-test:

➤ Instruct the patient to resume usual diet, fluids, medications, or activity, as directed by the health care practitioner.

➤ Monitor for reaction to iodinated contrast medium, including rash, urticaria, tachycardia, hyperpnea, hypertension, palpitations, nausea, or vomiting.

➤ Monitor urinary output after the procedure. Decreased urine output may indicate impending renal failure.

➤ Evaluate the patient for signs of infection, such as pain, fever, increased pulse rate, chills, flushing, abdominal pain, tachycardia, or muscle aches.

➤ Inform the patient that a vaginal discharge is common and that it may be bloody, lasting 1 to 2 days after the test.

➤ Inform the patient that dizziness and cramping may follow this procedure, and that analgesia may be given if there is persistent cramping. Instruct the patient to contact the health care practitioner in the event of severe cramping or profuse bleeding.

➤ A written report of the examination will be completed by a health care practitioner specializing in this branch of medicine. The report will be sent to the requesting health care practitioner, who will discuss the results with the patient.

➤ Recognize anxiety related to test results. Discuss the implications of abnormal test results on the patient's lifestyle. Provide teaching and information regarding the clinical implications of the test results, as appropriate.

➤ Reinforce information given by the patient's health care provider regarding further testing, treatment, or referral to another health care provider. Answer any questions or address any concerns voiced by the patient or family.

➤ Depending on the results of this procedure, additional testing may be needed to evaluate or monitor progression of the disease process and determine the need for a change in therapy. Evaluate test results in relation to the patient's symptoms and other tests performed.

Related diagnostic tests:

➤ Related diagnostic tests include computed tomography of the abdomen, kidney and urine bladder studies, magnetic resonance imaging of the abdomen, and ultrasound of the pelvis.

IMMUNOFIXATION ELECTROPHORESIS, BLOOD AND URINE

· ·

SYNONYM/ACRONYM: IFE.

SPECIMEN: Serum (1 mL) collected in a red-top tube. Urine (10 mL) from a random collection in a clean plastic container.

REFERENCE VALUE: (Method: Immunoprecipitation combined with electrophoresis) Test results are interpreted by a pathologist. Normal placement and intensity of staining provide information about the immunoglobulin bands.

DESCRIPTION & RATIONALE: Immunofixation electrophoresis (IFE) is a qualitative technique that provides a detailed separation of individual immunoglobulins according to their electrical charges. Abnormalities are revealed by changes produced in the individual bands, such as displacement, color, or absence of color. Urine IFE has replaced the Bence Jones screening test for light chains. IFE has replaced immunoelectrophoresis because it is more sensitive and easier to interpret. ■

INDICATIONS:

• Assist in the diagnosis of multiple myeloma and amyloidosis

• Assist in the diagnosis of suspected immunodeficiency

• Assist in the diagnosis of suspected immunoproliferative disorders, such as multiple myeloma and Waldenström's macroglobulinemia

• Identify biclonal or monoclonal gammopathies

• Identify cryoglobulinemia

• Monitor the effectiveness of chemotherapy or radiation therapy

RESULT: See monograph titled "Immunoglobulins A, D, G, and M."

CRITICAL VALUES: N/A

INTERFERING FACTORS:

• Drugs that may increase immunoglobulin levels include asparaginase, cimetidine, and narcotics.

• Drugs that may decrease immunoglobulin levels include dextran, oral contraceptives, methylprednisolone (high doses), and phenytoin.

• Chemotherapy and radiation treatments may alter the width of the bands and make interpretation difficult.

Nursing Implications and Procedure ....

Pretest:

➤ Inform the patient that the test is used to assess the immune system

with respect to the type and quantity of immunoglobulins in blood and urine.

➤ Obtain a history of the patient's complaints, including a list of known allergens (especially allergies or sensitivities to latex), and inform the appropriate health care practitioner accordingly.

➤ Obtain a history of the patient's hematopoietic and immune systems, as well as results of previously performed laboratory tests, surgical procedures, and other diagnostic procedures. For related laboratory tests, refer to the Hematopoietic and Immune System tables.

➤ Note any recent procedures that can interfere with test results. Assess whether the patient received any vaccinations or immunizations within the last 6 months or any blood or blood components within the last 6 weeks.

➤ Obtain a list of medications the patient is taking, including herbs, nutritional supplements, and nutraceuticals. The requesting health care practitioner and laboratory should be advised if the patient regularly uses these products so that their effects can be taken into consideration when reviewing results.

➤ Review the procedure with the patient. Inform the patient that specimen collection takes approximately 5 to 10 minutes. Address concerns about pain related to the procedure. Explain to the patient that there may be some discomfort during the venipuncture.

➤ Provide a nonmetallic urinal, bedpan, or toilet-mounted collection device.

➤ Usually a 24-hour time frame for urine collection is ordered. Inform the patient that all urine must be saved during that 24-hour period. Instruct the patient not to void directly into the laboratory collection container. Instruct the patient to avoid defecating in the collection device and to keep toilet tissue out of the collection device to prevent contamination of the specimen.

Place a sign in the bathroom to remind the patient to save all urine.

➤ Instruct the patient to void all urine into the collection device and then to pour the urine into the laboratory collection container. Alternatively the specimen can be left in the collection device for a health care staff member to add to the laboratory collection container.

➤ *Sensitivity to cultural and social issues,* as well as concern for modesty, is important in providing psychological support before, during, and after the procedure.

➤ There are no food, fluid, or medication restrictions, unless by medical direction.

Intratest:

➤ If the patient has a history of severe allergic reaction to latex, care should be taken to avoid the use of equipment containing latex.

➤ Instruct the patient to cooperate fully and to follow directions. Direct the patient to breathe normally and to avoid unnecessary movement.

➤ Observe standard precautions, and follow the general guidelines in Appendix A. Positively identify the patient, and label the appropriate specimen containers with the corresponding patient demographics, date, and time of collection.

Blood:

➤ Perform a venipuncture; collect the specimen in a 5-mL red-top tube.

➤ Remove the needle, and apply a pressure dressing over the puncture site.

Urine:

Clean-catch specimen:

➤ Instruct the male patient to (1) thoroughly wash his hands, (2) cleanse the meatus, (3) void a small amount into the toilet, and (4) void directly into the specimen container.

➤ Instruct the female patient to (1)

thoroughly wash her hands; (2) cleanse the labia from front to back; (3) while keeping the labia separated, void a small amount into the toilet; and (4) without interrupting the urine stream, void directly into the specimen container.

Blood or urine:

➤ Promptly transport the specimen to the laboratory for processing and analysis.

➤ The results are recorded manually or in a computerized system for recall and postprocedure interpretation by the appropriate health care practitioner.

Post-test:

➤ Observe venipuncture site for bleeding or hematoma formation. Apply paper tape or other adhesive to hold pressure bandage in place, or replace with a plastic bandage.

➤ A written report of the examination will be sent to the requesting health care practitioner, who will discuss the results with the patient.

➤ Reinforce information given by the patient's health care provider regarding further testing, treatment, or referral to another health care provider. Answer any questions or address any concerns voiced by the patient or family.

➤ Depending on the results of this procedure, additional testing may be performed to evaluate or monitor progression of the disease process and determine the need for a change in therapy. Evaluate test results in relation to the patient's symptoms and other tests performed.

Related laboratory tests:

➤ Related laboratory tests include bone marrow biopsy, lymph node biopsy, complete blood count with examination of peripheral smear, quantitative immunoglobulin levels, protein quantitative (blood and urine) and fractions, and urinalysis.

IMMUNOGLOBULIN E

SYNONYM/ACRONYM: IgE.

SPECIMEN: Serum (1 mL) collected in a red- or tiger-top tube.

REFERENCE VALUE: (Method: Immunoassay)

Age	Conventional Units	SI Units (Conventional Units × 10)
Newborn	Less than 12 IU/mL	Less than 120 mg/L
Less than 1 y	Less than 50 IU/mL	Less than 500 mg/L
2–4 y	Less than 100 IU/mL	Less than 1000 mg/L
5 y and older	Less than 300 IU/mL	Less than 3000 mg/L

DESCRIPTION & RATIONALE: Immunoglobulin E (IgE) is an antibody whose primary response is to allergic reactions and parasitic infections. Most of the body's IgE is bound to specialized tissue cells; little is available in the circulating blood. IgE binds to the membrane of special granulocytes called *basophils* in the circulating blood and *mast cells* in the tissues. Basophil and mast cell membranes have receptors for IgE. Mast cells are abundant in the skin and the tissues lining the respiratory and alimentary tracts. When IgE antibody becomes cross-linked with antigen/allergen, the release of histamine, heparin, and other chemicals from the granules in the cells is triggered. A sequence of events follows activation of IgE that affects smooth muscle contraction, vascular permeability, and inflammatory reactions.

The inflammatory response allows proteins from the bloodstream to enter the tissues. Helminths (worm parasites) are especially susceptible to immunoglobulin-mediated cytotoxic chemicals. The inflammatory reaction proteins attract macrophages from the circulatory system and granulocytes, such as eosinophils, from circulation and bone marrow. Eosinophils also contain enzymes effective against the parasitic invaders. ▪

INDICATIONS: Assist in the evaluation of allergy and parasitic infection

RESULT

Increased in:
• Alcoholism

• Allergy

• Asthma

• Bronchopulmonary aspergillosis

- Dermatitis
- Eczema
- Hay fever
- IgE myeloma
- Parasitic infestation
- Rhinitis
- Sinusitis
- Wiskott-Aldrich syndrome

Decreased in:
- Advanced carcinoma
- Agammaglobulinemia
- Ataxia-telangiectasia
- IgE deficiency

CRITICAL VALUES: N/A

INTERFERING FACTORS:
- Drugs that may cause a decrease in IgE levels include phenytoin and tryptophan.
- Penicillin G has been associated with increased IgE levels in some patients with drug-induced acute interstitial nephritis.
- Normal IgE levels do not eliminate allergic disorders as a possible diagnosis.

Nursing Implications and Procedure . . . .

Pretest:

▶ Inform the patient that the test is used to assess IgE levels in order to identify the presence of an allergic or inflammatory immune system response.

▶ Obtain a history of the patient's complaints, including a list of known allergens (especially allergies or sensitivities to latex), and inform the appropriate health care practitioner accordingly.

▶ Obtain a history of the patient's immune and respiratory systems, as well as results of previously performed laboratory tests, surgical procedures, and other diagnostic procedures. For related laboratory tests, refer to the Immune and Respiratory System tables.

▶ Obtain a list of the medications the patient is taking, including herbs, nutritional supplements, and neutraceuticals. The requesting health care practitioner and laboratory should be advised if the patient regularly uses these products so that their effects can be taken into consideration when reviewing results.

▶ Review the procedure with the patient. Inform the patient that specimen collection takes approximately 5 to 10 minutes. Address concerns about pain related to the procedure. Explain to the patient that there may be some discomfort during the venipuncture.

▶ There are no food, fluid, or medication restrictions, unless by medical direction.

Intratest:

▶ If the patient has a history of severe allergic reaction to latex, care should be taken to avoid the use of equipment containing latex.

▶ Instruct the patient to cooperate fully and to follow directions. Direct the patient to breathe normally and to avoid unnecessary movement.

▶ Observe standard precautions, and follow the general guidelines in Appendix A. Positively identify the patient, and label the appropriate tubes with the corresponding patient demographics, date, and time of collection. Perform a venipuncture; collect the specimen in a 5-mL red- or tiger-top tube.

▶ Remove the needle, and apply a pressure dressing over the puncture site.

▶ Promptly transport the specimen to the laboratory for processing and analysis.

▶ The results are recorded manually

or in a computerized system for recall and postprocedure interpretation by the appropriate health care practitioner.

➤ Observe venipuncture site for bleeding or hematoma formation. Apply paper tape or other adhesive to hold pressure bandage in place, or replace with a plastic bandage.

➤ A written report of the examination will be sent to the requesting health care practitioner, who will discuss the results with the patient.

➤ *Nutritional considerations:* Increased IgE levels may be associated with allergy. Consideration should be given to diet if the patient has food allergies.

➤ Reinforce information given by the patient's health care provider regarding further testing, treatment, or referral to another health care provider. Answer any questions or address any concerns voiced by the patient or family.

➤ Depending on the results of this procedure, additional testing may be performed to evaluate or monitor progression of the patient's condition and determine the need for a change in therapy. Evaluate test results in relation to the patient's symptoms and other tests performed.

Related laboratory tests:

➤ Related laboratory tests include allergen-specific IgE, alveolar/arterial gradient and arterial/alveolar oxygen ratio, blood gases, complete blood count, eosinophil count, hypersensitivity pneumonitis, and theophylline.

IMMUNOGLOBULINS A, D, G, AND M

SYNONYMS/ACRONYMS: IgA, IgD, IgG, and IgM.

SPECIMEN: Serum (1 mL) collected in a red-top tube.

REFERENCE VALUE: (Method: Nephelometry)

Age	Conventional Units	SI Units
	Immunoglobulin A	
		(Conventional Units × 0.01)
Newborn	1–4 mg/dL	0.01–0.04 g/L
1–9 mo	2–80 mg/dL	0.02–0.80 g/L
10–12 mo	15–90 mg/dL	0.15–0.90 g/L
2–3 y	18–150 mg/dL	0.18–1.50 g/L
4–5 y	25–160 mg/dL	0.25–1.60 g/L
6–8 y	35–200 mg/dL	0.35–2.00 g/L
9–12 y	45–250 mg/dL	0.45–2.50 g/L
Older than 12 y	40–350 mg/dL	0.40–3.50 g/L

Age	Conventional Units	SI Units
	Immunoglobulin D	
		(Conventional Units × 10)
Newborn	Greater than 2 mg/dL	Greater than 20 mg/L
Adult	Less than 15 mg/dL	Less than 150 mg/L
	Immunoglobulin G	
		(Conventional Units × 0.01)
Newborn	650–1600 mg/dL	6.5–16 g/L
1–9 mo	250–900 mg/dL	2.5–9 g/L
10–12 mo	290–1070 mg/dL	2.9–10.7 g/L
2–3 y	420–1200 mg/dL	4.2–12 g/L
4–6 y	460–1240 mg/dL	4.6–12.4 g/L
Greater than 6 y	650–1600 mg/dL	6.5–16 g/L
	Immunoglobulin M	
		(Conventional Units × 0.01)
Newborn	Less than 25 mg/dL	Less than 0.25 g/L
1–9 mo	20–125 mg/dL	0.2–1.25 g/L
10–12 mo	40–150 mg/dL	0.4–1.5 g/L
2–8 y	45–200 mg/dL	0.45–2.0 g/L
9–12 y	50–250 mg/dL	0.5–2.5 g/L
Greater than 12 y	50–300 mg/dL	0.5–3.0 g/L

DESCRIPTION & RATIONALE: Immunoglobulins A, D, E, G, and M are made by plasma cells in response to foreign particles. Immunoglobulins neutralize toxic substances, support phagocytosis, and destroy invading microorganisms. They are made up of heavy and light chains. Immunoglobulins produced by the proliferation of a single plasma cell (clone) are called *monoclonal.* Polyclonal increases result when multiple cell lines produce antibody. IgA is found mainly in secretions such as tears, saliva, and breast milk. It is believed to protect mucous membranes from viruses and bacteria. The function of IgD is not well understood. For details on IgE, see the monograph titled "Immunoglobulin E." IgG is the predominant serum immunoglobulin and is important in long-term defense against disease. It is the only antibody that crosses the placenta. IgM is the largest immunoglobulin, and it is the first antibody to react to an antigenic stimulus. IgM also forms natural antibodies, such as ABO blood group antibodies. The presence of IgM in cord blood is an indication of congenital infection. ■

INDICATIONS:

• Assist in the diagnosis of multiple myeloma

• Evaluate humoral immunity status

• Monitor therapy for multiple myeloma

• IgA: Evaluate patients suspected of IgA deficiency prior to transfusion. Evaluate anaphylaxis associated with the transfusion of blood and blood products (anti-

IgA antibodies may develop in patients with low levels of IgA, possibly resulting in anaphylaxis when donated blood is transfused)

RESULT

Increases in:

IgA:

* Polyclonal:
   Chronic liver disease
   Immunodeficiency states, such as Wiskott-Aldrich syndrome
   Inflammatory bowel disease
   Lower GI cancer
   Rheumatoid arthritis

* Monoclonal:
   IgA-type multiple myeloma

IgD:

* Polyclonal:
   Certain liver diseases
   Chronic infections
   Connective tissue disorders

* Monoclonal:
   IgD-type multiple myeloma

IgG:

* Polyclonal:
   Autoimmune diseases, such as systemic lupus erythematosus, rheumatoid arthritis, and Sjögren's syndrome
   Chronic liver disease
   Chronic or recurrent infections
   Intrauterine devices
   Sarcoidosis

* Monoclonal:
   IgG-type multiple myeloma
   Leukemias
   Lymphomas

IgM:

* Polyclonal:
   Active sarcoidosis

Chronic hepatocellular disease
Collagen vascular disease
Early response to bacterial or parasitic infection
Hyper-IgM dysgammaglobulinemia
Rheumatoid arthritis
Variable in nephrotic syndrome
Viral infection (hepatitis or mononucleosis)

* Monoclonal:
   Cold agglutinin hemolysis disease
   Malignant lymphoma
   Neoplasms (especially GI tract)
   Reticulosis
   Waldenström's macroglobulinemia

Decreases in:

IgA:

* Ataxia-telangiectasia
* Chronic sinopulmonary disease
* Genetic IgA deficiency

IgD:

* Genetic IgD deficiency
* Malignant melanoma of the skin
* Pre-eclampsia

IgG:

* Burns
* Genetic IgG deficiency
* Nephrotic syndrome
* Pregnancy

IgM:

* Burns
* Secondary IgM deficiency associated with IgG or IgA gammopathies

CRITICAL VALUES: N/A

INTERFERING FACTORS:

* Drugs that may increase immunoglobulin levels include asparaginase, cimetidine, and narcotics.

- Drugs that may decrease immunoglobulin levels include dextran, oral contraceptives, methylprednisolone (high doses), and phenytoin.

- Chemotherapy, immunosuppressive therapy, and radiation treatments decrease immunoglobulin levels.

- Specimens with macroglobulins, cryoglobulins, or cold agglutinins tested at cold temperatures may give falsely low values.

Nursing Implications and Procedure

Pretest:

➤ Inform the patient that the test is used to assess the immune system with respect to the quantity of immunoglobulin levels present in the blood.

➤ Obtain a history of the patient's complaints, including a list of known allergens (especially allergies or sensitivities to latex), and inform the appropriate health care practitioner accordingly.

➤ Obtain a history of the patient's gastrointestinal, hematopoietic, immune, and musculoskeletal systems, as well as results of previously performed laboratory tests, surgical procedures, and other diagnostic procedures. For related laboratory tests, refer to the Gastrointestinal, Hematopoietic, Immune, and Musculoskeletal System tables.

➤ Obtain a list of medications the patient is taking, including herbs, nutritional supplements, and nutraceuticals. The requesting health care practitioner and laboratory should be advised if the patient regularly uses these products so that their effects can be taken into consideration when reviewing results.

➤ Note any recent procedures that can interfere with test results.

➤ Review the procedure with the patient. Inform the patient that specimen collection takes approximately 5 to 10 minutes. Address concerns about pain related to the procedure. Explain to the patient that there may be some discomfort during the venipuncture.

➤ There are no food, fluid, or medication restrictions, unless by medical direction.

Intratest:

➤ If the patient has a history of severe allergic reaction to latex, care should be taken to avoid the use of equipment containing latex.

➤ Instruct the patient to cooperate fully and to follow directions. Direct the patient to breathe normally and to avoid unnecessary movement.

➤ Observe standard precautions, and follow the general guidelines in Appendix A. Positively identify the patient, and label the appropriate tubes with the corresponding patient demographics, date, and time of collection. Perform a venipuncture; collect the specimen in a 5-mL red-top tube.

➤ Remove the needle, and apply a pressure dressing over the puncture site.

➤ Promptly transport the specimen to the laboratory for processing and analysis.

➤ The results are recorded manually or in a computerized system for recall and postprocedure interpretation by the appropriate health care practitioner.

Post-test:

➤ Observe venipuncture site for bleeding or hematoma formation. Apply paper tape or other adhesive to hold pressure bandage in place, or replace with a plastic bandage.

➤ A written report of the examination will be sent to the requesting health care practitioner, who will discuss the results with the patient.

➤ Reinforce information given by the patient's health care provider regard-

ing further testing, treatment, or referral to another health care provider. Answer any questions or address any concerns voiced by the patient or family.

➤ Depending on the results of this procedure, additional testing may be performed to evaluate or monitor progression of the disease process and determine the need for a change in therapy. Evaluate test results in relation to the patient's symptoms and other tests performed.

➤ Related laboratory tests include bone marrow biopsy, blood groups and antibodies, complete blood count with evaluation of peripheral smear, immunofixation electrophoresis (blood and urine), protein quantitative (blood and urine) and fractions, and urinalysis.

IMMUNOSUPPRESSANTS: CYCLOSPORINE, METHOTREXATE

· ·

SYNONYMS/ACRONYM: Cyclosporine (Sandimmune), methotrexate (MTX, amethopterin, Folex, Rheumatrex), methotrexate sodium (Mexate).

SPECIMEN: Whole blood (1 mL) collected in lavender-top tube for cyclosporine. Serum (1 mL) collected in a red-top tube for methotrexate.

Immunosuppressant	Route of Administration	Recommended Collection Time
Cyclosporine	Oral	12 h after dose
Methotrexate	Oral	Varies according to dosing protocol
	Intramuscular	Varies according to dosing protocol

Important note: This information must be clearly and accurately communicated to avoid misunderstanding of the dose time in relation to the collection time. Miscommunication between the individual administering the medication and the individual collecting the specimen is the most frequent cause of subtherapeutic levels, toxic levels, and misleading information used in calculation of future doses.

REFERENCE VALUE: (Method: Immunoassay)

	Therapeutic Dose		Half-Life	Volume of Distribution	Protein Binding	Excre-tion
	Conven-tional Units	*SI Units (Conven-(tional Units × 0.832)*				
Cyclo-sporine	100–250 ng/mL Renal transplant	83–208 nmol/L	8–24 h	4–6 L/kg	90%	Renal
	100–400 ng/mL Cardiac transplant	83–333 nmol/L	8–24 h	4–6 L/kg	90%	Renal
	100–300 ng/mL Bone marrow transplant	83–250 nmol/L	8–24 h	4–6 L/kg	90%	Renal
	100–400 ng/mL Liver transplant	83–333 nmol/L	8–24 h	4–6 L/kg	90%	Renal
Metho-trexate	0.01–5.00 μmol/L*		8–15 h	0.4–1.0 L/kg	50–70%	Renal

*Dependent on therapeutic approach.

DESCRIPTION & RATIONALE: Cyclosporine is an immunosuppressive drug used in the management of organ rejection, especially rejection of heart, liver, and kidney transplants. Its most serious side effect is renal impairment or renal failure. Methotrexate is a highly toxic drug that causes cell death by disrupting DNA synthesis.

Many factors must be considered in effective dosing and monitoring of therapeutic drugs, including patient age, weight, interacting medications, electrolyte balance, protein levels, water balance, and conditions that affect absorption and excretion; as well as foods, herbals, vitamins, and minerals that can either potentiate or inhibit the intended target concentration. ■

INDICATIONS

Cyclosporine:
• Assist in the management of treatments to prevent organ rejection

• Monitor for toxicity

Methotrexate:
• Monitor effectiveness of treatment of cancer and some autoimmune disorders

• Monitor for toxicity

RESULT

Normal levels	Therapeutic effect
Toxic levels	Adjust dose as indicated
Cyclosporine	Renal impairment
Methotrexate	Renal impairment

CRITICAL VALUES: ⚠️ It is important to note the adverse effects of toxic and subtherapeutic levels. Care must be taken to investigate signs and symptoms of too little and too much medication. Note and immediately report to the health care practitioner any critically increased values and related symptoms.

Cyclosporine: Greater than 400 ng/mL

Signs and symptoms of cyclosporine toxicity include increased severity of expected side effects, which include nausea, stomatitis, vomiting, anorexia, hypertension, infection, fluid retention, hypercalcemic metabolic acidosis, tremor, seizures, headache, and flushing. Possible interventions include close monitoring of blood levels to make dosing adjustments, inducing emesis (if orally ingested), performing gastric lavage (if orally ingested), withholding the drug, and initiating alternative therapy for a short time until the patient is stabilized.

Methotrexate: Greater than 5.00 μmol/L after 24 h; greater than 0.50 μmol/L after 48 h; greater than 0.05 μmol/L after 72 h

Signs and symptoms of methotrexate toxicity include increased severity of expected side effects, which include nausea, stomatitis, vomiting, anorexia, bleeding, infection, bone marrow depression, and, over a prolonged period of use, hepatotoxicity. The effect of methotrexate on normal cells can be reversed by administration of 5-formyltetrahydrofolate (citrovorum or leucovorin). 5-Formyltetrahydrofolate allows higher doses of methotrexate to be given.

INTERFERING FACTORS:

- Numerous drugs interact with cyclosporine and either increase cyclosporine levels or increase the risk of toxicity. These drugs include acyclovir, aminoglycosides, amiodarone, amphotericin B, anabolic steroids, cephalosporins, cimetidine, danazol, erythromycin, furosemide, ketoconazole, melphalan, methylprednisolone, miconazole, nonsteroidal anti-inflammatory drugs (NSAIDs), oral contraceptives, and trimethoprim-sulfamethoxazole.

- Drugs that may decrease cyclosporine levels include carbamazepine, ethotoin, mephenytoin, phenobarbital, phenytoin, primidone, and rifampin.

- Drugs that may increase methotrexate levels or increase the risk of toxicity include NSAIDs, probenecid, salicylate, and sulfonamides.

- Antibiotics may decrease the absorption of methotrexate.

Nursing Implications and Procedure ....

Pretest:

➤ Inform the patient that the test is used to monitor for therapeutic and toxic drug levels.

➤ Obtain a history of the patient's complaints, including a list of known allergens (especially allergies or sensitivities to latex), and inform the appropriate health care practitioner accordingly.

➤ Obtain a history of the patient's genitourinary and immune systems, as well as results of previously performed laboratory tests, surgical procedures, and other diagnostic procedures. For related laboratory tests, refer to the Genitourinary and Immune System and Therapeutic/Toxicology table.

➤ Obtain a list of the medications the patient is taking, including herbs, nutritional supplements, and nutraceuticals. Note the last time and dose of medication taken. The requesting health care practitioner and laboratory should be advised if the patient regularly uses these products so that their effects can be taken into consideration when reviewing results.

➤ Review the procedure with the patient. Inform the patient that specimen collection takes approximately 5 to 10 minutes. Address concerns about pain related to the procedure. Explain to the patient that there may be some discomfort during the venipuncture.

➤ *Sensitivity to cultural and social issues,* as well as concern for modesty, is important in providing psychological support before, during, and after the procedure.

➤ There are no food, fluid, or medication restrictions, unless by medical direction.

Intratest:

➤ If the patient has a history of severe allergic reaction to latex, care should be taken to avoid the use of equipment containing latex.

➤ Instruct the patient to cooperate fully and to follow directions. Direct the patient to breathe normally and to avoid unnecessary movement.

➤ Observe standard precautions, and follow the general guidelines in Appendix A. Consider recommended collection time with regard to dosing schedule. Positively identify the patient, and label the appropriate tubes with the corresponding patient demographics, date, and time of collection. Perform a venipuncture; collect the specimen in a lavender-top tube for cyclosporine and a red-top tube for methotrexate.

➤ Remove the needle, and apply a pressure dressing over the puncture site.

➤ Promptly transport the specimen to the laboratory for processing and analysis.

➤ The results are recorded manually or in a computerized system for recall and postprocedure interpretation by the appropriate health care practitioner.

Post-test:

➤ Observe venipuncture site for bleeding or hematoma formation. Apply paper tape or other adhesive to hold pressure bandage in place, or replace with a plastic bandage.

➤ *Nutritional considerations:* Patients taking immunosuppressant therapy tend to have decreased appetites due to the side effects of the medication. Instruct patients to consume a variety of foods within the basic food groups, maintain a healthy weight, be physically active, limit salt intake, limit alcohol intake, and be a nonsmoker.

➤ A written report of the examination will be sent to the requesting health care practitioner, who will discuss the results with the patient.

➤ Recognize anxiety related to test results, and offer support. Patients receiving these drugs usually have conditions that can be intermittently moderately to severely debilitating, resulting in significant lifestyle changes. Educate the patient regarding access to counseling services, as appropriate.

➤ Reinforce information given by the patient's health care provider regarding further testing, treatment, or referral to another health care provider. Explain to the patient the importance of following the medication regimen and give instructions regarding drug interactions. Answer any questions or address any concerns voiced by the patient or family.

➤ Instruct the patient to be prepared to provide the pharmacist with a list of other medications he or she is already taking in the event that the requesting health care practitioner prescribes a medication.

➤ Depending on the results of this procedure, additional testing may be performed to evaluate or monitor progression of the disease process

and determine the need for a change in therapy. Evaluate test results in relation to the patient's symptoms and other tests performed.

Related laboratory tests:

➤ Related laboratory tests include blood urea nitrogen and creatinine.

INFECTIOUS MONONUCLEOSIS SCREEN

SYNONYMS/ACRONYM: Monospot, heterophil antibody test, IM serology.

SPECIMEN: Serum (1 mL) collected in a red-top tube.

REFERENCE VALUE: (Method: Agglutination) Negative.

DESCRIPTION & RATIONALE: Infectious mononucleosis is caused by the Epstein-Barr virus (EBV). The incubation period is 10 to 50 days, and the symptoms last 1 to 4 weeks after the infection has fully developed. The hallmark of EBV infection is the presence of heterophil antibodies, also called *Paul-Bunnell-Davidsohn antibodies,* which are immunoglobulin M (IgM) antibodies that agglutinate sheep or horse red blood cells. The disease induces formation of abnormal lymphocytes in the lymph nodes; stimulates increased formation of heterophil antibodies; and is characterized by fever, cervical lymphadenopathy, tonsillopharyngitis, and hepatosplenomegaly. EBV is also thought to play a role in Burkitt's lym-

phoma, nasopharyngeal carcinoma, and chronic fatigue syndrome. If the results of the heterophil antibody screening test are negative and infectious mononucleosis is highly suspected, EBV-specific serology should be requested. ■

INDICATIONS: Assist in confirming infectious mononucleosis

RESULT

Positive findings in:
Infectious mononucleosis

CRITICAL VALUES: N/A

INTERFERING FACTORS:
• False-positive results may occur in the presence of narcotic addiction, serum sickness, lymphomas, hepatitis,

leukemia, cancer of the pancreas, and phenytoin therapy.

* A false-negative result may occur if treatment was begun before antibodies developed or if the test was done less than 6 days after exposure to the virus.

Nursing Implications and Procedure • • • • • • • • • • •

➤ Inform the patient that the test is used to assist in the diagnosis of mononucleosis infection.

➤ Obtain a history of the patient's complaints, including a list of known allergens (especially allergies or sensitivities to latex), and inform the appropriate health care practitioner accordingly. Obtain a history of exposure.

➤ Obtain a history of the patient's hepatobiliary and immune systems, as well as results of previously performed laboratory tests, surgical procedures, and other diagnostic procedures. For related laboratory tests, refer to the Hepatobiliary and Immune System tables.

➤ Note any recent therapies that can interfere with test results.

➤ Obtain a list of medications the patient is taking, including herbs, nutritional supplements, and nutraceuticals. The requesting health care practitioner and laboratory should be advised if the patient regularly uses these products so that their effects can be taken into consideration when reviewing results.

➤ Review the procedure with the patient. Inform the patient that specimen collection takes approximately 5 to 10 minutes. Address concerns about pain related to the procedure. Explain to the patient that there may be some discomfort during the venipuncture.

➤ There are no food, fluid, or medication restrictions, unless by medical direction.

Intratest:

➤ If the patient has a history of severe allergic reaction to latex, care should be taken to avoid the use of equipment containing latex.

➤ Instruct the patient to cooperate fully and to follow directions. Direct the patient to breathe normally and to avoid unnecessary movement.

➤ Observe standard precautions, and follow the general guidelines in Appendix A. Positively identify the patient, and label the appropriate tubes with the corresponding patient demographics, date, and time of collection. Perform a venipuncture; collect the specimen in a 5-mL red-top tube.

➤ Remove the needle, and apply a pressure dressing over the puncture site.

➤ Promptly transport the specimen to the laboratory for processing and analysis.

➤ The results are recorded manually or in a computerized system for recall and postprocedure interpretation by the appropriate health care practitioner.

Post-test:

➤ Observe venipuncture site for bleeding or hematoma formation. Apply paper tape or other adhesive to hold pressure bandage in place, or replace with a plastic bandage.

➤ Inform the patient that approximately 10% of all results are false-negative or false-positive. Inform the patient that signs and symptoms of infection include fever, chills, sore throat, enlarged lymph nodes, and fatigue. Self-care while the disease runs its course includes adequate fluid and nutritional intake along with sufficient rest. Activities that cause fatigue or stress should be avoided.

➤ A written report of the examination will be sent to the requesting health care practitioner, who will discuss the results with the patient.

➤ Reinforce information given by the patient's health care provider regarding further testing, treatment, or referral to another health care provider. Advise the patient to refrain from direct contact with others because the disease is transmitted through saliva. Answer any questions or address any concerns voiced by the patient or family.

➤ Depending on the results of this procedure, additional testing may be performed to evaluate or monitor progression of the disease process and determine the need for a change in therapy. Evaluate test results in relation to the patient's symptoms and other tests performed.

Related laboratory tests:

➤ Related laboratory tests include complete blood count with peripheral blood smear evaluation.

INSULIN AND INSULIN RESPONSE TO GLUCOSE

· ·

SYNONYM/ACRONYM: N/A.

SPECIMEN: Serum (1 mL) collected in a red-top tube.

REFERENCE VALUE: (Method: Radioimmunoassay)

	Insulin	SI Units (Conventional Units × 6.945)	Tolerance for Glucose (Hypoglycemia)
Fasting	Less than 25 mIU/L	Less than 174 pmol/L	65–115 mg/dL
30 min	30–230 mIU/L	208–1597 pmol/L	N/A
1 h	18–276 mIU/L	125–1917 pmol/L	Less than 200 mg/dL
2 h	16–166 mIU/L	111–1153 pmol/L	Less than 140 mg/dL
3 h	Less than 25 mIU/L	Less than 174 pmol/L	65–120 mg/dL
4 h	Less than 25 mIU/L	Less than 174 pmol/L	65–120 mg/dL
5 h	Less than 25 mIU/L	Less than 174 pmol/L	65–115 mg/dL

DESCRIPTION & RATIONALE: Insulin is secreted in response to elevated blood glucose, and its overall effect is to promote glucose use and energy storage. The insulin response test measures the rate of insulin secreted by the beta cells of the islets of Langerhans in the pancreas; it may be performed simultaneously with a 5-hour glucose tolerance test for hypoglycemia. ■

INDICATIONS:

- Assist in the diagnosis of early or developing non–insulin-dependent (type 2) diabetes, as indicated by excessive production of insulin in relation to blood glucose levels (best shown with glucose tolerance tests or 2-hour postprandial tests)

- Assist in the diagnosis of insulinoma, as indicated by sustained high levels of insulin and absence of blood glucose–related variations

- Confirm functional hypoglycemia, as indicated by circulating insulin levels appropriate to changing blood glucose levels

- Differentiate between insulin-resistant diabetes, in which insulin levels are high, and non–insulin-resistant diabetes, in which insulin levels are low

- Evaluate fasting hypoglycemia of unknown cause

- Evaluate postprandial hypoglycemia of unknown cause

- Evaluate uncontrolled insulin-dependent (type 1) diabetes

RESULT

Increased in:
- Acromegaly
- Alcohol use
- Cushing's syndrome
- Diabetes
- Excessive administration of insulin
- Insulin- and proinsulin-secreting tumors (insulinomas)
- Obesity
- Reactive hypoglycemia in developing diabetes
- Severe liver disease

Decreased in:
- Beta cell failure

CRITICAL VALUES: NA

INTERFERING FACTORS:

- Drugs and substances that may increase insulin levels include acetohexamide, alanine, albuterol, amino acids, beclomethasone, betamethasone, broxaterol, calcium gluconate, cannabis, chlorpropamide, cyclic AMP, glibornuride, glipizide, glisoxepide, glucagon, glyburide, ibopamine, insulin, insulin-like growth factor–I, oral contraceptives, pancreozymin, prednisolone, prednisone, rifampin, salbutamol, terbutaline, tolazamide, tolbutamide, trichlormethiazide, and verapamil.

- Drugs that may decrease insulin levels include acarbose, asparaginase, calcitonin, cimetidine, clofibrate, dexfenfluramine, diltiazem, doxazosin, enalapril, enprostil, ether, hydroxypropyl methylcellulose, insulin-like growth factor–I, metformin, niacin, nifedipine, nitrendipine, octreotide, phenytoin, propranolol, and psyllium.

- Administration of insulin or oral hypoglycemic agents within 8 hours of the test can lead to falsely elevated levels.

- Hemodialysis destroys insulin and affects test results.

- Recent radioactive scans or radiation can interfere with test results when radioimmunoassay is the test method.

Nursing Implications and Procedure . . . .

Pretest:

➤ Inform the patient that the test is used to assist in the evaluation of fasting hypoglycemia.

➤ Obtain a history of the patient's complaints, including a list of known allergens (especially allergies or sensitivities to latex), and inform the appropriate health care practitioner accordingly.

➤ Obtain a history of the patient's endocrine system and results of previously performed laboratory tests, surgical procedures, and other diagnostic procedures. For related laboratory tests, refer to the Endocrine System table.

➤ Note any recent procedures that can interfere with test results.

➤ Obtain a list of the medications the patient is taking, including herbs, nutritional supplements and nutraceuticals. Note the last time and dose of medication taken. The requesting health care practitioner and laboratory should be advised if the patient regularly uses these products so their effects can be taken into consideration when reviewing results.

➤ Review the procedure with the patient. Inform the patient that multiple specimens may be required. Inform the patient that specimen collection takes approximately 5 to 10 minutes. Address concerns about pain related to the procedure. Explain to the patient that there may be some discomfort during the venipuncture.

➤ *Sensitivity to cultural and social issues,* as well as concern for modesty, is important in providing psychological support before, during, and after the procedure.

➤ If a single sample is to be collected, the patient should have fasted and refrained, with medical direction, from taking insulin or other oral hypoglycemic agents for at least 8 hours before specimen collection.

➤ *Hypoglycemia:* Serial specimens for insulin levels are collected in conjunction with glucose levels after administration of a 100-g glucose load. The patient should be prepared as for a standard oral glucose tolerance test over a 5-hour period.

➤ There are no fluid restrictions, unless by medical direction.

Intratest:

➤ Ensure that the patient has complied with dietary or medication restrictions and other pretesting preparations; assure that food or medications have been restricted as instructed prior to the specific procedure's protocol.

➤ If the patient has a history of severe allergic reaction to latex, care should be taken to avoid the use of equipment containing latex.

➤ Instruct the patient to cooperate fully and to follow directions. Direct the patient to breathe normally and to avoid unnecessary movement.

➤ Observe standard precautions, and follow the general guidelines in Appendix A. Positively identify the patient, and label the appropriate tubes with the corresponding patient demographics, date, and time of collection. Perform a venipuncture; collect the specimen in a 5-mL redtop tube.

➤ Remove the needle, and apply a pressure dressing over the puncture site.

➤ Promptly transport the specimen to the laboratory for processing and analysis.

➤ The results are recorded manually or in a computerized system for recall and postprocedure interpretation by the appropriate health care practitioner.

Post-test:

➤ Observe venipuncture site for bleeding or hematoma formation. Apply paper tape or other adhesive to hold pressure bandage in place, or replace with a plastic bandage.

- Instruct the patient to resume usual diet and medication, as directed by the health care practitioner.

- *Nutritional considerations:* Increased insulin levels may be associated with diabetes. The nutritional needs of each diabetic patient need to be determined individually (especially during pregnancy) by a health care practitioner trained in nutrition. Patients who adhere to dietary recommendations report a better general feeling of health, better weight management, greater control of glucose and lipid values, and improved use of insulin. There is no "diabetic diet"; however, many meal-planning approaches with nutritional goals are endorsed by the American Dietetic Association.

- Impaired glucose tolerance may be associated with diabetes. Instruct the patient and caregiver to report signs and symptoms of hypoglycemia (weakness, confusion, diaphoresis, rapid pulse) or hyperglycemia (thirst, polyuria, hunger, lethargy).

- A written report of the examination will be sent to the requesting health care practitioner, who will discuss the results with the patient.

- Recognize anxiety related to test results, and be supportive of perceived loss of independence and fear of shortened life expectancy. Discuss the implications of abnormal test results on the patient's lifestyle. Provide teaching and information regarding the clinical implications of the test results, as appropriate. Emphasize, as appropriate, that good glycemic control delays the onset of and slows the progression of diabetic retinopathy, nephropathy, and neuropathy. Educate the patient regarding access to counseling services. Provide contact information, if desired, for the American Diabetes Association (*http://www.diabetes.org*).

- Reinforce information given by the patient's health care provider regarding further testing, treatment, or referral to another health care provider. Answer any questions or address any concerns voiced by the patient or family.

- Depending on the results of this procedure, additional testing may be performed to evaluate or monitor progression of the disease process and determine the need for a change in therapy. Evaluate test results in relation to the patient's symptoms and other tests performed.

Related laboratory tests:

- Related laboratory tests include C-peptide, fructosamine, glucose, glucose tolerance tests, glycated hemoglobin, insulin antibodies, and microalbumin.

INSULIN ANTIBODIES

. . . .

Synonym/Acronym: N/A.

Specimen: Serum (1 mL) collected in a red-top tube.

Reference value: (Method: Radioimmunoassay) Less than 3%; includes binding of human, beef, and pork insulin to antibodies in patient's serum.

DESCRIPTION & RATIONALE: The most common anti-insulin antibody is immunoglobulin (Ig) G, but IgA, IgM, IgD, and IgE antibodies also have anti-insulin properties. These antibodies usually do not cause clinical problems, but they may complicate insulin assay testing. IgM is thought to participate in insulin resistance and IgE in insulin allergy. Improvements in the purity of animal insulin and increased use of human insulin have resulted in a significant decrease in the incidence of insulin antibody formation. ■

INDICATIONS:

• Assist in confirming insulin resistance

• Assist in determining if hypoglycemia is caused by insulin abuse

• Assist in determining insulin allergy

RESULT

• Factitious hypoglycemia

• Insulin allergy or resistance

• Polyendocrine autoimmune syndromes

• Steroid-induced diabetes (a side effect of treatment for systemic lupus erythematosus)

Decreased in: N/A

CRITICAL VALUES: N/A

INTERFERING FACTORS: Recent radioactive scans or radiation can interfere with test results when radioimmunoassay is the test method.

Nursing Implications and Procedure ....

Pretest:

➤ Inform the patient that the test is used to assist in the prediction, diagnosis, and management of type I diabetes.

➤ Obtain a history of the patient's complaints, including a list of known allergens (especially allergies or sensitivities to latex), and inform the appropriate health care practitioner accordingly.

➤ Obtain a history of the patient's endocrine and immune systems, as well as results of previously performed laboratory tests, surgical procedures, and other diagnostic procedures. For related laboratory tests, refer to the Endocrine and Immune System tables.

➤ Note any recent procedures that can interfere with test results.

➤ Obtain a list of medications the patient is taking, including herbs, nutritional supplements, and nutraceuticals. Note the last time and dose of medication taken. The requesting health care practitioner and laboratory should be advised if the patient is regularly using these products so that their effects can be taken into consideration when reviewing results.

➤ Review the procedure with the patient. Inform the patient that specimen collection takes approximately 5 to 10 minutes. Address concerns about pain related to the procedure. Explain to the patient that there may be some discomfort during the venipuncture.

➤ *Sensitivity to cultural and social issues,* as well as concern for modesty, is important in providing psychological support before, during, and after the procedure.

➤ There are no food, fluid, or medication restrictions, unless by medical direction.

Intratest:

➤ If the patient has a history of severe allergic reaction to latex, care should be taken to avoid the use of equipment containing latex.

➤ Instruct the patient to cooperate fully and to follow directions. Direct the

patient to breathe normally and to avoid unnecessary movement.

➤ Observe standard precautions, and follow the general guidelines in Appendix A. Positively identify the patient, and label the appropriate tubes with the corresponding patient demographics, date, and time of collection. Perform a venipuncture; collect the specimen in a 5-mL red-top tube.

➤ Remove the needle, and apply a pressure dressing over the puncture site.

➤ Promptly transport the specimen to the laboratory for processing and analysis.

➤ The results are recorded manually or in a computerized system for recall and postprocedure interpretation by the appropriate health care practitioner.

Post-test:

➤ Observe venipuncture site for bleeding or hematoma formation. Apply paper tape or other adhesive to hold pressure bandage in place, or replace with a plastic bandage.

➤ Instruct the patient to resume usual diet and medication, as directed by the health care practitioner.

➤ *Nutritional considerations:* The nutritional needs of each diabetic patient need to be determined individually (especially during pregnancy) by a health care practitioner trained in nutrition. Patients who adhere to dietary recommendations report a better general feeling of health, better weight management, greater control of glucose and lipid values, and improved use of insulin. There is no "diabetic diet"; however, many meal-planning approaches with nutritional goals are endorsed by the American Dietetic Association.

➤ Impaired glucose tolerance may be associated with diabetes. Instruct the patient and caregiver to report signs and symptoms of hypoglycemia (weakness, confusion, diaphoresis, rapid pulse) or hyperglycemia (thirst, polyuria, hunger, lethargy).

➤ A written report of the examination will be sent to the requesting health care practitioner, who will discuss the results with the patient.

➤ Recognize anxiety related to test results, and be supportive of perceived loss of independence and fear of shortened life expectancy. Discuss the implications of abnormal test results on the patient's lifestyle. Provide teaching and information regarding the clinical implications of the test results, as appropriate. Emphasize, as appropriate, that good glycemic control delays the onset of and slows the progression of diabetic retinopathy, nephropathy, and neuropathy. Educate the patient regarding access to counseling services. Provide contact information, if desired, for the American Diabetes Association *(http://www. diabetes.org).*

➤ Reinforce information given by the patient's health care provider regarding further testing, treatment, or referral to another health care provider. Answer any questions or address any concerns voiced by the patient or family.

➤ Depending on the results of this procedure, additional testing may be performed to evaluate or monitor progression of the disease process and determine the need for a change in therapy. Evaluate test results in relation to the patient's symptoms and other tests performed.

Related laboratory tests:

➤ Related laboratory tests include C-peptide, glucose, glucose tolerance tests, and insulin.

INTRAOCULAR MUSCLE FUNCTION

SYNONYMS/ACRONYMS: IOM function.

AREA OF APPLICATION: Eyes.

CONTRAST: N/A.

DESCRIPTION & RATIONALE: Evaluation of ocular motility is performed to detect and measure muscle imbalance in conditions classified as heterotropias or heterophorias. This evaluation is performed in a manner to assess fixation of each eye, alignment of both eyes in all directions, and the ability of both eyes to work together binocularly. Heterophorias are latent ocular deviations kept in check by the binocular power of fusion, and made intermittent by disrupting fusion. Heterotropias are conditions that manifest constant ocular deviations. The prefixes eso- (tendency for the eye to turn in), exo- (tendency for the eye to turn out), and hyper- (tendency for one eye to turn up) indicate the direction in which the affected eye moves spontaneously. *Strabismus* is the failure of both eyes to spontaneously fixate on the same object because of a muscular imbalance (crossed eyes). *Amblyopia,* or lazy eye, is a term used for loss of vision in one or both eyes that cannot be attributed to an organic pathologic condition of the eye or optic nerve. There are six extraocular muscles in each eye whose movement is controlled by three nerves. The actions of the muscles vary depending on the position of the eye when they become innervated. The cover test is commonly used because it is reliable, easy to perform, and does not require special equipment. The cover test method is described in this monograph. Another method for evaluation of ocular muscle function is the corneal light reflex test. It is useful with patients who cannot cooperate for prism cover testing or for patients who have poor fixation. ∎

INDICATIONS:
- Detection and evaluation of extraocular muscle imbalance

RESULT
The examiner should determine the range of ocular movements in all gaze positions, usually to include up and out, in, down and out, up and in, down and in, and out. Limited movements in gaze position can be recorded semiquantitatively as –1 (minimal), –2 (moderate), –3 (severe), or –4 (total).

Normal Findings:
- Normal range of ocular movements in all gaze positions.

Abnormal Findings:

- Amblyopia

- Heterophorias

- Heterotropias

- Strabismus

CRITICAL VALUES: N/A

INTERFERING FACTORS:

Factors that may impair the results of the examination:

- Inability of the patient to cooperate and remain still during the test because of age, significant pain, or mental status may interfere with the test results.

- Rubbing or squeezing the eyes may affect results.

Nursing Implications and Procedure • • • • • • • • • • •

Pretest:

➤ Inform the patient that the procedure evaluates extraocular muscle function.

➤ Obtain a history of the patient's complaints, including a list of known allergens.

➤ Obtain a history of the patient's known or suspected vision loss, changes in visual acuity, including type and cause; use of glasses or contact lenses; eye conditions with treatment regimens; eye surgery; and other tests and procedures to assess and diagnose visual deficit.

➤ Obtain a history of results of previously performed laboratory tests, surgical procedures, and other diagnostic procedures.

➤ Obtain a list of the medications the patient is taking, including herbs, nutritional supplements, and nutraceuticals. The requesting health care practitioner should be advised if

the patient regularly uses these products so that their effects can be taken into consideration when reviewing results.

➤ Review the procedure with the patient. Address concerns about pain related to the procedure. Explain to the patient that no discomfort will be experienced during the test. Inform the patient that a technician, optometrist, orthoptist, or physician performs the test, in a quiet room, and that to evaluate both eyes, the test can take 2 to 4 minutes.

➤ Instruct the patient to remove contact lenses or glasses, as appropriate. Instruct the patient regarding the importance of keeping the eyes open for the test.

➤ There are no food, fluid, or medication restrictions, unless by medical direction.

Intratest:

➤ Instruct the patient to cooperate fully and to follow directions. Ask the patient to remain still during the procedure because movement produces unreliable results.

➤ One eye is tested at a time. The patient is given a fixation point, usually the testing personnel's index finger. An object, such as a small toy, can be used to ensure fixation in pediatric patients. The patient is asked to follow the fixation point with his or her gaze in the direction the fixation point moves. When testing is completed, the procedure is repeated using the other eye. The procedure is performed at distance and near, first with and then without corrective lenses.

➤ The results are recorded manually for recall and postprocedure interpretation by the appropriate health care practitioner.

Post-test:

➤ A written report of the examination will be completed by a health care practitioner specializing in this branch of medicine. The report will be sent to the requesting health care practitioner, who will discuss the results with the patient.

➤ Recognize anxiety related to test results, and be supportive of impaired activity related to vision loss, perceived loss of driving privileges, or the possibility of requiring corrective lenses (self-image).

➤ Reinforce information given by the patient's health care provider regarding further testing, treatment, or referral to another health care provider. Educate the patient, as appropriate, that he or she may be referred for special therapy to correct the anomaly, which may include glasses, prisms, eye exercises, eye patches, or chemical patching with drugs that modify the focusing power of the eye. The patient and family should be educated that the chosen therapy involves a process of mental

retraining. The mode of therapy in itself does not correct vision. It is the process by which the brain becomes readapted to accept, receive, and store visual images received by the eye that results in vision correction. Therefore, the patient must be prepared to be alert, cooperative, and properly motivated. Answer any questions or address any concerns voiced by the patient or family.

➤ Depending on the results of this procedure, additional testing may be performed to evaluate or monitor progression of the disease process and determine the need for a change in therapy. Evaluate test results in relation to the patient's symptoms and other tests performed.

Related diagnostic tests:

➤ Related diagnostic tests include refraction and slit-lamp biomicroscopy.

INTRAOCULAR PRESSURE

SYNONYMS/ACRONYMS: IOP.

AREA OF APPLICATION: Eyes.

CONTRAST: N/A.

DESCRIPTION & RATIONALE: The pressure of the eye depends on a number of factors. The two most significant are the amount of aqueous humor present in the eye and the circumstances by which it leaves the eye. Other physiologic variables that affect intraocular pressure (IOP) include respiration, pulse, and the degree of

hydration of the body. Individual eyes respond to intraocular pressures differently. Some can tolerate high pressures (20 to 30 mm Hg), and some will incur optic nerve damage at lower pressures. With respiration, variations of up to 4 mm Hg in IOP can occur, and changes of 1 to 2 mm Hg occur with every pulsation of the central retinal artery. IOP is measured with a tonometer; normal values indicate the pressure at which no damage is done to the intraocular contents.

The rate of fluid leaving the eye, or its ability to leave the eye unimpeded, is the most important factor regulating IOP. There are three primary conditions that result in occlusion of the outflow channels for fluid. The most common condition is open-angle glaucoma, in which the diameter of the openings of the trabecular meshwork becomes narrowed, resulting in an increased IOP due to an increased resistance of fluid moving out of the eye. In secondary glaucoma, the trabecular meshwork becomes occluded by tumor cells, pigment, red blood cells in hyphema, or other material. Additionally, the obstructing material may cover parts of the meshwork itself, as with scar tissue or other types of adhesions that form after severe iritis, an angle closure glaucoma attack, or a central retinal vein occlusion. The third condition impeding fluid outflow in the trabecular channels occurs with pupillary block, most commonly associated with primary angle-closure glaucoma. In eyes predisposed to this condition, dilation of the pupil causes the iris to fold up like an accordion against the narrow-angle structures of the eye. Fluid in the posterior chamber has difficulty circulating into the anterior chamber; therefore, pressure in the posterior chamber increases, causing the iris to bow forward and obstruct the outflow channels even more. Angle-closure attacks occur quite suddenly and therefore do not give the eye a chance to adjust itself to the sudden increase in pressure. The eye becomes very red, the cornea edematous (patient may report seeing halos), and the pupil fixed and dilated, accompanied by a complaint of moderate pain. Pupil dilation can be initiated by emotional arousal or fear, conditions in which the eye must adapt to darkness (movie theaters), or mydriatics. Angle-closure glaucoma is an ocular emergency that is resolved by a peripheral iridectomy to allow movement of fluid between the anterior and posterior chambers. This procedure constitutes removal of a portion of the peripheral iris either by surgery or by use of an argon or yttrium-aluminum-garnet (YAG) laser. ■

INDICATIONS:
- Diagnosis or ongoing monitoring of glaucoma
- Screening test included in a routine eye examination

RESULT

Normal Findings:
- Normal intraocular pressure is between 13 and 22 mm Hg.

Abnormal Findings:
- Open-angle glaucoma
- Primary angle closure glaucoma
- Secondary glaucoma

CRITICAL VALUES: N/A

INTERFERING FACTORS:
- Inability of the patient to remain still and cooperative during the test may interfere with the test results.

Nursing Implications and Procedure . . . .

Pretest:

▶ Inform the patient that the procedure measures the intraocular pressure of the eye.

➤ Obtain a history of the patient's complaints, including a list of known allergens, especially allergies or sensitivities to topical anesthetic eyedrops.

➤ Obtain a history of the patient's known or suspected vision loss, changes in visual acuity, including type and cause; use of glasses or contact lenses; eye conditions with treatment regimens; eye surgery; and other tests and procedures to assess and diagnose visual deficit.

➤ Obtain a history of results of previously performed laboratory tests, surgical procedures, and other diagnostic procedures.

➤ Obtain a list of the medications the patient is taking, including herbs, nutritional supplements, and nutraceuticals. The requesting health care practitioner should be advised if the patient regularly uses these products so that their effects can be taken into consideration when reviewing results.

➤ Review the procedure with the patient. Explain that the patient will be requested to fixate the eyes during the procedure. Address concerns about pain related to the procedure. Explain to the patient that he or she may feel coldness or a slight sting when the anesthetic drops are instilled at the beginning of the procedure, but that no discomfort will be experienced during the test. Instruct the patient as to what should be expected with the use of the tonometer. The patient will experience less anxiety if he or she understands that the tonometer tip will touch the tear film and not the eye directly. Inform the patient that a technician, optometrist, or physician performs the test, in a quiet, darkened room, and that to evaluate both eyes, the test can take 1 to 3 minutes.

➤ Instruct the patient to remove contact lenses or glasses, as appropriate. Instruct the patient regarding the importance of keeping the eyes open for the test.

➤ There are no food, fluid, or medica-

tion restrictions, unless by medical direction.

Intratest:

➤ Instruct the patient to cooperate fully and to follow directions. Ask the patient to remain still during the procedure because any movement, such as coughing, breath holding, or wandering eye movements, produces unreliable results.

➤ Seat the patient comfortably. Instruct the patient to look at directed target while the eyes are examined.

➤ Instill ordered topical anesthetic in each eye, as ordered, and allow time for it to work. Topical anesthetic drops are placed in the eye with the patient looking up and the solution directed at the six o'clock position of the sclera (white of the eye) near the limbus (grey, semitransparent area of the eyeball where the cornea and sclera meet). The dropper bottle should not touch the eyelashes.

➤ Instruct the patient to look straight ahead, keeping the eyes open and unblinking.

➤ A number of techniques are used to measure intraocular pres-sure. Intraocular pressure can be measured at the slit lamp or with a miniaturized, handheld applanation tonometer or an airpuff tonometer.

➤ When the applanation tonometer is positioned on the patient's cornea, place the instrument's headrest against the patient's forehead. The tonometer should be held at an angle with the handle slanted away from the patient's nose. The tonometer tip should not touch the eyelids.

➤ When the tip is properly aligned and in contact with the fluorescein-stained tear film, force is applied to the tip using an adjustment control to the desired endpoint. The tonometer is removed from the eye. The reading is taken a second time and, if the pressure is elevated, a third reading is taken. The procedure is repeated on the other eye.

➤ With the airpuff tonometer, an air

pump blows air onto the cornea, and the time it takes for the air puff to flatten the cornea is detected by infrared light and photoelectric cells. This time is directly related to the intraocular pressure.

➤ The results are recorded manually, taking care to denote left and right readings, for recall and postprocedure interpretation by the appropriate health care practitioner.

Post-test:

➤ A written report of the examination will be completed by a health care practitioner specializing in this branch of medicine. The report will be sent to the requesting health care practitioner, who will discuss the results with the patient.

➤ Recognize anxiety related to test results, and be supportive of impaired activity related to vision loss or perceived loss of driving privileges. Discuss the implications of abnormal test results on the patient's lifestyle. Provide teaching and information regarding the clinical implications of the test results, as appropriate.

➤ Reinforce information given by the patient's health care provider regarding further testing, treatment, or referral to another health care provider. Answer any questions or address any concerns voiced by the patient or family.

➤ Instruct the patient in the use of any ordered medications, usually eyedrops, that are intended to decrease intraocular pressure. Explain the importance of adhering to the therapy regimen, especially since increased intraocular pressure does not present symptoms. Instruct the patient in both the ocular side effects and systemic reactions associated with the prescribed medication. Encourage him or her to review corresponding literature provided by a pharmacist.

➤ Depending on the results of this procedure, additional testing may be performed to evaluate or monitor progression of the disease process and determine the need for a change in therapy. Evaluate test results in relation to the patient's symptoms and other tests performed.

Related diagnostic tests:

➤ Related diagnostic tests include fundus photography, gonioscopy, nerve fiber analysis, slit-lamp biomicroscopy, and visual field testing.

INTRAVENOUS PYELOGRAPHY

· ·

SYNONYMS/ACRONYMS: Excretory urography (EUG), intravenous urography (IVU, IUG), IVP.

AREA OF APPLICATION: Kidneys, ureters, bladder, and renal pelvis.

CONTRAST: Intravenous radiopaque iodine-based contrast medium.

DESCRIPTION & RATIONALE: Intravenous pyelography (IVP) is the most commonly performed test to determine urinary tract dysfunction or renal disease. IVP uses IV radiopaque contrast medium to visualize the kidneys, ureters, bladder, and renal pelvis. The contrast medium concentrates in the blood and is filtered out by the glomeruli; it passes out through the renal tubules and is concentrated in the urine. Renal function is reflected by the length of time it takes the contrast medium to appear and to be excreted by each kidney. A series of x-rays is performed during a 30-minute period to view passage of the medium through the kidneys and ureters into the bladder. A final film is taken after the patient empties the bladder (postvoiding film). Computed tomography may be employed during the examination to permit the examination of an individual layer or plane of the organ that may be obscured by surrounding overlying structures. ■

INDICATIONS:

- Aid in the diagnosis of renovascular hypertension

- Evaluate the cause of blood in the urine

- Evaluate the effects of urinary system trauma

- Evaluate function of the kidneys, ureters, and bladder

- Evaluate known or suspected ureteral obstruction

- Evaluate the presence of renal, ureter, or bladder calculi

- Evaluate space-occupying lesions or congenital anomalies of the urinary system

RESULT

Normal Findings:

- Normal size and shape of kidneys, ureters, and bladder

- Normal bladder and absence of masses or renal calculi, with prompt visualization of contrast medium through the urinary system

Abnormal Findings:

- Absence of a kidney (congenital malformation)

- Benign and malignant kidney tumors

- Bladder tumors

- Congenital renal or urinary tract abnormalities

- Glomerulonephritis

- Hydronephrosis

- Prostatic enlargement

- Pyelonephritis

- Renal cysts

- Renal hematomas

- Renal or ureteral calculi

- Soft-tissue masses

- Tumors of the collecting system

CRITICAL VALUES: N/A

INTERFERING FACTORS:

This procedure is contraindicated for:

- ⚠ Patients with allergies to shellfish or iodinated dye. The contrast medium used may cause a life-threatening allergic reaction. Patients with a known hypersensitivity to the contrast medium may benefit from premedication with corticosteroids or the use of nonionic contrast medium.

- Patients with bleeding disorders.

- Patients who are pregnant or suspected of being pregnant, unless the potential benefits of the procedure far outweigh the risks to the fetus and mother.

- ⚠ Elderly and other patients who are chronically dehydrated before the test, because of their risk of contrast-induced renal failure.

- ⚠ Patients who are in renal failure.

- Patients with renal insufficiency, indicated by a blood urea nitrogen value greater than 40 mg/dL, because contrast medium can complicate kidney function.

- Young patients (17 years old and younger), unless the benefits of the x-ray diagnosis outweigh the risks of exposure to high levels of radiation.

- Patients with multiple myeloma, who may experience decreased kidney function subsequent to administration of contrast medium.

Factors that may impair clear imaging:

- Gas or feces in the gastrointestinal tract resulting from inadequate cleansing or failure to restrict food intake before the study

- Retained barium from a previous radiologic procedure

- Metallic objects within the examination field (e.g., jewelry, body rings), which may inhibit organ visualization and can produce unclear images

- Improper adjustment of the radiographic equipment to accommodate obese or thin patients, which can cause overexposure or underexposure and a poor-quality study

- Patients who are very obese, who may exceed the weight limit for the equipment

- Incorrect positioning of the patient, which may produce poor visualization of the area to be examined

- Inability of the patient to cooperate or remain still during the procedure because of age, significant pain, or mental status

- End-stage renal disease, which may produce an examination of poor quality

Other considerations:

- The procedure may be terminated if chest pain or severe cardiac arrhythmias occur.

- Failure to follow dietary restrictions and other pretesting preparations may cause the procedure to be canceled or repeated.

- Consultation with a health care practitioner should occur before the procedure for radiation safety concerns regarding younger patients or patients who are lactating.

- Risks associated with radiographic overexposure can result from frequent x-ray procedures. Personnel in the room with the patient should wear a protective lead apron, stand behind a shield, or leave the area while the examination is being done. Personnel working in the area where the examination is being done should wear badges that reveal their level of exposure to radiation.

Nursing Implications and Procedure

Pretest:

➤ Inform the patient that the procedure assesses the kidneys, ureters, and bladder.

➤ Obtain a history of the patient's complaints or symptoms, including a list of known allergens, especially allergies or sensitivities to latex, iodine, seafood, contrast medium, and dyes.

➤ Obtain a history of the patient's gastrointestinal and genitourinary systems, and results of previously performed diagnostic procedures, surgical procedures, and laboratory tests. For related diagnostic tests, refer to the Gastrointestinal and Genitourinary System tables.

➤ Ensure that this procedure is performed before an upper gastrointestinal study or barium swallow.

➤ Record the date of the last menstrual period and determine the possibility of pregnancy in perimenopausal women.

➤ Obtain a list of the medications the patient is taking.

➤ Review the procedure with the patient. Address concerns about pain related to the procedure. Explain to the patient that some pain may be experienced during the test, and there may be moments of discomfort. Explain the purpose of the test and how the procedure is performed. Inform the patient that the procedure is performed in a radiology department, usually by a technologist and support staff, and takes approximately 30 to 60 minutes.

➤ *Sensitivity to cultural and social issues,* as well as concern for modesty, is important in providing psychological support before, during, and after the procedure.

➤ Instruct the patient to fast and restrict fluids for 8 hours prior to the procedure.

➤ Patients receiving metformin (Glucophage) for non–insulin-dependent (type 2) diabetes should discontinue the drug on the day of the test and continue to withhold it for 48 hours after the test. Failure to do so may result in lactic acidosis.

➤ Instruct the patient to take a laxative or a cathartic, as ordered, on the evening before the examination.

➤ Instruct the patient to remove jewelry (including watches), credit cards, and other metallic objects.

➤ *Make sure a written and informed consent has been signed prior to the procedure and before administering any medications.*

Intratest:

➤ Ensure that the patient has complied with dietary and medication restrictions and pretesting preparations for at least 8 hours prior to the procedure. Ensure that the patient has removed all external metallic objects prior to the procedure.

➤ Assess for completion of bowel preparation according to the institution's procedure. Administer enemas or suppositories on the morning of the test, as ordered.

➤ Have emergency equipment readily available.

➤ Patients are given a gown and robe to wear and instructed to void prior to the procedure.

➤ Instruct the patient to cooperate fully and to follow directions. Instruct the patient to remain still throughout the procedure because movement produces unreliable results.

➤ Observe standard precautions, and follow the general guidelines in Appendix A.

➤ Place the patient in the supine position on an exam table.

➤ For male patients, place lead protection over the testicles to prevent their irradiation but remove it for bladder exposures.

➤ A kidney, ureter, and bladder (KUB) or plain film is taken to ensure that no barium or stool obscures visualization of the urinary system.

➤ Insert an IV line, if one is not already in place, and inject the contrast medium.

➤ X-ray exposures are made at 1, 5, 10, 15, 20, and 30 minutes to follow the course of the contrast medium through the urinary system. Instruct the patient to exhale deeply and to hold his or her breath while the x-ray is taken, and then to breathe after the film is taken.

➤ Ask the patient to void; a postvoiding exposure is done to visualize the empty bladder.

The results are recorded manually, on film, or by automated equipment in a computerized system for recall and postprocedure interpretation by the appropriate health care practitioner.

Post-test:

➤ Instruct the patient to resume usual diet, fluids, medications, or activity, as directed by the health care practitioner.

➤ Monitor for reaction to iodinated contrast medium, including rash, urticaria, tachycardia, hyperpnea, hypertension, palpitations, nausea, or vomiting.

➤ Monitor urinary output after the procedure. Decreased urine output may indicate impending renal failure.

➤ A written report of the examination will be completed by a health care practitioner specializing in this branch of medicine. The report will be sent to the requesting health care practitioner, who will discuss the results with the patient.

➤ Recognize anxiety related to test results, and offer support. Discuss the implications of abnormal test results on the patient's lifestyle. Provide teaching and information regarding the clinical implications of the test results, as appropriate.

➤ Reinforce information given by the patient's health care provider regarding further testing, treatment, or referral to another health care provider. Answer any questions or address any concerns voiced by the patient or family.

➤ Depending on the results of this procedure, additional testing may be needed to evaluate or monitor progression of the disease process and determine the need for a change in therapy. Evaluate test results in relation to the patient's symptoms and other tests performed.

Related diagnostic tests:

➤ Related diagnostic tests include computed tomography of the abdomen, magnetic resonance imaging of the abdomen, renogram, and ultrasound of the kidney.

INTRINSIC FACTOR ANTIBODIES

. . . .

SYNONYM/ACRONYM: IF antibodies.

SPECIMEN: Serum (1 mL) collected in a red-top tube. Plasma (1 mL) collected in a lavender-top (EDTA) tube is also acceptable.

REFERENCE VALUE: (Method: Radioimmunoassay) None detected.

DESCRIPTION & RATIONALE: Intrinsic factor (IF) is produced by the parietal cells of the gastric mucosa and is required for the normal absorption of vitamin B_{12}. In some diseases, antibodies are produced that bind the cobalamin-IF complex, prevent the complex from binding to ileum receptors, and prevent vitamin B_{12} absorption. There are two types of antibodies: type 1, the more commonly present blocking antibody; and type 2, the binding antibody. The blocking antibody inhibits uptake of vitamin B_{12} at the binding site of IF. Binding antibody combines with either free or complexed IF. ∎

INDICATIONS:

- Assist in the diagnosis of pernicious anemia
- Evaluate patients with decreased vitamin B_{12} levels

RESULT

Increased in:
- Megaloblastic anemia
- Pernicious anemia
- Some patients with hyperthyroidism
- Some patients with insulin-dependent (type 1) diabetes

Decreased in: N/A

CRITICAL VALUES: N/A

INTERFERING FACTORS:

- Recent treatment with methotrexate or another folic acid antagonist can interfere with test results.
- Vitamin B_{12} injected or ingested within 48 hours of the test invalidates results.

- Recent radioactive scans or radiation can interfere with test results when radioimmunoassay is the test method.
- Failure to follow dietary restrictions before the procedure may cause the procedure to be canceled or repeated.

Nursing Implications and Procedure • • • • • • • • • • •

Pretest:

▶ Inform the patient that the test is used to assist in the investigation of suspected pernicious anemia.

▶ Obtain a history of the patient's complaints, including a list of known allergens (especially allergies or sensitivities to latex), and inform the appropriate health care practitioner accordingly.

▶ Obtain a history of the patient's hematopoietic and gastrointestinal systems, as well as results of previously performed laboratory tests, surgical procedures, and other diagnostic procedures. For related laboratory tests, refer to the Hematopoietic and Gastrointestinal System tables.

▶ Note any recent procedures that can interfere with test results.

▶ Obtain a list of the medications the patient is taking, including herbs, nutritional supplements, and nutraceuticals. The requesting health care practitioner and laboratory should be advised if the patient is regularly using these products so that their effects can be taken into consideration when reviewing results.

▶ Review the procedure with the patient. Inform the patient that specimen collection takes approximately 5 to 10 minutes. Address concerns about pain related to the procedure. Explain to the patient that there may be some discomfort during the venipuncture.

▶ There are no food or fluid restrictions, unless by medical direction.

Administration of vitamin B_{12} should be withheld within 48 hours before testing.

Intratest:

➤ Ensure that vitamin B_{12} has been withheld within 48 hours before testing.

➤ If the patient has a history of severe allergic reaction to latex, care should be taken to avoid the use of equipment containing latex.

➤ Instruct the patient to cooperate fully and to follow directions. Direct the patient to breathe normally and to avoid unnecessary movement.

➤ Observe standard precautions, and follow the general guidelines in Appendix A. Positively identify the patient, and label the appropriate tubes with the corresponding patient demographics, date, and time of collection. Perform a venipuncture; collect the specimen in a 5-mL red-top tube.

➤ Remove the needle, and apply a pressure dressing over the puncture site.

➤ Promptly transport the specimen to the laboratory for processing and analysis.

➤ The results are recorded manually or in a computerized system for recall and postprocedure interpreta-tion by the appropriate health care practitioner.

Post-test:

➤ Observe venipuncture site for bleeding or hematoma formation. Apply paper tape or other adhesive to hold pressure bandage in place, or replace with a plastic bandage.

➤ A written report of the examination will be sent to the requesting health care practitioner, who will discuss the results with the patient.

➤ Reinforce information given by the patient's health care provider regarding further testing, treatment, or referral to another health care provider. Answer any questions or address any concerns voiced by the patient or family.

➤ Depending on the results of this procedure, additional testing may be performed to evaluate or monitor progression of the disease process and determine the need for a change in therapy. Evaluate test results in relation to the patient's symptoms and other tests performed.

Related laboratory tests:

➤ Related laboratory tests include complete blood count, folic acid, red blood cell indices, and vitamin B_{12}.

IRON

. . . .

SYNONYM/ACRONYM: Fe.

SPECIMEN: Serum (1 mL) collected in a red- or tiger-top tube.

REFERENCE VALUE: (Method: Spectrophotometry)

Age	Conventional Units	SI Units (Conventional Units × 0.179)
Newborn	100–250 µg/dL	17.9–44.8 µmol/L
Infant–9 y	20–105 µg/dL	3.6–18.8 µmol/L
10–14 y	20–145 µg/dL	3.6–26.0 µmol/L
Adult		
Male	65–175 µg/dL	11.6–31.3 µmol/L
Female	50–170 µg/dL	9–30.4 µmol/L

DESCRIPTION & RATIONALE: Iron plays a principal role in erythropoiesis. Iron is necessary for the proliferation and maturation of red blood cells and is required for hemoglobin synthesis. Of the body's normal 4 g of iron, approximately 65% resides in hemoglobin and 3% in myoglobin. A small amount is also found in cellular enzymes that catalyze the oxidation and reduction of iron. The remainder of iron is stored in the liver, bone marrow, and spleen as ferritin or hemosiderin. Any iron present in the serum is in transit among the alimentary tract, the bone marrow, and available iron storage forms. Iron travels in the bloodstream bound to transferrin, a protein manufactured by the liver. Normally, iron enters the body by oral ingestion; only 10% is absorbed, but up to 20% can be absorbed in patients with iron-deficiency anemia. Unbound iron is highly toxic, but there is generally an excess of transferrin available to prevent the buildup of unbound iron in the circulation. Iron overload is as clinically significant as iron deficiency, especially in the accidental poisoning of children caused by excessive intake of iron-containing multivitamins. ■

INDICATIONS:
- Assist in the diagnosis of blood loss, as evidenced by decreased serum iron

- Assist in the diagnosis of hemochromatosis or other disorders of iron metabolism and storage
- Determine the differential diagnosis of anemia
- Determine the presence of disorders that involve diminished protein synthesis or defects in iron absorption
- Evaluate accidental iron poisoning
- Evaluate iron overload in dialysis patients or patients with transfusion-dependent anemias
- Evaluate thalassemia and sideroblastic anemia
- Monitor hematologic responses during pregnancy, when serum iron is usually decreased
- Monitor response to treatment for anemia

RESULT

Increased in:
- Acute iron poisoning (children)
- Acute leukemia
- Acute liver disease
- Aplastic anemia
- Excessive iron therapy
- Hemochromatosis
- Hemolytic anemias
- Lead toxicity
- Nephritis

- Pernicious anemias

- Sideroblastic anemias

- Thalassemia

- Transfusions (repeated)

- Vitamin B$_6$ deficiency

Decreased in:
- Acute and chronic infection

- Carcinoma

- Chronic blood loss (gastrointestinal, uterine)

- Hypothyroidism

- Iron-deficiency anemia

- Nephrosis

- Postoperative state

- Protein malnutrition (kwashiorkor)

- Remission of pernicious anemia

CRITICAL VALUES:
  Mild toxicity: greater than 350 μg/dL
  Serious toxicity: greater than 400 μg/dL
  Lethal: greater than 1000 μg/dL
  Note and immediately report to the health care practitioner any critically increased values and related symptoms. Intervention may include chelation therapy by administration of deferoxamine mesylate (Desferal).

INTERFERING FACTORS:

- Drugs that may increase iron levels include blood transfusions, chemotherapy drugs, iron (intramuscular), iron dextran, iron-protein-succinylate, methimazole, methotrexate, oral contraceptives, and rifampin.

- Drugs that may decrease iron levels include acetylsalicylic acid, allopurinol, cholestyramine, corticotropin, cortisone, deferoxamine, and metformin.

- Gross hemolysis can interfere with test results.

- Failure to withhold iron-containing medications 24 hours before the test may falsely increase values.

- Failure to follow dietary restrictions before the procedure may cause the procedure to be canceled or repeated.

Nursing Implications and Procedure • • • • • • • • • • •

Pretest:

▸ Inform the patient that the test is used in the differential diagnosis of anemia.

▸ Obtain a history of the patient's complaints, including a list of known allergens (especially allergies or sensitivities to latex), and inform the appropriate health care practitioner accordingly.

▸ Obtain a history of the patient's gastrointestinal and hematopoietic systems and results of previously performed laboratory tests, surgical procedures, and other diagnostic procedures. For related laboratory tests, refer to the Gastrointestinal and Hematopoietic System tables.

▸ Note any recent therapies that can interfere with test results. Specimen collection should be delayed for several days after blood transfusion.

▸ Obtain a list of medications the patient is taking, including herbs, nutritional supplements, and nutraceuticals. The requesting health care practitioner and laboratory should be advised if the patient regularly uses these products so that their effects can be taken into consideration when reviewing results.

▸ Review the procedure with the patient. Inform the patient that specimen collection takes approximately 5 to 10 minutes. Address concerns about pain related to the procedure. Explain to the patient that there may be some discomfort during the venipuncture.

▶ *Sensitivity to social and cultural issues,* as well as concern for modesty, is important in providing psychological support before, during, and after the procedure.

▶ Instruct the patient to fast for at least 12 hours before testing, and with medical direction, to refrain from taking iron-containing medicines before specimen collection.

▶ There are no fluid restrictions, unless by medical direction.

Intratest:

▶ Ensure that the patient has complied with dietary and medication restrictions; assure that food has been restricted for at least 12 hours prior to the procedure.

▶ If the patient has a history of severe allergic reaction to latex, care should be taken to avoid the use of equipment containing latex.

▶ Instruct the patient to cooperate fully and to follow directions. Direct the patient to breathe normally and to avoid unnecessary movement.

▶ Observe standard precautions, and follow the general guidelines in Appendix A. Positively identify the patient, and label the appropriate tubes with the corresponding patient demographics, date, and time of collection. Perform a venipuncture; collect the specimen in a 5-mL red- or tiger-top tube.

▶ Remove the needle, and apply a pressure dressing over the puncture site.

▶ Promptly transport the specimen to the laboratory for processing and analysis.

▶ The results are recorded manually or in a computerized system for recall and postprocedure interpretation by the appropriate health care practitioner.

Post-test:

▶ Observe venipuncture site for bleeding or hematoma formation. Apply paper tape or other adhesive to hold pressure bandage in place, or replace with a plastic bandage.

▶ Instruct the patient to resume usual diet, fluids, medications, or activity, as directed by the health care practitioner.

▶ *Nutritional considerations:* Educate the patient with abnormally elevated iron values, as appropriate, on the importance of reading food labels. Foods high in iron include meats (especially liver), eggs, grains, and green leafy vegetables. It is also important to explain that iron levels in foods can be increased if foods are cooked in cookware containing iron.

▶ *Nutritional considerations:* Educate the patient with abnormal iron values that numerous factors affect the absorption of iron, enhancing or decreasing absorption regardless of the original content of the iron-containing dietary source. Consumption of large amounts of alcohol damages the intestine and allows increased absorption of iron. A high intake of calcium and ascorbic acid also increases iron absorption. Iron absorption after a meal is also increased by factors in meat, fish, or poultry. Iron absorption is decreased by the absence (gastric resection) or diminished presence (use of antacids) of gastric acid. Phytic acids from cereals, tannins from tea and coffee, oxalic acid from vegetables, and minerals such as copper, zinc, and manganese interfere with iron absorption.

▶ A written report of the examination will be sent to the requesting health care practitioner, who will discuss the results with the patient.

▶ Reinforce information given by the patient's health care provider regarding further testing, treatment, or referral to another health care provider. Answer any questions or address any concerns voiced by the patient or family.

▶ Depending on the results of this procedure, additional testing may be performed to evaluate or monitor progression of the disease process and determine the need for a change in therapy. Evaluate test results in relation to the patient's symptoms and other tests performed.

IRON-BINDING CAPACITY (TOTAL), TRANSFERRIN, AND IRON SATURATION

SYNONYMS/ACRONYMS: TIBC, Fe Sat.

SPECIMEN: Serum (1 mL) collected in a red- or tiger-top tube.

REFERENCE VALUE: (Method: Spectrophotometry for TIBC and nephelometry for transferrin)

Test	Conventional Units	SI Units
TIBC	250–350 µg/dL	*(Conventional Units × 0.179)* 45–63 µmol/L
Transferrin	200–380 mg/dL	*(Conventional Units × 0.01)* 2–3.8 g/L
Iron saturation	20–50%	

TIBC = total iron-binding capacity.

DESCRIPTION & RATIONALE: Iron plays a principal role in erythropoiesis. It is necessary for proliferation and maturation of red blood cells and for hemoglobin synthesis. Of the body's normal 4 g of iron (less in women), about 65% is present in hemoglobin and about 3% in myoglobin. A small amount is also found in cellular enzymes that catalyze the oxidation and reduction of iron. The remainder of iron is stored in the liver, bone marrow, and spleen as ferritin or hemosiderin. Any iron present in the serum is in transit among the alimentary tract, the bone marrow, and available iron storage forms. Iron travels in the bloodstream bound to transport proteins. Transferrin is the major iron-transport protein, carrying 60% to 70% of the body's iron. For this reason, total iron-binding capacity (TIBC) and transferrin are sometimes referred to interchangeably, even though other proteins carry iron and contribute to the TIBC. Unbound iron is highly toxic, but there is generally an excess of transferrin available to prevent the buildup of unbound iron in the circulation. The percentage of iron saturation is calculated by dividing the serum iron value by the TIBC value and multiplying by 100. ■

INDICATIONS:
- Assist in the diagnosis of iron-deficiency anemia
- Differentiate between iron-deficiency anemia and anemia secondary to chronic disease
- Monitor hematologic response to therapy during pregnancy and iron-deficiency anemias
- Provide support for diagnosis of hemochromatosis or diseases of iron metabolism and storage

RESULT

Increased in:
- Acute liver disease
- Hypochromic (iron-deficiency) anemias
- Late pregnancy

Decreased in:
- Chronic infections
- Cirrhosis
- Hemochromatosis
- Hemolytic anemias

- Neoplastic diseases
- Protein depletion
- Renal disease
- Sideroblastic anemias
- Thalassemia

CRITICAL VALUES: N/A

INTERFERING FACTORS:
- Drugs that may increase TIBC levels include mestranol and oral contraceptives.
- Drugs that may decrease TIBC levels include asparaginase, chloramphenicol, corticotropin, cortisone, and testosterone.

Nursing Implications and Procedure ● ● ● ● ● ● ● ● ● ● ●

Pretest:
➤ Inform the patient that the test is used in the differential diagnosis of anemia.

➤ Obtain a history of the patient's complaints, including a list of known allergens (especially allergies or sensitivities to latex) and inform the appropriate health care practitioner accordingly.

➤ Obtain a history of the patient's hematopoietic system and results of previously performed laboratory tests, surgical procedures, and other diagnostic procedures. For related laboratory tests, refer to the Hematopoietic System table.

➤ Obtain a list of the medications the patient is taking, including herbs, nutritional supplements, and nutraceuticals. The requesting health care practitioner and laboratory should be advised if the patient is regularly using these products so that their effects can be taken into consideration when reviewing results.

➤ Review the procedure with the patient. Inform the patient that specimen collection takes approximately 5 to 10 minutes. Address concerns about pain related to the procedure. Explain to the patient that there may be some discomfort during the venipuncture.

➤ There are no food, fluid, or medication restrictions, unless by medical direction.

Intratest:

➤ If the patient has a history of severe allergic reaction to latex, care should be taken to avoid the use of equipment containing latex.

➤ Instruct the patient to cooperate fully and to follow directions. Direct the patient to breathe normally and to avoid unnecessary movement.

➤ Observe standard precautions, and follow the general guidelines in Appendix A. Positively identify the patient, and label the appropriate tubes with the corresponding patient demographics, date, and time of collection. Perform a venipuncture; collect the specimen in a 5-mL red- or tiger-top tube.

➤ Remove the needle, and apply a pressure dressing over the puncture site.

➤ Promptly transport the specimen to the laboratory for processing and analysis.

➤ The results are recorded manually or in a computerized system for recall and postprocedure interpreta-tion by the appropriate health care practitioner.

Post-test:

➤ Observe venipuncture site for bleeding or hematoma formation. Apply paper tape or other adhesive to hold pressure bandage in place, or replace with a plastic bandage.

➤ A written report of the examination will be sent to the requesting health care practitioner, who will discuss the results with the patient.

➤ Reinforce information given by the patient's health care provider regarding further testing, treatment, or referral to another health care provider. Answer any questions or address any concerns voiced by the patient or family.

➤ Depending on the results of this procedure, additional testing may be performed to evaluate or monitor progression of the disease process and determine the need for a change in therapy. Evaluate test results in relation to the patient's symptoms and other tests performed.

Related laboratory tests:

➤ Related laboratory tests include bone marrow biopsy, complete blood count, erythropoietin, ferritin, hemosiderin, iron, lead, and porphyrins.

KETONES, BLOOD AND URINE

SYNONYMS/ACRONYM: Ketone bodies, acetoacetate, acetone.

SPECIMEN: Serum (1 mL) collected from red- or tiger-top tube. Urine (5 mL), random or timed specimen, collected in a clean plastic collection container.

REFERENCE VALUE: (Method: Colorimetric nitroprusside reaction) Negative.

DESCRIPTION & RATIONALE: Ketone bodies refer to the three intermediate products of metabolism: acetone, acetoacetic acid, and β-hydroxybutyrate. Even though β-hydroxybutyrate is not a ketone, it is usually listed with the ketone bodies. In healthy individuals, ketones are produced and completely metabolized by the liver so that measurable amounts are not normally present in serum. Ketones appear in the urine before a significant serum level is detectable. If the patient has excessive fat metabolism, ketones are found in blood and urine. Excessive fat metabolism may occur if the patient has impaired ability to metabolize carbohydrates, inadequate carbohydrate intake, inadequate insulin levels, excessive carbohydrate loss, or increased carbohydrate demand. A strongly positive acetone result without severe acidosis, accompanied by normal glucose, electrolyte, and bicarbonate levels, is strongly suggestive of isopropyl alcohol poisoning. A low-carbohydrate or low-fat diet may cause a positive acetone test. Ketosis in diabetics is usually accompanied by increased glucose and decreased bicarbonate and pH. Extremely elevated levels of ketone bodies can result in coma. This situation is particularly life-threatening in children younger than 10 years old. ■

INDICATIONS:

- Assist in the diagnosis of starvation, stress, alcoholism, suspected isopropyl alcohol ingestion, glycogen storage disease, and other metabolic disorders

- Detect and monitor treatment of diabetic ketoacidosis

- Monitor the control of diabetes

- Screen for ketonuria due to acute illness or stress in nondiabetic patients

- Screen for ketonuria to assist in the assessment of inborn errors of metabolism

- Screen for ketonuria to assist in the diagnosis of suspected isopropyl alcohol poisoning

RESULT

Increased in:
- Acidosis
- Branched-chain ketonuria
- Carbohydrate deficiency
- Eclampsia
- Fasting or starvation
- Gestational diabetes
- Glycogen storage diseases
- High-fat or high-protein diet
- Hyperglycemia
- Ketoacidosis of alcoholism and diabetes
- Illnesses with marked vomiting and diarrhea
- Isopropyl alcohol ingestion
- Methylmalonic aciduria
- Postanesthesia period
- Propionyl coenzyme A carboxylase deficiency

Decreased in: N/A

CRITICAL VALUES:

Strongly positive test results for glucose and ketones

Note and immediately report to the health care practitioner strongly positive results in urine and related symptoms. An elevated level of ketone bodies is evidenced by fruity-smelling breath, acidosis, ketonuria, and decreased level of consciousness. Administration of insulin and frequent blood glucose measurement may be indicated.

INTERFERING FACTORS:

- Drugs that may cause an increase in serum ketone levels include acetylsalicylic acid (if therapy results in acidosis, especially in children), albuterol, fenfluramine, levodopa, nifedipine, and paraldehyde.

- Drugs that may cause a decrease in serum ketone levels include acetylsalicylic acid and valproic acid. Increases have been shown in hyperthyroid patients receiving propranolol and propylthiouracil.

- Drugs that may increase urine ketone levels include acetylsalicylic acid (if therapy results in acidosis, especially in children), captopril, dimercaprol, ether, ifosfamide, insulin, levodopa, mesna, metformin, methyldopa, *N*-acetylcysteine, niacin, paraldehyde, penicillamine, phenazopyridine, phenolphthalein, phenolsulfonphthalein, pyrazinamide, streptozocin, sulfobromophthalein, and valproic acid.

- Drugs that may decrease urine ketone levels include acetylsalicylic acid and phenazopyridine.

- Urine should be checked within 60 minutes of collection.

- Bacterial contamination of urine can cause false-negative results.

- Failure to keep reagent strip container tightly closed can cause false-negative results. Light and moisture affect the ability of the chemicals in the strip to perform as expected.

- False-negative or weakly false-positive test results can be obtained when β-hydroxybutyrate is the predominating ketone body in cases of lactic acidosis.

Nursing Implications and Procedure • • • • • • • • • • •

Pretest:

➤ Inform the patient that the test is most commonly used to investigate diabetes as the cause of ketoacidosis.

➤ Obtain a history of the patient's complaints, including a list of known allergens (especially allergies or sensitivities to latex), and inform the appropriate health care practitioner accordingly.

➤ Obtain a history of the patient's endocrine system and results of previously performed laboratory tests, surgical procedures, and other diagnostic procedures. For related laboratory tests, refer to the Endocrine System table.

➤ Obtain a list of the medications the patient is taking, including herbs, nutritional supplements, and nutraceuticals. The requesting health care practitioner and laboratory should be advised if the patient regularly uses these products so that their effects can be taken into consideration when reviewing results.

➤ Review the procedure with the patient. Inform the patient that blood specimen collection takes approximately 5 to 10 minutes. The amount of time required to collect a urine specimen depends on the level of cooperation from the patient. Address concerns about pain related to the procedure. Explain to the patient that there may be some discomfort during the venipuncture.

➤ *Sensitivity to social and cultural issues,* as well as concern for modesty, is important in providing psychological support before, during, and after the procedure.

➤ There are no food, fluid, or medication restrictions, unless by medical direction.

Intratest:

➤ Observe standard precautions, and follow the general guidelines in Appendix A.

Blood:

➤ If the patient has a history of severe allergic reaction to latex, care should be taken to avoid the use of equipment containing latex.

➤ Instruct the patient to cooperate fully and to follow directions. Direct the patient to breathe normally and to avoid unnecessary movement.

➤ Positively identify the patient, and label the appropriate tubes with the corresponding patient demographics, date, and time of collection. Perform a venipuncture; collect the specimen in a 5-mL red- or tiger-top tube. Alternatively, a finger- or heel-stick method of specimen collection can be used.

➤ Remove the needle, and apply a pressure dressing over the puncture site.

Urine:

➤ Review the procedure with the patient. Explain to the patient how to collect a second-voided midstream specimen: (1) void, then drink a glass of water; and (2) wait 30 minutes, and then try to void again.

➤ Instruct the patient to avoid excessive exercise and stress before specimen collection.

Clean-catch specimen:

➤ Instruct the male patient to (1) thoroughly wash his hands, (2) cleanse the meatus, (3) void a small amount into the toilet, and (4) void directly into the specimen container.

➤ Instruct the female patient to (1) thoroughly wash her hands; (2) cleanse the labia from front to back; (3) while keeping the labia separated, void a small amount into the toilet; and (4) without interrupting the urine stream, void directly into the specimen container.

Blood or urine:

➤ Promptly transport the specimen to the laboratory for processing and analysis.

➤ The results are recorded manually or in a computerized system for recall and postprocedure interpretation by the appropriate health care practitioner.

Post-test:

➤ Observe venipuncture site for bleeding or hematoma formation. Apply paper tape or other adhesive to hold pressure bandage in place, or replace with a plastic bandage.

➤ *Nutritional considerations:* Increased levels of ketone bodies may be associated with diabetes. The nutritional needs of each diabetic patient need to be determined individually (especially during pregnancy) by a health care practitioner trained in nutrition. Patients who adhere to dietary recommendations report a better general feeling of health, better weight management, greater control of glucose and lipid values, and improved use of insulin. There is no "diabetic diet"; however, many meal-planning approaches with nutritional goals are endorsed by the American Dietetic Association.

➤ Impaired glucose tolerance may be associated with diabetes. Instruct the patient and caregiver to report signs and symptoms of hypoglycemia (weakness, confusion, diaphoresis, rapid pulse) or hyperglycemia (thirst, polyuria, hunger, lethargy).

➤ *Nutritional considerations:* Increased levels of ketone bodies may be associated with poor carbohydrate intake; therefore, the body breaks down fat instead of carbohydrate for energy. Increasing carbohydrate intake in the patient's diet reduces the levels of ketone bodies. Carbohydrates can be found in starches and sugars. Starch is a complex carbohydrate that can be found in foods such as grains (breads, cereals, pasta, rice) and starchy vegetables (corn, peas, potatoes). Sugar is a simple carbohydrate that can be found in natural foods (fruits and natural honey) and processed foods (desserts and candy).

➤ A written report of the examination will be sent to the requesting health care practitioner, who will discuss the results with the patient.

➤ Recognize anxiety related to test results, and be supportive of perceived loss of independence and fear of shortened life expectancy. Discuss the implications of abnormal test results on the patient's lifestyle. Provide teaching and information regarding the clinical implications of the test results, as appropriate. Emphasize, as appropriate, that good glycemic control delays the onset of and slows the progression of diabetic retinopathy, nephropathy, and neuropathy. Educate the patient regarding access to counseling services. Provide contact information, if desired, for the American Diabetes Association *(http://www. diabetes.org)*.

➤ Reinforce information given by the patient's health care provider regarding further testing, treatment, or referral to another health care provider. Answer any questions or address any concerns voiced by the patient or family.

➤ Depending on the results of this procedure, additional testing may be performed to evaluate or monitor progression of the disease process and determine the need for a change in therapy. Evaluate test results in relation to the patient's symptoms and other tests performed.

Related laboratory tests:

➤ Related laboratory tests include anion gap, blood gases, electrolytes, glucose, glycated hemoglobin, lactic acid, osmolality (blood and urine), phosphorus, and routine urinalysis.

KIDNEY, URETER, AND BLADDER STUDY

SYNONYMS/ACRONYM: Flat plate of the abdomen, plain film of the abdomen, scout film, KUB.

AREA OF APPLICATION: Kidneys, ureters, bladder, and abdomen.

CONTRAST: None.

DESCRIPTION & RATIONALE: A kidney, ureter, and bladder (KUB) x-ray examination provides information regarding the structure, size, and position of the abdominal organs; it also indicates whether there is any obstruction or abnormality of the abdomen caused by disease or congenital malformation. Calcifications of the renal calyces or renal pelvis, as well as any radiopaque calculi present in the urinary tract or surrounding organs, may be visualized. Patterns of air and gas appear light and bright on the image. Air normally remains contained within the intestinal tract; perforation of either the stomach or the intestines causes air to escape into the abdominal cavity. When there is an intestinal obstruction, air and fluid collect above the area of obstruction, distending the lumen of the intestine. KUB x-rays are among the first examinations done to diagnose intra-abdominal diseases such as intestinal obstruction, masses, tumors, ruptured organs, abnormal gas accumulation, and ascites. ■

INDICATIONS:

- Determine the cause of acute abdominal pain or palpable mass
- Evaluate the effects of lower abdominal trauma, such as internal hemorrhage
- Evaluate known or suspected intestinal obstruction
- Evaluate the presence of renal, ureter, or other organ calculi
- Evaluate the size, shape, and position of the liver, kidneys, and spleen
- Evaluate suspected abnormal fluid, air, or metallic object or obstruction in the abdomen

RESULT

Normal Findings:
- Normal size and shape of kidneys
- Normal bladder, absence of masses and renal calculi, and no abnormal accumulation of air or fluid

Abnormal Findings:
- Abnormal accumulation of bowel gas
- Ascites

- Bladder distention
- Congenital renal anomaly
- Hydronephrosis
- Intestinal obstruction
- Organomegaly
- Renal calculi
- Renal hematomas
- Ruptured viscus
- Soft-tissue masses
- Trauma to liver, spleen, kidneys, and bladder
- Vascular calcification

CRITICAL VALUES: N/A

INTERFERING FACTORS:

This procedure is contraindicated for:
- Patients who are pregnant or suspected of being pregnant, unless the potential benefits of the procedure far outweigh the risks to the fetus and mother

Factors that may impair clear imaging:
- Inability of the patient to cooperate or remain still during the procedure because of age, significant pain, or mental status
- Metallic objects within the examination field (e.g., jewelry, body rings), which may inhibit organ visualization and can produce unclear images
- Improper adjustment of the radiographic equipment to accommodate obese or thin patients, which can cause overexposure or underexposure and a poor-quality study
- Patients who are very obese, who may exceed the weight limit for the equipment
- Incorrect positioning of the patient, which may produce poor visualization of the area to be examined, especially

for oblique and decubitus views and for films done by portable equipment

- Retained barium from a previous radiologic procedure

- Gas or feces in the gastrointestinal tract resulting from inadequate cleansing or failure to restrict food intake before the study

- Ascites, uterine tumors, and ovarian tumors, which can interfere with the quality of the procedure

Other considerations:

- Consultation with a health care practitioner should occur before the procedure for radiation safety concerns regarding younger patients or patients who are lactating.

- Risks associated with radiographic overexposure can result from frequent x-ray procedures. Personnel in the room with the patient should wear a protective lead apron, stand behind a shield, or leave the area while the examination is being done. Personnel working in the area where the examination is being done should wear badges that reveal their level of exposure to radiation.

Nursing Implications and Procedure • • • • • • • • • • •

Pretest:

- ➤ Inform the patient that the procedure assesses the status of the abdomen.

- ➤ Obtain a history of the patient's complaints and symptoms.

- ➤ Obtain a history of the patient's gastrointestinal and genitourinary systems, and results of previously performed diagnostic procedures, surgical procedures, and laboratory tests. For related diagnostic tests, refer to the Gastrointestinal and Genitourinary System tables.

- ➤ Schedule intravenous pyelography (IVP) or gastrointestinal studies after this study.

- ➤ Record the date of the last menstrual period and determine the possibility of pregnancy in perimenopausal women.

- ➤ Obtain a list of the medications the patient is taking.

- ➤ Review the procedure with the patient. Address concerns about pain related to the procedure. Explain to the patient that little or no pain is expected during the test, but there may be moments of discomfort. Inform the patient that the procedure is performed in the radiology department or at the bedside, by a registered radiologic techologist, and takes approximately 5 to 15 minutes to complete.

- ➤ *Sensitivity to cultural and social issues,* as well as concern for modesty, is important in providing psychological support before, during, and after the procedure.

- ➤ There are no food, fluid, or medication, restrictions unless by medical direction.

- ➤ Instruct the patient to remove jewelry (including watches), credit cards, and other metallic objects.

Intratest:

- ➤ Ensure that jewelry, watches, chains, belts, and any other metallic objects have been removed from the abdominal area.

- ➤ Patients are given a gown, robe, and foot coverings to wear and instructed to void prior to the procedure.

- ➤ Instruct the patient to cooperate fully and to follow directions. Instruct the patient to remain still throughout the procedure because movement produces unreliable results.

- ➤ Observe standard precautions, and follow the general guidelines in Appendix A.

- ➤ Remove any wires connected to electrodes, if allowed.

- ➤ Place the patient on the table in a supine position with hands over the head or relaxed at the side.

- ➤ For male patients, place lead protection over the testicles to prevent their irradiation.

➤ For portable examinations, elevate the head of the bed to the high Fowler's position.

➤ Ask the patient to inhale deeply and hold his or her breath while the x-ray images are taken, and then to exhale after the images are taken.

➤ The results are recorded on a sheet of x-ray film or electronically, in a computerized system, for recall and postprocedure interpretation by the appropriate health care practitioner.

Post-test:

➤ A written report of the examination will be completed by a health care practitioner specializing in this branch of medicine. The report will be sent to the requesting health care practitioner, who will discuss the results with the patient.

➤ Reinforce information given by the patient's health care provider regarding further testing, treatment, or referral to another health care provider. Answer any questions or address any concerns voiced by the patient or family.

➤ Depending on the results of this procedure, additional testing may be performed to evaluate or monitor progression of the disease process and determine the need for a change in therapy. Evaluate test results in relation to the patient's symptoms and other tests performed.

Related diagnostic tests:

➤ Related diagnostic tests include IVP as well as computed tomography, ultrasound, and magnetic resonance imaging of the abdomen.

KLEIHAUER-BETKE TEST

SYNONYMS/ACRONYM: Fetal hemoglobin, hemoglobin F, acid elution slide test.

SPECIMEN: Whole blood (1 mL) collected in a lavender-top (EDTA) tube. Freshly prepared blood smears are also acceptable. Cord blood may be requested for use as a positive control.

REFERENCE VALUE: (Method: Microscopic examination of treated and stained peripheral blood smear) Less than 1%.

DESCRIPTION & RATIONALE: The Kleihauer-Betke test is used to determine the degree of fetal-maternal hemorrhage and to help calculate the dosage of RhoGAM to be given in some cases of Rh-negative mothers.

The test can also be used to distinguish some forms of thalassemia from the hereditary persistence of fetal hemoglobin, but hemoglobin electrophoresis and flow cytometry methods are more commonly used for this purpose. ■

INDICATIONS:

- Assist in the diagnosis of certain types of anemia

- Calculating dosage of RhoGAM

- Screening postpartum maternal blood for the presence of fetal-maternal hemorrhage

RESULT

Positive in:
- Fetal-maternal hemorrhage

- Hereditary persistence of fetal hemoglobin

Negative in: N/A

CRITICAL VALUES: N/A

INTERFERING FACTORS: Specimens must be obtained before transfusion.

Nursing Implications and Procedure • • • • • • • • • •

Pretest:

➤ Inform the patient that the test is used to determine occurrence and extent of fetal-maternal bleed. It is also used to calculate Rh immune globulin dosage.

➤ Obtain a history of the patient's complaints, including a list of known allergens (especially allergies or sensitivities to latex), and inform the appropriate health care practitioner accordingly.

➤ Obtain a history of the patient's hematopoietic and reproductive systems, as well as results of previously performed laboratory tests, surgical procedures, and other diagnostic procedures. For related laboratory tests, refer to the Hematopoietic and Reproductive System tables.

➤ Note any recent procedures that can interfere with test results.

➤ Obtain a list of medications the patient is taking, including herbs, nutritional supplements, and nutraceuticals. The requesting health care practitioner and laboratory should be advised if the patient regularly uses these products so that their effects can be taken into consideration when reviewing results.

➤ Review the procedure with the patient. Inform the patient that specimen collection takes approximately 5 to 10 minutes. Address concerns about pain related to the procedure. Explain to the patient that there may be some discomfort during the venipuncture.

➤ There are no food, fluid, or medication restrictions, unless by medical direction.

Intratest:

➤ If the patient has a history of severe allergic reaction to latex, care should be taken to avoid the use of equipment containing latex.

➤ Instruct the patient to cooperate fully and to follow directions. Direct the patient to breathe normally and to avoid unnecessary movement.

➤ Observe standard precautions, and follow the general guidelines in Appendix A. Positively identify the patient, and label the appropriate tubes with the corresponding patient demographics, date, and time of collection. Perform a venipuncture; collect the specimen in a 5-mL lavender-top tube.

➤ Remove the needle and apply a pressure dressing over the puncture site.

➤ Promptly transport the specimen to the laboratory for processing and analysis. Sample must be less than 6 hours old.

➤ The results are recorded manually or in a computerized system for recall and postprocedure interpretation by the appropriate health care practitioner.

Post-test:

➤ Observe venipuncture site for bleeding or hematoma formation. Apply paper tape or other adhesive to hold pressure bandage in place, or replace with a plastic bandage.

➤ A written report of the examination will be sent to the requesting health care practitioner, who will discuss the results with the patient.

➤ Reinforce information given by the patient's health care provider regarding further testing, treatment, or referral to another health care provider. Answer any questions or address any concerns voiced by the patient or family.

➤ Depending on the results of this procedure, additional testing may be performed to evaluate or monitor progression of the disease process and determine the need for a change in therapy. Evaluate test results in relation to the patient's symptoms and other tests performed.

Related laboratory tests:

➤ Related laboratory tests include blood group and type and hemoglobin electrophoresis.

LACTATE DEHYDROGENASE AND ISOENZYMES

SYNONYMS/ACRONYMS: LDH and isos, LD and isos.

SPECIMEN: Serum (1 mL) collected in a red- or tiger-top tube.

REFERENCE VALUE: (Method: Enzymatic [L to P] for lactate dehydrogenase, electrophoretic analysis for isoenzymes) Reference ranges are method dependent and may vary from laboratory to laboratory.

Lactate Dehydrogenase

Age	Conventional & SI Units
0–2 y	125–275 U/L
2–3 y	166–232 U/L
4–6 y	104–206 U/L
7–12 y	90–203 U/L
13–14 y	90–199 U/L
15–43 y	90–156 U/L
Greater than 43 y	90–176 U/L

LDH Fraction	% of Total	Fraction of Total
LDH$_1$	14–26	0.14–0.26
LDH$_2$	29–39	0.29–0.39
LDH$_3$	20–26	0.20–0.26
LDH$_4$	8–16	0.08–0.16
LDH$_5$	6–16	0.06–0.16

DESCRIPTION & RATIONALE: Lactate dehydrogenase (LDH) is an enzyme that catalyzes the reversible conversion of lactate to pyruvate within cells. Because many tissues contain LDH, elevated total LDH is considered a nonspecific indicator of cellular damage unless other clinical data make the tissue origin obvious. Determining tissue origin is aided by electrophoretic analysis of the five isoenzymes specific to certain tissues. The heart and erythrocytes are rich sources of LDH$_1$, LDH$_2$, and LDH$_3$; the kidneys contain large amounts of LDH$_3$ and LDH$_4$; and the liver and skeletal muscles are high in LDH$_4$ and LDH$_5$. Certain glands (e.g., thyroid, adrenal, thymus), the pancreas, spleen, lungs, lymph nodes, and white blood cells contain LDH$_3$, whereas the ilium is an additional source of LDH$_5$. There have been documented reports of a sixth isoenzyme of LDH. It is seen in patients with severe liver disease and is an indicator of a very poor prognosis. LDH is found in every tissue of the body. It is of no use as a specific diagnostic marker. Testing for the presence of LDH and isoenzymes is rarely used anymore to confirm acute myocardial infarction (MI), having been replaced by more sensitive and specific creatine kinase (CK-MB) and troponin assays. Acute myocardial infarction releases LDH into the serum within the first 12 hours, causing a "flip" isoenzyme pattern within 48 hours of MI, and levels remain elevated 1 to 2 weeks after CK and aspartate aminotransferase have returned to normal levels. ∎

INDICATIONS:

• Differentiate acute MI, as evidenced by elevated LDH$_1$ and LDH$_2$, from pulmonary infarction and liver problems, which elevate LDH$_4$ and LDH$_5$

• Evaluate the degree of muscle wasting in muscular dystrophy (LDH levels rise early in this disorder and approach normal as muscle mass is reduced by atrophy)

• Evaluate the effectiveness of cancer chemotherapy (LDH levels should fall with successful treatment)

• Evaluate red cell hemolysis or renal infarction, especially as indicated by reversal of the LDH$_1$:LDH$_2$ ratio

• Investigate acute MI or extension thereof, as indicated by elevation (usually) of total LDH, elevation of LDH$_1$ and LDH$_2$, and reversal of the LDH$_1$:LDH$_2$ ratio within 48 hours of the infarction

• Investigate chronicity of liver, lung, and kidney disorders, as evidenced by LDH levels that remain persistently high

RESULT

Total LDH increased in:

• Carcinoma of the liver

• Chronic alcoholism

- Cirrhosis
- Congestive heart failure
- Hemolytic anemias
- Hypoxia
- Leukemias
- Megaloblastic and pernicious anemia
- MI or pulmonary infarction
- Musculoskeletal disease
- Obstructive jaundice
- Pancreatitis
- Renal disease (severe)
- Shock
- Viral hepatitis

Total LDH decreased in: N/A

LDH Isoenzymes:
- LDH_1 fraction increased over LDH_2 can be seen in acute MI, anemias (pernicious, hemolytic, acute sickle cell, megaloblastic, hemolytic), and acute renal cortical injury due to any cause. The LDH_1 fraction in particular is elevated in cases of germ cell tumors.

- Increases in the middle fractions are associated with conditions in which massive platelet destruction has occurred (e.g., pulmonary embolism, post-transfusion period), and in lymphatic system disorders (e.g., infectious mononucleosis, lymphomas, lymphocytic leukemias).

- An increase in LDH_5 occurs with musculoskeletal damage and many types of liver damage (e.g., cirrhosis, cancer, hepatitis).

CRITICAL VALUES: N/A

INTERFERING FACTORS:
- Drugs that may increase total LDH levels include amiodarone, etretinate, fluosol-DA, methotrexate, oxacillin, plicamycin, propoxyphene, and streptokinase.

- Drugs that may decrease total LDH levels include ascorbic acid, cefotaxime, enalapril, fluorides, naltrexone, and oxylate.

- Hemolysis will cause significant false elevations in total LDH and a false "flip" pattern of the isoenzymes because LDH_1 fraction is of red blood cell origin.

- Some isoenzymes are temperature sensitive; therefore, prolonged storage at refrigerated temperatures may cause false decreases.

Nursing Implications and Procedure

Pretest:

➤ Inform the patient that the test is primarily used to monitor MI.

➤ Obtain a history of the patient's complaints, including a list of known allergens (especially allergies or sensitivities to latex), and inform the appropriate health care practitioner accordingly.

➤ Obtain a history of the patient's cardiovascular, hematopoietic, hepatobiliary, and musculoskeletal systems, as well as results of previously performed laboratory tests, surgical procedures, and other diagnostic procedures. For related laboratory tests, refer to the Cardiovascular, Hematopoietic, Hepatobiliary, and Musculoskeletal System tables.

➤ Obtain a list of the medications the patient is taking, including herbs, nutritional supplements, and nutraceuticals. The requesting health care practitioner and laboratory should be advised if the patient regularly uses these products so that their effects can be taken into consideration when reviewing results.

➤ Review the procedure with the

patient. (Samples at time of admission, 2 to 4 hours, 6 to 8 hours, and 12 hours after admission are the minimal recommendations. Additional samples may be requested.) Inform the patient that specimen collection takes approximately 5 to 10 minutes. Address concerns about pain related to the procedure. Explain to the patient that there may be some discomfort during the venipuncture.

➤ There are no food, fluid, or medication restrictions, unless by medical direction.

Intratest:

➤ If the patient has a history of severe allergic reaction to latex, care should be taken to avoid the use of equipment containing latex.

➤ Instruct the patient to cooperate fully and to follow directions. Direct the patient to breathe normally and to avoid unnecessary movement.

➤ Observe standard precautions, and follow the general guidelines in Appendix A. Positively identify the patient, and label the appropriate tubes with the corresponding patient demographics, date, and time of collection. Perform a venipuncture; collect the specimen in a 5-mL red- or tiger-top tube.

➤ Remove the needle, and apply a pressure dressing over the puncture site.

➤ Promptly transport the specimen to the laboratory for processing and analysis.

➤ The results are recorded manually or in a computerized system for recall and postprocedure interpretation by the appropriate health care practitioner.

Post-test:

➤ Observe venipuncture site for bleeding or hematoma formation. Apply paper tape or other adhesive to hold pressure bandage in place, or replace with a plastic bandage.

➤ *Nutritional considerations:* Increased LDH levels may be associated with coronary artery disease (CAD). Nutritional therapy is recommended for individuals identified to be at high risk for developing CAD. If overweight, the patient should be encouraged to achieve a normal weight. The American Heart Association Step 1 and Step 2 diets may be helpful in achieving a goal of lowering total cholesterol and triglyceride levels. The Step 1 diet emphasizes a reduction in foods high in saturated fats and cholesterol. Red meats, eggs, and dairy products are the major sources of saturated fats and cholesterol. If triglycerides are also elevated, the patient should be advised to eliminate or reduce alcohol and simple carbohydrates from the diet. The Step 2 diet recommends stricter reductions.

➤ A written report of the examination will be sent to the requesting health care practitioner, who will discuss the results with the patient.

➤ Recognize anxiety related to test results, and be supportive of fear of shortened life expectancy. Discuss the implications of abnormal test results on the patient's lifestyle. Provide teaching and information regarding the clinical implications of the test results, as appropriate. Educate the patient regarding access to counseling services. Provide contact information, if desired, for the American Heart Association *(http://www.americanheart.org)*.

➤ Reinforce information given by the patient's health care provider regarding further testing, treatment, or referral to another health care provider. Answer any questions or address any concerns voiced by the patient or family.

➤ Depending on the results of this procedure, additional testing may be performed to evaluate or monitor progression of the disease process and determine the need for a change in therapy. Evaluate test results in relation to the patient's symptoms and other tests performed.

LACTIC ACID

SYNONYM/ACRONYM: Lactate.

SPECIMEN: Plasma (1 mL) collected in a gray-top (sodium fluoride) or green-top (lithium heparin) tube. Specimen should be transported tightly capped and in an ice slurry.

REFERENCE VALUE: (Method: Spectrophotometry/enzymatic analysis)

Conventional Units	SI Units (Conventional Units × 0.111)
3–23 mg/dL	0.3–2.6 mmol/L

DESCRIPTION & RATIONALE: Lactic acid (present in blood as lactate) is a byproduct of carbohydrate metabolism. Normally metabolized in the liver, lactate concentration is based on the rate of production and metabolism. Levels increase during strenuous exercise, which results in insufficient oxygen delivery to the tissues. Pyruvate, the normal end product of glucose metabolism, is converted to lactate in emergency situations when energy is needed but there is insufficient oxygen in the system to favor the aerobic and customary energy cycle. When hypoxia or circulatory collapse increases production of lactate, or when the hepatic system does not metabolize lactate sufficiently, lactate levels become elevated. The lactic acid test can be performed in conjunction with pyruvic acid testing to monitor tissue oxygenation. Lactic acidosis can be differentiated from ketoacidosis by the absence of ketosis and grossly elevated glucose levels. ■

INDICATIONS:
• Assess tissue oxygenation

• Evaluate acidosis

RESULT

Increased in:
- Cardiac failure
- Diabetes
- Hemorrhage
- Hepatic coma
- Ingestion of large doses of ethanol or acetaminophen
- Lactic acidosis
- Pulmonary embolism
- Pulmonary failure
- Reye's syndrome
- Shock
- Strenuous exercise

Decreased in: N/A

CRITICAL VALUES:

Greater than or equal to 31 mg/dL
Note and immediately report to the health care practitioner any critically increased values and related symptoms. Observe the patient for signs and symptoms of elevated levels, such as Kussmaul's breathing and increased pulse rate. In general, there is an inverse relationship between critically elevated lactate levels and survival.

INTERFERING FACTORS:

- Drugs that may increase lactate levels include albuterol, anticonvulsants (long-term use), epinephrine, intravenous glucose, isoniazid, lactose, metformin, oral contraceptives, sodium bicarbonate, and sorbitol.

- Falsely low lactate levels are obtained in samples with elevated levels of the enzyme lactate dehydrogenase (LDH) because this enzyme reacts with the available lactate substrate.

- Using a tourniquet or instructing the patient to clench his or her fist during a venipuncture can cause elevated levels.

- Engaging in strenuous physical activity (i.e., activity in which blood flow and oxygen distribution cannot keep pace with increased energy needs) before specimen collection can cause an elevated result.

- Delay in transport of the specimen to the laboratory must be avoided. Specimens not processed by centrifugation in a tightly stoppered collection container within 15 minutes of collection should be rejected for analysis. It is preferable to transport specimens to the laboratory in an ice slurry to further retard cellular metabolism that might shift lactate levels in the sample before analysis.

- Failure to follow dietary restrictions before the procedure may cause the procedure to be canceled or repeated.

Nursing Implications and Procedure ● ● ● ● ● ● ● ● ● ● ●

Pretest:

▶ Inform the patient that the test is used to investigate suspected lactic acidosis, most commonly caused by hypoperfusion.

▶ Obtain a history of the patient's complaints, including a list of known allergens (especially allergies or sensitivities to latex), and inform the appropriate health care practitioner accordingly.

▶ Obtain a history of the patient's cardiovascular, endocrine, hepatobiliary, musculoskeletal, and respiratory systems, as well as results of previously performed laboratory tests, surgical procedures, and other diagnostic procedures. For related laboratory tests, refer to the Cardiovascular, Endocrine, Hepatobiliary, Musculoskeletal, and Respiratory System tables.

➤ Obtain a list of the medications the patient is taking, including herbs, nutritional supplements, and nutraceuticals. The requesting health care practitioner and laboratory should be advised if the patient regularly uses these products so that their effects can be taken into consideration when reviewing results.

➤ Review the procedure with the patient. Instruct the patient to rest for 1 hour before specimen collection. Inform the patient that specimen collection takes approximately 5 to 10 minutes. Address concerns about pain related to the procedure. Explain to the patient that there may be some discomfort during the venipuncture.

➤ Instruct the patient to fast and to restrict fluids overnight. Instruct the patient not to ingest alcohol for 12 hours before the test.

➤ *Sensitivity to social and cultural issues,* as well as concern for modesty, is important in providing psychological support before, during, and after the procedure.

➤ There are no medication restrictions, unless by medical direction.

➤ Prepare an ice slurry in a cup or plastic bag to have on hand for immediate transport of the specimen to the laboratory.

Intratest:

➤ Ensure that the patient has complied with dietary restrictions and other pretesting preparations; assure that food and liquids have been restricted for at least 12 hours prior to the procedure.

➤ If the patient has a history of severe allergic reaction to latex, care should be taken to avoid the use of equipment containing latex.

➤ Instruct the patient to cooperate fully and to follow directions. Direct the patient to breathe normally and to avoid unnecessary movement.

➤ Observe standard precautions, and follow the general guidelines in

Appendix A. Positively identify the patient, and label the appropriate tubes with the corresponding patient demographics, date, and time of collection. Instruct the patient *not* to clench and unclench fist immediately before or during specimen collection. Do not use a tourniquet. Perform a venipuncture; collect the specimen in a 5-mL gray- or green-top tube. The tightly capped sample should be placed in an ice slurry immediately after collection. Information on the specimen label can be protected from water in the ice slurry if the specimen is first placed in a protective plastic bag.

➤ Remove the needle, and apply a pressure dressing over the puncture site.

➤ Promptly transport the specimen to the laboratory for processing and analysis.

➤ The results are recorded manually or in a computerized system for recall and postprocedure interpretation by the appropriate health care practitioner.

Post-test:

➤ Observe venipuncture site for bleeding or hematoma formation. Apply paper tape or other adhesive to hold pressure bandage in place, or replace with a plastic bandage.

➤ *Nutritional considerations:* Instruct patients to consume water when exercising. Dehydration may occur when the body loses water during exercise. Early signs of dehydration include dry mouth, thirst, and concentrated dark yellow urine. If replacement fluids are not consumed at this time, the patient may become moderately dehydrated and exhibit symptoms of extreme thirst, dry oral mucus membranes, inability to produce tears, decreased urinary output, and light-headedness. Severe dehydration manifests as confusion, lethargy, vertigo, tachycardia, anuria, diaphoresis, and loss of consciousness.

➤ Instruct the patient to resume usual diet and fluids, as directed by the health care practitioner.

➤ A written report of the examination will be sent to the requesting health care practitioner, who will discuss the results with the patient.

➤ Reinforce information given by the patient's health care provider regarding further testing, treatment, or referral to another health care provider. Answer any questions or address any concerns voiced by the patient or family.

➤ Depending on the results of this procedure, additional testing may be performed to evaluate or monitor progression of the disease process and determine the need for a change in therapy. Evaluate test results in relation to the patient's symptoms and other tests performed.

Related laboratory tests:

➤ Related laboratory tests include anion gap, arterial/alveolar oxygen ratio, blood gases, electrolytes, glucose, and ketones.

LACTOSE TOLERANCE TEST

· ·

SYNONYM/ACRONYM: LTT.

SPECIMEN: Plasma (1 mL) collected in gray-top (fluoride/oxalate) tube.

REFERENCE VALUE: (Method: Spectrophotometry)

Change in Glucose Value	Conventional Units	SI Units (Conventional Units × 0.0555)
Normal*	Greater than 30 mg/dL	Greater than 1.7 mmol/L
Inconclusive*	20–30 mg/dL	1.1–1.7 mmol/L
Abnormal*	Less than 20 mg/dL	Less than 1.1 mmol/L

*Compared to fasting sample.

DESCRIPTION & RATIONALE: Lactose is a disaccharide found in dairy products. When ingested, lactose is broken down in the intestine, by the sugar-splitting enzyme lactase, into glucose and galactose. When sufficient lactase is not available, intestinal bacteria metabolize the lactose, resulting in abdominal bloating, pain, flatus, and diarrhea. The lactose tolerance test screens for lactose intolerance by monitoring glucose levels after ingestion of a dose of lactose. ■

INDICATIONS: Evaluate patients for suspected lactose intolerance

RESULT

Glucose levels increased in: N/A

Glucose levels decreased in:
Lactose intolerance

CRITICAL VALUES:

Less than 40 mg/dL
Greater than 400 mg/dL
Note and immediately report to the health care practitioner any critically increased or decreased values and symptoms.

Symptoms of decreased glucose levels include headache, confusion, hunger, irritability, nervousness, restlessness, sweating, and weakness. Possible interventions include oral or intravenous (IV) administration of glucose, IV or intramuscular injection of glucagon, and continuous glucose monitoring.

Symptoms of elevated glucose levels include abdominal pain, fatigue, muscle cramps, nausea, vomiting, polyuria, and thirst. Possible interventions include subcutaneous or IV injection of insulin with continuous glucose monitoring.

INTERFERING FACTORS:

- Numerous medications may alter glucose levels (see monograph titled "Glucose").

- Delayed gastric emptying may decrease glucose levels.

- Smoking may falsely increase glucose levels.

- Failure to follow dietary and activity restrictions before the procedure may cause the procedure to be canceled or repeated.

Nursing Implications and Procedure • • • • • • • • • • •

Pretest:

➤ Inform the patient that the test is used to evaluate lactose intolerance and other malabsorption disorders.

➤ Obtain a history of the patient's complaints, including a list of known allergens (especially allergies or sensitivities to latex), and inform the appropriate health care practitioner accordingly.

➤ Obtain a history of the patient's gastrointestinal system and results of previously performed laboratory tests, surgical procedures, and other diagnostic procedures. For related laboratory tests, refer to the Gastrointestinal System table.

➤ Obtain a list of the medications the patient is taking, including herbs, nutritional supplements, and nutraceuticals. The requesting health care practitioner and laboratory should be advised if the patient regularly uses these products so that their effects can be taken into consideration when reviewing results.

➤ Review the procedure with the patient. Obtain the pediatric patient's weight to calculate dose of lactose to be administered. Inform the patient that multiple samples will be collected over a 90-minute interval. Inform the patient that each specimen collection takes approximately 5 to 10 minutes. Address concerns about pain related to the procedure. Inform the patient that the test may produce symptoms such as cramps and diarrhea. Instruct the patient not to smoke cigarettes or chew gum during the test. Explain to the patient that there may be some discomfort during the venipuncture.

➤ *Sensitivity to social and cultural issues,* as well as concern for modesty, is important in providing psychological support before, during, and after the procedure.

➤ Inform the patient that fasting for at least 12 hours before the test is required and that strenuous activity should also be avoided for at least 12 hours before the test.

➤ There are no medication restrictions, unless by medical direction.

Intratest:

➤ Ensure that the patient has complied with dietary and activity restrictions as well as other pretesting preparations; assure that food has been restricted for at least 12 hours prior to the procedure.

➤ If the patient has a history of severe allergic reaction to latex, care should be taken to avoid the use of equipment containing latex.

➤ Administer 50 g of lactose dissolved in a small amount of water to adults over a 5- to 10-minute period. Pediatric dosage is based on weight: 0.6 to 1.3 g lactose per kilogram of body weight for infants less than 12 months old; 1.7 g lactose per kilogram of body weight for children 1 to 12 years old. Record time of ingestion. Encourage the patient to drink one to two glasses of water.

➤ Instruct the patient to cooperate fully and to follow directions. Direct the patient to breathe normally and to avoid unnecessary movement.

➤ Observe standard precautions, and follow the general guidelines in Appendix A. Positively identify the patient, and label the appropriate tubes with the corresponding patient demographics, date, and time of collection. Perform a venipuncture; collect the specimen in a 5-mL red- or tiger-top tube or red pediatric Microtainer. Samples should be collected at baseline, 30, 45, 60, and 90 minutes. Record any symptoms the patient reports throughout the course of the test.

➤ Remove the needle, and apply a pressure dressing over the puncture site.

➤ Promptly transport the specimen to the laboratory for processing and analysis. Glucose values change rapidly in an unprocessed, unpreserved specimen; therefore, if a Microtainer is used, each sample should be transported immediately after collection.

➤ The results are recorded manually or in a computerized system for recall and postprocedure interpretation by the appropriate health care practitioner.

Post-test:

➤ Observe venipuncture site for bleeding or hematoma formation. Apply paper tape or other adhesive to hold pressure bandage in place, or replace with a plastic bandage.

➤ Instruct the patient that resuming his or her usual diet may not be possible if lactose intolerance is identified. Educate patients on the importance of following the dietary advice of a nutritionist to ensure proper nutritional balance.

➤ *Nutritional considerations:* Instruct the patient with lactose intolerance to avoid milk products and to carefully read labels on prepared products. Yogurt, which contains inactive lactase enzyme, may be ingested. The lactase in yogurt is activated by the temperature and pH of the duodenum and substitutes for the lack of endogenous lactase. Advise the patient that products such as Lactaid tablets or drops may allow ingestion of milk products without sequelae. Many lactose-free food products are now available in grocery stores.

➤ A written report of the examination will be sent to the requesting health care practitioner, who will discuss the results with the patient.

➤ Recognize anxiety related to test results, and be supportive of concerns related to a perceived change in lifestyle. Discuss the implications of abnormal test results on the patient's lifestyle. Provide teaching and information regarding the clinical implications of the test results, as appropriate.

➤ Reinforce information given by the patient's health care provider regarding further testing, treatment, or referral to another health care provider. Answer any questions or address any concerns voiced by the patient or family.

➤ Depending on the results of this procedure, additional testing may be performed to evaluate or monitor

progression of the disease process and determine the need for a change in therapy. Evaluate test results in relation to the patient's symptoms and other tests performed.

LAPAROSCOPY, ABDOMINAL

SYNONYM/ACRONYM: Abdominal peritoneoscopy.

AREA OF APPLICATION: Pelvis.

CONTRAST: Carbon dioxide (CO_2).

DESCRIPTION & RATIONALE: Abdominal or gastrointestinal laparoscopy provides direct visualization of the liver, gallbladder, spleen, and stomach after insufflation of carbon dioxide (CO_2). In this procedure, a rigid laparoscope is introduced into the body cavity through a 1- to 2-cm abdominal incision. The endoscope has a microscope to allow visualization of the organs, and it can be used to insert instruments for performing certain procedures, such as biopsy and tumor resection. Under general anesthesia, the peritoneal cavity is inflated with 2 to 3 L of CO_2. The gas distends the abdominal wall so that the instruments can be inserted safely. Advantages of this procedure compared to an open laparotomy include reduced pain, reduced length of stay at the hospital or surgical center, and reduced time off from work. ■

INDICATIONS:
- Assist in performing surgical procedures such as cholecystectomy, appendectomy, hernia repair, hiatal hernia repair, and bowel resection
- Detect cirrhosis of the liver
- Detect pancreatic disorders
- Evaluate abdominal pain or abdominal mass of unknown origin
- Evaluate abdominal trauma in an emergency
- Evaluate and treat appendicitis
- Evaluate the extent of splenomegaly due to portal hypertension
- Evaluate jaundice of unknown origin
- Obtain biopsy specimens of benign or cancerous tumors
- Stage neoplastic disorders such as lymphomas, Hodgkin's disease, and hepatic carcinoma

RESULT

Normal Findings:
- Normal appearance of the liver, spleen, gallbladder, pancreas, and other abdominal contents

Abnormal Findings:
- Abdominal adhesions
- Appendicitis
- Ascites
- Cancer of any of the organs
- Cirrhosis of the liver
- Gangrenous gallbladder
- Intra-abdominal bleeding
- Portal hypertension
- Splenomegaly

CRITICAL VALUES: N/A

INTERFERING FACTORS:

This procedure is contraindicated for:
- Patients who are pregnant or suspected of being pregnant, unless the potential benefits of the procedure far outweigh the risk of radiation exposure to the fetus
- Patients with bleeding disorders, especially those associated with uremia and cytotoxic chemotherapy
- Patients with cardiac conditions or dysrhythmias
- Patients with advanced respiratory or cardiovascular disease
- Patients with intestinal obstruction, abdominal mass, abdominal hernia, or suspected intra-abdominal hemorrhage
- Patients with a history of peritonitis or multiple abdominal operations causing dense adhesions

Factors that may impair clear visualization:
- Gas or feces in the gastrointestinal tract resulting from inadequate cleansing or failure to restrict food intake before the study
- Retained barium from a previous radiologic procedure
- Patients who are very obese, who may exceed the weight limit for the equipment
- Incorrect positioning of the patient, which may produce poor visualization of the area to be examined
- Inability of the patient to cooperate or remain still during the procedure because of age, significant pain, or mental status

Other considerations:
- The procedure may be terminated if chest pain or severe cardiac arrhythmias occur.
- Failure to follow dietary restrictions and other pretesting preparations may cause the procedure to be canceled or repeated.
- Patients who are in a hypoxemic or hypercapnic state will require continuous oxygen administration.
- Patients with acute infection or advanced malignancy involving the abdominal wall are at increased risk because organisms may be introduced into the normally sterile peritoneal cavity.

Nursing Implications and Procedure • • • • • • • • • • •

Pretest:

➤ Inform the patient that the procedure assesses the abdominal organs.

➤ Obtain a history of the patient's complaints, including a list of known allergens, especially allergies or sensitivities to latex, iodine, seafood, contrast medium, and dyes. Assess if the patient has an allergy to local anesthetics, and inform the health care practitioner accordingly.

➤ Obtain a history of the patient's gastrointestinal, genitourinary, reproductive, and hepatobiliary systems, as well as results of previously performed diagnostic procedures, surgical procedures, and laboratory tests. For related diagnostic tests, refer to the Gastrointestinal, Genitourinary, Reproductive, and Hepatobiliary System tables.

➤ Ensure that this procedure is performed before an upper gastrointestinal study or barium swallow.

➤ Record the date of the last menstrual period and determine the possibility of pregnancy in perimenopausal women.

➤ Obtain a list of the medications the patient is taking.

➤ Review the procedure with the patient. Address concerns about pain related to the procedure. Explain to the patient that some pain may be experienced during the test, and there may be moments of discomfort. Explain the purpose of the test and how the procedure is performed. Inform the patient that the procedure is performed in a surgery department, usually by a health care practitioner and support staff, and takes approximately 30 to 60 minutes.

➤ Explain that an intravenous (IV) line may be inserted to allow infusion of IV fluids, anesthetics, analgesics, or IV sedation.

➤ *Sensitivity to cultural and social issues, as well as concern for modesty, is important in providing psychological support before, during, and after the procedure.*

➤ Instruct the patient to fast and restrict fluids for 8 hours prior to the procedure.

➤ Inform the patient that a laxative and cleansing enema may be needed the day before the procedure, with cleansing enemas on the morning of the procedure, depending on the institution's policy.

➤ Instruct the patient to remove jewelry (including watches), credit cards, and other metallic objects.

➤ *Make sure a written and informed consent has been signed prior to the procedure and before administering any medications.*

Intratest:

➤ Ensure that the patient has complied with dietary and medication restrictions and pretesting preparations for at least 8 hours prior to the procedure. Ensure that the patient has removed all external metallic objects prior to the procedure.

➤ Ensure that nonallergy to anesthesia is confirmed before the procedure is performed under general anesthesia.

➤ Assess for completion of bowel preparation according to the institution's procedure.

➤ Have emergency equipment readily available.

➤ Patients are given a gown, robe, and foot coverings to wear and instructed to void prior to the procedure.

➤ Instruct the patient to cooperate fully and to follow directions. Instruct the patient to remain still throughout the procedure because movement produces unreliable results.

➤ Obtain and record baseline vital signs.

➤ Observe standard precautions, and follow the general guidelines in Appendix A.

➤ Administer medications, as ordered, to reduce discomfort and to promote relaxation and sedation.

➤ Insert an IV line or venous access device at a low "keep open" rate.

➤ Place the patient on the laparoscopy table. If general anesthesia is to be used, it is administered at this time. Then place the patient in a modified lithotomy position with the head tilted downward. Cleanse the abdomen with an antiseptic solution, and drape and catheterize the patient, if ordered.

➤ The physician identifies the site for the scope insertion, and administers local anesthesia if that is to be used. After deeper layers are anesthetized, a pneumoperitoneum needle is placed between the visceral and parietal peritoneum.

➤ CO_2 is insufflated through the pneumoperitoneum needle to separate the abdominal wall from the viscera and to aid in visualization of the abdominal structures. The pneumoperitoneum needle is removed, and the trocar and laparoscope are inserted through the incision.

➤ After the examination, collection of tissue samples, and performance of therapeutic procedures, the scope is withdrawn. All possible CO_2 is evacuated via the trocar, which is then removed. The skin incision is closed with sutures, clips, or sterile strips, and a small dressing or adhesive strip is applied.

Post-test:

➤ Monitor vital signs and neurologic status every 15 minutes for 1 hour, then every 2 hours for 4 hours, and as ordered. Take temperature every 4 hours for 24 hours. Compare with baseline values. Notify the health care practitioner if temperature is elevated. Protocols may vary from facility to facility.

➤ Instruct the patient to resume usual diet, fluids, and medication, as directed by the health care practitioner.

➤ Instruct the patient to restrict activity for 2 to 7 days after the procedure.

➤ If indicated, inform the patient of a follow-up appointment for the removal of sutures.

➤ Inform the patient that shoulder discomfort may be experienced for 1 or 2 days after the procedure as a result of abdominal distention caused by insufflation of CO_2 into the abdomen, and that mild analgesics and cold compresses, as ordered, can be used to relieve the discomfort.

➤ Emphasize that any persistent shoulder pain, abdominal pain, vaginal bleeding, fever, redness, or swelling of the incisional area must be reported to the health care practitioner immediately.

➤ A written report of the examination will be completed by a health care practitioner specializing in this branch of medicine. The report will be sent to the requesting health care practitioner, who will discuss the results with the patient.

➤ Recognize anxiety related to test results. Discuss the implications of abnormal test results on the patient's lifestyle. Provide teaching and information regarding the clinical implications of the test results, as appropriate.

➤ Reinforce information given by the patient's health care provider regarding further testing, treatment, or referral to another health care provider. Answer any questions or address any concerns voiced by the patient or family.

➤ Depending on the results of this procedure, additional testing may be needed to evaluate or monitor progression of the disease process and determine the need for a change in therapy. Evaluate test results in relation to the patient's symptoms and other tests performed.

Related diagnostic tests:

➤ Related diagnostic tests include computed tomography of the abdomen; hepatobiliary scan; kidney, ureter, and bladder study; magnetic resonance imaging of the abdomen; and ultrasound of the abdomen.

LAPAROSCOPY, GYNECOLOGIC

SYNONYMS/ACRONYM: Gynecologic pelviscopy, gynecologic laparoscopy, pelvic endoscopy, peritoneoscopy.

AREA OF APPLICATION: Pelvis.

CONTRAST: Carbon dioxide (CO_2).

DESCRIPTION & RATIONALE: Gynecologic laparoscopy provides direct visualization of the internal pelvic contents, including the ovaries, fallopian tubes, and uterus, after insufflation of carbon dioxide (CO_2). It is done to diagnose and treat pelvic organ disorders, as well as to perform surgical procedures on the organs. In this procedure, a rigid laparoscope is introduced into the body cavity through a 1- to 2-cm periumbilical incision. The endoscope has a microscope to allow visualization of the organs, and it can be used to insert instruments for performing certain procedures, such as biopsy and tumor resection. Under general or local anesthesia, the peritoneal cavity is inflated with 2 to 3 L of CO_2. The gas distends the abdominal wall so that the instruments can be inserted safely. Advantages of this procedure compared to an open laparotomy include reduced pain, reduced length of stay at the hospital or surgical center, and reduced time off from work. ■

INDICATIONS:
- Detect ectopic pregnancy and determine the need for surgery
- Detect pelvic inflammatory disease or abscess

- Detect uterine fibroids, ovarian cysts, and uterine malformations (ovarian cysts may be aspirated during the procedure)
- Evaluate amenorrhea and infertility
- Evaluate fallopian tubes and anatomic defects to determine the cause of infertility
- Evaluate known or suspected endometriosis, salpingitis, and hydrosalpinx
- Evaluate pelvic pain or masses of unknown cause
- Evaluate reproductive organs after therapy for infertility
- Obtain biopsy specimens to confirm suspected pelvic malignancies or metastasis
- Perform tubal sterilization and ovarian biopsy
- Perform vaginal hysterectomy
- Remove adhesions or foreign bodies such as intrauterine devices (IUDs)
- Treat endometriosis through electrocautery or laser vaporization

RESULT

Normal Findings:
- Normal appearance of uterus, ovaries, fallopian tubes, and other pelvic contents

Abnormal Findings:
- Ectopic pregnancy
- Endometriosis
- Ovarian cyst
- Ovarian tumor
- Pelvic adhesions
- Pelvic inflammatory disease
- Pelvic tumor
- Salpingitis
- Uterine fibroids

CRITICAL VALUES: N/A

INTERFERING FACTORS:

This procedure is contraindicated for:
- Patients who are pregnant or suspected of being pregnant, unless the potential benefits of the procedure far outweigh the risks to the fetus and mother
- Patients with bleeding disorders, especially those associated with uremia and cytotoxic chemotherapy
- Patients with cardiac conditions or dysrhythmias
- Patients with advanced respiratory or cardiovascular disease
- Patients with intestinal obstruction, abdominal mass, abdominal hernia, or suspected intra-abdominal hemorrhage

Factors that may impair clear visualization:
- Gas or feces in the gastrointestinal tract resulting from inadequate cleansing or failure to restrict food intake before the study
- Retained barium from a previous radiologic procedure
- Patients who are very obese, who may exceed the weight limit for the equipment

- Incorrect positioning of the patient, which may produce poor visualization of the area to be examined
- Inability of the patient to cooperate or remain still during the procedure because of age, significant pain, or mental status

Other considerations:
- The procedure may be terminated if chest pain or severe cardiac arrhythmias occur.
- Failure to follow dietary restrictions and other pretesting preparations may cause the procedure to be canceled or repeated.
- Patients who are in a hypoxemic or hypercapnic state will require continuous oxygen administration.
- Patients with acute infection or advanced malignancy involving the abdominal wall are at increased risk because organisms may be introduced into the normally sterile peritoneal cavity

Nursing Implications and Procedure

Pretest:

▶ Inform the patient that the procedure assesses the abdominal and pelvic organs.

▶ Obtain a history of the patient's complaints, including a list of known allergens, especially allergies or sensitivities to latex, iodine, seafood, contrast medium, and dyes. Assess if the patient has an allergy to local anesthetics, and inform the health care practitioner accordingly.

▶ Obtain a history of the patient's gastrointestinal, genitourinary, and reproductive systems, as well as results of previously performed diagnostic procedures, surgical procedures, and laboratory tests. For related diagnostic tests, refer to the

Gastrointestinal, Genitourinary, and Reproductive System tables.

➤ Ensure that this procedure is performed before an upper gastrointestinal study or barium swallow.

➤ Record the date of the last menstrual period and determine the possibility of pregnancy in perimenopausal women.

➤ Obtain a list of the medications the patient is taking.

➤ Review the procedure with the patient. Address concerns about pain related to the procedure. Explain to the patient that some pain may be experienced during the test, and there may be moments of discomfort. Explain the purpose of the test and how the procedure is performed. Inform the patient that the procedure is performed in a surgery department, usually by a health care practitioner and support staff and takes approximately 30 to 60 minutes.

➤ *Sensitivity to cultural and social issues,* as well as concern for modesty, is important in providing psychological support before, during, and after the procedure.

➤ Explain that an intravenous (IV) line may be inserted to allow infusion of IV fluids, anesthetics, analgesics, or IV sedation.

➤ Instruct the patient to fast and restrict fluids for 8 hours prior to the procedure.

➤ Inform the patient that a laxative and cleansing enema may be needed the day before the procedure, with cleansing enemas on the morning of the procedure, depending on the institution's policy.

➤ Instruct the patient to remove jewelry (including watches), credit cards, and other metallic objects.

➤ *Make sure a written and informed consent has been signed prior to the procedure and before administering any medications.*

Intratest:

➤ Ensure that the patient has complied with dietary, and medication restric-

tions and pretesting preparations for at least 8 hours prior to the procedure. Ensure the patient has removed all external metallic objects prior to the procedure.

➤ Ensure that nonallergy to anesthesia is confirmed before the procedure is performed under general anesthesia.

➤ Assess for completion of bowel preparation according to the institution's procedure.

➤ Have emergency equipment readily available.

➤ Patients are given a gown, robe, and foot coverings to wear and instructed to void prior to the procedure.

➤ Instruct the patient to cooperate fully and to follow directions. Instruct the patient to remain still throughout the procedure because movement produces unreliable results.

➤ Obtain and record baseline vital signs.

➤ Observe standard precautions, and follow the general guidelines in Appendix A.

➤ Administer medications, as ordered, to reduce discomfort and to promote relaxation and sedation.

➤ Insert an IV line or venous access device at a low "keep open" rate.

➤ Place the patient on the laparoscopy table. If general anesthesia is to be used, it is administered at this time. Then place the patient in a modified lithotomy position with the head tilted downward. Cleanse the abdomen with an antiseptic solution, and drape and catheterize the patient, if ordered.

➤ The physician identifies the site for the scope insertion, and administers local anesthesia if that is to be used. After deeper layers are anesthetized, a pneumoperitoneum needle is placed between the visceral and parietal peritoneum.

➤ CO_2 is insufflated through the pneumoperitoneum needle to separate the abdominal wall from the viscera and to aid in visualization of the abdominal structures. The pneumoperitoneum needle is removed, and the trocar and laparoscope are inserted through the incision.

> The physician inserts a uterine manipulator through the vagina and cervix and into the uterus so that the uterus, fallopian tubes, and ovaries can be moved to permit better visualization.

> After the examination, collection of tissue samples, and performance of therapeutic procedures (e.g., tubal ligation), the scope is withdrawn. All possible CO_2 is evacuated via the trocar, which is then removed. The skin incision is closed with sutures, clips, or sterile strips, and a small dressing or adhesive strip is applied. After the perineum is cleansed, the uterine manipulator is removed and a sterile pad applied.

Post-test:

> Monitor vital signs and neurologic status every 15 minutes for 1 hour, then every 2 hours for 4 hours, and as ordered. Take temperature every 4 hours for 24 hours. Compare with baseline values. Notify the health care practitioner if temperature is elevated. Protocols may vary from facility to facility.

> Instruct the patient to resume usual diet, fluids, and medication, as directed by the health care practitioner.

> Instruct the patient to restrict activity for 2 to 7 days after the procedure.

> If indicated, inform the patient of a follow-up appointment for the removal of sutures.

> Inform the patient that shoulder discomfort may be experienced for 1 or 2 days after the procedure as a result of abdominal distention caused by insufflation of CO_2 into the abdomen,

and that mild analgesics and cold compresses, as ordered, can be used to relieve the discomfort.

> Emphasize that any persistent shoulder pain, abdominal pain, vaginal bleeding, fever, redness, or swelling of the incisional area must be reported to the health care practitioner immediately.

> A written report of the examination will be completed by a health care practitioner specializing in this branch of medicine. The report will be sent to the requesting health care practitioner, who will discuss the results with the patient.

> Recognize anxiety related to test results. Discuss the implications of abnormal test results on the patient's lifestyle. Provide teaching and information regarding the clinical implications of the test results, as appropriate.

> Reinforce information given by the patient's health care provider regarding further testing, treatment, or referral to another health care provider. Answer any questions or address any concerns voiced by the patient or family.

> Depending on the results of this procedure, additional testing may be needed to evaluate or monitor progression of the disease process and determine the need for a change in therapy. Evaluate test results in relation to the patient's symptoms and other tests performed.

Related diagnostic tests:

> Related diagnostic tests include computed tomography of the abdomen; hepatobiliary scan; kidney, ureter, and bladder study; magnetic resonance imaging of the abdomen; and ultrasound of the abdomen.

LATEX ALLERGY

· ·

SYNONYM/ACRONYM: N/A.

SPECIMEN: Serum (1 mL) collected in a red-top tube.

REFERENCE VALUE: (Method: Immunoassay) Negative.

DESCRIPTION & RATIONALE: Latex is found in numerous medical supplies, such as gloves, catheters, and bandages. Some individuals who are routinely exposed to latex products, particularly as part of their occupation, have become highly allergic to latex. Health care workers are classified as high risk, especially since the 1987 mandate of standard/universal precautions that resulted in increased use of latex gloves. It is estimated that 8% to 17% of health care workers have become allergic to latex. There are two types of allergic reactions. Type IV allergic contact dermatitis is caused by chemicals used in the process of manufacturing latex. It is a delayed reaction occurring within 6 to 48 hours of direct skin or mucous membrane contact with latex products. The type I allergic reaction occurs in response to proteins in the natural latex products by direct skin or mucous membrane contact or by inhaling aerosolized powder from a latex glove. Other high-risk individuals include people with spina bifida, spinal cord injury, myelodysplasia, atopic dermatitis, eczema, history of allergies (personal or family), history of chronic illness, or multiple surgeries. ■

INDICATIONS: Suspected latex allergy

RESULT

Positive findings in: Latex allergy

Negative findings in: N/A

CRITICAL VALUES: N/A

INTERFERING FACTORS: N/A

Nursing Implications and Procedure · · · · · · · · · · · ·

Pretest:

➤ Inform the patient that the test is used to detect latex sensitivity.

➤ Obtain a history of the patient's complaints, including a list of known allergens, and inform the appropriate health care practitioner accordingly.

➤ Obtain a history of the patient's immune system, a history of latex exposure, and results of previously performed laboratory tests, surgical procedures, and other diagnostic procedures. For related laboratory tests, refer to the Immune System table.

➤ Obtain a list of the medications the patient is taking, including herbs, nutritional supplements, and nutraceuticals. The requesting health care practitioner and laboratory should be advised if the patient regularly uses these products so that their effects can be taken into consideration when reviewing results.

➤ Review the procedure with the patient. Inform the patient that specimen collection takes approximately 5 to 10 minutes. Address concerns about pain related to the procedure. Explain to the patient that there may be some discomfort during the venipuncture.

➤ There are no food, fluid, or medication restrictions, unless by medical direction.

Intratest:

➤ If the patient has a history of severe allergic reaction to latex, care should be taken to avoid the use of equipment containing latex.

➤ Instruct the patient to cooperate fully and to follow directions. Direct the patient to breathe normally and to avoid unnecessary movement.

➤ Observe standard precautions, and follow the general guidelines in Appendix A. Positively identify the patient, and label the appropriate tubes with the corresponding patient demographics, date, and time of collection. Perform a venipuncture; collect the specimen in a 5-mL red-top tube.

➤ Remove the needle, and apply a pressure dressing over the puncture site.

➤ Promptly transport the specimen to the laboratory for processing and analysis.

➤ The results are recorded manually or in a computerized system for recall and postprocedure interpretation by the appropriate health care practitioner.

Post-test:

➤ Observe venipuncture site for bleeding or hematoma formation. Apply paper tape or other adhesive to hold pressure bandage in place, or replace with a plastic bandage.

➤ Assist the patient, as appropriate, in identifying sources of exposure in order for the patient to eliminate or reduce the opportunity for continued exposure.

➤ A written report of the examination will be sent to the requesting health care practitioner, who will discuss the results with the patient.

➤ Reinforce information given by the patient's health care provider regarding further testing, treatment, or referral to another health care provider. Answer any questions or address any concerns voiced by the patient or family.

➤ Depending on the results of this procedure, additional testing may be performed to evaluate or monitor progression of the disease process and determine the need for a change in therapy. Evaluate test results in relation to the patient's symptoms and other tests performed.

Related laboratory tests:

➤ Related laboratory tests include complete blood count, eosinophil count, and immunoglobulin E.

LEAD

SYNONYM/ACRONYM: Pb.

SPECIMEN: Whole blood (1 mL) collected in a special lead-free royal blue– or tan-top tube. Plasma (1 mL) collected in lavender-top (EDTA) tube is also acceptable.

REFERENCE VALUE: (Method: Atomic absorption spectrophotometry)

	Conventional Units	SI Units (Conventional Units × 0.0483)
Children	0–9.9 μg/dL	0–0.48 μmol/L
Adults	0–25.0 μg/dL	0–1.20 μmol/L
OSHA action limit for occupational exposure	Up to 40 μg/dL	Up to 1.93 μmol/L

OSHA = Occupational Safety and Health Administration.

DESCRIPTION & RATIONALE: Lead is a heavy metal and trace element. It is absorbed through the respiratory and gastrointestinal systems. It can also be transported from mother to fetus through the placenta. When there is frequent exposure to lead-containing items (e.g., paint, batteries, gasoline, pottery, bullets, printing materials) or occupations (mining, automobile, printing, and welding industries), many organs of the body are affected. Lead poisoning can cause severe behavioral and neurologic effects. The blood test is considered the best indicator of lead poisoning, and confirmation is made by the lead mobilization test performed on a 24-hour urine specimen. ▪

INDICATIONS: Assist in the diagnosis and treatment of lead poisoning

RESULT

Increased in:

• Anemia of lead intoxication

• Lead encephalopathy

• Metal poisoning

Decreased in: N/A

CRITICAL VALUES:

Levels greater than 30 μg/dL indicate significant exposure.

Levels greater than 60 μg/dL require chelation therapy.

Note and immediately report to the health care practitioner any critically increased values and related symptoms.

INTERFERING FACTORS: Contamination of the collection site and/or specimen with lead in dust can be avoided by taking special care to have the surfaces surrounding the collection location cleaned. Extra care should also be used to avoid contamination during the actual venipuncture.

Nursing Implications and Procedure . . . .

Pretest:

➤ Inform the patient that the test is used to detect lead toxicity and monitor exposure to lead.

➤ Obtain a history of the patient's complaints, including a list of known allergens (especially allergies or sensitivities to latex), and inform the appropriate health care practitioner accordingly.

➤ Obtain a history of the patient's hematopoietic system and results of previously performed laboratory tests, surgical procedures, and other diagnostic procedures. For related laboratory tests, refer to the Hematopoietic System and Therapeutic/Toxicology tables.

➤ Obtain a history of the patient's exposure to lead.

➤ Obtain a list of the medications the patient is taking, including herbs, nutritional supplements, and nutraceuticals. The requesting health care practitioner and laboratory should be advised if the patient regularly uses these products so that their effects can be taken into consideration when reviewing results.

➤ Review the procedure with the patient. Inform the patient that specimen collection takes approximately 5 to 10 minutes. Address concerns about pain related to the procedure. Explain to the patient that there may be some discomfort during the venipuncture.

➤ There are no food, fluid, or medica-

tion restrictions, unless by medical direction.

Intratest:

➤ If the patient has a history of severe allergic reaction to latex, care should be taken to avoid the use of equipment containing latex.

➤ Instruct the patient to cooperate fully and to follow directions. Direct the patient to breathe normally and to avoid unnecessary movement.

➤ Observe standard precautions, and follow the general guidelines in Appendix A. Positively identify the patient, and label the appropriate tubes with the corresponding patient demographics, date, and time of collection. Perform a venipuncture; collect the specimen in a 5-mL royal blue– or tan-top tube.

➤ Remove the needle, and apply a pressure dressing over the puncture site.

➤ Promptly transport the specimen to the laboratory for processing and analysis.

➤ The results are recorded manually or in a computerized system for recall and postprocedure interpretation by the appropriate health care practitioner.

Post-test:

➤ Observe venipuncture site for bleeding or hematoma formation. Apply paper tape or other adhesive to hold pressure bandage in place, or replace with a plastic bandage.

➤ A written report of the examination will be sent to the requesting health care practitioner, who will discuss the results with the patient.

➤ Reinforce information given by the patient's health care practitioner regarding further testing, treatment, or referral to another health care practitioner. Answer any questions or address any concerns voiced by the patient or family.

➤ Depending on the results of this procedure, additional testing may be

performed to evaluate or monitor progression of the disease process and determine the need for a change in therapy. Evaluate test results in relation to the patient's symptoms and other tests performed.

LECITHIN/SPHINGOMYELIN RATIO

SYNONYM/ACRONYM: L/S ratio.

SPECIMEN: Amniotic fluid (10 mL) collected in a sterile, brown glass or plastic tube or bottle protected from light.

REFERENCE VALUE: (Method: Thin-layer chromatography)
Mature (nondiabetic): Greater than 2:1 in the presence of phosphatidyl glycerol
Borderline: 1.5 to 1.9:1
Immature: Less than 1.5:1

DESCRIPTION & RATIONALE: Respiratory distress syndrome (RDS) is the most common problem encountered in the care of premature infants. RDS, also called hyaline membrane disease, results from a deficiency of phospholipid lung surfactants. The phospholipids in surfactant are produced by specialized alveolar cells and stored in granular lamellar bodies in the lung. In normally developed lungs, surfactant coats the surface of the alveoli. Surfactant reduces the surface tension of the alveolar wall during breathing. When there is an insufficient quantity of surfactant, the alveoli are unable to expand normally and gas exchange is inhibited. Amniocentesis, a procedure by which fluid is removed from the amniotic sac, is used to assess fetal lung maturity.

Lecithin is the primary surfactant phospholipid, and it is a stabilizing factor for the alveoli. It is produced at a low but constant rate until the 35th week of gestation, after which its production sharply increases. Sphingomyelin, another phospholipid component of surfactant, is also produced at a constant rate after the 26th week of gestation. Before the 35th week, the lecithin/sphingomyelin (L/S) ratio is usually less than 1.6:1. The ratio increases to 2.0 or greater when the rate of lecithin production increases after the 35th week of gestation. Other phospholipids, such as phosphatidyl glycerol (PG) and phosphatidyl inositol (PI), increase over time in amniotic fluid as well. The presence of PG indicates that the fetus is within 2 to 6 weeks of lung maturity (i.e., at full term). Simultaneous measurement of PG with the L/S ratio improves diagnostic accuracy. Production of phospholipid surfactant is delayed in diabetic mothers. Therefore, caution must be used when interpreting the results obtained from a diabetic patient, and a higher ratio is expected to predict maturity. ■

INDICATIONS:

• Assist in the evaluation of fetal lung maturity

• Determine the optimal time for obstetric intervention in cases of threatened fetal survival caused by stresses related to maternal diabetes, toxemia, hemolytic diseases of the newborn, or postmaturity

• Identify fetuses at risk of developing RDS

RESULT

Increased in:

• Hypertension

• Intrauterine growth retardation

• Malnutrition

• Maternal diabetes

• Placenta previa

• Placental infarction

• Premature rupture of the membranes

Decreased in:

• Advanced maternal age

• Immature fetal lungs

• Multiple gestation

• Polyhydramnios

CRITICAL VALUES:

An L/S ratio less than 1.5:1 is predictive of RDS at the time of delivery.

Note and immediately report to the health care practitioner any critically increased or decreased values and related symptoms. Infants known to be at risk for RDS can be treated with surfactant by intratracheal administration at birth.

INTERFERING FACTORS:

• Fetal blood falsely elevates the L/S ratio.

• Exposing the specimen to light may cause falsely decreased values.

• There is some risk to having an amniocentesis performed, and this should be weighed against the need to obtain the desired diagnostic information. A small percentage (0.5%) of patients have experienced complications including premature rupture of the membranes, premature labor, spontaneous abortion, and stillbirth.

Nursing Implications and Procedure . . . .

Pretest:

➤ Inform the patient that the test is primarily used to obtain an estimate of fetal age.

➤ Obtain a history of the patient's complaints, including a list of known allergens (especially allergies or sensitivities to latex), and inform the appropriate health care practitioner accordingly.

➤ Obtain a history of the patient's reproductive and respiratory systems and results of previously performed laboratory tests, surgical procedures, and other diagnostic procedures. Include any family history of genetic disorders such as cystic fibrosis, Duchenne's muscular dystrophy, hemophilia, sickle cell disease, Tay-Sachs disease, thalassemia, and trisomy 21. Obtain maternal Rh type.

If Rh-negative, check for prior sensitization. A standard RhoGAM dose is indicated after amniocentesis; repeat doses should be considered if repeated amniocentesis is performed. For related laboratory tests, refer to the Reproductive and Respiratory System tables.

➤ Record the date of the last menstrual period, and determine that the pregnancy is in the third trimester between the 28th and 40th weeks.

➤ Obtain a list of the medications the patient is taking, including herbs, nutritional supplements, and nutraceuticals. The requesting health care practitioner and laboratory should be advised if the patient regularly uses these products so that their effects can be taken into consideration when reviewing results.

➤ Review the procedure with the patient. Warn the patient that normal results do not guarantee a normal fetus. Assure the patient that precautions to avoid injury to the fetus will be taken by localizing the fetus with ultrasound. Address concerns about pain related to the procedure. Explain that during the transabdominal procedure, any discomfort with a needle biopsy will be minimized with local anesthetics. Patients who are at 20 weeks' gestation or beyond should void before the test, because an empty bladder is less likely to be accidentally punctured during specimen collection. Encourage relaxation and controlled breathing during the procedure to aid in reducing any mild discomfort. Inform the patient that specimen collection is performed by health care practitioner specializing in this procedure and usually takes approximately 20 to 30 minutes to complete.

➤ *Sensitivity to social and cultural issues,* as well as concern for modesty, is important in providing psychological support before, during, and after the procedure.

➤ There are no food, fluid, or medication restrictions, unless by medical direction.

➤ *Make sure a written and informed consent has been signed prior to the procedure and before administering any medications.*

Intratest:

➤ Ensure that the patient has voided before the procedure if gestation is 21 weeks or more.

➤ Have emergency equipment readily available.

➤ Have patient remove clothes below the waist. Assist the patient to a supine position on the exam table with abdomen exposed. Drape the patient's legs, leaving the abdomen exposed. Raise her head or legs slightly to promote comfort and to relax abdominal muscles. If the uterus is large, place a pillow or rolled blanket under the patient's right side to prevent hypertension caused by great-vessel compression.

➤ Instruct the patient to cooperate fully and to follow directions. Direct the patient to breathe normally and to avoid unnecessary movement during the local anesthetic and the procedure.

➤ Record maternal and fetal baseline vital signs and continue to monitor throughout the procedure. Monitor for uterine contractions. Monitor fetal vital signs using ultrasound. Protocols may vary from facility to facility.

➤ Observe standard precautions, and follow the general guidelines in Appendix A. Positively identify the patient, and label the appropriate collection containers with the corresponding patient demographics, date and time of collection, and site location.

➤ Assess the position of the amniotic fluid, fetus, and placenta using ultrasound.

➤ Assemble the necessary equipment, including an amniocentesis tray with solution for skin preparation, local anesthetic, 10- or 20-mL syringe, needles of various sizes (including a 22-gauge, 5-inch spinal needle), sterile drapes, sterile gloves, and foil-covered or amber specimen collection containers.

➤ Cleanse suprapubic area with an antiseptic solution and protect with sterile drapes. A local anesthetic is injected. Explain that this may cause a stinging sensation.

➤ A 22-gauge, 5-inch spinal needle is inserted through the abdominal and uterine walls. Explain that a sensation of pressure may be experienced when the needle is inserted. Explain to the patient how to use focusing and controlled breathing for relaxation during the procedure.

➤ After the fluid is collected and the needle withdrawn, apply slight pressure to the site. Apply a sterile adhesive bandage to the site.

➤ Monitor the patient for complications related to the procedure (e.g., premature labor, allergic reaction, anaphylaxis).

➤ Place samples in properly labeled specimen container and promptly transport the specimen to the laboratory for processing and analysis.

➤ The results are recorded manually or in a computerized system for recall and postprocedure interpretation by the appropriate health care practitioner.

Post-test:

➤ ⚠ Fetal heart rate and maternal vital signs (i.e., heart rate, blood pressure, pulse, and respiration) must be compared to baseline values and closely monitored every 15 minutes for 30 to 60 minutes after the amniocentesis procedure. Protocols may vary from facility to facility

➤ Observe for delayed allergic reactions, such as rash, urticaria, tachycardia, hyperpnea, hypertension, palpitations, nausea, or vomiting.

➤ Observe the amniocentesis site for bleeding, inflammation, or hematoma formation.

➤ Instruct the patient in the care and assessment of the amniocentesis site. Instruct the patient to report any redness, edema, bleeding, or pain at the site. Instruct the patient to keep the site clean and change the dressing as needed.

➤ Instruct the patient to expect mild cramping, leakage of small amount of amniotic fluic, and vaginal spotting for up to 2 days following the procedure. Instruct the patient to immediately report moderate to severe abdominal pain or cramps, change in fetal activity, increased or prolonged leaking of amniotic fluid from abdominal needle site, vaginal bleeding that is heavier than spotting, and either chills or fever to the health care practitioner.

➤ Instruct the patient to rest until all symptoms have disappeared before resuming normal levels of activity.

➤ Administer standard RhoGAM dose to maternal Rh-negative patients to prevent maternal Rh sensitization should the fetus be Rh-positive.

➤ Administer mild analgesic and antibiotic therapy as ordered. Remind the patient of the importance of completing the entire course of antibiotic therapy, even if signs and symptoms disappear before completion of therapy.

➤ A written report of the examination will be completed by a health care practitioner specializing in this branch of medicine. The report will be sent to the requesting health care practitioner, who will discuss the results with the patient.

➤ Recognize anxiety related to test results, and offer support. Provide teaching and information regarding the clinical implications of the test results, as appropriate. Encourage the family to seek counseling if concerned with pregnancy termination or to seek genetic counseling if a chromosomal abnormality is determined. Provide teaching and information regarding the clinical implications of the test results, as appropriate. Decisions regarding elective abortion should take place in the presence of both parents. Provide a nonjudgmental, nonthreatening atmosphere for discussing the risks and difficulties of delivering and raising a developmentally challenged infant, as well as exploring other options (termination of pregnancy or adoption). It is also important to discuss feelings the mother and father may experience (e.g., guilt, depression, anger) if fetal abnormalities are detected.

➤ Reinforce information given by the patient's health care provider regarding further testing, treatment, or referral to another health care provider. Answer any questions or address any concerns voiced by the patient or family.

➤ Instruct the patient in the use of any ordered medications. Explain the importance of adhering to the therapy regimen. As appropriate, instruct the patient in significant side effects and systemic reactions associated with the prescribed medication. Encourage her to review corresponding literature provided by a pharmacist.

➤ Depending on the results of this procedure, additional testing may be performed to evaluate or monitor progression of the disease process and determine the need for a change in therapy. Evaluate test results in relation to the patient's symptoms and other tests performed.

Related laboratory tests:

➤ Related laboratory tests include amniotic fluid analysis, blood groups and antibodies, chromosome analysis, α-fetoprotein, and Kleihauer-Betke test.

LEUKOCYTE ALKALINE PHOSPHATASE

SYNONYMS/ACRONYM: LAP, LAP score, LAP smear.

SPECIMEN: Whole blood (1 mL) collected in a lavender-top (EDTA) tube.

REFERENCE VALUE: (Method: Microscopic evaluation of specially stained blood smears) 32 to 182 (score based on 0 to 4+ rating of 100 neutrophils).

DESCRIPTION & RATIONALE: Alkaline phosphatase is an enzyme important for intracellular metabolic processes. It is present in the cytoplasm of neutrophilic granulocytes from the metamyelocyte to the segmented stage. Leukocyte alkaline phosphatase (LAP) concentrations may be altered by the presence of infection, stress, chronic inflammatory diseases, Hodgkin's disease, and hematologic disorders. Levels are low in leukemic leukocytes and high in normal white blood cells (WBCs), making this test useful as a supportive test in the differential diagnosis of leukemia. It should be noted that test results must be correlated with the patient's condition because LAP levels increase toward normal in response to therapy. ■

INDICATIONS:

* Differentiate chronic myelocytic leukemia from other disorders that increase the WBC count
* Monitor response of Hodgkin's disease to therapy

RESULT

Increased in:

* Aplastic leukemia
* Chronic inflammation
* Down syndrome
* Hairy cell leukemia
* Hodgkin's disease
* Leukemia (acute and chronic lymphoblastic)
* Myelofibrosis with myeloid metaplasia
* Multiple myeloma
* Polycythemia vera
* Pregnancy
* Stress
* Thrombocytopenia

Decreased in:

* Chronic myelogenous leukemia
* Hereditary hypophosphatemia
* Idiopathic thrombocytopenia purpura
* Nephrotic syndrome
* Paroxysmal nocturnal hemoglobinuria
* Sickle cell anemia
* Sideroblastic anemia

CRITICAL VALUES: N/A

INTERFERING FACTORS: Drugs that may increase the LAP score include steroids.

Nursing Implications and Procedure • • • • • • • • • •

Pretest:

➤ Inform the patient that the test is used to evaluate disorders of the hematologic system.

➤ Obtain a history of the patient's complaints, including a list of known allergens (especially allergies or sensitivities to latex), and inform the appropriate health care practitioner accordingly.

➤ Obtain a history of the patient's hematopoietic and immune systems, as well as results of previously performed laboratory tests, surgical procedures, and other diagnostic procedures. For related laboratory tests, refer to the Hematopoietic and Immune System tables.

➤ Obtain a list of the medications the patient is taking, including herbs, nutritional supplements, and nutraceuticals. The requesting health care practitioner and laboratory should be advised if the patient regularly uses these products so that their effects can be taken into consideration when reviewing results.

➤ Review the procedure with the patient. Inform the patient that specimen collection takes approximately 5 to 10 minutes. Address concerns about pain related to the procedure. Explain to the patient that there may be some discomfort during the venipuncture.

➤ There are no food, fluid, or medication restrictions, unless by medical direction.

Intratest:

➤ If the patient has a history of severe allergic reaction to latex, care should be taken to avoid the use of equipment containing latex.

➤ Instruct the patient to cooperate fully and to follow directions. Direct the patient to breathe normally and to avoid unnecessary movement.

➤ Observe standard precautions, and follow the general guidelines in Appendix A. Positively identify the patient, and label the appropriate tubes with the corresponding patient demographics, date, and time of collection. Perform a venipuncture; collect the specimen in a 5-mL lavender-top tube.

➤ Remove the needle, and apply a pressure dressing over the puncture site.

➤ Promptly transport the specimen to the laboratory for processing and analysis.

➤ The results are recorded manually or in a computerized system for recall and postprocedure interpretation by the appropriate health care practitioner.

Post-test:

➤ Observe venipuncture site for bleeding or hematoma formation. Apply paper tape or other adhesive to hold pressure bandage in place, or replace with a plastic bandage.

➤ Instruct the patient to avoid exposure to infection if WBC count is decreased.

➤ A written report of the examination will be sent to the requesting health care practitioner, who will discuss the results with the patient.

➤ Recognize anxiety related to test results, and be supportive of perceived loss of independence and fear of shortened life expectancy. Discuss the implications of abnormal test results on the patient's lifestyle. Provide teaching and information regarding the clinical implications of the test results, as appropriate. Educate the patient regarding access to counseling services.

➤ Reinforce information given by the patient's health care provider regarding further testing, treatment, or referral to another health care provider. Answer any questions or address any concerns voiced by the patient or family.

➤ Depending on the results of this procedure, additional testing may be performed to evaluate or monitor progression of the disease process and determine the need for a change in therapy. Evaluate test results in relation to the patient's symptoms and other tests performed.

Related laboratory tests:

➤ Related laboratory tests include bone marrow biopsy and WBC count.

LIPASE

. . . .

SYNONYM/ACRONYM: Triacylglycerol acylhydrolase.

SPECIMEN: Serum (1 mL) collected in a red- or tiger-top tube. Plasma (1 mL) collected in green-top (heparin) tube is also acceptable.

REFERENCE VALUE: (Method: Spectrophotometry) Plasma values may be 15% lower than serum values.

Conventional & SI Units
40–375 U/L

DESCRIPTION & RATIONALE: Lipases are digestive enzymes secreted by the pancreas into the duodenum. Different lipolytic enzymes have specific substrates, but overall activity is collectively described as lipase. Lipase participates in fat digestion by breaking down triglycerides into fatty acids and glycerol. Lipase is released into the bloodstream when damage occurs to the pancreatic acinar cells. Its presence in the blood indicates pancreatic disease because the pancreas is the only organ that secretes this enzyme. ■

INDICATIONS:

• Assist in the diagnosis of acute and chronic pancreatitis

• Assist in the diagnosis of pancreatic carcinoma

RESULT

Increased in:

• Acute cholecystitis

• Obstruction of the pancreatic duct

• Pancreatic carcinoma (early)

• Pancreatic cyst or pseudocyst

• Pancreatic inflammation

• Pancreatitis (acute and chronic)

• Renal failure (early)

Decreased in: N/A

CRITICAL VALUES: N/A

INTERFERING FACTORS:

• Drugs that may increase lipase levels include asparaginase, azathioprine, cholinergics, codeine, deoxy-cholate, didanosine, glycocholate, indomethacin, methacholine, methyl-prednisolone, morphine, narcotics, pancreozymin, pentazocine, and tauro-cholate.

• Drugs that may decrease lipase levels include protamine and saline (intravenous infusions).

• Endoscopic retrograde cholangiopancreatography may increase lipase levels.

• Serum lipase levels increase with hemodialysis. Therefore, predialysis specimens should be collected for lipase analysis.

Nursing Implications and Procedure • • • • • • • • • • •

Pretest:

➤ Inform the patient that the test is primarily used to diagnose pancreatitis.

➤ Obtain a history of the patient's complaints, including a list of known allergens (especially allergies or sensitivities to latex), and inform the appropriate health care practitioner accordingly.

➤ Obtain a history of the patient's gastrointestinal and hepatobiliary systems, as well as results of previously performed laboratory tests, surgical procedures, and other diagnostic procedures. For related laboratory tests, refer to the Gastrointestinal and Hepatobiliary System tables.

➤ Note any recent procedures that can interfere with test results.

➤ Obtain a list of the medications the patient is taking, including herbs, nutritional supplements, and nutraceuticals. The requesting health care practitioner and laboratory should be advised if the patient regularly uses these products so that their effects can be taken into consideration when reviewing results.

➤ Review the procedure with the patient. Inform the patient that specimen collection takes approximately

5 to 10 minutes. Address concerns about pain related to the procedure. Explain to the patient that there may be some discomfort during the venipuncture.

➤ There are no food, fluid, or medication restrictions, unless by medical direction.

Intratest:

➤ If the patient has a history of severe allergic reaction to latex, care should be taken to avoid the use of equipment containing latex.

➤ Instruct the patient to cooperate fully and to follow directions. Direct the patient to breathe normally and to avoid unnecessary movement.

➤ Observe standard precautions, and follow the general guidelines in Appendix A. Positively identify the patient, and label the appropriate tubes with the corresponding patient demographics, date, and time of collection. Perform a venipuncture; collect the specimen in a 5-mL red- or tiger-top tube.

➤ Remove the needle, and apply a pressure dressing over the puncture site.

➤ Promptly transport the specimen to the laboratory for processing and analysis.

➤ The results are recorded manually or in a computerized system for recall and postprocedure interpretation by the appropriate health care practitioner.

Post-test:

➤ Observe venipuncture site for bleeding or hematoma formation. Apply paper tape or other adhesive to hold pressure bandage in place, or replace with a plastic bandage.

➤ *Nutritional considerations:* Instruct the patient to ingest small, frequent meals if he or she has a gastrointestinal disorder; advise the patient to consider other dietary alterations as well. After acute symptoms subside and bowel sounds return, patients are usually prescribed a clear liquid diet, progressing to a low-fat, high-carbohydrate diet.

➤ Administer vitamin B_{12}, as ordered, to the patient with decreased lipase levels, especially if his or her disease prevents adequate absorption of the vitamin.

➤ Encourage the alcoholic patient to avoid alcohol and to seek appropriate counseling for substance abuse.

➤ A written report of the examination will be sent to the requesting health care practitioner, who will discuss the results with the patient.

➤ Reinforce information given by the patient's health care provider regarding further testing, treatment, or referral to another health care provider. Answer any questions or address any concerns voiced by the patient or family.

➤ Depending on the results of this procedure, additional testing may be performed to evaluate or monitor progression of the disease process and determine the need for a change in therapy. Evaluate test results in relation to the patient's symptoms and other tests performed.

Related laboratory tests:

➤ Related laboratory tests include alanine aminotransferase, alkaline phosphatase, amylase, aspartate aminotransferase, bilirubin, CA 19-9, calcium, fecal fat, γ-glutamyltranspeptidase, magnesium, mumps serology, pleural fluid amylase, triglycerides, and white blood cell count.

LIPOPROTEIN ELECTROPHORESIS

. . . .

SYNONYMS/ACRONYMS: Lipid fractionation; lipoprotein phenotyping; $3ga_1$-lipoprotein cholesterol, high-density lipoprotein (HDL); β-lipoprotein cholesterol, low-density lipoprotein (LDL); pre-β-lipoprotein cholesterol, very-low-density lipoprotein (VLDL).

SPECIMEN: Serum (3 mL) collected in a red- or tiger-top tube.

REFERENCE VALUE: (Method: Electrophoresis and 4°C test for specimen appearance) There is no quantitative interpretation of this test. The specimen appearance and electrophoretic pattern is visually interpreted.

Hyperlipoproteinemia: Fredrickson Type	Specimen Appearance	Electrophoretic Pattern
Type I	Clear with creamy top layer	Heavy chylomicron band
Type IIa	Clear	Heavy β band
Type IIb	Clear or faintly turbid	Heavy β and pre-β band
Type III	Slightly to moderately turbid	Heavy β band
Type IV	Slightly to moderately turbid	Heavy pre-β band
Type V	Slightly to moderately turbid with creamy top layer	Intense chylomicron band and heavy pre-β band

DESCRIPTION & RATIONALE: Lipoprotein electrophoresis measures lipoprotein fractions to determine abnormal distribution and concentration of lipoproteins in the serum, an important risk factor in the development of coronary artery disease (CAD). The lipoprotein fractions, in order of increasing density, are (1) chylomicrons, (2) very-low-density lipoprotein (VLDL), (3) low-density lipoprotein (LDL), and (4) high-density lipoprotein (HDL). Chylomicrons and VLDL contain the highest levels of triglycerides and lower amounts of cholesterol and protein. LDL and HDL contain the lowest amounts of triglycerides and relatively higher amounts of cholesterol and protein. ▪

INDICATIONS:
- Evaluate known or suspected disorders associated with altered lipoprotein levels

- Evaluate patients with serum cholesterol levels greater than 250 mg/dL, which indicate a high risk for CAD

• Evaluate the response to treatment for high cholesterol, and determine the need for drug therapy

RESULT:

Type I: Hyperlipoproteinemia or increased chylomicrons can be primary, resulting from an inherited deficiency of lipoprotein lipase; or secondary, caused by uncontrolled diabetes, systemic lupus erythematosus, and dysgammaglobulinemia. Total cholesterol is normal to moderately elevated and triglycerides (mostly exogenous chylomicrons) are grossly elevated. If the condition is inherited, symptoms will appear in childhood.

Type IIa: Hyperlipoproteinemia can be primary, resulting from inherited characteristics, or secondary, caused by hypothyroidism, nephrotic syndrome, and dysgammaglobulinemia. Total cholesterol is elevated, triglycerides are normal, and LDL cholesterol (LDLC) is elevated. If the condition is inherited, symptoms will appear in childhood.

Type IIb: Hyperlipoproteinemia can occur for the same reasons as in type IIa. Total cholesterol, triglycerides, and LDLC are all elevated.

Type III: Hyperlipoproteinemia can be primary, resulting from inherited characteristics; or secondary, caused by hypothyroidism, uncontrolled diabetes, alcoholism, and dysgammaglobulinemia. Total cholesterol and triglycerides are elevated, whereas LDLC is normal.

Type IV: Hyperlipoproteinemia can be primary, resulting from

inherited characteristics; or secondary, caused by poorly controlled diabetes, alcoholism, nephrotic syndrome, chronic renal failure, and dysgammaglobulinemia. Total cholesterol is normal to moderately elevated, triglycerides are moderately to grossly elevated, and LDLC is normal.

Type V: Hyperlipoproteinemia can be primary, resulting from inherited characteristics; or secondary, caused by uncontrolled diabetes, alcoholism, nephrotic syndrome, and dysgammaglobulinemia. Total cholesterol is normal to moderately elevated, triglycerides are grossly elevated, and LDLC is normal.

CRITICAL VALUES: N/A

INTERFERING FACTORS:

• Failure to follow usual diet for 2 weeks before the test can yield results that do not accurately reflect the patient's cholesterol values.

• Ingestion of alcohol 24 hours before the test, ingestion of food 12 hours before the test, and excessive exercise 12 hours before the test can alter results.

• Numerous drugs can alter results (see monographs titled "Cholesterol, Total" and "Triglycerides").

• Failure to follow dietary restrictions before the procedure may cause the procedure to be canceled or repeated.

Nursing Implications and Procedure • • • • • • • • • • •

Pretest:

➤ Inform the patient that the test is used to assist in evaluating risk for cardiovascular disease.

➤ Obtain a history of the patient's complaints, including a list of known allergens (especially allergies or sensitivities to latex), and inform the appropriate health care practitioner accordingly.

➤ Obtain a history of the patient's cardiovascular system and risk for heart disease, as well as results of previously performed laboratory tests, surgical procedures, and other diagnostic procedures. For related laboratory tests, refer to the Cardiovascular System table.

➤ Obtain a list of the medications the patient is taking, including herbs, nutritional supplements, and nutraceuticals. The requesting health care practitioner and laboratory should be advised if the patient regularly uses these products so that their effects can be taken into consideration when reviewing results.

➤ Review the procedure with the patient. Inform the patient that specimen collection takes approximately 5 to 10 minutes. Address concerns about pain related to the procedure. Explain to the patient that there may be some discomfort during the venipuncture.

➤ Instruct the patient to follow his or her usual diet for 2 weeks before testing.

➤ Instruct the patient to fast and to avoid excessive exercise for at least 12 hours before testing, and to refrain from alcohol consumption for 24 hours before testing.

➤ There are no medication restrictions, unless by medical direction.

Intratest:

➤ Ensure that the patient has complied with dietary and activity restrictions as well as other pretesting preparations; assure that food, fluids, and activity have been restricted for at least 12 hours prior to the procedure.

➤ If the patient has a history of severe allergic reaction to latex, care should be taken to avoid the use of equipment containing latex.

➤ Instruct the patient to cooperate fully and to follow directions. Direct the patient to breathe normally and to avoid unnecessary movement.

➤ Observe standard precautions, and follow the general guidelines in Appendix A. Positively identify the patient, and label the appropriate tubes with the corresponding patient demographics, date, and time of collection. Perform a venipuncture; collect the specimen in a 5-mL red- or tiger-top tube.

➤ Remove the needle, and apply a pressure dressing over the puncture site.

➤ Promptly transport the specimen to the laboratory for processing and analysis.

➤ The results are recorded manually or in a computerized system for recall and postprocedure interpretation by the appropriate health care practitioner.

Post-test:

➤ Observe venipuncture site for bleeding or hematoma formation. Apply paper tape or other adhesive to hold pressure bandage in place, or replace with a plastic bandage.

➤ Instruct the patient to resume usual diet, fluids, and activity, as directed by the health care practitioner.

➤ *Nutritional considerations:* Abnormal lipoprotein electrophoresis patterns may be associated with cardiovascular disease. Nutritional therapy is recommended for the patient identified to be at high risk for developing CAD. If overweight, the patient should be encouraged to achieve a normal weight. The American Heart Association Step 1 and Step 2 diets may be helpful in achieving a goal of lowering total cholesterol and triglyceride levels. The Step 1 diet emphasizes a reduction in foods high in saturated fats and cholesterol. Red meats, eggs, and dairy products are the major sources of saturated fats and cholesterol. If triglycerides also are elevated, the patient should be advised to eliminate or reduce alcohol and simple carbohydrates from the diet. The Step 2 diet recommends stricter reductions.

➤ *Social and cultural considerations:* Numerous studies point to the prevalence of excess body weight in American children and adolescents. Experts estimate that obesity is present in 25% of the population ages 6 to 11 years. The medical, social, and emotional consequences of excess body weight are significant. Special attention should be given to instructing the child and caregiver regarding health risks and weight control education.

➤ A written report of the examination will be sent to the requesting health care practitioner, who will discuss the results with the patient.

➤ Recognize anxiety related to test results, and be supportive of fear of shortened life expectancy. Discuss the implications of abnormal test results on the patient's lifestyle. Provide teaching and information regarding the clinical implications of the test results, as appropriate. Educate the patient regarding access to counseling services. Provide contact information, if desired, for the American Heart Association *(http://www.americanheart.org)*.

➤ Reinforce information given by the patient's health care provider regarding further testing, treatment, or referral to another health care provider. Answer any questions or address any concerns voiced by the patient or family.

➤ Depending on the results of this procedure, additional testing may be performed to evaluate or monitor progression of the disease process and determine the need for a change in therapy. Evaluate test results in relation to the patient's symptoms and other tests performed.

Related laboratory tests:

➤ Related laboratory tests include antiarrhythmic drugs, apolipoprotein A, apolipoprotein B, aspartate aminotransferase, atrial natriuretic peptide, blood gases, B-type natriuretic peptide, calcium (blood and ionized), cholesterol (total, HDL, and LDL), C-reactive protein, creatine kinase and isoenzymes, glucose, glycated hemoglobin, homocysteine, ketones, lactate dehydrogenase and isoenzymes, magnesium, myoglobin, potassium, triglycerides, and troponin.

LIVER AND SPLEEN SCAN

SYNONYMS/ACRONYM: Liver and spleen scintigraphy, liver-spleen scan, radionuclide liver scan, spleen scan.

AREA OF APPLICATION: Abdomen.

CONTRAST: Intravenous radioactive technetium-99m sulfur colloid.

DESCRIPTION & RATIONALE: The liver and spleen scan is performed to help diagnose abnormalities in the function and structure of the liver and spleen. It is often performed in combination with lung scanning to help diagnose masses or inflammation in the diaphragmatic area. This procedure is useful for evaluating right-upper-quadrant pain, metastatic disease, jaundice, cirrhosis, ascites, traumatic infarction, and radiation-induced organ cellular necrosis. Technetium-99m (Tc-99m) sulfur colloid is injected intravenously and rapidly taken up through phagocytosis by the reticuloendothelial cells, which normally function to remove particulate matter, including radioactive colloids in the liver and spleen. False-negative results may occur in patients with space-occupying lesions (e.g., tumors, cysts, abscesses) smaller than 2 cm. This scan can detect portal hypertension, demonstrated by a greater uptake of the radionuclide in the spleen than in the liver. Single-photon emission computed tomography (SPECT) has significantly improved the resolution and accuracy of liver scanning. SPECT enables images to be recorded from multiple angles around the body and reconstructed by a computer to produce images or "slices" representing the organ at different levels. For evaluation of a suspected hemangioma, the patient's red blood cells are combined with Tc-99m and images are recorded over the liver. To confirm the diagnosis, liver and spleen scans are done in conjunction with computed tomography (CT), magnetic resonance imaging (MRI), ultrasonography, and SPECT scans and interpreted in light of the results of liver function tests. ■

INDICATIONS:

- Assess the condition of the liver and spleen after abdominal trauma

- Detect a bacterial or amebic abscess

- Detect and differentiate between primary and metastatic tumor focal disease

- Detect benign tumors, such as adenoma and cavernous hemangioma

- Detect cystic focal disease

- Detect diffuse hepatocellular disease, such as hepatitis and cirrhosis

- Detect infiltrative processes that affect the liver, such as sarcoidosis and amyloidosis

- Determine superior vena cava obstruction or Budd-Chiari syndrome

- Differentiate between splenomegaly and hepatomegaly

- Evaluate the effects of lower abdominal trauma, such as internal hemorrhage

- Evaluate jaundice

- Evaluate liver and spleen damage caused by radiation therapy or toxic drug therapy

- Evaluate palpable abdominal masses

RESULT

Normal Findings:

- Normal size, contour, position, and function of the liver and spleen

Abnormal Findings:

- Abscesses
- Cirrhosis
- Cysts
- Hemangiomas
- Hematoma
- Hepatitis
- Hodgkin's disease
- Infarction

- Infection
- Infiltrative process (amyloidosis and sarcoidosis)
- Inflammation of the diaphragmatic area
- Metastatic tumors
- Nodular hyperplasia
- Portal hypertension
- Primary benign or malignant tumors
- Traumatic lesions

CRITICAL VALUES: N/A

INTERFERING FACTORS:

This procedure is contraindicated for:
- Patients who are pregnant or suspected of being pregnant, unless the potential benefits of the procedure far outweigh the risks to the fetus and mother

Factors that may impair clear imaging:
- Inability of the patient to cooperate or remain still during the procedure because of age, significant pain, or mental status
- Metallic objects within the examination field (e.g., jewelry, body rings), which may inhibit organ visualization and can produce unclear images
- Patients who are very obese, who may exceed the weight limit for the equipment
- Incorrect positioning of the patient, which may produce poor visualization of the area to be examined, especially for oblique and decubitus views
- Other nuclear scans done within the preceding 24 to 48 hours

Other considerations:
- The scan may fail to detect focal lesions smaller than 2 cm in diameter.

- Improper injection of the radionuclide may allow the tracer to seep deep into the muscle tissue, producing erroneous hot spots.
- Consultation with a health care practitioner should occur before the procedure for radiation safety concerns regarding younger patients or patients who are lactating.
- Risks associated with radiologic overexposure can result from frequent x-ray procedures. Personnel in the room with the patient should wear a protective lead apron, stand behind a shield, or leave the area while the examination is being done. Personnel working in the area where the examination is being done should wear badges that reveal their level of exposure to radiation.

Nursing Implications and Procedure • • • • • • • • • •

Pretest:

➤ Inform the patient that the procedure assesses liver and spleen function.

➤ Obtain a history of the patient's complaints and symptoms, including a list of known allergens.

➤ Obtain a history of the patient's gastrointestinal and hepatobiliary systems, signs and symptoms of liver and spleen dysfunction, and results of previously performed diagnostic procedures, surgical procedures, and laboratory tests. For related diagnostic tests, refer to the Gastrointestinal and Hepatobiliary System tables.

➤ Note any recent procedures that can interfere with test results, including examinations using iodine-based contrast medium.

➤ Record the date of the last menstrual period and determine the possibility of pregnancy in perimenopausal women.

➤ Obtain a list of the medications the patient is taking, including anticoagulant therapy, aspirin and other salicylates, herbs, nutritional supplements, and nutraceuticals, especially those known to affect coagulation (see Appendix F). It is recommended that use be discontinued 14 days before surgical procedures. The requesting health care practitioner and laboratory should be advised if the patient regularly uses these products so that their effects can be taken into consideration when reviewing results.

> Review the procedure with the patient. Address concerns about pain related to the procedure. Explain to the patient that some pain may be experienced during the test, or there may be moments of discomfort. Reassure the patient that the radionuclide poses no radioactive hazard and rarely produces side effects. Inform the patient that the procedure is performed in a special department, usually in a radiology department, by a health care practitioner and support staff and takes approximately 30 to 60 minutes.

> *Sensitivity to social and cultural issues,* as well as concern for modesty, is important in providing psychological support before, during, and after the procedure.

> The patient should fast and restrict fluids for 8 hours prior to the procedure. Instruct the patient to avoid taking anticoagulant medication or to reduce dosage as ordered prior to the procedure.

> Instruct the patient to remove dentures, jewelry (including watches), hairpins, credit cards, and other metallic objects in the area to be examined.

Intratest:

> Ensure that the patient has complied with dietary, fluids, and medication restrictions and pretesting preparations; assure that food, fluids, and medications have been restricted for at least 8 hours prior to the procedure. Ensure that the patient has removed all external metallic objects

(jewelry, dentures, etc.) prior to the procedure.

> Have emergency equipment readily available.

> If the patient has a history of severe allergic reactions to any substance or drug, administer ordered prophylactic steroids or antihistamines before the procedure. Use nonionic contrast medium for the procedure.

> Patients are given a gown, robe, and foot coverings to wear and instructed to void prior to the procedure.

> Record baseline vital signs and assess neurologic status. Protocols may vary from facility to facility.

> Instruct the patient to cooperate fully and to follow directions. Instruct the patient to remain still throughout the procedure because movement produces unreliable results.

> Observe standard precautions, and follow the general guidelines in Appendix A.

> Administer an antianxiety agent, as ordered, if the patient has claustrophobia. Administer a sedative to a child or to an uncooperative adult, as ordered.

> Place the patient in a supine position on a flat table with foam wedges, which help maintain position and immobilization. The radionuclide is administered intravenously and the abdomen is scanned immediately for 1 minute to screen for vascular lesions. Then images are taken in the anterior, oblique, lateral, and posterior oblique positions.

> Wear gloves during the radionuclide injection and while handling the patient's urine.

> Instruct the patient to take slow, deep breaths if nausea occurs during the procedure. Monitor and administer an antiemetic agent if ordered. Ready an emesis basin for use.

> Monitor the patient for complications related to the procedure (e.g., allergic reaction, anaphylaxis, bronchospasm).

> The needle or catheter is removed,

and a pressure dressing is applied over the puncture site.

➤ The results are recorded on x-ray film or electronically, in a computerized system, for recall and postprocedure interpretation by the appropriate health care practitioner.

➤ The patient may be imaged by SPECT techniques to further clarify areas of suspicious radionuclide localization.

Post-test:

➤ Instruct the patient to resume usual diet, fluids, medication, or activity, as directed by the health care practitioner.

➤ Monitor vital signs and neurologic status every 15 minutes for 1 hour, then every 2 hours for 4 hours, and then as ordered by the health care practitioner. Compare with baseline values. Protocols may vary from facility to facility.

➤ Observe for delayed allergic reactions, such as rash, urticaria, tachycardia, hyperpnea, hypertension, palpitations, nausea, or vomiting.

➤ Instruct the patient to immediately report symptoms such as fast heart rate, difficulty breathing, skin rash, itching, or decreased urinary output.

➤ Observe the needle/catheter insertion site for bleeding, inflammation, or hematoma formation.

➤ Instruct the patient to apply cold compresses to the puncture site, as needed, to reduce discomfort or edema.

➤ Instruct patient to drink increased amounts of fluids for 24 to 48 hours to eliminate the radionuclide from the body, unless contraindicated. Tell the patient that radionuclide is eliminated from the body within 6 to 24 hours.

➤ Instruct the patient to flush the toilet immediately after each voiding following the procedure, and to wash hands meticulously with soap and water after each voiding for 24 hours after the procedure.

➤ Instruct all caregivers to wear gloves when discarding urine for 24 hours after the procedure. Wash gloved hands with soap and water before removing gloves. Then wash hands after the gloves are removed.

➤ If a woman who is breast-feeding must have a nuclear scan, she should not breast-feed the infant until the radionuclide has been eliminated. This could take as long as 3 days. She should be instructed to express the milk and discard it during the 3-day period to prevent cessation of milk production.

➤ *Nutritional considerations:* A low-fat, low-cholesterol, and low-sodium diet should be consumed to reduce current disease processes. High fat consumption increases the amount of bile acids in the colon and should be avoided.

➤ No other radionuclide tests should be scheduled for 24 to 48 hours after this procedure.

➤ A written report of the examination will be completed by a health care practitioner specializing in this branch of medicine. The report will be sent to the requesting health care practitioner, who will discuss the results with the patient.

➤ Recognize anxiety related to test results, and be supportive of perceived loss of independent function. Discuss the implications of abnormal test results on the patient's lifestyle. Provide teaching and information regarding the clinical implications of the test results, as appropriate.

➤ Reinforce information given by the patient's health care provider regarding further testing, treatment, or referral to another health care provider. Answer any questions or address any concerns voiced by the patient or family.

➤ Instruct the patient in the use of any ordered medications. Explain the importance of adhering to the therapy regimen. As appropriate, instruct the patient in significant side effects and systemic reactions associated with the prescribed medication.

Encourage him or her to review corresponding literature provided by a pharmacist.

➤ Depending on the results of this procedure, additional testing may be needed to evaluate or monitor progression of the disease process and determine the need for a change in therapy. Evaluate test results in relation to the patient's symptoms and other tests performed.

Related diagnostic tests:

➤ Related diagnostic tests include computed tomography of the abdomen, hepatobiliary scan, liver ultrasound, and magnetic resonance imaging of the abdomen.

LUNG PERFUSION SCAN

· ·

SYNONYMS/ACRONYM: Radioactive perfusion scan, lung scintiscan, lung perfusion scintigraphy, ventilation-perfusion scan, pulmonary scan, radionuclide perfusion lung scan, V/Q scan.

AREA OF APPLICATION: Chest/thorax.

CONTRAST: Intravenous radioactive material, usually macroaggregated albumin (MAA).

DESCRIPTION & RATIONALE: The lung perfusion scan is a nuclear medicine study performed to evaluate a patient for pulmonary embolus (PE) or other pulmonary disorders. Technetium (Tc-99m) is injected intravenously and distributed throughout the pulmonary vasculature because of the gravitational effect on perfusion. The scan, which produces a visual image of pulmonary blood flow, is useful in diagnosing or confirming pulmonary vascular obstruction. The diameter of the intravenously injected macroaggregated albumin (MAA) is larger than that of the pulmonary capillaries; therefore, the MAA temporarily becomes lodged in the pulmonary vasculature. A gamma camera detects the radiation emitted from the injected radioactive material, and a representative image of the lung is obtained. This procedure is often done in conjunction with the lung ventilation scan to obtain clinical information that assists in differentiating among the many possible pathologic conditions revealed by the procedure. The results are correlated with other diagnostic studies, such as pulmonary function, chest x-ray, pulmonary angiography, and arterial blood gases. A recent chest x-ray is essential for accurate interpretation of the lung perfusion scan. An area of nonperfusion seen in the same area as a pulmonary parenchymal abnormality on the chest x-ray indicates that a PE is not present; the defect may represent some other pathologic condition, such as pneumonia. ■

INDICATIONS:

- Aid in the diagnosis of PE in a patient with a normal chest x-ray
- Detect malignant tumor
- Differentiate between PE and other pulmonary diseases, such as pneumonia, pulmonary effusion, atelectasis, asthma, bronchitis, emphysema, and tumors
- Evaluate perfusion changes associated with congestive heart failure and pulmonary hypertension
- Evaluate pulmonary function preoperatively in a patient with pulmonary disease

RESULT

Normal Findings:
- Diffuse and homogeneous uptake of the radioactive material by the lungs

Abnormal Findings:
- Asthma
- Atelectasis
- Bronchitis
- Chronic obstructive pulmonary disease
- Emphysema
- Left atrial or pulmonary hypertension
- Lung displacement by fluid or chest masses
- Pneumonia
- Pneumonitis
- Pulmonary embolism
- Tuberculosis

CRITICAL VALUES: N/A

INTERFERING FACTORS:

This procedure is contraindicated for:
- Patients who are pregnant or suspected of being pregnant, unless the potential benefits of the procedure far outweigh the risks to the fetus and mother
- Patients with atrial and ventricular septal defects, because the MAA particles will not reach the lungs
- Patients with pulmonary hypertension

Factors that may impair clear imaging:
- Inability of the patient to cooperate or remain still during the procedure because of age, significant pain, or mental status
- Metallic objects within the examination field (e.g., jewelry, body rings), which may inhibit organ visualization and can produce unclear images
- Patients who are very obese, who may exceed the weight limit for the equipment
- Incorrect positioning of the patient, which may produce poor visualization of the area to be examined, especially for oblique and decubitus views and for films done by portable equipment
- Other nuclear scans done on the same day

Other considerations:
- Improper injection of the radionuclide may allow the tracer to seep deep into the muscle tissue, producing erroneous hot spots.
- Consultation with a health care practitioner should occur before the procedure for radiation safety concerns regarding younger patients or patients who are lactating.

• Risks associated with radiologic overexposure can result from frequent x-ray procedures. Personnel in the room with the patient should wear a protective lead apron, stand behind a shield, or leave the area while the examination is being done. Personnel working in the area where the examination is being done should wear badges that reveal their level of exposure to radiation.

Nursing Implications and Procedure • • • • • • • • • • •

Pretest:

➤ Inform the patient that the procedure assesses blood flow to the lungs.

➤ Obtain a history of the patient's complaints and symptoms, including a list of known allergens.

➤ Obtain a history of the patient's respiratory system, as well as results of previously performed diagnostic procedures, surgical procedures, and laboratory tests. For related diagnostic tests, refer to the Respiratory System table.

➤ Obtain a history of signs and symptoms of pulmonary embolism, such as sudden sharp chest pain, shortness of breath, chest pain that worsens with deep breathing/coughing, coughing up blood, rapid heart rate, sweating, and/or anxiety.

➤ Note any recent procedures that can interfere with test results, including examinations using iodine-based contrast medium.

➤ Record the date of the last menstrual period and determine the possibility of pregnancy in perimenopausal women.

➤ Obtain a list of the medications the patient is taking, including anticoagulant therapy, aspirin and other salicylates, herbs, nutritional supplements, and nutraceuticals, especially those known to affect coagulation (see Appendix F). It is recommended that use be discontinued 14 days before surgical procedures. The requesting health care practitioner and laboratory should be advised if the patient regularly uses these products so that their effects can be taken into consideration when reviewing results.

➤ Review the procedure with the patient. Address concerns about pain related to the procedure. Explain to the patient that some pain may be experienced during the test, or there may be moments of discomfort. Reassure the patient that the radionuclide poses no radioactive hazard and rarely produces side effects. Inform the patient that the procedure is performed in a special department, usually in a radiology department, by a health care practitioner and support staff and takes approximately 60 minutes.

➤ *Sensitivity to social and cultural issues,* as well as concern for modesty, is important in providing psychological support before, during, and after the procedure.

➤ Instruct the patient to remove dentures, jewelry (including watches), hairpins, credit cards, and other metallic objects in the area to be examined.

Intratest:

➤ Ensure that the patient has complied with dietary, fluids, and medication restrictions and pretesting preparations; assure that food, fluids, and medications have been restricted for at least 8 hours prior to the procedure. Ensure that the patient has removed all external metallic objects (jewelry, dentures, etc.) prior to the procedure.

➤ Have emergency equipment readily available.

➤ If the patient has a history of severe allergic reactions to any substance or drug, administer ordered prophylactic steroids or antihistamines before the procedure. Use nonionic contrast medium for the procedure.

➤ Patients are given a gown, robe, and foot coverings to wear and instructed to void prior to the procedure.

➤ Record baseline vital signs and assess neurologic status. Protocols may vary from facility to facility.

➤ Instruct the patient to cooperate fully and to follow directions. Instruct the patient to remain still throughout the procedure because movement produces unreliable results.

➤ Observe standard precautions, and follow the general guidelines in Appendix A.

➤ Administer an antianxiety agent, as ordered, if the patient has claustrophobia. Administer a sedative to a child or to an uncooperative adult, as ordered.

➤ Place the patient in a supine position on a flat table with foam wedges, which help maintain position and immobilization. The radionuclide is administered intravenously after the syringe is shaken to resuspend the particles. Images of the lungs are obtained in the anterior, posterior, both lateral, and both oblique views.

➤ Wear gloves during the radionuclide administration and while handling the patient's urine.

➤ Instruct the patient to take slow, deep breaths if nausea occurs during the procedure. Monitor and administer an antiemetic agent if ordered. Ready an emesis basin for use.

➤ Monitor the patient for complications related to the procedure (e.g., allergic reaction, anaphylaxis, bronchospasm).

➤ The needle or catheter is removed, and a pressure dressing is applied over the puncture site.

➤ The results are recorded on x-ray film or electronically, in a computerized system, for recall and postprocedure interpretation by the appropriate health care practitioner.

Post-test:

➤ Instruct the patient to resume usual diet, fluids, medication, or activity, as directed by the health care practitioner.

➤ Monitor vital signs and neurologic status every 15 minutes for 1 hour, then every 2 hours for 4 hours, and then as ordered health care practitioner. Compare with baseline values. Protocols may vary from facility to facility.

➤ Observe for delayed allergic reactions, such as rash, urticaria, tachycardia, hyperpnea, hypertension, palpitations, nausea, or vomiting.

➤ Instruct the patient to immediately report symptoms such as fast heart rate, difficulty breathing, skin rash, itching, or decreased urinary output.

➤ Observe the needle/catheter insertion site for bleeding, inflammation, or hematoma formation.

➤ Instruct the patient to apply cold compresses to the puncture site, as needed, to reduce discomfort or edema.

➤ Instruct patient to drink increased amounts of fluids for 24 to 48 hours to eliminate the radionuclide from the body, unless contraindicated. Tell the patient that radionuclide is eliminated from the body within 24 to 48 hours.

➤ Instruct the patient to flush the toilet immediately after each voiding following the procedure, and to wash hands meticulously with soap and water after each voiding for 24 hours after the procedure.

➤ Instruct all caregivers to wear gloves when discarding urine for 24 hours after the procedure. Wash gloved hands with soap and water before removing gloves. Then wash hands after the gloves are removed.

➤ If a woman who is breast-feeding must have a nuclear scan, she should not breast-feed the infant until the radionuclide has been eliminated. This could take as long as 3 days. She should be instructed to express the milk and discard it during the 3-day period to prevent cessation of milk production.

➤ *Nutritional considerations:* A low-fat, low-cholesterol, and low-sodium diet should be consumed to reduce current disease processes and/or decrease risk of hypertension and coronary artery disease.

> No other radionuclide tests should be scheduled for 24 to 48 hours after this procedure.

> A written report of the examination will be completed by a health care practitioner specializing in this branch of medicine. The report will be sent to the requesting health care practitioner, who will discuss the results with the patient.

> Recognize anxiety related to test results, and be supportive of perceived loss of independent function. Discuss the implications of abnormal test results on the patient's lifestyle. Provide teaching and information regarding the clinical implications of the test results, as appropriate.

> Reinforce information given by the patient's health care provider regarding further testing, treatment, or referral to another health care provider. Answer any questions or address any concerns voiced by the patient or family.

> Instruct the patient in the use of any ordered medications. Explain the importance of adhering to the therapy regimen. As appropriate, instruct the patient in significant side effects and systemic reactions associated with the prescribed medication. Encourage him or her to review corresponding literature provided by a pharmacist.

> Depending on the results of this procedure, additional testing may be needed to evaluate or monitor progression of the disease process and determine the need for a change in therapy. Evaluate test results in relation to the patient's symptoms and other tests performed.

Related diagnostic tests:

> Related diagnostic tests include chest x-ray, computed tomography of the thorax and magnetic resonance imaging of the chest.

LUNG VENTILATION SCAN

SYNONYMS/ACRONYM: Radioactive ventilation scan, VQ lung scan, aerosol lung scan, ventilation scan, xenon lung scan.

AREA OF APPLICATION: Chest/thorax.

CONTRAST: Done with inhaled radioactive material (xenon gas or technetium-DTPA).

DESCRIPTION & RATIONALE: The lung ventilation scan is a nuclear medicine study performed to evaluate a patient for pulmonary embolus (PE) or other pulmonary disorders. It can evaluate respiratory function (i.e., demonstrating areas of the lung that are patent and capable of ventilation) and dysfunction (e.g., parenchymal abnormalities affecting ventilation, such as pneumonia). The procedure is performed after the patient inhales air mixed with a radioactive gas through a face mask and mouthpiece. The radioactive gas delineates areas of the lung during ventilation. The distribution of the gas throughout the lung is measured in three phases:

Wash-in phase: Phase during buildup of the radioactive gas

Equilibrium phase: Phase after the patient rebreathes from a closed delivery system

Wash-out phase: Phase after the radioactive gas has been removed

This procedure is usually performed along with a lung perfusion scan. When PE is present, ventilation scans display a normal wash-in and wash-out of radioactivity from the lung areas. Parenchymal disease responsible for perfusion abnormalities will produce abnormal wash-in and wash-out phases. This test can be used to quantify regional ventilation in patients with pulmonary disease. ■

INDICATIONS:

• Aid in the diagnosis of PE

• Differentiate between PE and other pulmonary diseases, such as pneumonia, pulmonary effusion, atelectasis, asthma, bronchitis, emphysema, and tumors

• Evaluate regional respiratory function

• Identify areas of the lung that are capable of ventilation

• Locate hypoventilation (regional), which can result from chronic obstructive pulmonary disease (COPD) or excessive smoking

RESULT

Normal Findings:

• Equal distribution of radioactive gas throughout both lungs and a normal wash-out phase

Abnormal Findings:

• Atelectasis

• Bronchitis

• Bronchogenic carcinoma

• COPD

• Emphysema

• PE

• Pneumonia

• Regional hypoventilation

• Sarcoidosis

• Tuberculosis

• Tumor

CRITICAL VALUES: N/A

INTERFERING FACTORS:

This procedure is contraindicated for:

• Patients who are pregnant or suspected of being pregnant, unless the potential benefits of the procedure far outweigh the risks to the fetus and mother

Factors that may impair clear imaging:

• Inability of the patient to cooperate or remain still during the procedure because of age, significant pain, or mental status

- Metallic objects within the examination field (e.g., jewelry, body rings), which may inhibit organ visualization and can produce unclear images

- Patients who are very obese, who may exceed the weight limit for the equipment

- Incorrect positioning of the patient, which may produce poor visualization of the area to be examined, especially for oblique and decubitus views and for films done by portable equipment

- Other nuclear scans done within the preceding 24 to 48 hours

Other considerations:

- The presence of conditions that affect perfusion or ventilation (e.g., tumors that obstruct the pulmonary artery, vasculitis, pulmonary edema, sickle cell disease, parasitic disease, emphysema, effusion, infection) can simulate a perfusion defect similar to PE.

- Consultation with a health care practitioner should occur before the procedure for radiation safety concerns regarding younger patients or patients who are lactating.

- Risks associated with radiographic overexposure can result from frequent x-ray procedures. Personnel in the room with the patient should wear a protective lead apron, stand behind a shield, or leave the area while the examination is being done. Personnel working in the area where the examination is being done should wear badges that reveal their level of exposure to radiation.

Nursing Implications and Procedure . . . .

Pretest:

➤ Inform the patient that the procedure assesses airflow to the lungs.

➤ Obtain a history of the patient's complaints and symptoms, including a list of known allergens.

➤ Obtain a history of the patient's respiratory system, as well as results of previously performed diagnostic procedures, surgical procedures, and laboratory tests. For related diagnostic tests, refer to the Respiratory System table.

➤ Record the date of the last menstrual period and determine the possibility of pregnancy in perimenopausal women.

➤ Obtain a list of the patient's current medications.

➤ Review the procedure with the patient. Address concerns about pain related to the procedure. Explain to the patient that some pain may be experienced during the test, and there may be moments of discomfort. Explain the purpose of the test and how the procedure is performed. Reassure the patient that the radionuclide poses no radioactive hazard and rarely produces side effects. Inform the patient that the procedure is performed in a nuclear medicine department, usually by a technologist and support staff, and takes approximately 30 to 60 minutes.

➤ *Sensitivity to cultural and social issues,* as well as concern for modesty, is important in providing psychological support before, during, and after the procedure.

➤ There are no food, fluid, or medication restrictions, unless by medical direction.

➤ Instruct the patient to remove dentures, jewelry (including watches), hairpins, credit cards, and other metallic objects in the area to be examined.

Intratest:

➤ Make sure jewelry, chains, and any other metallic objects have been removed from the chest area.

➤ Patients are given a gown, robe, and foot coverings to wear and instructed to void prior to the procedure.

➤ Obtain and record baseline vital signs.

➤ Instruct the patient to cooperate fully and to follow directions. Instruct the patient to remain still throughout the procedure because movement produces unreliable results.

➤ Observe standard precautions, and follow the general guidelines in Appendix A.

➤ Administer an antianxiety agent, as ordered, if the patient has claustrophobia. Administer sedative to a child or to an uncooperative adult, as ordered.

➤ Place the patient in a supine position on a flat table with foam wedges, which help maintain position and immobilization. The radionuclide is administered through a mask, which is placed over the patient's nose and mouth. The patient is asked to hold his or her breath for a short period of time while the scan is taken. The distribution of the radioactive gas is monitored and measured on a nuclear scanner. The patient's chest is imaged while the gas is in the lungs. Images of the lungs are obtained in the posterior and, when possible, both oblique views.

➤ Wear gloves during the radionuclide administration and while handling the patient's urine.

➤ Instruct the patient to take slow, deep breaths if nausea occurs during the procedure. Monitor and administer an antiemetic agent if ordered. Ready an emesis basin for use.

➤ Monitor the patient for complications related to the procedure (e.g., allergic reaction, anaphylaxis, bronchospasm).

➤ The results are recorded on film or in a computerized system for recall and postprocedure interpretation by the appropriate health care practitioner.

Post-test:

➤ Evaluate the patient's vital signs. Monitor vital signs every 15 to 30 minutes and compare with baseline readings until the patient is stable.

➤ Observe for delayed allergic reactions, such as rash, urticaria, tachy-

cardia, hyperpnea, hypertension, palpitations, nausea, or vomiting.

➤ Instruct the patient to immediately report symptoms such as fast heart rate, difficulty breathing, skin rash, itching, or decreased urinary output.

➤ Advise patient to drink increased amounts of fluids for 24 to 48 hours to eliminate the radionuclide from the body, unless contraindicated. Tell the patient that radionuclide is eliminated from the body within 6 to 24 hours.

➤ Instruct the patient to flush the toilet immediately after each voiding following the procedure, and to wash hands meticulously with soap and water after each voiding for 24 hours after the procedure.

➤ Tell all caregivers to wear gloves when discarding urine for 24 hours after the procedure. Wash gloved hands with soap and water before removing gloves. Then wash hands after the gloves are removed.

➤ If a woman who is breast-feeding must have a nuclear scan, she should not breast-feed the infant until the radionuclide has been eliminated. This could take as long as 3 days. She should be instructed to express the milk and discard it during the 3-day period to prevent cessation of milk production.

➤ A written report of the examination will be completed by a health care practitioner specializing in this branch of medicine. The report will be sent to the requesting health care practitioner, who will discuss the results with the patient.

➤ Recognize anxiety related to test results, and be supportive of perceived loss of independent function. Discuss the implications of abnormal test results on the patient's lifestyle. Provide teaching and information regarding the clinical implications of the test results, as appropriate.

➤ Reinforce information given by the patient's health care provider regarding further testing, treatment, or referral to another health care provider. Answer any questions or address any concerns voiced by the patient or family.

➤ Depending on the results of this procedure, additional testing may be needed to evaluate or monitor progression of the disease process and determine the need for a change in therapy. Evaluate test results in rela-

tion to the patient's symptoms and other tests performed.

Related diagnostic tests:

➤ Related diagnostic tests include chest x-ray, computed tomography of the thorax, and magnetic resonance imaging of the chest.

LUPUS ANTICOAGULANT ANTIBODIES

SYNONYMS/ACRONYM: Lupus inhibitor phospholipid type, lupus antiphospholipid antibodies.

SPECIMEN: Plasma (1 mL) collected in blue-top (sodium citrate) tube.

REFERENCE VALUE: (Method: Dilute Russell venom viper test time) Negative.

DESCRIPTION & RATIONALE: Lupus anticoagulant antibodies are immunoglobulins, usually of the immunoglobulin G class. They are also referred to as lupus antiphospholipid antibodies because they interfere with phospholipid-dependent coagulation tests such as activated partial thromboplastin time by reacting with the phospholipids in the test system. They are not associated with a bleeding disorder unless thrombocytopenia or antiprothrombin antibodies are already present. They are associated with an increased risk of thrombosis. ■

INDICATIONS:
• Evaluate prolonged activated partial thromboplastin times
• Investigate reasons for fetal death

RESULT

Positive in:
• Fetal loss
• Raynaud's disease
• Rheumatoid arthritis
• Systemic lupus erythematosus
• Thromboembolism

Negative in: N/A

CRITICAL VALUES: N/A

INTERFERING FACTORS:
• Drugs that may cause a positive lupus anticoagulant test result include chlorpromazine and heparin.
• Placement of a tourniquet for longer than 1 minute can result in venous stasis and changes in the concentration

of plasma proteins to be measured. Platelet activation may also occur under these conditions, causing erroneous results.

- Vascular injury during phlebotomy can activate platelets and coagulation factors, causing erroneous results.

- Hemolyzed specimens must be rejected because hemolysis is an indication of platelet and coagulation factor activation.

- Incompletely filled tubes contaminated with heparin or clotted specimens must be rejected.

- Icteric or lipemic specimens interfere with optical testing methods, producing erroneous results.

Nursing Implications and Procedure • • • • • • • • • • •

Pretest:

➤ Inform the patient that the test is used to evaluate coagulation disorders.

➤ Obtain a history of the patient's complaints, including a list of known allergens (especially allergies or sensitivities to latex), and inform the appropriate health care practitioner accordingly.

➤ Obtain a history of the patient's hematopoietic, immune, musculoskeletal, and reproductive systems, as well as results of previously performed laboratory tests, surgical procedures, and other diagnostic procedures. For related laboratory tests, refer to the Hematopoietic, Immune, Musculoskeletal, and Reproductive System tables.

➤ Obtain a list of the medications the patient is taking, including herbs, nutritional supplements, and nutraceuticals. The requesting health care practitioner and laboratory should be advised if the patient regularly uses these products so that their effects can be taken into consideration when reviewing results.

➤ Review the procedure with the patient. Inform the patient that specimen collection takes approximately 5 to 10 minutes. Address concerns about pain related to the procedure. Explain to the patient that there may be some discomfort during the venipuncture.

➤ Heparin therapy should be discontinued 2 days before specimen collection, with medical direction. Coumarin therapy should be discontinued 2 weeks before specimen collection, with medical direction.

➤ There are no food or fluid restrictions, unless by medical direction.

Intratest:

➤ Ensure that the patient has complied with pretesting preparations; assure that anticoagulent therapy has been restricted as required prior to the procedure.

➤ If the patient has a history of severe allergic reaction to latex, care should be taken to avoid the use of equipment containing latex.

➤ Instruct the patient to cooperate fully and to follow directions. Direct the patient to breathe normally and to avoid unnecessary movement.

➤ Observe standard precautions, and follow the general guidelines in Appendix A. Positively identify the patient, and label the appropriate tubes with the corresponding patient demographics, date, and time of collection. Perform a venipuncture; collect the specimen in a 5-mL blue-top tube. *Important note:* Two different concentrations of sodium citrate preservative are currently added to blue-top tubes for coagulation studies: 3.2% and 3.8%. The Clinical and Laboratory Standards Institute/CLSI (formerly the National Committee for Clinical Laboratory Standards/ NCCLS) guideline for sodium citrate is 3.2%. Laboratories establish reference ranges for coagulation testing based on numerous factors, including sodium citrate concentration, test equipment, and test reagents. It is important to inquire from the laboratory which concentration it recommends, because each concentration will have its own specific reference range.

> When multiple specimens are drawn, the blue-top tube should be collected after sterile (i.e., blood culture) and red-top tubes. When coagulation testing is the only test to be done, an extra red-top tube should be collected before the blue-top tube to avoid contaminating the specimen with tissue thromboplastin, which can falsely decrease values.

> Remove the needle, and apply a pressure dressing over the puncture site.

> Promptly transport the specimen to the laboratory for processing and analysis. The CLSI recommendation for processed and unprocessed samples stored in unopened tubes is that testing should be completed within 1 to 4 hours of collection.

> The results are recorded manually or in a computerized system for recall and postprocedure interpretation by the appropriate health care practitioner.

Post-test:

> Observe venipuncture site for bleeding or hematoma formation. Apply paper tape or other adhesive to hold pressure bandage in place, or replace with a plastic bandage.

> Instruct the patient to resume usual medications, as directed by the health care practitioner.

> A written report of the examination will be sent to the requesting health care practitioner, who will discuss the results with the patient.

> Reinforce information given by the patient's health care provider regarding further testing, treatment, or referral to another health care provider. Answer any questions or address any concerns voiced by the patient or family.

> Depending on the results of this procedure, additional testing may be performed to evaluate or monitor progression of the disease process and determine the need for a change in therapy. Evaluate test results in relation to the patient's symptoms and other tests performed.

Related laboratory tests:

> Related laboratory tests include anticardiolipin antibody, antinuclear antibody, activated partial thromboplastin time, protein S, and rheumatoid factor.

LUTEINIZING HORMONE

SYNONYMS/ACRONYMS: LH, luteotropin, interstitial cell–stimulating hormone (ICSH).

SPECIMEN: Serum (1 mL) collected in a red- or tiger-top tube. Plasma (1 mL) collected in green-top (heparin) tube is also acceptable.

REFERENCE VALUE: (Method: Immunoassay)

Concentration by Sex and by Phase (in Women)	Conventional Units	SI Units (Conversion Factor ×1)
Male		
Less than 2 y	0.5–1.9 mIU/mL	0.5–1.9 IU/L
2–10 y	Less than 0.5 mIU/mL	Less than 0.5 IU/L
11–20 y	0.5–5.3 mIU/mL	0.5–5.3 IU/L
Adult	1.2–7.8 mIU/mL	1.2–7.8 IU/L
Female		
Less than 2–10 y	Less than 0.5 mIU/mL	Less than 0.5 IU/L
11–20 y	0.5–9.0 mIU/mL	0.5–9.0 IU/L
Phase in Women		
Follicular	1.7–15.0 mIU/mL	1.7–15.0 IU/L
Ovulatory	21.9–56.6 mIU/mL	21.9–56.6 IU/L
Luteal	0.6–16.3 mIU/mL	0.6–16.3 IU/L
Postmenopausal	14.2–52.3 mIU/mL	14.2–52.3 IU/L

DESCRIPTION & RATIONALE:

Luteinizing hormone (LH) is secreted by the anterior pituitary gland in response to stimulation by gonadotropin-releasing hormone, the same hypothalamic releasing factor that stimulates follicle-stimulating hormone release. LH affects gonadal function in both men and women. In women, a surge of LH normally occurs at the midpoint of the menstrual cycle (ovulatory phase); this surge is believed to be induced by high estrogen levels. LH causes the ovum to be expelled from the ovary and stimulates development of the corpus luteum and progesterone production. As progesterone levels rise, LH production decreases. In males, LH stimulates the interstitial cells of Leydig, located in the testes, to produce testosterone. For this reason, in reference to males, LH is sometimes called interstitial cell–stimulating hormone. Secretion of LH is pulsatile and follows a circadian rhythm in response to the normal intermittent secretion of gonadotropin-releasing hormone. ■

INDICATIONS:

* Distinguish between primary and secondary causes of gonadal failure

* Evaluate children with precocious puberty

* Evaluate male and female infertility, as indicated by decreased LH levels

* Evaluate response to therapy to induce ovulation

* Support diagnosis of infertility caused by anovulation, as evidenced by lack of LH surge at the midpoint of the menstrual cycle

RESULT

Increased in:
* Anorchia

* Gonadal failure

* Menopause

* Primary gonadal dysfunction

Decreased in:

- Anorexia nervosa
- Kallmann's syndrome
- Malnutrition
- Pituitary or hypothalamic dysfunction
- Severe stress

CRITICAL VALUES: N/A

INTERFERING FACTORS:

- Drugs and hormones that may increase LH levels include clomiphene, gonadotropin-releasing hormone, goserelin, ketoconazole, mestranol, nafarelin, naloxone, nilutamide, spironolactone, and tamoxifen.

- Drugs and hormones that may decrease LH levels include anabolic steroids, anticonvulsants, conjugated estrogens, danazol, digoxin, D-Trp-6-LHRH, estrogen/progestin therapy, goserelin, megestrol, norethindrone, octreotide, oral contraceptives, phenothiazine, pimozide, pravastatin, progesterone, stanozolol, and tamoxifen.

- In menstruating women, values vary in relation to the phase of the menstrual cycle.

- LH secretion follows a circadian rhythm, with higher levels occurring during sleep.

Nursing Implications and Procedure

Pretest:

- Inform the patient that the test is used to evaluate disorders of the hypothalmic-pituitary-gonadal axis.

- Obtain a history of the patient's complaints, including a list of known allergens (especially allergies or sensitivities to latex), and inform the appropriate health care practitioner accordingly.

- Obtain a history of the patient's endocrine and reproductive systems, as well as results of previously performed laboratory tests, surgical procedures, and other diagnostic procedures. For related laboratory tests, refer to the Endocrine and Reproductive System tables.

- Record the date of the last menstrual period and determine the possibility of pregnancy in perimenopausal women.

- Obtain a list of the medications the patient is taking, including herbs, nutritional supplements, and nutraceuticals. The requesting health care practitioner and laboratory should be advised if the patient regularly uses these products so that their effects can be taken into consideration when reviewing results.

- Review the procedure with the patient. If the test is being performed to detect ovulation, inform the patient that it may be necessary to obtain a series of samples over a period of several days to detect peak LH levels. Inform the patient that specimen collection takes approximately 5 to 10 minutes. Address concerns about pain related to the procedure. Explain to the patient that there may be some discomfort during the venipuncture.

- There are no food, fluid, or medication restrictions, unless by medical direction.

Intratest:

- If the patient has a history of severe allergic reaction to latex, care should be taken to avoid the use of equipment containing latex.

- Instruct the patient to cooperate fully and to follow directions. Direct the patient to breathe normally and to avoid unnecessary movement.

- Observe standard precautions, and follow the general guidelines in Appendix A. Positively identify the patient, and label the appropriate tubes with the corresponding patient demographics, date, and time of collection. Perform a venipuncture; collect the specimen in a 5-mL red- or tiger-top tube.

➤ Remove the needle, and apply a pressure dressing over the puncture site.

➤ Promptly transport the specimen to the laboratory for processing and analysis.

➤ The results are recorded manually or in a computerized system for recall and postprocedure interpretation by the appropriate health care practitioner.

Post-test:

➤ Observe venipuncture site for bleeding or hematoma formation. Apply paper tape or other adhesive to hold pressure bandage in place, or replace with a plastic bandage.

➤ A written report of the examination will be sent to the requesting health care practitioner, who will discuss the results with the patient.

➤ Reinforce information given by the patient's health care provider regarding further testing, treatment, or referral to another health care provider. Answer any questions or address any concerns voiced by the patient or family.

➤ Depending on the results of this procedure, additional testing may be performed to evaluate or monitor progression of the disease process and determine the need for a change in therapy. Evaluate test results in relation to the patient's symptoms and other tests performed.

Related laboratory tests:

➤ Related laboratory tests include adrenocorticotropic hormone, antisperm antibody, estradiol, folliclestimulating hormone, progesterone, prolactin, and testosterone.

LYME ANTIBODY

SYNONYM/ACRONYM: N/A.

SPECIMEN: Serum (1 mL) collected in a red-top tube.

REFERENCE VALUE: (Method: Indirect immunofluorescence) Negative.

DESCRIPTION & RATIONALE: *Borrelia burgdorferi*, a deer tick–borne spirochete, is the organism that causes Lyme disease. Lyme disease affects multiple systems and is characterized by fever, arthralgia, and arthritis. The circular, red rash characterizing erythema migrans can appear 3 to 30 days after the tick bite. About one-half of patients in the early stage of Lyme disease (stage 1) and generally all of those in the advanced stage (stage 2)—with cardiac, neurologic, and rheumatoid manifestations—will have a positive test result. Patients in remission will also have a positive test response. The presence of immunoglobulin M (IgM) antibodies indicates acute infection. The presence of IgG antibodies indicates current or past infection. ▪

INDICATIONS: Assist in establishing a diagnosis of Lyme disease

RESULT

Positive findings in: Lyme disease

Negative findings in: N/A

CRITICAL VALUES: N/A

INTERFERING FACTORS:
• High rheumatoid-factor titers as well as cross-reactivity with Epstein-Barr virus and other spirochetes (e.g., *Rickettsia, Treponema*) may cause false-positive results.

• Positive test results should be confirmed by the Western blot method.

Nursing Implications and Procedure ● ● ● ● ● ● ● ● ● ● ●

Pretest:

➤ Inform the patient that the test is used to detect antibodies to *Borrrelia burgdorferi*.

➤ Obtain a history of the patient's complaints, including a list of known allergens (especially allergies or sensitivities to latex), and inform the appropriate health care practitioner accordingly.

➤ Obtain a history of the patient's immune and musculoskeletal systems and a history of exposure, as well as results of previously performed laboratory tests, surgical procedures, and other diagnostic procedures. For related laboratory tests,

refer to the Immune and Musculoskeletal System tables.

➤ Obtain a list of the medications the patient is taking, including herbs, nutritional supplements, and nutraceuticals. The requesting health care practitioner and laboratory should be advised if the patient regularly uses these products so that their effects can be taken into consideration when reviewing results.

➤ Review the procedure with the patient. Inform the patient that several tests may be necessary to confirm diagnosis. Inform the patient that specimen collection takes approximately 5 to 10 minutes. Address concerns about pain related to the procedure. Explain to the patient that there may be some discomfort during the venipuncture.

➤ There are no food, fluid, or medication restrictions, unless by medical direction.

Intratest:

➤ If the patient has a history of severe allergic reaction to latex, care should be taken to avoid the use of equipment containing latex.

➤ Instruct the patient to cooperate fully and to follow directions. Direct the patient to breathe normally and to avoid unnecessary movement.

➤ Observe standard precautions, and follow the general guidelines in Appendix A. Positively identify the patient, and label the appropriate tubes with the corresponding patient demographics, date, and time of collection. Perform a venipuncture; collect the specimen in a 5-mL redtop tube.

➤ Remove the needle, and apply a pressure dressing over the puncture site.

➤ Promptly transport the specimen to the laboratory for processing and analysis.

➤ The results are recorded manually or in a computerized system for recall and postprocedure interpretation by the appropriate health care practitioner.

Post-test:

➤ Observe venipuncture site for bleeding or hematoma formation. Apply paper tape or other adhesive to hold pressure bandage in place, or replace with a plastic bandage.

➤ Advise the patient to wear light-colored clothing that covers extremities when in areas infested by deer ticks, and to check body for ticks after returning from infested area.

➤ A written report of the examination will be sent to the requesting health care practitioner, who will discuss the results with the patient.

➤ Recognize anxiety related to test results, and be supportive of impaired activity related to perceived loss of independence and fear of shortened life expectancy. Lyme disease can be debilitating and can result in significant changes in lifestyle. Discuss the implications of abnormal test results on the patient's lifestyle. Provide teaching and information regarding the clinical implications of the test results, as appropriate. Educate the patient regarding access to counseling services.

➤ Reinforce information given by the patient's health care provider regarding further testing, treatment, or referral to another health care provider. Warn the patient that false-positive test results can occur and that false-negative test results frequently occur. Answer any questions or address any concerns voiced by the patient or family.

➤ Depending on the results of this procedure, additional testing may be performed to evaluate or monitor progression of the disease process and determine the need for a change in therapy. Evaluate test results in relation to the patient's symptoms and other tests performed.

Related laboratory tests:

➤ A related test is synovial fluid analysis.

LYMPHANGIOGRAPHY

· ·

SYNONYM/ACRONYM: Lymphangiogram.

AREA OF APPLICATION: Lymphatic system.

CONTRAST: Intravenous iodine based.

DESCRIPTION: Lymphangiography involves visualization of the lymphatic system after the injection of an iodinated oil–based contrast medium into a lymphatic vessel in the hand or foot. The lymphatic system consists of lymph vessels and nodes. Assessment of this system is important because cancer (lymphomas and Hodgkin's disease) often spreads via the lymphatic system. When the lymphatic system becomes obstructed, painful edema of the extremities usually results. The procedure is usually performed for cancer staging in patients with an established diagnosis of lymphoma or metastatic tumor. Injection into the hand allows visualization of the axillary and supraclavicular nodes. Injection into the foot allows visualization of the lymphatics of the leg, inguinal and iliac regions, and retroperitoneum up to the thoracic duct. Less commonly, injection into the foot can be used to visualize the cervical region (retroauricular area). This procedure can assess progression of the disease, assist in planning surgery, and monitor the effectiveness of chemotherapy or radiation treatment. ■

INDICATIONS:

- Determine the extent of adenopathy
- Determine lymphatic cancer staging
- Distinguish primary from secondary lymphedema
- Evaluate edema of an extremity without known cause
- Evaluate effects of chemotherapy or radiation therapy
- Plan surgical treatment or evaluate effectiveness of chemotherapy or radiation therapy in controlling malignant tumors

RESULT

Normal Findings:

- Normal lymphatic vessels and nodes that fill completely with contrast medium on the initial films. On the 24-hour films, the lymph nodes are fully opacified and well circumscribed. The lymphatic channels are emptied a few hours after injection of the contrast medium.

Abnormal Findings:

- Abnormal lymphatic vessels
- Hodgkin's disease
- Metastatic tumor involving the lymph glands
- Nodal lymphoma
- Retroperitoneal lymphomas associated with Hodgkin's disease

CRITICAL VALUES: N/A

INTERFERING FACTORS:

This procedure is contraindicated for:

- Patients with pulmonary insufficiencies, cardiac diseases, or severe renal or hepatic disease.

- ⚠ Patients with allergies to shellfish or iodinated dye. The contrast medium used may cause a life-threatening allergic reaction. Patients with a known hypersensitivity to the contrast medium may benefit from premedication with corticosteroids or the use of nonionic contrast medium.

- Patients who are pregnant or suspected of being pregnant, unless the potential benefits of the procedure far outweigh the risks to the fetus and mother

- ⚠ Elderly and other patients who are chronically dehydrated before the test, because of their risk of contrast-induced renal failure.

- ⚠ Patients who are in renal failure.

- Young patients (17 years old and younger), unless the benefits of the x-ray diagnosis outweigh the risks of exposure to high levels of radiation.

Factors that may impair clear imaging:

- Inability of the patient to cooperate or remain still during the procedure because of age, significant pain, or mental status

• Metallic objects within the examination field (e.g., jewelry, body rings), which may inhibit organ visualization and can produce unclear images

• Improper adjustment of the radiographic equipment to accommodate obese or thin patients, which can cause overexposure or underexposure and a poor-quality study

• Patients who are very obese, who may exceed the weight limit for the equipment

• Incorrect positioning of the patient, which may produce poor visualization of the area to be examined

• Gas or feces in the gastrointestinal tract resulting from inadequate cleansing or failure to restrict food intake before the study

• Retained barium from a previous radiologic procedure

• Inability to cannulate the lymphatic vessels

Other considerations:

• ⚠ Be aware of risks associated with the contrast medium. The oil-based contrast medium may embolize into the lungs and will temporarily diminish pulmonary function. This can produce lipid pneumonia, which is a life-threatening complication.

• Consultation with a health care practitioner should occur before the procedure for radiation safety concerns regarding younger patients or patients who are lactating.

• Risks associated with radiographic overexposure can result from frequent x-ray procedures. Personnel in the room with the patient should wear a protective lead apron, stand behind a shield, or leave the area while the examination is being done. Personnel working in the area where the examination is being done should wear badges that reveal their level of exposure to radiation.

Nursing Implications and Procedure

Pretest:

➤ Inform the patient that the procedure assesses the lymphatic system.

➤ Obtain a history of the patient's complaints or clinical symptoms, including a list of known allergens, especially allergies or sensitivities to iodine, seafood, or other contrast mediums.

➤ Obtain a history of the patient's lymphatic system and previously performed diagnostic procedures, surgical procedures, and laboratory tests. Include specific tests as they apply (e.g., blood urea nitrogen [BUN], creatinine, coagulation tests, platelets, bleeding time). Ensure that the results of blood tests are obtained and recorded before the procedure, especially BUN and creatinine, if contrast medium is to be used. For related diagnostic tests, refer to the Endocrine and Immunologic System tables.

➤ Note any recent procedures that can interfere with test results, including examinations using iodine-based contrast medium or barium.

➤ Record the date of the last menstrual period and determine the possibility of pregnancy in perimenopausal women.

➤ Obtain a list of the medications the patient is taking, including anticoagulant therapy, acetylsalicylic acid, herbs, nutritional supplements, and nutraceuticals, especially those known to affect coagulation (see Appendix F). It is recommended that use be discontinued 14 days before surgical procedures. The requesting health care practitioner and laboratory should be advised if the patient regularly uses these products so that their effects can be taken into consideration when reviewing results.

➤ Review the procedure with the patient. Address concerns about pain related to the procedure. Inform the patient that he or she may feel some discomfort when the contrast medium and anesthesia are injected. Reassure the patient that the radionuclide poses no radioactive hazard and rarely produces side effects. Inform the patient that the procedure is performed by a health care practitioner and takes 1 to 2 hours. Inform the patient that he or she may have to return the next day, but that this set of images will take only 30 minutes.

➤ Instruct the patient to remove dentures, jewelry (including watches), hairpins, credit cards, and other metallic objects.

➤ There are no food or fluid restrictions, unless by medical direction.

➤ Instruct patient to withhold anticoagulant medication or to reduce dosage before the procedure, as ordered by the health care practitioner.

➤ *Make sure a written and informed consent has been signed prior to the procedure and before administering any medications.*

Intratest:

➤ Ensure that the patient has complied with medication restrictions and pretesting preparations. Ensure that the patient has removed all external metallic objects (jewelry, dentures, etc.) prior to the procedure.

➤ Have emergency equipment readily accessible.

➤ If the patient has a history of severe allergic reactions to any substance or drug, administer ordered prophylactic steroids or antihistamines before the procedure. Use nonionic contrast medium for the procedure.

➤ Patients are given a gown, robe, and foot coverings to wear and instructed to void prior to the procedure.

➤ Obtain and record baseline vital signs, and assess neurologic status.

➤ Instruct the patient to cooperate fully and to follow directions. Instruct the patient to remain still throughout the procedure because movement produces unreliable results.

➤ Observe standard precautions, and follow the general guidelines in Appendix A.

➤ Administer a mild sedative, as ordered.

➤ Place the patient in a supine position on an x-ray table. Cleanse the selected vein and cover with a sterile drape.

➤ A local anesthetic is injected at the site, and a small incision is made or a needle inserted. The contrast medium is injected intradermally into the area between the toes or fingers. The lymphatic vessels are identified as the contrast medium moves. A local anesthetic is then injected into the dorsum of each foot or hand, and a small incision is made and cannulated for injection of the contrast medium.

➤ The contrast medium is then injected, and the flow of the contrast medium is followed by fluoroscopy. When the contrast medium reaches the upper lumbar level, the infusion of contrast medium is discontinued. X-ray images are taken of the chest, abdomen, and pelvis to determine the extent of filling of the lymphatic vessels. Twenty-four–hour delayed images may be taken to examine the lymphatic system after a period of time has elapsed and to monitor the progress of delayed flow.

➤ Ask the patient to inhale deeply and hold his or her breath while the x-ray images are taken, and then to exhale after the images are taken.

➤ Monitor the patient for complications related to the contrast medium (e.g., allergic reaction, anaphylaxis, bronchospasm).

➤ When the procedure is complete, the cannula is removed and the incision sutured.

➤ The results are recorded on film or by automated equipment in a computerized system for recall and postprocedure interpretation by the appropriate health care practitioner.

Post-test:

➤ Monitor vital signs and neurologic status every 15 minutes for 30 minutes. Compare with baseline values. Protocols may vary from facility to facility.

➤ Observe for a delayed allergic reaction to contrast medium or pulmonary embolus, which may include shortness of breath, increased heart rate, pleuritic pain, hypotension, low-grade fever, and cyanosis.

➤ Instruct the patient to resume usual medications, as directed by the health care practitioner.

➤ Instruct the patient to maintain bed rest up to 24 hours to reduce extremity swelling after the procedure, or as ordered.

➤ Advise the patient to drink increased amounts of fluids for 24 to 48 hours to eliminate the radionuclide from the body, unless contraindicated. Tell the patient that radionuclide is eliminated from the body within 6 to 24 hours.

➤ Advise the patient to immediately report symptoms such as fast heart rate, difficulty breathing, skin rash, itching, nausea, vomiting, or decreased urinary output.

➤ Observe the cannula insertion site for bleeding, inflammation, or hematoma formation.

➤ Instruct the patient to apply cold compresses to the cannulated site, as needed, to reduce discomfort or edema.

➤ Monitor for signs of infection, such as pain, fever, increased pulse rate, and muscle aches.

➤ A written report of the examination will be completed by a health care practitioner specializing in this branch of medicine. The report will be sent to the requesting health care practitioner, who will discuss the results with the patient.

➤ Reinforce information given by the patient's health care provider regarding further testing, treatment, or referral to another health care provider. Answer any questions or address any concerns voiced by the patient or family.

➤ Depending on the results of this procedure, additional testing may be needed to evaluate or monitor progression of the disease process and determine the need for a change in therapy. Evaluate test results in relation to the patient's symptoms and other tests performed.

Related diagnostic tests:

➤ Related diagnostic tests include computed tomography of the abdomen and pelvis.

MAGNESIUM, BLOOD

SYNONYM/ACRONYM: Mg^{2+}.

SPECIMEN: Serum (1 mL) collected in a red- or tiger-top tube.

REFERENCE VALUE: (Method: Spectrophotometry)

Age	Conventional Units	Alternative Units (Conventional Units × 0.8229)	SI Units (Conventional Units × 0.4114)
Newborn	1.5–2.2 mg/dL	1.23–1.81 mEq/L	0.62–0.91 mmol/L
Child	1.7–2.1 mg/dL	1.40–1.73 mEq/L	0.70–0.86 mmol/L
Adult	1.6–2.6 mg/dL	1.32–2.14 mEq/L	0.66–1.07 mmol/L

DESCRIPTION & RATIONALE: Magnesium is required as a cofactor in numerous crucial enzymatic processes, such as protein synthesis, nucleic acid synthesis, and muscle contraction. Magnesium is also required for the use of adenosine diphosphate as a source of energy. It is the fourth most abundant cation and the second most abundant intracellular ion. Magnesium is needed for the transmission of nerve impulses and muscle relaxation. It controls absorption of sodium, potassium, calcium, and phosphorus; utilization of carbohydrate, lipid, and protein; and activation of enzyme systems that enable the B vitamins to function. Magnesium is also essential for oxidative phosphorylation, nucleic acid synthesis, and blood clotting. Urine magnesium levels reflect magnesium deficiency before serum levels. Magnesium deficiency severe enough to cause hypocalcemia and cardiac arrhythmias can exist despite normal serum magnesium levels. ∎

INDICATIONS:
- Determine electrolyte balance in renal failure and chronic alcoholism
- Evaluate cardiac arrhythmias (decreased magnesium levels can lead to excessive ventricular irritability)
- Evaluate known or suspected disorders associated with altered magnesium levels
- Monitor the effects of various drugs on magnesium levels

RESULT

Increased in:
- Addison's disease
- Adrenocortical insufficiency
- Dehydration
- Diabetic acidosis (severe)
- Hypothyroidism
- Multiple myeloma
- Overuse of antacids
- Renal insufficiency
- Systemic lupus erythematosus
- Tissue trauma

Decreased in:
- Alcoholism
- Diabetic acidosis
- Glomerulonephritis (chronic)
- Hemodialysis
- Hyperaldosteronism
- Hypercalcemia
- Hypoparathyroidism
- Inadequate intake
- Inappropriate secretion of antidiuretic hormone
- Long-term hyperalimentation
- Malabsorption
- Pancreatitis
- Pregnancy
- Severe loss of body fluids (diarrhea, lactation, sweating, laxative abuse)

CRITICAL VALUES:
Less than 1.2 mg/dL
Greater than 4.9 mg/dL

Note and immediately report to the health care practitioner any critically increased or decreased values and related symptoms.

Symptoms such as tetany, weakness, dizziness, tremors, hyperactivity, nausea, vomiting, and convulsions occur at decreased (less than 1.2 mg/dL) concentrations. Electrocardiographic (ECG) changes (prolonged P-R and Q-T intervals, broad flat T waves, and ventricular tachycardia) may also occur. Treatment may include administration of magnesium salts, monitoring for respiratory depression and areflexia (intravenous [IV] administration of magnesium salts), monitoring for diarrhea and metabolic alkalosis (oral administration to replace magnesium).

Respiratory paralysis, decreased reflexes, and cardiac arrest occur at grossly elevated (greater than 15 mg/dL) levels. ECG changes, such as prolonged P-R and Q-T intervals, and bradycardia may be seen. Toxic levels of magnesium may be reversed with the administration of calcium, dialysis treatments, and removal of the source of excessive intake.

INTERFERING FACTORS:

• Drugs that may increase magnesium levels include acetylsalicylic acid and progesterone.

• Drugs that may decrease magnesium levels include albuterol, aminoglycosides, amphotericin B, bendroflumethiazide, chlorthalidone, cisplatin, citrates, cyclosporines, digoxin, gentamicin, glucagon, and oral contraceptives.

• Hemolysis results in a false elevation in values; such specimens should be rejected for analysis.

• Specimens should never be collected above an IV line because of the potential for dilution when the specimen and the IV solution combine in the collection container, falsely decreasing the result. There is also the potential of contaminating the sample with the substance of interest, if it is present in the IV solution, falsely increasing the result.

Nursing Implications and Procedure

Pretest:

➤ Inform the patient that the test is used to assist in the evaluation of electrolyte balance.

➤ Obtain a history of the patient's complaints, including a list of known allergens (especially allergies or sensitivities to latex), and inform the appropriate health care practitioner accordingly.

➤ Obtain a history of the patient's cardiovascular, endocrine, gastrointestinal, genitourinary, and reproductive systems, as well as results of previously performed laboratory tests, surgical procedures, and other diagnostic procedures. For related laboratory tests, refer to the Cardiovascular, Endocrine, Gastrointestinal, Genitourinary, and Reproductive System tables.

➤ Obtain a list of medications the patient is taking, including herbs, nutritional supplements, and nutraceuticals. The requesting health care practitioner and laboratory should be advised if the patient regularly uses these products so that their effects can be taken into consideration when reviewing results.

➤ Review the procedure with the patient. Inform the patient that specimen collection takes approximately 5 to 10 minutes. Address concerns about pain related to the procedure. Explain to the patient that there may be some discomfort during the venipuncture.

➤ There are no food, fluid, or medication restrictions, unless by medical direction.

Intratest:

➤ If the patient has a history of severe allergic reaction to latex, care should be taken to avoid the use of equipment containing latex.

➤ Instruct the patient to cooperate fully and to follow directions. Direct the patient to breathe normally and to avoid unnecessary movement.

➤ Observe standard precautions, and follow the general guidelines in Appendix A. Positively identify the patient, and label the appropriate tubes with the corresponding patient demographics, date, and time of collection. Perform a venipuncture; collect the specimen in a 5-mL red- or tiger-top tube.

➤ Remove the needle, and apply a pressure dressing over the puncture site.

➤ Promptly transport the specimen to the laboratory for processing and analysis.

➤ The results are recorded manually or in a computerized system for recall and postprocedure interpretation by the appropriate health care practitioner.

Post-test:

➤ Observe venipuncture site for bleeding or hematoma formation. Apply paper tape or other adhesive to hold pressure bandage in place, or replace with a plastic bandage.

➤ *Nutritional considerations:* Educate the magnesium-deficient patient regarding good dietary sources of magnesium, such as green vegetables, seeds, legumes, shrimp, and some bran cereals. Advise the patient that high intake of substances such as phosphorus, calcium, fat, and protein interferes with the absorption of magnesium.

➤ Instruct the patient to report any signs or symptoms of electrolyte imbalance, such as dehydration, diarrhea, vomiting, or prolonged anorexia.

➤ A written report of the examination will be sent to the requesting health care practitioner, who will discuss the results with the patient.

➤ Reinforce information given by the patient's health care provider regarding further testing, treatment, or referral to another health care provider. Answer any questions or address any concerns voiced by the patient or family.

➤ Depending on the results of this procedure, additional testing may be performed to evaluate or monitor progression of the disease process and determine the need for a change in therapy. Evaluate test results in relation to the patient's symptoms and other tests performed.

Related laboratory tests:

➤ Related laboratory tests include antiarrhythmic drugs, aspartate aminotransferase, calcium, C-reactive protein, creatine kinase and isoenzymes, homocysteine, kidney stone analysis, lactate dehydrogenase and isoenzymes, urine magnesium, myoglobin, potassium, troponin, and vitamin D.

MAGNESIUM, URINE

Synonyms/Acronym: Urine Mg^{2+}.

Specimen: Urine (5 mL) from a random or timed specimen collected in a clean plastic collection container with 6N hydrochloride as a preservative.

Reference value: (Method: Spectrophotometry)

Conventional Units	Alternative Units (Conventional Units × 0.8229)	SI Units (Conventional Units × 0.4114)
7.3–12.2 mg/24 h	6.0–10.0 mEq/24 h	3.0–5.0 mmol/24 h

Description & Rationale: Magnesium is required as a cofactor in numerous crucial enzymatic processes, such as protein synthesis, nucleic acid synthesis, and muscle contraction. Magnesium is also required for the use of adenosine diphosphate as a source of energy. It is the fourth most abundant cation and the second most abundant intracellular ion. Magnesium is needed for the transmission of nerve impulses and muscle relaxation. It controls absorption of sodium, potassium, calcium, and phosphorus; utilization of carbohydrate, lipid, and protein; and activation of enzyme systems that enable the B vitamins to function. Magnesium is also essential for oxidative phosphorylation, nucleic acid synthesis, and blood clotting. Urine magnesium levels reflect magnesium deficiency before serum levels. Magnesium deficiency severe enough to cause hypocalcemia and cardiac arrhythmias can exist despite normal serum magnesium levels.

Regulating electrolyte balance is one of the major functions of the kidneys. In normally functioning kidneys, urine levels increase when serum levels are high and decrease when serum levels are low to maintain homeostasis. Analyzing these urinary levels can provide important clues as to the functioning of the kidneys and other major organs. Tests for electrolytes, such as magnesium, in urine usually involve timed urine collections over a 12- or 24-hour period. Measurement of random specimens may also be requested. ■

Indications:
• Determine the potential cause of renal calculi

• Evaluate known or suspected endocrine disorder

- Evaluate known or suspected renal disease

- Evaluate magnesium imbalance

- Evaluate a malabsorption problem

RESULT

Increased in:
- Alcoholism
- Bartter's syndrome
- Transplant recipients on cyclosporine and prednisone
- Use of corticosteroids
- Use of diuretics

Decreased in:
- Abnormal renal function
- Crohn's disease
- Inappropriate secretion of antidiuretic hormone
- Salt-losing conditions

CRITICAL VALUES: N/A

INTERFERING FACTORS:

- Drugs that may increase urine magnesium levels include cisplatin, cyclosporine, ethacrynic acid, furosemide, mercaptomerin, mercurial diuretics, and thiazides.

- Drugs that may decrease urine magnesium levels include amiloride, angiotensin, oral contraceptives, parathyroid extract, and phosphates.

- Magnesium levels follow a circadian rhythm, and for this reason 24-hour collections are recommended.

- All urine voided for the timed collection period must be included in the collection, or else falsely decreased values may be obtained. Compare output records with volume collected to verify that all voids were included in the collection.

Nursing Implications and Procedure • • • • • • • • • •

Pretest:

➤ Inform the patient that the test is used to evaluate magnesium balance.

➤ Obtain a history of the patient's complaints, including a list of known allergens (especially allergies or sensitivities to latex), and inform the appropriate health care practitioner accordingly.

➤ Obtain a history of the patient's endocrine, gastrointestinal, and genitourinary systems, as well as results of previously performed laboratory tests, surgical procedures, and other diagnostic procedures. For related laboratory tests, refer to the Endocrine, Gastrointestinal, and Genitourinary System tables.

➤ Obtain a list of medications the patient is taking, including herbs, nutritional supplements, and nutraceuticals. The requesting health care practitioner and laboratory should be advised if the patient regularly uses these products so that their effects can be taken into consideration when reviewing results.

➤ Review the procedure with the patient. Provide a nonmetallic urinal, bedpan, or toilet-mounted collection device. Address concerns about pain related to the procedure. Explain to the patient that there should be no discomfort during the procedure.

➤ Usually a 24-hour time frame for urine collection is ordered. Inform the patient that all urine must be saved during that 24-hour period. Instruct the patient not to void directly into the laboratory collection container. Instruct the patient to avoid defecating in the collection device and to keep toilet tissue out of the collection device to prevent contamination of the specimen. Place a sign in the bathroom to remind the patient to save all urine.

➤ Instruct the patient to void all urine into the collection device and then to pour the urine into the laboratory collection container. Alternatively, the specimen can be left in the collection device for a health care staff member to add to the laboratory collection container.

➤ *Sensitivity to social and cultural issues,* as well as concern for modesty, is important in providing psychological support before, during, and after the procedure.

➤ Instruct the patient to avoid excessive exercise and stress during the 24-hour collection of urine.

➤ There are no food, fluid, or medication restrictions, unless by medical direction.

Intratest:

➤ Ensure that the patient has complied with activity restrictions during the procedure.

➤ If the patient has a history of severe allergic reaction to latex, care should be taken to avoid the use of equipment containing latex.

➤ Instruct the patient to cooperate fully and to follow directions.

➤ Observe standard precautions, and follow the general guidelines in Appendix A. Positively identify the patient, and label the appropriate tubes with the corresponding patient demographics, date, and time of collection.

Random specimen (collect in early morning):

Clean-catch specimen:

➤ Instruct the male patient to (1) thoroughly wash his hands, (2) cleanse the meatus, (3) void a small amount into the toilet, and (4) void directly into the specimen container.

➤ Instruct the female patient to (1) thoroughly wash her hands; (2) cleanse the labia from front to back; (3) while keeping the labia separated, void a small amount into the toilet; and (4) without interrupting the urine

stream, void directly into the specimen container.

Indwelling catheter:

➤ Put on gloves. Empty drainage tube of urine. It may be necessary to clamp off the catheter for 15 to 30 minutes before specimen collection. Cleanse specimen port with antiseptic swab, and then aspirate 5 mL of urine with a 21- to 25-gauge needle and syringe. Transfer urine to a sterile container.

Timed specimen:

➤ Obtain a clean 3-L urine specimen container, toilet-mounted collection device, and plastic bag (for transport of the specimen container). The specimen must be refrigerated or kept on ice throughout the entire collection period. If an indwelling urinary catheter is in place, the drainage bag must be kept on ice.

➤ Begin the test between 6 and 8 a.m., if possible. Collect first voiding and discard. Record the time the specimen was discarded as the beginning of the timed collection period. The next morning, ask the patient to void at the same time the collection was started and add this last voiding to the container.

➤ If an indwelling catheter is in place, replace the tubing and container system at the start of the collection time. Keep the container system on ice during the collection period, or empty the urine into a larger container periodically during the collection period; monitor to ensure continued drainage, and conclude the test the next morning at the same hour the collection was begun.

➤ At the conclusion of the test, compare the quantity of urine with the urinary output record for the collection; if the specimen contains less than what was recorded as output, some urine may have been discarded, invalidating the test.

➤ Include on the collection container's label the amount of urine, test start and stop times, and ingestion of any foods or medications that can affect test results.

➤ Promptly transport the specimen to the laboratory for processing and analysis.

➤ The results are recorded manually or in a computerized system for recall and postprocedure interpretation by the appropriate health care practitioner.

Post-test:

➤ *Nutritional considerations:* Educate the magnesium-deficient patient regarding good dietary sources of magnesium, such as green vegetables, seeds, legumes, shrimp, and some bran cereals. Advise the patient that high intake of substances such as phosphorus, calcium, fat, and protein interferes with the absorption of magnesium.

➤ Instruct the patient to report any signs or symptoms of electrolyte imbalance, such as dehydration, diarrhea, vomiting, or prolonged anorexia.

➤ A written report of the examination will be sent to the requesting health care practitioner, who will discuss the results with the patient.

➤ Recognize anxiety related to test results. Discuss the implications of abnormal test results on the patient's lifestyle. Provide teaching and information regarding the clinical implications of the test results, as appropriate.

➤ Reinforce information given by the patient's health care provider regarding further testing, treatment, or referral to another health care provider. Answer any questions or address any concerns voiced by the patient or family.

➤ Depending on the results of this procedure, additional testing may be performed to evaluate or monitor progression of the disease process and determine the need for a change in therapy. Evaluate test results in relation to the patient's symptoms and other tests performed.

Related laboratory tests:

➤ Related laboratory tests include calcium, kidney stone analysis, magnesium, phosphorus, potassium, and vitamin D.

MAGNETIC RESONANCE ANGIOGRAPHY

SYNONYM/ACRONYM: MRA.

AREA OF APPLICATION: Vascular.

CONTRAST: Can be done with or without intravenous (IV) contrast (gadolinium).

DESCRIPTION & RATIONALE: Magnetic resonance imaging (MRI) uses a magnet and radio waves to produce an energy field that can be displayed as an image. The magnetic field causes the hydrogen atoms in tissue to line up, and when radio waves are directed toward the magnetic field, the atoms absorb the radio waves and change their position. When the radio waves are turned off, the atoms go back to their original position, this change in the energy field is sensed by the equipment, and an image is generated by the attached computer system. MRI produces cross-sectional images of the vessels in multiple planes without the use of ionizing radiation or the interference of bone or surrounding tissue.

Magnetic resonance angiography (MRA) is an application of MRI that provides images of blood flow and diseased and normal blood vessels. In patients who are allergic to iodinated contrast medium, MRA is used in place of angiography. MRA is particularly useful for visualizing vascular abnormalities, dissections, and other pathology. Special imaging sequences allow the visualization of moving blood within the vascular system. Two common techniques to obtain images of flowing blood are time-of-flight and phase-contrast MRA. In time-of-flight imaging, incoming blood makes the vessels appear bright and surrounding tissue is suppressed. Phase-contrast images are produced by subtracting the stationary tissue surrounding the vessels where the blood is moving through vessels during the imaging, producing high-contrast images. MRA is the most accurate technique for imaging blood flowing in veins and small arteries (*laminar flow*), but it does not accurately depict blood flow in tortuous sections of vessels and distal to bifurcations and stenosis. Swirling blood may cause a signal loss and result in inadequate images, and the degree of vessel stenosis may be overestimated. Images can be obtained in two-dimensional (series of slices) or three-dimensional sequences. ■

INDICATIONS:
- Detect pericardial abnormalities
- Detect peripheral vascular disease
- Detect thoracic and abdominal vascular diseases
- Determine renal artery stenosis
- Differentiate aortic aneurysms from tumors near the aorta
- Evaluate cardiac chambers and pulmonary vessels
- Evaluate postoperative angioplasty sites and bypass grafts
- Identify congenital vascular diseases
- Monitor and evaluate the effectiveness of medical or surgical treatment

RESULT

Normal Findings:
- Normal blood flow in the area being examined, including blood flow rate

Abnormal Findings:
- Coarctations
- Dissections
- Thrombosis within a vessel
- Tumor invasion of a vessel
- Vascular abnormalities
- Vessel occlusion
- Vessel stenosis

CRITICAL VALUES: N/A

INTERFERING FACTORS

This procedure is contraindicated for:

- Patients with certain ferrous metal prosthetics, valves, aneurysm clips, inner ear prostheses, or other metallic objects

- Patients with metal in their body, such as shrapnel or ferrous metal in the eye

- ⚠ Patients with cardiac pacemakers, because the pacemaker can be deactivated by MRI

- Patients who are claustrophobic

- Patients who are pregnant or suspected of being pregnant, unless the potential benefits of the procedure far outweigh the risks to the fetus and mother

Factors that may impair clear imaging:

- Metallic objects within the examination field (e.g., jewelry, body rings, dental amalgams), which may inhibit organ visualization and can produce unclear images

- Patients who are very obese, who may exceed the weight limit for the equipment

- Incorrect positioning of the patient, which may produce poor visualization of the area to be examined

- Inability of the patient to cooperate or remain still during the procedure because of age, significant pain, or mental status

- Patients with extreme cases of claustrophobia, unless sedation is given before the study

Other considerations:

- If contrast medium is allowed to seep deep into the muscle tissue, vascular visualization will be impossible.

Nursing Implications and Procedure • • • • • • • • • • •

Pretest:

➤ Inform the patient that the procedure assesses the vascular system.

➤ Obtain a history of the patient's complaints, including a list of known allergens (especially allergies or sensitivities to contrast medium), and inform the appropriate health care practitioner accordingly.

➤ Obtain a history of the patient's cardiovascular system, as well as results of previously performed diagnostic procedures, surgical procedures, and laboratory tests. For related diagnostic tests, refer to the Cardiovascular System table.

➤ Determine if the patient has ever had any device implanted into his or her body, including copper intrauterine devices, pacemakers, ear implants, and heart valves.

➤ Obtain occupational history to determine the presence of metal in the body, such as shrapnel or flecks of ferrous metal in the eye (which can cause retinal hemorrhage).

➤ Note any recent procedures that can interfere with test results.

➤ Record the date of the last menstrual period and determine the possibility of pregnancy in perimenopausal women.

➤ Obtain a list of the medications the patient is taking.

➤ Review the procedure with the patient. Address concerns about pain related to the procedure. Explain to the patient that no pain will be experienced during the test, but there may be moments of discomfort. Inform the patient that the procedure is performed in an MRI department, usually by a technologist and support staff, and takes approximately 30 to 60 minutes.

➤ Inform the patient that the technologist will place him or her in a supine position on a flat table in a large cylindrical scanner.

➤ Tell the patient to expect to hear loud banging from the scanner and possibly to see magnetophosphenes (flickering lights in the visual field); these will stop when the procedure is over.

➤ *Sensitivity to cultural and social issues,* as well as concern for modesty, is important in providing psychological support before, during, and after the procedure.

➤ Explain that an IV line may be inserted to allow infusion of IV fluids, contrast medium, dye, or sedatives. Usually normal saline is infused.

➤ There are no food, fluid, or medication restrictions, unless by medical direction.

➤ Instruct the patient to remove dentures, jewelry (including watches), hairpins, credit cards, and other metallic objects.

Intratest:

➤ Ensure that the patient has removed jewelry, dentures, all external metallic objects etc. prior to the procedure.

➤ Have emergency equipment readily available.

➤ If the patient has a history of severe allergic reactions to any substance or drug, administer ordered prophylactic steroids or antihistamines before the procedure.

➤ Patients are given a gown, robe, and foot coverings to wear and instructed to void prior to the procedure.

➤ Instruct the patient to cooperate fully and to follow directions. Instruct the patient to remain still throughout the procedure because movement produces unreliable results.

➤ Observe standard precautions, and follow the general guidelines in Appendix A.

➤ Supply earplugs to the patient to block out the loud, banging sounds that occur during the test.

➤ If an electrocardiogram or respiratory

gating is to be performed in conjunction with the scan, apply MRI-safe electrodes to the appropriate sites.

➤ The patient can communicate with the technologist during the examination via a microphone within the machine.

➤ Establish intravenous fluid line for the injection of emergency drugs, and sedatives.

➤ Administer an antianxiety agent, as ordered, if the patient has claustrophobia. Administer a sedative to a child or to an uncooperative adult, as ordered.

➤ Place the patient in the supine position on an exam table.

➤ If ordered with contrast, the contrast medium is injected, and a series of images is taken during and after the filling of the vessels to be examined. Delayed images may be taken to monitor the venous phase of the procedure.

➤ Instruct the patient to take slow, deep breaths if nausea occurs during the procedure.

➤ Monitor the patient for complications related to the procedure (e.g., allergic reaction, anaphylaxis, bronchospasm).

➤ The results are recorded on film or on automated equipment in a computerized system for recall and post-procedure interpretation by the appropriate health care practitioner.

Post-test:

➤ If contrast is administered, observe for delayed allergic reactions, such as rash, urticaria, tachycardia, hyperpnea, hypertension, palpitations, nausea, or vomiting.

➤ Advise the patient to immediately report symptoms such as fast heart rate, difficulty breathing, skin rash, itching or decreased urinary output

➤ Observe the needle/catheter insertion site for bleeding, inflammation, or hematoma formation.

➤ Instruct the patient to apply cold compresses to the puncture site, as

➤ needed, to reduce discomfort or edema.

➤ A written report of the examination will be completed by a health care practitioner specializing in this branch of medicine. The report will be sent to the requesting health care practitioner, who will discuss the results with the patient.

➤ Reinforce information given by the patient's health care provider regarding further testing, treatment, or referral to another health care provider. Explain the importance of adhering to the therapy regimen. Answer any questions or address any concerns voiced by the patient or family.

➤ Depending on the results of this procedure, additional testing may be performed to evaluate or monitor progression of the disease process and determine the need for a change in therapy. Evaluate test results in relation to the patient's symptoms and other tests performed.

Related diagnostic tests:

➤ Related diagnostic tests include angiography of the body area of interest, computed tomography angiography, and ultrasound arterial Doppler carotid and venous Doppler ultrasound.

MAGNETIC RESONANCE IMAGING, ABDOMEN

SYNONYM/ACRONYM: Abdominal MRI.

AREA OF APPLICATION: Liver/abdominal area.

CONTRAST: Can be done with or without intravenous (IV) contrast medium (gadolinium).

DESCRIPTION & RATIONALE: Magnetic resonance imaging (MRI) uses a magnet and radio waves to produce an energy field that can be displayed as an image. Use of magnetic fields with the aid of radiofrequency energy produces images primarily based on water content of tissue. The magnetic field causes the hydrogen atoms in tissue to line up, and when radio waves are directed toward the magnetic field, the atoms absorb the radio waves and change their position. When the radio waves are turned off, the atoms go back to their original position; this change in the energy field is sensed by the equipment, and an image is generated by the attached computer system.

MRI produces cross-sectional images of the abdomen in multiple planes without the use of ionizing radiation or the interference of bone.

Abdominal MRI is performed to assist in diagnosing abnormalities of abdominal and hepatic structures. Contrast-enhanced imaging is effective for distinguishing peritoneal metastases from primary tumors of the gastrointestinal tract. Primary tumors of the stomach, pancreas, colon, and appendix often spread by intraperitoneal tumor shedding and subsequent peritoneal carcinomatosis. MRI uses the noniodinated contrast medium gadopentetate dimeglumine (Magnevist), which is administered intravenously to enhance contrast differences between normal and abnormal tissues.

Magnetic resonance angiography (MRA) is an application of MRI that provides images of blood flow and diseased and normal blood vessels. In patients who are allergic to iodinated contrast medium, MRA is used in place of angiography (see monograph titled "Magnetic Resonance Angiography"). When the Food and Drug Administration approves gastrointestinal contrast agents, these agents would assist in identifying areas of bowel wall thickening, stricture, and intraluminal abnormalities, such as tumors, sites of perforation, and fistula. ∎

INDICATIONS:

- Detect abdominal aortic diseases

- Detect and stage cancer (primary or metastatic tumors of liver, pancreas, prostate, uterus, and bladder)

- Detect chronic pancreatitis

- Detect renal vein thrombosis

- Detect soft tissue abnormalities

- Determine and monitor tissue damage in renal transplant patients

- Determine the presence of blood clots, cysts, fluid or fat accumulation in tissues, hemorrhage, and infarctions

- Determine vascular complications of pancreatitis, venous thrombosis, or pseudoaneurysm

- Differentiate aortic aneurysms from tumors near the aorta

- Differentiate liver tumors from liver abnormalities, such as cysts, cavernous hemangiomas, and hepatic amebic abscesses

- Evaluate postoperative angioplasty sites and bypass grafts

- Monitor and evaluate the effectiveness of medical or surgical interventions and the course of the disease

RESULT

Normal Findings:
- Normal anatomic structures, soft tissue density, and biochemical constituents of body tissues, including blood flow

Abnormal Findings:
- Acute tubular necrosis

- Aneurysm

- Cholangitis

- Glomerulonephritis

- Hydronephrosis

- Internal bleeding

- Masses, lesions, infections, or inflammations

- Renal vein thrombosis

- Vena cava obstruction

CRITICAL VALUES: N/A

INTERFERING FACTORS:

This procedure is contraindicated for:

- Patients with certain ferrous metal prostheses, valves, aneurysm clips, inner ear prostheses, or other metallic objects

- Patients with metal in their body, such as shrapnel or ferrous metal in the eye

- ⚠️ Patients with cardiac pacemakers, because the pacemaker can be deactivated by MRI

- Patients with intrauterine devices

- Patients with iron pigments in tattoos

- Patients who are claustrophobic

- Patients who are pregnant or suspected of being pregnant, unless the potential benefits of the procedure far outweigh the risks to the fetus and mother

Factors that may impair clear imaging:

- Metallic objects within the examination field (e.g., jewelry, body rings, dental amalgams), which may inhibit organ visualization and can produce unclear images

- Patients who are very obese, who may exceed the weight limit for the equipment

- Incorrect positioning of the patient, which may produce poor visualization of the area to be examined

- Inability of the patient to cooperate or remain still during the procedure because of age, significant pain, or mental status

- Patients with extreme cases of claustrophobia, unless sedation is given before the study or an open MRI is utilized

Other considerations:

- If contrast medium is allowed to seep deep into the muscle tissue, vascular visualization will be impossible.

Nursing Implications and Procedure • • • • • • • • • • •

Pretest:

➤ Inform the patient that the procedure assesses the organs and structures inside the abdomen.

➤ Obtain a history of the patient's complaints, including a list of known allergens (especially allergies or sensitivities to contrast medium), and inform the appropriate health care practitioner accordingly.

➤ Obtain a history of the patient's gastrointestinal, genitourinary, and hepatobiliary systems, as well as results of previously performed diagnostic procedures, surgical procedures, and laboratory tests. Ensure that the results of blood tests are obtained and recorded before the procedure, especially coagulation tests, blood urea nitrogen, and creatinine, if contrast medium is to be used. For related diagnostic tests, refer to the Gastrointestinal, Genitourinary, and Hepatobiliary System tables.

➤ Determine if the patient has ever had any device implanted into his or her body, including copper intrauterine devices, pacemakers, ear implants, and heart valves.

➤ Obtain occupational history to determine the presence of metal in the body, such as shrapnel or flecks of ferrous metal in the eye (which can cause retinal hemorrhage).

➤ Note any recent procedures that can interfere with test results, including examinations using iodine-based contrast medium or barium.

➤ Record the date of the last menstrual period and determine the possibility of pregnancy in perimenopausal women.

➤ Obtain a list of the medications the patient is taking.

➤ Review the procedure with the patient. Address concerns about pain related to the procedure. Explain to the patient that no pain will be experienced during the test, but there may be moments of discomfort. Reassure the patient that, if contrast is used, the radionuclide poses no radioactive hazard and rarely produces side effescts. Inform the patient that the procedure is performed in an MRI department, usually by a technologist and support staff, and takes approximately 30 to 60 minutes.

➤ Inform the patient that the technologist will place him or her in a supine position on a flat table in a large cylindrical scanner.

➤ Tell the patient to expect to hear loud banging from the scanner and possibly to see magnetophosphenes (flickering lights in the visual field); these will stop when the procedure is over.

➤ *Sensitivity to social and cultural issues,* as well as concern for modesty, is important in providing psychological support before, during, and after the procedure.

➤ Explain that an IV line may be inserted to allow infusion of IV fluids, contrast medium, dye, or sedatives. Usually normal saline is infused.

➤ Inform the patient that a burning and flushing sensation may be felt throughout the body during injection of the contrast medium. After injection of the contrast medium, the patient may experience an urge to cough, flushing, nausea, or a salty or metallic taste.

➤ There are no food, fluid, or medication restrictions, unless by medical direction.

➤ Instruct the patient to remove dentures, jewelry (including watches), hairpins, credit cards, and other metallic objects.

➤ *Make sure a written and informed consent has been signed prior to the procedure and before administering any medications.*

Intratest:

➤ Ensure that the patient has removed all external metallic objects (jew-

elry, dentures, etc.) prior to the procedure.

➤ Have emergency equipment readily available.

➤ If the patient has a history of severe allergic reactions to any substance or drug, administer ordered prophylactic steroids or antihistamines before the procedure.

➤ Patients are given a gown, robe, and foot coverings to wear and instructed to void prior to the procedure.

➤ Instruct the patient to cooperate fully and to follow directions. Instruct the patient to remain still throughout the procedure because movement produces unreliable results.

➤ Observe standard precautions, and follow the general guidelines in Appendix A.

➤ Supply earplugs to the patient to block out the loud, banging sounds that occur during the test.

➤ The patient can communicate with the technologist during the examination via a microphone within the machine.

➤ Establish an IV fluid line for the injection of emergency drugs and of sedatives.

➤ Administer an antianxiety agent, as ordered, if the patient has claustrophobia. Administer a sedative to a child or to an uncooperative adult, as ordered.

➤ Place the patient in the supine position on an exam table.

➤ If ordered with contrast, the contrast medium is injected, and a series of images is taken during and after the filling of the vessels to be examined. Delayed images may be taken to monitor the venous phase of the procedure.

➤ Instruct the patient to take slow, deep breaths if nausea occurs during the procedure.

➤ Monitor the patient for complications related to the procedure (e.g., allergic reaction, anaphylaxis, bronchospasm).

➤ The needle or catheter is removed,

and a pressure dressing is applied over the puncture site.

➤ The results are recorded on film or on automated equipment in a computerized system for recall and postprocedure interpretation by the appropriate health care practitioner.

Post-test:

➤ Observe for delayed allergic reactions, such as rash, urticaria, tachycardia, hyperpnea, hypertension, palpitations, nausea, or vomiting, if contrast medium was used.

➤ Instruct the patient to immediately report symptoms such as fast heart rate, difficulty breathing, skin rash, itching or decreased urinary output

➤ Observe the needle/catheter insertion site for bleeding, inflammation, or hematoma formation.

➤ Instruct the patient to apply cold compresses to the puncture site, as needed, to reduce discomfort or edema.

➤ No other radionuclide tests should be scheduled for 24 to 48 hours after this procedure.

➤ A written report of the examination will be completed by a health care practitioner specializing in this branch of medicine. The report will be sent to the requesting health care practitioner, who will discuss the results with the patient.

➤ Recognize anxiety related to test results, and be supportive of perceived loss of independent function. Discuss the implications of abnormal test results on the patient's lifestyle. Provide teaching and information regarding the clinical implications of the test results, as appropriate.

➤ Reinforce information given by the patient's health care provider regarding further testing, treatment, or referral to another health care provider. Explain the importance of adhering to the therapy regimen. Answer any questions or address any concerns voiced by the patient or family.

➤ Depending on the results of this procedure, additional testing may be performed to evaluate or monitor progression of the disease process and determine the need for a change in therapy. Evaluate test results in relation to the patient's symptoms and other tests performed.

Related diagnostic tests:

➤ Related diagnostic tests include angiography of the abdomen; computed tomography of the abdomen; kidney, ureter, and bladder (KUB) study; and ultrasound of the liver and biliary system.

MAGNETIC RESONANCE IMAGING, BRAIN

• •

SYNONYM/ACRONYM: Brain MRI.

AREA OF APPLICATION: Brain area.

CONTRAST: Can be done with or without intravenous (IV) contrast medium (gadolinium).

DESCRIPTION & RATIONALE: Magnetic resonance imaging (MRI) uses a magnet and radio waves to produce an energy field that can be displayed as an image. Use of magnetic fields with the aid of radiofrequency energy produces images primarily based on water content of tissue. The magnetic field causes the hydrogen atoms in tissue to line up, and when radio waves are directed toward the magnetic field, the atoms absorb the radio waves and change their position. When the radio waves are turned off, the atoms go back to their original position, this change in the energy field is sensed by the equipment, and an image is generated by the attached computer system. MRI produces cross-sectional images of pathologic lesions of the brain in multiple planes without the use of ionizing radiation or the interference of bone or surrounding tissue.

Brain MRI can distinguish solid, cystic, and hemorrhagic components of lesions. This procedure is done to aid in the diagnosis of intracranial abnormalities, including tumors, ischemia, infection, and multiple sclerosis, and in assessment of brain maturation in pediatric patients. Rapidly flowing blood on spin-echo MRI appears as an absence of signal or a void in the vessel's lumen. Blood flow can be evaluated in the cavernous and carotid arteries. Aneurysms may be diagnosed without traditional iodine-based contrastangiography, and old clotted blood in the walls of the aneurysms appears white. MRI uses the noniodinated contrast medium gadopentetate dimeglumine (Magnevist), which is administered intravenously to enhance contrast differences between normal and abnormal tissues.

Magnetic resonance angiography (MRA) is an application of MRI that provides images of blood flow and diseased and normal blood vessels. In patients who are allergic to iodinated contrast medium, MRA is used in place of angiography (see monograph titled "Magnetic Resonance Angiography"). ∎

INDICATIONS:

• Detect and locate brain tumors

• Detect cause of cerebrovascular accident, cerebral infarct, or hemorrhage

• Detect cranial bone, face, throat, and neck soft tissue lesions

• Evaluate the cause of seizures, such as intracranial infection, edema, or increased intracranial pressure

• Evaluate cerebral changes associated with dementia

• Evaluate demyelinating disorders

• Evaluate intracranial infections

• Evaluate optic and auditory nerves

• Evaluate the potential causes of headache, visual loss, and vomiting

• Evaluate shunt placement and function in patients with hydrocephalus

• Evaluate the solid, cystic, and hemorrhagic components of lesions

• Evaluate vascularity of the brain and vascular integrity

• Monitor and evaluate the effectiveness of medical or surgical interventions, chemotherapy, and radiation therapy and the course of disease

RESULT

Normal Findings:

• Normal anatomic structures, soft tissue density, blood flow rate, face, nasopharynx, neck, tongue, and brain

Abnormal Findings:

- Abscess
- Acoustic neuroma
- Alzheimer's disease
- Aneurysm
- Arteriovenous malformation
- Benign meningioma
- Cerebral aneurysm
- Cerebral infarction
- Craniopharyngioma or meningioma
- Granuloma
- Intraparenchymal hematoma or hemorrhage
- Lipoma
- Metastasis
- Multiple sclerosis
- Optic nerve tumor
- Parkinson's disease
- Pituitary microadenoma
- Subdural empyema
- Ventriculitis

CRITICAL VALUES: N/A

INTERFERING FACTORS:

This procedure is contraindicated for:

- Patients with certain ferrous metal prostheses, valves, aneurysm clips, inner ear prostheses, or other metallic objects
- Patients with metal in their body, such as shrapnel or ferrous metal in the eye
- ⚠ Patients with cardiac pacemakers, because the pacemaker can be deactivated by MRI
- Patients with intrauterine devices
- Patients with iron pigments in tattoos

- Patients who are claustrophobic
- Patients who are pregnant or suspected of being pregnant, unless the potential benefits of the procedure far outweigh the risks to the fetus and mother

Factors that may impair clear imaging:

- Metallic objects within the examination field (e.g., jewelry, body rings, dental amalgams), which may inhibit organ visualization and can produce unclear images
- Patients who are very obese, who may exceed the weight limit for the equipment
- Incorrect positioning of the patient, which may produce poor visualization of the area to be examined
- Inability of the patient to cooperate or remain still during the procedure because of age, significant pain, or mental status
- Patients with extreme cases of claustrophobia, unless sedation is given before the study or an open MRI is utilized

Other considerations:

- If contrast medium is allowed to seep deep into the muscle tissue, vascular visualization will be impossible.

Nursing Implications and Procedure • • • • • • • • • •

Pretest:

➤ Inform the patient that the procedure assesses the brain.

➤ Obtain a history of the patient's complaints, including a list of known allergens (especially allergies or sensitivities to contrast medium), and inform the appropriate health care practitioner accordingly.

➤ Obtain a history of the patient's cardiovascular and endocrine systems, as well as results of previously performed diagnostic procedures, surgical procedures, and laboratory tests. For related diagnostic tests, refer to the Cardiovascular and Endocrine System tables.

➤ Determine if the patient has ever had any device implanted into his or her body, including copper intrauterine devices, pacemakers, ear implants, and heart valves.

➤ Obtain occupational history to determine the presence of metal in the body, such as shrapnel or flecks of ferrous metal in the eye (which can cause retinal hemorrhage).

➤ Note any recent procedures that can interfere with test results, including examinations using iodine-based contrast medium or barium.

➤ Record the date of the last menstrual period and determine the possibility of pregnancy in perimenopausal women.

➤ Obtain a list of the medications the patient is taking.

➤ Review the procedure with the patient. Address concerns about pain related to the procedure. Explain to the patient that no pain will be experienced during the test, but there may be moments of discomfort. Inform the patient that the procedure is performed in an MRI department, usually by a technologist and support staff, and takes approximately 30 to 60 minutes.

➤ Inform the patient that the technologist will place him or her in a supine position on a flat table in a large cylindrical scanner.

➤ Tell the patient to expect to hear loud banging from the scanner and possibly to see magnetophosphenes (flickering lights in the visual field); these will stop when the procedure is over.

➤ *Sensitivity to social and cultural issues,* as well as concern for modesty, is important in providing psychological support before, during, and after the procedure.

➤ Explain that an IV line may be

inserted to allow infusion of IV fluids, contrast medium, dye, or sedatives. Usually normal saline is infused.

➤ There are no food, fluid, or medication restrictions, unless by medical direction.

➤ Instruct the patient to remove dentures, jewelry (including watches), hairpins, credit cards, and other metallic objects.

Intratest:

➤ Ensure that the patient has removed all external metallic objects (jewelry, dentures, etc.) prior to the procedure.

➤ Have emergency equipment readily available.

➤ If the patient has a history of severe allergic reactions to any substance or drug, administer ordered prophylactic steroids or antihistamines before the procedure.

➤ Patients are given a gown, robe, and foot coverings to wear and instructed to void prior to the procedure.

➤ Instruct the patient to cooperate fully and to follow directions. Instruct the patient to remain still throughout the procedure because movement produces unreliable results.

➤ Observe standard precautions, and follow the general guidelines in Appendix A.

➤ Supply earplugs to the patient to block out the loud, banging sounds that occur during the test.

➤ If an electrocardiogram or respiratory gating is to be performed in conjunction with the scan, apply MRI-safe electrodes to the appropriate sites.

➤ The patient can communicate with the technologist during the examination via a microphone within the machine.

➤ Establish an IV fluid line for the injection of emergency drugs and of sedatives.

➤ Administer an antianxiety agent, as ordered, if the patient has claustrophobia. Administer a sedative to a child or to an uncooperative adult, as ordered.

➤ Place the patient in the supine position on an exam table.

➤ If ordered with contrast, the contrast medium is injected, and a series of images is taken during and after the filling of the vessels to be examined. Delayed images may be taken to monitor the venous phase of the procedure.

➤ Instruct the patient to take slow, deep breaths if nausea occurs during the procedure.

➤ Monitor the patient for complications related to the procedure (e.g., allergic reaction, anaphylaxis, bronchospasm).

➤ The needle or catheter is removed, and a pressure dressing is applied over the puncture site.

➤ The results are recorded on film or on automated equipment in a computerized system for recall and postprocedure interpretation by the appropriate health care practitioner.

Post-test:

➤ Observe for delayed allergic reactions, such as rash, urticaria, tachycardia, hyperpnea, hypertension, palpitations, nausea, or vomiting, if contrast medium was used.

➤ Instruct the patient to immediately report symptoms such as fast heart rate, difficulty breathing, skin rash, itching or decreased urinary output

➤ Observe the needle/catheter insertion site for bleeding, inflammation, or hematoma formation.

➤ Instruct the patient to apply cold compresses to the puncture site, as needed, to reduce discomfort or edema.

➤ A written report of the examination will be completed by a health care practitioner specializing in this branch of medicine. The report will be sent to the requesting health care practitioner, who will discuss the results with the patient.

➤ Recognize anxiety related to test results, and be supportive of perceived loss of independent function. Discuss the implications of abnormal test results on the patient's lifestyle. Provide teaching and information regarding the clinical implications of the test results, as appropriate.

➤ Reinforce information given by the patient's health care provider regarding further testing, treatment, or referral to another health care provider. Explain the importance of adhering to the therapy regimen. Answer any questions or address any concerns voiced by the patient or family.

➤ Depending on the results of this procedure, additional testing may be performed to evaluate or monitor progression of the disease process and determine the need for a change in therapy. Evaluate test results in relation to the patient's symptoms and other tests performed.

Related diagnostic tests:

➤ Related diagnostic tests include angiography of the carotids, computed tomography of the brain, and positron emission tomography scan of the brain.

MAGNETIC RESONANCE IMAGING, BREAST

- -

SYNONYM/ACRONYM: Breast MRI.

AREA OF APPLICATION: Breast area.

CONTRAST: Can be done with or without intravenous (IV) contrast medium (gadolinium).

DESCRIPTION & RATIONALE: Magnetic resonance imaging (MRI) uses a magnet and radio waves to produce an energy field that can be displayed as an image. Use of magnetic fields with the aid of radiofrequency energy produces images primarily based on water content of tissue. The magnetic field causes the hydrogen atoms in tissue to line up, and when radio waves are directed toward the magnetic field, the atoms absorb the radio waves and change their position. When the radio waves are turned off, the atoms go back to their original position, this change in the energy field is sensed by the equipment, and an image is generated by the attached computer system. MRI produces cross-sectional images of the pathologic lesions in multiple planes without the use of ionizing radiation or the interference of surrounding tissue, breast implants, or surgically implanted clips.

MRI imaging of the breast is not a replacement for traditional mammography, ultrasound, or biopsy. This exam is extremely helpful in evaluating mammogram abnormalities and identifying early breast cancer in women at high risk. High-risk women include those who have had breast cancer, have an abnormal mutated breast cancer gene (*BRCA1* or *BRCA2*), or have a mother or sister who has been diagnosed with breast cancer. Breast MRI is used most commonly in high-risk women when findings of a mammogram or ultrasound are inconclusive because of dense breast tissue or there is a suspected abnormality that requires further evaluation. MRI is also an excellent exam in the augmented breast, including both the breast implant itself and the breast tissue surrounding the implant. This same exam is also useful for staging breast cancer and determining the most appropriate treatment. MRI uses the noniodinated contrast medium gadopentetate dimeglumine (Magnevist), which is administered intravenously to enhance contrast differences between normal and abnormal tissues. ∎

INDICATIONS:

- Evaluate breast implants

- Evaluate dense breasts

- Evaluate for residual cancer after lumpectomy

- Evaluate inverted nipples

- Evaluate small abnormalities

- Evaluate tissue after lumpectomy or mastectomy

- Evaluate women at high risk for breast cancer

RESULT

Normal Findings:

- Normal anatomic structures, soft tissue density, and blood flow rate

Abnormal Findings:

- Breast abscess or cyst

- Breast cancer

- Breast implant rupture

- Hematoma

- Soft tissue masses

- Vascular abnormalities

CRITICAL VALUES: N/A

INTERFERING FACTORS:

This procedure is contraindicated for:

- Patients with certain ferrous metal prostheses, valves, aneurysm clips, inner ear prostheses, or other metallic objects

- Patients with metal in their body, such as shrapnel or ferrous metal in the eye

- ⚠ Patients with cardiac pacemakers, because the pacemaker can be deactivated by MRI

- Patients with intrauterine devices

- Patients with iron pigments in tattoos

- Patients who are claustrophobic

- Patients who are pregnant or suspected of being pregnant, unless the potential benefits of the procedure far outweigh the risks to the fetus and mother

Factors that may impair clear imaging:

- Metallic objects within the examination field (e.g., jewelry, body rings), which may inhibit organ visualization and can produce unclear images

- Patients who are very obese, who may exceed the weight limit for the equipment

- Incorrect positioning of the patient, which may produce poor visualization of the area to be examined

- Inability of the patient to cooperate or remain still during the procedure because of age, significant pain, or mental status, may interfere with the test results.

- Patients with extreme cases of claustrophobia, unless sedation is given before the study or an open MRI is utilized

Other considerations:

- The procedure may take 30 to 60 minutes to complete, and may require the injection of contrast material.

- If contrast medium is allowed to seep deep into the muscle tissue, vascular visualization will be impossible.

- The procedure can be nonspecific; the exam is unable to image calcifications that can indicate breast cancer, and there may be difficulty distinguishing between cancerous and noncancerous tumors.

- The procedure is not widely available, and costs significantly more than a mammogram or ultrasound.

Nursing Implications and Procedure • • • • • • • • • • •

Pretest:

➤ Inform the patient that the procedure assesses the breast.

➤ Obtain a history of the patient's complaints, including a list of known allergens (especially allergies or sensitivities to contrast medium), and inform the appropriate health care practitioner accordingly.

➤ Obtain a history of the patient's reproductive system, as well as results of previously performed diagnostic procedures, surgical procedures, and laboratory tests. For related diagnostic tests, refer to the Reproductive System table.

➤ Determine if the patient has ever had any device implanted into his or her body, including copper intrauterine devices, pacemakers, ear implants, and heart valves.

➤ Obtain occupational history to determine the presence of metal in the body, such as shrapnel or flecks of ferrous metal in the eye (which can cause retinal hemorrhage).

➤ Note any recent procedures that can interfere with test results, including examinations using iodine-based contrast medium or barium.

➤ Record the date of the last menstrual period and determine the possibility of pregnancy in perimenopausal women.

➤ Obtain a list of the medications the patient is taking.

➤ Review the procedure with the patient. Address concerns about pain related to the procedure. Explain to the patient that no pain will be experienced during the test, but there may be moments of discomfort. Inform the patient that the procedure is performed in an MRI department, usually by a technologist and support staff, and takes approximately 30 to 60 minutes.

➤ Inform the patient that the technologist will place him or her in a prone position on a special imaging table in a large cylindrical scanner.

➤ Tell the patient to expect to hear loud banging from the scanner and possibly to see magnetophosphenes (flickering lights in the visual field); these will stop when the procedure is over.

➤ *Sensitivity to social and cultural issues,* as well as concern for modesty, is important in providing psychological support before, during, and after the procedure.

➤ Explain that an IV line may be inserted to allow infusion of IV fluids, contrast medium, dye, or sedatives. Usually normal saline is infused.

➤ There are no food, fluid, or medication restrictions, unless by medical direction.

➤ Instruct the patient to remove dentures, jewelry (including watches), hairpins, credit cards, and other metallic objects.

Intratest:

➤ Ensure that the patient has removed all external metallic objects (jewelry, dentures, etc.) prior to the procedure.

➤ Have emergency equipment readily available.

➤ If the patient has a history of severe allergic reactions to any substance or drug, administer ordered prophylactic steroids or antihistamines before the procedure.

➤ Patients are given a gown, robe, and foot coverings to wear and instructed to void prior to the procedure.

➤ Instruct the patient to cooperate fully and to follow directions. Instruct the patient to remain still throughout the procedure because movement produces unreliable results.

➤ Observe standard precautions, and follow the general guidelines in Appendix A.

➤ Supply earplugs to the patient to block out the loud, banging sounds that occur during the test.

➤ The patient can communicate with the technologist during the examination via a microphone within the machine.

➤ Establish an IV fluid line for the injection of emergency drugs and of sedatives.

➤ Administer an antianxiety agent, as ordered, if the patient has claustrophobia. Administer a sedative to a child or to an uncooperative adult, as ordered.

➤ Place the patient in the prone position on a special exam table designed for breast imaging.

➤ If ordered with contrast, the contrast medium is injected, and a series of images is taken during and after the filling of the vessels to be examined. Delayed images may be taken to monitor the venous phase of the procedure.

➤ Instruct the patient to take slow, deep breaths if nausea occurs during the procedure.

➤ Monitor the patient for complications related to the procedure (e.g., allergic reaction, anaphylaxis, bronchospasm).

➤ The needle or catheter is removed, and a pressure dressing is applied over the puncture site.

➤ The results are recorded on film or on automated equipment in a computerized system for recall and postprocedure interpretation by the appropriate health care practitioner.

Post-test:

➤ Observe for delayed allergic reactions, such as rash, urticaria, tachycardia, hyperpnea, hypertension, palpitations, nausea, or vomiting, if contrast medium was used.

➤ Instruct the patient to immediately report symptoms such as fast heart rate, difficulty breathing, skin rash, itching or decreased urinary output

➤ Observe the needle/catheter insertion site for bleeding, inflammation, or hematoma formation.

➤ Instruct the patient to apply cold compresses to the puncture site, as needed, to reduce discomfort or edema.

➤ A written report of the examination will be completed by a health care practitioner specializing in this branch of medicine. The report will be sent to the requesting health care practitioner, who will discuss the results with the patient.

➤ Recognize anxiety related to test results, and be supportive of perceived loss of independent function. Discuss the implications of abnormal test results on the patient's lifestyle. Provide teaching and information regarding the clinical implications of the test results, as appropriate.

➤ Reinforce information given by the patient's health care provider regarding further testing, treatment, or referral to another health care provider. Explain the importance of adhering to the therapy regimen. Answer any questions or address any concerns voiced by the patient or family.

➤ Depending on the results of this procedure, additional testing may be performed to evaluate or monitor progression of the disease process and determine the need for a change in therapy. Evaluate test results in relation to the patient's symptoms and other tests performed.

Related diagnostic tests:

➤ Related diagnostic tests include bone scan, computed tomography of the thorax, mammogram, sterotatic biopsy of the breast, and ultrasound of the breast.

MAGNETIC RESONANCE IMAGING, CHEST

· ·

SYNONYM/ACRONYM: Chest MRI.

AREA OF APPLICATION: Chest/thorax.

CONTRAST: Can be done with or without intravenous (IV) contrast medium (gadolinium).

DESCRIPTION & RATIONALE: Magnetic resonance imaging (MRI) uses a magnet and radio waves to produce an energy field that can be displayed as an image. Use of magnetic fields with the aid of radiofrequency energy produces images primarily based on water content of tissue. The magnetic field causes the hydrogen atoms in tissue to line up, and when radio waves are directed toward the magnetic field, the atoms absorb the radio waves and change their position. When the radio waves are turned off, the atoms go back to their original position, this change in the energy field is sensed by the equipment, and an image is generated by the attached computer system. MRI produces cross-sectional images of pathologic lesions in multiple planes without the use of ionizing radiation or the interference of bone or surrounding tissue.

Chest MRI scanning is performed to assist in diagnosing abnormalities of cardiovascular and pulmonary structures. Two special techniques are available for evaluation of cardiovascular structures. One is the electrocardiograph (ECG)–gated multislice spin-echo sequence, used to diagnose anatomic abnormalities of the heart and aorta, and the other is the ECG-referenced gradient refocused sequence, used to diagnose heart function and analyze blood flow patterns.

Magnetic resonance angiography (MRA) is an application of MRI that provides images of blood flow and diseased and normal blood vessels. In patients who are allergic to iodinated contrast medium, MRA is used in place of angiography (see monograph titled "Magnetic Resonance Angiography"). ■

INDICATIONS:
- Confirm diagnosis of cardiac and pericardiac masses

- Detect aortic aneurysms

- Detect myocardial infarction and cardiac muscle ischemia

- Detect pericardial abnormalities

- Detect pleural effusion

- Detect thoracic aortic diseases

- Determine blood, fluid, or fat accumulation in tissues, pleuritic space, or vessels

- Determine cardiac ventricular function

- Differentiate aortic aneurysms from tumors near the aorta

- Evaluate cardiac chambers and pulmonary vessels

- Evaluate postoperative angioplasty sites and bypass grafts

- Identify congenital heart diseases

- Monitor and evaluate the effectiveness of medical or surgical therapeutic regimen

RESULT

Normal Findings:
- Normal heart and lung structures, soft tissue, and function, including blood flow rate

Abnormal Findings:
- Aortic dissection

- Congenital heart diseases, including pulmonary atresia, aortic coarctation, agenesis of the pulmonary artery, and transposition of the great vessels

- Constrictive pericarditis

- Intramural and periaortic hematoma

- Myocardial infarction

- Pericardial hematoma or effusion

- Pleural effusion

CRITICAL VALUES: N/A

INTERFERING FACTORS:

This procedure is contraindicated for:
- Patients with certain ferrous metal prostheses, valves, aneurysm clips, inner ear prostheses, or other metallic objects

- Patients with metal in their body, such as shrapnel or ferrous metal in the eye

- ⚠ Patients with cardiac pacemakers, because the pacemaker can be deactivated by MRI

- Patients with intrauterine devices

- Patients with iron pigments in tattoos

- Patients who are claustrophobic

- Patients who are pregnant or suspected of being pregnant, unless the potential benefits of the procedure far outweigh the risks to the fetus and mother

Factors that may impair clear imaging:
- Metallic objects within the examination field (e.g., jewelry, body rings, dental amalgams), which may inhibit organ visualization and can produce unclear images

- Patients who are very obese, who may exceed the weight limit for the equipment

- Incorrect positioning of the patient, which may produce poor visualization of the area to be examined

- Inability of the patient to cooperate or remain still during the procedure because of age, significant pain, or mental status

- Patients with extreme cases of claustrophobia, unless sedation is given before the study or an open MRI is utilized

Other considerations:
- If contrast medium is allowed to seep deep into the muscle tissue, vascular visualization will be impossible.

Nursing Implications and Procedure . . . .

Pretest:
▶ Inform the patient that the procedure assesses the organs and structures inside the chest.

▶ Obtain a history of the patient's complaints, including a list of known allergens (especially allergies or sensitivities to contrast medium), and inform the appropriate health care practitioner accordingly.

➤ Obtain a history of the patient's cardiovascular and respiratory systems, as well as results of previously performed diagnostic procedures, surgical procedures, and laboratory tests. For related diagnostic tests, refer to the Cardiovascular and Respiratory System tables.

➤ Determine if the patient has ever had any device implanted into his or her body, including copper intrauterine devices, pacemakers, ear implants, and heart valves.

➤ Obtain occupational history to determine the presence of metal in the body, such as shrapnel or flecks of ferrous metal in the eye (which can cause retinal hemorrhage).

➤ Note any recent procedures that can interfere with test results, including examinations using iodine-based contrast medium or barium.

➤ Record the date of the last menstrual period and the determine possibility of pregnancy in perimenopausal women.

➤ Obtain a list of the medications the patient is taking.

➤ Review the procedure with the patient. Address concerns about pain related to the procedure. Explain to the patient that no pain will be experienced during the test, but there may be moments of discomfort. Inform the patient that the procedure is performed in an MRI department, usually by a technologist and support staff, and takes approximately 30 to 60 minutes.

➤ Inform the patient that the technologist will place him or her in a supine position on a flat table in a large cylindrical scanner.

➤ Tell the patient to expect to hear loud banging from the scanner and possibly to see magnetophosphenes (flickering lights in the visual field); these will stop when the procedure is over.

➤ *Sensitivity to social and cultural issues,* as well as concern for modesty, is important in providing psychological support before, during, and after the procedure.

➤ Explain that an IV line may be inserted to allow infusion of IV fluids, contrast medium, dye, or sedatives. Usually normal saline is infused.

➤ There are no food, fluid, or medication restrictions, unless by medical direction.

➤ Instruct the patient to remove dentures, jewelry (including watches), hairpins, credit cards, and other metallic objects.

Intratest: ■

➤ Ensure that the patient has removed all external metallic objects (jewelry, dentures, etc.) prior to the procedure.

➤ Have emergency equipment readily available.

➤ If the patient has a history of severe allergic reactions to any substance or drug, administer ordered prophylactic steroids or antihistamines before the procedure.

➤ Patients are given a gown, robe, and foot coverings to wear and instructed to void prior to the procedure.

➤ Instruct the patient to cooperate fully and to follow directions. Instruct the patient to remain still throughout the procedure because movement produces unreliable results.

➤ Observe standard precautions, and follow the general guidelines in Appendix A.

➤ Supply earplugs to the patient to block out the loud, banging sounds that occur during the test.

➤ If an electrocardiogram or respiratory gating is to be performed in conjunction with the scan, apply MRI-safe electrodes to the appropriate sites.

➤ The patient can communicate with the technologist during the examination via a microphone within the machine.

➤ Establish an IV fluid line for the injection of emergency drugs and of sedatives.

➤ Administer an antianxiety agent, as ordered, if the patient has claustrophobia. Administer a sedative to a child or to an uncooperative adult, as ordered.

➤ Place the patient in the supine position on an exam table.

➤ If ordered with contrast, the contrast medium is injected, and a series of images is taken during and after the filling of the vessels to be examined. Delayed images may be taken to monitor the venous phase of the procedure.

➤ Instruct the patient to take slow, deep breaths if nausea occurs during the procedure.

➤ Monitor the patient for complications related to the procedure (e.g., allergic reaction, anaphylaxis, bronchospasm).

➤ The needle or catheter is removed, and a pressure dressing is applied over the puncture site.

➤ The results are recorded on film or on automated equipment in a computerized system for recall and postprocedure interpretation by the appropriate health care practitioner.

Post-test:

➤ Observe for delayed allergic reactions, such as rash, urticaria, tachycardia, hyperpnea, hypertension, palpitations, nausea, or vomiting, if contrast medium was used.

➤ Instruct the patient to immediately report symptoms such as fast heart rate, difficulty breathing, skin rash, itching or decreased urinary output

➤ Observe the needle/catheter insertion site for bleeding, inflammation, or hematoma formation.

➤ Instruct the patient to apply cold compresses to the puncture site, as needed, to reduce discomfort or edema.

➤ A written report of the examination will be completed by a health care practitioner specializing in this branch of medicine. The report will be sent to the requesting health care practitioner, who will discuss the results with the patient.

➤ Recognize anxiety related to test results, and be supportive of perceived loss of independent function. Discuss the implications of abnormal test results on the patient's lifestyle. Provide teaching and information regarding the clinical implications of the test results, as appropriate.

➤ Reinforce information given by the patient's health care provider regarding further testing, treatment, or referral to another health care provider. Explain the importance of adhering to the therapy regimen. Answer any questions or address any concerns voiced by the patient or family.

➤ Depending on the results of this procedure, additional testing may be performed to evaluate or monitor progression of the disease process and determine the need for a change in therapy. Evaluate test results in relation to the patient's symptoms and other tests performed.

Related diagnostic tests:

➤ Related diagnostic tests include chest x-ray, computed tomography of the thorax, echocardiography, myocardial infarct scan, mycardial perfusion heart scan, and positron emission tomography scan of the heart.

MAGNETIC RESONANCE IMAGING, MUSCULOSKELETAL

SYNONYM/ACRONYM: Musculoskeletal (knee, shoulder, hand, wrist, foot, elbow, hip) MRI.

AREA OF APPLICATION: Bones, joints, soft tissues.

CONTRAST: Can be done with or without intravenous (IV) contrast medium (gadolinium).

DESCRIPTION & RATIONALE: Magnetic resonance imaging (MRI) uses a magnet and radio waves to produce an energy field that can be displayed as an image. Use of magnetic fields with the aid of radiofrequency energy produces images primarily based on water content of tissue. The magnetic field causes the hydrogen atoms in tissue to line up, and when radio waves are directed toward the magnetic field, the atoms absorb the radio waves and change their position. When the radio waves are turned off, the atoms go back to their original position, this change in the energy field is sensed by the equipment, and an image is generated by the attached computer system. MRI produces cross-sectional images of bones and joints in multiple planes without the use of ionizing radiation or the interference of bone or surrounding tissue.

Musculoskeletal MRI is performed to assist in diagnosing abnormalities of bones and joints and surrounding soft tissue structures, including cartilage, synovium, ligaments, and tendons. MRI eliminates the risks associated with exposure to x-rays and causes no harm to cells. Contrast-enhanced imaging is effective for evaluating scarring from previous surgery, vascular abnormalities, and differentiation of metastases from primary tumors. MRI uses the noniodinated contrast medium gadopentetate dimeglumine (Magnevist), which is administered intravenously to enhance contrast differences between normal and abnormal tissues.

Magnetic resonance angiography (MRA) is an application of MRI that provides images of blood flow and diseased and normal blood vessels. In patients who are allergic to iodinated contrast medium, MRA is used in place of angiography (see monograph titled "Magnetic Resonance Angiography"). ▪

INDICATIONS:

• Confirm diagnosis of osteomyelitis

• Detect avascular necrosis of the femoral head or knee

• Detect benign and cancerous tumors and cysts of the bone or soft tissue

- Detect bone infarcts in the epiphyseal or diaphyseal sites

- Detect changes in bone marrow

- Detect tears or degeneration of ligaments, tendons, and menisci resulting from trauma or pathology

- Determine cause of low back pain, including herniated disk and spinal degenerative disease

- Differentiate between primary and secondary malignant processes of the bone marrow

- Differentiate between a stress fracture and a tumor

- Evaluate meniscal detachment of the temporomandibular joint

RESULT

Normal Findings:

- Normal bones, joints, and surrounding tissue structures; no articular disease, bone marrow disorders, tumors, infections, or trauma to the bones, joints, or muscles

Abnormal Findings:

- Avascular necrosis of femoral head or knee, as found in Legg-Calvé-Perthes disease

- Bone marrow disease, such as Gaucher's disease, aplastic anemia, sickle cell disease, or polycythemia

- Degenerative spinal disease, such as spondylosis or arthritis

- Fibrosarcoma

- Hemangioma (muscular or osseous)

- Herniated disk

- Infection

- Meniscal tears or degeneration

- Osteochondroma

- Osteogenic sarcoma

- Osteomyelitis

- Rotator cuff tears

- Spinal stenosis

- Stress fracture

- Synovitis

- Tumor

CRITICAL VALUES: N/A

INTERFERING FACTORS:

This procedure is contraindicated for:

- ⚠ Patients with cardiac pacemakers, because the pacemaker can be deactivated by MRI

- Patients with certain ferrous metal prostheses, valves, aneurysm clips, inner ear prostheses, or other metallic objects

- Patients with metal in their body, such as shrapnel or ferrous metal in the eye

- Patients with intrauterine devices

- Patients with iron pigments in tattoos

- Patients who are claustrophobic

- Patients who are pregnant or suspected of being pregnant, unless the potential benefits of the procedure far outweigh the risks to the fetus and mother

Factors that may impair clear imaging:

- Metallic objects within the examination field (e.g., jewelry, body rings, dental amalgams), which may inhibit organ visualization and can produce unclear images

- Patients who are very obese, who may exceed the weight limit for the equipment

- Incorrect positioning of the patient, which may produce poor visualization of the area to be examined

• Inability of the patient to cooperate or remain still during the procedure because of age, significant pain, or mental status

• Patients with extreme cases of claustrophobia, unless sedation is given before the study or an open MRI is utilized

Other considerations:
• If contrast medium is allowed to seep deep into the muscle tissue, vascular visualization will be impossible.

Nursing Implications and Procedure . . . .

Pretest:

➤ Inform the patient that the procedure assesses muscles, bones, and joints.

➤ Obtain a history of the patient's complaints, including a list of known allergens (especially allergies or sensitivities to contrast medium), and inform the appropriate health care practitioner accordingly.

➤ Obtain a history of the patient's cardiovascular and musculoskeletal systems, as well as results of previously performed diagnostic procedures, surgical procedures, and laboratory tests. For related diagnostic tests, refer to the Cardiovascular and Musculoskeletal System tables.

➤ Determine if the patient has ever had any device implanted into his or her body, including copper intrauterine devices, pacemakers, ear implants, and heart valves.

➤ Obtain occupational history to determine the presence of metal in the body, such as shrapnel or flecks of ferrous metal in the eye (which can cause retinal hemorrhage).

➤ Note any recent procedures that can interfere with test results, including examinations using iodine-based contrast medium or barium.

➤ Record the date of the last menstrual period and determine the possibility of pregnancy in perimenopausal women.

➤ Obtain a list of the medications the patient is taking.

➤ Review the procedure with the patient. Address concerns about pain related to the procedure. Explain to the patient that no pain will be experienced during the test, but there may be moments of discomfort. Inform the patient that the procedure is performed in an MRI department, usually by a technologist and support staff, and takes approximately 30 to 60 minutes.

➤ Inform the patient that the technologist will place him or her in a supine position on a flat table in a large cylindrical scanner.

➤ Tell the patient to expect to hear loud banging from the scanner and possibly to see magnetophosphenes (flickering lights in the visual field); these will stop when the procedure is over.

➤ *Sensitivity to social and cultural issues,* as well as concern for modesty, is important in providing psychological support before, during, and after the procedure.

➤ Explain that an IV line may be inserted to allow infusion of IV fluids, contrast medium, dye, or sedatives. Usually normal saline is infused.

➤ There are no food, fluid, or medication restrictions, unless by medical direction.

➤ Instruct the patient to remove dentures, jewelry (including watches), hairpins, credit cards, and other metallic objects.

Intratest:

➤ Ensure that the patient has removed all external metallic objects (jewelry, dentures, etc.) prior to the procedure.

➤ Have emergency equipment readily available.

➤ If the patient has a history of severe allergic reactions to any substance or drug, administer ordered prophylactic steroids or antihistamines before the procedure.

➤ Patients are given a gown, robe, and foot coverings to wear and instructed to void prior to the procedure.

➤ Instruct the patient to cooperate fully and to follow directions. Instruct the patient to remain still throughout the procedure because movement produces unreliable results.

➤ Observe standard precautions, and follow the general guidelines in Appendix A.

➤ Supply earplugs to the patient to block out the loud, banging sounds that occur during the test.

➤ The patient can communicate with the technologist during the examination via a microphone within the machine.

➤ Establish an IV fluid line for the injection of emergency drugs and of sedatives.

➤ Administer an antianxiety agent, as ordered, if the patient has claustrophobia. Administer a sedative to a child or to an uncooperative adult, as ordered.

➤ Place the patient in the supine position on an exam table.

➤ If ordered with contrast, the contrast medium is injected, and a series of images is taken during and after the filling of the vessels to be examined. Delayed images may be taken to monitor the venous phase of the procedure.

➤ Instruct the patient to take slow, deep breaths if nausea occurs during the procedure.

➤ Monitor the patient for complications related to the procedure (e.g., allergic reaction, anaphylaxis, bronchospasm).

➤ The needle or catheter is removed, and a pressure dressing is applied over the puncture site.

➤ The results are recorded on film or on automated equipment in a computerized system for recall and postprocedure interpretation by the appropriate health care practitioner.

Post-test:

➤ Observe for delayed allergic reactions, such as rash, urticaria, tachycardia, hyperpnea, hypertension, palpitations, nausea, or vomiting, if contrast medium was used.

➤ Instruct the patient to immediately report symptoms such as fast heart rate, difficulty breathing, skin rash, itching or decreased urinary output

➤ Observe the needle/catheter insertion site for bleeding, inflammation, or hematoma formation.

➤ Instruct the patient to apply cold compresses to the puncture site, as needed, to reduce discomfort or edema.

➤ A written report of the examination will be completed by a health care practitioner specializing in this branch of medicine. The report will be sent to the requesting health care practitioner, who will discuss the results with the patient.

➤ Recognize anxiety related to test results, and be supportive of perceived loss of independent function. Discuss the implications of abnormal test results on the patient's lifestyle. Provide teaching and information regarding the clinical implications of the test results, as appropriate.

➤ Reinforce information given by the patient's health care provider regarding further testing, treatment, or referral to another health care provider. Explain the importance of adhering to the therapy regimen. Answer any questions or address any concerns voiced by the patient or family.

➤ Depending on the results of this procedure, additional testing may be performed to evaluate or monitor progression of the disease process and determine the need for a change in therapy. Evaluate test results in relation to the patient's symptoms and other tests performed.

Related diagnostic tests:

➤ Related diagnostic tests include arthroscopy, bone mineral densitometry, bone scan, and radiography of the bone.

MAGNETIC RESONANCE IMAGING, PANCREAS

SYNONYM/ACRONYM: Pancreatic MRI.

AREA OF APPLICATION: Pancreatic/upper abdominal area.

CONTRAST: Can be done with or without intravenous (IV) contrast medium (gadolinium).

DESCRIPTION & RATIONALE: Magnetic resonance imaging (MRI) uses a magnet and radio waves to produce an energy field that can be displayed as an image. Use of magnetic fields with the aid of radiofrequency energy produces images primarily based on water content of tissue. The magnetic field causes the hydrogen atoms in tissue to line up, and when radio waves are directed toward the magnetic field, the atoms absorb the radio waves and change their position. When the radio waves are turned off, the atoms go back to their original position, this change in the energy field is sensed by the equipment, and an image is generated by the attached computer system. MRI produces cross-sectional images of the abdominal area in multiple planes without the use of ionizing radiation or the interference of bone or surrounding tissue.

MRI of the pancreas is employed to evaluate small pancreatic adenocarcinomas, islet cell tumors, ductal abnormalities and calculi, or parenchymal abnormalities. A T1-weighted, fat-saturation series of images is probably best for evaluating the pancreatic parenchyma. This sequence is ideal for showing fat planes between the pancreas and peripancreatic structures and for identifying abnormalities, such as fatty infiltration of the pancreas, hemorrhage, adenopathy, and carcinomas. T2-weighted images are most useful for depicting intrapancreatic or peripancreatic fluid collections, pancreatic neoplasms, and calculi. Imaging sequences can be adjusted to display fluid in the biliary tree and pancreatic ducts. MRI uses the noniodinated contrast medium gadopentetate dimeglumine (Magnevist), which is administered intravenously to enhance contrast differences between normal and abnormal tissues.

Magnetic resonance angiography (MRA) is an application of MRI that provides images of blood flow and diseased and normal blood vessels. In patients who are allergic to iodinated contrast medium, MRA is used in place of angiography (see monograph titled "Magnetic Resonance Angiography"). When the Food and Drug Administration approves gastrointestinal contrast agents, they may be useful for delineating the exact relationship among the stomach, duodenum, and proximal jejunum and the pancreas. These agents would assist in identifying areas of bowel wall thickening, stricture, and intraluminal abnormalities, such as tumors, sites of perforation, and fistula. ∎

INDICATIONS:
- Detect pancreatic fatty infiltration, hemorrhage, and adenopathy
- Detect a pancreatic mass
- Detect pancreatitis
- Detect primary or metastatic tumors of the pancreas and provide cancer staging
- Detect soft tissue abnormalities
- Determine vascular complications of pancreatitis, venous thrombosis, or pseudoaneurysm
- Differentiate tumors from other abnormalities, such as cysts, cavernous hemangiomas, and pancreatic abscesses
- Monitor and evaluate the effectiveness of medical or surgical interventions and course of disease

RESULT

Normal Findings:
- Normal anatomic structures and soft tissue density and biochemical constituents of the pancreatic parenchyma, including blood flow

Abnormal Findings:
- Islet cell tumor
- Metastasis
- Pancreatic duct obstruction or calculi
- Pancreatic fatty infiltration, hemorrhage, and adenopathy
- Pancreatic mass
- Pancreatitis

CRITICAL VALUES: N/A

INTERFERING FACTORS:

This procedure is contraindicated for:
- Patients with certain ferrous metal prostheses, valves, aneurysm clips, inner ear prostheses, or other metallic objects
- Patients with metal in their body, such as shrapnel or ferrous metal in the eye
- ⚠ Patients with cardiac pacemakers, because the pacemaker can be deactivated by MRI
- Patients with intrauterine devices
- Patients with iron pigments in tattoos
- Patients who are claustrophobic
- Patients who are pregnant or suspected of being pregnant, unless the potential benefits of the procedure far outweigh the risks to the fetus and mother

Factors that may impair clear imaging:
- Metallic objects within the examination field (e.g., jewelry, body rings, dental amalgams), which may inhibit organ visualization and can produce unclear images
- Patients who are very obese, who may exceed the weight limit for the equipment
- Incorrect positioning of the patient, which may produce poor visualization of the area to be examined
- Inability of the patient to cooperate or remain still during the procedure because of age, significant pain, or mental status
- Patients with extreme cases of claustrophobia, unless sedation is given before the study or an open MRI is utilized

Other considerations:
- If contrast medium is allowed to seep deep into the muscle tissue, vascular visualization will be impossible.

Nursing Implications and Procedure

➤ Inform the patient that the procedure assesses the pancreas and the organs and structures inside the abdomen.

➤ Obtain a history of the patient's complaints, including a list of known allergens (especially allergies or sensitivities to contrast medium), and inform the appropriate health care practitioner accordingly.

➤ Obtain a history of the patient's hepatobiliary and endocrine systems, as well as results of previously performed diagnostic procedures, surgical procedures, and laboratory tests. For related diagnostic tests, refer to the Hepatobiliary and Endocrine System tables.

➤ Determine if the patient has ever had any device implanted into his or her body, including copper intrauterine devices, pacemakers, ear implants, and heart valves.

➤ Obtain occupational history to determine the presence of metal in the body, such as shrapnel or flecks of ferrous metal in the eye (which can cause retinal hemorrhage).

➤ Note any recent procedures that can interfere with test results, including examinations using iodine-based contrast medium or barium.

➤ Record the date of the last menstrual period and determine the possibility of pregnancy in perimenopausal women.

➤ Obtain a list of the medications the patient is taking.

➤ Review the procedure with the patient. Address concerns about pain related to the procedure. Explain to the patient that no pain will be experienced during the test, but there may be moments of discomfort. Inform the patient that the procedure is performed in an MRI department, usually by a technologist and support staff, and takes approximately 30 to 60 minutes.

➤ Inform the patient that the technologist will place him or her in a supine position on a flat table in a large cylindrical scanner.

➤ Tell the patient to expect to hear loud banging from the scanner and possibly to see magnetophosphenes (flickering lights in the visual field); these will stop when the procedure is over.

➤ *Sensitivity to social and cultural issues,* as well as concern for modesty, is important in providing psychological support before, during, and after the procedure.

➤ Explain that an IV line may be inserted to allow infusion of IV fluids, contrast medium, dye, or sedatives. Usually normal saline is infused.

➤ There are no food, fluid, or medication restrictions, unless by medical direction.

➤ Instruct the patient to remove dentures, jewelry (including watches), hairpins, credit cards, and other metallic objects.

➤ Ensure that the patient has removed all external metallic objects (jewelry, dentures, etc.) prior to the procedure.

➤ Have emergency equipment readily available.

➤ If the patient has a history of severe allergic reactions to any substance or drug, administer ordered prophylactic steroids or antihistamines before the procedure.

➤ Patients are given a gown, robe, and foot coverings to wear and instructed to void prior to the procedure.

➤ Instruct the patient to cooperate fully and to follow directions. Instruct the patient to remain still throughout the procedure because movement produces unreliable results.

➤ Observe standard precautions, and follow the general guidelines in Appendix A.

➤ Supply earplugs to the patient to block out the loud, banging sounds that occur during the test.

➤ The patient can communicate with the technologist during the examination via a microphone within the machine.

➤ Establish an IV fluid line for the injection of emergency drugs and of sedatives.

➤ Administer an antianxiety agent, as ordered, if the patient has claustrophobia. Administer a sedative to a child or to an uncooperative adult, as ordered.

➤ Place the patient in the supine position on an exam table.

➤ If ordered with contrast, the contrast medium is injected, and a series of images is taken during and after the filling of the vessels to be examined. Delayed images may be taken to monitor the venous phase of the procedure.

➤ Instruct the patient to take slow, deep breaths if nausea occurs during the procedure.

➤ Monitor the patient for complications related to the procedure (e.g., allergic reaction, anaphylaxis, bronchospasm).

➤ The needle or catheter is removed, and a pressure dressing is applied over the puncture site.

➤ The results are recorded on film or on automated equipment in a computerized system for recall and postprocedure interpretation by the appropriate health care practitioner.

Post-test:

➤ Observe for delayed allergic reactions, such as rash, urticaria, tachycardia, hyperpnea, hypertension, palpitations, nausea, or vomiting, if contrast medium was used.

➤ Instruct the patient to immediately report symptoms such as fast heart rate, difficulty breathing, skin rash, itching or decreased urinary output

➤ Observe the needle/catheter insertion site for bleeding, inflammation, or hematoma formation.

➤ Instruct the patient to apply cold compresses to the puncture site, as needed, to reduce discomfort or edema.

➤ A written report of the examination will be completed by a health care practitioner specializing in this branch of medicine. The report will be sent to the requesting health care practitioner, who will discuss the results with the patient.

➤ Recognize anxiety related to test results, and be supportive of perceived loss of independent function. Discuss the implications of abnormal test results on the patient's lifestyle. Provide teaching and information regarding the clinical implications of the test results, as appropriate.

➤ Reinforce information given by the patient's health care provider regarding further testing, treatment, or referral to another health care provider. Explain the importance of adhering to the therapy regimen. Answer any questions or address any concerns voiced by the patient or family.

➤ Depending on the results of this procedure, additional testing may be performed to evaluate or monitor progression of the disease process and determine the need for a change in therapy. Evaluate test results in relation to the patient's symptoms and other tests performed.

Related diagnostic tests:

➤ Related diagnostic and laboratory tests include amylase, angiography of the abdomen, computed tomography of the abdomen, hepatobiliary scan; 5-hydroxyindoleacetic acid, lipase, ultrasound of the liver and biliary system, and ultrasound of the pancreas.

MAGNETIC RESONANCE IMAGING, PELVIS

SYNONYM/ACRONYM: Pelvic MRI.

AREA OF APPLICATION: Pelvic area.

CONTRAST: Can be done with or without intravenous (IV) contrast (gadolinium).

DESCRIPTION & RATIONALE: Magnetic resonance imaging (MRI) uses a magnet and radio waves to produce an energy field that can be displayed as an image. Use of magnetic fields with the aid of radiofrequency energy produces images primarily based on water content of tissue. The magnetic field causes the hydrogen atoms in tissue to line up, and when radio waves are directed toward the magnetic field, the atoms absorb the radio waves and change their position. When the radio waves are turned off, the atoms go back to their original position, this change in the energy field is sensed by the equipment, and an image is generated by the attached computer system. MRI produces cross-sectional images of the pelvic area in multiple planes without the use of ionizing radiation or the interference of bone or surrounding tissue.

Pelvic MRI is performed to assist in diagnosing abnormalities of the pelvis and associated structures. Contrast-enhanced MRI is effective for evaluating metastases from primary tumors. MRI is highly effective for depicting small-volume peritoneal tumors, carcinomatosis, and peritonitis and for determining the response to surgical and chemical therapies. MRI uses the noniodinated contrast medium gadopentetate dimeglumine (Magnevist), which is administered intravenously to enhance contrast differences between normal and abnormal tissues. Oral and rectal contrast administration may be used to isolate the bowel from adjacent pelvic organs and improve organ visualization.

Magnetic resonance angiography (MRA) is an application of MRI that provides images of blood flow and diseased and normal blood vessels. In patients who are allergic to iodinated contrast medium, MRA is used in place of angiography (see monograph titled "Magnetic Resonance Angiography"). When the Food and Drug Administration approves gastrointestinal contrast agents, these agents would assist in identifying areas of bowel wall thickening, stricture, and intraluminal abnormalities, such as tumors, sites of perforation, and fistula. ▪

INDICATIONS:

- Detect cancer (primary or metastatic tumors of ovary, prostate, uterus, and bladder) and provide cancer staging

- Detect pelvic vascular diseases

- Detect peritonitis

- Detect soft tissue abnormalities

- Determine blood clots, cysts, fluid or fat accumulation in tissues, hemorrhage, and infarctions

- Differentiate tumors from tissue abnormalities, such as cysts, cavernous hemangiomas, and abscesses

- Monitor and evaluate the effectiveness of medical or surgical interventions and course of the disease

RESULT

Normal Findings:

- Normal pelvic structures and soft tissue density and biochemical constituents of pelvic tissues, including blood flow

Abnormal Findings:

- Adenomyosis

- Ascites

- Fibroids

- Masses, lesions, infections, or inflammations

- Peritoneal tumor or carcinomatosis

- Peritonitis

- Pseudomyxoma peritonei

CRITICAL VALUES: N/A

INTERFERING FACTORS:

This procedure is contraindicated for:

- Patients with certain ferrous metal prostheses, valves, aneurysm clips, inner ear prostheses, or other metallic objects

- Patients with metal in their body, such as shrapnel or ferrous metal in the eye

- ⚠ Patients with cardiac pacemakers, because the pacemaker can be deactivated by MRI

- Patients with intrauterine devices

- Patients with iron pigments in tattoos

- Patients who are claustrophobic

- Patients who are pregnant or suspected of being pregnant, unless the potential benefits of the procedure far outweigh the risks to the fetus and mother

Factors that may impair clear imaging:

- Metallic objects within the examination field (e.g., jewelry, body rings, dental amalgams), which may inhibit organ visualization and can produce unclear images

- Patients who are very obese, who may exceed the weight limit for the equipment

- Incorrect positioning of the patient, which may produce poor visualization of the area to be examined

- Inability of the patient to cooperate or remain still during the procedure because of age, significant pain, or mental status

- Patients with extreme cases of claustrophobia, unless sedation is given before the study or an open MRI is utilized

Other considerations:

- If contrast medium is allowed to seep deep into the muscle tissue, vascular visualization will be impossible.

Nursing Implications and Procedure • • • • • • • • • • •

Pretest:

▶ Inform the patient that the procedure assesses the organs and structures inside the pelvis and lower abdomen.

➤ Obtain a history of the patient's complaints, including a list of known allergens (especially allergies or sensitivities to contrast medium), and inform the appropriate health care practitioner accordingly.

➤ Obtain a history of the patient's gastrointestinal and genitourinary systems, as well as results of previously performed diagnostic procedures, surgical procedures, and laboratory tests. For related diagnostic tests, refer to the Gastrointestinal and Genitourinary System tables.

➤ Determine if the patient has ever had any device implanted into his or her body, including copper intrauterine devices, pacemakers, ear implants, and heart valves.

➤ Obtain occupational history to determine the presence of metal in the body, such as shrapnel or flecks of ferrous metal in the eye (which can cause retinal hemorrhage).

➤ Note any recent procedures that can interfere with test results, including examinations using iodine-based contrast medium or barium.

➤ Record the date of the last menstrual period and determine the possibility of pregnancy in perimenopausal women.

➤ Obtain a list of the medications the patient is taking.

➤ Review the procedure with the patient. Address concerns about pain related to the procedure. Explain to the patient that no pain will be experienced during the test, but there may be moments of discomfort. Inform the patient that the procedure is performed in an MRI department, usually by a technologist and support staff, and takes approximately 30 to 60 minutes.

➤ Inform the patient that the technologist will place him or her in a supine position on a flat table in a large cylindrical scanner.

➤ Tell the patient to expect to hear loud banging from the scanner and possibly to see magnetophosphenes (flickering lights in the visual field); these will stop when the procedure is over.

➤ *Sensitivity to social and cultural issues,* as well as concern for modesty, is important in providing psychological support before, during, and after the procedure.

➤ Explain that an IV line may be inserted to allow infusion of IV fluids, contrast medium, dye, or sedatives. Usually normal saline is infused.

➤ There are no food, fluid, or medication restrictions, unless by medical direction.

➤ Instruct the patient to remove dentures, jewelry (including watches), hairpins, credit cards, and other metallic objects.

Intratest:

➤ Ensure that the patient has removed all external metallic objects (jewelry, dentures, etc.) prior to the procedure.

➤ Have emergency equipment readily available.

➤ If the patient has a history of severe allergic reactions to any substance or drug, administer ordered prophylactic steroids or antihistamines before the procedure.

➤ Patients are given a gown, robe, and foot coverings to wear and instructed to void prior to the procedure.

➤ Instruct the patient to cooperate fully and to follow directions. Instruct the patient to remain still throughout the procedure because movement produces unreliable results.

➤ Observe standard precautions, and follow the general guidelines in Appendix A.

➤ Supply earplugs to the patient to block out the loud, banging sounds that occur during the test.

➤ The patient can communicate with the technologist during the examination via a microphone within the machine.

➤ Establish an IV fluid line for the injection of emergency drugs and of sedatives.

➤ Administer an antianxiety agent, as ordered, if the patient has claustrophobia. Administer a sedative to a

➤ child or to an uncooperative adult, as ordered.

➤ Place the patient in the supine position on an exam table.

➤ If ordered with contrast, the contrast medium is injected, and a series of images is taken during and after the filling of the vessels to be examined. Delayed images may be taken to monitor the venous phase of the procedure.

➤ Instruct the patient to take slow, deep breaths if nausea occurs during the procedure.

➤ Monitor the patient for complications related to the procedure (e.g., allergic reaction, anaphylaxis, bronchospasm).

➤ The needle or catheter is removed, and a pressure dressing is applied over the puncture site.

➤ The results are recorded on film or on automated equipment in a computerized system for recall and postprocedure interpretation by the appropriate health care practitioner.

Post-test:

➤ Observe for delayed allergic reactions, such as rash, urticaria, tachycardia, hyperpnea, hypertension, palpitations, nausea, or vomiting, if contrast medium was used.

➤ Instruct the patient to immediately report symptoms such as fast heart rate, difficulty breathing, skin rash, itching or decreased urinary output.

➤ Observe the needle/catheter insertion site for bleeding, inflammation, or hematoma formation.

➤ Instruct the patient to apply cold compresses to the puncture site, as needed, to reduce discomfort or edema.

➤ A written report of the examination will be completed by a health care practitioner specializing in this branch of medicine. The report will be sent to the requesting health care practitioner, who will discuss the results with the patient.

➤ Recognize anxiety related to test results, and be supportive of perceived loss of independent function. Discuss the implications of abnormal test results on the patient's lifestyle. Provide teaching and information regarding the clinical implications of the test results, as appropriate.

➤ Reinforce information given by the patient's health care provider regarding further testing, treatment, or referral to another health care provider. Explain the importance of adhering to the therapy regimen. Answer any questions or address any concerns voiced by the patient or family.

➤ Depending on the results of this procedure, additional testing may be performed to evaluate or monitor progression of the disease process and determine the need for a change in therapy. Evaluate test results in relation to the patient's symptoms and other tests performed.

Related diagnostic tests:

➤ Related diagnostic tests include computed tomography of the pelvis; kidney, ureter, and bladder (KUB) study; and ultrasound of the pelvis.

MAGNETIC RESONANCE IMAGING, PITUITARY

· ·

SYNONYMS/ACRONYM: Pituitary MRI, MRI of the perisellar region.

AREA OF APPLICATION: Brain/pituitary area.

CONTRAST: Can be done with or without intravenous (IV) contrast medium (gadolinium).

DESCRIPTION & RATIONALE: Magnetic resonance imaging (MRI) uses a magnet and radio waves to produce an energy field that can be displayed as an image. Use of magnetic fields with the aid of radiofrequency energy produces images primarily based on water content of tissue. The magnetic field causes the hydrogen atoms in tissue to line up, and when radio waves are directed toward the magnetic field, the atoms absorb the radio waves and change their position. When the radio waves are turned off, the atoms go back to their original position, this change in the energy field is sensed by the equipment, and an image is generated by the attached computer system. MRI produces cross-sectional images of the pituitary and perisellar region in multiple planes without the use of ionizing radiation or the interference of bone or surrounding tissue.

Pituitary MRI shows the relationship of pituitary lesions to the optic chiasm and cavernous sinuses. MRI has the capability of distinguishing the solid, cystic, and hemorrhagic components of lesions. Rapidly flowing blood on spin-echo MRI appears as an absence of signal or a void in the vessel's lumen. Blood flow can be evaluated in the cavernous and carotid arteries. Suprasellar aneurysms may be diagnosed without angiography, and old clotted blood in the walls of the aneurysms appears white. MRI uses the noniodinated contrast medium gadopentetate dimeglumine (Magnevist), which is administered intravenously to enhance contrast differences between normal and abnormal tissues.

Magnetic resonance angiography (MRA) is an application of MRI that provides images of blood flow and diseased and normal blood vessels. In patients who are allergic to iodinated contrast medium, MRA is used in place of angiography (see monograph titled "Magnetic Resonance Angiography"). ▪

INDICATIONS:
• Detect microadenoma or macroadenoma of the pituitary

• Detect perisellar abnormalities

• Detect tumors of the pituitary

- Evaluate potential cause of headache, visual loss, and vomiting
- Evaluate the solid, cystic, and hemorrhagic components of lesions
- Evaluate vascularity of the pituitary
- Monitor and evaluate the effectiveness of medical or surgical interventions and course of disease

RESULT

Normal Findings:
- Normal anatomic structures, density, and biochemical constituents of the pituitary, including blood flow

Abnormal Findings:
- Abscess
- Aneurysm
- Choristoma
- Craniopharyngioma or meningioma
- Empty sella
- Granuloma
- Infarct or hemorrhage
- Macroadenoma or microadenoma
- Metastasis
- Parasitic infection

CRITICAL VALUES: N/A

INTERFERING FACTORS:

This procedure is contraindicated for:
- Patients with certain ferrous metal prostheses, valves, aneurysm clips, inner ear prostheses, or other metallic objects
- Patients with metal in their body, such as shrapnel or ferrous metal in the eye
- ⚠ Patients with cardiac pacemakers, because the pacemaker can be deactivated by MRI
- Patients with intrauterine devices

- Patients with iron pigments in tattoos
- Patients who are claustrophobic
- Patients who are pregnant or suspected of being pregnant, unless the potential benefits of the procedure far outweigh the risks to the fetus and mother

Factors that may impair clear imaging:
- Metallic objects within the examination field (e.g., jewelry, body rings, dental amalgams), which may inhibit organ visualization and can produce unclear images
- Patients who are very obese, who may exceed the weight limit for the equipment
- Incorrect positioning of the patient, which may produce poor visualization of the area to be examined
- Inability of the patient to cooperate or remain still during the procedure because of age, significant pain, or mental status
- Patients with extreme cases of claustrophobia, unless sedation is given before the study or an open MRI is utilized

Other considerations:
- If contrast medium is allowed to seep deep into the muscle tissue, vascular visualization will be impossible.

Nursing Implications and Procedure • • • • • • • • • • •

Pretest:

➤ Inform the patient that the procedure assesses the pituitary and surrounding brain tissue.

➤ Obtain a history of the patient's complaints, including a list of known allergens (especially allergies or sensitivities to contrast medium), and inform the appropriate health care practitioner accordingly.

➤ Obtain a history of the patient's cardiovascular and endocrine systems, as well as results of previously performed diagnostic procedures, surgical procedures, and laboratory tests. For related diagnostic tests, refer to the Cardiovascular and Endocrine System tables.

➤ Determine if the patient has ever had any device implanted into his or her body, including copper intrauterine devices, pacemakers, ear implants, and heart valves.

➤ Obtain occupational history to determine the presence of metal in the body, such as shrapnel or flecks of ferrous metal in the eye (which can cause retinal hemorrhage).

➤ Note any recent procedures that can interfere with test results, including examinations using iodine-based contrast medium or barium.

➤ Record the date of the last menstrual period and determine the possibility of pregnancy in perimenopausal women.

➤ Obtain a list of the medications the patient is taking.

➤ Review the procedure with the patient. Address concerns about pain related to the procedure. Explain to the patient that no pain will be experienced during the test, but there may be moments of discomfort. Inform the patient that the procedure is performed in an MRI department, usually by a technologist and support staff, and takes approximately 30 to 60 minutes.

➤ Inform the patient that the technologist will place him or her in a supine position on a flat table in a large cylindrical scanner.

➤ Tell the patient to expect to hear loud banging from the scanner and possibly to see magnetophosphenes (flickering lights in the visual field); these will stop when the procedure is over.

➤ *Sensitivity to social and cultural issues*, as well as concern for modesty, is important in providing psychological support before, during, and after the procedure.

➤ Explain that an IV line may be inserted to allow infusion of IV fluids, contrast medium, dye, or sedatives. Usually normal saline is infused.

➤ There are no food, fluid, or medication restrictions, unless by medical direction.

➤ Instruct the patient to remove dentures, jewelry (including watches), hairpins, credit cards, and other metallic objects.

Intratest:

➤ Ensure that the patient has removed all external metallic objects (jewelry, dentures, etc.) prior to the procedure.

➤ Have emergency equipment readily available.

➤ If the patient has a history of severe allergic reactions to any substance or drug, administer ordered prophylactic steroids or antihistamines before the procedure.

➤ Patients are given a gown, robe, and foot coverings to wear and instructed to void prior to the procedure.

➤ Instruct the patient to cooperate fully and to follow directions. Instruct the patient to remain still throughout the procedure because movement produces unreliable results.

➤ Observe standard precautions, and follow the general guidelines in Appendix A.

➤ Supply earplugs to the patient to block out the loud, banging sounds that occur during the test.

➤ The patient can communicate with the technologist during the examination via a microphone within the machine.

➤ Establish an IV fluid line for the injection of emergency drugs and of sedatives.

➤ Administer an antianxiety agent, as ordered, if the patient has claustrophobia. Administer a sedative to a child or to an uncooperative adult, as ordered.

➤ Place the patient in the supine position on an exam table.

➤ If ordered with contrast, the contrast medium is injected, and a series of images is taken during and after the filling of the vessels to be examined. Delayed images may be taken to monitor the venous phase of the procedure.

➤ Instruct the patient to take slow, deep breaths if nausea occurs during the procedure.

➤ Monitor the patient for complications related to the procedure (e.g., allergic reaction, anaphylaxis, bronchospasm).

➤ The needle or catheter is removed, and a pressure dressing is applied over the puncture site.

➤ The results are recorded on film or on automated equipment in a computerized system for recall and postprocedure interpretation by the appropriate health care practitioner.

Post-test:

➤ Observe for delayed allergic reactions, such as rash, urticaria, tachycardia, hyperpnea, hypertension, palpitations, nausea, or vomiting, if contrast medium was used.

➤ Instruct the patient to immediately report symptoms such as fast heart rate, difficulty breathing, skin rash, itching or decreased urinary output

➤ Observe the needle/catheter insertion site for bleeding, inflammation, or hematoma formation.

➤ Instruct the patient to apply cold compresses to the puncture site, as needed, to reduce discomfort or edema.

➤ A written report of the examination will be completed by a health care practitioner specializing in this branch of medicine. The report will be sent to the requesting health care practitioner, who will discuss the results with the patient.

➤ Recognize anxiety related to test results, and be supportive of perceived loss of independent function. Discuss the implications of abnormal test results on the patient's lifestyle. Provide teaching and information regarding the clinical implications of the test results, as appropriate.

➤ Reinforce information given by the patient's health care provider regarding further testing, treatment, or referral to another health care provider. Explain the importance of adhering to the therapy regimen. Answer any questions or address any concerns voiced by the patient or family.

➤ Depending on the results of this procedure, additional testing may be performed to evaluate or monitor progression of the disease process and determine the need for a change in therapy. Evaluate test results in relation to the patient's symptoms and other tests performed.

Related diagnostic tests:

➤ Related diagnostic tests include computed tomography of the brain, electroencephalography, magnetic resonance imaging of the brain, and positron emission tomography of the brain.

MAMMOGRAPHY

· ·

SYNONYMS/ACRONYM: Mammogram, breast x-ray.

AREA OF APPLICATION: Breast.

CONTRAST: None.

DESCRIPTION & RATIONALE: Mammography, an x-ray examination of the breast, is most commonly used to detect breast cancer; however, it can also be used to detect and evaluate symptomatic changes associated with other breast diseases, including mastitis, abscess, cystic changes, cysts, benign tumors, masses, and lymph nodes. Mammography is usually performed with traditional x-ray film, but totally electronic image recording is becoming commonplace. This type of radiologic procedure reduces the amount of radiation exposure to the patient and produces detailed images with excellent contrast. Two views of each breast are usually taken. Benign cysts appear as clearly defined, regular, clear spots that are bilateral; cancer appears as irregular, poorly defined, unilateral opaque areas or clusters of calcifications. Mammography can be used to locate a nonpalpable lesion for biopsy. Mammography cannot detect breast cancer with 100% accuracy: In approximately 15% of breast cancer cases, the cancer is not detected with mammography. To assist in early detection of nonpalpable breast lesions, computer-assisted diagnosis is currently being used. With this technique, a computer performs automated scanning of the mammogram before the physician interprets the findings.

When a mass is detected, additional studies are performed to help differentiate the nature of the mass, as follows:

Magnification views of the area in question

Focal or "spot" views of the area in question, done with a specialized paddle-style compression device

Ultrasound images of the area in question, which help differentiate between a fluid-filled cystic lesion and a solid lesion indicative of cancer

The American Cancer Society recommends that all women follow a personal breast-care plan according to age:

Women ages 20 to 39: Clinical breast examination performed by a health care professional every 3 years and a monthly breast self-examination

Women ages 40 and older: Annual mammogram, clinical breast examination every year by a health care professional (near time of the mammogram), and monthly breast self-examination. ■

INDICATIONS:

- Differentiate between benign and neoplastic breast disease

- Evaluate breast pain, skin retraction, nipple erosion, or nipple discharge

- Evaluate known or suspected breast cancer

- Evaluate nonpalpable breast masses

- Evaluate opposite breast after mastectomy

- Monitor postoperative and post–radiation treatment status of the breast

- Evaluate size, shape, and position of breast masses

RESULT

Normal Findings:

- Normal breast tissue, with no cysts, tumors, or calcifications

Abnormal Findings:

- Breast calcifications

- Breast cysts or abscesses

- Breast tumors

- Hematoma resulting from trauma

- Mastitis

- Soft-tissue masses

- Vascular calcification

CRITICAL VALUES: N/A

INTERFERING FACTORS:

This procedure is contraindicated for:

- Patients who are pregnant or suspected of being pregnant, unless the potential benefits of the procedure far outweigh the risks to the fetus and mother

- Patients younger than age 25, because the density of the breast tissue is such that diagnostic x-rays are of limited value

Factors that may impair clear imaging:

- Inability of the patient to cooperate or remain still during the procedure because of age, significant pain, or mental status

- Metallic objects within the examination field (e.g., jewelry, body rings), which may inhibit organ visualization and can produce unclear images

- Improper adjustment of the radiographic equipment to accommodate obese or thin patients, which can cause overexposure or underexposure and a poor-quality study

- Incorrect positioning of the patient, which may produce poor visualization of the area to be examined

- Application of substances such as talcum powder or creams to the skin of breasts or underarms, which may alter test results

- Previous breast surgery, breast augmentation, or the presence of breast implants, which may decrease the readability of the examination

Other considerations:

- Consultation with a health care practitioner should occur before the procedure for radiation safety concerns regarding infants of patients who are lactating.

- Risks associated with radiographic overexposure can result from frequent x-ray procedures. Personnel in the room with the patient should wear a protective lead apron, stand behind a shield, or leave the area while the examination is being done. Personnel working in the area where the examination is being done should wear badges that reveal their level of exposure to radiation.

Nursing Implications and Procedure ....

➤ Inform the patient that the procedure assesses breast status.

➤ Obtain a history of the patient's symptoms and complaints.

➤ Obtain a history of known or suspected breast disease, and family history of breast disease, or breast biopsies.

➤ Obtain a history of results of previously performed diagnostic procedures and surgical procedures. For related diagnostic tests, refer to the Reproductive System table.

➤ Record the date of the last menstrual period and determine the possibility of pregnancy in perimenopausal women.

➤ Obtain a list of the medications the patient is taking.

➤ Review the procedure with the patient. Address concerns about pain related to the procedure. Inform the patient there may be discomfort associated with the study, while the breast is being compressed, but that the compression allows for better visualization of the breast tissue. Explain to the patient that the radiation dose will be kept to an absolute minimum. Inform the patient that the procedure is performed in the mammography department by a registered radiologic techologist and takes approximately 15 to 30 minutes to complete.

➤ Inform the patient that the best time to schedule the examination is 1 week after menses, when breast tenderness is decreased.

➤ *Sensitivity to cultural and social issues,* as well as concern for modesty, is important in providing psychological support before, during and after the procedure.

➤ There are no food, fluid, or medication restrictions, unless by medical direction.

➤ Inform the patient not to apply deodorant, body creams, or powders on the day of the procedure.

➤ Instruct the patient to remove jewelry and other metallic objects from the field of examination.

➤ Patients are given a gown, robe, and foot coverings to wear and instructed to void prior to the procedure.

➤ Make sure jewelry, chains, and any other metallic objects have been removed from the chest area.

➤ Instruct the patient to cooperate fully and to follow directions. Instruct the patient to remain still throughout the procedure because movement produces unreliable results.

➤ Observe standard precautions and follow the general guidelines in Appendix A.

➤ Assist the patient to a standing or sitting position in front of the x-ray machine, which is adjusted to the level of the breasts. Position the patient's arms out of the range of the area to be filmed.

➤ Place breasts, one at a time, between the compression apparatus. Usually two views or exposures are taken of each breast. Ask the patient to hold her breath during exposures.

➤ The results are recorded on a sheet of x-ray film or electronically, in a computerized system, for recall and postprocedure interpretation by the appropriate health care practitioner.

➤ Determine if patient or family members have any further questions or concerns.

➤ Educate the patient regarding the techniques for breast self-examination.

➤ A written report of the examination will be completed by a health care practitioner specializing in this branch of medicine. The report will be sent to the requesting health care practitioner, who will discuss the results with the patient.

➤ Recognize anxiety related to test results, and be supportive of perceived loss of independence and fear of shortened life expectancy. Discuss the implications of abnormal test results on the patient's lifestyle. Provide teaching and information regarding the clinical implications of the test results, as appropriate.

➤ Reinforce information given by the patient's health care provider regarding further testing, treatment, or referral to another health care provider. Answer any questions or address any concerns voiced by the patient or family.

➤ Depending on the results of this procedure, additional testing may be performed to evaluate or monitor progression of the disease process and determine the need for a change in therapy. Evaluate test results in relation to the patient's symptoms and other tests performed.

Related diagnostic tests:

➤ Related diagnostic tests include breast biopsy, bone scan, computed tomography scan of the thorax, and ultrasound of the breast.

MECKEL'S DIVERTICULUM SCAN

SYNONYMS/ACRONYM: Meckel's scan, Meckel's scintigraphy, ectopic gastric mucosa scan.

AREA OF APPLICATION: Abdomen.

CONTRAST: Intravenous radioactive technetium-99m pertechnetate.

DESCRIPTION & RATIONALE:

Meckel's diverticulum scan is a nuclear medicine study performed to assist in diagnosing the cause of abdominal pain or occult gastrointestinal (GI) bleeding, and to assess the presence and size of a congenital anomaly of the GI tract. After intravenous injection of technetium-99m pertechnetate, immediate and delayed imaging is performed, with various views of the abdomen obtained. The radionuclide is taken up and concentrated by parietal cells of the gastric mucosa, whether located in the stomach or in a Meckel's diverticulum. Up to 25% of Meckel's diverticulum is lined internally with ectopic gastric mucosal tissue. This tissue is usually located in the ileum and right lower quadrant of the abdomen; it secretes acid that causes ulceration of intestinal tissue, which results in abdominal pain and occult blood in stools. ∎

INDICATIONS:

- Aid in the diagnosis of unexplained abdominal pain and GI bleeding caused by hydrochloric acid and pepsin secreted by ectopic gastric mucosa, which ulcerates nearby mucosa
- Detect sites of ectopic gastric mucosa

RESULT

Normal Findings:

- Normal distribution of radionuclide by gastric mucosa at normal sites

Abnormal Findings:

- Meckel's diverticulum, as evidenced by focally increased radioactive uptake in areas other than normal structures

CRITICAL VALUES: N/A

INTERFERING FACTORS:

This procedure is contraindicated for:

- Patients who are pregnant or suspected of being pregnant, unless the potential benefits of the procedure far outweigh the risks to the fetus and mother

Factors that may impair clear imaging:

- Inability of the patient to cooperate or remain still during the procedure because of age, significant pain, or mental status
- Metallic objects within the examination field (e.g., jewelry, body rings), which may inhibit organ visualization and can produce unclear images
- Patients who are very obese, who may exceed the weight limit for the equipment
- Incorrect positioning of the patient, which may produce poor visualization of the area to be examined
- Retained barium from a previous radiologic procedure
- Other nuclear scans done within the preceding 24 hours

Other considerations:

- False-positive results may occur from nondiverticular bleeding, intussusception, duplication cysts, inflammatory bowel disease, hemangioma of the bowel, and other organ infections.
- Inadequate amount of gastric mucosa within Meckel's diverticulum can affect the ability to visualize abnormalities.
- Inaccurate timing for imaging after the radionuclide injection can affect the results.
- Failure to follow dietary restrictions before the procedure may cause the procedure to be canceled or repeated.
- Improper injection of the radionuclide that allows the tracer to seep deep into the muscle tissue produces erroneous hot spots.
- Consultation with a health care practitioner should occur before the procedure for radiation safety concerns regarding younger patients or patients who are lactating.
- Risks associated with radiographic overexposure can result from frequent x-ray procedures. Personnel in the room with the patient should wear a protective lead apron, stand behind a shield, or leave the area while the examination is being done. Personnel working in the area where the examination is being done should wear badges that reveal their level of exposure to radiation.

Nursing Implications and Procedure • • • • • • • • • • •

Pretest:

▶ Inform the patient that the procedure assesses GI bleeding.

▶ Obtain a history of the patient's complaints and symptoms, including a list of known allergens.

> Obtain a history of the patient's gastrointestinal and cardiovascular systems, as well as results of previously performed diagnostic procedures, surgical procedures, and laboratory tests. For related diagnostic tests, refer to the Gastrointestinal and Cardiovascular System tables.

> Obtain a history of signs and symptoms of Meckel's diverticulum, such as bleeding, pain, intussusception, volvulus, or diverticulitis.

> Note any recent procedures that can interfere with test results.

> Record the date of the last menstrual period and determine the possibility of pregnancy in perimenopausal women.

> Obtain a list of the medications the patient is taking, including anticoagulant therapy, aspirin and other salicylates, herbs, nutritional supplements, and nutraceuticals, especially those known to affect coagulation (see Appendix F). It is recommended that use be discontinued 14 days before surgical procedures. The requesting health care practitioner and laboratory should be advised if the patient regularly uses these products so that their effects can be taken into consideration when reviewing results.

> Review the procedure with the patient. Address concerns about pain related to the procedure. Explain to the patient that some pain may be experienced during the test, or there may be moments of discomfort. Reassure the patient that the radionuclide poses no radioactive hazard and rarely produces side effects. Inform the patient that the procedure is performed in a special department, usually in a radiology department, by a health care practitioner and support staff, and takes approximately 60 minutes.

> *Sensitivity to social and cultural issues,* as well as concern for modesty, is important in providing psychological support before, during, and after the procedure.

> Explain that an intravenous (IV) line may be inserted to allow infusion of IV fluids, contrast medium, dye, or sedatives. Usually normal saline is infused.

> Ensure that a histamine blocker is administered, as ordered, 2 days before the study to block GI secretion, as appropriate.

> Occasionally, gastrin is given to increase the uptake of the radionuclide by the ectopic gastric mucosa.

> The patient should fast and restrict fluids for 8 hours prior to the procedure. Instruct the patient to avoid taking anticoagulant medication or to reduce dosage as ordered prior to the procedure.

> Instruct the patient to remove dentures, jewelry (including watches), hairpins, credit cards, and other metallic objects in the area to be examined.

Intratest:

> Ensure that the patient has complied with dietary, fluids, and medication restrictions and pretesting preparations; assure that food and medications have been restricted for at least 8 hours prior to the procedure. Ensure that the patient has removed all external metallic objects (jewelry, dentures, etc.) prior to the procedure.

> Have emergency equipment readily available.

> Patients are given a gown, robe, and foot coverings to wear and instructed to void prior to the procedure.

> Record baseline vital signs and assess neurologic status. Protocols may vary from facility to facility.

> Instruct the patient to cooperate fully and to follow directions. Instruct the patient to remain still throughout the procedure because movement produces unreliable results.

> Observe standard precautions, and follow the general guidelines in Appendix A.

> Place the patient in a supine position on a flat table with foam wedges,

which help maintain position and immobilization. The radionuclide is administered intravenously, and the abdomen is scanned immediately for 1 minute to screen for vascular lesions that cause bleeding. Then images are taken every 5 minutes for the next 60 minutes in the anterior, oblique, and lateral views, and then in a single postvoid anterior view.

➤ Wear gloves during the radionuclide injection and while handling the patient's urine.

➤ Instruct the patient to take slow, deep breaths if nausea occurs during the procedure. Monitor and administer an antiemetic agent if ordered. Ready an emesis basin for use.

➤ Monitor the patient for complications related to the procedure (e.g., allergic reaction, anaphylaxis, bronchospasm).

➤ The needle or catheter is removed, and a pressure dressing is applied over the puncture site.

➤ The results are recorded on x-ray film or electronically, in a computerized system, for recall and postprocedure interpretation by the appropriate health care practitioner.

Post-test:

➤ Instruct the patient to resume usual diet, fluids, and medications, as directed by the health care practitioner.

➤ Monitor vital signs and neurologic status every 15 minutes for 1 hour, then every 2 hours for 4 hours, and then as ordered by the health care practitioner. Compare with baseline values. Protocols may vary from facility to facility.

➤ Observe for delayed allergic reactions, such as rash, urticaria, tachycardia, hyperpnea, hypertension, palpitations, nausea, or vomiting.

➤ Instruct the patient to immediately report symptoms such as fast heart rate, difficulty breathing, skin rash, itching, or decreased urinary output.

➤ Observe the needle/catheter insertion site for bleeding, inflammation, or hematoma formation.

➤ Instruct the patient to apply cold compresses to the puncture site, as needed, to reduce discomfort or edema.

➤ Instruct patient to drink increased amounts of fluids for 24 to 48 hours to eliminate the radionuclide from the body, unless contraindicated. Tell the patient that radionuclide is eliminated from the body within 6 to 24 hours.

➤ Instruct the patient to flush the toilet immediately after each voiding following the procedure, and to wash hands meticulously with soap and water after each voiding for 24 hours after the procedure.

➤ Instruct all caregivers to wear gloves when discarding urine for 24 hours after the procedure. Wash gloved hands with soap and water before removing gloves. Then wash hands after the gloves are removed.

➤ If a woman who is breast-feeding must have a nuclear scan, she should not breast-feed the infant until the radionuclide has been eliminated. This could take as long as 3 days. She should be instructed to express the milk and discard it during the 3-day period to prevent cessation of milk production.

➤ *Nutritional considerations:* A low-fat, low-cholesterol, and low-sodium diet should be consumed to reduce current disease processes. High fat consumption increases the amount of bile acids in the colon and should be avoided.

➤ No other radionuclide tests should be scheduled for 24 to 48 hours after this procedure.

➤ A written report of the examination will be completed by a health care practitioner specializing in this branch of medicine. The report will be sent to the requesting health care practitioner, who will discuss the results with the patient.

➤ Recognize anxiety related to test results, and be supportive of perceived loss of independent function. Discuss the implications of abnormal test results on the patient's lifestyle. Provide teaching and information

regarding the clinical implications of the test results, as appropriate.

➤ Reinforce information given by the patient's health care provider regarding further testing, treatment, or referral to another health care provider. Answer any questions or address any concerns voiced by the patient or family.

➤ Instruct the patient in the use of any ordered medications. Explain the importance of adhering to the therapy regimen. As appropriate, instruct the patient in significant side effects and systemic reactions associated with the prescribed medication. Encourage him or her to review corresponding literature provided by a pharmacist.

➤ Depending on the results of this procedure, additional testing may be needed to evaluate or monitor progression of the disease process and determine the need for a change in therapy. Evaluate test results in relation to the patient's symptoms and other tests performed.

Related diagnostic tests:

➤ Related diagnostic tests include computed tomography of the abdomen or pelvis, and magnetic resonance imaging of the abdomen or pelvis.

MEDIASTINOSCOPY

· ·

SYNONYM/ACRONYM: N/A.

AREA OF APPLICATION: Mediastinum.

CONTRAST: None.

DESCRIPTION & RATIONALE: Mediastinoscopy provides direct visualization of the structures that lie beneath the mediastinum, which is the area behind the sternum and between the lungs. The test is performed under general anesthesia by means of a mediastinoscope inserted through a surgical incision at the suprasternal notch. Structures that can be viewed include the trachea, the esophagus, the heart and its major vessels, the thymus gland, and the lymph nodes that receive drainage from the lungs. The procedure is performed primarily to visualize and obtain biopsy specimens of the mediastinal lymph nodes, and to determine the extent of metastasis into the mediastinum for the determination of treatment planning in cancer patients. ■

INDICATIONS:
• Confirm radiologic evidence of a thoracic infectious process of an indeterminate nature, coccidioidomycosis, or histoplasmosis

• Confirm radiologic or cytologic evidence of carcinoma or sarcoidosis

• Detect Hodgkin's disease

• Detect metastasis into the anterior mediastinum or extrapleurally into the chest

• Determine stage of known bronchogenic carcinoma, as indicated by the extent of mediastinal lymph node involvement

• Evaluate a patient with signs and symptoms of obstruction of mediastinal lymph flow and a history of head or neck cancer to determine recurrence or spread

RESULT

Normal Findings:
• Normal appearance of mediastinal structures

• No abnormal lymph node tissue

Abnormal Findings:
• Bronchogenic carcinoma

• Coccidioidomycosis

• Granulomatous infections

• Histoplasmosis

• Hodgkin's disease

• *Pneumocystis carinii* infection

• Sarcoidosis

• Tuberculosis

CRITICAL VALUES: N/A

INTERFERING FACTORS:

This procedure is contraindicated for:
• Patients who have had a previous mediastinoscopy, because scarring can make insertion of the scope and biopsy of lymph nodes difficult

• Patients who have superior vena cava obstruction, because this condition causes increased venous collateral circulation in the mediastinum

• Patients who are pregnant or suspected of being pregnant, unless the potential benefits of the procedure far outweigh the risks to the fetus and mother

Other considerations:
• Failure to follow dietary restrictions before the procedure may cause the procedure to be canceled or repeated.

Nursing Implications and Procedure • • • • • • • • • • •

Pretest:

➤ Inform the patient that the procedure assesses the mediastinum.

➤ Obtain a history of the patient's complaints or symptoms, including a list of known allergens (especially allergies or sensitivities to latex), and inform the appropriate health care practitioner accordingly.

➤ Obtain a history of the patient's immune and respiratory systems, any bleeding disorders, and results of previously performed laboratory tests (especially bleeding time, complete blood count, partial thromboplastin time, platelets, and prothrombin time), surgical procedures, and other diagnostic procedures. For related laboratory tests, refer to the Immune and Respiratory System tables.

➤ Note any recent procedures that can interfere with test results. Ensure that this procedure is performed before an upper gastrointestinal study or barium swallow.

➤ Record the date of the last menstrual period and determine the possibility of pregnancy in perimenopausal women.

➤ Obtain a list of the medications the patient is taking, including anticoagulant therapy, acetylsalicylic acid, herbs, nutritional supplements, and nutraceuticals, especially those known to affect coagulation. It is recommended that use be discontinued 14 days before dental or surgical procedures. The requesting health care practitioner and laboratory should be

advised if the patient regularly uses these products so that their effects can be taken into consideration when reviewing results.

> Review the procedure with the patient. Inform the patient that prophylactic antibiotics may be administered prior to the procedure. Address concerns about pain related to the procedure. Explain that a general anesthesia will be administered to promote relaxation and reduce discomfort prior to the mediastinoscopy. Explain to the patient that some pain may be experienced after the test. Meperidine (Demerol) or morphine may be given as a sedative. Inform the patient that the procedure is performed in the operating room, under sterile conditions, by a health care practitioner specializing in this procedure. The procedure usually takes about 30 to 60 minutes to complete.

> Explain that an intravenous (IV) line will be inserted to allow infusion of IV fluids, antibiotics, anesthetics, and analgesics.

> *Sensitivity to cultural and social issues,* as well as concern for modesty, is important in providing psychological support before, during, and after the procedure.

> The patient should fast and restrict fluids for 8 hours prior to the procedure. Instruct the patient to avoid taking anticoagulant medication or to reduce dosage as ordered prior to the procedure. Number of days to withhold medication is dependent on the type of anticoagulant.

> Instruct the patient to remove dentures, jewelry (including watches), hairpins, credit cards, and other metallic objects in the area to be examined.

> Ensure that the results of blood typing and cross-matching are obtained and recorded before the procedure in the event that an emergency thoracotomy is required.

> *Make sure a written and informed consent has been signed prior to the procedure and before administering any medications.*

Intratest: ▮

> Ensure that the patient has complied with dietary, fluids, and medication restrictions and pretesting preparations; assure that food and fluids have been restricted for at least 8 hours prior to the procedure. Ensure that the patient has removed all external metallic objects (jewelry, dentures, etc.) prior to the procedure.

> Ensure that anticoagulant therapy has been withheld for the appropriate amount of days prior to the procedure. Notify the health care practitioner if patient anticoagulant therapy has not been withheld.

> Have emergency equipment readily available. Keep resuscitation equipment on hand in the case of respiratory impairment or laryngospasm after the procedure.

> Avoid using morphine sulfate in patients with asthma or other pulmonary disease. This drug can further exacerbate bronchospasms and respiratory impairment.

> Patients are given a gown, robe, and foot coverings to wear and instructed to void prior to the procedure.

> Instruct the patient to cooperate fully and to follow directions. Instruct the patient to remain still throughout the procedure because movement produces unreliable results.

> Record baseline vital signs and assess neurologic status. Protocols may vary from facility to facility.

> Observe standard precautions, and follow the general guidelines in Appendix A.

> Establish IV fluid line for the injection of emergency drugs and of sedatives.

> Place electrocardiographic electrodes on the patient for cardiac monitoring. Establish baseline rhythm; determine if the patient has ventricular arrhythmias.

> Place the patient in the supine position. General anesthesia is administered via an endotracheal tube.

> An incision is made at the suprasternal notch, and a path for the medi-

astinoscope is made using finger dissection. The lymph nodes can be palpated at this time. The lymph nodes on the right side of the mediastinum are most accessible and safest to biopsy by medastinoscopy; the lymph nodes on the left side are more difficult to explore and biopsy because of their proximity to the aorta. Biopsy specimens of nodes on the left side of the mediastinum may need to be obtained by mediastinotomy, which involves performing a left anterior thoracotomy.

➤ Place tissue samples in properly labeled specimen containers, and promptly transport the specimen to the laboratory for processing and analysis.

➤ The scope is removed, and the incision is closed.

➤ If the patient is stable and if no further surgery is immediately indicated, the patient is extubated.

Post-test:

➤ The patient should remain in a semi-Fowler's position on either side until vital signs revert to preprocedure levels.

➤ Monitor vital signs and neurologic status every 15 minutes for 1 hour, then every 2 hours for 4 hours, and then as ordered by the health care practitioner. Take temperature every 4 hours for 24 hours. Compare with baseline values. Notify the health care practitioner if temperature is elevated. Protocols may vary from facility to facility.

➤ Do not allow the patient to eat or drink for 12 to 24 hours. Instruct the patient to resume normal activity, medication, and diet in 24 hours or as tolerated after the examination, unless otherwise indicated.

➤ Observe for delayed allergic reactions, such as rash, urticaria, tachycardia, hyperpnea, hypertension, palpitations, nausea, or vomiting.

➤ Instruct the patient to immediately report symptoms such as fast heart rate, difficulty breathing, skin rash, itching, or decreased urinary output.

➤ Instruct the patient in the care and assessment of the site. Observe the site for bleeding, hematoma formation, and inflammation. Note any pleuritic pain, persistent right shoulder pain, or chest pain.

➤ *Nutritional considerations:* A low-fat, low-cholesterol, and low-sodium diet should be consumed to reduce current disease processes and/or decrease risk of hypertension and coronary artery disease.

➤ Emphasize that any excessive bleeding, difficulty breathing, excessive coughing after biopsy, or pain must be reported to the health care practitioner immediately.

➤ A written report of the examination will be completed by a health care practitioner specializing in this branch of medicine. The report will be sent to the requesting health care practitioner, who will discuss the results with the patient.

➤ Recognize anxiety related to test results, and be supportive of perceived loss of independent function. Discuss the implications of abnormal test results on the patient's lifestyle. Provide teaching and information regarding the clinical implications of the test results, as appropriate.

➤ Reinforce information given by the patient's health care provider regarding further testing, treatment, or referral to another health care provider. Answer any questions or address any concerns voiced by the patient or family.

➤ Instruct the patient in the use of any ordered medications. Explain the importance of adhering to the therapy regimen. As appropriate, instruct the patient in significant side effects and systemic reactions associated with the prescribed medication. Encourage him or her to review corresponding literature provided by a pharmacist.

➤ Depending on the results of this procedure, additional testing may be

needed to evaluate or monitor progression of the disease process and determine the need for a change in therapy. Evaluate test results in relation to the patient's symptoms and other tests performed.

➤ Related diagnostic tests include chest x-ray, computed tomography of the thorax, lung scan, and magnetic resonance imaging of the chest.

METANEPHRINES

. . . .

SYNONYM/ACRONYM: N/A.

SPECIMEN: Urine (25 mL) from a timed specimen collected in a clean amber plastic collection container with 6N hydrochloride as a preservative.

REFERENCE VALUE: (Method: High-pressure liquid chromatography)

Age	Conventional Units	SI Units
	Normetanephrines	
		(Conventional Units × 5.46)
0–3 mo	47–156 μg/24 h	257–852 nmol/24 h
4–6 mo	31–111 μg/24 h	171–607 nmol/24 h
7–9 mo	42–109 μg/24 h	230–595 nmol/24 h
10–12 mo	23–103 μg/24 h	127–562 nmol/24 h
1–2 y	32–118 μg/24 h	175–647 nmol/24 h
2–6 y	50–111 μg/24 h	274–604 nmol/24 h
6–10 y	47–176 μg/24 h	255–964 nmol/24 h
10–16 y	53–290 μg/24 h	289–1586 nmol/24 h
Adult	82–500 μg/24 h	448–2730 nmol/24 h
	Metanephrines	
		(Conventional Units × 5.07)
0–3 mo	5.9–37 μg/24 h	30–188 nmol/24 h
4–6 mo	6.1–42 μg/24 h	31–213 nmol/24 h
7–9 mo	12–41 μg/24 h	61–210 nmol/24 h
10–12 mo	8.5–101 μg/24 h	43–510 nmol/24 h
1–2 y	6.7–52 μg/24 h	34–264 nmol/24 h
2–6 y	11–99 μg/24 h	56–501 nmol/24 h
6–10 y	54–138 μg/24 h	275–701 nmol/24 h
10–16 y	39–243 μg/24 h	200–1231 nmol/24 h
Adult	45–290 μg/24 h	228–1470 nmol/24 h

DESCRIPTION & RATIONALE:

Metanephrines are the inactive metabolites of epinephrine and norepinephrine. Metanephrines are either excreted or further metabolized into vanillylmandelic acid. Release of metanephrines in the urine is indicative of disorders associated with excessive catecholamine production, particularly pheochromocytoma. Vanillylmandelic acid and catecholamines are normally measured with urinary metanephrines. Creatinine is usually measured simultaneously to ensure adequate collection and to calculate an excretion ratio of metabolite to creatinine. ■

INDICATIONS:

• Assist in the diagnosis of suspected pheochromocytoma

• Assist in identifying the cause of hypertension

• Verify suspected tumors associated with excessive catecholamine secretion

RESULT

Increased in:
• Ganglioneuroma
• Neuroblastoma
• Pheochromocytoma
• Severe stress

Decreased in: N/A

CRITICAL VALUES: N/A

INTERFERING FACTORS:

• Drugs that may increase metanephrine levels include labetalol, monoamine oxidase inhibitors, oxprenolol, oxytetracycline, and prochlorperazine.

• Methylglucamine in x-ray contrast medium may cause false-negative results.

Nursing Implications and Procedure

Pretest:

➤ Inform the patient that the test is used to assist in the diagnosis of pheochromocytoma, neuroblastoma, and ganglioblastoma.

➤ Obtain a history of the patient's complaints, including a list of known allergens (especially allergies or sensitivities to latex), and inform the appropriate health care practitioner accordingly.

➤ Obtain a history of the patient's endocrine system, as well as results of previously performed laboratory tests, surgical procedures, and other diagnostic procedures. For related laboratory tests, refer to the Endocrine System table.

➤ Note any recent procedures that can interfere with test results.

➤ Obtain a list of the medications the patient is taking, including herbs, nutritional supplements, and nutraceuticals. The requesting health care practitioner and laboratory should be advised if the patient regularly uses these products so that their effects can be taken into consideration when reviewing results.

➤ Review the procedure with the patient. Provide a nonmetallic urinal, bedpan, or toilet-mounted collection device. Address concerns about pain related to the procedure. Explain to the patient that there should be no discomfort during the procedure.

➤ Usually a 24-hour time frame for urine collection is ordered. Inform the patient that all urine must be saved during that 24-hour period. Instruct the patient not to void directly into the laboratory collection container. Instruct the patient to avoid defecating in the collection device and to keep toilet tissue out of the collection device to prevent contamination of the specimen. Place a sign in the bathroom to remind the patient to save all urine.

➤ Instruct the patient to void all urine

into the collection device and then to pour the urine into the laboratory collection container. Alternatively, the specimen can be left in the collection device for a health care staff member to add to the laboratory collection container.

➤ *Sensitivity to social and cultural issues,* as well as concern for modesty, is important in providing psychological support before, during, and after the procedure.

➤ Instruct the patient to avoid excessive exercise and stress during the 24-hour collection of urine.

➤ There are no food, fluid, or medication restrictions, unless by medical direction.

Intratest:

➤ Ensure that the patient has complied with activity restrictions during the procedure.

➤ If the patient has a history of severe allergic reaction to latex, care should be taken to avoid the use of equipment containing latex.

➤ Instruct the patient to cooperate fully and to follow directions.

➤ Observe standard precautions, and follow the general guidelines in Appendix A. Positively identify the patient, and label the appropriate collection container with the corresponding patient demographics, date, and time of collection.

Timed specimen:

➤ Obtain a clean 3-L urine specimen container, toilet-mounted collection device, and plastic bag (for transport of the specimen container). The specimen must be refrigerated or kept on ice throughout the entire collection period. If an indwelling urinary catheter is in place, the drainage bag must be kept on ice.

➤ Begin the test between 6 and 8 a.m., if possible. Collect first voiding and discard. Record the time the specimen was discarded as the beginning of the timed collection period. The next morning, ask the patient to void

at the same time the collection was started and add this last voiding to the container.

➤ If an indwelling catheter is in place, replace the tubing and container system at the start of the collection time. Keep the container system on ice during the collection period, or empty the urine into a larger container periodically during the collection period; monitor to ensure continued drainage, and conclude the test the next morning at the same hour the collection was begun.

➤ At the conclusion of the test, compare the quantity of urine with the urinary output record for the collection; if the specimen contains less than what was recorded as output, some urine may have been discarded, invalidating the test.

➤ Include on the collection container's label the amount of urine and test start and stop times.

➤ Promptly transport the specimen to the laboratory for processing and analysis.

➤ The results are recorded manually or in a computerized system for recall and postprocedure interpretation by the appropriate health care practitioner.

Post-test:

➤ Instruct the patient to resume usual activity, as directed by the health care practitioner.

➤ A written report of the examination will be sent to the requesting health care practitioner, who will discuss the results with the patient.

➤ Recognize anxiety related to test results, and be supportive of fear of shortened life expectancy. Discuss the implications of abnormal test results on the patient's lifestyle. Provide teaching and information regarding the clinical implications of the test results, as appropriate. Educate the patient regarding access to counseling services.

➤ Reinforce information given by the

patient's health care provider regarding further testing, treatment, or referral to another health care provider. Answer any questions or address any concerns voiced by the patient or family.

➤ Depending on the results of this procedure, additional testing may be performed to evaluate or monitor progression of the disease process

and determine the need for a change in therapy. Evaluate test results in relation to the patient's symptoms and other tests performed.

➤ Related laboratory tests include catecholamines, homovanillic acid, and vanillylmandelic acid.

METHEMOGLOBIN

- -

SYNONYMS/ACRONYM: Hemoglobin, hemoglobin M, MetHb, Hgb M.

SPECIMEN: Whole blood (1 mL) collected in green-top (heparin) tube. Specimen should be transported tightly capped and in an ice slurry.

REFERENCE VALUE: (Method: Spectrophotometry)

Conventional Units	SI Units (Conventional Units × 155)
0.06–0.24 g/dL*	9.3–37.2 μmol/L*

* Percentage of total hemoglobin = 0.41–1.15%.
Note: The conversion factor of ×155 is based on the molecular weight of hemoglobin of 64,500 daltons (d), or 64.5 kd.

DESCRIPTION & RATIONALE: Methemoglobin is a structural hemoglobin variant formed when the heme portion of the deoxygenated hemoglobin is oxidized to a ferric state that renders it incapable of combining with and transporting oxygen to tissues. Visible cyanosis can result as levels approach 10% to 15% of total hemoglobin. ∎

INDICATIONS:

• Assist in the detection of acquired methemoglobinemia caused by the toxic effects of chemicals and drugs

• Assist in the detection of congenital methemoglobinemia, indicated by deficiency of red blood cell nicotinamide adenine dinucleotide (NADH)-methemoglobin reductase or presence of methemoglobin.

• Evaluate cyanosis in the presence of normal blood gases

RESULT

Increased in:

• Acquired methemoglobinemia (drugs, tobacco smoking, or ionizing radiation)

• Carbon monoxide poisoning

- Hereditary methemoglobinemia (deficiency of NADH-methemoglobin reductase or hemoglobinopathy)

Decreased in: N/A

CRITICAL VALUES:

Cyanosis can occur at levels greater than 10%.

Dizziness, fatigue, headache, and tachycardia can occur at levels greater than 30%.

Signs of central nervous system depression can occur at levels greater than 45%.

Death may occur at levels greater than 70%.

Note and immediately report to the health care practitioner any critically increased or decreased values and related symptoms. Possible interventions include airway protection, administration of oxygen, monitoring neurologic status every hour, continuous pulse oximetry, hyperbaric oxygen therapy, and exchange transfusion. Administration of activated charcoal or gastric lavage may be effective if performed soon after the toxic agent is ingested. Emesis should never be induced in patients with no gag reflex because of the risk of aspiration. Methylene blue may be used to reverse the process of methemoglobin formation, but it should be used cautiously when methemoglobin levels are greater than 30%. Use of methylene blue is contraindicated in the presence of glucose-6-phosphate dehydrogenase deficiency.

INTERFERING FACTORS:

- Drugs that may increase methemoglobin levels include acetanilid, amyl nitrate, aniline derivatives, benzocaine, chlorates, chloroquine, dapsone, glucosulfone, isoniazid, lidocaine, nitroglycerin, phenacetin, phenytoin, primaquine, resorcinol, sulfonamides, and thiazolsulfone.

- Well water containing nitrate is the most common cause of methemoglobinemia in infants.

- Breast-feeding infants are capable of converting inorganic nitrate from common topical anesthetic applications containing nitrate to the nitrite ion, causing nitrite toxicity and increased methemoglobin.

- Prompt and proper specimen processing, storage, and analysis are important to achieve accurate results. Methemoglobin is unstable and should be transported on ice within a few hours of collection, or else the specimen should be rejected.

Nursing Implications and Procedure

Pretest:

➤ Inform the patient that the test is used to investigate cyanosis associated with polycythemia, hemoglobinopathies, and drug toxicity (inhaled substances).

➤ Obtain a history of the patient's complaints, including a list of known allergens (especially allergies or sensitivities to latex), and inform the appropriate health care practitioner accordingly.

➤ Obtain a history of the patient's hematopoietic and respiratory systems and results of previously performed laboratory tests, surgical procedures, and other diagnostic procedures. For related laboratory tests, refer to the Hematopoietic and Respiratory System tables.

➤ Note any recent procedures that can interfere with test results.

➤ Obtain a list of medications the patient is taking, including herbs, nutritional supplements, and nutraceuticals. The requesting health care practitioner and laboratory should be advised if the patient regularly uses these products so that their effects can be taken into consideration when reviewing results.

➤ Review the procedure with the patient. Inform the patient that specimen collection takes approximately 5 to 10 minutes. Address concerns about pain related to the procedure. Explain to the patient that there may be some discomfort during the venipuncture.

➤ There are no food, fluid, or medication restrictions, unless by medical direction.

➤ Prepare an ice slurry in a cup or plastic bag to have on hand for immediate transport of the specimen to the laboratory.

Intratest:

➤ If the patient has a history of severe allergic reaction to latex, care should be taken to avoid the use of equipment containing latex.

➤ Instruct the patient to cooperate fully and to follow directions. Direct the patient to breathe normally and to avoid unnecessary movement.

➤ Observe standard precautions, and follow the general guidelines in Appendix A. Positively identify the patient, and label the appropriate tubes with the corresponding patient demographics, date, and time of collection. Perform a venipuncture; collect the specimen in a 5-mL green-top tube.

➤ Remove the needle, and apply a pressure dressing over the puncture site.

➤ Promptly transport the specimen to the laboratory for processing and analysis. The specimen should be placed in an ice slurry immediately after collection. Information on the specimen label can be protected from water in the ice slurry if the specimen is first placed in a protective plastic bag.

➤ The results are recorded manually or in a computerized system for recall and postprocedure interpretation by the appropriate health care practitioner.

Post-test:

➤ Observe venipuncture site for bleeding or hematoma formation. Apply paper tape or other adhesive to hold pressure bandage in place, or replace with a plastic bandage.

➤ Teach the patient to avoid carbon monoxide from first- or second-hand smoking, to have home gas furnace checked yearly for leaks, and to utilize gas appliances such as gas grills in a well-ventilated area.

➤ A written report of the examination will be sent to the requesting health care practitioner, who will discuss the results with the patient.

➤ Reinforce information given by the patient's health care provider regarding further testing, treatment, or referral to another health care provider. Answer any questions or address any concerns voiced by the patient or family.

➤ Depending on the results of this procedure, additional testing may be performed to evaluate or monitor progression of the disease process and determine the need for a change in therapy. Evaluate test results in relation to the patient's symptoms and other tests performed.

Related laboratory tests:

➤ Related laboratory tests include arterial/alveolar oxygen ratio, blood gases, carboxyhemoglobin, and hemoglobin electrophoresis.

MICROALBUMIN

Sʏɴᴏɴʏᴍs/Aᴄʀᴏɴʏᴍ: Albumin, urine.

Sᴘᴇᴄɪᴍᴇɴ: Urine (10 mL) from a random or timed specimen collected in a clean plastic collection container.

Rᴇꜰᴇʀᴇɴᴄᴇ ᴠᴀʟᴜᴇ: (Method: Nephelometry immunoassay)

Test	Conventional & SI Units
24-h Urine, Microalbumin	Less than 30 mg/24h
Random Urine, Microalbumin/ Creatinine Ratio	Less than 30 µg/mg creatinine

Simultaneous measurement of urine creatinine or creatinine clearance may be requested. Normal ratio of microalbumin to creatinine is less than 15.

Dᴇsᴄʀɪᴘᴛɪᴏɴ & Rᴀᴛɪᴏɴᴀʟᴇ: The term *microalbumin* is used to describe concentrations of albumin in urine that are greater than normal but undetectable by dipstick or traditional spectrophotometry methods. Microalbuminuria precedes the nephropathy associated with diabetes and is often elevated years before creatinine clearance shows abnormal values. Studies have shown that the median duration from onset of microalbuminuria to development of nephropathy is 5 to 7 years. ∎

Iɴᴅɪᴄᴀᴛɪᴏɴs:
• Evaluate renal disease
• Screen diabetic patients for early signs of nephropathy

Rᴇsᴜʟᴛ

Increased in:
• Cardiomyopathy

• Diabetic nephropathy
• Exercise
• Hypertension (uncontrolled)
• Pre-eclampsia
• Renal disease
• Urinary tract infections

Decreased in: N/A

Cʀɪᴛɪᴄᴀʟ ᴠᴀʟᴜᴇs: N/A

Iɴᴛᴇʀꜰᴇʀɪɴɢ ꜰᴀᴄᴛᴏʀs:
• Drugs that may decrease microalbumin levels include captopril, dipyridamole, enalapril, furosemide, indapamide, perindopril, quinapril, ramipril, tolrestat, and triflusal.

• All urine voided for the timed collection period must be included in the collection or else falsely decreased values may be obtained. Compare output records with volume collected to verify that all voids were included in the collection.

Nursing Implications and Procedure • • • • • • • • • • •

➤ Inform the patient that the test is used to assist in the mangement of early diabetes in order to avoid or delay the onset of renal disease associated with diabetes.

➤ Obtain a history of the patient's complaints, including a list of known allergens (especially allergies or sensitivities to latex), and inform the appropriate health care practitioner accordingly.

➤ Obtain a history of the patient's endocrine and genitourinary systems as well as results results of previously performed laboratory tests, surgical procedures, and other diagnostic procedures. For related laboratory tests, refer to the Endocrine and Genitourinary System tables.

➤ Obtain a list of medications the patient is taking, including herbs, nutritional supplements, and nutraceuticals. The requesting health care practitioner and laboratory should be advised if the patient regularly uses these products so that their effects can be taken into consideration when reviewing results.

➤ Review the procedure with the patient. Provide a nonmetallic urinal, bedpan, or toilet-mounted collection device. Address concerns about pain related to the procedure. Explain to the patient that there should be no discomfort during the procedure.

➤ Usually a 24-hour time frame for urine collection is ordered. Inform the patient that all urine must be saved during that 24-hour period. Instruct the patient not to void directly into the laboratory collection container. Instruct the patient to avoid defecating in the collection device and to keep toilet tissue out of the collection device to prevent contamination of the specimen. Place a sign in the bathroom to remind the patient to save all urine.

➤ Instruct the patient to void all urine into the collection device and then to pour the urine into the laboratory collection container. Alternatively, the specimen can be left in the collection device for a health care staff member to add to the laboratory collection container.

➤ *Sensitivity to social and cultural issues,* as well as concern for modesty, is important in providing psychological support before, during, and after the procedure.

➤ Instruct the patient to avoid excessive exercise and stress during the 24-hour collection of urine.

➤ There are no food, fluid, or medication restrictions, unless by medical direction.

➤ Ensure that the patient has complied with activity restrictions during the procedure.

➤ If the patient has a history of severe allergic reaction to latex, care should be taken to avoid the use of equipment containing latex.

➤ Instruct the patient to cooperate fully and to follow directions.

➤ Observe standard precautions, and follow the general guidelines in Appendix A. Positively identify the patient, and label the appropriate collection container with the corresponding patient demographics, date, and time of collection.

Random specimen (collect in early morning):

Clean-catch specimen:

➤ Instruct the male patient to (1) thoroughly wash his hands, (2) cleanse the meatus, (3) void a small amount into the toilet, and (4) void directly into the specimen container.

➤ Instruct the female patient to (1) thoroughly wash her hands; (2) cleanse the labia from front to back; (3) while keeping the labia separated, void a small amount into the toilet; and (4) without interrupting the urine stream, void directly into the specimen container.

Indwelling catheter:

➤ Put on gloves. Empty drainage tube of urine. It may be necessary to clamp off the catheter for 15 to 30 minutes before specimen collection. Cleanse specimen port with antiseptic swab, and then aspirate 5 mL of urine with a 21- to 25-gauge needle and syringe. Transfer urine to a sterile container.

Timed specimen:

➤ Obtain a clean 3-L urine specimen container, toilet-mounted collection device, and plastic bag (for transport of the specimen container). The specimen must be refrigerated or kept on ice throughout the entire collection period. If an indwelling urinary catheter is in place, the drainage bag must be kept on ice.

➤ Begin the test between 6 and 8 a.m., if possible. Collect first voiding and discard. Record the time the specimen was discarded as the beginning of the timed collection period. The next morning, ask the patient to void at the same time the collection was started and add this last voiding to the container.

➤ If an indwelling catheter is in place, replace the tubing and container system at the start of the collection time. Keep the container system on ice during the collection period, or empty the urine into a larger container periodically during the collection period; monitor to ensure continued drainage, and conclude the test the next morning at the same hour the collection was begun.

➤ At the conclusion of the test, compare the quantity of urine with the urinary output record for the collection; if the specimen contains less than what was recorded as output, some urine may have been discarded, invalidating the test.

➤ Include on the collection container's label the amount of urine and test start and stop times.

General:

➤ Promptly transport the specimen to the laboratory for processing and analysis.

➤ The results are recorded manually or in a computerized system for recall and postprocedure interpretation by the appropriate health care practitioner.

Post-test:

➤ Instruct the patient to resume usual activity, as directed by the health care practitioner.

➤ Instruct the patient and caregiver to report signs and symptoms of hypoglycemia or hyperglycemia.

➤ *Nutritional considerations:* Instruct the patient, as appropriate, in nutritional management of diabetes. Patients who adhere to dietary recommendations report a better general feeling of health, better weight management, greater control of glucose and lipid values, and improved use of insulin. There is no "diabetic diet"; however, there are many meal-planning approaches with nutritional goals endorsed by the American Dietetic Association. The nutritional needs of each diabetic patient need to be determined individually with the appropriate health care professionals, particularly professionals trained in nutrition.

➤ Recognize anxiety related to test results, and be supportive of perceived loss of independence and fear of shortened life expectancy. Discuss the implications of abnormal test results on the patient's lifestyle. Provide teaching and information regarding the clinical implications of the test results, as appropriate. Emphasize, if indicated, that good glycemic control delays the onset and slows the progression of diabetic retinopathy, nephropathy, and neuropathy. Educate the patient regarding access to counseling services, as appropriate. Provide contact information, if desired, for the American Diabetes Association (http://www.diabetes.org).

> A written report of the examination will be sent to the requesting health care practitioner who will discuss the results with the patient.

> Reinforce information given by the patient's health care provider regarding further testing, treatment, or referral to another health care provider. Answer any questions or address any concerns voiced by the patient or family.

> Depending on the results of this procedure, additional testing may be performed to evaluate or monitor progression of the disease process and determine the need for a change in therapy. Evaluate test results in relation to the patient's symptoms and other tests performed.

Related laboratory tests:

> Related laboratory tests include cortisol, urine creatinine, creatinine clearance, glucose, glucose tolerance test, glycated hemoglobin, insulin, insulin antibodies, urinalysis, and urine protein and fractions.

β₂-MICROGLOBULIN

SYNONYM/ACRONYM: β_2-M.

SPECIMEN: Serum (1 mL) collected in a red-top tube or 5 mL urine from a timed collection in a clean plastic container with 1N NaOH as a preservative.

REFERENCE VALUE: (Method: Immunoassay for serum sample, radioimmunoassay for urine sample)

Sample	Conventional Units	SI Units (Conventional Units × 10)
Serum		
Newborn	Less than 0.3 mg/dL	Less than 3 mg/L
Adult	Less than 0.2 mg/dL	Less than 2 mg/L
Urine	0.03–0.37 mg/24 h	

DESCRIPTION & RATIONALE: β_2-Microglobulin is an amino acid peptide component of human leukocyte antigen (HLA) complexes. β_2-Microglobulin increases in inflammatory conditions and when lymphocyte turnover increases, such as in lymphocytic leukemia or when T-lymphocyte helper (OKT4) cells are attacked by human immunodeficiency virus

(HIV). Serum β2-microglobulin becomes elevated with malfunctioning glomeruli, but decreases with malfunctioning tubules because it is metabolized by the renal tubules. Conversely, urine β2-microglobulin decreases with malfunctioning glomeruli, but becomes elevated with malfunctioning tubules. ▪

INDICATIONS:
- Detect aminoglycoside toxicity (becomes elevated before creatinine)
- Detect chronic lymphocytic leukemia, multiple myeloma, lung cancer, hepatoma, or breast cancer
- Detect HIV infection (*note:* levels do not correlate with stages of infection)
- Evaluate renal disease to differentiate glomerular from tubular dysfunction
- Monitor antiretroviral therapy

RESULT

Increased in:
- Acquired immunodeficiency syndrome (AIDS)
- Aminoglycoside toxicity
- Amyloidosis
- Autoimmune disorders
- Breast cancer
- Crohn's disease
- Felty's syndrome
- Hepatitis
- Hepatoma
- Hyperthyroidism
- Inflammation of all types
- Leukemia (chronic lymphocytic)
- Lung cancer
- Lymphoma
- Multiple myeloma
- Poisoning with heavy metals, such as mercury or cadmium
- Renal dialysis
- Renal disease (glomerular): serum only
- Renal disease (tubular): urine only
- Sarcoidosis
- Systemic lupus erythematosus
- Vasculitis
- Viral infections (e.g., cytomegalovirus)

Decreased in:
- Renal disease (glomerular): urine only
- Renal disease (tubular): serum only
- Response to zidovudine (AZT)

CRITICAL VALUES: N/A

INTERFERING FACTORS:
- Drugs and proteins that may increase serum β2-microglobulin levels include cefuroxime, cyclosporin A, gentamicin, interferon alfa, pentoxifylline, and tumor necrosis factor.
- Drugs that may decrease serum β2-microglobulin levels include zidovudine.
- Drugs that may increase urine β2-microglobulin levels include azathioprine, cisplatin, cyclosporin A, furosemide, gentamicin, mannitol, nifedipine, sisomicin, and tobramycin.
- Drugs that may decrease urine β2-microglobulin levels include cilostazol.
- Urinary β2-microglobulin is unstable at pH less than 5.5.
- Recent radioactive scans or radiation within 1 week before the test can interfere with test results when radioimmunoassay is the test method.

Nursing Implications and Procedure • • • • • • • • • • •

➤ Inform the patient that the test is used to evaluate renal disease, AIDS, and certain malignancies.

➤ Obtain a history of the patient's complaints, including a list of known allergens (especially allergies or sensitivities to latex), and inform the appropriate health care practitioner accordingly.

➤ Obtain a history of the patient's genitourinary and immune system, as well as results of previously performed laboratory tests, surgical procedures, and other diagnostic procedures. For related laboratory tests, refer to the Genitourinary and Immune System tables.

➤ Note any recent procedures that can interfere with test results.

➤ Obtain a list of medications the patient is taking, including herbs, nutritional supplements, and nutraceuticals. The requesting health care practitioner and laboratory should be advised if the patient regularly uses these products so their effects can be taken into consideration when reviewing results.

➤ *Sensitivity to social and cultural issues,* as well as concern for modesty, is important in providing psychological support before, during, and after the procedure.

➤ There are no food, fluid, or medication restrictions, unless by medical direction.

Blood:

➤ Review the procedure with the patient. Inform the patient that specimen collection takes approximately 5 to 10 minutes. Address concerns about pain related to the procedure. Explain to the patient that there may be some discomfort during the venipuncture.

Urine:

➤ Review the procedure with the patient. Provide a nonmetallic urinal, bedpan, or toilet-mounted collection device.

➤ Usually a 24-hour urine collection is ordered. Inform the patient that all urine over a 24-hour period must be saved; instruct the patient to avoid defecating in the collection device and to keep toilet tissue out of the collection device to prevent contamination of the specimen. Place a sign in the bathroom as a reminder to save all urine.

➤ Instruct the patient to void all urine into the collection device and then pour the urine into the laboratory collection container. Alternatively, the specimen can be left in the collection device for a health care staff member to add to the laboratory collection container.

➤ Instruct the patient to cooperate fully and to follow directions. Direct the patient to breathe normally and to avoid unnecessary movement during the venipuncture.

➤ Observe standard precautions, and follow the general guidelines in Appendix A. Positively identify the patient, and label the appropriate tubes or collection containers with the corresponding patient demographics, date, and time of collection.

Blood:

➤ If the patient has a history of severe allergic reaction to latex, care should be taken to avoid the use of equipment containing latex.

➤ Perform a venipuncture; collect the specimen in a 5-mL red-top tube.

➤ Remove the needle, and apply a pressure dressing over the puncture site.

Urine:

➤ Obtain a clean 3-L urine specimen container, toilet-mounted collection device, and plastic bag (for transport of the specimen container). The specimen must be refrigerated or kept on ice throughout the entire collection period. If an indwelling urinary catheter is in place, the drainage bag must be kept on ice.

➤ If possible, begin the test between 6 and 8 a.m. Collect first voiding and discard. Record the time the specimen was discarded as the beginning of the timed collection period. At the same time the next morning, ask the patient to void and add this last voiding to the container.

➤ If an indwelling catheter is in place, replace the tubing and container system at the start of the collection time. Keep the container system on ice during the collection period, or empty the urine into a larger container periodically during the collection period; monitor to ensure continued drainage, and conclude the test the next morning at the same hour the collection started.

➤ At the conclusion of the test, compare the quantity of urine with the urinary output record for the collection. If the specimen contains less than what was recorded as output, some urine may have been discarded, thus invalidating the test.

Blood or urine:

➤ Promptly transport the specimen to the laboratory for processing and analysis. Include on the urine specimen label the amount of urine and ingestion of any medications that can affect test results.

➤ The results are recorded manually or in a computerized system for recall and postprocedure interpretation by the appropriate health care practitioner.

Post-test: ▪

➤ Observe venipuncture site for bleeding or hematoma formation. Apply paper tape or other adhesive to hold pressure bandage in place, or replace with a plastic bandage.

➤ Educate the patient regarding the risk of infection related to immunosuppressed inflammatory response and fatigue related to decreased energy production.

➤ *Nutritional considerations:* Stress the importance of good nutrition, and suggest that the patient meet with a nutritional specialist. Also, stress the importance of following the care plan for medications and follow-up visits.

➤ A written report of the examination will be sent to the requesting health care practitioner, who will discuss the results with the patient.

➤ *Social and cultural considerations:* Recognize anxiety related to test results, and be supportive of impaired activity related to weakness, perceived loss of independence, and fear of shortened life expectancy. Discuss the implications of abnormal test results on the patient's lifestyle. Provide teaching and information regarding the clinical implications of the test results, as appropriate. Educate the patient regarding access to counseling services. Provide contact information, if desired, for AIDS information provided by the National Institutes of Health *(http://www. aidsinfo.nih.gov)*.

➤ *Social and cultural considerations:* Counsel the patient, as appropriate, regarding risk of transmission and proper prophylaxis, and reinforce the importance of strict adherence to the treatment regimen.

➤ *Social and cultural considerations:* Offer support, as appropriate, to patients who may be the victims of rape or sexual assault. Educate the patient regarding access to counseling services. Provide a nonjudgmental, nonthreatening atmosphere for a discussion during which risks of sexually transmitted diseases are explained. It is also important to discuss problems the patient may experience (e.g., guilt, depression, anger).

➤ Reinforce information given by the patient's health care provider regarding further testing, treatment, or referral to another health care provider. Inform the patient that retesting may be necessary. Answer any questions or address any concerns voiced by the patient or family.

➤ Depending on the results of this procedure, additional testing may be performed to evaluate or monitor progression of the disease process and determine the need for a change in therapy. Evaluate test results in relation to the patient's symptoms and other tests performed.

➤ Related laboratory tests include biopsy of the suspect tissue; CD4/CD8 enumeration; complete blood count; creatinine; erythrocyte sedimentation rate; gentamicin; hepatitis serology; HIV-1/HIV-2 serology; immunofixation electrophoresis; immunoglobulins A, G, and M; protein fraction electrophoresis; total protein; tobramycin; and urinalysis.

MUMPS SEROLOGY

· ·

SYNONYMS/ACRONYM: N/A.

SPECIMEN: Serum (1 mL) collected in a red-top tube.

REFERENCE VALUE: (Method: Indirect immunofluorescence) Negative or less than a fourfold increase in titer.

DESCRIPTION & RATIONALE: Mumps serology is done to determine the presence of mumps antibody, indicating exposure to or active presence of mumps. Mumps, also known as *parotitis,* is an infectious viral disease of the parotid glands caused by a myxovirus that is transmitted by direct contact with or droplets spread from the saliva of an infected person. The incubation period averages 3 weeks. Virus can be shed in saliva for 2 weeks after infection and in urine for 2 weeks after the onset of symptoms. Complications of infection include aseptic meningitis, encephalitis, and inflammation of the testes, ovaries, and pancreas. The presence of immunoglobulin M (IgM) antibodies indicates acute infection. The presence of IgG antibodies indicates current or past infection. ∎

INDICATIONS:
• Determine resistance to or protection against the mumps virus by a positive reaction, or susceptibility to mumps by a negative reaction

• Document immunity

• Evaluate mumps-like diseases and differentiate between these and actual mumps

RESULT

Positive findings in: Past or current mumps infection.

CRITICAL VALUES: N/A

INTERFERING FACTORS: N/A

Nursing Implications and Procedure • • • • • • • • • •

➤ Inform the patient that the test is used to confirm acute infection with or immunity to the mumps virus.

➤ Obtain a history of the patient's complaints, including a list of known allergens (especially allergies or sensitivities to latex), and inform the appropriate health care practitioner accordingly. Obtain a history of exposure.

➤ Obtain a history of the patient's immune system as well as results of previously performed laboratory tests, surgical procedures, and other diagnostic procedures. For related laboratory tests, refer to the Immune System table.

➤ Obtain a list of medications the patient is taking, including herbs, nutritional supplements, and nutraceuticals. The requesting health care practitioner and laboratory should be advised if the patient regularly uses these products so that their effects can be taken into consideration when reviewing results.

➤ Review the procedure with the patient. Inform the patient that several tests may be necessary to confirm diagnosis. Any individual positive result should be repeated in 7 to 14 days to monitor a change in titer. Inform the patient that specimen collection takes approximately 5 to 10 minutes. Address concerns about pain related to the procedure. Explain to the patient that there may be some discomfort during the venipuncture.

➤ There are no food, fluid, or medication restrictions, unless by medical direction.

➤ If the patient has a history of severe allergic reaction to latex, care should be taken to avoid the use of equipment containing latex.

➤ Instruct the patient to cooperate fully and to follow directions. Direct the patient to breathe normally and to avoid unnecessary movement.

➤ Observe standard precautions, and follow the general guidelines in Appendix A. Positively identify the patient, and label the appropriate tubes with the corresponding patient demographics, date, and time of collection. Perform a venipuncture; collect the specimen in a 5-mL red-top tube.

➤ Remove the needle, and apply a pressure dressing over the puncture site.

➤ Promptly transport the specimen to the laboratory for processing and analysis.

➤ The results are recorded manually or in a computerized system for recall and postprocedure interpretation by the appropriate health care practitioner.

➤ Observe venipuncture site for bleeding or hematoma formation. Apply paper tape or other adhesive to hold pressure bandage in place, or replace with a plastic bandage.

➤ Instruct the patient in isolation precautions during the time of communicability or contagion.

➤ Emphasize that the patient must return to have a convalescent blood sample taken in 7 to 14 days.

➤ Inform the patient that the presence of mumps antibodies ensures lifelong immunity.

➤ A written report of the examination will be sent to the requesting health care practitioner, who will discuss the results with the patient.

▶ Reinforce information given by the patient's health care provider regarding further testing, treatment, or referral to another health care provider. Answer any questions or address any concerns voiced by the patient or family.

▶ Depending on the results of this procedure, additional testing may be performed to evaluate or monitor progression of the disease process and determine the need for a change in therapy. Evaluate test results in relation to the patient's symptoms and other tests performed.

MYOCARDIAL INFARCT SCAN

SYNONYMS/ACRONYM: PYP cardiac scan, infarct scan, pyrophosphate cardiac scan, acute myocardial infarction scan.

AREA OF APPLICATION: Heart, chest/thorax.

CONTRAST: Intravenous contrast medium.

DESCRIPTION & RATIONALE: Technetium-99m stannous pyrophosphate (PYP) scanning, also known as *myocardial infarct imaging*, reveals the presence of myocardial perfusion and the extent of myocardial infarction (MI). This procedure can distinguish new from old infarcts when a patient has had abnormal electrocardiograms (ECGs) and cardiac enzymes have returned to normal. PYP uptake by acutely infarcted tissue may be related to the influx of calcium through damaged cell membranes, which accompanies myocardial necrosis; that is, the radionuclide may be binding to calcium phosphates or to hydroxyapatite. The PYP in these damaged cells can be viewed as spots of increased radionuclide uptake that appear in 12 hours at the earliest.

PYP uptake usually takes place 24 to 72 hours after MI, and the radionuclide remains detectable for approximately 10 to 14 days after the MI. PYP uptake is proportional to the blood flow to the affected area; with large areas of necrosis, PYP uptake may be maximal around the periphery of a necrotic area, with little uptake being detectable in the poorly perfused center. Most of the PYP is concentrated in regions that have 20% to 40% of the normal blood flow.

Single-photon emission computed tomography (SPECT) can be used to visualize the heart from multiple angles and planes, enabling areas of

MI to be viewed with greater accuracy and resolution. This technique removes overlying structures that may confuse interpretation of the results. With the availability of assays of troponins, myocardial infarct imaging has become less important in the diagnosis of acute MI. ∎

INDICATIONS:

- Aid in the diagnosis of (or confirm and locate) acute MI when ECG and enzyme testing do not provide a diagnosis
- Aid in the diagnosis of perioperative MI
- Differentiate between a new and old infarction
- Evaluate possible reinfarction or extension of the infarct
- Obtain baseline information about infarction before cardiac surgery

RESULT

Normal Findings:

- Normal coronary blood flow and tissue perfusion, with no PYP localization in the myocardium
- No uptake above background activity in the myocardium (*note:* when PYP uptake is present, it is graded in relation to adjacent rib activity)

Abnormal Findings:

- MI, indicated by increased PYP uptake in the myocardium

CRITICAL VALUES: N/A

INTERFERING FACTORS:

This procedure is contraindicated for:

- Patients who are pregnant or suspected of being pregnant, unless the potential benefits of the procedure far outweigh the risk of radiation exposure to the fetus
- Patients with hypersensitivity to the radionuclide

Factors that may impair clear imaging:

- Inability of the patient to cooperate or remain still during the procedure because of age, significant pain, or mental status
- Metallic objects within the examination field (e.g., jewelry, earrings, and/or dental amalgams), which may inhibit organ visualization and can produce unclear images
- Improper adjustment of the radiographic equipment to accommodate obese or thin patients, which can cause overexposure or underexposure and poor-quality study
- Patients who are very obese, who may exceed the weight limit for the equipment
- Incorrect positioning of the patient, which may produce poor visualization of the area to be examined
- Other nuclear scans done within the previous 24 to 48 hours
- Conditions such as chest wall trauma, cardiac trauma, or recent cardioversion procedure
- Myocarditis
- Pericarditis
- Left ventricular aneurysm
- Metastasis
- Valvular and coronary artery calcifications
- Cardiac neoplasms
- Aneurysms

Other considerations:

- Improper injection of the radionuclide may allow the tracer to seep deep into the muscle tissue, producing erroneous hot spots.

• Consultation with a health care practitioner should occur before the procedure for radiation safety concerns regarding younger patients or patients who are lactating.

• Risks associated with radiologic overexposure can result from frequent x-ray procedures. Personnel in the room with the patient should wear a protective lead apron, stand behind a shield, or leave the area while the examination is being done. Badges that reveal the level of exposure to radiation should be worn by persons working in the area where the examination is being done.

Nursing Implications and Procedure • • • • • • • • • • •

Pretest:

➤ Inform the patient that the procedure assesses blood flow to the heart.

➤ Obtain a history of the patient's complaints and symptoms, including a list of known allergens.

➤ Obtain a history of the patient's cardiovascular system, as well as results of previously performed laboratory tests, surgical procedures, and diagnostic procedures. For related diagnostic tests, refer to the Cardiovascular System table.

➤ Record the date of the last menstrual period and determine the possibility of pregnancy in perimenopausal women.

➤ Obtain a list of the patient's current medications.

➤ Review the procedure with the patient. Address concerns about pain related to the procedure. Explain to the patient that some pain may be experienced during the test, and there may be moments of discomfort. Explain the purpose of the test and how the procedure is performed. Inform the patient that the procedure

is performed in a nuclear medicine department, usually by a technologist and support staff, and takes approximately 30 to 60 minutes. Inform the patient that the technologist will administer an intravenous injection of the radionuclide and that he or she will need to return 2 to 3 hours later for the scan.

➤ *Sensitivity to cultural and social issues,* as well as concern for modesty, is important in providing psychological support before, during, and after the procedure.

➤ Instruct the patient to fast for 4 hours, refrain from smoking for 4 to 6 hours, and withhold medications for 24 hours before the procedure.

➤ Instruct the patient to remove dentures, jewelry (including watches), hairpins, credit cards, and other metallic objects.

Intratest:

➤ Ensure that the patient has complied with dietary and medication restrictions and other pretesting preparations. Ensure that the patient has removed all external metallic objects (jewelry, dentures, etc.) prior to the procedure.

➤ Have emergency equipment readily available.

➤ Patients are given a gown, robe, and foot coverings to wear and instructed to void prior to the procedure.

➤ Instruct the patient to cooperate fully and to follow directions. Instruct the patient to lie very still during the procedure because movement will produce unclear images.

➤ Observe standard precautions, and follow the general guidelines in Appendix A.

➤ Place the patient in a supine position on a flat table with foam wedges to help maintain position and immobilization.

➤ Wear gloves during the radionuclide injection and while handling the patient's urine.

➤ Imaging of the patient's heart begin

2 to 4 hours after injection of the radionuclide.

➤ Images of the heart are taken from a minimum of three angles: anterior, left anterior oblique, and left lateral. In most circumstances, however, SPECT is done so that the heart can be viewed from multiple angles and planes.

➤ The results are recorded on film or in a computerized system for recall and postprocedure interpretation by the appropriate health care practitioner.

Post-test:

➤ Instruct the patient to resume normal activity and diet, unless otherwise indicated.

➤ If the patient must return for additional imaging, advise the patient to rest in the interim and restrict diet to liquids before redistribution studies.

➤ Advise patient to drink increased amounts of fluids for 24 to 48 hours to eliminate the radionuclide from the body, unless contraindicated. Tell the patient that radionuclide is eliminated from the body within 6 to 24 hours.

➤ Observe the injection site for redness, swelling, or hematoma.

➤ Observe patient for up to 60 minutes after the study for a possible anaphylactic reaction to the radionuclide, such as rash, tightening of throat, or difficulty breathing.

➤ Instruct the patient to flush the toilet immediately after each voiding following the procedure, and to wash hands meticulously with soap and water after each voiding for 24 hours after the procedure.

➤ Tell all caregivers to wear gloves when discarding urine for 24 hours

after the procedure. Wash gloved hands with soap and water before removing gloves. Then wash hands after the gloves are removed.

➤ If a woman who is breast-feeding must have a nuclear scan, she should not breast-feed the infant until the radionuclide has been eliminated. This could take as long as 3 days. She should be instructed to express the milk and discard it during the 3-day period to prevent cessation of milk production.

➤ No other radionuclide tests should be scheduled for 24 to 48 hours after this procedure.

➤ A written report of the examination will be completed by a health care practitioner specializing in this branch of medicine. The report will be sent to the requesting health care practitioner, who will discuss the results with the patient.

➤ Reinforce information given by the patient's health care provider regarding further testing, treatment, or referral to another health care provider. Answer any questions or address any concerns voiced by the patient or family.

➤ Depending on the results of this procedure, additional testing may be needed to evaluate or monitor progression of the disease process and determine the need for a change in therapy. Evaluate test results in relation to the patient's symptoms and other tests performed.

Related diagnostic tests:

➤ Related diagnostic tests include computed tomography of the thorax, echocardiography, electrocardiogram, magnetic resonance imaging of the chest, and myocardial perfusion scan.

MYOCARDIAL PERFUSION HEART SCAN

SYNONYMS/ACRONYM: Thallium scan, sestamibi scan, stress thallium.

AREA OF APPLICATION: Heart, chest/thorax.

CONTRAST: Intravenous contrast medium.

DESCRIPTION & RATIONALE: Cardiac scanning is a nuclear medicine study that reveals clinical information about coronary blood flow, ventricular size, and cardiac function. Thallium-201 chloride rest or stress studies are used to evaluate myocardial blood flow to assist in diagnosing or determining the risk for ischemic cardiac disease, coronary artery disease (CAD), and myocardial infarction (MI). This procedure is an alternative to angiography or cardiac catheterization in cases in which these procedures may pose a risk to the patient. Thallium-201 is a potassium analogue and is taken up by myocardial cells proportional to blood flow to the cell and cell viability. During stress studies, the radionuclide is injected at peak exercise, after which the patient continues to exercise for several minutes. During exercise, areas of heart muscle supplied by normal arteries increase their blood supply, as well as the supply of thallium-201 delivery to the heart muscle, to a greater extent than regions of the heart muscle supplied by stenosed coronary arteries. This discrepancy in blood flow becomes apparent and quantifi-

able in subsequent imaging. Comparison of early stress images with images taken after 3 to 4 hours' redistribution (delayed images) enables differentiation between normally perfused, healthy myocardium (which is normal at rest but ischemic on stress) and infarcted myocardium.

Technetium-99m agents such as sestamibi (2-methoxyisobutylisonitrile) are delivered similarly to thallium-201 during myocardial perfusion imaging, but they are extracted to a lesser degree on the first pass through the heart and are taken up by the mitochondria. Over a short period, the radionuclide concentrates in the heart to the same degree as thallium-201. The advantage to technetium-99m agents is that immediate imaging is unnecessary because the radionuclide remains fixed to the heart muscle for several hours. The examination requires two separate injections, one for the rest portion and one for the stress portion of the procedure. These injections can take place on the same day or preferably over a 2-day period. Examination quality is improved if the patient is given a light, fatty meal after the radionuclide is injected to facilitate hepatobiliary clearance of the radioactivity.

If stress testing cannot be performed by exercising, dipyridamole (Persantine) or adenosine, a vasodilator, can be administered orally or intravenously. A coronary vasodilator is administered before the thallium-201, or other radionuclide, and the scanning procedure is then performed. Vasodilators increase blood flow in normal coronary arteries twofold to threefold without exercise, and they reveal perfusion defects when blood flow is compromised by vessel pathology. Vasodilator-mediated myocardial perfusion scanning is reserved for patients who are unable to participate in treadmill, bicycle, or handgrip exercises for stress testing because of lung disease, neurologic disorders (e.g., multiple sclerosis, spinal cord injury), morbid obesity, and orthopedic disorders (e.g., arthritis, limb amputation).

Single-photon emission computed tomography can be used to visualize the heart from multiple angles and planes, enabling areas of MI to be viewed with greater accuracy and resolution. This technique removes overlying structures that may confuse interpretation of the results. ■

INDICATIONS:
- Aid in the diagnosis of CAD or risk for CAD
- Determine rest defects and reperfusion with delayed imaging in unstable angina
- Evaluate the extent of CAD and determine cardiac function
- Assess the function of collateral coronary arteries
- Evaluate bypass graft patency and general cardiac status after surgery

- Evaluate the site of an old MI to determine obstruction to cardiac muscle perfusion
- Evaluate the effectiveness of medication regimen and balloon angioplasty procedure on narrow coronary arteries

RESULT

Normal Findings:
- Normal wall motion, coronary blood flow, tissue perfusion, and ventricular size and function

Abnormal Findings:
- Abnormal stress and resting images, indicating previous MI
- Abnormal stress images with normal resting images, indicating transient ischemia
- Cardiac hypertrophy, indicated by increased radionuclide uptake in the myocardium
- Enlarged left ventricle
- Heart chamber disorder
- Ventricular septal defects

CRITICAL VALUES: N/A

INTERFERING FACTORS:

This procedure is contraindicated for:
- ⚠ Patients who have taken sildenafil (Viagra) within the previous 48 hours, as this test may require the use of nitrates (nitroglycerin) that can precipitate life-threatening low blood pressure
- Patients with bleeding disorders
- Patients who are pregnant or suspected of being pregnant, unless the potential benefits of the procedure far outweigh the risk of radiation exposure to the fetus
- Patients with hypersensitivity to the radionuclide

- Patients with left ventricular hypertrophy, right and left bundle branch block, or hypokalemia, and patients receiving cardiotonic therapy

- Patients with anginal pain at rest or patients with severe atherosclerotic coronary vessels, in whom dipyridamole testing cannot be performed

- Patients with asthma, because chemical stress with vasodilators can cause bronchospasms

***Factors that may
impair clear imaging:***

- Inability of the patient to cooperate or remain still during the procedure because of age, significant pain, or mental status

- Medications such as digitalis and quinidine, which can alter cardiac contractility; and nitrates, which can affect cardiac performance

- Single-vessel disease, which can produce false-negative thallium-201 scanning results

- Conditions such as chest wall or cardiac trauma, angina that is difficult to control, significant cardiac arrhythmias, and recent cardioversion procedure

- Suboptimal cardiac stress or patient exhaustion preventing maximum heart rate testing

- Excessive eating or exercising between initial and redistribution imaging 4 hours later, which produces false-positive results

- Improper adjustment of the radiologic equipment to accommodate obese or thin patients, which can cause overexposure or underexposure and a poor-quality study

- Patients who are very obese, who may exceed the weight limit for the equipment

- Incorrect positioning of the patient, which may produce poor visualization of the area to be examined

- Metallic objects within the examination field (e.g., jewelry, body rings), which may inhibit organ visualization and can produce unclear images

Other considerations:

- Failure to follow dietary restrictions before the procedure may cause the procedure to be canceled or repeated.

- Improper injection of the radionuclide that allows the tracer to seep deep into the muscle tissue produces erroneous hot spots.

- Inaccurate timing for imaging after radionuclide injection can affect the results.

- Consultation with a health care practitioner should occur before the procedure for radiation safety concerns regarding younger patients or patients who are lactating.

- Risks associated with radiographic overexposure can result from frequent x-ray procedures. Personnel in the room with the patient should wear a protective lead apron, stand behind a shield, or leave the area while the examination is being done. Personnel working in the area where the examination is being done should wear badges that reveal their level of exposure to radiation.

Nursing Implications and Procedure

Pretest:

➤ Inform the patient that the procedure assesses blood flow to the heart.

➤ Obtain a history of the patient's complaints and symptoms, including a list of known allergens.

➤ Obtain a history of the patient's cardiovascular system, as well as results of previously performed laboratory tests, surgical procedures, and diagnostic procedures. For related laboratory tests, refer to the Cardiovascular System table.

➤ Record the date of the last menstrual period and determine the possibility of pregnancy in perimenopausal women.

➤ Obtain a list of the medications the patient is taking, including anticoagulant therapy, aspirin and other salicylates, herbs, nutritional supplements, and nutraceuticals, especially those known to affect coagulation (see Appendix F). It is recommended that use be discontinued 14 days before surgical procedures. The requesting health care practitioner and laboratory should be advised if the patient regularly uses these products so that their effects can be taken into consideration when reviewing results.

➤ Review the procedure with the patient. Address concerns about pain related to the procedure. Explain to the patient that some pain may be experienced during the test, or there may be moments of discomfort. Inform the patient that the procedure is performed in a special department, usually in a radiology or vascular suite, by a health care practitioner and support staff, and takes approximately 30 to 60 minutes.

➤ *Sensitivity to social and cultural issues,* as well as concern for modesty, is important in providing psychological support before, during, and after the procedure.

➤ Explain that an intravenous (IV) line may be inserted to allow infusion of IV fluids, contrast medium, dye, or sedatives. Usually normal saline is infused.

➤ Instruct the patient to fast for 4 hours, refrain from smoking for 4 to 6 hours, and withhold medications for 24 hours before the test. Instruct the patient to avoid taking anticoagulant medication or to reduce dosage as ordered prior to the procedure.

➤ Instruct the patient to wear walking shoes (if treadmill exercise testing is to be performed), and emphasize the importance of the patient reporting fatigue, pain, or shortness of breath.

➤ Instruct the patient to remove dentures, jewelry (including watches), hairpins, credit cards, and other metallic objects in the area to be examined.

➤ *Make sure a written and informed consent has been signed prior to the procedure and before administering any medications.*

➤ This procedure may be terminated if chest pain, severe cardiac arrhythmias, or signs of a cerebrovascular accident occur.

Intratest:

➤ Ensure that the patient has complied with dietary and medication restrictions and other pretesting preparations. Ensure that the patient has removed all external metallic objects (jewelry, dentures, etc.) prior to the procedure.

➤ Have emergency equipment readily available.

➤ If the patient has a history of severe allergic reactions to any substance or drug, administer ordered prophylactic steroids or antihistamines before the procedure. Use nonionic contrast medium for the procedure.

➤ Patients are given a gown, robe, and foot coverings to wear and instructed to void prior to the procedure.

➤ Record baseline vital signs and assess neurologic status. Protocols may vary from facility to facility.

➤ Instruct the patient to cooperate fully and to follow directions.

➤ Observe standard precautions, and follow the general guidelines in Appendix A.

➤ Establish IV fluid line for the injection of emergency drugs and of sedatives.

➤ Place electrocardiographic (ECG) electrodes on the patient for cardiac monitoring. Establish baseline rhythm; determine if the patient has ventricular arrhythmias. Monitor the patient's blood pressure throughout the procedure by using an automated blood pressure machine.

➤ Assist the patient onto the treadmill or bicycle ergometer and ask the patient to exercise to a calculated 80% to 85% of the maximum heart rate, as determined by the protocol selected.

➤ Wear gloves during the radionuclide injection and while handling the patient's urine.

➤ Thallium-201 is injected 60 to 90 seconds before exercise is terminated, and imaging is done immediately in the supine position and repeated in 4 hours.

➤ Patients who cannot exercise are given dipyridamole 4 minutes before thallium-201 is injected.

➤ Inform the patient that movement during the resting procedure affects the results and makes interpretation difficult.

➤ The results are recorded on film or in a computerized system for recall and postprocedure interpretation by the appropriate health care practitioner.

Post-test:

➤ Instruct the patient to resume usual diet, fluids, medications, or activity, as directed by the health care practitioner. If the patient must return for further thallium-201 imaging, advise the patient to rest in the interim and to restrict diet to liquids before redistribution studies.

➤ Monitor vital signs and ECG tracings every 15 minutes for 60 minutes after the procedure. Compare with baseline values. Protocols may vary from facility to facility.

➤ Observe for delayed allergic reactions, such as rash, urticaria, tachycardia, hyperpnea, hypertension, palpitations, nausea, or vomiting.

➤ Instruct the patient to immediately report symptoms such as fast heart rate, difficulty breathing, skin rash, itching or decreased urinary output.

➤ Observe the needle/catheter insertion site for bleeding, inflammation, or hematoma formation.

➤ Instruct the patient to drink increased amounts of fluids for 24 to 48 hours to eliminate the radionuclide from the body, unless contraindicated. Educate the patient that radionuclide is eliminated from the body within 6 to 24 hours.

➤ Instruct the patient to flush the toilet immediately after each voiding following the procedure, and to wash hands meticulously with soap and water after each voiding for 24 hours after the procedure.

➤ Instruct all caregivers to wear gloves when discarding urine for 24 hours after the procedure. Wash gloved hands with soap and water before removing gloves. Then wash hands after the gloves are removed.

➤ If a woman who is breast-feeding must have a nuclear scan, she should not breast-feed the infant until the radionuclide has been eliminated. This could take as long as 3 days. She should be instructed to express the milk and discard it during the 3-day period to prevent cessation of milk production.

➤ *Nutritional considerations:* A low-fat, low-cholesterol, and low-sodium diet should be consumed to reduce current disease processes and/or decrease risk of hypertension and coronary artery disease.

➤ No other radionuclide tests should be scheduled for 24 to 48 hours after this procedure.

➤ A written report of the examination will be completed by a health care practitioner specializing in this branch of medicine. The report will be sent to the requesting health care practitioner, who will discuss the results with the patient.

➤ Recognize anxiety related to test results, and be supportive of perceived loss of independent function. Discuss the implications of abnormal test results on the patient's lifestyle. Provide teaching and information

regarding the clinical implications of the test results, as appropriate.

➤ Reinforce information given by the patient's health care provider regarding further testing, treatment, or referral to another health care provider. Answer any questions or address any concerns voiced by the patient or family.

➤ Instruct the patient in the use of any ordered medications. Explain the importance of adhering to the therapy regimen. As appropriate, instruct the patient in significant side effects and systemic reactions associated with the prescribed medication. Encourage him or her to review cor- responding literature provided by a pharmacist.

➤ Depending on the results of this procedure, additional testing may be needed to evaluate or monitor progression of the disease process and determine the need for a change in therapy. Evaluate test results in relation to the patient's symptoms and other tests performed.

Related diagnostic tests:

➤ Related diagnostic tests include computed tomography of the thorax, echocardiogram, electrocardiography, Holter monitoring, and magnetic resonance imaging of the chest.

MYOGLOBIN

SYNONYM/ACRONYM: MB.

SPECIMEN: Serum (1 mL) collected in a red- or tiger-top tube.

REFERENCE VALUE: (Method: Nephelometry)

Conventional & SI Units
5–70 µg/dL

DESCRIPTION & RATIONALE: Myoglobin is an oxygen-binding muscle protein normally found in skeletal and cardiac muscle. It is released into the bloodstream after muscle damage from ischemia, trauma, or inflammation. Although myoglobin testing is more sensitive than creatinine kinase and isoenzymes, it does not indicate the specific site involved. ■

INDICATIONS:
• Assist in predicting a flare-up of polymyositis
• Estimate damage from skeletal muscle injury or myocardial infarction

RESULT

Increased in:
• Cardiac surgery
• Cocaine use

- Exercise
- Malignant hyperthermia
- Myocardial infarction
- Progressive muscular dystrophy
- Renal failure
- Rhabdomyolysis
- Shock
- Thrombolytic therapy

Decreased in:
- Myasthenia gravis
- Presence of antibodies to myoglobin, as seen in patients with polymyositis
- Rheumatoid arthritis

CRITICAL VALUES: N/A

INTERFERING FACTORS: N/A

Nursing Implications and Procedure ⋯⋯⋯⋯⋯

Pretest:

➤ Inform the patient that the test is used to assist in the diagnosis of skeletal or myocardial muscle damage.

➤ Obtain a history of the patient's complaints, including a list of known allergens (especially allergies or sensitivities to latex), and inform the appropriate health care practitioner accordingly.

➤ Obtain a history of the patient's cardiovascular and musculoskeletal system as well as results of previously performed laboratory tests, surgical procedures, and other diagnostic procedures. For related laboratory tests, refer to the Cardiovascular and Musculoskeletal System tables.

➤ Obtain a list of medications the patient is taking, including herbs, nutritional supplements, and nutra-

ceuticals. The requesting health care practitioner and laboratory should be advised if the patient regularly uses these products so that their effects can be taken into consideration when reviewing results.

➤ Review the procedure with the patient. Inform the patient that specimen collection takes approximately 5 to 10 minutes. Address concerns about pain related to the procedure. Explain to the patient that there may be some discomfort during the venipuncture.

➤ There are no food, fluid, or medication restrictions, unless by medical direction.

Intratest:

➤ If the patient has a history of severe allergic reaction to latex, care should be taken to avoid the use of equipment containing latex.

➤ Instruct the patient to cooperate fully and to follow directions. Direct the patient to breathe normally and to avoid unnecessary movement.

➤ Observe standard precautions, and follow the general guidelines in Appendix A. Positively identify the patient, and label the appropriate tubes with the corresponding patient demographics, date, and time of collection. Perform a venipuncture; collect the specimen in a 5-mL red- or tiger-top tube.

➤ Remove the needle, and apply a pressure dressing over the puncture site.

➤ Promptly transport the specimen to the laboratory for processing and analysis.

➤ The results are recorded manually or in a computerized system for recall and postprocedure interpretation by the appropriate health care practitioner.

Post-test:

➤ Observe venipuncture site for bleeding or hematoma formation. Apply paper tape or other adhesive to hold pressure bandage in place, or replace with a plastic bandage.

➤ A written report of the examination will be sent to the requesting health care practitioner, who will discuss the results with the patient.

➤ Reinforce information given by the patient's health care provider regarding further testing, treatment, or referral to another health care provider. Answer any questions or address any concerns voiced by the patient or family.

➤ Depending on the results of this procedure, additional testing may be performed to evaluate or monitor progression of the disease process and determine the need for a change in therapy. Evaluate test results in relation to the patient's symptoms and other tests performed.

Related laboratory tests:

➤ Related laboratory tests include antiarrhythmic drugs, apolipoprotein A, apolipoprotein B, aspartate aminotransferase, atrial natriuretic peptide, blood gases, B-type natriuretic peptide, calcium (blood and ionized), cholesterol (total, HDL, and LDL), C-reactive protein, creatine kinase and isoenzymes, glucose, glycated hemoglobin, homocysteine, ketones, lactate dehydrogenase and isoenzymes, lipoprotein electrophoresis, magnesium, pericardial fluid, potassium, triglycerides, and troponin.

NERVE FIBER ANALYSIS

· ·

SYNONYMS/ACRONYMS: NFA.

AREA OF APPLICATION: Eyes.

CONTRAST: N/A.

DESCRIPTION & RATIONALE: There are over 1 million ganglion nerve cells in the retina of each eye. Each nerve cell has a long fiber that travels through the nerve fiber layer of the retina and exits the eye through the optic nerve. The optic nerve is made up of all the ganglion nerve fibers and connects the eye to the brain for vision to occur. As the ganglion cells die, the nerve fiber layer becomes thinner and an empty space in the optic nerve, called the cup, becomes larger. The thinning of the nerve fiber layer and the enlargement of the nerve fiber cup are measurements used to gauge the extent of damage to the retina. Significant damage to the nerve fiber layer occurs before loss of vision is noticed by the patient. Damage can be caused by glaucoma or by aging or occlusion of the vessels in the retina. Ganglion cell loss due to glaucoma begins in the periphery of the retina, thereby first affecting peripheral vision. This change in vision can also be detected by visual field testing. There are several different techniques for measuring nerve fiber layer thickness. One of the most common employs the use of a laser that emits polarizing light waves. The laser's computer measures the change in direction of alignment of the light beam after it passes through the nerve fiber layer tissue. The amount of change in polarization correlates to the thickness of the retinal nerve fiber layer. ■

INDICATIONS:

• Assist in the diagnosis of eye diseases

• Determine retinal nerve fiber layer thickness

• Monitor the effects of various therapies or the progression of conditions resulting in loss of vision

RESULT

Normal Findings:
• Normal nerve fiber layer thickness

Abnormal Findings:
• Glaucoma or suspicion of glaucoma

• Ocular hypertension

CRITICAL VALUES: N/A

INTERFERING FACTORS:

Factors that may impair the results of the examination:
• Inability of the patient to fixate on focal point

• Corneal disorder that prevents proper alignment of the retinal nerve fibers

• Dense cataract that prevents visualization of a clear nerve fiber image

• Inability of the patient to cooperate or remain still during the test because of age, significant pain, or mental status

Nursing Implications and Procedure • • • • • • • • • • •

Pretest:

➤ Inform the patient that the procedure measures the thickness of the retinal nerve fiber layer.

➤ Obtain a history of the patient's complaints, including a list of known allergens.

➤ Obtain a history of narrow-angle glaucoma. Obtain a history of known or suspected visual impairment, changes in visual acuity, and use of glasses or contact lenses.

➤ Obtain a history of the patient's known or suspected vision loss, including type and cause; eye conditions with treatment regimens; eye surgery; and other tests and procedures to assess and diagnose visual deficit. For related diagnostic tests, refer to the table of tests associated with the Ocular System.

➤ Obtain a history of results of previously performed laboratory tests, surgical procedures, and other diagnostic procedures.

➤ Obtain a list of the medications the patient is taking, including herbs, nutritional supplements, and nutraceuticals. The requesting health care practitioner should be advised if the patient regularly uses these products so that their effects can be taken into consideration when reviewing results.

➤ Instruct the patient to remove contact lenses or glasses, as appropriate. Instruct the patient regarding the importance of keeping the eyes open for the test.

➤ Review the procedure with the patient. Explain that the patient will be requested to fixate the eyes during the procedure. Address concerns about pain related to the procedure. Explain to the patient that no pain will be experienced during the test, but there may be moments of discomfort. Explain to the patient that some discomfort may be experienced after the test when the numbness wears off from anesthetic drops administered prior to the test. Inform the patient that a technician, optometrist, or physician performs the test, and that to evaluate both eyes, the test can take 10 to 15 minutes.

➤ There are no food, fluid, or medication restrictions, unless by medical direction.

Intratest:

➤ Instruct the patient to cooperate fully and to follow directions. Ask the patient to remain still during the procedure because movement produces unreliable results.

➤ Seat the patient comfortably. Instruct the patient to look straight ahead, keeping the eyes open and unblinking.

➤ Instill topical anesthetic in each eye, as ordered, and allow time for it to work. Topical anesthetic drops are placed in the eye with the patient looking up and the solution directed at the six o'clock position of the sclera (white of the eye) near the limbus (grey, semitransparent area of the eyeball where the cornea and sclera meet). The dropper bottle should not touch the eyelashes.

➤ The equipment used to perform the test determines whether dilation of the pupils is required (OCT) or avoided (GDX).

➤ Request that the patient look straight ahead at a fixation light with the chin in the chin rest and forehead against the support bar. The patient should be reminded not to move the eyes or blink the eyelids as the measurement is taken. The person performing the test can store baseline data or retrieve previous images from the equipment. The equipment can create the mean image from current and previous data, and its computer can make a comparison against previous images.

➤ The results are recorded manually or in a computerized system for recall and postprocedure interpretation by the appropriate health care practitioner.

Post-test:

➤ A written report of the examination will be completed by a health care practitioner specializing in this branch of medicine. The report will be sent to the requesting health care practitioner, who will discuss the results with the patient.

➤ Recognize anxiety related to test results, and be supportive of impaired activity related to vision loss or perceived loss of driving privileges. Discuss the implications of abnormal test results on the patient's lifestyle. Provide teaching and information regarding the clinical implications of the test results, as appropriate.

➤ Reinforce information given by the patient's health care provider regarding further testing, treatment, or referral to another health care provider. Instruct the patient in the use of any ordered medications, usually eyedrops. Explain the importance of adhering to the therapy regimen, especially since glaucoma does not present symptoms. Instruct the patient in both the ocular side effects and systemic reactions associated with the prescribed medication. Encourage him or her to review corresponding literature provided by a pharmacist. Answer any questions or address any concerns voiced by the patient or family.

➤ Depending on the results of this procedure, additional testing may be performed to evaluate or monitor progression of the disease process and determine the need for a change in therapy. Evaluate test results in relation to the patient's symptoms and other tests performed.

Related diagnostic tests:

➤ Related diagnostic tests include fundus photography, gonioscopy, pachymetry, slit-lamp biomicroscopy, and visual field testing.

OSMOLALITY, BLOOD AND URINE

SYNONYM/ACRONYM: Osmo.

SPECIMEN: Serum (1 mL) collected in a red- or tiger-top tube; urine (5 mL) from an unpreserved random specimen collected in a clean plastic collection container.

REFERENCE VALUE: (Method: Freezing point depression)

	Conventional Units	SI Units (Conventional Units × 1)
Serum	275–295 mOsm/kg	275–295 mmol/kg
Urine		
Newborn	75–300 mOsm/kg	75–300 mmol/kg
Children and adults	250–900 mOsm/kg	250–900 mmol/kg

DESCRIPTION & RATIONALE: Osmolality refers to the number of particles in solution; it is independent of particle size, shape, and charge. Measurement of osmotic concentration in serum provides clinically useful information about water and dissolved-particle transport across fluid compartment membranes. Osmolality is used to assist in the diagnosis of metabolic, renal, and endocrine disorders. The simultaneous determination of serum and urine osmolality provides the opportunity to compare values between the two fluids. A normal urine-to-serum ratio is approximately 0.2 to 4.7 for random samples and greater than 3.0 for first-morning samples (dehydration normally occurs overnight). The major dissolved particles that contribute to osmolality are sodium, chloride, bicarbonate, urea, and glucose. Some of these substances are used in the following calculated estimate:

$$\text{Serum osmolality} = \{[2\,(Na^+)] + [\text{glucose}/18] + [BUN/2.8]\}$$

Measured osmolality is higher than the estimated value. The osmolal gap is the difference between the measured and calculated values and is normally 5 to 10 mOsm/kg. If the difference is greater than 15 mOsm/kg, consider ethylene glycol, isopropanol, methanol, or ethanol toxicity. These substances behave like antifreeze, lowering the freezing point in the blood, and provide misleadingly high results. ■

INDICATIONS

Serum:

- Assist in the evaluation of antidiuretic hormone (ADH) function

- Assist in rapid screening for toxic substances, such as ethylene glycol, ethanol, isopropanol, and methanol

- Evaluate electrolyte and acid-base balance

- Evaluate state of hydration

Urine:

- Evaluate concentrating ability of the kidneys

- Evaluate diabetes insipidus

- Evaluate neonatal patients with protein or glucose in the urine

- Perform workup for renal disease

RESULT

Increased in:

- Serum:
  Azotemia
  Dehydration
  Diabetes insipidus
  Diabetic ketoacidosis
  Hypercalcemia
  Hypernatremia

- Urine:
  Amyloidosis
  Azotemia
  Congestive heart failure
  Dehydration
  Hyponatremia
  Syndrome of inappropriate antidiuretic hormone production (SIADH)

Decreased in:

- Serum:
  Adrenocorticoid insufficiency
  Hyponatremia
  SIADH
  Water intoxication

- Urine:
  Diabetes insipidus
  Hypernatremia
  Hypokalemia
  Primary polydipsia

CRITICAL VALUES: Serum:

Less than 265 mOsm/kg
Greater than 320 mOsm/kg

Note and immediately report to the health care practitioner any critically increased or decreased values and related symptoms.

Serious clinical conditions may be associated with elevated or decreased serum osmolality. The following conditions are associated with elevated serum osmolality:

Respiratory arrest: 360 mOsm/kg

Stupor of hyperglycemia: 385 mOsm/kg

Grand mal seizures: 420 mOsm/kg

Death: greater than 420 mOsm/kg

Symptoms of critically high levels include poor skin turgor, listlessness, acidosis (decreased pH), shock, seizures, coma, and cardiopulmonary arrest. Intervention may include close monitoring of electrolytes, administering intravenous fluids with the appropriate composition to shift water either into or out of the intravascular space as needed, monitoring cardiac signs, continuing neurologic checks, and taking seizure precautions.

INTERFERING FACTORS:

- Drugs that may increase serum osmolality include citrates (as an anticoagulant), corticosteroids, ethylene glycol, glycerin, inulin, ioxithalamic acid, mannitol, and methoxyflurane.

- Drugs that may decrease serum osmolality include bendroflumethiazide, carbamazepine, chlorpromazine, chlorthalidone, cyclophosphamide, cyclothiazide, hydrochlorothiazide, lorcainide, methyclothiazide, and polythiazide.

- Drugs that may increase urine osmolality include anesthetic agents, chlorpropamide, cyclophosphamide, furosemide, mannitol, metolazone, octreotide, phloridzin, and vincristine.

- Drugs that may decrease urine osmolality include captopril, demeclocycline, glyburide, lithium, methoxyflurane, octreotide, tolazamide, and verapamil.

Nursing Implications and Procedure • • • • • • • • • • • •

Pretest:

➤ Inform the patient that the test is used to evaluate electrolyte and water balance.

➤ Obtain a history of the patient's complaints, including a list of known allergens (especially allergies or sensitivities to latex), and inform the appropriate health care practitioner accordingly.

➤ Obtain a history of the patient's endocrine and genitourinary systems, as well as results of previously performed laboratory tests, surgical procedures, and other diagnostic procedures. For related laboratory tests, refer to the Endocrine and Genitourinary System tables.

➤ Obtain a list of the medications the patient is taking, including herbs, nutritional supplements, and nutraceuticals. The requesting health care practitioner and laboratory should be advised if the patient regularly uses these products so that their effects can be taken into consideration when reviewing results.

➤ Review the procedure with the patient. Inform the patient that blood specimen collection takes approximately 5 to 10 minutes; random urine collection takes approximately 5 minutes and depends on the cooperation of the patient. Urine specimen collection may also be timed. Address concerns about pain related to the procedure. Explain to the patient that there may be some dis-

comfort during the venipuncture; there will be no discomfort during urine collection.

➤ *Sensitivity to social and cultural issues,* as well as concern for modesty, is important in providing psychological support before, during, and after the procedure.

➤ There are no food, fluid, or medication restrictions, unless by medical direction.

Intratest:

➤ Direct the patient to breathe normally and to avoid unnecessary movement during the venipuncture.

➤ Observe standard precautions, and follow the general guidelines in Appendix A. Positively identify the patient, and label the appropriate tubes or collection containers with the corresponding patient demographics, date, and time of collection.

Blood:

➤ If the patient has a history of severe allergic reaction to latex, care should be taken to avoid the use of equipment containing latex.

➤ Perform a venipuncture; collect the specimen in a 5-mL red- or tiger-top tube.

➤ Remove the needle, and apply a pressure dressing over the puncture site.

Urine:

➤ Provide a nonmetallic urinal, bedpan, or toilet-mounted collection device.

➤ Either a random specimen or a timed collection may be requested. For timed specimens, a 12- or 24-hour time frame for urine collection may be ordered. Inform the patient that all urine must be saved during that 12 or 24-hour period. Instruct the patient not to void directly into the laboratory collection container. Instruct the patient to avoid defecating in the collection device and to keep toilet tissue out of the collection device to prevent contamination of the specimen. Place a sign in the bathroom to remind the patient to save all urine.

➤ Instruct the patient to void all urine into the collection device and then to pour the urine into the laboratory collection container. Alternatively, the specimen can be left in the collection device for a health care staff member to add to the laboratory collection container.

Clean-catch specimen:

➤ Instruct the male patient to (1) thoroughly wash his hands, (2) cleanse the meatus, (3) void a small amount into the toilet, and (4) void directly into the specimen container.

➤ Instruct the female patient to (1) thoroughly wash her hands; (2) cleanse the labia from front to back; (3) while keeping the labia separated, void a small amount into the toilet; and (4) without interrupting the urine stream, void directly into the specimen container.

Indwelling catheter:

➤ Put on gloves. Empty drainage tube of urine. It may be necessary to clamp off the catheter for 15 to 30 minutes before specimen collection. Cleanse specimen port with antiseptic swab, and then aspirate 5 mL of urine with a 21- to 25-gauge needle and syringe. Transfer urine to a sterile container.

Blood or urine:

➤ Promptly transport the specimen to the laboratory for processing and analysis.

➤ The results are recorded manually or in a computerized system for recall and postprocedure interpretation by the appropriate health care practitioner.

➤ Observe venipuncture site for bleeding or hematoma formation. Apply paper tape or other adhesive to hold pressure bandage in place, or replace with a plastic bandage.

➤ *Nutritional considerations:* Decreased osmolality may be associated with overhydration. Observe the patient for signs and symptoms of fluid-volume excess related to excess electrolyte intake, fluid-volume deficit related to active loss, or risk of injury related to an alteration in body chemistry. (For electrolyte-specific dietary references, see monographs titled "Chloride," "Potassium," and "Sodium.")

➤ Increased osmolality may be associated with dehydration. Evaluate the patient for signs and symptoms of dehydration. Dehydration is a significant and common finding in geriatric and other patients in whom renal function has deteriorated.

➤ A written report of the examination will be sent to the requesting health care practitioner, who will discuss the results with the patient.

➤ Recognize anxiety related to test results. Discuss the implications of abnormal test results on the patient's lifestyle. Provide teaching and information regarding the clinical implications of the test results, as appropriate. Educate the patient regarding access to counseling services. Provide contact information, if desired, for the National Kidney Foundation (*http://www.kidney.org*).

➤ Reinforce information given by the patient's health care provider regarding further testing, treatment, or referral to another health care provider. Answer any questions or address any concerns voiced by the patient or family.

➤ Depending on the results of this procedure, additional testing may be performed to evaluate or monitor progression of the disease process and determine the need for a change in therapy. Evaluate test results in relation to the patient's symptoms and other tests performed.

Related laboratory tests:

➤ Related laboratory tests include antidiuretic hormone, ammonia, blood and urine urea nitrogen, blood and urine creatinine, blood and urine electrolytes, ethanol, glucose, and blood and urine ketones.

OSMOTIC FRAGILITY

SYNONYM/ACRONYM: Red blood cell osmotic fragility, OF.

SPECIMEN: Whole blood (1 mL) collected in a green-top (heparin) tube and two peripheral blood smears.

REFERENCE VALUE: (Method: Spectrophotometry) Hemolysis begins at 0.5 w/v sodium chloride (NaCl) solution and is complete at 0.3 w/v NaCl solution. Results are compared to a normal curve.

DESCRIPTION & RATIONALE: Osmotic fragility (OF) is an indication of the ability of red blood cells (RBCs) to take on water without lysing. In this test, RBCs are placed in graded dilutions of sodium chloride. Swelling of the cells occurs at lower concentrations of NaCl as they take on water in the hypotonic solution. Thicker cells, such as spherocytes, have an increased OF; thinner cells have a decreased OF. ■

INDICATIONS: Evaluate hemolytic anemia

RESULT

Increased in:
• Acquired immune hemolytic anemias
• Hemolytic disease of the newborn
• Hereditary spherocytosis
• Malaria
• Pyruvate kinase deficiency

Decreased in:
• Asplenia
• Hemoglobinopathies

• Iron-deficiency anemia
• Liver disease
• Reticulocytosis
• Thalassemias

CRITICAL VALUES: N/A

INTERFERING FACTORS:
• Drugs that may increase osmotic fragility include dapsone.

• Parasitic infestations, such as malaria, may independently cause cell hemolysis.

• Specimens should be submitted for analysis immediately after collection.

Nursing Implications and Procedure

Pretest:

➤ Inform the patient that the test is primarily used to assist in the diagnosis of hereditary spherocytosis.

➤ Obtain a history of the patient's complaints, including a list of known allergens (especially allergies or sensitivities to latex), and inform the appropriate health care practitioner accordingly.

➤ Obtain a history of the patient's hematopoietic system and results of previously performed laboratory tests, surgical procedures, and other diagnostic procedures. For related laboratory tests, refer to the Hematopoietic System table.

➤ Obtain a list of the medications the patient is taking, including herbs, nutritional supplements, and nutraceuticals. The requesting health care practitioner and laboratory should be advised if the patient regularly uses these products so that their effects can be taken into consideration when reviewing results.

➤ Review the procedure with the patient. Inform the patient that specimen collection takes approximately 5 to 10 minutes. Address concerns about pain related to the procedure. Explain to the patient that there may be some discomfort during the venipuncture.

➤ There are no food, fluid, or medication restrictions, unless by medical direction.

Intratest:

➤ If the patient has a history of severe allergic reaction to latex, care should be taken to avoid the use of equipment containing latex.

➤ Instruct the patient to cooperate fully and to follow directions. Direct the patient to breathe normally and to avoid unnecessary movement.

➤ Observe standard precautions, and follow the general guidelines in Appendix A. Positively identify the patient, and label the appropriate tubes with the corresponding patient demographics, date, and time of collection. Perform a venipuncture;

collect the specimen in a 5-mL green-top tube.

➤ Remove the needle, and apply a pressure dressing over the puncture site.

➤ Promptly transport the specimen to the laboratory for processing and analysis.

➤ The results are recorded manually or in a computerized system for recall and postprocedure interpretation by the appropriate health care practitioner.

Post-test:

➤ Observe venipuncture site for bleeding or hematoma formation. Apply paper tape or other adhesive to hold pressure bandage in place, or replace with a plastic bandage.

➤ A written report of the examination will be sent to the requesting health care practitioner, who will discuss the results with the patient.

➤ Reinforce information given by the patient's health care provider regarding further testing, treatment, or referral to another health care provider. Answer any questions or address any concerns voiced by the patient or family.

➤ Depending on the results of this procedure, additional testing may be performed to evaluate or monitor progression of the disease process and determine the need for a change in therapy. Evaluate test results in relation to the patient's symptoms and other tests performed.

Related laboratory tests:

➤ Related laboratory tests include complete blood count, glucose-6-phosphate dehydrogenase, Ham's test, hemoglobin electrophoresis, total iron, pyruvate kinase, and red blood cell morphology and inclusions.

OSTEOCALCIN

. . . .

SYNONYMS/ACRONYMS: Bone GLA protein, BGP.

SPECIMEN: Serum (1 mL) collected in a red-top tube.

REFERENCE VALUE: (Method: Radioimmunoassay)

Age and Sex	Conventional Units	SI Units (Conventional Units × 1)
Newborn	20–40 ng/mL	20–40 µg/L
1–17 y	2.8–41 ng/mL	2.8–41 µg/L
Adult		
Male	3–13 ng/mL	3–13 µg/L
Female		
Premenopausal	0.4–8.2 ng/mL	0.4–8.2 µg/L
Postmenopausal	1.5–11 ng/mL	1.5–11 µg/L

DESCRIPTION & RATIONALE: Osteocalcin is an important bone cell matrix protein and a sensitive marker in bone metabolism. It is produced by osteoblasts during the matrix mineralization phase of bone formation and is the most abundant noncollagenous bone cell protein. Synthesis of osteocalcin is dependent on vitamin K. Osteocalcin levels parallel alkaline phosphatase levels. Osteocalcin levels are affected by a number of factors, including the hormone estrogen. Assessment of osteocalcin levels permits indirect measurement of osteoblast activity and bone formation. Because it is released into the bloodstream during bone resorption, there is some question as to whether osteocalcin might also be considered a marker for bone matrix degradation and turnover. ∎

INDICATIONS:
- Assist in the diagnosis of bone cancer
- Evaluate bone disease
- Evaluate bone metabolism
- Monitor effectiveness of estrogen replacement therapy

RESULT

Increased in:
- Adolescents undergoing a growth spurt
- Chronic renal failure
- Hyperthyroidism (primary and secondary)
- Metastatic skeletal disease

- Paget's disease
- Renal osteodystrophy
- Some patients with osteoporosis

Decreased in:
- Growth hormone deficiency
- Pregnancy
- Primary biliary cirrhosis

CRITICAL VALUES: N/A

INTERFERING FACTORS:
- Drugs that may increase calcitonin levels include anticonvulsants, calcitriol, and estrogens.

- Drugs that may decrease calcitonin levels include glucocorticoids.

- Recent radioactive scans or radiation within 1 week before the serum osteocalcin test can interfere with test results when radioimmunoassay is the test method.

Nursing Implications and Procedure

Pretest:

➤ Inform the patient that the test is used to evaluate bone disease.

➤ Obtain a history of the patient's complaints, including a list of known allergens (especially allergies or sensitivities to latex), and inform the appropriate health care practitioner accordingly.

➤ Obtain a history of the patient's musculoskeletal system and results of previously performed laboratory tests, surgical procedures, and other diagnostic procedures. For related laboratory tests, refer to the Musculoskeletal System table.

➤ Note any recent procedures that can interfere with test results.

➤ Obtain a list of the medications the patient is taking, including herbs, nutritional supplements, and nutra-

ceuticals. The requesting health care practitioner and laboratory should be advised if the patient regularly uses these products so that their effects can be taken into consideration when reviewing results.

➤ Review the procedure with the patient. Inform the patient that specimen collection takes approximately 5 to 10 minutes. Address concerns about pain related to the procedure. Explain to the patient that there may be some discomfort during the venipuncture.

➤ There are no food, fluid, or medication restrictions, unless by medical direction.

Intratest:

➤ If the patient has a history of severe allergic reaction to latex, care should be taken to avoid the use of equipment containing latex.

➤ Instruct the patient to cooperate fully and to follow directions. Direct the patient to breathe normally and to avoid unnecessary movement.

➤ Observe standard precautions, and follow the general guidelines in Appendix A. Positively identify the patient, and label the appropriate tubes with the corresponding patient demographics, date, and time of collection. Perform a venipuncture; collect the specimen in a 5-mL red-top tube.

➤ Remove the needle, and apply a pressure dressing over the puncture site.

➤ Promptly transport the specimen to the laboratory for processing and analysis.

➤ The results are recorded manually or in a computerized system for recall and postprocedure interpretation by the appropriate health care practitioner.

Post-test:

➤ Observe venipuncture site for bleeding or hematoma formation. Apply paper tape or other adhesive to hold pressure bandage in place, or replace with a plastic bandage.

➤ *Nutritional considerations:* Increased osteocalcin levels may be associated with skeletal disease. Nutritional therapy is indicated for individuals identified as being at high risk for developing osteoporosis. Educate the patient regarding the National Osteoporosis Foundation's guidelines, which include a regular regimen of weight-bearing exercises, limited alcohol intake, avoidance of tobacco products, and adequate dietary intake of vitamin D (400 to 800 IU/day) and calcium (120 mg/day). Dietary calcium can be obtained from animal or plant sources. Milk and milk products, sardines, clams, oysters, salmon, rhubarb, spinach, beet greens, broccoli, kale, tofu, legumes, and fortified orange juice are high in calcium. Milk and milk products also contain vitamin D and lactose, which assist calcium absorption. Cooked vegetables yield more absorbable calcium than raw vegetables. Patients should be informed of the substances that can inhibit calcium absorption by irreversibly binding to some of the calcium, making it unavailable for absorption, such as oxalates, which naturally occur in some vegetables; phytic acid, found in some cereals; and insoluble dietary fiber (in excessive amounts). Excessive protein intake can also negatively affect calcium absorption, especially if it is combined with foods high in phosphorus. Vitamin D is synthesized by the skin and is also available in fortified dairy foods and cod liver oil.

➤ A written report of the examination will be sent to the requesting health care practitioner, who will discuss the results with the patient.

➤ Reinforce information given by the patient's health care provider regarding further testing, treatment, or referral to another health care provider. Answer any questions or address any concerns voiced by the patient or family.

➤ Depending on the results of this procedure, additional testing may be performed to evaluate or monitor progression of the disease process and determine the need for a change in therapy. Evaluate test results in relation to the patient's symptoms and other tests performed.

Related laboratory tests:

➤ Related laboratory tests include alkaline phosphatase, calcium (blood and urine), collagen cross-linked N-telopeptide, parathyroid hormone, phosphorus, and vitamin D.

OTOSCOPY

SYNONYMS/ACRONYMS: N/A.

AREA OF APPLICATION: Ears.

CONTRAST: N/A.

DESCRIPTION & RATIONALE: This noninvasive procedure is used to inspect the external ear, auditory canal, and tympanic membrane. Otoscopy is an essential part of any general physical examination, but is also done before any other audiologic studies when symptoms of ear pain or hearing loss are present. ■

INDICATIONS:

• Detect causes of deafness, obstruction, stenosis, or swelling of the pinna or canal causing a narrowing or closure that prevents sound from entering

• Detect ear abnormalities during routine physical examination

• Diagnose cause of ear pain

• Remove impacted cerumen (with a dull ring curette) or foreign bodies (with a forceps) that are obstructing the entrance of sound waves into the ear

• Evaluate acute or chronic otitis media and effectiveness of therapy in controlling infections

RESULT

Normal Findings:

• Normal structure and appearance of the external ear, auditory canal, and tympanic membrane.
   Pinna: funnel-shaped cartilaginous structure; no evidence of infection, pain, dermatitis with swelling, redness, or itching
   External auditory canal: S-shaped canal lined with fine hairs, sebaceous and ceruminous glands; no evidence of redness, lesions, edema, scaliness, pain, accumulation of cerumen, drainage, or presence of foreign bodies
   Tympanic membrane: shallow, circular cone that is shiny and pearl gray in color, semi-transparent whitish cord

crossing from front to back just under the upper edge, cone of light on the right side at the 4 o'clock position; no evidence of bulging, retraction, lusterless membrane, or obliteration of the cone of light

Abnormal Findings:

• Cerumen accumulation

• Ear trauma

• Foreign bodies

• Otitis externa

• Otitis media

• Tympanic membrane perforation or rupture

CRITICAL VALUES: N/A

INTERFERING FACTORS:

Factors that may impair the results of the examination:

• Obstruction of the auditory canal with cerumen, dried drainage, or foreign bodies that prevent introduction of the otoscope

Nursing Implications and Procedure • • • • • • • • • • •

Pretest:

➤ Inform the patient that the procedure is performed to investigate suspected ear disorders.

➤ Obtain a history of the patient's complaints, including a list of known allergens.

➤ Obtain a history of the patient's known or suspected hearing loss, including type and cause; ear conditions with treatment regimens; ear surgery; and other tests and procedures to assess and diagnose auditory deficit. Obtain a history of the patient's complaints of pain, itching, drainage, deafness, or presence of tympanotomy tube.

➤ Obtain a history of results of previously performed laboratory tests, surgical procedures, and other diagnostic procedures.

➤ Obtain a list of the medications the patient is taking, especially antibiotic regimen, as well as herbs, nutritional supplements, and nutraceuticals. The requesting health care practitioner should be advised if the patient regularly uses these products so that their effects can be taken into consideration when reviewing results.

➤ Review the procedure with the patient. Inform the caregiver that he or she may need to restrain a child in order to prevent damage to the ear if the child cannot remain still. Address concerns about pain related to the procedure. Explain to the patient that no discomfort will be experienced during the test. Inform the patient that a physician, nurse or health care practitioner specializing in this field performs the test, and that to evaluate both ears, the test can take 5 to 10 minutes.

➤ Ensure that the external auditory canal is clear of impacted cerumen.

Intratest:

➤ Instruct the patient to cooperate fully and to follow directions. Ask the patient to remain still during the procedure because movement produces unreliable results.

➤ Administer ear drops or irrigation to prepare for cerumen removal, if ordered.

➤ Place adult patient in a sitting position; place a child in a supine position on the caregiver's lap. Request that the patient remain very still during the examination; a child can be restrained by the caregiver if needed.

➤ Assemble the otoscope with the correct-size speculum to fit the size of the patient's ear and check the light source. For the adult, tilt the head slightly away and, with the nondominant hand, pull the pinna upward and backward. For a child, hold the head steady or have the caregiver hold the child's head steady, depending on the

age, and pull the pinna downward. Gently and slowly insert the speculum into the ear canal downward and forward with the handle of the otoscope held downward. For the child, hold the handle upward while placing the edge of the hand holding the otoscope on the head to steady it during insertion. If the speculum resists insertion, withdraw and attach a smaller one.

➤ Place an eye to the lens of the otoscope, turn on the light source, and advance the speculum into the ear canal until the tympanic membrane is visible. Examine the posterior and anterior membrane, cone of light, outer rim (annulus), umbo, handle of the malleus, folds, and pars tensa.

➤ Culture any effusion with a sterile swab and culture tube (see "Culture, Bacterial, Ear," monograph); or a health care practitioner will perform needle aspiration from the middle ear through the tympanic membrane during the examination. Other procedures such as cerumen and foreign body removal can also be performed.

➤ Pneumatic otoscopy can be done to determine tympanic membrane flexibility. This test permits the introduction of air into the canal that reveals a reduction in movement of the membrane in otitis media and absence of movement in chronic otitis media.

➤ The results are recorded manually for recall and postprocedure interpretation by a health care professional specializing in this field.

Post-test:

➤ Administer ear drops of a soothing oil, and as ordered, if the canal is irritated by removal of cerumen or foreign bodies.

➤ A written report of the examination will be completed by a health care practitioner specializing in this branch of medicine. The report will be sent to the requesting health care practitioner, who will discuss the results with the patient.

➤ Recognize anxiety related to test

results, and be supportive of impaired activity related to hearing loss. Discuss the implications of abnormal test results on the patient's lifestyle. Provide teaching and information regarding the clinical implications of the test results, as appropriate.

➤ Reinforce information given by the patient's health care provider regarding further testing, treatment, or referral to another health care provider. Answer any questions or address any concerns voiced by the patient or family.

➤ Depending on the results of this procedure, additional testing may be performed to evaluate or monitor progression of the disease process and determine the need for a change in therapy. Evaluate test results in relation to the patient's symptoms and other tests performed.

Related diagnostic tests:

➤ Related diagnostic tests include audiometry and bacterial culture of the ear.

OVA AND PARASITES, STOOL

SYNONYM/ACRONYM: O & P.

SPECIMEN: Stool collected in a clean plastic, tightly capped container.

REFERENCE VALUE: (Method: Macroscopic and microscopic examination) No presence of parasites, ova, or larvae.

DESCRIPTION & RATIONALE: This test evaluates stool for the presence of intestinal parasites and their eggs. Some parasites are nonpathogenic; others, such as protozoa and worms, can cause serious illness. ■

INDICATIONS: Assist in the diagnosis of parasitic infestation

RESULT

Positive findings in:
• Amebiasis—*Entamoeba histolytica* infection
• Ascariasis—*Ascaris lumbricoides* infection

• Blastocystis—*Blastocystis hominis* infection
• Cryptosporidiosis—*Cryptosporidium parvum* infection
• Enterobiasis—*Enterobius vermicularis* (pinworm) infection
• Giardiasis—*Giardia lamblia* infection
• Hookworm disease—*Ancylostoma duodenale, Necator americanus* infection
• Isospora—*Isospora belli* infection
• Schistosomiasis—*Schistosoma haematobium, Schistosoma japonicum, Schistosoma mansoni* infection
• Strongyloidiasis—*Strongyloides stercoralis* infection

- Tapeworm disease—*Diphyllobothrium, Hymenolepiasis, Taenia saginata, Taenia solium* infection

- Trematode disease—*Clonorchis sinensis, Fasciola hepatica, Fasciolopsis buski* infection

- Trichuriasis—*Trichuris trichiura* infection

CRITICAL VALUES: N/A

INTERFERING FACTORS:
- Failure to test a fresh specimen may yield a false-negative result.

- Antimicrobial or antiamebic therapy within 10 days of test may yield a false-negative result.

- Failure to wait 1 week after a gastrointestinal study using barium or after laxative use can affect test results.

- Medications such as antacids, antibiotics, antidiarrheal compounds, bismuth, castor oil, iron, magnesia, or psyllium fiber (Metamucil) may interfere with analysis.

Nursing Implications and Procedure • • • • • • • • • • •

Pretest:

➤ Inform the patient that the test is used to assist in the diagnosis of parasitic infection.

➤ Obtain a history of the patient's complaints, including a list of known allergens, and inform the appropriate health care practitioner accordingly. Document any travel to foreign countries.

➤ Obtain a history of the patient's gastrointestinal and immune systems, and results of previously performed laboratory tests, surgical procedures, and other diagnostic procedures. For related laboratory tests, refer to the Gastrointestinal and Immune System tables.

➤ Note any recent therapies that can interfere with test results.

➤ Obtain a list of the medications the patient is taking, including herbs, nutritional supplements, and nutraceuticals. The requesting health care practitioner and laboratory should be advised if the patient regularly uses these products so their effects can be taken into consideration when reviewing results.

➤ Review the procedure with the patient. Instruct the patient on handwashing procedures, and inform the patient that the infection may be contagious. Warn the patient not to contaminate the specimen with urine, toilet paper, or toilet water. Address concerns about pain related to the procedure. Explain to the patient that there should be no discomfort during the procedure.

➤ *Sensitivity to social and cultural issues,* as well as concern for modesty, is important in providing psychological support before, during, and after the procedure.

➤ Instruct the patient to avoid medications that interfere with test results.

➤ There are no food or fluid restrictions, unless by medical direction.

Intratest:

➤ Instruct the patient to cooperate fully and to follow directions.

➤ Observe standard precautions, and follow the general guidelines in Appendix A. Positively identify the patient, and label the appropriate collection container with the corresponding patient demographics, date, and time of collection.

➤ Collect a stool specimen directly into the container. If the patient is bedridden, use a clean bedpan and transfer the specimen into the container using a tongue depressor.

➤ Specimens to be examined for the presence of pinworms are collected by the "Scotch tape" method in the morning before bathing or defecation. A small paddle with a piece of cellophane tape (sticky side facing out) is pressed against the perianal area. The tape is placed in a collection container and submitted to determine if ova are present. Sometimes adult worms are observed protruding from the rectum.

➤ Promptly transport the specimen to the laboratory for processing and analysis.

➤ The results are recorded manually or in a computerized system for recall and postprocedure interpretation by the appropriate health care practitioner.

Post-test:

➤ A written report of the examination will be sent to the requesting health care practitioner, who will discuss the results with the patient.

➤ Recognize anxiety related to test results. Discuss the implications of abnormal test results on the patient's lifestyle. Provide teaching and information regarding the clinical implications of the test results, as appropriate.

➤ Reinforce information given by the patient's health care provider regarding further testing, treatment, or referral to another health care provider. Educate the patient with positive findings on the transmission of the parasite, as indicated. Warn the patient that one negative result does not rule out parasitic infestation and that additional specimens may be required. Answer any questions or address any concerns voiced by the patient or family.

➤ Depending on the results of this procedure, additional testing may be performed to evaluate or monitor progression of the disease process and determine the need for a change in therapy. Evaluate test results in relation to the patient's symptoms and other tests performed.

Related laboratory tests:

➤ Related laboratory tests include fecal analysis, immunoglobulin E, and stool culture.

OXALATE, URINE

SYNONYM/ACRONYM: N/A.

SPECIMEN: Urine (25 mL) from a timed specimen collected in a clean plastic collection container with hydrogen chloride (HCl) as a preservative.

REFERENCE VALUE: (Method: Spectrophotometry)

Conventional Units	SI Units (Conventional Units × 11.4)
0–40 mg/24 h	0–456 μmol/24 h

DESCRIPTION & RATIONALE: Oxalate is derived from the metabolism of oxalic acid, glycine, and ascorbic acid. Some individuals with malabsorption disorders absorb and excrete abnormally high amounts of oxalate, resulting in *hyperoxaluria*. Hyperoxaluria may be seen in patients who consume large amounts of animal protein, certain fruits and vegetables, or megadoses of vitamin C (ascorbic acid). Hyperoxaluria is also associated with ethylene glycol poisoning (oxalic acid is used in cleaning and bleaching agents). Patients who absorb and excrete large amounts of oxalate may form calcium oxalate kidney stones. Simultaneous measurement of serum and urine calcium is often requested. ■

INDICATIONS:
- Assist in the evaluation of patients with ethylene glycol poisoning
- Assist in the evaluation of patients with a history of kidney stones
- Assist in the evaluation of patients with malabsorption syndromes or patients who have had jejunoileal bypass surgery

RESULT

Increased in:
- Bacterial overgrowth
- Biliary tract disease
- Bowel disease
- Celiac disease
- Cirrhosis
- Crohn's disease
- Diabetes
- Ethylene glycol poisoning
- Ileal resection
- Jejunal shunt
- Pancreatic disease

- Primary hereditary hyperoxaluria (rare)
- Pyridoxine (vitamin B_6) deficiency
- Sarcoidosis

Decreased in:
- Hypercalciuria
- Renal failure

CRITICAL VALUES: N/A

INTERFERING FACTORS:
- Drugs and vitamins that may increase oxalate levels include methoxyflurane, ascorbic acid, and calcium.
- Drugs that may decrease oxalate levels include nifedipine and pyridoxine.
- Failure to follow dietary restrictions before the procedure may cause the procedure to be canceled or repeated.

Nursing Implications and Procedure . . . .

Pretest:

➤ Inform the patient that the test is used to identify patients at risk for renal calculus formation, specifically calcium oxalate calculi. Hyperoxaluria is also commonly observed in patients with malabsorption conditions.

➤ Obtain a history of the patient's complaints, including a list of known allergens (especially allergies or sensitivities to latex), and inform the appropriate health care practitioner accordingly.

➤ Obtain a history of the patient's gastrointestinal and genitourinary systems, as well as results of previously performed laboratory tests, surgical procedures, and other diagnostic procedures. For related laboratory tests, refer to the Gastrointestinal and Genitourinary System tables.

➤ Obtain a list of the medications the patient is taking, including herbs, nutritional supplements and nutraceuticals. The requesting health care practitioner and laboratory should be advised if the patient regularly uses these products so that their effects can be taken into consideration when reviewing results.

➤ Review the procedure with the patient. Provide a nonmetallic urinal, bedpan, or toilet-mounted collection device. Address concerns about pain related to the procedure. Explain to the patient that there should be no discomfort during the procedure.

➤ Usually a 24-hour time frame for urine collection is ordered. Inform the patient that all urine must be saved during that 24-hour period. Instruct the patient not to void directly into the laboratory collection container. Instruct the patient to avoid defecating in the collection device and to keep toilet tissue out of the collection device to prevent contamination of the specimen. Place a sign in the bathroom to remind the patient to save all urine.

➤ Instruct the patient to void all urine into the collection device and then to pour the urine into the laboratory collection container. Alternatively, the specimen can be left in the collection device for a health care staff member to add to the laboratory collection container.

➤ *Sensitivity to social and cultural issues,* as well as concern for modesty, is important in providing psychological support before, during, and after the procedure.

➤ There are no fluid or medication restrictions, unless by medical direction.

➤ Calcium supplements, gelatin, rhubarb, spinach, strawberries, tomatoes, and vitamin C should be restricted for at least 24 hours before the test. High-protein meals should also be avoided 24 hours before specimen collection.

Intratest:

➤ Ensure that the patient has complied with dietary restrictions; assure that restricted foods have been avoided for at least 24 hours prior to the procedure.

➤ If the patient has a history of severe allergic reaction to latex, care should be taken to avoid the use of equipment containing latex.

➤ Instruct the patient to cooperate fully and to follow directions.

➤ Observe standard precautions, and follow the general guidelines in Appendix A. Positively identify the patient, and label the appropriate tubes with the corresponding patient demographics, date, and time of collection.

Random specimen (collect in early morning):

Clean-catch specimen:

➤ Instruct the male patient to (1) thoroughly wash his hands, (2) cleanse the meatus, (3) void a small amount into the toilet, and (4) void directly into the specimen container.

➤ Instruct the female patient to (1) thoroughly wash her hands; (2) cleanse the labia from front to back; (3) while keeping the labia separated, void a small amount into the toilet; and (4) without interrupting the urine stream, void directly into the specimen container.

Indwelling catheter:

➤ Put on gloves. Empty drainage tube of urine. It may be necessary to clamp off the catheter for 15 to 30 minutes before specimen collection. Cleanse specimen port with antiseptic swab, and then aspirate 5 mL of urine with a 21- to 25-gauge needle and syringe. Transfer urine to a sterile container.

Timed specimen:

➤ Obtain a clean 3-L urine specimen container, toilet-mounted collection device, and plastic bag (for transport of the specimen container). The specimen must be refrigerated or kept on ice throughout the entire collection period. If an indwelling urinary catheter is in place, the drainage bag must be kept on ice.

➤ Begin the test between 6 and 8 a.m.,

if possible. Collect first voiding and discard. Record the time the specimen was discarded as the beginning of the timed collection period. The next morning, ask the patient to void at the same time the collection was started and add this last voiding to the container.

➤ If an indwelling catheter is in place, replace the tubing and container system at the start of the collection time. Keep the container system on ice during the collection period, or empty the urine into a larger container periodically during the collection period; monitor to ensure continued drainage, and conclude the test the next morning at the same hour the collection was begun.

➤ At the conclusion of the test, compare the quantity of urine with the urinary output record for the collection; if the specimen contains less than what was recorded as output, some urine may have been discarded, invalidating the test.

➤ Include on the collection container's label the amount of urine, test start and stop times, and ingestion of any foods or medications that can affect test results.

General:

➤ Promptly transport the specimen to the laboratory for processing and analysis.

➤ The results are recorded manually or in a computerized system for recall and postprocedure interpretation by the appropriate health care practitioner.

Post-test:

➤ Instruct the patient to resume usual diet, as directed by the health care practitioner.

➤ *Nutritional considerations:* Consider-

ation may be given to lessening dietary intake of oxalate if urine levels are increased. Encourage patients with abnormal results to seek advice regarding dietary modifications from a trained nutritionist. Magnesium supplementation may be recommended for patients with gastrointestinal disease to prevent the development of calcium oxalate kidney stones.

➤ A written report of the examination will be sent to the requesting health care practitioner, who will discuss the results with the patient.

➤ Recognize anxiety related to test results, and be supportive of fear of shortened life expectancy. Discuss the implications of abnormal test results on the patient's lifestyle. Provide teaching and information regarding the clinical implications of the test results, as appropriate. Educate the patient regarding access to counseling services.

➤ Reinforce information given by the patient's health care provider regarding further testing, treatment, or referral to another health care provider. Answer any questions or address any concerns voiced by the patient or family.

➤ Depending on the results of this procedure, additional testing may be performed to evaluate or monitor progression of the disease process and determine the need for a change in therapy. Evaluate test results in relation to the patient's symptoms and other tests performed.

Related laboratory tests:

➤ Related laboratory tests include serum and urine calcium, kidney stone analysis, serum and urine magnesium, urinalysis, urine uric acid, and vitamin C.

PACHYMETRY

SYNONYMS/ACRONYMS: N/A.

AREA OF APPLICATION: Eyes.

CONTRAST: N/A.

DESCRIPTION & RATIONALE: Pachymetry is the measurement of the thickness of the cornea using an ultrasound device called a pachymeter. Refractive surgery procedures such as LASIK remove tissue from the cornea. Pachymetry is used to ensure that there will be enough central corneal tissue remaining after surgery to prevent ectasia, or abnormal bowing, of thin corneas. Also, recently published ophthalmology studies point to a correlation between increased risk of glaucoma and decreased corneal thickness. This correlation has influenced some health care practitioners to include pachymetry as a part of a regular eye health examination for patients who have a family history of glaucoma or who are part of a high-risk population. African Americans have a higher incidence of glaucoma than any other ethnic group. ▪

INDICATIONS:
- Assist in the diagnosis of glaucoma (*note:* the intraocular pressure in glaucoma patients with a thin cornea, 530 μ or less, may be higher than in patients whose corneal thickness is within normal limits)
- Determine corneal thickness in potential refractive surgery candidates
- Monitor the effects of various therapies using eyedrops, laser, or filtering surgery

RESULT

Normal Findings:
- 535 to 555 μ

Abnormal Findings:
- Bullous keratopathy
- Corneal rejection after penetrating keratoplasty
- Fuchs endothelial dystrophy
- Glaucoma

CRITICAL VALUES: N/A

INTERFERING FACTORS:

Factors that may impair the results of the examination:
- Inability of the patient to cooperate or remain still during the test because of age, significant pain, or mental status
- Improper technique during application of the probe tip to the cornea

Nursing Implications and Procedure • • • • • • • • • • • •

➤ Inform the patient that the procedure measures corneal thickness.

➤ Obtain a history of the patient's complaints, including a list of known allergens.

➤ Obtain a history of narrow-angle glaucoma. Obtain a history of known or suspected visual impairment, changes in visual acuity, use of glasses or contact lenses.

➤ Obtain a history of the patient's known or suspected vision loss, including type and cause; eye conditions with treatment regimens; eye surgery; and other tests and procedures to assess and diagnose visual deficit. For related diagnostic tests, refer to the table of tests associated with the Ocular System.

➤ Obtain a history of results of previously performed laboratory tests, surgical procedures, and other diagnostic procedures.

➤ Obtain a list of the medications the patient is taking, including herbs, nutritional supplements, and nutraceuticals. The requesting health care practitioner should be advised if the patient regularly uses these products so that their effects can be taken into consideration when reviewing results.

➤ Instruct the patient to remove contact lenses or glasses, as appropriate. Instruct the patient regarding the importance of keeping the eyes open for the test.

➤ Review the procedure with the patient. Explain that the patient will be requested to fixate the eyes during the procedure. Address concerns about pain related to the procedure. Explain to the patient that no pain will be experienced during the test, but there may be moments of discomfort. Explain to the patient that some discomfort may be experienced after the test when the numbness wears off from anesthetic drops administered prior to the test, or discomfort may occur if too much pressure is used during the test. Inform the patient that a technician, optometrist, or physician performs the test, and that to evaluate both eyes, the test can take 3 to 5 minutes.

➤ There are no food, fluid, or medication restrictions, unless by medical direction.

➤ Instruct the patient to cooperate fully and to follow directions. Ask the patient to remain still during the procedure because movement produces unreliable results.

➤ Seat the patient comfortably. Instruct the patient to look straight ahead, keeping the eyes open and unblinking.

➤ Instill topical anesthetic in each eye, as ordered, and allow time for it to work. Topical anesthetic drops are placed in the eye with the patient looking up and the solution directed at the six o'clock position of the sclera (white of the eye) near the limbus (grey, semitransparent area of the eyeball where the cornea and sclera meet). The dropper bottle should not touch the eyelashes.

➤ Request that the patient look straight ahead while the probe of the pachymeter is applied directly on the cornea of the eye. Take an average of three readings for each eye. Individual readings should be within 10 μ. Results on both eyes should be similar.

➤ The results are recorded manually for recall and postprocedure interpretation by the appropriate health care practitioner.

➤ A written report of the examination will be completed by a health care practitioner specializing in this branch of medicine. The report will be sent to the requesting health care practitioner, who will discuss the results with the patient.

Recognize anxiety related to test results. Encourage the family to recognize and be supportive of impaired activity related to vision loss, perceived loss of driving privileges, or the possibility of requiring corrective lenses (self-image). Discuss the implications of test results on the patient's lifestyle. Reassure the patient regarding concerns related to their impending cataract surgery. Provide teaching and information regarding the clinical implications of the test results, as appropriate.

Reinforce information given by the patient's health care provider regarding further testing, treatment, or referral to another health care provider. Answer any questions or address any concerns voiced by the patient or family.

Depending on the results of this procedure, additional testing may be performed to evaluate or monitor progression of the disease process and determine the need for a change in therapy. Evaluate test results in relation to the patient's symptoms and other tests performed.

Related diagnostic tests:

Related diagnostic tests include fundus photography, gonioscopy, intraocular pressure, and visual field testing.

PAPANICOLAOU SMEAR

· ·

SYNONYMS/ACRONYM: Pap smear, cervical smear.

SPECIMEN: Cervical and endocervical cells.

REFERENCE VALUE: (Method: Microscopic examination of fixed and stained smear) Reporting of Pap smear findings may follow one of several formats and may vary from laboratory to laboratory. Simplified content of the two most common formats for interpretation are listed in the table.

Bethesda System	Description
Specimen type	Conventional, liquid based or other
Specimen adequacy	*Satisfactory* for evaluation— (endocervical/transformation zone component is described as present/absent along with other quality indicators, e.g., partially obscuring blood, inflammation) *Unsatisfactory* for evaluation—either the specimen is rejected and the reason given or the specimen is processed and examined but not evaluated for epithelial abnormalities and the reason is given

(Continued on the following page)

Bethesda System	Description
General categorization	*Negative* for intraepithelial lesion or malignancy *Epithelial cell abnormality* (abnormality is specified in the interpretation section of the report) *Other comments*
Automated review	Indicates the case was examined by an automated device and the results are listed along with the name of the device
Ancillary testing	Describes the test method and result
Interpretation/result	Organisms—*Trichomonas vaginalis*, fungal organisms consistent with *Candida* spp., shift in flora suggestive of bacterial vaginosis, bacteria morphologically consistent with *Actinomyces* spp., cellular changes consistent with Herpes simplex virus *Other nonneoplastic findings*—reactive cellular changes associated with inflammation, radiation, intrauterine device; glandular cell status post-hysterectomy; atrophy; endometrial cells (in a woman of 40 years or greater)
Epithelial cell abnormalities	*Squamous cell* *Atypical squamous cells*—of undetermined significance (ASC-US) -cannot exclude HSIL (ASC-H) *Low grade squamous intraepithelial lesion (LSIL)*—encompassing: HPV/mild dysplasia/CIN 1 *High grade squamous intraepithelial lesion (HSIL)*—encompassing: moderate and severe dysplasia, CIS/CIN 2 and CIN 3 –with features suspicious for invasion (if invasion is suspected) *Squamous cell carcinoma* *Glandular cell* Atypical—endocervical cells (NOS or specify otherwise) –endometrial cells (NOS or specify otherwise) –glandular cells (NOS or specify otherwise) Atypical—endocervical cells, favor neoplastic –glandular cells – favor neoplastic Endocervical carcinoma in situ Adenocarcinoma—endocervical –endometrial –extrauterine –not otherwise specified (NOS) Other malignant neoplasms Should be consistent with clinical followup guidelines published by professional organizations with references included
Educational notes and suggestions	

DESCRIPTION & RATIONALE: The Papanicolaou (Pap) smear is primarily used for the early detection of cervical cancer. The interpretation of Pap smears is as heavily dependent on the collection and fixation technique as it is on the completeness and accuracy of the clinical information provided with the specimen. The patient's age, date of last menstrual period, parity, surgical status, postmenopausal status, use of hormone therapy (including use of oral contraceptives), history of radiation or chemotherapy, history of abnormal vaginal bleeding, and history of previous Pap smears are essential for proper interpretation.

A Schiller's test entails applying an iodine solution to the cervix. Normal cells pick up the iodine and stain brown. Abnormal cells do not pick up any color.

Improvements in specimen preparation have added to the increased quality of screening procedures. The Cytyc ThinPrep PapTest (Cytyc Corporation, Boxborough, MA), ap-proved by the U.S. Food and Drug Administration in 1996, is a technique that provides a uniform monolayer of cells free of debris such as blood and mucus. Computerized scanning systems are also being used to reduce the number of smears that require manual review by a cytotechnologist or pathologist.

There are now some alternatives to cone biopsy and cryosurgery for the treatment of cervical dysplasia. Patients with abnormal Pap smear results may have a cervical loop electrosurgical excision procedure (LEEP) performed to remove or destroy abnormal cervical tissue. In the LEEP procedure, a speculum is inserted into the vagina, the cervix is numbed, and a special electrically charged wire loop is used to painlessly remove the suspicious area. Postprocedure cramping and bleeding can occur. Laser ablation is another technique that can be employed for the precise removal of abnormal cervical tissue. ∎

INDICATIONS:
- Assist in the diagnosis of cervical dysplasia
- Assist in the diagnosis of endometriosis, condyloma, and vaginal adenosis
- Assist in the diagnosis of genital infections (herpes, *Candida* spp., *Trichomonas vaginalis,* cytomegalovirus, *Chlamydia,* lymphogranuloma venereum, human papillomavirus, and *Actinomyces* spp.)
- Assist in the diagnosis of primary and metastatic neoplasms
- Evaluate hormonal function

RESULT

Positive findings in: (See table [Bethesda system], presented earlier under "Reference Value")

Decreased in: N/A

CRITICAL VALUES: N/A

INTERFERING FACTORS:
- The smear should not be allowed to air dry before fixation.
- Lubricating jelly should not be used on the speculum.
- Improper collection site may result in specimen rejection. Samples for cancer screening are obtained from the posterior vaginal fornix and from the cervix. Samples for hormonal evaluation are obtained from the vagina.
- Douching, sexual intercourse, using tampons, or using vaginal medication within 24 hours prior to specimen collection can interfere with the specimen's results.

- Collection of other specimens prior to the collection of the Pap smear may be cause for specimen rejection.
- Contamination with blood from samples collected during the patient's menstrual period may be cause for specimen rejection.

Nursing Implications and Procedure • • • • • • • • • • •

Pretest:

➤ Inform the patient that the test is primarily used to establish a histologic diagnosis of cervical and vaginal disease and identify the presence of genital infections.

➤ Obtain a history of the patient's complaints, including a list of known allergens (especially allergies or sensitivities to latex), and inform the appropriate health care practitioner accordingly.

➤ Obtain a history of the patient's immune and reproductive systems and results of previously performed laboratory tests, surgical procedures, and other diagnostic procedures. For related tests, refer to the Immune and Reproductive System tables.

➤ Record the date of the last menstrual period and determine the possibility of pregnancy in perimenopausal women.

➤ Note any recent procedures that can interfere with test results.

➤ Obtain a list of the medications the patient is taking, including herbs, nutritional supplements, and nutraceuticals. The requesting health care practitioner and laboratory should be advised if the patient regularly uses these products so that their effects can be taken into consideration when reviewing results.

➤ Review the procedure with the patient. Instruct the patient to avoid douching or sexual intercourse for 24 hours before specimen collection. Verify that the patient is not menstruating. Address concerns about pain related to the procedure. Explain to

the patient that there may be some discomfort during the procedure. Inform the patient that specimen collection is performed by a health care practitioner specializing in this procedure and takes approximately 5 to 10 minutes.

➤ *Sensitivity to social and cultural issues,* as well as concern for modesty, is important in providing psychological support before, during, and after the procedure.

➤ There are no food, fluid, or medication restrictions, unless by medical direction.

➤ If the patient is taking vaginal antibiotic medication, testing should be delayed for 1 month after the treatment has been completed.

➤ *Make sure a written and informed consent has been signed prior to the procedure and before administering any medications.*

Intratest:

➤ Have the patient void before the procedure.

➤ Have the patient remove clothes below the waist.

➤ Instruct the patient to cooperate fully and to follow directions. Direct the patient to breathe normally and to avoid unnecessary movement during the procedure.

➤ Observe standard precautions, and follow the general guidelines in Appendix A. Positively identify the patient, and label the appropriate collection containers with the corresponding patient demographics, date and time of collection, and site location.

➤ Assist the patient into a lithotomy position on a gynecologic examination table (with feet in stirrups). Drape the patient's legs.

➤ A plastic or metal speculum is inserted into the vagina and is opened to gently spread apart the vagina for inspection of the cervix. The speculum may be dipped in warm water to aid in comfortable insertion.

➤ After the speculum is properly positioned, the cervical and vaginal specimens are obtained. A synthetic fiber brush is inserted deep enough into the cervix to reach the endocervical canal. The brush is then rotated one turn and removed. The plastic or wooden spatula is used to lightly scrape the cervix and vaginal wall.

Conventional collection:

➤ Both specimens that are on the brush and spatula are then plated on the glass slide. The brush specimen is plated using a gentle rolling motion, whereas the spatula specimen is plated using a light gliding motion across the slide. The specimens are immediately fixed to the slide with a liquid or spray containing 95% ethanol. The speculum is removed from the vagina. A pelvic and/or rectal exam is usually performed after specimen collection is completed.

ThinPrep collection:

➤ The ThinPrep bottle lid is opened and removed, exposing the solution. The brush and spatula specimens are then gently swished in the ThinPrep solution to remove the adhering cells. The brush and spatula are then removed from the ThinPrep solution, and the bottle lid is replaced and secured.

General:

➤ Place samples in properly labeled specimen container and promptly transport the specimen to the laboratory for processing and analysis.

➤ The results are recorded manually or in a computerized system for recall and postprocedure interpretation by the appropriate health care practitioner.

Post-test:

➤ Cleanse or allow the patient to cleanse secretions or excess lubricant (if a pelvic and/or rectal examination is also performed) from the perineal area. Provide a sanitary pad if cervical bleeding occurs.

➤ A written report of the examination will be completed by a health care practitioner specializing in this branch of medicine. The report will be sent to the requesting health care practitioner, who will discuss the results with the patient.

➤ Recognize anxiety related to test results, and offer support. Discuss the implications of abnormal test results on the patient's lifestyle. Provide teaching and information regarding the clinical implications of the test results, as appropriate. Educate the patient regarding access to counseling services.

➤ Reinforce information given by the patient's health care provider regarding further testing, treatment, or referral to another health care provider. Inform the patient, as appropriate, that repeat testing may be requested in the event of specimen rejection or abnormal findings. Inform the patient that non–sexually active women should begin yearly Pap smears at 18 years of age, and younger sexually active women should begin yearly Pap smears earlier. Pap smears should be repeated more frequently if the results return abnormal. After a hysterectomy, a vaginal cuff Pap smear is used to monitor the cells lining the terminal end of the vagina. Several guidelines differ in their recommendations on when to cease Pap smear testing. Encourage patients to discuss their Pap smear result history and women's health history with their health care provider to determine at what age testing may be terminated. Answer any questions or address any concerns voiced by the patient or family.

➤ Depending on the results of this procedure, additional testing may be performed to evaluate or monitor progression of the disease process and determine the need for a change in therapy. Evaluate test results in relation to the patient's symptoms and other tests performed.

Related laboratory tests:

➤ Related laboratory tests include bacterial throat culture for gonorrhea, cervical biopsy, and *Chlamydia* group antibody.

PARATHYROID HORMONE: INTACT, C-TERMINAL, AND N-TERMINAL

SYNONYM/ACRONYM: Parathormone, PTH.

SPECIMEN: Serum (1 mL) collected in a red- or tiger-top tube. Specimen should be transported tightly capped and in an ice slurry.

REFERENCE VALUE: (Method: Immunoassay)

	Conventional Units	SI Units (Conventional Units × 1)
C-terminal		
1–16 y	51–217 pg/mL	51–217 ng/L
Adults	50–330 pg/mL	50–330 ng/L
N-terminal		
2–13 y	14–21 pg/mL	14–21 ng/L
Adult	8–24 pg/mL	8–24 ng/L
Intact		
Cord blood	Less than 3 pg/mL	Less than 3 ng/L
2–20 y	9–52 pg/mL	9–52 ng/L
Adult	10–65 pg/mL	10–65 ng/L

DESCRIPTION & RATIONALE: Parathyroid hormone (PTH) is secreted by the parathyroid glands in response to decreased levels of circulating calcium. PTH assists in the mobilization of calcium from bone into the bloodstream, promoting renal tubular reabsorption of calcium and depression of phosphate reabsorption, thereby reducing calcium excretion and increasing phosphate excretion by the kidneys. PTH also decreases the renal secretion of hydrogen ions, which leads to increased renal excretion of bicarbonate and chloride. PTH enhances renal production of active vitamin D metabolites, causing increased calcium absorption in the small intestine. The net result of PTH action is maintenance of adequate serum calcium levels. In normal individuals, intact PTH has a circulating half-life of about 5 minutes. N-terminal PTH has a circulating half-life of about 2 minutes and is found in very small quantities. Intact and N-terminal PTH are the only biologically active forms of the hormone. Ninety percent of circulating PTH is composed of inactive C-terminal and midregion fragments. PTH is cleared from the body by the kidneys. ∎

INDICATIONS:

- Assist in the diagnosis of hyperparathyroidism

- Assist in the diagnosis of suspected secondary hyperparathyroidism due to chronic renal failure, malignant tumors that produce ectopic PTH, and malabsorption syndromes

- Detect incidental damage or inadvertent removal of the parathyroid glands during thyroid or neck surgery

- Differentiate parathyroid and nonparathyroid causes of hypercalcemia

- Evaluate autoimmune destruction of the parathyroid glands

- Evaluate parathyroid response to altered serum calcium levels, especially those that result from malignant processes, leading to decreased PTH production

- Evaluate source of altered calcium metabolism

RESULT

Increased in:

- Fluorosis

- Primary, secondary, or tertiary hyperparathyroidism

- Pseudogout

- Pseudohypoparathyroidism

- Spinal cord trauma

- Zollinger-Ellison syndrome

Decreased in:

- Autoimmune destruction of the parathyroids

- DiGeorge syndrome

- Hyperthyroidism

- Hypomagnesemia

- Nonparathyroid hypercalcemia (in the absence of renal failure)

- Sarcoidosis

- Secondary hypoparathyroidism due to surgery

CRITICAL VALUES: N/A

INTERFERING FACTORS:

- Drugs that may increase PTH levels include clodronate, dopamine, estrogen/progestin therapy, foscarnet, furosemide, hydrocortisone, isoniazid, lithium, octreotide, pamidronate, phosphates, prednisone, tamoxifen, and verapamil.

- Drugs and vitamins that may decrease PTH levels include alfacalcidol, aluminum hydroxide, calcitriol, cimetidine (C-terminal only), diltiazem, magnesium sulfate, pindolol, prednisone (intact), and vitamin D.

- PTH levels are subject to diurnal variation, with highest levels occurring in the morning.

- PTH levels should always be measured in conjunction with calcium for proper interpretation.

- Failure to follow dietary restrictions before the procedure may cause the procedure to be canceled or repeated.

Nursing Implications and Procedure • • • • • • • • • •

Pretest:

➤ Inform the patient that the test is used to assist in the diagnosis of parathyroid disease and disorders of calcium balance. It is also used to monitor patients undergoing renal dialysis.

➤ Obtain a history of the patient's complaints, including a list of known allergens (especially allergies or sensitivities to latex), and inform the appropriate health care practitioner accordingly.

➤ Obtain a history of the patient's endocrine system and results of previously performed laboratory tests, surgical procedures, and other diagnostic procedures. For related laboratory tests, refer to the Endocrine System table.

➤ Obtain a list of the medications the patient is taking, including herbs, nutritional supplements, and nutraceuticals. The requesting health care practitioner and laboratory should be advised if the patient regularly uses these products so that their effects can be taken into consideration when reviewing results.

➤ Review the procedure with the patient. Early-morning specimen collection is recommended because of the diurnal variation in PTH levels. Inform the patient that specimen collection takes approximately 5 to 10 minutes. Address concerns about pain related to the procedure. Explain to the patient that there may be some discomfort during the venipuncture.

➤ The patient should fast for 12 hours before specimen collection.

➤ There are no fluid or medication restrictions, unless by medical direction.

➤ Prepare an ice slurry in a cup or plastic bag to have on hand for immediate transport of the specimen to the laboratory.

Intratest:

➤ Ensure that the patient has complied with dietary restrictions; assure that food has been restricted for at least 12 hours prior to the procedure.

➤ If the patient has a history of severe allergic reaction to latex, care should be taken to avoid the use of equipment containing latex.

➤ Instruct the patient to cooperate fully and to follow directions. Direct the patient to breathe normally and to avoid unnecessary movement.

➤ Observe standard precautions, and follow the general guidelines in Appendix A. Positively identify the patient, and label the appropriate tubes with the corresponding patient demographics, date, and time of collection. Perform a venipuncture; collect the specimen in a 5-mL red-top tube.

➤ Remove the needle, and apply a pressure dressing over the puncture site.

➤ Promptly transport the specimen to the laboratory for processing and analysis. The sample should be placed in an ice slurry immediately after collection. Information on the specimen label can be protected from water in the ice slurry if the specimen is first placed in a protective plastic bag.

➤ The results are recorded manually or in a computerized system for recall and postprocedure interpretation by the appropriate health care practitioner.

Post-test:

➤ Observe venipuncture site for bleeding or hematoma formation. Apply paper tape or other adhesive to hold pressure bandage in place, or replace with a plastic bandage.

➤ Instruct the patient to resume usual diet, as directed by the health care practitioner.

➤ *Nutritional considerations:* Patients with abnormal parathyroid levels are also likely to experience the effects of calcium level imbalances. Instruct the patient to report signs and symptoms of hypocalcemia and hypercalcemia to the health care practitioner. (For critical values, signs and symptoms of calcium imbalance, and nutritional information, see monographs titled "Calcium.")

➤ A written report of the examination will be sent to the requesting health care practitioner, who will discuss the results with the patient.

➤ Reinforce information given by the patient's health care provider regarding further testing, treatment, or referral to another health care provider. Answer any questions or address any concerns voiced by the patient or family.

➤ Depending on the results of this procedure, additional testing may be performed to evaluate or monitor progression of the disease process and determine the need for a change in therapy. Evaluate test results in relation to the patient's symptoms and other tests performed.

Related laboratory tests:

➤ Related laboratory tests include calcium (blood and ionized), blood and urine phosphorus, and vitamin D.

PARATHYROID SCAN

SYNONYM/ACRONYM: Parathyroid scintiscan.

AREA OF APPLICATION: Parathyroid.

CONTRAST: Intravenous technetium-99m (Tc-99m) pertechnetate, Tc-99m sestamibi, oral iodine-123, and thallium.

DESCRIPTION & RATIONALE: Parathyroid scanning is performed to assist in the preoperative localization of parathyroid adenomas in clinically proven primary hyperparathyroidism; it is useful for distinguishing between intrinsic and extrinsic parathyroid adenomas. It is also performed after surgery to verify the presence of the parathyroid gland in children, and it is done after thyroidectomy as well.

The radionuclide is administered 10 to 20 minutes before the imaging is performed. The thyroid and surrounding tissues should be carefully palpated.

Fine-needle aspiration biopsy guided by ultrasound is occasionally necessary to differentiate thyroid pathology, as well as pathology of other tissues, from parathyroid neoplasia. ■

INDICATIONS:
- Aid in the diagnosis of hyperparathyroidism
- Differentiate between extrinsic and intrinsic parathyroid adenoma, but not between benign and malignant conditions
- Evaluate the parathyroid in patients with severe hypercalcemia or in patients before parathyroidectomy

RESULT

Normal Findings:
- No areas of increased perfusion or uptake in the thyroid or parathyroid

Abnormal Findings:
- Intrinsic and extrinsic parathyroid adenomas

CRITICAL VALUES: N/A

INTERFERING FACTORS:

This procedure is contraindicated for:
- Patients who are pregnant or suspected of being pregnant, unless the potential benefits of the procedure far outweigh the risks to the fetus and mother

Factors that may impair clear imaging:
- Inability of the patient to cooperate or remain still during the procedure because of age, significant pain, or mental status

- Ingestion of foods containing iodine (e.g., iodized salt) and medications containing iodine (e.g., cough syrup, potassium iodide, vitamins, Lugol's solution, thyroid replacement medications), which can decrease uptake of the radionuclide

- Recent use of iodinated contrast medium for radiographic studies or recently performed nuclear medicine procedures, which can affect the uptake of the radionuclide

- Patients who are very obese, who may exceed the weight limit for the equipment

- Incorrect positioning of the patient, which may produce poor visualization of the area to be examined

- Metallic objects within the examination field (e.g., jewelry, body rings), which may inhibit organ visualization and can produce unclear images

Other considerations:

- Improper injection of the radionuclide that allows the tracer to seep deep into the muscle tissue produces erroneous hot spots.

- Consultation with a health care practitioner should occur before the procedure for radiation safety concerns regarding younger patients or patients who are lactating.

- Risks associated with radiographic overexposure can result from frequent x-ray procedures. Personnel in the room with the patient should stand behind a shield or leave the area while the examination is being done. Personnel working in the area where the examination is being done should wear badges that reveal their level of exposure to radiation.

Nursing Implications and Procedure • • • • • • • • • • •

Pretest:

➤ Inform the patient that the procedure assesses the parathyroid glands.

➤ Obtain a history of the patient's complaints and symptoms, including a list of known allergens.

➤ Obtain a history of the patient's immune system, as well as results of previously performed diagnostic procedures, surgical procedures, and laboratory tests. For related diagnostic tests, refer to the Immune System table.

➤ Record the date of the last menstrual period and determine the possibility of pregnancy in perimenopausal women.

➤ Obtain a list of the medications the patient is taking.

➤ Determine whether the patient has had any recent intake of iodine.

➤ Review the procedure with the patient. Address concerns about pain related to the procedure. Explain to the patient that some pain may be experienced during the test, and there may be moments of discomfort. Explain the purpose of the test and how the procedure is performed. Inform the patient that the procedure is performed in a nuclear medicine department, usually by a technologist and support staff, and takes approximately 30 to 60 minutes. Inform the patient that the technologist will administer an intravenous injection of the radionuclide and that he or she will need to return 2 to 3 hours later for the scan.

➤ Record the date of the last menstrual period. Note any recent procedures that can interfere with test results, including examinations using iodine-based contrast mediums or barium.

➤ Ensure that the patient has not been scheduled for more than one radionuclide scan on the same day. Multiple procedures on the same day may interfere with interpretation of results.

➤ *Sensitivity to cultural and social issues,* as well as concern for modesty, is important in providing psychological support before, during, and after the procedure.

➤ There are no food, fluid, or medication restrictions, unless by medical direction.

➤ Instruct the patient to remove dentures, jewelry (including watches), hairpins, credit cards, and other metallic objects.

Intratest:

➤ Make sure jewelry, chains, and any other metallic objects have been removed from the neck area.

➤ Patients are given a gown, robe, and foot coverings to wear and instructed to void prior to the procedure.

➤ Instruct the patient to cooperate fully and to follow directions. Instruct the patient to remain still throughout the procedure because movement produces unreliable results.

➤ Observe standard precautions, and follow the general guidelines in Appendix A.

➤ Wear gloves during the radionuclide injection and while handling the patient's urine.

➤ Administer technetium-99m (Tc-99m) pertechnetate intravenously before scanning.

➤ To scan the parathyroid gland, the patient is placed in a supine position under a radionuclide gamma camera 15 minutes after the radionuclide injection. Imaging is performed over the anterior neck area.

➤ With the patient in the same position, Tc-99m sestamibi is injected, and after 10 minutes a second image is obtained and stored in the computer. The computer subtracts the technetium-visualized thyroid structures from the thallium accumulation in a parathyroid adenoma.

➤ Iodine-123 may be administered orally in place of Tc-99m pertechnetate; the imaging sequence, as described previously, is performed 24 hours later.

➤ The images are recorded on film or stored electronically for recall and postprocedure interpretation by the appropriate health care practitioner.

Post-test:

➤ Assess injection site for bleeding, hematoma formation, and inflammation. Apply warm soaks to promote comfort if a hematoma develops.

➤ Advise patient to drink increased amounts of fluids for 24 to 48 hours to eliminate the radionuclide from the body, unless contraindicated. Tell the patient that radionuclide is eliminated from the body within 6 to 24 hours.

➤ Instruct the patient to flush the toilet immediately after each voiding following the procedure, and to wash hands meticulously with soap and water after each voiding for 24 hours after the procedure.

➤ Tell all caregivers to wear gloves when discarding urine for 24 hours after the procedure. Wash gloved hands with soap and water before removing gloves. Then wash hands after the gloves are removed.

➤ A written report of the examination will be completed by a health care practitioner specializing in this branch of medicine. The report will be sent to the requesting health care practitioner, who will discuss the results with the patient.

➤ Reinforce information given by the patient's health care provider regarding further testing, treatment, or referral to another health care provider. Answer any questions or address any concerns voiced by the patient or family.

➤ Depending on the results of this procedure, additional testing may be needed to evaluate or monitor progression of the disease process and determine the need for a change in therapy. Evaluate test results in relation to the patient's symptoms and other tests performed.

Related diagnostic tests:

➤ Related diagnostic tests include computed tomography of the thorax and magnetic resonance imaging of the chest.

PARTIAL THROMBOPLASTIN TIME, ACTIVATED

SYNONYM/ACRONYM: APTT.

SPECIMEN: Plasma (1 mL) collected in a completely filled blue-top (sodium citrate) tube.

REFERENCE VALUE: (Method: Clot detection) 25 to 39 seconds. Reference ranges vary with respect to the equipment and reagents used to perform the assay.

DESCRIPTION & RATIONALE: The activated partial thromboplastin time (APTT) coagulation test evaluates the function of the intrinsic (factors XII, XI, IX, and VIII) and common (factors V, X, II, and I) pathways of the coagulation sequence, specifically the intrinsic thromboplastin system. It represents the time required for a firm fibrin clot to form after tissue thromboplastin or phospholipid reagents similar to thromboplastin and calcium are added to the specimen. The APTT is abnormal in 90% of patients with coagulation disorders and is useful in monitoring the inactivation of factor II effect of heparin therapy. The test is prolonged when there is a 30% to 40% deficiency in one of the factors required, or when factor inhibitors (e.g., antithrombin III, protein C, or protein S) are present. The APTT has additional activators, such as kaolin, Celite, or elegiac acid, that more rapidly activate factor XII, making this test faster and more reliably reproducible than the partial thromboplastin time (PTT). A comparison between the results of APTT and prothrombin time (PT) tests can allow some inferences to be made that a factor deficiency exists. A normal APTT with a prolonged PT can only occur with factor VII deficiency. A prolonged APTT with a normal PT could indicate a deficiency in factors XII, XI, IX, VIII, and VIII:C (von Willebrand factor). Factor deficiencies can also be identified by correction or substitution studies using normal serum. These studies are easy to perform and are accomplished by adding plasma from a normal patient to a sample from a patient suspected to be factor deficient. When the APTT is repeated and is corrected, or within the reference range, it can be assumed that the prolonged APTT is caused by a factor deficiency. The administration of prophylactic low-dose heparin does not require serial monitoring of APTT. (For more information on factor deficiencies, see monograph titled "Fibrinogen.") ■

INDICATIONS:

- Detect congenital deficiencies in clotting factors, as seen in diseases such as hemophilia A (factor VIII) and hemophilia B (factor IX)
- Evaluate response to anticoagulant therapy with heparin or coumarin derivatives
- Identify individuals who may be prone to bleeding during surgical, obstetric, dental, or invasive diagnostic procedures
- Identify the possible cause of abnormal bleeding, such as epistaxis, hematoma, gingival bleeding, hematuria, and menorrhagia
- Monitor the hemostatic effects of conditions such as liver disease, protein deficiency, and fat malabsorption

RESULT

Prolonged in:

- Afibrinogenemia
- Circulating products of fibrin and fibrinogen degradation
- Disseminated intravascular coagulation
- Factor deficiencies
- Hemodialysis patients
- Polycythemia
- Severe liver disease
- Vitamin K deficiency
- Von Willebrand's disease

CRITICAL VALUES: N/A

Greater than 70 seconds.

The requesting health care practitioner should also be notified if the APTT is less than 53 seconds in a patient receiving heparin therapy. Low values indicate that the therapy is providing inadequate anticoagulation.

Note and immediately report to the health care practitioner any critically increased or decreased values and related symptoms. Important signs to note are prolonged bleeding, hematoma at the puncture site, hemorrhage, blood in the stool, bleeding gums, and shock. Monitoring vital signs and neurologic changes until values are within normal range is indicated. Administration of protamine sulfate may be requested.

INTERFERING FACTORS:

- Drugs and vitamins such as anistreplase, antihistamines, chlorpromazine, salicylates, and ascorbic acid may cause prolonged APTT.
- Anticoagulant therapy with heparin will prolong the APTT.
- Copper is a component of factor V, and severe copper deficiencies may result in prolonged APTT values.
- Traumatic venipunctures can activate the coagulation sequence by contamination of the sample with tissue thromboplastin and can produce falsely shortened results.
- Failure to fill the tube sufficiently to yield a proper blood-to-anticoagulant ratio invalidates the results and is reason for specimen rejection.
- Excessive agitation that causes sample hemolysis can falsely shorten the APTT because the hemolyzed cells activate plasma-clotting factors.
- Inadequate mixing of the tube can produce erroneous results.
- Specimens left unprocessed for longer than 4 hours should be rejected for analysis.
- High platelet count or inadequate centrifugation will result in decreased values.
- Hematocrit greater than 55% may cause falsely prolonged results because of anticoagulant excess. The excess anticoagulant chelates the calcium reagent in the test system, making it unavailable to react properly with the patient sample.

Nursing Implications and Procedure • • • • • • • • • • •

➤ Inform the patient that the test is used to evaluate coagulation disorders and monitor therapy.

➤ Obtain a history of the patient's complaints, including a list of known allergens (especially allergies or sensitivities to latex), and inform the appropriate health care practitioner accordingly.

➤ Obtain a history of the patient's hematopoietic and hepatobiliary systems, history of any bleeding disorders, and results of previously performed laboratory tests (especially bleeding time, complete blood count, PTT, platelets, and PT), surgical procedures, and other diagnostic procedures. For related laboratory tests, refer to the Hematopoietic and Hepatobiliary System tables.

➤ Obtain a list of the medications the patient is taking, including anticoagulant therapy, acetylsalicylic acid, herbs, nutritional supplements, and nutraceuticals, especially those known to affect coagulation. It is recommended that use of these products be discontinued 14 days before dental or surgical procedures. The requesting health care practitioner and laboratory should be advised if the patient regularly uses these products so that their effects can be taken into consideration when reviewing results. If the patient is receiving anticoagulant therapy, note the time and amount of the last dose.

➤ Review the procedure with the patient. Inform the patient that specimen collection takes approximately 5 to 10 minutes. Address concerns about pain related to the procedure. Explain to the patient that there may be some discomfort during the venipuncture.

➤ There are no food, fluid, or medication restrictions, unless by medical direction.

➤ Instruct the patient to cooperate fully and to follow directions. Direct the patient to breathe normally and to avoid unnecessary movement.

➤ Observe standard precautions, and follow the general guidelines in Appendix A. Positively identify the patient, and label the appropriate tubes with the corresponding patient demographics, date, and time of collection. Perform a venipuncture; collect the specimen in a 5-mL blue-top tube. Fill the tube completely. *Important note:* Two different concentrations of sodium citrate preservative are currently added to blue-top tubes for coagulation studies: 3.2% and 3.8%. The Clinical and Laboratory Standards Institute/CLSI (formerly the National Committee for Clinical Laboratory Standards/NCCLS) guideline for sodium citrate is 3.2%. Laboratories establish reference ranges for coagulation testing based on numerous factors, including sodium citrate concentration, test equipment, and test reagents. It is important to inquire from the laboratory which concentration it recommends, because each concentration will have its own specific reference range.

➤ When multiple specimens are drawn, the blue-top tube should be collected after sterile (i.e., blood culture) and red-top tubes. When coagulation testing is the only work to be done, an extra red-top tube should be collected before the blue-top tube to avoid contaminating the specimen with tissue thromboplastin.

➤ Promptly transport the specimen to the laboratory for processing and analysis. The CLSI recommendation for processed and unprocessed specimens stored in unopened tubes is that testing should be completed within 1 to 4 hours of collection.

➤ The results are recorded manually or in a computerized system for recall and postprocedure interpretation by the appropriate health care practitioner.

Post-test:

➤ Observe venipuncture site for bleeding or hematoma formation. Apply paper tape or other adhesive to hold pressure bandage in place, or replace with a plastic bandage.

➤ Instruct the patient to report severe bruising or bleeding from any areas of the skin or mucous membranes.

➤ Inform the patient with prolonged APTT values of the importance of taking precautions against bruising and bleeding, including the use of a soft bristle toothbrush, use of an electric razor, avoidance of constipation, avoidance of acetylsalicylic acid and similar products, and avoidance of intramuscular injections.

➤ Inform the patient of the importance of periodic laboratory testing while taking an anticoagulant.

➤ A written report of the examination will be sent to the requesting health care practitioner, who will discuss the results with the patient.

➤ Reinforce information given by the patient's health care provider regarding further testing, treatment, or referral to another health care provider. Answer any questions or address any concerns voiced by the patient or family.

➤ Depending on the results of this procedure, additional testing may be performed to evaluate or monitor progression of the disease process and determine the need for a change in therapy. Evaluate test results in relation to the patient's symptoms and other tests performed.

Related laboratory tests:

➤ Related laboratory tests include antithrombin III, bleeding time, coagulation factors, complete blood count, copper, fibrin degradation products, platelet count, protein C, protein S, prothrombin time and International Normalized Ratio, and vitamin K.

PARVOVIRUS B19 IMMUNOGLOBULIN G AND IMMUNOGLOBULIN M ANTIBODIES

• •

SYNONYM/ACRONYM: N/A.

SPECIMEN: Serum (2 mL) collected in a red- or tiger-top tube.

REFERENCE VALUE: (Method: Immunoassay)

| Negative | Less than 0.8 |
| Equivocal | 0.8–1.2 |

DESCRIPTION & RATIONALE: Parvovirus B19, a single-stranded DNA virus transmitted by respiratory secretions, is the only parvovirus known to infect humans. Its primary site of replication is in red blood cell precursors in the bone marrow. It is capable of causing disease along a wide spectrum ranging from a self-limited erythema (fifth disease) to bone marrow failure or aplastic crisis in patients with sickle cell anemia, spherocytosis, or thalassemia. Fetal hydrops and spontaneous abortion may also occur as a result of infection during pregnancy. The incubation period is approximately 1 week after exposure. B19-specific antibodies appear in the serum approximately 3 days after the onset of symptoms. The presence of immunoglobulin M (IgM) antibodies indicates acute infection. The presence of IgG antibodies indicates past infection and is believed to confer lifelong immunity. Parvovirus can also be detected by DNA hybridization using a polymerase chain reaction. ▪

INDICATIONS: Assist in establishing a diagnosis of parvovirus B19 infection

RESULT

Positive findings in:
• Arthritis

• Erythema infectiosum (fifth disease)

• Erythrocyte aplasia

• Hydrops fetalis

Negative findings in: N/A

CRITICAL VALUES: N/A

INTERFERING FACTORS: Immunocompromised patients may not develop sufficient antibody to be detected.

Nursing Implications and Procedure

Pretest:

➤ Inform the patient that the test is used to assist in confirming past or present parvovirus infection.

➤ Obtain a history of the patient's complaints, including a list of known allergens (especially allergies or sensitivities to latex), and inform the appropriate health care practitioner accordingly.

➤ Obtain a history of the patient's immune system and results of previously performed laboratory tests, surgical procedures, and other diagnostic procedures. For related laboratory tests, refer to the Immune System table.

➤ Obtain a list of the medications the patient is taking, including herbs, nutritional supplements, and nutraceuticals. The requesting health care practitioner and laboratory should be advised if the patient regularly uses these products so that their effects can be taken into consideration when reviewing results.

➤ Review the procedure with the patient. Inform the patient that specimen collection takes approximately 5 to 10 minutes. Inform the patient that a subsequent sample will be required in 7 to 14 days. Address concerns about pain related to the procedure. Explain to the patient that there may be some discomfort during the venipuncture.

➤ There are no food, fluid, or medication restrictions, unless by medical direction.

Intratest:

➤ If the patient has a history of severe allergic reaction to latex, care should

be taken to avoid the use of equipment containing latex.

➤ Instruct the patient to cooperate fully and to follow directions. Direct the patient to breathe normally and to avoid unnecessary movement.

➤ Observe standard precautions, and follow the general guidelines in Appendix A. Positively identify the patient, and label the appropriate tubes with the corresponding patient demographics, date, and time of collection. Perform a venipuncture; collect the specimen in a 5-mL red- or tiger-top tube.

➤ Remove the needle, and apply a pressure dressing over the puncture site.

➤ Promptly transport the specimen to the laboratory for processing and analysis.

➤ The results are recorded manually or in a computerized system for recall and postprocedure interpretation by the appropriate health care practitioner.

Post-test:

➤ Observe venipuncture site for bleeding or hematoma formation. Apply paper tape or other adhesive to hold pressure bandage in place, or replace with a plastic bandage.

➤ A written report of the examination will be sent to the requesting health care practitioner, who will discuss the results with the patient.

➤ Recognize anxiety related to test results, and be supportive of impaired activity related to lack of neuromuscular control, perceived loss of independence, and fear of shortened life expectancy. Discuss the implications of abnormal test results on the patient's lifestyle. Provide teaching and information regarding the clinical implications of the test results, as appropriate. Educate the patient regarding access to counseling services. Provide contact information, if desired, for the Myasthenia Gravis Foundation of America *(http://www.myasthenia. org)* and Muscular Dystrophy Association *(http://www.mdausa.org).*

➤ Reinforce information given by the patient's health care provider regarding further testing, treatment, or referral to another health care provider. Emphasize the need for the patient to return to have a convalescent blood sample taken in 7 to 14 days. Answer any questions or address any concerns voiced by the patient or family.

➤ Depending on the results of this procedure, additional testing may be performed to evaluate or monitor progression of the disease process and determine the need for a change in therapy. Evaluate test results in relation to the patient's symptoms and other tests performed.

Related laboratory tests:

➤ Related laboratory tests include bone marrow biopsy, complete blood count, hemoglobin electrophoresis, red blood cell morphology, and sickle cell screen.

PERICARDIAL FLUID ANALYSIS

SYNONYM/ACRONYM: None.

SPECIMEN: Pericardial fluid (5 mL) collected in a red- or green-top (heparin) tube for glucose, a lavender-top (EDTA) tube for cell count, and sterile containers for microbiology specimens; 200 to 500 mL of fluid in a clear container for cytology. Ensure that there is an equal amount of fluid relative to fixative in the container for cytology.

REFERENCE VALUE: (Method: Spectrophotometry for glucose; automated or manual cell count, macroscopic examination of cultured organisms, and microscopic examination of specimen for microbiology and cytology; microscopic examination of cultured microorganisms)

Pericardial Fluid	Reference Value
Appearance	Clear
Color	Pale yellow
Glucose	Parallel serum values
Red blood cell count	None seen
White blood cell count	Less than 1000/mm^3
Culture	No growth
Gram stain	No organisms seen
Cytology	No abnormal cells seen

DESCRIPTION & RATIONALE: The heart is located within a protective membrane called the *pericardium*. The fluid between the pericardial membranes is called *serous fluid*. Normally only a small amount of fluid is present because the rates of fluid production and absorption are about the same. Many abnormal conditions can result in the buildup of fluid within the pericardium. Specific tests are usually ordered in addition to a common battery of tests used to distinguish a transudate from an exudate. *Transudates* are effusions that form as a result of a systemic disorder that disrupts the regulation of fluid balance, such as a suspected perforation. *Exudates* are caused by conditions involving the tissue of the membrane itself, such as an infection or malignancy. Fluid is withdrawn from the pericardium by needle aspiration and tested as listed in the previous and following tables. ■

Characteristic	Transudate	Exudate
Appearance	Clear	Cloudy or turbid
Specific gravity	Less than 1.015	Greater than 1.015
Total protein	Less than 2.5 g/dL	Greater than 3.0 g/dL
Fluid–to–serum protein ratio	Less than 0.5	Greater than 0.5
LDH	Parallels serum value	Less than 200 U/L
Fluid–to–serum LDH ratio	Less than 0.6	Greater than 0.6
Fluid cholesterol	Less than 55 mg/dL	Greater than 55 mg/dL
White blood cell count	Less than 100/mm^3	Greater than 1000/mm^3

LDH = lactate dehydrogenase.

INDICATIONS:
- Evaluate effusion of unknown etiology
- Investigate suspected hemorrhage, immune disease, malignancy, or infection

RESULT

Increased in (condition/test showing increased result):
- Bacterial pericarditis (red blood cell [RBC] count, white blood cell [WBC] count with a predominance of neutrophils)
- Hemorrhagic pericarditis (RBC count, WBC count)
- Malignancy (RBC count, abnormal cytology)
- Post–myocardial infarction syndrome, also called Dressler's syndrome (RBC count, WBC count with a predominance of neutrophils)
- Rheumatoid disease or systemic lupus erythematosus (RBC count, WBC count)
- Tuberculous or fungal pericarditis (RBC count, WBC count with a predominance of lymphocytes)
- Viral pericarditis (RBC count, WBC count with a predominance of neutrophils)

Decreased in (condition/test showing decreased result):
- Bacterial pericarditis (glucose)
- Malignancy (glucose)
- Rheumatoid disease or systemic lupus erythematosus (glucose)

CRITICAL VALUES:
Note and immediately report to the health care practitioner positive culture results, if ordered, and related symptoms.

INTERFERING FACTORS:
- Bloody fluid may be the result of a traumatic tap.
- Unknown hyperglycemia or hypoglycemia may be misleading in the comparison of fluid and serum glucose levels. Therefore, it is advisable to collect comparative serum samples a few hours before performing pericardiocentesis.
- Failure to follow dietary restrictions before the procedure may cause the procedure to be canceled or repeated.

Nursing Implications and Procedure • • • • • • • • • • • •

Pretest:

> Inform the patient that the test is primarily used to classify the type of

effusion being produced and identify the cause of its accumulation.

➤ Obtain a history of the patient's complaints, including a list of known allergens (especially allergies or sensitivities to latex), and inform the appropriate health care practitioner accordingly.

➤ Obtain a history of the patient's cardiovascular and immune systems, any bleeding disorders, and results of previously performed laboratory tests (especially bleeding time, complete blood count, partial thromboplastin time, platelets, and prothrombin time), surgical procedures, and other diagnostic procedures. For related laboratory tests, refer to the Cardiovascular and Immune System tables.

➤ Note any recent procedures that can interfere with test results.

➤ Record the date of the last menstrual period and determine the possibility of pregnancy in perimenopausal women.

➤ Obtain a list of the medications the patient is taking, including anticoagulant therapy, acetylsalicylic acid, herbs, nutritional supplements, and nutraceuticals, especially those known to affect coagulation. The requesting health care practitioner and laboratory should be advised if the patient regularly uses these products so that their effects can be taken into consideration when reviewing results.

➤ Review the procedure with the patient. Inform the patient that it may be necessary to shave the site before the procedure. Address concerns about pain related to the procedure. Explain that a sedative and/or analgesia will be administered to promote relaxation and reduce discomfort prior to needle insertion through the chest wall. Explain to the patient that any discomfort with the needle insertion will be minimized with local anesthetics and systemic analgesics. Explain that the anesthetic injection may cause a stinging sensation. Explain that, after the skin has been anesthetized, a large needle will be inserted through the chest to obtain the fluid. Inform the patient that specimen collection is performed under sterile conditions by a health care practitioner specializing in this procedure. The procedure usually takes approximately 30 minutes to complete.

➤ Explain that an intravenous (IV) line will be inserted to allow infusion of IV fluids, antibiotics, anesthetics, and analgesics.

➤ *Sensitivity to social and cultural issues,* as well as concern for modesty, is important in providing psychological support before, during, and after the procedure.

➤ Food and fluids should be restricted for 6 to 8 hours before the procedure, as directed by the health care practitioner, unless the procedure is performed in an emergency situation to correct pericarditis. The requesting health care practitioner may request that anticoagulants and aspirin be withheld. The amount of days to withhold medication is dependent on the type of anticoagulant.

➤ *Make sure a written and informed consent has been signed prior to the procedure and before administering any medications.*

Intratest:

➤ Ensure that the patient has complied with dietary and fluids restrictions; assure that food has been restricted for at least 6 to 8 hours prior to the procedure.

➤ Ensure that anticoagulant therapy has been withheld for the appropriate amount of days prior to the procedure. Notify health care practitioner if patient anticoagulant therapy has not been withheld.

➤ Have emergency equipment readily available.

➤ Have the patient void before the procedure.

➤ Have the patient remove clothes above the waist and put on a gown.

➤ Instruct the patient to cooperate fully and to follow directions. Direct the patient to breathe normally and to avoid unnecessary movement during the local anesthetic and the procedure.

➤ Record baseline vital signs, and continue to monitor throughout the procedure. Protocols may vary from facility to facility.

➤ Observe standard precautions, and follow the general guidelines in Appendix A. Positively identify the patient, and label the appropriate collection containers with the corresponding patient demographics, date and time of collection, and site location.

➤ Establish an IV line to allow infusion of IV fluids, anesthetics, analgesics, or IV sedation.

➤ Assist the patient into a comfortable supine position with the head elevated 45° to 60°.

➤ Prior to the administration of local anesthesia, cleanse the site with an antiseptic solution, and drape the area with sterile towels. The skin at the injection site is then anesthetized.

➤ The precordial (V) cardiac lead wire is attached to the cardiac needle with an alligator clip. The cardiac needle is inserted just below and to the left of the breastbone, and fluid is removed.

➤ Monitor vital signs every 15 minutes for signs of hypovolemia or shock. Monitor electrocardiogram for needle-tip positioning to indicate accidental puncture of the right atrium.

➤ The needle is withdrawn, and slight pressure is applied to the site. Apply a sterile dressing to the site.

➤ Monitor the patient for complications related to the procedure (e.g., allergic reaction, anaphylaxis).

➤ Place samples in properly labeled specimen container, and promptly transport the specimen to the laboratory for processing and analysis.

➤ The results are recorded manually or in a computerized system for recall and postprocedure interpretation by the appropriate health care practitioner.

Post-test:

➤ Instruct the patient to resume usual diet and medications, as directed by the health care practitioner.

➤ Monitor vital signs and cardiac status every 15 minutes for the first hour, every 30 minutes for the next 2 hours, every hour for the next 4 hours, and every 4 hours for the next 24 hours. Take the patient's temperature every 4 hours for 24 hours. Monitor intake and output for 24 hours. Notify the health care practitioner if temperature is elevated. Protocols may vary from facility to facility.

➤ Observe the patient for signs of respiratory and cardiac distress, such as shortness of breath, cyanosis, or rapid pulse.

➤ Continue IV fluids until vital signs are stable and the patient can resume fluid intake independently.

➤ Inform the patient that 1 hour or more of bed rest is required after the procedure.

➤ Assess the puncture site for bleeding or drainage and signs of inflammation each time vital signs are taken and daily thereafter for several days. Report to health care practitioner if bleeding is present.

➤ Assess for nausea and pain. Administer antiemetic and analgesic medications as needed and as directed by the health care practitioner.

➤ Administer antibiotics, as ordered, and instruct the patient in the importance of completing the entire course of antibiotic therapy even if no symptoms are present.

➤ A written report of the examination will be completed by a health care practitioner specializing in this branch of medicine. The report will be sent to the requesting health care practitioner, who will discuss the results with the patient.

▶ Recognize anxiety related to test results, and offer support. Discuss the implications of abnormal test results on the patient's lifestyle. Provide teaching and information regarding the clinical implications of the test results, as appropriate. Educate the patient regarding access to counseling services, if appropriate.

▶ Reinforce information given by the patient's health care provider regarding further testing, treatment, or referral to another health care provider. Answer any questions or address any concerns voiced by the patient or family.

▶ Depending on the results of this procedure, additional testing may be performed to evaluate or monitor progression of the disease process and determine the need for a change in therapy. Evaluate test results in relation to the patient's symptoms and other tests performed.

Related laboratory tests:

▶ Related laboratory tests include aspartate aminotransferase, atrial natriuretic peptide, bacterial culture, blood gases, B-type natriuretic peptide, CA 15–3, CA 19–9, CA 125, carcinoembryonic antigen, creatine kinase and isoenzymes, α_1-fetoprotein, fungal culture, homocysteine, lactate dehydrogenase and isoenzymes, magnesium, mycobacterial culture, myoglobin, troponin, and viral culture.

PERITONEAL FLUID ANALYSIS

SYNONYM/ACRONYM: Ascites fluid analysis.w

SPECIMEN: Peritoneal fluid (5 mL) collected in a red- or green-top (heparin) tube for amylase, glucose, and alkaline phosphatase; lavender-top (EDTA) tube for cell count; sterile containers for microbiology specimens; 200 to 500 mL of fluid in a clear container with anticoagulant for cytology. Ensure that there is an equal amount of fluid relative to fixative in the container for cytology.

REFERENCE VALUE: (Method: Spectrophotometry for glucose, amylase, and alkaline phosphatase; automated or manual cell count, macroscopic examination of cultured organisms, and microscopic examination of specimen for microbiology and cytology; microscopic examination of cultured microorganisms)

Peritoneal Fluid	Reference Value
Appearance	Clear
Color	Pale yellow
Amylase	Parallel serum values

Peritoneal Fluid	Reference Value
Alkaline phosphatase	Parallel serum values
Glucose	Parallel serum values
Red blood cell count	Less than 100,000/mm^3
White blood cell count	Less than 300/mm^3
Culture	No growth
Acid-fast stain	No organisms seen
Gram stain	No organisms seen
Cytology	No abnormal cells seen

DESCRIPTION & RATIONALE: The peritoneal cavity and organs within it are lined with a protective membrane. The fluid between the membranes is called *serous fluid*. Normally only a small amount of fluid is present because the rates of fluid production and absorption are about the same. Many abnormal conditions can result in the buildup of fluid within the peritoneal cavity. Specific tests are usually ordered in addition to a common battery of tests used to distinguish a transudate from an exudate.

Transudates are effusions that form as a result of a systemic disorder that disrupts the regulation of fluid balance, such as a suspected perforation. *Exudates* are caused by conditions involving the tissue of the membrane itself, such as an infection or malignancy. Fluid is withdrawn from the peritoneal cavity by needle aspiration and tested as listed in the previous and following tables. ∎

INDICATIONS:
• Evaluate ascites of unknown cause

Characteristic	Transudate	Exudate
Appearance	Clear	Cloudy or turbid
Specific gravity	Less than 1.015	Greater than 1.015
Total protein	Less than 2.5 g/dL	Greater than 3.0 g/dL
Fluid-to–serum protein ratio	Less than 0.5	Greater than 0.5
LDH	Parallels serum value	Less than 200 U/L
Fluid-to–serum LDH ratio	Less than 0.6	Greater than 0.6
Fluid cholesterol	Less than 55 mg/dL	Greater than 55 mg/dL
White blood cell count	Less than 100/mm^3	Greater than 1000/mm^3

LDH = lactate dehydrogenase.

• Investigate suspected peritoneal rupture, perforation, malignancy, or infection

RESULT

Increased in (condition/test showing increased result):

• Abdominal malignancy (red blood cell [RBC] count, carcinoembryonic antigen, abnormal cytology)

• Abdominal trauma (RBC count greater than 100,000/mm^3)

• Ascites caused by cirrhosis (white blood cell [WBC] count, neutrophils greater than 25% but less than 50%, absolute granulocyte count greater than 250/mm³)

• Bacterial peritonitis (WBC count, neutrophils greater than 50%, absolute granulocyte count greater than 250/mm³)

• Peritoneal effusion due to gastric strangulation, perforation, or necrosis (amylase, ammonia, alkaline phosphatase)

• Peritoneal effusion due to pancreatitis, pancreatic trauma, or pancreatic pseudocyst (amylase)

• Rupture or perforation of urinary bladder (ammonia, creatinine, urea)

• Tuberculous effusion (elevated lymphocyte count, positive acid-fast bacillus smear and culture [25% to 50% of cases])

Decreased in (condition/test showing decreased result):
• Abdominal malignancy (glucose)

• Tuberculous effusion (glucose)

CRITICAL VALUES:
Note and immediately report to the health care practitioner positive culture results, if ordered, and related symptoms.

INTERFERING FACTORS:
• Bloody fluids may result from a traumatic tap.

• Unknown hyperglycemia or hypoglycemia may be misleading in the comparison of fluid and serum glucose levels. Therefore, it is advisable to collect comparative serum samples a few hours before performing paracentesis.

Nursing Implications and Procedure

Pretest:

➤ Inform the patient that the test is primarily used to classify the type of

effusion being produced and identify the cause of its accumulation.

➤ Obtain a history of the patient's complaints, including a list of known allergens (especially allergies or sensitivities to latex), and inform the appropriate health care practitioner accordingly.

➤ Obtain a history of the patient's gastrointestinal and immune systems, any bleeding disorders, and results of previously performed laboratory tests (especially bleeding time, complete blood count, partial thromboplastin time, platelets, and prothrombin time), surgical procedures, and other diagnostic procedures. For related laboratory tests, refer to the Gastrointestinal and Immune System tables.

➤ Note any recent procedures that can interfere with test results.

➤ Record the date of the last menstrual period and determine the possibility of pregnancy in perimenopausal women.

➤ Obtain a list of the medications the patient is taking, including anticoagulant therapy, acetylsalicylic acid, herbs, nutritional supplements, and nutraceuticals, especially those known to affect coagulation. The requesting health care practitioner and laboratory should be advised if the patient regularly uses these products so that their effects can be taken into consideration when reviewing results.

➤ Review the procedure with the patient. If patient has ascites, obtain weight and measure abdominal girth. Inform the patient that it may be necessary to shave the site before the procedure. Address concerns about pain related to the procedure. Explain that a sedative and/or analgesia will be administered to promote relaxation and reduce discomfort prior to needle insertion through the abdomen wall. Explain to the patient that any discomfort with the needle insertion will be minimized with local anesthetics and systemic analgesics. Explain that the anesthetic injection may cause an initial stinging sensation. Explain that, after the skin has been anesthetized, a large needle will be inserted through the abdominal wall and a "popping" sensation may be experienced as the needle penetrates the peritoneum. Inform the patient that specimen collection is performed under sterile conditions by a health care practitioner specializing in this procedure. The procedure usually takes approximately 30 minutes to complete.

➤ Explain that an intravenous (IV) line will be inserted to allow infusion of IV fluids, antibiotics, anesthetics, and analgesics.

➤ *Sensitivity to social and cultural issues,* as well as concern for modesty, is important in providing psychological support before, during, and after the procedure.

➤ There are no food or fluid restrictions, unless by medical direction. The requesting health care practitioner may request that anticoagulants and aspirin be withheld. The amount of days to withhold medication is dependent on the type of anticoagulant.

➤ *Make sure a written and informed consent has been signed prior to the procedure and before administering any medications.*

Intratest:

➤ Ensure that anticoagulant therapy has been withheld for the appropriate amount of days prior to the procedure. Notify the health care practitioner if patient anticoagulant therapy has not been withheld.

➤ Have emergency equipment readily available.

➤ Have the patient void or catheterize the patient to avoid accidental puncture of the bladder if he or she is unable to void.

➤ Have the patient remove clothing and change into a gown for the procedure.

➤ Instruct the patient to cooperate fully and to follow directions. Direct the patient to breathe normally and to avoid unnecessary movement during the local anesthetic and the procedure.

➤ Observe standard precautions, and follow the general guidelines in Appendix A. Positively identify the patient, and label the appropriate collection containers with the corresponding patient demographics, date and time of collection, and site location.

➤ Record baseline vital signs and continue to monitor throughout the procedure. Protocols may vary from facility to facility.

➤ Establish an IV line to allow infusion of IV fluids, anesthetics, analgesics, or IV sedation.

➤ Assist the patient to a comfortable seated position with feet and back supported or in high Fowler's position.

➤ Prior to the administration of local anesthesia, shave and cleanse the site with an antiseptic solution, and drape the area with sterile towels. The skin at the injection site is then anesthetized.

➤ The paracentesis needle is inserted 1 to 2 inches below the umbilicus, and fluid is removed. If lavage fluid is required (helpful if malignancy is suspected), saline or Ringer's lactate can be infused via the needle over a 15- to 20-minute period before the lavage fluid is removed. Monitor vital signs every 15 minutes for signs of hypovolemia or shock.

➤ No more than 1500 to 2000 mL of fluid should be removed at a time, even in the case of a therapeutic paracentesis, because of the risk of hypovolemia and shock.

➤ The needle is withdrawn, and slight pressure applied to the site. Apply a sterile dressing to the site.

➤ Monitor the patient for complications related to the procedure (e.g., allergic reaction, anaphylaxis).

➤ Place samples in properly labeled specimen container, and promptly transport the specimen to the laboratory for processing and analysis.

▶ The results are recorded manually or in a computerized system for recall and postprocedure interpretation by the appropriate health care practitioner.

Post-test:

▶ Instruct the patient to resume usual medications, as directed by the health care practitioner.

▶ Monitor vital signs every 15 minutes for the first hour, every 30 minutes for the next 2 hours, every hour for the next 4 hours, and every 4 hours for the next 24 hours. Take the patient's temperature every 4 hours for 24 hours. Monitor intake and output for 24 hours. Notify the health care practitioner if temperature is elevated. Protocols may vary from facility to facility.

▶ Assess the puncture site for bleeding or drainage and signs of inflammation each time vital signs are taken and daily thereafter for several days. Report to health care practitioner if bleeding is present.

▶ If a large amount of fluid was removed, obtain weight and measure abdominal girth.

▶ Inform the patient that 1 hour or more of bed rest is required after the procedure.

▶ Instruct the patient to immediately report severe abdominal pain (*note:* rigidity of abdominal muscles indicates developing peritonitis). Report to health care practitioner if abdominal rigidity or pain is present.

▶ Assess for nausea and pain. Administer antiemetic and analgesic medications as needed and as directed by the health care practitioner.

▶ Administer antibiotics, as ordered, and instruct the patient in the importance of completing the entire course of antibiotic therapy even if no symptoms are present.

▶ A written report of the examination will be completed by a health care practitioner specializing in this branch of medicine. The report will be sent to the requesting health care practitioner, who will discuss the results with the patient.

▶ Recognize anxiety related to test results, and offer support. Discuss the implications of abnormal test results on the patient's lifestyle. Provide teaching and information regarding the clinical implications of the test results, as appropriate. Educate the patient regarding access to counseling services, if appropriate.

▶ Reinforce information given by the patient's health care provider regarding further testing, treatment, or referral to another health care provider. Answer any questions or address any concerns voiced by the patient or family.

▶ Depending on the results of this procedure, additional testing may be performed to evaluate or monitor progression of the disease process and determine the need for a change in therapy. Evaluate test results in relation to the patient's symptoms and other tests performed.

Related laboratory tests:

▶ Related laboratory tests include bacterial culture, CA 15-3, CA 19-9, CA 125, carcinoembryonic antigen, fungal culture, mycobacterial culture, and viral culture.

PHOSPHORUS, BLOOD

- -

SYNONYMS/ACRONYM: Inorganic phosphorus, phosphate, PO_4.

SPECIMEN: Serum (1 mL) collected in a red- or tiger-top tube. Plasma (1 mL) collected in green-top (heparin) tube is also acceptable.

REFERENCE VALUE: (Method: Spectrophotometry)

Age	Conventional Units	SI Units (Conventional Units × 0.323)
0–5 d	4.6–8.0 mg/dL	1.5–2.6 mmol/L
1–3 y	3.9–6.5 mg/dL	1.3–2.1 mmol/L
4–6 y	4.0–5.4 mg/dL	1.3–1.7 mmol/L
7–11 y	3.7–5.6 mg/dL	1.2–1.8 mmol/L
12–13 y	3.3–5.4 mg/dL	1.1–1.7 mmol/L
14–15 y	2.9–5.4 mg/dL	0.9–1.7 mmol/L
16–19 y	2.8–4.6 mg/dL	0.9–1.5 mmol/L
Adult	2.5–4.5 mg/dL	0.8–1.4 mmol/L

DESCRIPTION & RATIONALE: Phosphorus, in the form of phosphate, is distributed throughout the body. Approximately 85% of the body's phosphorus is stored in bones; the remainder is found in cells and body fluids. It is the major intracellular anion and plays a crucial role in cellular metabolism, maintenance of cellular membranes, and formation of bones and teeth. Phosphorus also indirectly affects the release of oxygen from hemoglobin by affecting the formation of 2,3-bisphosphoglycerate. Levels of phosphorus are dependent on dietary intake.

Phosphorus excretion is regulated by the kidneys. Calcium and phosphorus are interrelated with respect to absorption and metabolic function. They have an inverse relationship with respect to concentration: serum phosphorus is increased when serum calcium is decreased. Hyperphosphatemia can result in an infant fed only cow's milk during the first few weeks of life because of the combination of a high phosphorus content in cow's milk and the inability of infants' kidneys to clear the excess phosphorus. ■

INDICATIONS:
- Assist in establishing a diagnosis of hyperparathyroidism

- Assist in the evaluation of renal failure

RESULT

Increased in:
- Acromegaly
- Bone metastases
- Diabetic ketoacidosis
- Excessive levels of vitamin D
- Hyperthermia
- Hypocalcemia
- Hypoparathyroidism
- Lactic acidosis
- Milk alkali syndrome
- Pseudohypoparathyroidism
- Pulmonary embolism
- Renal failure
- Respiratory acidosis

Decreased in:
- Acute gout
- Alcohol withdrawal
- Gram-negative bacterial septicemia
- Growth hormone deficiency
- Hyperalimentation therapy
- Hypercalcemia
- Hyperinsulinism
- Hyperparathyroidism
- Hypokalemia
- Impaired renal absorption
- Malabsorption syndromes
- Malnutrition
- Osteomalacia
- Parathyroid hormone–producing tumors
- Primary hyperparathyroidism
- Renal tubular acidosis
- Renal tubular defects

- Respiratory alkalosis
- Respiratory infections
- Rickets
- Salicylate poisoning
- Severe burns
- Severe vomiting and diarrhea
- Vitamin D deficiency

CRITICAL VALUES:

Values less than 1.0 mg/dL may have significant effects on the neuromuscular, gastrointestinal, cardiopulmonary, and skeletal systems.

Note and immediately report to the health care practitioner any critically increased or decreased values and related symptoms. Interventions including intravenous (IV) replacement therapy with sodium or potassium phosphate may be necessary. Close monitoring of both phosphorus and calcium is important during replacement therapy.

INTERFERING FACTORS:

- Drugs that may increase phosphorus levels include anabolic steroids, β-adrenergic blockers, ergocalciferol, furosemide, hydrochlorothiazide, methicillin (occurs with nephrotoxicity), oral contraceptives, parathyroid extract, phosphates, sodium etidronate, tetracycline (occurs with nephrotoxicity), and vitamin D.

- Drugs that may decrease phosphorus levels include acetazolamide, albuterol, aluminum salts, amino acids (via IV hyperalimentation), anesthetic agents, anticonvulsants, calcitonin, epinephrine, fibrin hydrolysate, fructose, glucocorticoids, glucose, insulin, mannitol, oral contraceptives, pamidronate, phenothiazine, phytate, and plicamycin.

- Serum phosphorus levels are subject to diurnal variation: They are highest in late morning and lowest in the evening;

therefore, serial samples should be collected at the same time of day for consistency in interpretation.

- Hemolysis will falsely increase phosphorus values.

- Specimens should never be collected above an IV line because of the potential for dilution when the specimen and the IV solution combine in the collection container, thereby falsely decreasing the result. There is also the potential of contaminating the sample with the substance of interest, if it is present in the IV solution, thereby falsely increasing the result.

Nursing Implications and Procedure • • • • • • • • • •

➤ Inform the patient that the test is used to assist in the general evaluation of multiple body systems.

➤ Obtain a history of the patient's complaints, including a list of known allergens (especially allergies or sensitivities to latex), and inform the appropriate health care practitioner accordingly.

➤ Obtain a history of the patient's endocrine, gastrointestinal, genitourinary, and musculoskeletal systems, as well as results of previously performed laboratory tests, surgical procedures, and other diagnostic procedures. For related laboratory tests, refer to the Endocrine, Gastrointestinal, Genitourinary, and Musculoskeletal System tables.

➤ Obtain a list of the medications the patient is taking, including herbs, nutritional supplements, and nutraceuticals. The requesting health care practitioner and laboratory should be advised if the patient regularly uses these products so that their effects can be taken into consideration when reviewing results.

➤ Review the procedure with the patient. Inform the patient that specimen collection takes approximately 5 to 10 minutes. Address concerns about pain related to the procedure. Explain to the patient that there may be some discomfort during the venipuncture.

➤ There are no food, fluid, or medication restrictions, unless by medical direction.

Intratest:

➤ If the patient has a history of severe allergic reaction to latex, care should be taken to avoid the use of equipment containing latex.

➤ Instruct the patient to cooperate fully and to follow directions. Direct the patient to breathe normally and to avoid unnecessary movement.

➤ Observe standard precautions, and follow the general guidelines in Appendix A. Positively identify the patient, and label the appropriate tubes with the corresponding patient demographics, date, and time of collection. Perform a venipuncture; collect the specimen in a 5-mL red- or tiger-top tube.

➤ Remove the needle, and apply a pressure dressing over the puncture site.

➤ Promptly transport the specimen to the laboratory for processing and analysis.

➤ The results are recorded manually or in a computerized system for recall and postprocedure interpretation by the appropriate health care practitioner.

Post-test:

➤ Observe venipuncture site for bleeding or hematoma formation. Apply paper tape or other adhesive to hold pressure bandage in place, or replace with a plastic bandage.

➤ *Nutritional considerations:* Severe hypophosphatemia is common in elderly patients or patients who have been hospitalized for long periods of time. Good dietary sources of phosphorus include meat, dairy products, nuts, and legumes.

➤ *Nutritional considerations:* To decrease phosphorus levels to normal in the patient with hyperphosphatemia, dietary restriction may be recommended. Other interventions may include the administration of phosphate binders or administration of calcitriol (the activated form of vitamin D).

➤ A written report of the examination will be sent to the requesting health care practitioner, who will discuss the results with the patient.

➤ Reinforce information given by the patient's health care provider regarding further testing, treatment, or referral to another health care provider.

Answer any questions or address any concerns voiced by the patient or family.

➤ Depending on the results of this procedure, additional testing may be performed to evaluate or monitor progression of the disease process and determine the need for a change in therapy. Evaluate test results in relation to the patient's symptoms and other tests performed.

Related laboratory tests:

➤ Related laboratory tests include calcitonin, calcium, collagen cross-linked N-telopeptides, growth hormone, kidney stone analysis, osteocalcin, parathyroid hormones, urine phosphorus, and vitamin D.

PHOSPHORUS, URINE

· ·

SYNONYM/ACRONYM: Urine phosphate.

SPECIMEN: Urine (5 mL) from an unpreserved random or timed specimen collected in a clean plastic collection container.

REFERENCE VALUE: (Method: Spectrophotometry) Reference values are dependent on phosphorus and calcium intake. Phosphate excretion exhibits diurnal variation and is significantly higher at night.

Conventional Units	SI Units (Conventional Units × 32.3)
0.4–1.3 g/24 h	12.9–42.0 g/24 h

DESCRIPTION & RATIONALE: Phosphorus, in the form of phosphate, is distributed throughout the body. Approximately 85% of the body's

phosphorus is stored in bones; the remainder is found in cells and body fluids. It is the major intracellular anion and plays a crucial role in cellular metabolism, maintenance of cellular membranes, and formation of bones and teeth. Phosphorus also indirectly affects the release of oxygen from hemoglobin by affecting the formation of 2,3-bisphosphoglycerate. Levels of phosphorus are dependent on dietary intake.

Analyzing urinary phosphorus levels can provide important clues to the functioning of the kidneys and other major organs. Tests for phosphorus in urine usually involve timed urine collections over a 12- or 24-hour period. Measurement of random specimens may also be requested. Children with thalassemia may have normal phosphorus absorption but increased excretion, which may result in a phosphorus deficiency. ■

INDICATIONS:
• Assist in the diagnosis of hyperparathyroidism

• Assist in the evaluation of calcium and phosphorus balance

• Assist in the evaluation of nephrolithiasis

• Assist in the evaluation of renal tubular disease

RESULT

Increased in:
• Abuse of diuretics

• Primary hyperparathyroidism

• Renal tubular acidosis

• Vitamin D deficiency

Decreased in:
• Hypoparathyroidism

• Pseudohypoparathyroidism

• Vitamin D intoxication

CRITICAL VALUES: N/A

INTERFERING FACTORS:
• Drugs and vitamins that can cause an increase in urine phosphorus levels include acetazolamide, acetylsalicylic acid, alanine, bismuth salts, calcitonin, corticosteroids, dihydrotachysterol, glycine, hydrochlorothiazide, metolazone, parathyroid extract, parathyroid hormone, phosphates, tryptophan, valine, and vitamin D.

• Drugs that can cause a decrease in urine phosphorus levels include aluminum-containing antacids.

• Urine phosphorus levels are subject to diurnal variation: Output is highest in the afternoon, which is why 24-hour urine collections are recommended.

• All urine voided for the timed collection period must be included in the collection or else falsely decreased values may be obtained. Compare output records with volume collected to verify that all voids were included in the collection.

Nursing Implications and Procedure • • • • • • • • • • •

Pretest:

➤ Inform the patient that the test is used to evaluate calcium and phosphorus balance.

➤ Obtain a history of the patient's complaints, including a list of known allergens (especially allergies or sensitivities to latex), and inform the appropriate health care practitioner accordingly.

➤ Obtain a history of the patient's endocrine and genitourinary systems, as well as results results of previously performed laboratory tests, surgical procedures, and other diagnostic procedures. For related laboratory tests, refer to the Endocrine and Genitourinary System tables.

➤ Obtain a list of the medications the patient is taking, including herbs, nutritional supplements, and nutraceuticals. The requesting health care practitioner and laboratory should be advised if the patient regularly uses these products so that their effects can be taken into consideration when reviewing results.

➤ Review the procedure with the patient. Provide a nonmetallic urinal, bedpan, or toilet-mounted collection device. Address concerns about pain related to the procedure. Explain to the patient that there should be no discomfort during the procedure.

➤ Usually a 24-hour time frame for urine collection is ordered. Inform the patient that all urine must be saved during that 24-hour period. Instruct the patient not to void directly into the laboratory collection container. Instruct the patient to avoid defecating in the collection device and to keep toilet tissue out of the collection device to prevent contamination of the specimen. Place a sign in the bathroom to remind the patient to save all urine.

➤ Instruct the patient to void all urine into the collection device and then to pour the urine into the laboratory collection container. Alternatively, the specimen can be left in the collection device for a health care staff member to add to the laboratory collection container.

➤ *Sensitivity to social and cultural issues,* as well as concern for modesty, is important in providing psychological support before, during, and after the procedure.

➤ Instruct the patient to avoid excessive exercise and stress during the 24-hour collection of urine.

➤ There are no food, fluid, or medication restrictions, unless by medical direction.

Intratest:

➤ Ensure that the patient has complied with activity restrictions and pretesting preparations; assure that excessive exercise and stress have been restricted during the 24-hour procedure.

➤ If the patient has a history of severe allergic reaction to latex, care should be taken to avoid the use of equipment containing latex.

➤ Instruct the patient to cooperate fully and to follow directions.

➤ Observe standard precautions, and follow the general guidelines in Appendix A. Positively identify the patient, and label the appropriate tubes with the corresponding patient demographics, date, and time of collection.

Random specimen (collect in early morning):

Clean-catch specimen:

➤ Instruct the male patient to (1) thoroughly wash his hands, (2) cleanse the meatus, (3) void a small amount into the toilet, and (4) void directly into the specimen container.

➤ Instruct the female patient to (1) thoroughly wash her hands; (2) cleanse the labia from front to back; (3) while keeping the labia separated, void a small amount into the toilet; and (4) without interrupting the urine stream, void directly into the specimen container.

Indwelling catheter:

➤ Put on gloves. Empty drainage tube of urine. It may be necessary to clamp off the catheter for 15 to 30 minutes before specimen collection. Cleanse specimen port with antiseptic swab, and then aspirate 5 mL of urine with a 21- to 25-gauge needle and syringe. Transfer urine to a sterile container.

Timed specimen:

➤ Obtain a clean 3-L urine specimen container, toilet-mounted collection device, and plastic bag (for transport of the specimen container). The specimen must be refrigerated or kept on ice throughout the entire collection period. If an indwelling urinary catheter is in place, the drainage bag must be kept on ice.

➤ Begin the test between 6 and 8 a.m.,

if possible. Collect first voiding and discard. Record the time the specimen was discarded as the beginning of the timed collection period. The next morning, ask the patient to void at the same time the collection was started and add this last voiding to the container.

➤ If an indwelling catheter is in place, replace the tubing and container system at the start of the collection time. Keep the container system on ice during the collection period, or empty the urine into a larger container periodically during the collection period; monitor to ensure continued drainage, and conclude the test the next morning at the same hour the collection was begun.

➤ At the conclusion of the test, compare the quantity of urine with the urinary output record for the collection; if the specimen contains less than what was recorded as output, some urine may have been discarded, invalidating the test.

➤ Include on the collection container's label the amount of urine, test start and stop times, and ingestion of any foods or medications that can affect test results.

General:

➤ Promptly transport the specimen to the laboratory for processing and analysis.

➤ The results are recorded manually or in a computerized system for recall and postprocedure interpretation by the appropriate health care practitioner.

➤ *Nutritional considerations:* Vitamin D is necessary for the body to absorb phosphorus. Vitamin D is added to food products such as milk, cheese, and orange juice. The recommended daily intake of vitamin D is 200 IU per day.

➤ Increased urine phosphorus levels may be associated with the formation of kidney stones. Educate the patient, if appropriate, on the importance of drinking a sufficient amount of water when kidney stones are suspected.

➤ A written report of the examination will be sent to the requesting health care practitioner, who will discuss the results with the patient.

➤ Recognize anxiety related to test results. Discuss the implications of abnormal test results on the patient's lifestyle. Provide teaching and information regarding the clinical implications of the test results, as appropriate.

➤ Reinforce information given by the patient's health care provider regarding further testing, treatment, or referral to another health care provider. Answer any questions or address any concerns voiced by the patient or family.

➤ Depending on the results of this procedure, additional testing may be performed to evaluate or monitor progression of the disease process and determine the need for a change in therapy. Evaluate test results in relation to the patient's symptoms and other tests performed.

➤ Related laboratory tests include calcitonin, blood and urine calcium, kidney stone analysis, parathyroid hormone, blood phosphorus, and urinalysis.

PLASMINOGEN

. . . .

SYNONYM/ACRONYM: Profibrinolysin, PMG.

SPECIMEN: Plasma (1 mL) collected in blue-top (sodium citrate) tube.

REFERENCE VALUE: (Method: Chromogenic substrate) 80% to 120% of normal for plasma.

DESCRIPTION & RATIONALE: Plasminogen is a plasma glycoprotein. It is the circulating, inactive precursor to plasmin. Damaged tissues release a substance called *plasminogen activator* that initiates the conversion of plasminogen to plasmin. Plasmin participates in fibrinolysis and is capable of degrading fibrin, factor I (fibrinogen), factor V, and factor VIII. (For more information on fibrin degradation, see monograph titled "Fibrinogen.") ∎

INDICATIONS: Evaluate the level of circulating plasminogen in patients with thrombosis or disseminated intravascular coagulation (DIC)

RESULT

Increased in:
• Pregnancy (late)

Decreased in:
• DIC
• Fibrinolytic therapy with tissue plasminogen activators such as streptokinase or urokinase
• Hereditary deficiency
• Liver disease
• Neonatal hyaline membrane disease
• Postsurgical period

CRITICAL VALUES: N/A

INTERFERING FACTORS: Drugs that may decrease plasminogen levels include streptokinase and urokinase.

Nursing Implications and Procedure . . . .

Pretest:

▶ Inform the patient that the test is used to evaluate thrombotic disorders and monitor thrombolytic therapy.

▶ Obtain a history of the patient's complaints, including a list of known allergens (especially allergies or sensitivities to latex), and inform the appropriate health care practitioner accordingly.

▶ Obtain a history of the patient's hematopoietic system and results of previously performed laboratory tests, surgical procedures, and other diagnostic procedures. For related laboratory tests, refer to the Hematopoietic System table.

▶ Obtain a list of the medications the patient is taking, including herbs, nutritional supplements, and nutraceuticals. The requesting health care practitioner and laboratory should be advised if the patient regularly uses these products so that their effects can be taken into consideration when reviewing results.

> Review the procedure with the patient. Inform the patient that specimen collection takes approximately 5 to 10 minutes. Address concerns about pain related to the procedure. Explain to the patient that there may be some discomfort during the venipuncture.

> There are no food, fluid, or medication restrictions, unless by medical direction.

Intratest:

> If the patient has a history of severe allergic reaction to latex, care should be taken to avoid the use of equipment containing latex.

> Instruct the patient to cooperate fully and to follow directions. Direct the patient to breathe normally and to avoid unnecessary movement.

> Observe standard precautions and follow the general guidelines in Appendix A. Positively identify the patient and label the appropriate tubes with the corresponding patient demographics, date, and time of collection. Perform a venipuncture; collect the specimen in a 5-mL blue-top tube. *Important note:* Two different concentrations of sodium citrate preservative are currently added to blue-top tubes for coagulation studies: 3.2% and 3.8%. The Clinical and Laboratory Standards Institute/CLSI (formerly the National Committee for Clinical Laboratory Standards/ NCCLS) guideline for sodium citrate is 3.2%. Laboratories establish reference ranges for coagulation testing based on numerous factors, including sodium citrate concentration, test equipment, and test reagents. It is important to inquire from the laboratory which concentration it recommends, because each concentration will have its own specific reference range.

> When multiple specimens are drawn, the blue-top tube should be collected after sterile (i.e., blood culture) and red-top tubes. When coagulation testing is the only work to be done, an extra red-top tube should be collected before the blue-top tube to avoid contaminating the specimen with tissue thromboplastin, which can falsely decrease values.

> Remove the needle, and apply a pressure dressing over the puncture site.

> Promptly transport the specimen to the laboratory for processing and analysis. The CLSI recommendation for processed and unprocessed specimens stored in unopened tubes is that testing should be completed within 1 to 4 hours of collection.

> The results are recorded manually or in a computerized system for recall and postprocedure interpretation by the appropriate health care practitioner.

Post-test:

> Observe venipuncture site for bleeding or hematoma formation. Apply paper tape or other adhesive to hold pressure bandage in place, or replace with a plastic bandage.

> A written report of the examination will be sent to the requesting health care practitioner, who will discuss the results with the patient.

> Reinforce information given by the patient's health care provider regarding further testing, treatment, or referral to another health care provider. Answer any questions or address any concerns voiced by the patient or family.

> Depending on the results of this procedure, additional testing may be performed to evaluate or monitor progression of the disease process and determine the need for a change in therapy. Evaluate test results in relation to the patient's symptoms and other tests performed.

Related laboratory tests:

> Related laboratory tests include coagulation factors, fibrin degradation products, and fibrinogen.

PLATELET ANTIBODIES

SYNONYMS/ACRONYMS: Antiplatelet antibody; platelet-bound IgG/IgM, direct and indirect.

SPECIMEN: Serum (1 mL) collected in a red-top tube for indirect immunoglobulin G (IgG) antibody. Whole blood (7 mL) collected in lavender-top (EDTA) tube for direct antibody.

REFERENCE VALUE: (Method: Solid-phase hemagglutination and flow cytometry) Negative.

DESCRIPTION & RATIONALE: Platelet antibodies can be formed by autoimmune response, or they can be acquired in reaction to transfusion products. Platelet autoantibodies are immunoglobulins of autoimmune origin (i.e., immunoglobulin G), and they are present in various autoimmune disorders, including thrombocytopenias. Platelet alloantibodies develop in patients who become sensitized to platelet antigens of transfused blood. As a result, destruction of both donor and native platelets occurs along with a shortened survival time of platelets in the transfusion recipient. The platelet antibody detection test is also used for platelet typing, which allows compatible platelets to be transfused to patients with disorders such as aplastic anemia and cancer. Platelet typing decreases the alloimmunization risk resulting from repeated transfusions from random donors. Platelet typing may also provide additional support for a diagnosis of post-transfusional purpura. ∎

INDICATIONS:
- Assist in the detection of platelet alloimmune disorders
- Determine platelet type for refractory patients

RESULT

Increased in:
- Acquired immunodeficiency syndrome
- Acute myeloid leukemia
- Idiopathic thrombocytopenic purpura
- Immune complex diseases
- Multiple blood transfusions
- Multiple myeloma
- Neonatal immune thrombocytopenia
- Paroxysmal hemoglobinuria
- Rheumatoid arthritis
- Systemic lupus erythematosus
- Thrombocytopenias provoked by drugs (see monograph titled "Platelet Count")

Decreased in: N/A

CRITICAL VALUES: N/A

INTERFERING FACTORS: Hemolyzed or clotted specimens will affect results.

Nursing Implications and Procedure • • • • • • • • • • •

➤ Inform the patient that the test is used to evaluate thrombocytopenia.

➤ Obtain a history of the patient's complaints, including a list of known allergens (especially allergies or sensitivities to latex), and inform the appropriate health care practitioner accordingly.

➤ Obtain a history of the patient's hematopoietic and immune systems, a history of any bleeding disorders, and results of previously performed laboratory tests (especially bleeding time, complete blood count, partial thromboplastin time, prothrombin time, and platelets), surgical procedures, and other diagnostic procedures. For related laboratory tests, refer to the Hematopoietic and Immune System tables.

➤ Obtain a list of the medications the patient is taking, including include anticoagulant therapy, acetylsalicylic acid, herbs, nutritional supplements, and nutraceuticals, especially those known to affect coagulation. It is recommended that use be discontinued 14 days before dental or surgical procedures. The requesting health care practitioner and laboratory should be advised if the patient regularly uses these products so that their effects can be taken into consideration when reviewing results.

➤ Review the procedure with the patient. Inform the patient that specimen collection takes approximately 5 to 10 minutes. Address concerns about pain related to the procedure. Explain to the patient that there may be some discomfort during the venipuncture.

➤ There are no food, fluid, or medication restrictions, unless by medical direction.

➤ If the patient has a history of severe allergic reaction to latex, care should be taken to avoid the use of equipment containing latex.

➤ Instruct the patient to cooperate fully and to follow directions. Direct the patient to breathe normally and to avoid unnecessary movement.

➤ Observe standard precautions, and follow the general guidelines in Appendix A. Positively identify the patient, and label the appropriate tubes with the corresponding patient demographics, date, and time of collection. Perform a venipuncture; collect the specimen in a 5-mL red-top and a 7-mL lavender-top tube.

➤ Remove the needle, and apply a pressure dressing over the puncture site.

➤ Promptly transport the specimen to the laboratory for processing and analysis.

➤ The results are recorded manually or in a computerized system for recall and postprocedure interpretation by the appropriate health care practitioner.

➤ Observe venipuncture site for bleeding or hematoma formation. Apply paper tape or other adhesive to hold pressure bandage in place, or replace with a plastic bandage.

➤ Note the patient's response to platelet transfusions.

➤ Instruct the patient to report severe bruising or bleeding from any areas of the skin or mucous membranes.

➤ Inform the patient who has developed platelet antibodies of the importance of taking precautions against bruising and bleeding, including the use of a soft bristle toothbrush, use of an electric razor, avoidance of constipation, avoidance of acetylsalicylic acid and similar products, and avoidance of intramuscular injections.

➤ A written report of the examination will be sent to the requesting health

care practitioner, who will discuss the results with the patient.

➤ Reinforce information given by the patient's health care provider regarding further testing, treatment, or referral to another health care provider. Answer any questions or address any concerns voiced by the patient or family.

➤ Depending on the results of this procedure, additional testing may be performed to evaluate or monitor progression of the disease process and determine the need for a change in therapy. Evaluate test results in relation to the patient's symptoms and other tests performed.

Related laboratory tests:

➤ Related laboratory tests include bleeding time, clot retraction, and platelet count.

PLATELET COUNT

SYNONYM/ACRONYM: Thrombocytes.

SPECIMEN: Whole blood from one full lavender-top (EDTA) tube.

REFERENCE VALUE: (Method: Automated, computerized multichannel analyzers that sort and size cells on the basis of either changes in electrical impedance or light pulses as the cells pass in front of a laser)

Age	Platelet Count*	SI Units (Conventional Units × 10⁶)	MPV (fL)
1–5 y	217–497 × 10^3/µL or 217,000–497,000/mm^3 or 217–497 × 10^3/mm^3	217–497 × 10^9/L	7.2–10.0
Adult	150–450 × 10^3/µL or 150,000–400,000/mm^3 or 150–400 × 10^3/mm^3	150–450 × 10^9/L	7.0–10.2

Note: Platelet counts decrease with age.
*Conventional units.
MPV = mean platelet volume.

DESCRIPTION & RATIONALE: *Platelets* are non-nucleated, cytoplasmic, round or oval disks formed by budding off of large, multinucleated cells (megakaryocytes). Platelets have an essential function in coagulation, hemostasis, and blood thrombus formation. *Thrombocytosis* is an increase in platelet count. In reactive thrombocytosis, the increase is transient and short lived, and it usually does not pose a health risk. One exception may be reactive thrombocytosis occurring after coronary bypass surgery. This circumstance has been identified as an important risk factor for postoperative infarction and thrombosis. The term *thrombocythemia* is used to describe platelet increases associated with chronic myeloproliferative disorders; *thrombocytopenia* is used to describe platelet counts of less than $140 \times 10^3/\mu L$. Decreased platelet counts occur whenever the body's need for platelets exceeds the rate of platelet production; this circumstance will arise if production rate decreases or platelet loss increases. The severity of bleeding is related to platelet count as well as platelet function. Platelet counts can be within normal limits, but the patient may exhibit signs of internal bleeding; this circumstance usually indicates an anomaly in platelet function. Abnormal scatterplot findings by automated cell counters may indicate the need to review a smear of peripheral blood for platelet estimate. Abnormally large or giant platelets may result in underestimation of automated counts by 30% to 50%. A large discrepancy between the automated count and the estimate requires that a manual count be performed.

The significance of platelet sizing is becoming more widely known, as modern cell counters are capable of reporting platelet indexes that are analogous to red blood cell (RBC) indices. Platelet size, reflected by mean platelet volume (MPV), and cellular age are inversely related; that is, younger platelets tend to be larger. An increase in MPV indicates an increase in platelet turnover. Therefore, in a normal patient the platelet count and MPV have an inverse relationship. Abnormal platelet size may also indicate the presence of a disorder. MPV and platelet distribution width (PDW) are both increased in idiopathic thrombocytopenic purpura. MPV is also increased in May-Hegglin anomaly, Bernard-Soulier syndrome, myeloproliferative disorders, hyperthyroidism, and pre-eclampsia. MPV is decreased in Wiskott-Aldrich syndrome, septic thrombocytopenia, and hypersplenism. ∎

INDICATIONS:
- Confirm an elevated platelet count (thrombocytosis), which can cause increased clotting
- Confirm a low platelet count (thrombocytopenia), which can be associated with bleeding
- Identify the possible cause of abnormal bleeding, such as epistaxis, hematoma, gingival bleeding, hematuria, and menorrhagia
- Provide screening as part of a complete blood count in a general physical examination, especially upon admission to a health care facility or before surgery

RESULT

Increased in:
- Acute infections
- After exercise (transient)
- Anemias (posthemorrhagic, hemolytic, iron-deficiency)
- Chronic heart disease
- Cirrhosis
- Essential thrombocythemia
- Leukemias (chronic)

- Malignancies (carcinoma, Hodgkin's, lymphomas)
- Pancreatitis (chronic)
- Polycythemia vera
- Rebound recovery from thrombocytopenia
- Rheumatic fever (acute)
- Rheumatoid arthritis
- Splenectomy (2 months postprocedure)
- Surgery (2 weeks postprocedure)
- Trauma
- Tuberculosis
- Ulcerative colitis

Decreased in (as a result of megakaryocytic hypoproliferation):
- Alcohol toxicity
- Aplastic anemia
- Congenital states (Fanconi's syndrome, May Hegglin anomaly, Bernard-Soulier syndrome, Wiskott-Aldrich syndrome, Gaucher's disease, Chédiak-Higashi syndrome)
- Drug toxicity
- Prolonged hypoxia

Decreased in (as a result of ineffective thrombopoiesis):
- Ethanol abuse without malnutrition
- Iron-deficiency anemia
- Megaloblastic anemia (B_{12}/folate deficiency)
- Paroxysmal nocturnal hemoglobinuria
- Thrombopoietin deficiency
- Viral infection

Decreased in (as a result of bone marrow replacement):
- Lymphoma
- Granulomatous infections

- Metastatic carcinoma
- Myelofibrosis

Increased destruction in (as a result of increased loss/consumption):
- Contact with foreign surfaces (dialysis membranes, artificial organs, grafts, prosthetic devices)
- Disseminated intravascular coagulation
- Extensive transfusion
- Severe hemorrhage
- Thrombotic thrombocytopenic purpura
- Uremia

Increased destruction in (as a result of immune reaction):
- Antibody/human leukocyte antigen reactions
- Hemolytic disease of the newborn (target is platelets instead of RBCs)
- Idiopathic thrombocytopenic purpura
- Refractory reaction to platelet transfusion

Increased destruction in (as a result of immune reaction secondary to infection):
- Bacterial infections
- Burns
- Congenital infections (cytomegalovirus, herpes, syphilis, toxoplasmosis)
- Histoplasmosis
- Malaria
- Rocky Mountain spotted fever

Increased destruction in (as a result of other causes):
- Radiation
- Splenomegaly caused by liver disease

CRITICAL VALUES:
Less than 50,000 × 10^3/µL (or 50 × 10^3/mm³ or 50,000/mm³)

Greater than 1,000 × 10³/μL (or 1,000,000/mm³)

Note and immediately report to the health care practitioner any critically increased or decreased values and related symptoms. Possible interventions for decreased platelet count may include transfusion of platelets.

INTERFERING FACTORS:
- Drugs that may decrease platelet counts include acetohexamide, acetophenazine, amphotericin B, antazoline, anticonvulsants, antimony compounds, apronalide, arsenicals, azathioprine, barbiturates, benzene, busulfan, butaperazine, chlordane, chlorophenothane, chlortetracycline, dactinomycin, dextromethorphan, diethylstilbestrol, ethinamate, ethoxzolamide, floxuridine, hexachlorobenzene, hydantoin derivatives, hydroflumethiazide, hydroxychloroquine, iproniazid, mechlorethamine, mefenamic acid, mepazine, miconazole, mitomycin, nitrofurantoin, novobiocin, nystatin, phenolphthalein, phenothiazine, pipamazine, plicamycin, procarbazine, pyrazolones, streptomycin, sulfonamides, tetracycline, thiabendazole, thiouracil, tolazamide, tolazoline, tolbutamide, trifluoperazine, and urethane.

- Drugs that may increase platelet counts include glucocorticoids.

- X-ray therapy may also decrease platelet counts.

- The results of blood counts may vary depending on the patient's position. Platelet counts can decrease when the patient is recumbent, as a result of hemodilution, and can increase when the patient rises, as a result of hemoconcentration.

- Platelet counts normally increase under a variety of stressors, such as high altitudes or strenuous exercise.

- Platelet counts are normally decreased before menstruation and during pregnancy.

- Leaving the tourniquet in place for longer than 60 seconds can affect the results.

- Traumatic venipunctures may lead to erroneous results as a result of activation of the coagulation sequence.

- Failure to fill the tube sufficiently (i.e., tube less than three-quarters full) may yield inadequate sample volume for automated analyzers and may be a reason for specimen rejection.

- Hemolysis or clotted specimens are reasons for rejection.

- Complete blood count should be carefully evaluated after transfusion or acute blood loss because the value may appear to be normal.

- A white blood cell count greater than 100,000/mm³, severe RBC fragmentation, and extraneous particles in the fluid used to dilute the sample can alter test results.

Nursing Implications and Procedure

Pretest:

➤ Inform the patient that the test is used to evaluate, diagnose, and monitor bleeding disorders.

➤ Obtain a history of the patient's complaints, including a list of known allergens (especially allergies or sensitivities to latex), and inform the appropriate health care practitioner accordingly.

➤ Obtain a history of the patient's hematopoietic and immune systems, a history of any bleeding disorders, and results of previously performed laboratory tests (especially bleeding time, complete blood count, partial thromboplastin time, prothrombin time, and platelets), surgical procedures, and other diagnostic procedures. For related laboratory tests, refer to the Hematopoietic and Immune System tables.

➤ Note any recent procedures that can interfere with test results.

➤ Obtain a list of the medications the patient is taking, including antico-agulant therapy, acetylsalicylic acid, herbs, nutritional supplements, and nutraceuticals, especially those known to affect coagulation. It is recommended that use be discontinued 14 days before dental or surgical procedures. The requesting health care practitioner and laboratory should be advised if the patient regularly uses these products so that their effects can be taken into consideration when reviewing results.

➤ Review the procedure with the patient. Inform the patient that specimen collection takes approximately 5 to 10 minutes. Address concerns about pain related to the procedure. Explain to the patient that there may be some discomfort during the venipuncture.

➤ *Sensitivity to social and cultural issues,* as well as concern for modesty, is important in providing psychological support before, during, and after the procedure.

➤ There are no food, fluid, or medication restrictions, unless by medical direction.

Intratest:

➤ If the patient has a history of severe allergic reaction to latex, care should be taken to avoid the use of equipment containing latex.

➤ Instruct the patient to cooperate fully and to follow directions. Direct the patient to breathe normally and to avoid unnecessary movement.

➤ Observe standard precautions, and follow the general guidelines in Appendix A. Positively identify the patient, and label the appropriate tubes with the corresponding patient demographics, date, and time of collection. Perform a venipuncture; collect the specimen in a 5-mL lavender-top tube. The specimen should be mixed gently by inverting the tube 10 times. The specimen should be analyzed within 6 hours when stored at room temperature or within 24 hours if stored at refrigerated temperature. If it is anticipated the specimen will not be analyzed within 4 to 6 hours, two blood smears should be made immediately after the venipuncture and submitted with the blood sample.

➤ Remove the needle, and apply a pressure dressing over the puncture site.

➤ Promptly transport the specimen to the laboratory for processing and analysis.

➤ The results are recorded manually or in a computerized system for recall and postprocedure interpretation by the appropriate health care practitioner.

Post-test:

➤ Observe venipuncture site for bleeding or hematoma formation. Apply paper tape or other adhesive to hold pressure bandage in place, or replace with a plastic bandage.

➤ Instruct the patient to report bleeding from any areas of the skin or mucous membranes.

➤ Inform the patient with a decreased platelet count of the importance of taking precautions against bruising and bleeding, including the use of a soft bristle toothbrush, use of an electric razor, avoidance of constipation, avoidance of acetylsalicylic acid and similar products, and avoidance of intramuscular injections.

➤ Inform the patient of the importance of periodic laboratory testing if he or she is taking an anticoagulant.

➤ *Nutritional considerations:* Instruct patients to consume a variety of foods within the basic food groups, maintain a healthy weight, be physically active, limit salt intake, limit alcohol intake, and be a nonsmoker.

➤ A written report of the examination will be sent to the requesting health care practitioner, who will discuss the results with the patient.

➤ Recognize anxiety related to test

results. Discuss the implications of abnormal test results on the patient's lifestyle. Provide teaching and information regarding the clinical implications of the test results, as appropriate.

➤ Reinforce information given by the patient's health care provider regarding further testing, treatment, or referral to another health care provider. Answer any questions or address any concerns voiced by the patient or family.

➤ Depending on the results of this procedure, additional testing may be performed to evaluate or monitor progression of the disease process and determine the need for a change in therapy. Evaluate test results in relation to the patient's symptoms and other tests performed.

Related laboratory tests:

➤ Related laboratory tests include antiarrhythmic drugs (quinidine), bleeding time, clot retraction, complete blood count, platelet antibodies, RBC morphology and inclusions, and white blood cell count and differential.

PLETHYSMOGRAPHY

· ·

SYNONYM/ACRONYM: Impedance plethysmography, PVR.

AREA OF APPLICATION: Veins, arteries, and lungs.

CONTRAST: Done without contrast.

DESCRIPTION & RATIONALE: Plethysmography is a noninvasive diagnostic manometric study used to measure changes in the size of blood vessels by determining volume changes in the blood vessels of the eye, extremities, and neck; or to measure gas volume changes in the lungs.

Arterial plethysmography assesses arterial circulation in an upper or lower limb; it is used to diagnose extremity arteriosclerotic disease and to rule out occlusive disease. The test requires a normal extremity for comparison of results. The test is performed by applying a series of three blood pressure cuffs to the extremity. The amplitude of each pulse wave is then recorded.

Venous plethysmography, done with a series of cuffs, measures changes in venous capacity and outflow (volume and rate of outflow); it is used to diagnose a thrombotic condition that causes obstruction of the major veins of the extremity. When the cuffs are applied to an extremity in patients with venous obstruction, no initial increase in leg volume is recorded because the venous volume of the leg cannot dissipate quickly.

Body plethysmography measures the total amount (volume) of air within the thorax, whether or not the air is in ventilatory communication with the lung; the elasticity (compliance) of the lungs; and the resistance to airflow in the respiratory tree. It is used in conjunction with pulmonary stress testing and pulmonary function testing.

Impedance plethysmography is widely used to detect acute deep vein thrombosis (DVT) of the leg, but it can also be used in the arm, abdomen, neck, or thorax. Doppler flow studies now are used to identify DVT, but ultrasound studies are less accurate in examinations below the knee. ∎

INDICATIONS

Arterial Plethysmography:

- Confirm suspected acute arterial embolization

- Detect vascular changes associated with Raynaud's phenomenon and disease

- Determine changes in toe or finger pressures when ankle pressures are elevated as a result of arterial calcifications

- Determine the effect of trauma on the arteries in an extremity

- Determine peripheral small-artery changes (ischemia) caused by diabetes, and differentiate these changes from neuropathy

- Evaluate suspected arterial occlusive disease

- Locate and determine the degree of arterial atherosclerotic obstruction and vessel patency in peripheral atherosclerotic disease, as well as inflammatory changes causing obliteration in the vessels in thromboangiitis obliterans

Venous Plethysmography:

- Detect partial or total venous thrombotic obstruction

- Determine valve competency in conjunction with Doppler ultrasonography in the diagnosis of varicose veins

Body Plethysmography:

- Detect acute pulmonary disorders, such as atelectasis

- Detect or determine the status of chronic obstructive pulmonary disease (COPD), such as emphysema, asthma, or chronic bronchitis

- Detect or determine the status of restrictive pulmonary disease, such as fibrosis

- Detect infectious pulmonary diseases, such as pneumonia

- Determine baseline pulmonary status before pulmonary rehabilitation to determine potential therapeutic benefit

- Differentiate between obstructive and restrictive pulmonary pathology

Impedance Plethysmography:

- Act as a diagnostic screen for patients at risk for DVT

- Detect and evaluate DVT

- Evaluate degree of resolution of DVT after treatment

- Evaluate patients with suspected pulmonary embolism (most pulmonary emboli are complications of DVT in the leg)

RESULT

Normal Findings:

- Arterial plethysmography:

  Normal arterial pulse waves: steep upslope, more gradual downslope with narrow pointed peaks

  Normal pressure: less than 20 mm Hg systolic difference between the lower and upper extremities;

toe pressure greater than or equal to 80% of ankle pressure, and finger pressure greater than or equal to 80% of wrist pressure

- Venous plethysmography:
  Normal venous blood flow in the extremities
  Venous filling times greater than 20 seconds

- Body plethysmography:
  Thoracic gas volume: 2400 mL
  Compliance: 0.2 L/cm H_2O
  Airway resistance: 0.6 to 2.5 cm H_2O/L per second

- Impedance plethysmography:
  Sharp rise in volume with temporary occlusion
  Rapid venous outflow with release of the occlusion

Abnormal Findings:

- COPD, restrictive lung disease, lung infection, or atelectasis (body plethysmography)
- DVT (arterial, venous, or impedance plethysmography)
- Incompetent valves, thrombosis, or thrombotic obstruction in a major vein in an extremity
- Small-vessel diabetic changes
- Vascular disease (Raynaud's phenomenon)
- Vascular trauma

CRITICAL VALUES: N/A

INTERFERING FACTORS

Arterial Plethysmography:

Factors that may impair results of the examination:
- Cigarette smoking 2 hours before the study, which causes inaccurate results

because the nicotine constricts the arteries

- Alcohol consumption
- Low cardiac output
- Shock
- Compression of pelvic veins (tumors or external compression by dressings)
- Environmental temperatures (hot or cold)
- Arterial occlusion proximal to the extremity to be examined, which can prevent blood flow to the limb

Venous Plethysmography:

Factors that may impair results of the examination:
- Low environmental temperature or cold extremity, which constricts the vessels
- High anxiety level or muscle tenseness
- Venous thrombotic occlusion proximal to the extremity to be examined, which can affect blood flow to the limb

Body Plethysmography:

Factors that may impair results of the examination:
- Inability of the patient to follow breathing instructions during the procedure

Impedance Plethysmography:

Factors that may impair results of the examination:
- Movement of the extremity during electrical impedance recording, poor electrode contact, or nonlinear electrical output, which can cause false-positive impedance plethysmography results
- Constricting clothing or bandages

Nursing Implications and Procedure • • • • • • • • • • •

Pretest:

> Inform the patient that the test is used to measure changes in blood vessel size or changes in gas volume in the lungs.

> Obtain a history of the patient's cardiovascular system, including signs and symptoms of vascular disorders, known or suspected peripheral vascular disease (for arterial and vascular plethysmography), known or suspected diseases of the pulmonary system (for body plethysmography), and signs or symptoms of DVT or circulatory changes (for impedance plethysmography), as well as results of previously performed diagnostic procedures, surgical procedures, and laboratory tests. For related diagnostic tests, refer to the Cardiovascular System table.

> Record the date of the last menstrual period and determine the possibility of pregnancy in perimenopausal women.

> Obtain a list of the medications the patient is taking.

> Review the procedure with the patient. Explain the purpose of the test and how the procedure is performed. Address concerns about pain related to the procedure. Explain to the patient that no discomfort will be experienced during the test. For body plethysmography, explain that the procedure measures the amount of air contained in the chest, the elasticity of the lungs, and the occurrence of restrictive breathing in the bronchioles. Explain that there may be some discomfort during insertion of the nasoesophageal catheter if compliance testing is done. Inform the patient that the procedure is generally performed in a specialized area or at the bedside, by a technologist, and usually takes 30 to 60 minutes.

> Assess the patient's ability to comply with directions given for rest, positioning, and activity before and during the procedure.

> For body plethysmography, record the patient's weight, height, and gender. Determine whether the patient is claustrophobic.

> *Sensitivity to cultural and social issues,* as well as concern for modesty, is important in providing psychological support before, during, and after the procedure.

> The patient should refrain from smoking for 2 hours prior to the procedure.

> There are no food, fluid, or medication restrictions, unless by medical direction.

Intratest:

> Ensure that the patient has refrained from smoking for 2 hours before the procedure.

> Ask the patient to notify medical personnel if he or she has ill effects or unexpected symptoms during the test.

> Patients are given a gown, robe, and foot coverings to wear and instructed to void prior to the procedure.

> Obtain and record baseline vital signs.

> Observe standard precautions, and follow the general guidelines in Appendix A.

Arterial plethysmography:

> Explain to the patient that cuffs are applied to the extremity to measure and compare blood flow.

> Explain to the patient that it is essential to remain still during the procedure.

> Place the patient in a semi-Fowler position on an examining table or in bed.

> Apply three blood pressure cuffs to the extremity and attach a pulse volume recorder (plethysmograph), which records the amplitude of each pulse wave.

> Inflate the cuffs to 65 mm Hg to measure the pulse waves of each

cuff. When compared with a normal limb, these measurements determine the presence of arterial occlusive disease.

Venous plethysmography:

➤ Explain to the patient that cuffs are applied to the extremity to measure and compare blood flow.

➤ Explain to the patient that it is essential to remain still during the procedure.

➤ Place the patient in a semi-Fowler position on an examining table or in bed.

➤ Apply two blood pressure cuffs to the extremity, one on the proximal part of the extremity (occlusion cuff) and the other on the distal part of the extremity (recorder cuff). Attach a third cuff to the pulse volume recorder.

➤ Inflate the recorder cuff to 10 mm Hg, and evaluate the effects of respiration on venous volume: Absence of changes during respirations indicates venous thrombotic occlusion.

➤ Inflate the occlusion cuff to 50 mm Hg, and record venous volume on the pulse monitor. Deflate the occlusion cuff after the highest volume is recorded in the recorder cuff. A delay in the return to preocclusion volume indicates venous thrombotic occlusion.

Body plethysmography:

➤ Place the patient in a sitting position on a chair in the body box. Explain to the patient that the cuffs are applied to the extremities to measure and compare blood flow.

➤ Position a nose clip to prevent breathing through the nose, and connect a mouthpiece to a measuring instrument.

➤ Ask the patient to breathe through the mouthpiece.

➤ Close the door to the box, and record the start time of the procedure. At the beginning of the study, ask the patient to pant rapidly and shallowly, without allowing the glottis to close.

➤ For compliance testing, a double-lumen nasoesophageal catheter is inserted, and the bag is inflated with air. Intraesophageal pressure is recorded during normal breathing.

Impedance plethysmography:

➤ Explain to the patient that cuffs are applied to the extremity to measure and compare blood flow.

➤ Place the patient on his or her back with the leg being tested above the heart level.

➤ Flex the patient's knee slightly, and rotate the hips by shifting weight to the same side as the leg being tested.

➤ Apply conductive gel and electrodes to the legs, near the cuffs.

➤ Apply a blood pressure cuff to the thigh.

➤ Inflate the pressure cuff attached to the thigh temporarily to occlude venous return without interfering with arterial blood flow. Expect the blood volume in the other calf to increase.

➤ A tracing of changes in electrical impedance occurring during inflation and for 15 seconds after cuff deflation is recorded.

➤ With DVT, blood volume increases less than expected because the veins are already at capacity.

Post-test:

➤ Remove conductive gel and electrodes, as applied.

➤ Instruct the patient to resume usual activity and diet, as directed by the health care practitioner.

➤ Note severe ischemia, ulcers, and pain of the extremity after arterial, venous, or impedance plethysmography, and handle the extremity gently.

➤ Note respiratory pattern after body plethysmography, and allow the patient time to resume a normal breathing pattern. Monitor vital signs every 15 minutes until they return to baseline levels.

> A written report of the examination will be completed by a health care practitioner specializing in this branch of medicine. The report will be sent to the requesting health care practitioner, who will discuss the results with the patient.

> Reinforce information given by the patient's health care provider regarding further testing, treatment, or referral to another health care provider. Answer any questions or address any concerns voiced by the patient or family.

> Depending on the results of this pro-

cedure, additional testing may be needed to evaluate or monitor progression of the disease process and determine the need for a change in therapy. Evaluate test results in relation to the patient's symptoms and other tests performed.

Related diagnostic tests:

> Related diagnostic tests include computed tomography angiography, echocardiography, magnetic resonance angiography, and ultrasound arterial and venous Doppler of the extremities.

PLEURAL FLUID ANALYSIS

· ·

SYNONYM/ACRONYM: Thoracentesis fluid analysis.

SPECIMEN: Pleural fluid (5 mL) collected in a green-top (heparin) tube for amylase, cholesterol, glucose, lactate dehydrogenase (LDH), pH, protein, and triglycerides; lavender-top (EDTA) tube for cell count; sterile containers for microbiology specimens; 200 to 500 mL of fluid in a clear container with anticoagulant for cytology. Ensure that there is an equal amount of fixative and fluid in the container for cytology.

REFERENCE VALUE: (Method: Spectrophotometry for amylase, cholesterol, glucose, LDH, protein, and triglycerides; ion-selective electrode for pH; automated or manual cell count; macroscopic and microscopic examination of cultured microorganisms; microscopic examination of specimen for microbiology and cytology.)

Pleural Fluid	Reference Value
Appearance	Clear
Color	Pale yellow
Amylase	Parallel serum values
Cholesterol	Parallel serum values
Glucose	Parallel serum values
LDH	Less than 200 U/L

Pleural Fluid	Reference Value
Fluid LDH–to–serum LDH ratio	0.6 or less
Protein	3.0 g/dL
Fluid protein–to–serum protein ratio	0.5 or less
Triglycerides	Parallel serum values
pH	7.37–7.43
RBC count	Less than 1000/mm^3
WBC count	Less than 1000/mm^3
Culture	No growth
Gram stain	No organisms seen
Cytology	No abnormal cells seen

LDH = lactate dehydrogenase; RBC = red blood cell; WBC = white blood cell.

DESCRIPTION & RATIONALE: The pleural cavity and organs within it are lined with a protective membrane. The fluid between the membranes is called *serous fluid.* Normally only a small amount of fluid is present because the rates of fluid production and absorption are about the same. Many abnormal conditions can result in the buildup of fluid within the pleural cavity. Specific tests are usually ordered in addition to a common battery of tests used to distinguish a transudate from an exudate. *Transudates* are effusions that form as a result of a systemic disorder that disrupts the regulation of fluid balance, such as a suspected perforation. *Exudates* are caused by conditions involving the tissue of the membrane itself, such as an infection or malignancy. Fluid is withdrawn from the pleural cavity by needle aspiration and tested as listed in the previous and following tables. ∎

Characteristic	Transudate	Exudate
Appearance	Clear	Cloudy or turbid
Specific gravity	Less than 1.015	Greater than 1.015
Total protein	Less than 2.5 g/dL	Greater than 3.0 g/dL
Fluid protein–to–serum protein ratio	Less than 0.5	Greater than 0.5
LDH	Parallels serum value	Less than 200 U/L
Fluid LDH–to–serum LDH ratio	Less than 0.6	Greater than 0.6
Fluid cholesterol	Less than 55 mg/dL	Greater than 55 mg/dL
WBC count	Less than 100/mm^3	Greater than 1000/mm^3

LDH = lactate dehydrogenase; WBC = white blood cell.

INDICATIONS:
- Differentiate transudates from exudates
- Evaluate effusion of unknown cause
- Investigate suspected rupture, immune disease, malignancy, or infection

RESULT:
- *Bacterial or tuberculous empyema:* Red blood cell (RBC) count 5000/mm^3, white blood cell (WBC) count 25,000 to 100,000/mm^3 with a predominance of neutrophils, increased fluid protein–

to–serum protein ratio, increased fluid LDH–to–serum LDH ratio, decreased glucose, pH less than 7.3

- *Chylous pleural effusion:* Marked increase in both triglycerides (two to three times serum level) and chylomicrons

- *Effusion caused by pneumonia:* RBC count less than 5000/mm³, WBC count 5000 to 25,000/mm³ with a predominance of neutrophils and some eosinophils, increased fluid protein–to–serum protein ratio, increased fluid LDH–to–serum LDH ratio, pH less than 7.4 (and decreased glucose if bacterial pneumonia)

- *Esophageal rupture:* Significantly decreased pH (6.0) and elevated amylase

- *Hemothorax:* Bloody appearance, increased RBC count, elevated hematocrit

- *Malignancy:* RBC count 1000 to 100,000/mm³, WBC count 5000 to 10,000/mm³ with a predominance of lymphocytes, abnormal cytology, increased fluid protein–to–serum protein ratio, increased fluid LDH–to–serum LDH ratio, deceased glucose, pH less than 7.3

- *Pancreatitis:* RBC count 1000 to 10,000/mm³, WBC count 5000 to 20,000/mm³ with a predominance of neutrophils, pH greater than 7.3, increased fluid protein–to–serum protein ratio, increased fluid LDH–to–serum LDH ratio, increased amylase

- *Pulmonary infarction:* RBC count 10,000 to 100,000/mm³, WBC count 5000 to 15,000/mm³ with a predominance of neutrophils, pH greater than 7.3, normal glucose, increased fluid protein–to–serum protein ratio, and increased fluid LDH–to–serum LDH ratio.

- *Pulmonary tuberculosis:* RBC count 10,000/mm³, WBC count 5000 to 10,000/mm³ with a predominance of lymphocytes, positive acid-fast bacillus

stain and culture, increased protein, decreased glucose, pH less than 7.3

- *Rheumatoid disease:* Normal RBC count, WBC count 1000 to 20,000/mm³ with a predominance of either lymphocytes or neutrophils, pH less than 7.3, decreased glucose, increased fluid protein–to–serum protein ratio, increased fluid LDH–to–serum LDH ratio, increased immunoglobulins

- *Systemic lupus erythematosus:* Similar findings as with rheumatoid disease, except that glucose is usually not decreased

CRITICAL VALUES:
Note and immediately report to the health care practitioner positive culture results, if ordered, and related symptoms.

INTERFERING FACTORS:

- Bloody fluids may be the result of a traumatic tap.

- Unknown hyperglycemia or hypoglycemia may be misleading in the comparison of fluid and serum glucose levels. Therefore, it is advisable to collect comparative serum samples a few hours before performing thoracentesis.

Nursing Implications and Procedure . . . .

Pretest:

➤ Inform the patient that the test is primarily used to classify the type of effusion being produced and identify the cause of its accumulation.

➤ Obtain a history of the patient's complaints, including a list of known allergens (especially allergies or sensitivities to latex), and inform the appropriate health care practitioner accordingly.

➤ Obtain a history of the patient's immune and reproductive systems, any bleeding disorders, and results of previously performed laboratory tests (especially bleeding time, complete blood count, partial thromboplastin time, platelets, and prothrombin time), surgical procedures, and other diagnostic procedures. For related laboratory tests, refer to the Immune and Reproductive System tables.

➤ Note any recent procedures that can interfere with test results.

➤ Record the date of the last menstrual period and determine the possibility of pregnancy in perimenopausal women.

➤ Obtain a list of medications the patient is taking, including anticoagulant therapy, acetylsalicylic acid, herbs, nutritional supplements, and nutraceuticals, especially those known to affect coagulation. The requesting health care practitioner and laboratory should be advised if the patient regularly uses these products so that their effects can be taken into consideration when reviewing results.

➤ Review the procedure with the patient. Inform the patient that it may be necessary to shave the site before the procedure. Discuss with the patient that the requesting health care practitioner may request that a cough suppressant be given before the thoracentesis. Address concerns about pain related to the procedure. Explain that a sedative and/or analgesia will be administered to promote relaxation and reduce discomfort prior to needle insertion through the chest wall into the pleural space. Explain to the patient that any discomfort with the needle insertion will be minimized with local anesthetics and systemic analgesics. Explain that the local anesthetic injection may cause an initial stinging sensation. Meperidine (Demerol) or morphine may be given as a sedative. Inform the patient that the needle insertion is performed under sterile conditions by a health care practitioner specializing in this procedure. The procedure usually takes about 20 minutes to complete.

➤ Explain that an intravenous (IV) line will be inserted to allow infusion of IV fluids, antibiotics, anesthetics, and analgesics.

➤ *Sensitivity to social and cultural issues,* as well as concern for modesty, is important in providing psychological support before, during, and after the procedure.

➤ There are no food or fluid restrictions, unless by medical direction. The requesting health care practitioner may request that anticoagulants and aspirin be withheld. The amount of days to withhold medication is dependent on the type of anticoagulant.

➤ *Make sure a written and informed consent has been signed prior to the procedure and before administering any medications.*

Intratest:

➤ Ensure that anticoagulant therapy has been withheld for the appropriate amount of days prior to the procedure. Notify the health care practitioner if patient anticoagulant therapy has not been withheld.

➤ Have emergency equipment readily available. Keep resuscitation equipment on hand in the case of respiratory impairment or laryngospasm after the procedure.

➤ Avoid using morphine sulfate in those with asthma or other pulmonary disease. This drug can further exacerbate bronchospasms and respiratory impairment.

➤ Have the patient remove clothing and change into a gown for the procedure.

➤ Instruct the patient to cooperate fully and to follow directions. Direct the patient to breathe normally and to avoid unnecessary movement during the local anesthetic and the procedure.

➤ Observe standard precautions, and follow the general guidelines in Appendix A. Positively identify the patient, and label the appropriate collection containers with the corresponding patient demographics, date and time of collection, and site location.

➤ Record baseline vital signs and continue to monitor throughout the procedure. Protocols may vary from facility to facility.

➤ Establish an IV line to allow infusion of IV fluids, anesthetics, analgesics, or IV sedation.

➤ Assist the patient into a comfortable sitting or side-lying position.

➤ Prior to the administration of local anesthesia, shave and cleanse the site with an antiseptic solution, and drape the area with sterile towels. The skin at the injection site is then anesthetized.

➤ The thoracentesis needle is inserted, and fluid is removed.

➤ The needle is withdrawn, and pressure is applied to the site with a vaseline gauze. A pressure dressing is applied over the vaseline gauze.

➤ Monitor the patient for complications related to the procedure (e.g., allergic reaction, anaphylaxis).

➤ Place samples in properly labeled specimen container, and promptly transport the specimen to the laboratory for processing and analysis.

➤ The results are recorded manually or in a computerized system for recall and postprocedure interpretation by the appropriate health care practitioner.

Post-test:

➤ Instruct the patient to resume usual medications, as directed by the health care practitioner.

➤ Monitor vital signs every 15 minutes for the first hour, every 30 minutes for the next 2 hours, every hour for the next 4 hours, and every 4 hours for the next 24 hours. Take the patient's temperature every 4 hours for 24 hours. Monitor intake and output for 24 hours. Notify the health care practitioner if temperature is elevated. Protocols may vary from facility to facility.

➤ Observe the patient for signs of respiratory distress or skin color changes.

➤ Observe the thoracentesis site for bleeding, inflammation, or hematoma formation each time vital signs are taken and daily thereafter for several days.

➤ Observe the patient for hemoptysis, difficulty breathing, cough, air hunger, pain, or absent breathing sounds over the affected area. Report to health care provider.

➤ Inform the patient that 1 hour or more of bed rest (lying on the unaffected side) is required after the procedure. Elevate the patient's head for comfort.

➤ Evaluate the patient for symptoms indicating the development of pneumothorax, such as dyspnea, tachypnea, anxiety, decreased breathing sounds, or restlessness. Prepare the patient for a chest x-ray, if ordered, to ensure that a pneumothorax has not occurred as a result of the procedure.

➤ Assess for nausea and pain. Administer antiemetic and analgesic medications as needed and as directed by the health care practitioner.

➤ Administer antibiotics, as ordered, and instruct the patient in the importance of completing the entire course of antibiotic therapy even if no symptoms are present.

➤ A written report of the examination will be completed by a health care practitioner specializing in this branch of medicine. The report will be sent to the requesting health care practitioner, who will discuss the results with the patient.

➤ Recognize anxiety related to test results, and offer support. Discuss the implications of abnormal test results on the patient's lifestyle. Provide teaching and information regarding the clinical implications of the test results, as appropriate. Educate the patient regarding access to counseling services, if appropriate.

➤ Reinforce information given by the patient's health care provider regard-

ing further testing, treatment, or referral to another health care provider. Answer any questions or address any concerns voiced by the patient or family.

➤ Depending on the results of this procedure, additional testing may be performed to evaluate or monitor progression of the disease process and determine the need for a change in therapy. Evaluate test results in relation to the patient's symptoms and other tests performed.

➤ Related laboratory tests include bacterial culture, CA 15–3, CA 19–9, CA 125, carcinoembryonic antigen, fungal culture, mycobacterial culture, and viral culture.

PORPHYRINS, URINE

. . . .

SYNONYMS/ACRONYM: Coproporphyrin, porphobilinogen, urobilinogen, and other porphyrins.

SPECIMEN: Urine (10 mL) from a random or timed specimen collected in a clean, amber-colored plastic collection container with sodium carbonate as a preservative.

REFERENCE VALUE: (Method: Chromatography for uroporphyrins; spectrophotometry for δ-aminolevulinic acid, urobilinogen, and porphobilinogen)

Test	Conventional Units	SI Units
Total porphyrins	Less than 320 μg/24 h	
		(Conventional Units × 1.53)
Coproporphyrin *Tetracarboxyl- coproporphyrin*		
Male	Less than 96 μg/24 h	Less than 147 nmol/24 h
Female	Less than 60 μg/24 h	Less than 92 nmol/24 h
		(Conversion Factor × 1.43)
Uroporphyrins *Pentacarboxyl- porphyrin*		
Male	Less than 4 μg/24 h	Less than 6 nmol/24 h
Female	Less than 3 μg/24 h	Less than 4 nmol/24 h

(Continued on the following page)

Test	Conventional Units	SI Units
		(Conventional Units × 1.34)
Hexacarboxyl-porphyrin		
Male	Less than 5 μg/24 h	Less than 7 nmol/24 h
Female	Less than 3 μg/24 h	Less than 4 nmol/24 h
		(Conventional Units × 1.27)
Heptacarboxyl-porphyrin		
Male	Less than 13 μg/24 h	Less than 17 nmol/24 h
Female	Less than 9 μg/24 h	Less than 11 nmol/24 h
		(Conventional Units × 4.42)
Porphobilinogen	Less than 2.0 mg/24 h	Less than 8.8 μmol/24 h
		(Conversion Factor × 1)
Urobilinogen	0.5–4.0 EU/24 h	0.5–4.0 EU/24 h
		(Conventional Units × 7.626)
δ-Aminolevulinic acid	1.5–7.5 mg/24 h	11.4–57.2 μmol/24 h

DESCRIPTION & RATIONALE: Porphyrins are produced during the synthesis of heme. If heme synthesis is disturbed, these precursors accumulate and are excreted in the urine in excessive amounts. Conditions producing increased levels of heme precursors are called *porphyrias*. The two main categories of genetically determined porphyrias are erythropoietic porphyrias, in which major abnormalities occur in red blood cell chemistry, and hepatic porphyrias, in which heme precursors are found in urine and feces. Erythropoietic and hepatic porphyrias are rare. Acquired porphyrias are characterized by greater accumulation of precursors in urine and feces than in red blood cells. Lead poisoning is the most common cause of acquired porphyrias. Porphyrins are reddish fluorescent compounds. Depending on the type of porphyrin present, the urine may be reddish,

resembling port wine. Porphobilinogen is excreted as a colorless compound. A color change may occur in an acidic sample containing porphobilinogen if the sample is exposed to air for several hours. ▪

INDICATIONS:
- Assist in the diagnosis of congenital or acquired porphyrias, characterized by abdominal pain, tachycardia, emesis, fever, leukocytosis, and neurologic abnormalities
- Detect suspected lead poisoning, as indicated by elevated porphyrins

RESULT

Increased in:
- Acute hepatic porphyrias
- Congenital or acquired porphyrias
- Heavy metal, benzene, or carbon tetrachloride toxicity
- Variegated porphyrias

Decreased in: N/A

CRITICAL VALUES: N/A

INTERFERING FACTORS:

- Drugs that may increase urine porphyrin levels include acriflavine, aminopyrine, ethoxazene, griseofulvin, hexachlorobenzene, oxytetracycline, and sulfonmethane.

- Numerous drugs are suspected as potential initiators of acute attacks, but drugs classified as unsafe for high-risk individuals include aminopyrine, aminoglutethimide, antipyrine, barbiturates, N-butylscopolammoniumine bromide, carbamazepine, carbromal, chlorpropamide, danazol, dapsone, diclofenac, diphenylhydantoin, ergot preparations, ethchlorvynol, ethinamate, glutethimide, griseofulvin, N-isopropyl meprobamate, mephenytoin, meprobamate, methyprylon, novobiocin, phenylbutazone, primidone, pyrazolone preparations, succinimides, sulfonamide antibiotics, sulfonethylmethane, sulfonmethane, synthetic estrogens and progestins, tolazamide, tolbutamide, trimethadione, and valproic acid.

- Exposure of the specimen to light can falsely decrease values.

- Screening methods are not well standardized and can produce false-negative results.

- Failure to collect all urine and store specimen properly during the 24-hour test period will interfere with results.

Nursing Implications and Procedure

Pretest:

- Inform the patient that the test is used to evaluate porphyrias.

- Obtain a history of the patient's complaints, including a list of known allergens (especially allergies or sensitivities to latex), and inform the appropriate health care practitioner accordingly.

- Obtain a history of the patient's hematopoietic system and results of previously performed laboratory tests, surgical procedures, and other diagnostic procedures. For related laboratory tests, refer to the Hematopoietic System table.

- Obtain a list of medications the patient is taking, including herbs, nutritional supplements, and nutraceuticals. The requesting health care practitioner and laboratory should be advised if the patient regularly uses these products so that their effects can be taken into consideration when reviewing results.

- Review the procedure with the patient. Provide a nonmetallic urinal, bedpan, or toilet-mounted collection device. Address concerns about pain related to the procedure. Explain to the patient that there should be no discomfort during the procedure.

- Usually a 24-hour time frame for urine collection is ordered. Inform the patient that all urine must be saved during that 24-hour period. Instruct the patient not to void directly into the laboratory collection container. Instruct the patient to avoid defecating in the collection device and to keep toilet tissue out of the collection device to prevent contamination of the specimen. Place a sign in the bathroom to remind the patient to save all urine.

- Instruct the patient to void all urine into the collection device and then to pour the urine into the laboratory collection container. Alternatively, the specimen can be left in the collection device for a health care staff member to add to the laboratory collection container.

- *Sensitivity to social and cultural issues,* as well as concern for modesty, is important in providing psychological support before, during, and after the procedure.

- There are no food, fluid, or medication restrictions, unless by medical direction.

➤ If the patient has a history of severe allergic reaction to latex, care should be taken to avoid the use of equipment containing latex.

➤ Instruct the patient to cooperate fully and to follow directions.

➤ Observe standard precautions, and follow the general guidelines in Appendix A. Positively identify the patient, and label the appropriate tubes with the corresponding patient demographics, date, and time of collection.

Random specimen (collect in early morning):

Clean-catch specimen:

➤ Instruct the male patient to (1) thoroughly wash his hands, (2) cleanse the meatus, (3) void a small amount into the toilet, and (4) void directly into the specimen container.

➤ Instruct the female patient to (1) thoroughly wash her hands; (2) cleanse the labia from front to back; (3) while keeping the labia separated, void a small amount into the toilet; and (4) without interrupting the urine stream, void directly into the specimen container.

Indwelling catheter:

➤ Put on gloves. Empty drainage tube of urine. It may be necessary to clamp off the catheter for 15 to 30 minutes before specimen collection. Cleanse specimen port with antiseptic swab, and then aspirate 5 mL of urine with a 21- to 25-gauge needle and syringe. Transfer urine to a sterile container.

Timed specimen:

➤ Obtain a clean 3-L urine specimen container, toilet-mounted collection device, and plastic bag (for transport of the specimen container). The specimen must be refrigerated or kept on ice throughout the entire collection period. If an indwelling urinary catheter is in place, the drainage bag must be kept on ice.

➤ Begin the test between 6 and 8 a.m., if possible. Collect first voiding and discard. Record the time the specimen was discarded as the beginning of the timed collection period. The next morning, ask the patient to void at the same time the collection was started and add this last voiding to the container.

➤ If an indwelling catheter is in place, replace the tubing and container system at the start of the collection time. Keep the container system on ice during the collection period, or empty the urine into a larger container periodically during the collection period; monitor to ensure continued drainage, and conclude the test the next morning at the same hour the collection was begun.

➤ At the conclusion of the test, compare the quantity of urine with the urinary output record for the collection; if the specimen contains less than what was recorded as output, some urine may have been discarded, invalidating the test.

➤ Include on the collection container's label the amount of urine, test start and stop times, and ingestion of any foods or medications that can affect test results.

General:

➤ Promptly transport the specimen to the laboratory for processing and analysis.

➤ The results are recorded manually or in a computerized system for recall and postprocedure interpretation by the appropriate health care practitioner.

➤ A written report of the examination will be sent to the requesting health care practitioner, who will discuss the results with the patient.

➤ Recognize anxiety related to test results. Discuss the implications of abnormal test results on the patient's lifestyle. Provide teaching and information regarding the clinical implications of the test results, as appropriate.

➤ Reinforce information given by the patient's health care provider regarding further testing, treatment, or referral to another health care provider. Answer any questions or address any concerns voiced by the patient or family.

➤ Depending on the results of this procedure, additional testing may be performed to evaluate or monitor progression of the disease process and determine the need for a change in therapy. Evaluate test results in relation to the patient's symptoms and other tests performed.

Related laboratory tests:

➤ Related laboratory tests include include δ-aminolevulinic acid, erythrocyte protoporphyrin, and lead.

POSITRON EMISSION TOMOGRAPHY, BRAIN

SYNONYM/ACRONYM: PET scan of the brain.

AREA OF APPLICATION: Brain.

CONTRAST: Intravenous radioactive material (fluorodeoxyglucose [FDG]).

DESCRIPTION & RATIONALE: Positron emission tomography (PET) combines the biochemical properties of nuclear medicine with the accuracy of computed tomography (CT). PET uses positron emissions from specific radionuclides (oxygen, nitrogen, carbon, and fluorine) to produce detailed functional images within the body. After the radionuclide becomes concentrated in the brain, PET images of blood flow or metabolic processes at the cellular level can be obtained. Fluorine-18, in the form of fluorodeoxyglucose (FDG), is one of the more commonly used radionuclides. FDG is a glucose analogue, and because every cell uses glucose, the metabolic activity occurring in neurologic conditions can be measured. There is little localization of FDG in normal tissue, allowing rapid detection of abnormal disease states. The brain uses oxygen and glucose almost exclusively to meet its energy needs, and therefore the brain's metabolism has been studied widely with PET.

The positron radiopharmaceuticals generally have short half-lives, ranging from a few seconds to a few hours, and therefore they must be produced in a cyclotron located near where the test is being done. The PET scanner translates the emissions from the radioactivity as the positron combines with the negative electrons from the tissues and forms gamma rays that can be detected by the scanner. This information is transmitted to the computer, which determines the location and its distribution and translates the emissions as color-coded images for viewing, quantitative measurements, activity changes in relation to time, and three-dimensional computer-aided analysis. Each radionuclide tracer is designed to measure a specific body process, such as glucose metabolism, blood flow, or brain tissue perfusion. The radionuclide can be administered intravenously or inhaled as a gas. PET has had the greatest clinical impact in patients with epilepsy, dementia, neurodegenerative diseases, inflammation, cerebrovascular disease (indirectly), and brain tumors.

The expense of the study and the limited availability of radiopharmaceuticals limit the use of PET, even though it is more sensitive than traditional nuclear scanning and single-photon emission computed tomography. Changes in reimbursement and the advent of mobile technology have increased the availability of this procedure in the community setting. ■

INDICATIONS:
- Detect Parkinson's disease and Huntington's disease, as evidenced by decreased metabolism
- Determine the effectiveness of therapy, as evidenced by biochemical activity of normal and abnormal tissues
- Determine physiologic changes in psychosis and schizophrenia
- Differentiate between tumor recurrence and radiation necrosis

- Evaluate Alzheimer's disease and differentiate it from other causes of dementia, as evidenced by decreased cerebral flow and metabolism
- Evaluate cranial tumors preoperatively and postoperatively and determine stage and appropriate treatment or procedure
- Identify cerebrovascular accident or aneurysm, as evidenced by decreased blood flow and oxygen use
- Identify focal seizures, as evidenced by decreased metabolism between seizures

RESULT

Normal Findings:
- Normal patterns of tissue metabolism, blood flow, and radionuclide distribution

Abnormal Findings:
- Alzheimer's disease
- Cerebral metastases
- Cerebrovascular accident
- Creutzfeldt-Jakob disease
- Dementia
- Head trauma
- Huntington's disease
- Migraine
- Parkinson's disease
- Schizophrenia
- Seizure disorders
- Tumors

CRITICAL VALUES: N/A

INTERFERING FACTORS

This procedure is contraindicated for:
- Patients who are pregnant or suspected of being pregnant, unless the potential

benefits of the procedure far outweigh the risks to the fetus and mother

Factors that may impair clear imaging:

- Inability of the patient to cooperate or remain still during the procedure because of age, significant pain, or mental status

- Patients who are very obese, who may exceed the weight limit for the equipment

- Incorrect positioning of the patient, which may produce poor visualization of the area to be examined

- Drugs that alter glucose metabolism, such as tranquilizers or insulin, because hypoglycemia can alter PET results

- The use of alcohol, tobacco, or caffeine-containing drinks at least 24 hours before the study, because the effects of these substances would make it difficult to evaluate the patient's true physiologic state (e.g., alcohol is a vasoconstrictor and would decrease blood flow to the target organ)

- Metallic objects within the examination field (e.g., jewelry, body rings), which may inhibit organ visualization and can produce unclear images

Other considerations:

- Failure to follow dietary restrictions before the procedure may cause the procedure to be canceled or repeated.

- Improper injection of the radionuclide that allows the tracer to seep deep into the muscle tissue produces erroneous hot spots.

- False-positive findings may occur as a result of normal gastrointestinal tract uptake and uptake in areas of infection or inflammation.

- Consultation with a health care practitioner should occur before the procedure for radiation safety concerns

regarding younger patients or patients who are lactating.

- Risks associated with radiologic overexposure can result from frequent x-ray procedures. Personnel in the room with the patient should stand behind a shield or leave the area while the examination is being done. Personnel working in the area where the examination is being done should wear badges that reveal their level of exposure to radiation.

Nursing Implications and Procedure · · · · · · · · · · ·

Pretest:

➤ Inform the patient that the procedure assesses blood flow to the brain and brain tissue metabolism.

➤ Obtain a history of the patient's complaints and symptoms, including a list of known allergens.

➤ Obtain a history of the patient's musculoskeletal system, as well as results of previously performed laboratory tests, surgical procedures, and other diagnostic procedures. For related diagnostic tests, refer to the Musculoskeletal System table.

➤ Note any recent procedures that can interfere with test results, including examinations using iodine-based contrast medium or barium.

➤ Record the date of the last menstrual period and determine the possibility of pregnancy in perimenopausal women.

➤ Obtain a list of the medications the patient is taking, including anticoagulant therapy, aspirin and other salicylates, herbs, nutritional supplements, and nutraceuticals, especially those known to affect coagulation (see Appendix F). It is recommended that use be discontinued 14 days before surgical procedures. The requesting health care practitioner and laboratory should be advised if the patient regularly uses these products so that their effects can be taken into consideration when reviewing results.

➤ Review the procedure with the patient. Address concerns about pain related to the procedure. Explain to the patient that some pain may be experienced during the test, or there may be moments of discomfort. Reassure the patient that radioactive material poses minimal radioactive hazard because of its short half-life and rarely produces side effects. Inform the patient that the procedure is performed in a special department, usually in a radiology suite, by a health care practitioner and support staff, and takes approximately 60 to 120 minutes.

➤ *Sensitivity to social and cultural issues*, as well as concern for modesty, is important in providing psychological support before, during, and after the procedure.

➤ The patient should restrict food for 4 hours; restrict alcohol, nicotine, or caffeine-containing drinks for 24 hours; and withhold medications for 24 hours before the test. Instruct the patient to avoid taking anticoagulant medication or to reduce dosage as ordered prior to the procedure.

➤ Instruct the patient to remove dentures, jewelry (including watches), hairpins, credit cards, and other metallic objects in the area to be examined.

➤ Sometimes fluorodeoxyglucose (FDG) examinations are done after blood has been drawn to determine circulating blood glucose levels. If blood glucose levels are high, insulin may be given.

Intratest:

➤ Ensure that the patient has complied with dietary and medication restrictions and pretesting preparations; assure that food and medications have been restricted as directed prior to the procedure. Ensure the patient has removed all external metallic objects (jewelry, dentures, etc.) prior to the procedure.

➤ Have emergency equipment readily available.

➤ Patients are given a gown, robe, and foot coverings to wear and instructed to void prior to the procedure.

➤ Instruct the patient to cooperate fully and to follow directions. Instruct the patient to remain still throughout the procedure because movement produces unreliable results

➤ Record baseline vital signs and assess neurologic status. Protocols may vary from facility to facility.

➤ Observe standard precautions, and follow the general guidelines in Appendix A.

➤ The radionuclide is injected, and imaging is started 30 minutes later. If comparative studies are indicated, additional injections may be needed. Patient is placed in a supine position on the table.

➤ The patient may be asked to perform different cognitive activities (e.g., reading) to measure changes in brain activity during reasoning or remembering.

➤ The patient may be blindfolded or asked to use earplugs to decrease auditory and visual stimuli.

➤ Wear gloves during the radionuclide injection and while handling the patient's urine.

➤ Monitor the patient for complications related to the procedure (e.g., allergic reaction, anaphylaxis, bronchospasm).

➤ The results are recorded on film or in a computerized system for recall and postprocedure interpretation by the appropriate health care practitioner.

Post-test:

➤ Instruct the patient to resume usual diet, fluids, medications, or activity, as directed by the health care practitioner.

➤ Advise the patient to immediately report symptoms such as fast heart rate, difficulty breathing, skin rash, itching, or decreased urinary output.

➤ Observe the needle/catheter insertion site for bleeding, inflammation, or hematoma formation.

➤ Instruct the patient to apply cold compresses to the puncture site, as needed, to reduce discomfort or edema.

➤ Instruct the patient to drink increased amounts of fluids for 24 to 48 hours to eliminate the radionuclide from the body, unless contraindicated. Educate the patient that radionuclide is eliminated from the body within 6 to 24 hours.

➤ Instruct the patient to flush the toilet immediately after each voiding following the procedure, and to wash hands meticulously with soap and water after each voiding for 24 hours after the procedure.

➤ Instruct all caregivers to wear gloves when discarding urine for 24 hours after the procedure. Wash gloved hands with soap and water before removing gloves. Then wash hands after the gloves are removed.

➤ If a woman who is breast-feeding must have a nuclear scan, she should not breast-feed the infant until the radionuclide has been eliminated. This could take as long as 3 days. She should be instructed to express the milk and discard it during the 3-day period to prevent cessation of milk production.

➤ *Nutritional considerations:* A low-fat, low-cholesterol, and low-sodium diet should be consumed to reduce current disease processes and/or decrease risk of hypertension and coronary artery disease.

➤ No other radionuclide tests should be scheduled for 24 to 48 hours after this procedure.

➤ A written report of the examination will be completed by a health care practitioner specializing in this branch of medicine. The report will be sent to the requesting health care practitioner, who will discuss the results with the patient.

➤ Recognize anxiety related to test results, and be supportive of perceived loss of independent function. Discuss the implications of abnormal test results on the patient's lifestyle. Provide teaching and information regarding the clinical implications of the test results, as appropriate.

➤ Reinforce information given by the patient's health care provider regarding further testing, treatment, or referral to another health care provider. Answer any questions or address any concerns voiced by the patient or family.

➤ Instruct the patient in the use of any ordered medications. Explain the importance of adhering to the therapy regimen. As appropriate, instruct the patient in significant side effects and systemic reactions associated with the prescribed medication. Encourage him or her to review corresponding literature provided by a pharmacist.

➤ Depending on the results of this procedure, additional testing may be needed to evaluate or monitor progression of the disease process and determine the need for a change in therapy. Evaluate test results in relation to the patient's symptoms and other tests performed.

Related diagnostic tests:

➤ Related diagnostic tests include computed tomography of the brain, electroencephalogram, magnetic resonance imaging of the brain, and ultrasound arterial Doppler of the carotids.

POSITRON EMISSION TOMOGRAPHY, HEART

SYNONYMS/ACRONYM: PET scan of the heart.

AREA OF APPLICATION: Heart, chest/thorax, vascular system.

CONTRAST: Intravenous radioactive material (fluorodeoxyglucose [FDG]).

DESCRIPTION & RATIONALE: Positron emission tomography (PET) combines the biochemical properties of nuclear medicine with the accuracy of computed tomography (CT). PET uses positron emissions from specific radionuclides (oxygen, nitrogen, carbon, and fluorine) to produce detailed functional images within the body. After the radionuclide becomes concentrated in the heart, PET images of blood flow or metabolic processes at the cellular level can be obtained. Fluorine-18, in the form of fluorodeoxyglucose (FDG), is one of the more commonly used radionuclides. FDG is a glucose analogue, and because every cell uses glucose, the metabolic activity occurring in heart conditions such as myocardial viability can be measured. There is little localization of FDG in normal tissue, allowing rapid detection of abnormal disease states.

The positron radiopharmaceuticals generally have short half-lives, ranging from a few seconds to a few hours, and therefore they must be produced in a cyclotron located near where the test is being done. The PET scanner translates the emissions from the radioactivity as the positron combines with the negative electrons from the tissues and forms gamma rays that can be detected by the scanner. This information is transmitted to the computer, which determines the location and its distribution and translates the emissions as color-coded images for viewing, quantitative measurements, activity changes in relation to time, and three-dimensional computer-aided analysis. Each radionuclide tracer is designed to measure a specific body process, such as glucose metabolism, blood flow, or tissue perfusion. The radionuclide can be administered intravenously or inhaled as a gas.

The expense of the study and the limited availability of radiopharmaceuticals limit the use of PET, even though it is more sensitive than traditional nuclear scanning and single-photon emission computed tomography. Changes in reimbursement and the advent of mobile technology have increased the availability of this procedure in the community setting. ■

INDICATIONS:

- Assess tissue permeability

- Determine the effects of therapeutic drugs on malfunctioning or diseased tissue

- Determine localization of areas of heart metabolism

- Determine the presence of coronary artery disease, as evidenced by metabolic state during ischemia and after angina

- Determine the size of heart infarcts

- Identify cerebrovascular accident or aneurysm, as evidenced by decreasing blood flow and oxygen use

RESULT

Normal Findings:

- Normal patterns of tissue metabolism, blood flow, and radionuclide distribution

Abnormal Findings:

- Chronic obstructive pulmonary disease

- Decreased blood flow and decreased glucose concentration, indicating necrotic, scarred tissue

- Enlarged left ventricle

- Heart chamber disorder

- Myocardial infarction, indicating increased radionuclide uptake in the myocardium

- Pulmonary edema

- Reduced blood flow but increased glucose concentration, indicating ischemia

CRITICAL VALUES: N/A

INTERFERING FACTORS:

This procedure is contraindicated for:

- Patients who are pregnant or suspected of being pregnant, unless the potential benefits of the procedure far outweigh the risks to the fetus and mother

- Patients with hypersensitivity to the radionuclide

Factors that may impair clear imaging:

- Inability of the patient to cooperate or remain still during the procedure because of age, significant pain, or mental status

- Patients who are very obese, who may exceed the weight limit for the equipment

- Incorrect positioning of the patient, which may produce poor visualization of the area to be examined

- Drugs that alter glucose metabolism, such as tranquilizers or insulin, because hypoglycemia can alter PET results

- The use of alcohol, tobacco, or caffeine-containing drinks at least 24 hours before the study, because the effects of these substances would make it difficult to evaluate the patient's true physiologic state (e.g., alcohol is a vasoconstrictor and would decrease blood flow to the target organ)

- Metallic objects within the examination field (e.g., jewelry, body rings), which may inhibit organ visualization and can produce unclear images

Other considerations:

- Failure to follow dietary restrictions before the procedure may cause the procedure to be canceled or repeated.

- Improper injection of the radionuclide that allows the tracer to seep deep into the muscle tissue produces erroneous hot spots.

- False-positive findings may occur as a result of normal gastrointestinal tract uptake and uptake in areas of infection or inflammation.

- Consultation with a health care practitioner should occur before the procedure for radiation safety concerns regarding younger patients or patients who are lactating.

• Risks associated with radiologic overexposure can result from frequent x-ray procedures. Personnel in the room with the patient should stand behind a shield or leave the area while the examination is being done. Personnel working in the area where the examination is being done should wear badges that reveal their level of exposure to radiation.

Nursing Implications and Procedure • • • • • • • • • • • •

Pretest:

➤ Inform the patient that the procedure assesses blood flow to the heart.

➤ Obtain a history of the patient's complaints and symptoms, including a list of known allergens.

➤ Obtain a history of the patient's cardiovascular system, as well as results of previously performed laboratory tests, surgical procedures, and other diagnostic procedures. For related diagnostic tests, refer to the Cardiovascular System table.

➤ Note any recent procedures that can interfere with test results, including examinations using iodine-based contrast medium or barium.

➤ Record the date of the last menstrual period and determine the possibility of pregnancy in perimenopausal women.

➤ Obtain a list of the medications the patient is taking, including anticoagulant therapy, aspirin and other salicylates, herbs, nutritional supplements, and nutraceuticals, especially those known to affect coagulation (see Appendix F). It is recommended that use be discontinued 14 days before surgical procedures. The requesting health care practitioner and laboratory should be advised if the patient regularly uses these products so that their effects can be taken into consideration when reviewing results.

➤ Review the procedure with the patient. Address concerns about pain related to the procedure. Explain to the patient that some pain may be experienced during the test, or there may be moments of discomfort. Reassure the patient that radioactive material poses minimal radioactive hazard because of its short half-life and rarely produces side effects. Inform the patient that the procedure is performed in a special department, usually in a radiology or vascular suite, by a health care practitioner and support staff, and takes approximately 60 to 120 minutes.

➤ *Sensitivity to social and cultural issues,* as well as concern for modesty, is important in providing psychological support before, during, and after the procedure.

➤ The patient should restrict food for 4 hours; restrict alcohol, nicotine, or caffeine-containing drinks for 24 hours; and withhold medications for 24 hours before the test. Instruct the patient to avoid taking anticoagulant medication or to reduce dosage as ordered prior to the procedure.

➤ Instruct the patient to remove dentures, jewelry (including watches), hairpins, credit cards, and other metallic objects in the area to be examined.

➤ Sometimes fluorodeoxyglucose (FDG) examinations are done after blood has been drawn to determine circulating blood glucose levels. If blood glucose levels are high, insulin may be given.

Intratest:

➤ Ensure that the patient has complied with dietary and medication restrictions and pretesting preparations; assure that food and medications have been restricted as directed prior to the procedure. Ensure the patient has removed all external metallic objects (jewelry, dentures, etc.) prior to the procedure.

➤ Have emergency equipment readily available.

➤ Patients are given a gown, robe, and

foot coverings to wear and instructed to void prior to the procedure.

➤ Instruct the patient to cooperate fully and to follow directions. Instruct the patient to remain still throughout the procedure because movement produces unreliable results.

➤ Record baseline vital signs and assess neurologic status. Protocols may vary from facility to facility.

➤ Observe standard precautions, and follow the general guidelines in Appendix A.

➤ The radionuclide is injected while the patient is in the supine position; imaging is done at periodic intervals, and continuous scanning is done for 1 hour. If comparative studies are indicated, additional injections may be needed.

➤ Wear gloves during the radionuclide injection and while handling the patient's urine.

➤ Monitor the patient for complications related to the procedure (e.g., allergic reaction, anaphylaxis, bronchospasm).

➤ The results are recorded on film or in a computerized system for recall and postprocedure interpretation by the appropriate health care practitioner.

Post-test:

➤ Instruct the patient to resume usual diet, fluids, medications, or activity, as directed by the health care practitioner.

➤ Observe for delayed allergic reactions, such as rash, urticaria, tachycardia, hyperpnea, hypertension, palpitations, nausea, or vomiting.

➤ Instruct the patient to immediately report symptoms such as fast heart rate, difficulty breathing, skin rash, itching, or decreased urinary output.

➤ Observe the needle/catheter insertion site for bleeding, inflammation, or hematoma formation.

➤ Instruct the patient to apply cold compresses to the puncture site, as needed, to reduce discomfort or edema.

➤ Instruct the patient to drink increased amounts of fluids for 24 to 48 hours to eliminate the radionuclide from the body, unless contraindicated. Educate the patient that radionuclide is eliminated from the body within 6 to 24 hours.

➤ Instruct the patient to flush the toilet immediately after each voiding following the procedure, and to wash hands meticulously with soap and water after each voiding for 24 hours after the procedure.

➤ Instruct all caregivers to wear gloves when discarding urine for 24 hours after the procedure. Wash gloved hands with soap and water before removing gloves. Then wash hands after the gloves are removed.

➤ If a woman who is breast-feeding must have a nuclear scan, she should not breast-feed the infant until the radionuclide has been eliminated. This could take as long as 3 days. She should be instructed to express the milk and discard it during the 3-day period to prevent cessation of milk production.

➤ *Nutritional considerations:* A low-fat, low-cholesterol, and low-sodium diet should be consumed to reduce current disease processes and/or decrease risk of hypertension and coronary artery disease.

➤ No other radionuclide tests should be scheduled for 24 to 48 hours after this procedure.

➤ A written report of the examination will be completed by a health care practitioner specializing in this branch of medicine. The report will be sent to the requesting health care practitioner, who will discuss the results with the patient.

➤ Recognize anxiety related to test results, and be supportive of perceived loss of independent function. Discuss the implications of abnormal test results on the patient's lifestyle. Provide teaching and information regarding the clinical implications of the test results, as appropriate.

➤ Reinforce information given by the patient's health care provider regard-

ing further testing, treatment, or referral to another health care provider. Answer any questions or address any concerns voiced by the patient or family.

➤ Instruct the patient in the use of any ordered medications. Explain the importance of adhering to the therapy regimen. As appropriate, instruct the patient in significant side effects and systemic reactions associated with the prescribed medication. Encourage him or her to review corresponding literature provided by a pharmacist.

➤ Depending on the results of this procedure, additional testing may be needed to evaluate or monitor progression of the disease process and determine the need for a change in therapy. Evaluate test results in relation to the patient's symptoms and other tests performed.

Related diagnostic tests:

➤ Related diagnostic tests include computed tomography of the thorax, echocardiogram, electrocardiography, magnetic resonance imaging of the chest, and myocardial perfusion scan.

POSITRON EMISSION TOMOGRAPHY, PELVIS

SYNONYM/ACRONYM: PET scan of the pelvis.

AREA OF APPLICATION: Pelvis.

CONTRAST: Intravenous radioactive material (fluorodeoxyglucose [FDG]).

DESCRIPTION & RATIONALE: Positron emission tomography (PET) combines the biochemical properties of nuclear medicine with the accuracy of computed tomography (CT). PET uses positron emissions from specific radionuclides (oxygen, nitrogen, carbon, and fluorine) to produce detailed functional images within the body. After the radionuclide becomes concentrated in the pelvis, PET images of blood flow or metabolic processes at the cellular level can be obtained. Colorectal tumor detection, tumor staging, evaluation of the effects of therapy, detection of recurrent disease,

and detection of metastases are the main reasons to do a pelvic PET scan. Fluorine-18, in the form of fluorodeoxyglucose (FDG), is one of the more commonly used radionuclides. FDG is a glucose analogue, and because every cell uses glucose, the metabolic activity occurring in pelvic conditions such as colorectal cancer can be measured. There is little localization of FDG in normal tissue, allowing rapid detection of abnormal disease states.

The positron radiopharmaceuticals generally have short half-lives, ranging from a few seconds to a few hours, and therefore they must be produced in a cyclotron located near where the test is being done. The PET scanner translates the emissions from the radioactivity as the positron combines with the negative electrons from the tissues and forms gamma rays that can be detected by the scanner. This information is transmitted to the computer, which determines the location and its distribution and translates the emissions as color-coded images for viewing, quantitative measurements, activity changes in relation to time, and three-dimensional computer-aided analysis. Each radionuclide tracer is designed to measure a specific body process, such as glucose metabolism, blood flow, or tissue perfusion.

The expense of the study and the limited availability of radiopharmaceuticals limit the use of PET, even though it is more sensitive than traditional nuclear scanning and single-photon emission computed tomography. Changes in reimbursement and the advent of mobile technology have increased the availability of this procedure in the community setting. ∎

INDICATIONS:
- Determine the effects of therapy
- Determine the presence of colorectal cancer
- Determine the presence of metastases of a cancerous tumor
- Determine the recurrence of tumor or cancer
- Identify the site for biopsy

RESULT

Normal Findings:
- Normal patterns of tissue metabolism, blood flow, and radionuclide distribution
- No focal uptake of radionuclide

Abnormal Findings:
- Focal uptake of the radionuclide in pelvis
- Focal uptake in abnormal lymph nodes
- Focal uptake in tumor
- Focal uptake in metastases

CRITICAL VALUES: N/A

INTERFERING FACTORS:

This procedure is contraindicated for:
- Patients who are pregnant or suspected of being pregnant, unless the potential benefits of the procedure far outweigh the risks to the fetus and mother

Factors that may impair clear imaging:
- Inability of the patient to cooperate or remain still during the procedure because of age, significant pain, or mental status
- Incorrect positioning of the patient, which may produce poor visualization of the area to be examined
- Patients who are very obese, who may exceed the weight limit for the equipment
- Drugs that alter glucose metabolism, such as tranquilizers or insulin, because hypoglycemia can alter PET results
- The use of alcohol, tobacco, or caffeine-containing drinks at least 24 hours before the study, because the effects of these substances would make it difficult to evaluate the patient's true physiologic state (e.g., alcohol is a vasoconstrictor and would decrease blood flow to the target organ)
- Metallic objects within the examination field (e.g., jewelry, body rings), which may inhibit organ visualization and can produce unclear images

Other considerations:
- Failure to follow dietary restrictions before the procedure may cause the procedure to be canceled or repeated.

- Improper injection of the radionuclide that allows the tracer to seep deep into the muscle tissue produces erroneous hot spots.

- False-positive findings may occur as a result of normal gastrointestinal tract uptake and uptake in areas of infection or inflammation.

- Consultation with a health care practitioner should occur before the procedure for radiation safety concerns regarding younger patients or patients who are lactating.

- Risks associated with radiologic overexposure can result from frequent x-ray procedures. Personnel in the room with the patient should wear a protective lead apron, stand behind a shield, or leave the area while the examination is being done. Personnel working in the area where the examination is being done should wear badges that reveal their level of exposure to radiation.

Nursing Implications and Procedure ···········

Pretest:

➤ Inform the patient that the procedure assesses the pelvis and its contents for abnormal organ function.

➤ Obtain a history of the patient's complaints and symptoms, including a list of known allergens.

➤ Obtain a history of the patient's gastrointestinal system, as well as results of previously performed laboratory tests, surgical procedures, and other diagnostic procedures. For related diagnostic tests, refer to the Gastrointestinal System table.

➤ Note any recent procedures that can interfere with test results, including examinations using iodine-based contrast medium or barium.

➤ Record the date of the last menstrual period and determine the possibility of pregnancy in perimenopausal women.

➤ Obtain a list of the medications the patient is taking, including anticoagulant therapy, aspirin and other salicylates, herbs, nutritional supplements, and nutraceuticals, especially those known to affect coagulation (see Appendix F). It is recommended that use be discontinued 14 days before surgical procedures. The requesting health care practitioner and laboratory should be advised if the patient regularly uses these products so that their effects can be taken into consideration when reviewing results.

➤ Review the procedure with the patient. Address concerns about pain related to the procedure. Explain to the patient that some pain may be experienced during the test, and there may be moments of discomfort. Explain the purpose of the test and how the procedure is performed. Reassure the patient that radioactive material poses minimal radioactive hazard because of its short half-life and rarely produces side effects. Inform the patient that the procedure is performed in a special department, usually in a radiology suite, by a health care practitioner and support staff, and takes approximately 30 to 60 minutes.

➤ *Sensitivity to cultural and social issues,* as well as concern for modesty, is important in providing psychological support before, during, and after the procedure.

➤ The patient should restrict food for 4 hours; restrict alcohol, nicotine, or caffeine-containing drinks for 24 hours; and withhold medications for 24 hours before the test. Instruct the patient to avoid taking anticoagulant medication or to reduce dosage as ordered prior to the procedure.

➤ Instruct the patient to remove dentures, jewelry (including watches), hairpins, credit cards, and other metallic objects in the area to be examined.

➤ Sometimes fluorodeoxyglucose (FDG) examinations are done after blood has been drawn to determine circulating blood glucose levels. If blood glucose levels are high, insulin may be given.

Intratest:

> Ensure that the patient has complied with dietary and medication restrictions and pretesting preparations; assure that food and medications have been restricted as directed prior to the procedure. Ensure the patient has removed all external metallic objects (jewelry, dentures, etc.) prior to the procedure.

> Have emergency equipment readily available.

> Patients are given a gown, robe, and foot coverings to wear and instructed to void prior to the procedure.

> Instruct the patient to cooperate fully and to follow directions. Instruct the patient to remain still throughout the procedure because movement produces unreliable results.

> Record baseline vital signs and assess neurologic status. Protocols may vary from facility to facility.

> Observe standard precautions, and follow the general guidelines in Appendix A.

> The radionuclide is injected, and imaging is started after a 45-minute delay. Continuous scanning may be done for 1 hour after the patient is placed in the supine position on a scanning table. If comparative studies are indicated, additional injections of radionuclide may be needed.

> If required, the bladder may need to be lavaged via a urinary catheter with 2 L of 0.9% saline solution to remove concentrated radionuclide.

> Wear gloves during the radionuclide injection and while handling the patient's urine.

> Monitor the patient for complications related to the procedure (e.g., allergic reaction, anaphylaxis, bronchospasm).

> The results are recorded on film or in a computerized system for recall and postprocedure interpretation by the appropriate health care practitioner.

Post-test:

> Instruct the patient to resume usual diet, fluids, medications, or activity, as directed by the health care practitioner.

> Observe for delayed allergic reactions, such as rash, urticaria, tachycardia, hyperpnea, hypertension, palpitations, nausea, or vomiting.

> Instruct the patient to immediately report symptoms such as fast heart rate, difficulty breathing, skin rash, itching, or decreased urinary output.

> Observe the needle/catheter insertion site for bleeding, inflammation, or hematoma formation.

> Instruct the patient to apply cold compresses to the puncture site, as needed, to reduce discomfort or edema.

> Instruct the patient to drink increased amounts of fluids for 24 to 48 hours to eliminate the radionuclide from the body, unless contraindicated. Tell the patient that radionuclide is eliminated from the body within 6 to 24 hours.

> Instruct the patient to flush the toilet immediately after each voiding following the procedure, and to wash hands meticulously with soap and water after each voiding for 24 hours after the procedure.

> Tell all caregivers to wear gloves when discarding urine for 24 hours after the procedure. Wash gloved hands with soap and water before removing gloves. Then wash hands after the gloves are removed.

> If a woman who is breast-feeding must have a nuclear scan, she should not breast-feed the infant until the radionuclide has been eliminated. This could take as long as 3 days. She should be instructed to express the milk and discard it during the 3-day period to prevent cessation of milk production.

> No other radionuclide tests should be scheduled for 24 to 48 hours after this procedure.

> A written report of the examination

will be completed by a health care practitioner specializing in this branch of medicine. The report will be sent to the requesting health care practitioner, who will discuss the results with the patient.

➤ Recognize anxiety related to test results, and be supportive of perceived loss of independent function. Discuss the implications of abnormal test results on the patient's lifestyle. Provide teaching and information regarding the clinical implications of the test results, as appropriate.

➤ Reinforce information given by the patient's health care provider regarding further testing, treatment, or referral to another health care provider. Answer any questions or address any concerns voiced by the patient or family.

➤ Instruct the patient in the use of any ordered medications. Explain the importance of adhering to the therapy regimen. As appropriate, instruct the patient in significant side effects and systemic reactions associated with the prescribed medication. Encourage him or her to review corresponding literature provided by a pharmacist.

➤ Depending on the results of this procedure, additional testing may be needed to evaluate or monitor progression of the disease process and determine the need for a change in therapy. Evaluate test results in relation to the patient's symptoms and other tests performed.

Related diagnostic tests:

➤ Related diagnostic tests include computed tomography of the abdomen; kidney, ureter, and bladder (KUB) study; and magnetic resonance imaging of the abdomen.

POTASSIUM, BLOOD

SYNONYM/ACRONYM: Serum K^+.

SPECIMEN: Serum (1 mL) collected in a red- or tiger-top tube. Plasma (1 mL) collected in green-top (heparin) tube is also acceptable.

REFERENCE VALUE: (Method: Ion-selective electrode)

Serum	Conventional Units	SI Units (Conventional Units × 1)
Newborn	3.7–5.9 mEq/L	3.7–5.9 mmol/L
Infant	4.1–5.3 mEq/L	4.1–5.3 mmol/L
Child	3.4–4.7 mEq/L	3.4–4.7 mmol/L
Adult	3.5–5.0 mEq/L	3.5–5.0 mmol/L

Note: Serum values are 0.1 mmol/L higher than plasma values, and reference ranges should be adjusted accordingly. It is important that serial measurements be collected using the same type of collection container to reduce variability of results from collection to collection.

DESCRIPTION & RATIONALE: Electrolytes dissociate into electrically charged ions when dissolved. Cations, including potassium, carry a positive charge. Body fluids contain approximately equal numbers of anions and cations, although the nature of the ions and their mobility differs between the intracellular and extracellular compartments. Both types of ions affect the electrical and osmolar functions of the body. Electrolyte quantities and the balance among them are controlled by oxygen and carbon dioxide exchange in the lungs; absorption, secretion, and excretion of many substances by the kidneys; and secretion of regulatory hormones by the endocrine glands. Potassium is the most abundant intracellular cation. It is essential for the transmission of electrical impulses in cardiac and skeletal muscle. It also functions in enzyme reactions that transform glucose into energy and amino acids into proteins. Potassium helps maintain acid-base equilibrium, and it has a significant and inverse relationship to pH: A decrease in pH of 0.1 increases the potassium level by 0.6 mEq/L.

Abnormal potassium levels can be caused by a number of contributing factors, which can be categorized as follows: ∎

Altered renal excretion: Normally, 80% to 90% of the body's potassium is filtered out through the kidneys each day (the remainder is excreted in sweat and stool); renal disease can result in abnormally high potassium levels.

Altered dietary intake: A severe potassium deficiency can be caused by an inadequate intake of dietary potassium.

Altered cellular metabolism: Damaged red blood cells (RBCs) release potassium into the circulating fluid, resulting in increased potassium levels.

INDICATIONS:
- Assess a known or suspected disorder associated with renal disease, glucose metabolism, trauma, or burns
- Assist in the evaluation of electrolyte imbalances; this test is especially indicated in elderly patients, patients receiving hyperalimentation supplements, patients on hemodialysis, and patients with hypertension
- Evaluate cardiac arrhythmia to determine whether altered potassium levels are contributing to the problem, especially during digitalis therapy, which leads to ventricular irritability
- Evaluate the effects of drug therapy, especially diuretics
- Evaluate the response to treatment for abnormal potassium levels
- Monitor known or suspected acidosis, because potassium moves from RBCs into the extracellular fluid in acidotic states
- Routine screen of electrolytes in acute and chronic illness

RESULT

Increased in:
- Acidosis
- Acute renal failure
- Addison's disease
- Asthma
- Burns
- Chronic interstitial nephritis
- Dehydration
- Dialysis
- Diet (excessive intake of salt substitutes or of potassium salts in medications)

- Excessive theophylline administration
- Exercise
- Hemolysis (massive)
- Hyperventilation
- Hypoaldosteronism
- Insulin deficiency
- Ketoacidosis
- Leukocytosis
- Muscle necrosis
- Near drowning
- Pregnancy
- Prolonged periods of standing
- Tissue trauma
- Transfusion of old banked blood
- Tubular unresponsiveness to aldosterone
- Uremia

Decreased in:
- Alcoholism
- Alkalosis
- Anorexia nervosa
- Bradycardia
- Chronic, excessive licorice ingestion (from licorice root)
- Congestive heart failure
- Crohn's disease
- Cushing's syndrome
- Diet deficient in meat and vegetables
- Excess insulin
- Familial periodic paralysis
- Gastrointestinal loss due to vomiting, diarrhea, nasogastric suction, or intestinal fistula
- Hyperaldosteronism
- Hypertension
- Hypomagnesemia

- Intravenous (IV) therapy with inadequate potassium supplementation
- Laxative abuse
- Malabsorption
- Pica (eating substances of no nutritional value, e.g., clay)
- Renal tubular acidosis
- Stress
- Sweating
- Thyrotoxicosis
- Toxic shock syndrome

CRITICAL VALUES: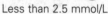
Less than 2.5 mmol/L
Greater than 6.5 mmol/L
Note and immediately report to the health care practitioner any critically increased or decreased values and related symptoms, especially symptoms of fluid imbalance.

Symptoms of hyperkalemia include irritability, diarrhea, cramps, oliguria, difficulty speaking, and cardiac arrhythmias (peaked T waves and ventricular fibrillation). Continuous cardiac monitoring is indicated. Administration of sodium bicarbonate or calcium chloride may be requested. If the patient is receiving an IV supplement, verify that the patient is voiding.

Symptoms of hypokalemia include malaise, thirst, polyuria, anorexia, weak pulse, low blood pressure, vomiting, decreased reflexes, and electrocardiographic changes (depressed T waves and ventricular ectopy). Replacement therapy is indicated.

INTERFERING FACTORS:
- Drugs that can cause an increase in potassium levels include dexamethasone, enalapril, mannitol, methicillin, metoprolol, nonsteroidal anti-inflammatory drugs, some drugs with potassium salts, propranolol, spironolactone, and succinylcholine.

- Drugs that can cause a decrease in potassium levels include acetazolamide, acetylsalicylic acid, alanine, albuterol, aldosterone, ammonium chloride, amphotericin B, bicarbonate, bisacodyl, captopril, carbenicillin, cathartics, cisplatin, clorexolone, desoxycorticosterone, dexamethasone, digoxin, diuretics, enalapril, furosemide, hydrocortisone, hydroflumethiazide, laxatives, moxalactam (common when coadministered with amikacin), large doses of any IV penicillin, phenolphthalein (with chronic laxative abuse), phosphates, IV theophylline, thiazides, and triamterene. A number of these medications initially increase the serum potassium level, but they also have a diuretic effect, which promotes potassium loss in the urine except in cases of renal insufficiency.

- Leukocytosis, as seen in leukemia, causes elevated potassium levels.

- False elevations can occur with vigorous pumping of the hand during venipuncture. Hemolysis of the sample and high platelet counts also increase potassium levels, as follows: (1) Because potassium is an intracellular ion and concentrations are approximately 150 times extracellular concentrations, even a slight amount of hemolysis can cause a significant increase in levels. (2) Platelets release potassium during the clotting process, and therefore serum samples collected from patients with elevated platelet counts may produce spuriously high potassium levels. Plasma would be the specimen of choice in patients known to have elevated platelet counts.

- False increases are seen in unprocessed samples left at room temperature because a significant amount of potassium leaks out of the cells within a few hours. Plasma or serum should be separated from cells within 4 hours of collection.

- Storage of unprocessed blood causes potassium levels to increase because a significant amount of potassium leaks out of the cells within a few hours. Plasma or serum should be separated from cells within 4 hours of collection.

- Specimens should never be collected above an IV line because of the potential for dilution when the specimen and the IV solution combine in the collection container, falsely decreasing the result. There is also the potential of contaminating the sample with the substance of interest, if it is present in the IV solution, falsely increasing the result.

Nursing Implications and Procedure • • • • • • • • • •

Pretest:

▶ Inform the patient that the test is used to assess electrolyte balance.

▶ Obtain a history of the patient's complaints, including a list of known allergens (especially allergies or sensitivities to latex), and inform the appropriate health care practitioner accordingly. Especially note complaints of weakness and confusion.

▶ Obtain a history of the patient's cardiovascular, endocrine, gastrointestinal, genitourinary, immune, and respiratory systems, as well as results of previously performed laboratory tests, surgical procedures, and other diagnostic procedures. For related laboratory tests, refer to the Cardiovascular, Endocrine, Gastrointestinal, Genitourinary, Immune, and Respiratory System tables.

▶ Obtain a list of medications the patient is taking, including herbs, nutritional supplements, and nutraceuticals. The requesting health care practitioner and laboratory should be advised if the patient regularly uses these products so that their effects can be taken into consideration when reviewing results.

▶ Review the procedure with the patient. Inform the patient that specimen collection takes approximately 5 to 10 minutes. Address concerns about pain related to the procedure. Explain to the patient that there may be some discomfort during the venipuncture.

➤ There are no food, fluid, or medication restrictions, unless by medical direction.

Intratest:

➤ If the patient has a history of severe allergic reaction to latex, care should be taken to avoid the use of equipment containing latex.

➤ Instruct the patient to cooperate fully and to follow directions. Direct the patient to breathe normally and to avoid unnecessary movement. Instruct patient not to clench and unclench the fist immediately before or during specimen collection.

➤ Observe standard precautions, and follow the general guidelines in Appendix A. Positively identify the patient, and label the appropriate tubes with the corresponding patient demographics, date, and time of collection. Perform a venipuncture; collect the specimen in a 5-mL red-, tiger-, or green-top (heparin) tube.

➤ Remove the needle, and apply a pressure dressing over the puncture site.

➤ Promptly transport the specimen to the laboratory for processing and analysis.

➤ The results are recorded manually or in a computerized system for recall and postprocedure interpretation by the appropriate health care practitioner.

Post-test:

➤ Observe venipuncture site for bleeding or hematoma formation. Apply paper tape or other adhesive to hold pressure bandage in place, or replace with a plastic bandage.

➤ *Nutritional considerations:* There are no recommended dietary allowances established for potassium, but the estimated minimum intake for adults is 200 mEq/d. Potassium is present in all plant and animal cells, making dietary replacement simple to achieve in the potassium-deficient patient.

➤ Observe the patient for signs and symptoms of fluid volume excess related to excess potassium intake, fluid volume deficit related to active loss, or risk of injury related to an alteration in body chemistry. Symptoms include dehydration, diarrhea, vomiting, or prolonged anorexia. Instruct the patient in electrolyte replacement therapy and changes in dietary intake that affect electrolyte levels.

➤ Increased potassium levels may be associated with dehydration. Evaluate the patient for signs and symptoms of dehydration. Dehydration is a significant and common finding in geriatric patients and other patients in whom renal function has deteriorated.

➤ Patients receiving digoxin or diuretics should have potassium levels monitored carefully because cardiac arrhythmias can occur.

➤ A written report of the examination will be sent to the requesting health care practitioner, who will discuss the results with the patient.

➤ Reinforce information given by the patient's health care provider regarding further testing, treatment, or referral to another health care provider. Answer any questions or address any concerns voiced by the patient or family.

➤ Depending on the results of this procedure, additional testing may be performed to evaluate or monitor progression of the disease process and determine the need for a change in therapy. Evaluate test results in relation to the patient's symptoms and other tests performed.

Related laboratory tests:

➤ Related laboratory tests include aldosterone, anion gap, antiarrhythmic drugs, arterial/alveolar oxygen ratio, blood gases, calcium, electrolytes, osmolality, potassium urine, and sodium (blood and urine).

POTASSIUM, URINE

SYNONYM/ACRONYM: Urine K^+.

SPECIMEN: Urine (5 mL) from an unpreserved random or timed specimen collected in a clean plastic collection container.

REFERENCE VALUE: (Method: Ion-selective electrode)

Age	Conventional Units	SI Units (Conventional Units × 1)
6–10 y		
Male	17–54 mEq/24 h	17–54 mmol/24 h
Female	8–37 mEq/24 h	8–37 mmol/24 h
10–14 y		
Male	22–57 mEq/24 h	22–57 mmol/24 h
Female	18–58 mEq/24 h	18–58 mmol/24 h
Adult	26–123 mEq/24 h	26–123 mmol/24 h

Note: Reference values depend on potassium intake and diurnal variation. Excretion is significantly higher at night.

DESCRIPTION & RATIONALE: Electrolytes dissociate into electrically charged ions when dissolved. Cations, including potassium, carry a positive charge. Body fluids contain approximately equal numbers of anions and cations, although the nature of the ions and their mobility differs between the intracellular and extracellular compartments. Both types of ions affect the electrical and osmolar functions of the body. Electrolyte quantities and the balance among them are controlled by oxygen and carbon dioxide exchange in the lungs; absorption, secretion, and excretion of many substances by the kidneys; and secretion of regulatory hormones by the endocrine glands. Potassium is the most abundant intracellular cation. It is essential for the transmission of electrical impulses in cardiac and skeletal muscle. It also functions in enzyme reactions that transform glucose into energy and amino acids into proteins. Potassium helps maintain acid-base equilibrium, and it has a significant and inverse relationship to pH: A decrease in pH of 0.1 increases the potassium level by 0.6 mEq/L.

Abnormal potassium levels can be caused by a number of contributing factors, which can be categorized as follows:

Altered renal excretion: Normally, 80% to 90% of the body's potassium is filtered out through the kidneys each day (the remainder is excreted in sweat and stool); renal disease can result in abnormally high potassium levels.

Altered dietary intake: A severe potassium deficiency can be caused by an inadequate intake of dietary potassium.

Altered cellular metabolism: Damaged red blood cells (RBCs) release potassium into the circulating fluid, resulting in increased potassium levels.

Regulating electrolyte balance is one of the major functions of the kidneys. In normally functioning kidneys, urine potassium levels increase when serum levels are high and decrease when serum levels are low to maintain homeostasis. The kidneys respond to alkalosis by excreting potassium to retain hydrogen ions and increase acidity. In acidosis, the body excretes hydrogen ions and retains potassium. Analyzing these urinary levels can provide important clues to the functioning of the kidneys and other major organs. Urine potassium tests usually involve timed urine collections over a 12- or 24-hour period. Measurement of random specimens also may be requested. ■

INDICATIONS:

* Determine the potential cause of renal calculi

* Evaluate known or suspected endocrine disorder

* Evaluate known or suspected renal disease

* Evaluate malabsorption disorders

RESULT

Increased in:
* Albright-type renal disease
* Cushing's syndrome
* Diabetic ketoacidosis
* Diuretic therapy
* Hyperaldosteronism
* Starvation (onset)
* Vomiting

Decreased in:
* Addison's disease
* Potassium deficiency (chronic)
* Renal failure with decreased urine flow

CRITICAL VALUES: N/A

INTERFERING FACTORS:
* Drugs and substances that can cause an increase in urine potassium levels include acetazolamide, acetylsalicylic acid, ammonium chloride, bendroflumethiazide, carbenoxolone, chlorthalidone, citrates, clopamide, corticosteroids, cortisone, desoxycorticosterone, dexamethasone, diuretics, dopamine, ethacrynic acid, glycyrrhiza, intra-amniotic saline, mefruside, niacinamide, some oral contraceptives, thiazides, triflocin, and viomycin.

* Drugs that can cause a decrease in urine potassium levels include alanine, amiloride, anesthetic agents, cyclosporine, felodipine, levarterenol, and ramipril.

* A dietary deficiency or excess of potassium can lead to spurious results.

* Diuretic therapy with excessive loss of electrolytes into the urine may falsely elevate results.

* All urine voided for the timed collection period must be included in the

collection or else falsely decreased values may be obtained. Compare output records with volume collected to verify that all voids were included in the collection.

- Potassium levels are subject to diurnal variation (output being highest at night), which is why 24-hour collections are recommended.

Nursing Implications and Procedure • • • • • • • • • • •

Pretest:

➤ Inform the patient that the test is used to evaluate electrolyte balance, acid-base balance, and hypokalemia.

➤ Obtain a history of the patient's complaints, including a list of known allergens (especially allergies or sensitivities to latex), and inform the appropriate health care practitioner accordingly.

➤ Obtain a history of the patient's endocrine, gastrointestinal, and genitourinary systems, as well as results of previously performed laboratory tests, surgical procedures, and other diagnostic procedures. For related laboratory tests, refer to the Endocrine, Gastrointestinal, and Genitourinary System tables.

➤ Obtain a list of the medications the patient is taking, including herbs, nutritional supplements, and nutraceuticals. The requesting health care practitioner and laboratory should be advised if the patient regularly uses these products so that their effects can be taken into consideration when reviewing results.

➤ Review the procedure with the patient. Provide a nonmetallic urinal, bedpan, or toilet-mounted collection device. Address concerns about pain related to the procedure. Explain to the patient that there should be no discomfort during the procedure.

➤ Usually a 24-hour time frame for urine collection is ordered. Inform the patient that all urine must be saved during that 24-hour period. Instruct the patient not to void directly into the laboratory collection container. Instruct the patient to avoid defecating in the collection device and to keep toilet tissue out of the collection device to prevent contamination of the specimen. Place a sign in the bathroom to remind the patient to save all urine.

➤ Instruct the patient to void all urine into the collection device and then to pour the urine into the laboratory collection container. Alternatively, the specimen can be left in the collection device for a health care staff member to add to the laboratory collection container.

➤ *Sensitivity to social and cultural issues*, as well as concern for modesty, is important in providing psychological support before, during, and after the procedure.

➤ There are no food, fluid, or medication restrictions, unless by medical direction.

Intratest:

➤ If the patient has a history of severe allergic reaction to latex, care should be taken to avoid the use of equipment containing latex.

➤ Instruct the patient to cooperate fully and to follow directions.

➤ Observe standard precautions, and follow the general guidelines in Appendix A. Positively identify the patient, and label the appropriate collection container with the corresponding patient demographics, date, and time of collection.

Random specimen (collect in early morning):

Clean-catch specimen:

➤ Instruct the male patient to (1) thoroughly wash his hands, (2) cleanse the meatus, (3) void a small amount into the toilet, and (4) void directly into the specimen container.

➤ Instruct the female patient to (1) thoroughly wash her hands; (2) cleanse the labia from front to back; (3) while keeping the labia separated, void a small amount into the toilet; and (4) without interrupting the urine stream, void directly into the specimen container.

Indwelling catheter:

➤ Put on gloves. Empty drainage tube of urine. It may be necessary to clamp off the catheter for 15 to 30 minutes before specimen collection. Cleanse specimen port with antiseptic swab, and then aspirate 5 mL of urine with a 21- to 25-gauge needle and syringe. Transfer urine to a sterile container.

Timed specimen:

➤ Obtain a clean 3-L urine specimen container, toilet-mounted collection device, and plastic bag (for transport of the specimen container). The specimen must be refrigerated or kept on ice throughout the entire collection period. If an indwelling urinary catheter is in place, the drainage bag must be kept on ice.

➤ Begin the test between 6 and 8 a.m., if possible. Collect first voiding and discard. Record the time the specimen was discarded as the beginning of the timed collection period. The next morning, ask the patient to void at the same time the collection was started and add this last voiding to the container.

➤ If an indwelling catheter is in place, replace the tubing and container system at the start of the collection time. Keep the container system on ice during the collection period, or empty the urine into a larger container periodically during the collection period; monitor to ensure continued drainage, and conclude the test the next morning at the same hour the collection was begun.

➤ At the conclusion of the test, compare the quantity of urine with the urinary output record for the collection; if the specimen contains less than what was recorded as output,

some urine may have been discarded, invalidating the test.

➤ Include on the collection container's label the amount of urine, test start and stop times, and ingestion of any foods or medications that can affect test results.

General:

➤ Promptly transport the specimen to the laboratory for processing and analysis.

➤ The results are recorded manually or in a computerized system for recall and postprocedure interpretation by the appropriate health care practitioner.

Post-test:

➤ *Nutritional considerations:* There are no recommended dietary allowances established for potassium, but the estimated minimum intake for adults is 200 mEq/d. Potassium is present in all plant and animal cells, making dietary replacement simple to achieve in the potassium-deficient patient.

➤ Observe the patient for signs and symptoms of fluid volume excess related to excess potassium intake, fluid volume deficit related to active loss, or risk of injury related to an alteration in body chemistry. Symptoms include dehydration, diarrhea, vomiting, or prolonged anorexia. Instruct the patient in electrolyte replacement therapy and changes in dietary intake that affect electrolyte levels.

➤ Increased potassium levels may be associated with dehydration. Evaluate the patient for signs and symptoms of dehydration. Dehydration is a significant and common finding in geriatric patients and other patients in whom renal function has deteriorated.

➤ Patients receiving digoxin or diuretics should have potassium levels monitored carefully because cardiac arrhythmias can occur.

➤ Increased urine potassium levels may be associated with the formation of kidney stones. Educate the patient, if appropriate, on the importance of drinking a sufficient amount of water when kidney stones are suspected.

➤ A written report of the examination will be sent to the requesting health care practitioner, who will discuss the results with the patient.

➤ Recognize anxiety related to test results. Discuss the implications of abnormal test results on the patient's lifestyle. Provide teaching and information regarding the clinical implications of the test results, as appropriate.

➤ Reinforce information given by the patient's health care provider regarding further testing, treatment, or re-ferral to another health care provider. Answer any questions or address any concerns voiced by the patient or family.

➤ Depending on the results of this procedure, additional testing may be performed to evaluate or monitor progression of the disease process and determine the need for a change in therapy. Evaluate test results in relation to the patient's symptoms and other tests performed.

Related laboratory tests:

➤ Related laboratory tests include aldosterone, kidney stone analysis, osmolality, blood potassium, renin, and blood and urine sodium.

PREALBUMIN

SYNONYM/ACRONYM: Transthyretin.

SPECIMEN: Serum (1 mL) collected in a red- or tiger-top tube.

REFERENCE VALUE: (Method: Nephelometry)

Age	Conventional Units	SI Units (Conventional Units × 10)
Newborn–1 mo	7.0–39.0 mg/dL	70–390 mg/L
1–6 mo	8.3–34.0 mg/dL	83–340 mg/L
6 mo–4 y	2.0–36.0 mg/dL	20–360 mg/L
5–6 y	12.0–30.0 mg/dL	120–300 mg/L
6 y–adult	12.0–42.0 mg/dL	120–420 mg/L

DESCRIPTION & RATIONALE: Prealbumin is a protein primarily produced by the liver. It is the major transport protein for triiodothyronine and thyroxine. It is also important in the metabolism of retinol-binding protein, which is needed for transporting vitamin A (retinol). Prealbumin has a short biologic half-life of 2 days. This makes it a good indicator of protein status and an excellent marker for malnutrition. Prealbumin is often measured simultaneously with transferrin and albumin. ■

INDICATIONS: Evaluate nutritional status

RESULT

Increased in:
• Alcoholism
• Chronic renal failure
• Patients receiving steroids

Decreased in:
• Acute-phase inflammatory response
• Diseases of the liver
• Hepatic damage
• Malnutrition
• Tissue necrosis

CRITICAL VALUES: N/A

INTERFERING FACTORS:

• Drugs that may increase prealbumin levels include anabolic steroids, anticonvulsants, danazol, oral contraceptives, prednisolone, prednisone, and propranolol.

• Drugs that may decrease prealbumin levels include amiodarone and diethylstilbestrol.

• Fasting 4 hours before specimen collection is highly recommended. Reference ranges are often based on fasting populations to provide some level of standardization for comparison. The presence of lipids in the blood may also interfere with the test method; fasting eliminates this potential source of error, especially if the patient has elevated lipid levels.

Nursing Implications and Procedure

Pretest:

➤ Inform the patient that the test is used to evaluate nutritional status and assess liver function.

➤ Obtain a history of the patient's complaints, including a list of known allergens (especially allergies or sensitivities to latex), and inform the appropriate health care practitioner accordingly.

➤ Obtain a history of the patient's endocrine, gastrointestinal, and hepatobiliary systems, as well as results of previously performed laboratory tests, surgical procedures, and other diagnostic procedures. For related laboratory tests, refer to the Endocrine, Gastrointestinal, and Hepatobiliary System tables.

➤ Obtain a list of medications the patient is taking, including herbs, nutritional supplements, and nutraceuticals. The requesting health care practitioner and laboratory should be advised if the patient regularly uses these products so that their effects can be taken into consideration when reviewing results.

➤ Review the procedure with the patient. Inform the patient that specimen collection takes approximately 5 to 10 minutes. Address concerns about pain related to the procedure. Explain to the patient that there may be some discomfort during the venipuncture.

➤ Instruct the patient to fast for 4 hours before specimen collection.

➤ There are no fluid or medication restrictions, unless by medical direction.

Intratest:

➤ Ensure that the patient has complied with dietary restrictions; assure that food has been restricted for at least 4 hours prior to the procedure.

➤ If the patient has a history of severe allergic reaction to latex, care should

be taken to avoid the use of equipment containing latex.

➤ Instruct the patient to cooperate fully and to follow directions. Direct the patient to breathe normally and to avoid unnecessary movement.

➤ Observe standard precautions, and follow the general guidelines in Appendix A. Positively identify the patient, and label the appropriate tubes with the corresponding patient demographics, date, and time of collection. Perform a venipuncture; collect the specimen in a 5-mL red- or tiger-top tube.

➤ Remove the needle, and apply a pressure dressing over the puncture site.

➤ Promptly transport the specimen to the laboratory for processing and analysis.

➤ The results are recorded manually or in a computerized system for recall and postprocedure interpretation by the appropriate health care practitioner.

Post-test:

➤ Observe venipuncture site for bleeding or hematoma formation. Apply paper tape or other adhesive to hold pressure bandage in place, or replace with a plastic bandage.

➤ Instruct the patient to resume usual diet, as directed by the health care practitioner.

➤ *Nutritional considerations:* Nutritional therapy may be indicated for patients with decreased prealbumin levels. Educate the patient, as appropriate, that good dietary sources of complete protein (containing all eight essential amino acids) include meat, fish, eggs, and dairy products; and that good sources of incomplete protein (lacking one or more of the eight essential amino acids) include grains, nuts, legumes, vegetables, and seeds.

➤ A written report of the examination will be sent to the requesting health care practitioner, who will discuss the results with the patient.

➤ Reinforce information given by the patient's health care provider regarding further testing, treatment, or referral to another health care provider. Answer any questions or address any concerns voiced by the patient or family.

➤ Depending on the results of this procedure, additional testing may be performed to evaluate or monitor progression of the disease process and determine the need for a change in therapy. Evaluate test results in relation to the patient's symptoms and other tests performed.

Related laboratory tests:

➤ Related laboratory tests include albumin, chloride, ferritin, iron/total iron-binding capacity, potassium, protein, sodium, and transferrin.

PROCTOSIGMOIDOSCOPY

SYNONYMS/ACRONYM: Anoscopy (anal canal), proctoscopy (rectum), sigmoidoscopy (sigmoid colon), flexible fiberoptic sigmoidoscopy, flexible proctosigmoidoscopy.

AREA OF APPLICATION: Anus, rectum, colon.

CONTRAST: Air.

DESCRIPTION & RATIONALE: Proctosigmoidoscopy allows direct visualization of the mucosa of the anal canal (anoscopy), rectum (proctoscopy), and distal sigmoid colon (sigmoidoscopy). The procedure can be performed using a rigid or flexible fiberoptic endoscope, but the flexible instrument is generally preferred. The endoscope is a multichannel device allowing visualization of the mucosal lining of the colon, instillation of air, removal of fluid and foreign objects, obtaining of tissue biopsy specimens, and use of a laser for the destruction of tissue and control of bleeding. The endoscope is advanced approximately 60 cm into the colon. This procedure is commonly used in patients with lower abdominal and perineal pain; changes in bowel habits; rectal prolapse during defecation; or passage of blood, mucus, or pus in the stool. Proctosigmoidoscopy can also be a therapeutic procedure, allowing removal of polyps or hemorrhoids or reduction of a volvulus. Biopsy specimens of suspicious sites may be obtained during the procedure. This procedure is recommended for patients who are more than 50 years old as part of a routine screening for colorectal cancer. ■

INDICATIONS:
- Confirm the diagnosis of diverticular disease
- Confirm the diagnosis of Hirschsprung's disease and colitis in children
- Determine the cause of pain and rectal prolapse during defecation
- Determine the cause of rectal itching, pain, or burning
- Evaluate the cause of blood, pus, or mucus in the stool
- Evaluate postoperative anastomosis of the colon
- Examine the distal colon before barium enema x-ray to obtain improved visualization of the area, and after a barium enema when x-ray findings are inconclusive
- Reduce volvulus of the sigmoid colon
- Remove hemorrhoids by laser therapy
- Screen for and excise polyps
- Screen for colon cancer

RESULT

Normal Findings:
- Normal mucosa of the anal canal, rectum, and sigmoid colon

Abnormal Findings:
- Anal fissure or fistula
- Anorectal abscess
- Benign lesions
- Bleeding sites
- Bowel infection or inflammation
- Crohn's disease
- Diverticula
- Hypertrophic anal papillae
- Internal and external hemorrhoids
- Polyps
- Rectal prolapse
- Tumors
- Ulcerative colitis
- Vascular abnormalities

CRITICAL VALUES: N/A

INTERFERING FACTORS:

This procedure is contraindicated for:

- Patients with bleeding disorders, especially disorders associated with uremia and cytotoxic chemotherapy

- Patients with cardiac conditions or arrhythmias

- Patients with bowel perforation, acute peritonitis, ischemic bowel necrosis, toxic megacolon, diverticulitis, recent bowel surgery, advanced pregnancy, severe cardiac or pulmonary disease, recent myocardial infarction, known or suspected pulmonary embolus, large abdominal aortic or iliac aneurysm, and coagulation abnormality

Factors that may impair clear imaging:

- Inability of the patient to cooperate or remain still during the procedure because of age, significant pain, or mental status

- Patients who are very obese, who may exceed the weight limit for the equipment

- Incorrect positioning of the patient, which may produce poor visualization of the area to be examined

- Strictures or other abnormalities preventing passage of the scope

- Barium swallow or upper gastrointestinal (GI) series within the preceding 48 hours

- Severe lower GI bleeding or the presence of feces, barium, blood, or blood clots

Other considerations:

- Failure to follow dietary restrictions before the procedure may cause the procedure to be canceled or repeated.

- Use of bowel preparations that include laxatives or enemas should be avoided in pregnant patients or patients with inflammatory bowel disease, unless specifically directed by a health care practitioner.

Nursing Implications and Procedure • • • • • • • • • •

Pretest:

▶ Inform the patient that the test is primarily used to examine the rectum and the distal portion of the colon.

▶ Obtain a history of the patient's complaints, including a list of known allergens (especially allergies or sensitivities to latex), and inform the appropriate health care practitioner accordingly.

▶ Obtain a history of the patient's gastrointestinal system, as well as results of previously performed diagnostic procedures, surgical procedures, and laboratory tests. For related diagnostic tests, refer to the Gastrointestinal System table.

▶ Ensure that this procedure is performed before an upper GI study or barium swallow.

▶ Record the date of the last menstrual period and determine the possibility of pregnancy in perimenopausal women.

▶ Obtain a list of the medications the patient is taking, including anticoagulant therapy, acetylsalicylic acid, herbs, nutritional supplements, and nutraceuticals, especially those known to affect coagulation. It is recommended that use be discontinued 14 days before dental or surgical procedures. The requesting health care practitioner and laboratory should be advised if the patient regularly uses these products so that their effects can be taken into consideration when reviewing results.

▶ Note intake of oral iron preparations within 1 week before the procedure because these cause black, sticky feces that are difficult to remove with bowel preparation.

➤ Review the procedure with the patient. Address concerns about pain related to the procedure. Explain to the patient that some pain may be experienced during the test, and there may be moments of discomfort. Explain that a sedative and/or analgesia will be administered to promote relaxation and reduce discomfort prior to insertion of the anoscope. Explain the purpose of the test and how the procedure is performed. Inform the patient that the procedure is performed in a GI lab, usually by a health care practitioner and support staff, and takes approximately 30 to 60 minutes.

➤ Inform the patient that the urge to defecate may be experienced when the scope is passed. Encourage slow, deep breathing through the mouth to help alleviate the feeling.

➤ Inform the patient that flatus may be expelled during and after the procedure owing to air that is injected into the scope to improve visualization.

➤ *Sensitivity to cultural and social issues,* as well as concern for modesty, is important in providing psychological support before, during, and after the procedure.

➤ Instruct the patient to eat a low-residue diet for several days before the procedure, to consume only clear liquids the evening before the test, and to fast and restrict fluids for 8 hours prior to the procedure.

➤ Inform the patient that it is important the bowel be cleaned thoroughly so that the physician can visualize the colon. Inform the patient that a laxative and cleansing enema may be needed the day before the procedure, with cleansing enemas on the morning of the procedure, depending on the institution's policy.

➤ *Make sure a written and informed consent has been signed prior to the procedure and before administering any medications.*

Intratest:

➤ Ensure that the patient has complied with dietary and fluid restrictions; assure that food and fluid have been restricted for at least 8 hours.

➤ Ensure that ordered laxative has been administered late in the afternoon of the day before the procedure. Two small-volume enemas are administered 1 hour before the procedure.

➤ Patients are given a gown, robe, and foot coverings to wear and instructed to void prior to the procedure.

➤ Instruct the patient to cooperate fully and to follow directions. Instruct the patient to remain still throughout the procedure because movement produces unreliable results.

➤ Observe standard precautions, and follow the general guidelines in Appendix A. Wear gloves and gown throughout the procedure.

➤ Place the patient an examination table in the left lateral decubitus position or the knee-chest position and drape with the buttocks exposed. The buttocks are placed at or extending slightly beyond the edge of the examination table or bed, preferably on a special examining table that tilts the patient into the desired position.

➤ The health care practitioner visually inspects the perianal area and then performs a digital rectal examination with a well-lubricated, gloved finger. A fecal specimen may be obtained from the glove when the finger is removed from the rectum.

➤ A lubricated anoscope (7 cm in length) is inserted, and the anal canal is inspected (anoscopy). The anoscope is removed, and a lubricated proctoscope (27 cm in length) or flexible sigmoidoscope (35 to 60 cm in length) is inserted.

➤ The scope is manipulated gently to facilitate passage, and air may be insufflated through the scope to improve visualization. Suction and cotton swabs also are used to remove materials that hinder visualization.

➤ The patient is instructed to take deep breaths to aid in movement of the scope downward through the ascending colon to the cecum and into the terminal portion of the ileum.

➤ Examination is done as the scope is gradually withdrawn. Photographs are obtained for future reference.

➤ At the end of the procedure, the scope is completely withdrawn, and residual lubricant is cleansed from the anal area.

➤ Place fecal or tissue samples and polyps in properly labeled specimen containers, and promptly transport the specimen to the laboratory for processing and analysis.

➤ The results are recorded manually, on film, or by automated equipment in a computerized system for recall and postprocedure interpretation by the appropriate health care practitioner.

Post-test:

➤ Instruct the patient to resume usual diet, medication, and activity, as directed by the health care practitioner.

➤ Monitor for any rectal bleeding. Instruct the patient to expect slight rectal bleeding for 2 days after removal of polyps or biopsy specimens, but that heavy rectal bleeding must be immediately reported to the health care practitioner.

➤ Emphasize that any abdominal pain, tenderness, or distention; pain on defecation; or fever must be reported to the health care practitioner immediately.

➤ Inform the patient that any bloating or flatulence is the result of air insufflation.

➤ Encourage the patient to drink several glasses of water to help replace fluid lost during test preparation.

➤ A written report of the examination will be completed by a health care practitioner specializing in this branch of medicine. The report will be sent to the requesting health care practitioner, who will discuss the results with the patient.

➤ Recognize anxiety related to test results, and be supportive of perceived loss of independence and fear of shortened life expectancy. Discuss the implications of abnormal test results on the patient's lifestyle. Provide teaching and information regarding the clinical implications of the test results, as appropriate. Educate the patient regarding access to counseling services.

➤ Reinforce information given by the patient's health care provider regarding further testing, treatment, or referral to another health care provider. Answer any questions or address any concerns voiced by the patient or family.

➤ Depending on the results of this procedure, additional testing may be needed to evaluate or monitor progression of the disease process and determine the need for a change in therapy. Evaluate test results in relation to the patient's symptoms and other tests performed.

Related diagnostic tests:

➤ Related diagnostic tests include barium enema, colonoscopy, computed tomography of the abdomen, and magnetic resonance imaging of the abdomen.

PROGESTERONE

SYNONYM/ACRONYM: N/A.

SPECIMEN: Serum (1 mL) collected in a red- or tiger-top tube.

REFERENCE VALUE: (Method: Immunochemiluminometric assay [ICMA])

Hormonal State	Conventional Units	SI Units (Conventional Units × 3.18)
Adult Male	Less than 0.3–1.2 ng/mL	Less than 0.9–3.8 nmol/L
Adult Female	Less than 0.5 ng/mL	Less than 1.6 nmol/L
Follicular phase	0.2–1.4 ng/mL	0.6–4.4 nmol/L
Luteal phase	3.3–25.6 ng/mL	10.5–81.4 nmol/L
Pregnancy, first trimester	11.2–90.0 ng/mL	35.6–286.2 nmol/L
Pregnancy, second trimester	25.5–89.4 ng/mL	81.1–284.3 nmol/L
Pregnancy, third trimester	48.4–422.5 ng/mL	153.9–1343.6 nmol/L
Postmenopausal period	0.0–0.7 ng/mL	0.0–2.2 nmol/L

DESCRIPTION & RATIONALE: Progesterone is a female sex hormone. Its function is to prepare the uterus for pregnancy and the breasts for lactation. Progesterone testing can be used to confirm that ovulation has occurred and to assess the functioning of the corpus luteum. Serial measurements can be performed to help determine the day of ovulation. ■

INDICATIONS:
• Assist in the diagnosis of luteal-phase defects (performed in conjunction with endometrial biopsy)

• Evaluate patients at risk for early or spontaneous abortion

• Identify patients at risk for ectopic pregnancy and assessment of corpus luteum function

• Monitor patients ovulating during human chorionic gonadotropin (HCG), human menopausal gonadotropin, follicle-stimulating hormone/luteinizing hormone–releasing hormone, or clomiphene induction (serial measurements can assist in pinpointing the day of ovulation)

• Monitor patients receiving progesterone replacement therapy

RESULT

Increased in:

- Chorioepithelioma of the ovary
- Congenital adrenal hyperplasia
- Hydatidiform mole
- Lipoid ovarian tumor
- Theca lutein cyst

Decreased in:

- Galactorrhea-amenorrhea syndrome
- Primary or secondary hypogonadism
- Short luteal phase syndrome
- Threatened abortion

CRITICAL VALUES: N/A

INTERFERING FACTORS:

- Drugs that may increase progesterone levels include clomiphene, corticotropin, hydroxyprogesterone, ketoconazole, mifepristone, progesterone, tamoxifen, and valproic acid.

- Drugs that may decrease progesterone levels include ampicillin, epostane, goserelin, leuprolide, and prostaglandin $F_{2\alpha}$.

Nursing Implications and Procedure • • • • • • • • • • •

Pretest:

▶ Inform the patient that the test is primarily used to assess ovarian function, assist in fertility workups, and monitor placental function during pregnancy.

▶ Obtain a history of the patient's complaints, including a list of known allergens (especially allergies or sensitivities to latex), and inform the appropriate health care practitioner accordingly.

▶ Obtain a history of the patient's endocrine and reproductive systems, as well as results of previously performed laboratory tests, surgical procedures, and other diagnostic procedures. For related laboratory tests, refer to the Endocrine and Reproductive System tables.

▶ Record the date of the last menstrual period and determine the possibility of pregnancy in perimenopausal women.

▶ Obtain a list of the medications the patient is taking, including herbs, nutritional supplements, and nutraceuticals. The requesting health care practitioner and laboratory should be advised if the patient regularly uses these products so that their effects can be taken into consideration when reviewing results.

▶ Review the procedure with the patient. Inform the patient that specimen collection takes approximately 5 to 10 minutes. Address concerns about pain related to the procedure. Explain to the patient that there may be some discomfort during the venipuncture.

▶ There are no food, fluid, or medication restrictions, unless by medical direction.

Intratest:

▶ If the patient has a history of severe allergic reaction to latex, care should be taken to avoid the use of equipment containing latex.

▶ Instruct the patient to cooperate fully and to follow directions. Direct the patient to breathe normally and to avoid unnecessary movement.

▶ Observe standard precautions, and follow the general guidelines in Appendix A. Positively identify the patient, and label the appropriate tubes with the corresponding patient demographics, date, and time of collection. Perform a venipuncture; collect the specimen in a 5-mL red- or tiger-top tube.

▶ Remove the needle, and apply a pressure dressing over the puncture site.

▶ Promptly transport the specimen to the laboratory for processing and analysis.

> The results are recorded manually or in a computerized system for recall and postprocedure interpretation by the appropriate health care practitioner.

Post-test:

> Observe venipuncture site for bleeding or hematoma formation. Apply paper tape or other adhesive to hold pressure bandage in place, or replace with a plastic bandage.

> A written report of the examination will be sent to the requesting health care practitioner, who will discuss the results with the patient.

> Recognize anxiety related to test results, and provide support. Provide teaching and information regarding the clinical implications of the test results, as appropriate. Provide a nonjudgmental, nonthreatening atmosphere for exploring other options (e.g., adoption). Educate the patient regarding access to counseling services, as appropriate.

> Reinforce information given by the patient's health care provider regarding further testing, treatment, or referral to another health care provider. Answer any questions or address any concerns voiced by the patient or family.

> Depending on the results of this procedure, additional testing may be performed to evaluate or monitor progression of the disease process and determine the need for a change in therapy. Evaluate test results in relation to the patient's symptoms and other tests performed.

Related laboratory tests:

> Related laboratory tests include cardiolipin antibodies, estradiol, fetal fibronectin, follicle-stimulating hormone, HCG, luteinizing hormone, and prolactin.

PROLACTIN

SYNONYMS/ACRONYMS: Luteotropic hormone, lactogenic hormone, lactogen, HPRL, PRL.

SPECIMEN: Serum (1 mL) collected in a red- or tiger-top tube. Specimen should be transported tightly capped and in an ice slurry.

REFERENCE VALUE: (Method: Immunoassay)

Age	Conventional Units	SI Units (Conventional Units × 1)
Prepubertal males and females	3.2–20.0 ng/mL	3.2–20.0 µg/L
Men	2.4–13.8 ng/mL	2.4–13.8 µg/L
Women	3.3–26.7 ng/mL	3.3–26.7 µg/L
Pregnant	5.3–215.3 ng/mL	5.3–215.3 µg/L
Postmenopausal	2.4–24.0 ng/mL	2.4–24.0 µg/L

DESCRIPTION & RATIONALE: Prolactin is secreted by the pituitary gland. It is unique among hormones in that it responds to inhibition by the hypothalamus rather than to stimulation. The only known function of prolactin is to induce milk production in female breasts that are already stimulated by high estrogen levels. When milk production is established, lactation can continue without elevated prolactin levels. Prolactin levels rise late in pregnancy, peak with the initiation of lactation, and surge each time a woman breast-feeds. The function of prolactin in males is unknown. ∎

INDICATIONS:
- Assist in the diagnosis of primary hypothyroidism, as indicated by elevated levels
- Assist in the diagnosis of suspected tumor involving the lungs or kidneys (elevated levels indicating ectopic prolactin production)
- Evaluate failure of lactation in the postpartum period
- Evaluate sexual dysfunction of unknown cause in men and women
- Evaluate suspected postpartum hypophyseal infarction (Sheehan's syndrome), as indicated by decreased levels

RESULT

Increased in:
- Adrenal insufficiency
- Amenorrhea
- Anorexia nervosa
- Breastfeeding
- Chiari-Frommel and Argonz–Del Castillo syndromes
- Chest wall injury
- Chronic renal failure
- Ectopic prolactin-secreting tumors (e.g., lung, kidney)
- Galactorrhea
- Hypothalamic and pituitary disorders
- Hypothyroidism (primary)
- Insulin-induced hypoglycemia
- Liver failure
- Pituitary tumor
- Polycystic ovary (Stein-Leventhal) syndrome
- Pregnancy
- Surgery (pituitary stalk section)

Decreased in:
- Sheehan's syndrome

CRITICAL VALUES: N/A

INTERFERING FACTORS:
- Drugs and hormones that may increase prolactin levels include amitryptyline, amoxapine, arginine, azosemide, benserazide, butaperazine, butorphanol, carbidopa, chlorophenylpiperazine, chlorpromazine, cimetidine, clomipramine, desipramine, diethylstilbestrol, β-endorphin, enflurane, fenfluramine, fenoldopam, flunarizine, fluphenazine, growth hormone–releasing hormone, imipramine, insulin, interferon-β, labetalol, loxapine, megestrol, mestranol, methyldopa, metoclopramide, molindone, morphine, nitrous oxide, oral contraceptives, oxcarbazepine, parathyroid hormone, pentagastrin, perphenazine, phenothiazines, phenytoin, pimozide, prochlorperazine, promazine, ranitidine, remoxipride, reserpine, sulpiride, sultopride, thiethylperazine, thioridazine, thiothixene, thyrotropin-releasing hormone, trifluoperazine, trimipramine, tumor necrosis factor, veralipride, verapamil, and zometapine.
- Drugs and hormones that may decrease prolactin levels include anticonvul-

sants, apomorphine, bromocriptine, cabergoline, calcitonin, cyclosporine, dexamethasone, dopamine, D-Trp-6-LHRH, levodopa, metoclopramide, morphine, nifedipine, octreotide, pergolide, ranitidine, rifampin, ritanserin, ropinirole, secretin, thyroid hormones, and terguride.

• Episodic elevations can occur in response to sleep, stress, exercise, hypoglycemia, and breast-feeding.

• Venipuncture can cause falsely elevated levels.

• Prolactin secretion is subject to diurnal variation, with highest levels occurring in the morning.

• Failure to follow dietary restrictions before the procedure may cause the procedure to be canceled or repeated.

Nursing Implications and Procedure • • • • • • • • • • •

Pretest:

➤ Inform the patient that the test is primarily used to evaluate lactation disorders and identify the presence of prolactin-secreting tumors.

➤ Obtain a history of the patient's complaints, including a list of known allergens (especially allergies or sensitivities to latex), and inform the appropriate health care practitioner accordingly.

➤ Obtain a history of the patient's endocrine and reproductive systems, as well as results of previously performed laboratory tests, surgical procedures, and other diagnostic procedures. For related laboratory tests, refer to the Endocrine and Reproductive System tables.

➤ Obtain a list of medications the patient is taking, including herbs, nutritional supplements, and nutraceuticals. The requesting health care practitioner and laboratory should be advised if the patient regularly uses

these products so that their effects can be taken into consideration when reviewing results.

➤ Review the procedure with the patient. Specimen collection should occur between 8 and 10 a.m. Inform the patient that specimen collection takes approximately 5 to 10 minutes. Address concerns about pain related to the procedure. Explain to the patient that there may be some discomfort during the venipuncture.

➤ The patient should fast for 12 hours before specimen collection.

➤ There are no fluid or medication restrictions, unless by medical direction.

➤ Prepare an ice slurry in a cup or plastic bag to have on hand for immediate transport of the specimen to the laboratory.

Intratest:

➤ Ensure that the patient has complied with dietary restrictions; assure that food has been restricted for at least 12 hours prior to the procedure.

➤ If the patient has a history of severe allergic reaction to latex, care should be taken to avoid the use of equipment containing latex.

➤ Instruct the patient to cooperate fully and to follow directions. Direct the patient to breathe normally and to avoid unnecessary movement.

➤ Observe standard precautions, and follow the general guidelines in Appendix A. Positively identify the patient, and label the appropriate tubes with the corresponding patient demographics, date, and time of collection. Perform a venipuncture; collect the specimen in a 5-mL red- or tiger-top tube.

➤ Remove the needle, and apply a pressure dressing over the puncture site.

➤ Promptly transport the specimen to the laboratory for processing and analysis. The specimen should be placed in an ice slurry immediately after collection. Information on the specimen label can be protected from water in the ice slurry if the specimen is first placed in a protective plastic bag.

➤ The results are recorded manually or in a computerized system for recall and postprocedure interpretation by the appropriate health care practitioner.

Post-test:

➤ Observe venipuncture site for bleeding or hematoma formation. Apply paper tape or other adhesive to hold pressure bandage in place, or replace with a plastic bandage.

➤ Instruct the patient to resume usual diet, as directed by the health care practitioner.

➤ A written report of the examination will be sent to the requesting health care practitioner, who will discuss the results with the patient.

➤ Reinforce information given by the patient's health care provider regarding further testing, treatment, or referral to another health care provider. Answer any questions or address any concerns voiced by the patient or family.

➤ Depending on the results of this procedure, additional testing may be performed to evaluate or monitor progression of the disease process and determine the need for a change in therapy. Evaluate test results in relation to the patient's symptoms and other tests performed.

Related laboratory tests:

➤ Related laboratory tests include dehydroepiandrosterone, estradiol, follicle-stimulating hormone, human chorionic gonadotropin, and luteinizing hormone.

PROSTATE-SPECIFIC ANTIGEN

SYNONYM/ACRONYM: PSA.

SPECIMEN: Serum (1 mL) collected in a red- or tiger-top tube.

REFERENCE VALUE: (Method: Immunoassay)

Sex	Conventional Units	SI Units (Conventional Units × 1)
Male	Less than 4 ng/mL	Less than 4 μg/L
Female	Less than 0.5 ng/mL	Less than 0.5 μg/L

DESCRIPTION & RATIONALE: Prostate-specific antigen (PSA) is produced exclusively by the epithelial cells of the prostate, periurethral, and perirectal glands. Used in conjunction with the digital rectal examination,

PSA is a useful test for monitoring adenocarcinoma of the prostate. PSA circulates in both free and bound (complexed) forms. A low ratio of free to complexed PSA (i.e., less than 10%) is suggestive of prostate cancer; a ratio of greater than 30% is rarely associated with prostate cancer. Serial measurements are often performed before and after surgery. *Important note:* When following patients using serial testing, use the same method of measurement consistently. ∎

INDICATIONS:

- Evaluate the effectiveness of treatment for prostate cancer (prostatectomy): Levels decrease if treatment is effective; rising levels are associated with recurrence and a poor prognosis.

- Investigate or evaluate an enlarged prostate gland, especially if prostate cancer is suspected.

- Stage prostate cancer.

RESULT

Increased in:

- Benign prostatic hypertrophy

- Prostate cancer

- Prostatic infarct

- Urinary retention

Decreased in: N/A

CRITICAL VALUES: N/A

INTERFERING FACTORS:

- Drugs that decrease PSA levels include buserelin, finasteride, and flutamide.

- There is growing evidence that rectal palpation does not cause elevated PSA. However, increases can occur due to prostatic needle biopsy, cytoscopy, or prostatic infarction.

Nursing Implications and Procedure • • • • • • • • • • •

Pretest:

➤ Inform the patient that the test is used to monitor status of prostate cancer and response to therapy.

➤ Obtain a history of the patient's complaints, including a list of known allergens (especially allergies or sensitivities to latex), and inform the appropriate health care practitioner accordingly.

➤ Obtain a history of the patient's genitourinary, immune, and reproductive systems, as well as results of previously performed laboratory tests, surgical procedures, and other diagnostic procedures. For related laboratory tests, refer to the Genitourinary, Immune, and Reproductive System tables.

➤ Note any recent procedures that can interfere with test results.

➤ Obtain a list of medications the patient is taking, including herbs, nutritional supplements, and nutraceuticals. The requesting health care practitioner and laboratory should be advised if the patient regularly uses these products so that their effects can be taken into consideration when reviewing results.

➤ Review the procedure with the patient. Inform the patient that specimen collection takes approximately 5 to 10 minutes. Address concerns about pain related to the procedure. Explain to the patient that there may be some discomfort during the venipuncture.

➤ There are no food, fluid, or medication restrictions, unless by medical direction.

Intratest:

➤ If the patient has a history of severe allergic reaction to latex, care should be taken to avoid the use of equipment containing latex.

➤ Instruct the patient to cooperate fully and to follow directions. Direct the

patient to breathe normally and to avoid unnecessary movement.

➤ Observe standard precautions, and follow the general guidelines in Appendix A. Positively identify the patient, and label the appropriate tubes with the corresponding patient demographics, date, and time of collection. Perform a venipuncture; collect the specimen in a 5-mL red- or tiger-top tube.

➤ Remove the needle, and apply a pressure dressing over the puncture site.

➤ Promptly transport the specimen to the laboratory for processing and analysis.

➤ The results are recorded manually or in a computerized system for recall and postprocedure interpretation by the appropriate health care practitioner.

Post-test:

➤ Observe venipuncture site for bleeding or hematoma formation. Apply paper tape or other adhesive to hold pressure bandage in place, or replace with a plastic bandage.

➤ A written report of the examination will be sent to the requesting health care practitioner, who will discuss the results with the patient.

➤ Recognize anxiety related to test results, and offer support. Counsel the patient, as appropriate, that sexual dysfunction related to altered body function, drugs, or radiation may occur. Discuss the implications of abnormal test results on the patient's lifestyle. Provide teaching and information regarding the clinical implications of the test results, as appropriate. Educate the patient regarding access to counseling services.

➤ Reinforce information given by the patient's health care provider regarding further testing, treatment, or referral to another health care provider. Answer any questions or address any concerns voiced by the patient or family.

➤ Depending on the results of this procedure, additional testing may be performed to evaluate or monitor progression of the disease process and determine the need for a change in therapy. Evaluate test results in relation to the patient's symptoms and other tests performed.

Related laboratory tests:

➤ Related laboratory tests include biopsy of the prostate and prostatic acid phosphatase.

PROTEIN, BLOOD, TOTAL AND FRACTIONS

· ·

SYNONYMS/ACRONYMS: TP, SPEP (fractions include albumin, α_1-globulin, α_2-globulin, β-globulin, and γ-globulin).

SPECIMEN: Serum (1 mL) collected in a red- or tiger-top tube.

REFERENCE VALUE: (Method: Spectrophotometry for total protein, electrophoresis for protein fractions)

Total Protein

Age	Conventional Units	SI Units (Conversion Factor × 10)
Newborn–5 d	3.8–6.2 g/dL	38–62 g/L
1–3 y	5.9–7.0 g/dL	59–70 g/L
4–6 y	5.9–7.8 g/dL	59–78 g/L
7–9 y	6.2–8.1 g/dL	62–81 g/L
10–19 y	6.3–8.6 g/dL	63–86 g/L
Adult	6.0–8.0 g/dL	60–80 g/L

Protein Fractions

	Conventional Units	SI Units (Conversion Factor × 10)
Albumin	3.4–4.8 g/dL	34–48 g/L
α_1-Globulin	0.2–0.4 g/dL	2–4 g/L
α_2-Globulin	0.4–0.8 g/dL	4–8 g/L
β-Globulin	0.5–1.0 g/dL	5–10 g/L
γ-Globulin	0.6–1.2 g/dL	6–12 g/L

DESCRIPTION & RATIONALE: Protein is essential to all physiologic functions. Proteins consist of amino acids, the building blocks of blood and body tissues. Protein is also required for the regulation of metabolic processes, immunity, and proper water balance. Total protein includes albumin and globulins. α_1-Globulin includes α_1-antitrypsin, α_1-fetoprotein, α_1-acid glycoprotein, α_1-antichymotrypsin, inter-α_1-trypsin inhibitor, high-density lipoproteins, and group-specific component (vitamin D–binding protein). α_2-Globulin includes haptoglobin, ceruloplasmin, and α_2-macroglobulin. β-Globulin includes transferrin, hemopexin, very-low-density lipoproteins, low-density lipoproteins, β_2-microglobulin, fibrinogen, complement, and C-reactive protein. γ-Globulin includes immunoglobulin (Ig) G, IgA, IgM, IgD, and IgE. After an acute infection or trauma, levels of many of the liver-derived proteins increase, whereas albumin level decreases; these conditions may not reflect an abnormal total protein determination. ■

INDICATIONS:

• Evaluation of edema, as seen in patients with low total protein and low albumin levels

• Evaluation of nutritional status

RESULT

Increased:

• α_1-Globulin proteins in acute and chronic inflammatory diseases

• α_2-Globulin proteins occasionally in diabetes, pancreatitis, and hemolysis

- β-Globulin proteins in hyperlipoproteinemias and monoclonal gammopathies

- γ-Globulin proteins in chronic liver diseases, chronic infections, autoimmune disorders, hepatitis, cirrhosis, and lymphoproliferative disorders

- Total protein:
  Dehydration
  Monoclonal and polyclonal
    gammopathies
  Myeloma
  Sarcoidosis
  Some types of chronic liver disease
  Tropical diseases (e.g., leprosy)
  Waldenström's macroglobulinemia

Decreased:

- α_1-Globulin proteins in hereditary deficiency

- α_2-Globulin proteins in nephrotic syndrome, malignancies, numerous subacute and chronic inflammatory disorders, and recovery stage of severe burns

- β-Globulin proteins in hypo-β-lipoproteinemias and IgA deficiency

- γ-Globulin proteins in immune deficiency or suppression

- Total protein
  Administration of intravenous fluids
  Burns
  Chronic alcoholism
  Chronic ulcerative colitis
  Cirrhosis
  Crohn's disease
  Glomerulonephritis
  Heart failure
  Hyperthyroidism
  Malabsorption
  Malnutrition
  Neoplasms
  Nephrotic syndrome
  Pregnancy
  Prolonged immobilization

Protein-losing enteropathies
Severe skin disease
Starvation

CRITICAL VALUES: N/A

INTERFERING FACTORS:

- Drugs that may increase protein levels include amino acids (if given intravenously), anabolic steroids, angiotensin, anticonvulsants, carbenicillin, corticosteroids, corticotropin, digitalis, furosemide, insulin, isotretinoin, levonorgestrel, oral contraceptives, progesterone, radiographic agents, and thyroid agents.

- Drugs and substances that may decrease protein levels include acetylsalicylic acid, arginine, benzene, carvedilol, citrates, floxuridine, laxatives, mercury compounds, oral contraceptives, pentastarch, phosgene, pyrazinamide, rifampin, trimethadione, and valproic acid.

- Values are significantly lower (5% to 10%) in recumbent patients.

- Hemolysis can falsely elevate results.

- Venous stasis can falsely elevate results; the tourniquet should not be left on the arm for longer than 60 seconds.

Nursing Implications and Procedure . . . .

Pretest:

➤ Inform the patient that the test is primarily used to evaluate nutritional status; abnormal values are found in numerous conditions and diseases.

➤ Obtain a history of the patient's complaints, including a list of known allergens (especially allergies or sensitivities to latex), and inform the appropriate health care practitioner accordingly.

➤ Obtain a history of the patient's gastrointestinal, hepatobiliary, and immune systems, as well as results of previously performed laboratory tests, surgical procedures, and other diagnostic procedures. For related laboratory tests, refer to the Gastrointestinal, Hepatobiliary, and Immune System tables.

➤ Obtain a list of medications the patient is taking, including herbs, nutritional supplements, and nutraceuticals. The requesting health care practitioner and laboratory should be advised if the patient regularly uses these products so that their effects can be taken into consideration when reviewing results.

➤ Review the procedure with the patient. Inform the patient that specimen collection takes approximately 5 to 10 minutes. Address concerns about pain related to the procedure. Explain to the patient that there may be some discomfort during the venipuncture.

➤ There are no food, fluid, or medication restrictions, unless by medical direction.

Intratest:

➤ If the patient has a history of severe allergic reaction to latex, care should be taken to avoid the use of equipment containing latex.

➤ Instruct the patient to cooperate fully and to follow directions. Direct the patient to breathe normally and to avoid unnecessary movement.

➤ Observe standard precautions, and follow the general guidelines in Appendix A. Positively identify the patient, and label the appropriate tubes with the corresponding patient demographics, date, and time of collection. Perform a venipuncture; collect the specimen in a 5-mL red- or tiger-top tube.

➤ Remove the needle, and apply a pressure dressing over the puncture site.

➤ Promptly transport the specimen to the laboratory for processing and analysis.

➤ The results are recorded manually or in a computerized system for recall and postprocedure interpretation by the appropriate health care practitioner.

Post-test:

➤ Observe venipuncture site for bleeding or hematoma formation. Apply paper tape or other adhesive to hold pressure bandage in place, or replace with a plastic bandage.

➤ *Nutritional considerations:* Educate the patient, as appropriate, that good dietary sources of complete protein (containing all eight essential amino acids) include meat, fish, eggs, and dairy products; and that good sources of incomplete protein (lacking one or more of the eight essential amino acids) include grains, nuts, legumes, vegetables, and seeds.

➤ A written report of the examination will be sent to the requesting health care practitioner, who will discuss the results with the patient.

➤ Reinforce information given by the patient's health care provider regarding further testing, treatment, or referral to another health care provider. Answer any questions or address any concerns voiced by the patient or family.

➤ Depending on the results of this procedure, additional testing may be performed to evaluate or monitor progression of the disease process and determine the need for a change in therapy. Evaluate test results in relation to the patient's symptoms and other tests performed.

Related laboratory tests:

➤ Related laboratory tests include albumin, complete blood count, IgA, IgG, IgM, blood and urine immunofixation electrophoresis, urine protein, and urine protein electrophoresis.

PROTEIN C

SYNONYMS/ACRONYM: Protein C antigen, protein C functional.

SPECIMEN: Plasma (1 mL) collected in blue-top (sodium citrate) tube.

REFERENCE VALUE: (Method: Chromogenic) 70% to 140% activity (0.7 to 1.4 U/mL). Values are significantly reduced in children (0.4 to 1.1 U/mL) because of liver immaturity.

DESCRIPTION & RATIONALE: Protein C is a vitamin K–dependent protein that originates in the liver and circulates in plasma. Protein C activation occurs on thrombomodulin receptors on the endothelial cell surface. Thrombin bound to thrombomodulin receptors preferentially activates protein C. Freely circulating thrombin mainly converts fibrinogen to fibrin. Other steps in the activation process require calcium and protein S cofactor binding (see monographs titled "Protein S" and "Fibrinogen"). Activated protein C exhibits potent anticoagulant effects by degrading activated factors V and VIII. There are two types of protein C deficiency:

Type I: Decreased antigen and function, detected by functional and antigenic assays

Type II: Normal antigen but decreased function, detected only by a functional assay

Functional assays are recommended for initial evaluation because of their greater sensitivity. ■

INDICATIONS:
• Differentiate inherited deficiency from acquired deficiency

• Investigate the mechanism of idiopathic venous thrombosis

RESULT

Increased in: N/A

Decreased in:
• Congenital deficiency
• Liver disease
• Oral anticoagulant therapy

CRITICAL VALUES: N/A

INTERFERING FACTORS:
• Drugs that may increase protein C levels include desmopressin and oral contraceptives.

• Drugs that may decrease protein C levels include coumarin and warfarin (Coumadin).

• Placement of tourniquet for longer than 1 minute can result in venous stasis and changes in the concentration of plasma proteins to be measured. Platelet activation may also occur under these conditions, causing erroneous results.

• Vascular injury during phlebotomy can activate platelets and coagulation factors, causing erroneous results.

• Hemolyzed specimens must be rejected because hemolysis is an indication of platelet and coagulation factor activation.

• Incompletely filled tubes contaminated with heparin or clotted specimens must be rejected.

• Icteric or lipemic specimens interfere with optical testing methods, producing erroneous results.

Nursing Implications and Procedure

➤ Inform the patient that the test is used to assess anticoagulant function.

➤ Obtain a history of the patient's complaints, including a list of known allergens (especially allergies or sensitivities to latex), and inform the appropriate health care practitioner accordingly.

➤ Obtain a history of the patient's hematopoietic and hepatobiliary systems, as well as results of previously performed laboratory tests, surgical procedures, and other diagnostic procedures. For related laboratory tests, refer to the Hematopoietic and Hepatobiliary System tables.

➤ Obtain a list of medications the patient is taking, including herbs, nutritional supplements, and nutraceuticals. The requesting health care practitioner and laboratory should be advised if the patient regularly uses these products so that their effects can be taken into consideration when reviewing results.

➤ Review the procedure with the patient. Inform the patient that specimen collection takes approximately 5 to 10 minutes. Address concerns about pain related to the procedure. Explain to the patient that there may be some discomfort during the venipuncture.

➤ There are no food, fluid, or medication restrictions, unless by medical direction.

➤ If the patient has a history of severe allergic reaction to latex, care should be taken to avoid the use of equipment containing latex.

➤ Instruct the patient to cooperate fully and to follow directions. Direct the patient to breathe normally and to avoid unnecessary movement.

➤ Observe standard precautions, and follow the general guidelines in Appendix A. Positively identify the patient, and label the appropriate tubes with the corresponding patient demographics, date, and time of collection. Perform a venipuncture, and collect the specimen in a 5-mL blue-top tube. *Important note:* Two different concentrations of sodium citrate preservative are currently added to blue-top tubes for coagulation studies: 3.2% and 3.8%. The Clinical and Laboratory Standards Institute/CLSI (formerly the National Committee for Clinical Laboratory Standards/ NCCLS) guideline for sodium citrate is 3.2%. Laboratories establish reference ranges for coagulation testing based on numerous factors, including sodium citrate concentration, test equipment, and test reagents. It is important to inquire from the laboratory which concentration it recommends, because each concentration will have its own specific reference range.

➤ When multiple specimens are drawn, the blue-top tube should be collected after sterile (i.e., blood culture) and red-top tubes. When coagulation testing is the only work to be done, an extra red-top tube should be collected before the blue-top tube to avoid contaminating the specimen with tissue thromboplastin, which can falsely decrease values.

➤ Remove the needle, and apply a pressure dressing over the puncture site.

➤ Promptly transport the specimen to the laboratory for processing and analysis. The CLSI recommendation for processed and unprocessed specimens stored in unopened tubes is that testing should be completed within 1 to 4 hours of collection.

➤ The results are recorded manually or in a computerized system for recall and postprocedure interpretation by the appropriate health care practitioner.

Post-test:

➤ Observe venipuncture site for bleeding or hematoma formation. Apply paper tape or other adhesive to hold pressure bandage in place, or replace with a plastic bandage.

➤ A written report of the examination will be sent to the requesting health care practitioner, who will discuss the results with the patient.

➤ Reinforce information given by the patient's health care provider regarding further testing, treatment, or referral to another health care provider. Answer any questions or address any concerns voiced by the patient or family.

➤ Depending on the results of this procedure, additional testing may be performed to evaluate or monitor progression of the disease process and determine the need for a change in therapy. Evaluate test results in relation to the patient's symptoms and other tests performed.

Related laboratory tests:

➤ Related laboratory tests include anticardiolipin antibody, antithrombin III, complete blood count, factor V, fibrin degradation products, fibrinogen, lupus anticoagulant, and protein S.

PROTEIN S

• •

SYNONYMS/ACRONYM: Protein S antigen, protein S functional.

SPECIMEN: Plasma (1 mL) collected in blue-top (sodium citrate) tube.

REFERENCE VALUE: (Method: Clot detection)

	Conventional Units	SI Units (Conventional Units × .01)
Total proteins	70–140% activity	0.7–1.4 U/mL
Free proteins	60–120% activity	0.6–1.2 U/mL

Note: The low end of "normal" is lower in children younger than age 16 years because of the immaturity of the liver.

DESCRIPTION & RATIONALE: Protein S is a vitamin K–dependent protein that originates in the liver and circulates in plasma. It is a cofactor required for the activation of protein C (see monographs titled "Protein C" and "Fibrinogen"). Protein S exists in two forms, free (biologically active) and bound. Approximately 40% of protein S circulates in the free form; the remainder is bound and is functionally inactive. There are two types of protein S deficiency:

Type I: Decreased antigen and function, detected by functional and antigenic assays

Type II: Normal antigen but decreased function, detected only by a functional assay

Functional assays are recommended for initial evaluation because of their greater sensitivity. ∎

INDICATIONS: Investigate the cause of hypercoagulable states

RESULT

> ***Increased in:*** N/A

> ***Decreased in:***
- Chronic renal failure due to hypertension
- Congenital deficiency
- Coumarin-induced skin necrosis
- Diabetic neuropathy
- Disseminated intravascular coagulation
- Liver disease
- Oral anticoagulant therapy

CRITICAL VALUES: N/A

INTERFERING FACTORS:
- Drugs that may decrease protein S levels include coumarin, oral contraceptives, and warfarin (Coumadin).
- Placement of tourniquet for longer than 1 minute can result in venous stasis and changes in the concentration of plasma proteins to be measured.

Platelet activation may also occur under these conditions, causing erroneous results.

- Vascular injury during phlebotomy can activate platelets and coagulation factors, causing erroneous results.

- Hemolyzed specimens must be rejected because hemolysis is an indication of platelet and coagulation factor activation.

- Incompletely filled tubes contaminated with heparin or clotted specimens must be rejected.

- Icteric or lipemic specimens interfere with optical testing methods, producing erroneous results.

Nursing Implications and Procedure • • • • • • • • • • •

Pretest:

➤ Inform the patient that the test is used to assess anticoagulant function.

➤ Obtain a history of the patient's complaints, including a list of known allergens (especially allergies or sensitivities to latex), and inform the appropriate health care practitioner accordingly.

➤ Obtain a history of the patient's hematopoietic and hepatobiliary systems, as well as results of previously performed laboratory tests, surgical procedures, and other diagnostic procedures. For related laboratory tests, refer to the Hematopoietic and Hepatobiliary System tables.

➤ Obtain a list of medications the patient is taking, including herbs, nutritional supplements, and nutraceuticals. The requesting health care practitioner and laboratory should be advised if the patient regularly uses these products so that their effects can be taken into consideration when reviewing results.

> Review the procedure with the patient. Inform the patient that specimen collection takes approximately 5 to 10 minutes. Address concerns about pain related to the procedure. Explain to the patient that there may be some discomfort during the venipuncture.

> There are no food, fluid, or medication restrictions, unless by medical direction.

Intratest:

> If the patient has a history of severe allergic reaction to latex, care should be taken to avoid the use of equipment containing latex.

> Instruct the patient to cooperate fully and to follow directions. Direct the patient to breathe normally and to avoid unnecessary movement.

> Observe standard precautions, and follow the general guidelines in Appendix A. Positively identify the patient, and label the appropriate tubes with the corresponding patient demographics, date, and time of collection. Perform a venipuncture, and collect the specimen in a 5-mL blue-top tube. *Important note:* Two different concentrations of sodium citrate preservative are currently added to blue-top tubes for coagulation studies: 3.2% and 3.8%. The Clinical and Laboratory Standards Institute/CLSI (formerly the National Committee for Clinical Laboratory Standards/NCCLS) guideline for sodium citrate is 3.2%. Laboratories establish reference ranges for coagulation testing based on numerous factors, including sodium citrate concentration, test equipment, and test reagents. It is important to inquire from the laboratory which concentration it recommends, because each concentration will have its own specific reference range.

> When multiple specimens are drawn, the blue-top tube should be collected after sterile (i.e., blood culture) and red-top tubes. When coagulation testing is the only work to be done, an extra red-top tube should be collected before the blue-top tube to avoid contaminating the specimen with tissue thromboplastin, which can falsely decrease values.

> Remove the needle, and apply a pressure dressing over the puncture site.

> Promptly transport the specimen to the laboratory for processing and analysis. The CLIS recommendation for processed and unprocessed specimens stored in unopened tubes is that testing should be completed within 1 to 4 hours of collection.

> The results are recorded manually or in a computerized system for recall and postprocedure interpretation by the appropriate health care practitioner.

Post-test:

> Observe venipuncture site for bleeding or hematoma formation. Apply paper tape or other adhesive to hold pressure bandage in place, or replace with a plastic bandage.

> A written report of the examination will be sent to the requesting health care practitioner, who will discuss the results with the patient.

> Reinforce information given by the patient's health care provider regarding further testing, treatment, or referral to another health care provider. Answer any questions or address any concerns voiced by the patient or family.

> Depending on the results of this procedure, additional testing may be performed to evaluate or monitor progression of the disease process and determine the need for a change in therapy. Evaluate test results in relation to the patient's symptoms and other tests performed.

Related laboratory tests:

> Related laboratory tests include anticardiolipin antibody, antithrombin III, complete blood count, fibrin degradation products, fibrinogen, lupus anticoagulant, and protein C.

PROTEIN, URINE: TOTAL QUANTITATIVE AND FRACTIONS

SYNONYM/ACRONYM: None.

SPECIMEN: Urine (5 mL) from an unpreserved random or timed specimen collected in a clean plastic collection container.

REFERENCE VALUE: (Method: Spectrophotometry for total protein, electrophoresis for protein fractions)

	Conventional Units	SI Units (Conventional Units × 0.001)
Total protein	10–140 mg/24 h	0.01–0.14 g/24 h

Electrophoresis for fractionation is qualitative: No monoclonal gammopathy detected. (Urine protein electrophoresis should be ordered along with serum protein electrophoresis.)

DESCRIPTION & RATIONALE: Most proteins, with the exception of the immunoglobulins, are synthesized and catabolized in the liver, where they are broken down into amino acids. The amino acids are converted to ammonia and ketoacids. Ammonia is converted to urea via the urea cycle. Urea is excreted in the urine. ∎

INDICATIONS:
- Assist in the detection of Bence Jones proteins (light chains)
- Assist in the diagnosis of myeloma, Waldenström's macroglobulinemia, lymphoma, and amyloidosis
- Evaluate kidney function

RESULT

Increased in:

- Diabetic nephropathy
- Fanconi's syndrome
- Heavy metal poisoning
- Malignancies of the urinary tract
- Monoclonal gammopathies
- Multiple myeloma
- Nephrotic syndrome
- Other myeloproliferative and lymphoproliferative disorders
- Postexercise period
- Sarcoidosis
- Sickle cell disease
- Urinary tract infections

Decreased in: N/A

CRITICAL VALUES: N/A

INTERFERING FACTORS:

- Drugs and substances that may increase urine protein levels include acetaminophen, aminosalicylic acid, amphotericin B, ampicillin, antimony compounds, antipyrine, arsenicals, ascorbic acid, bacitracin, bismuth subsalicylate, bromate, capreomycin, captopril, carbamazepine, carbarsone, carbenoxolone, carbutamide, cephaloglycin, cephaloridine, chlorpromazine, chlorpropamide, chlorthalidone, chrysarobin, colistimethate, colistin, corticosteroids, cyclosporine, demeclocycline, 1,2 diaminopropane, diatrizoic acid, dihydrotachysterol, doxycycline, enalapril, gentamicin, gold, hydrogen sulfide, iodoalphionic acid, iodopyracet, iopanoic acid, iophenoxic acid, ipodate, kanamycin, corn oil (Lipomul), lithium, mefenamic acid, melarsonyl, melarsoprol, mercury compounds, methicillin, methylbromide, meziocillin, mitomycin, nafcillin, naphthalene, neomycin, nonsteroidal anti-inflammatory drugs, oxacillin, paraldehyde, penicillamine, penicillin, phenolphthalein, phenols, phensuximide, phosphorus, picric acid, piperacillin, plicamycin, polymyxin, probenecid, promazine, pyrazolones, quaternary ammonium compounds, radiographic agents, rifampin, sodium bicarbonate, streptokinase, sulfisoxazole, suramin, tetracyclines, thallium, thiosemicarbazones, tolbutamide, tolmetin, triethylenemelamine, and vitamin D.

- Drugs that may decrease urine protein levels include captopril, cyclosporine, diltiazem, enalapril, fosinopril, interferon, lisinopril, prednisolone, and quinapril.

- All urine voided for the timed collection period must be included in the collection or else falsely decreased values may be obtained. Compare output records with volume collected to verify that all voids were included in the collection.

Nursing Implications and Procedure

Pretest:

▶ Inform the patient that the test is used to identify the underlying cause for proteinuria.

▶ Obtain a history of the patient's complaints, including a list of known allergens (especially allergies or sensitivities to latex), and inform the appropriate health care practitioner accordingly.

▶ Obtain a history of the patient's genitourinary and immune systems, as well as results of previously performed laboratory tests, surgical procedures, and other diagnostic procedures. For related laboratory tests, refer to the Genitourinary and Immune System tables.

▶ Obtain a list of medications the patient is taking, including herbs, nutritional supplements, and nutraceuticals. The requesting health care practitioner and laboratory should be advised if the patient regularly uses these products so that their effects can be taken into consideration when reviewing results.

▶ Review the procedure with the patient. Provide a nonmetallic urinal, bedpan, or toilet-mounted collection device. Address concerns about pain related to the procedure. Explain to the patient that there should be no discomfort during the procedure.

▶ Usually a 24-hour time frame for urine collection is ordered. Inform the patient that all urine must be saved during that 24-hour period. Instruct the patient not to void directly into the laboratory collection container. Instruct the patient to avoid defecating in the collection device and to keep toilet tissue out of the collection device to prevent contamination of the specimen. Place a sign in the bathroom to remind the patient to save all urine.

▶ Instruct the patient to void all urine into the collection device and then to pour the urine into the laboratory collection container. Alternatively, the specimen can be left in the collection device for a health care staff member to add to the laboratory collection container.

➤ *Sensitivity to social and cultural issues,* as well as concern for modesty, is important in providing psychological support before, during, and after the procedure.

➤ There are no food, fluid, or medication restrictions, unless by medical direction.

Intratest:

➤ If the patient has a history of severe allergic reaction to latex, care should be taken to avoid the use of equipment containing latex.

➤ Instruct the patient to cooperate fully and to follow directions.

➤ Observe standard precautions, and follow the general guidelines in Appendix A. Positively identify the patient, and label the appropriate collection container with the corresponding patient demographics, date, and time of collection.

Random specimen (collect in early morning):

Clean-catch specimen:

➤ Instruct the male patient to (1) thoroughly wash his hands, (2) cleanse the meatus, (3) void a small amount into the toilet, and (4) void directly into the specimen container.

➤ Instruct the female patient to (1) thoroughly wash her hands; (2) cleanse the labia from front to back; (3) while keeping the labia separated, void a small amount into the toilet; and (4) without interrupting the urine stream, void directly into the specimen container.

Indwelling catheter:

➤ Put on gloves. Empty drainage tube of urine. It may be necessary to clamp off the catheter for 15 to 30 minutes before specimen collection.

Cleanse specimen port with antiseptic swab, and then aspirate 5 mL of urine with a 21- to 25-gauge needle and syringe. Transfer urine to a sterile container.

Timed specimen:

➤ Obtain a clean 3-L urine specimen container, toilet-mounted collection device, and plastic bag (for transport of the specimen container). The specimen must be refrigerated or kept on ice throughout the entire collection period. If an indwelling urinary catheter is in place, the drainage bag must be kept on ice.

➤ Begin the test between 6 and 8 a.m., if possible. Collect first voiding and discard. Record the time the specimen was discarded as the beginning of the timed collection period. The next morning, ask the patient to void at the same time the collection was started and add this last voiding to the container.

➤ If an indwelling catheter is in place, replace the tubing and container system at the start of the collection time. Keep the container system on ice during the collection period, or empty the urine into a larger container periodically during the collection period; monitor to ensure continued drainage, and conclude the test the next morning at the same hour the collection was begun.

➤ At the conclusion of the test, compare the quantity of urine with the urinary output record for the collection; if the specimen contains less than the recorded output, some urine may have been discarded, invalidating the test.

➤ Include on the collection container's label the amount of urine collected and test start and stop times.

General:

➤ Promptly transport the specimen to the laboratory for processing and analysis.

➤ The results are recorded manually or in a computerized system for recall

and postprocedure interpretation by the appropriate health care practitioner.

Post-test:

> A written report of the examination will be sent to the requesting health care practitioner, who will discuss the results with the patient.

> Recognize anxiety related to test results. Discuss the implications of abnormal test results on the patient's lifestyle. Provide teaching and information regarding the clinical implications of the test results, as appropriate.

> Reinforce information given by the patient's health care provider regarding further testing, treatment, or re-

ferral to another health care provider. Answer any questions or address any concerns voiced by the patient or family.

> Depending on the results of this procedure, additional testing may be performed to evaluate or monitor progression of the disease process and determine the need for a change in therapy. Evaluate test results in relation to the patient's symptoms and other tests performed.

Related laboratory tests:

> Related laboratory tests include glucose, glycated hemoglobin, blood and urine immunofixation electrophoresis, microalbumin, blood and urine osmolality, blood protein and fractions, and urinalysis.

PROTHROMBIN TIME AND INTERNATIONAL NORMALIZED RATIO

SYNONYM/ACRONYM: Protime, PT.

SPECIMEN: Plasma (1 mL) collected in a completely filled blue-top (sodium citrate) tube.

REFERENCE VALUE: (Method: Clot detection) 10 to 13 seconds.

International Normalized Ratio (INR) = Less than 2.0 for patients not receiving anticoagulation therapy, 2.0 to 3.0 for patients receiving treatment for venous thrombosis, pulmonary embolism, and valvular heart disease.

INR = 2.5 to 3.5 for patients with mechanical heart valves and/or receiving treatment for recurrent systemic embolism.

DESCRIPTION & RATIONALE: Prothrombin time (PT) is a coagulation test performed to measure the time it takes for a firm fibrin clot to form after tissue thromboplastin (factor III) and calcium are added to the sample. It is used to evaluate the extrinsic pathway of the coagulation sequence in patients receiving oral warfarin or coumarin-type anticoagulants. Prothrombin is a vitamin K–dependent protein produced by the liver; measurement is reported as time in seconds or percentage of normal activity.

The goal of long-term anticoagulation therapy is to achieve a balance between in vivo thrombus formation and hemorrhage. It is a delicate clinical balance—and due to differences in instruments and reagents there is a wide variation in PT results between laboratories. Worldwide concern for the need to provide more consistency in monitoring patients receiving anticoagulant therapy led to the development of an international committee. In the early 1980s, manufacturers of instruments and reagents began comparing their measurement systems with a single reference material provided by the World Health Organization (WHO). The international effort successfully developed an algorithm to provide comparable PT values regardless of differences in laboratory methodology. Reagent and instrument manufacturers compare their results to the WHO reference and derive a factor called an International Sensitivity Index (ISI) that is applied to a mathematical formula to standardize the results. Laboratories convert their PT values into an International Normalized Ratio (INR) by using the following formula:

$$INR = (\text{patient PT result/normal patient average})^{(ISI)}$$

PT evaluation can now be based on an INR using a standardized thromboplastin reagent to assist in making decisions regarding oral anticoagulation therapy.

Some inferences of factor deficiency can be made by comparison of results obtained from the activated partial thromboplastin time (APTT) and PT tests. A normal APTT with a prolonged PT can occur only with factor VII deficiency. A prolonged APTT with a normal PT could indicate a deficiency in factors XII, XI, IX, and VIII as well as VIII:C (von Willebrand factor). Factor deficiencies can also be identified by correction or substitution studies using normal serum. These studies are easy to perform and are accomplished by adding plasma from a normal patient to a sample from a suspected factor-deficient patient. When the PT is repeated and corrected, or within the reference range, it can be assumed that the prolonged PT is due to a factor deficiency (see monograph titled "Coagulation Factors"). ■

INDICATIONS:

• Differentiate between deficiencies of clotting factors II, V, VII, and X, which prolong the PT; and congenital coagulation disorders, such as hemophilia A (factor VIII) and hemophilia B (factor IX), which do not alter the PT

• Evaluate the response to anticoagulant therapy with coumarin derivatives and determine dosage required to achieve therapeutic results

• Identify individuals who may be prone to bleeding during surgical, obstetric, dental, or invasive diagnostic procedures

• Identify the possible cause of abnormal bleeding, such as epistaxis, hematoma, gingival bleeding, hematuria, and menorrhagia

• Monitor the effects of conditions such as liver disease, protein deficiency, and fat malabsorption on hemostasis

- Screen for prothrombin deficiency
- Screen for vitamin K deficiency

RESULT

Increased in:
- Afibrinogenemia, dysfibrinogenemia, or hypofibrinogenemia
- Biliary obstruction
- Disseminated intravascular coagulation
- Hereditary deficiencies of factors II, V, VII, and X
- Intravascular coagulation
- Liver disease (cirrhosis)
- Poor fat absorption (tropical sprue, celiac disease, chronic diarrhea)
- Presence of circulating anticoagulant
- Systemic lupus erythematosus
- Vitamin K deficiency

Decreased in:
- Ovarian hyperfunction
- Regional enteritis or ileitis

CRITICAL VALUES:

INR:
Greater than 3 (in patients on anticoagulant therapy)

Prothrombin time:
Greater than 20 seconds (in patients not on anticoagulant therapy)

Three times normal control (in patients on anticoagulant therapy)

Note and immediately report to the health care practitioner any critically increased values and related symptoms. Important signs to note are prolonged bleeding from cuts or gums, hematoma at a puncture site, hemorrhage, blood in the stool, persistent epistaxis, heavy or prolonged menstrual flow, and shock. Monitor vital signs, unusual ecchymosis, occult blood, severe headache, unusual dizziness, and neurologic changes until PT is within normal range. Intramuscular administration of vitamin K, an anticoagulant reversal agent, may be requested by the health care practitioner.

INTERFERING FACTORS:
- Drugs that may increase the PT in patients receiving anticoagulation therapy include acetaminophen, acetylsalicylic acid, amiodarone, anabolic steroids, anisindione, anistreplase, antibiotics, antipyrine, carbenicillin, cathartics, chlorthalidone, cholestyramine, clofibrate, corticotropin, demeclocycline, dextrothyroxine, diazoxide, diflunisal, diuretics, doxycycline, erythromycin, glucagon, hydroxyzine, indomethacin, laxatives, mercaptopurine, miconazole, nalidixic acid, neomycin, niacin, oxyphenbutazone, phenytoin, quinine, sulfachlorpyridazine, and thyroxine.

- Drugs that may decrease the PT in patients receiving anticoagulation therapy include amobarbital, anabolic steroids, antacids, antihistamines, barbiturates, carbamazepine, chloral hydrate, chlordane, colchicine, corticosteroids, diuretics, oral contraceptives, penicillin, primidone, rifampin, simethicone, spironolactone, tolbutamide, and vitamin K.

- Traumatic venipunctures can activate the coagulation sequence by contaminating the sample with tissue thromboplastin, and producing falsely shortened PT.

- Failure to fill the tube sufficiently to yield proper blood-to-anticoagulant ratio may cause a falsely lengthened PT; an incompletely filled tube is reason for specimen rejection.

* Excessive agitation causing sample hemolysis can falsely shorten the PT because the hemolyzed cells activate plasma-clotting factors.

Nursing Implications and Procedure • • • • • • • • • • •

Pretest:

➤ Inform the patient that the test is used to evaluate the coagulation system and monitor anticoagulation therapy.

➤ Obtain a history of the patient's complaints, including a list of known allergens (especially allergies or sensitivities to latex), and inform the appropriate health care practitioner accordingly.

➤ Obtain a history of the patient's cardiovascular, hematopoietic, and hepatobiliary systems, any bleeding disorders, and results of previously performed laboratory tests (especially bleeding time, complete blood count, partial thromboplastin time, PT, and platelets), surgical procedures, and other diagnostic procedures. For related laboratory tests, refer to the Cardiovascular, Hematopoietic, and Hepatobiliary System tables.

➤ Obtain a list of medications the patient is taking, including anticoagulant therapy, acetylsalicylic acid, herbs, nutritional supplements, and nutraceuticals, especially those known to affect coagulation (see Appendix F). Note the last time and dose of medication taken. It is recommended that use be discontinued 14 days before dental or surgical procedures. The requesting health care practitioner and laboratory should be advised if the patient regularly uses these products so that their effects can be taken into consideration when reviewing results.

➤ Review the procedure with the patient. Inform the patient that specimen collection takes approximately 5 to 10 minutes. Address concerns about pain related to the procedure.

Explain to the patient that there may be some discomfort during the venipuncture.

➤ *Sensitivity to cultural and social issues,* as well as concern for modesty, is important in providing psychological support before, during, and after the procedure.

➤ There are no food, fluid, or medication restrictions, unless by medical direction.

Intratest:

➤ If the patient has a history of severe allergic reaction to latex, care should be taken to avoid the use of equipment containing latex.

➤ Instruct the patient to cooperate fully and to follow directions. Direct the patient to breathe normally and to avoid unnecessary movement.

➤ Observe standard precautions, and follow the general guidelines in Appendix A. Positively identify the patient, and label the appropriate tubes with the corresponding patient demographics, date, and time of collection. Perform a venipuncture, and collect the specimen in a 5-mL blue-top tube. Fill tube completely. *Important note:* Two different concentrations of sodium citrate preservative are currently added to blue-top tubes for coagulation studies: 3.2% and 3.8%. The Clinical and Laboratory Standards Institute/CLSI (formerly the National Committee for Clinical Laboratory Standards/NCCLS) guideline for sodium citrate is 3.2%. Laboratories establish reference ranges for coagulation testing based on numerous factors, including sodium citrate concentration, test equipment, and test reagents. It is important to inquire from the laboratory which concentration it recommends, because each concentration will have its own specific reference range.

➤ When multiple specimens are drawn, the blue-top tube should be collected after sterile (i.e., blood culture) and red-top tubes. When coagulation testing is the only work to be done, an extra red-top tube should be collected before the blue-top tube to avoid contaminating the specimen with tissue thromboplastin, which can falsely shorten PT.

➤ Remove the needle, and apply a pressure dressing over the puncture site.

➤ Promptly transport the specimen to the laboratory for processing and analysis. The CLSI recommendation for processed and unprocessed samples stored in unopened tubes is that testing should be completed within 1 to 4 hours of collection.

➤ The results are recorded manually or in a computerized system for recall and postprocedure interpretation by the appropriate health care practitioner.

Post-test:

➤ Observe venipuncture site for bleeding or hematoma formation. Apply paper tape or other adhesive to hold pressure bandage in place, or replace with a plastic bandage.

➤ Instruct the patient to report bleeding from any areas of the skin or mucous membranes.

➤ Inform the patient with prolonged PT of the importance of taking precautions against bruising and bleeding, including the use of a soft bristle toothbrush, use of an electric razor, avoidance of constipation, avoidance of aspirin products, and avoidance of intramuscular injections.

➤ Inform the patient of the importance of periodic laboratory testing while taking an anticoagulant.

➤ *Nutritional considerations:* Foods high in vitamin K should be avoided by the patient on anticoagulant therapy. Foods that contain vitamin K include cabbage, cauliflower, chickpeas, egg yolks, green tea, liver, milk, soybean products, tomatoes, and green leafy vegetables such as brussels sprouts, kale, spinach, and turnip greens.

➤ *Nutritional considerations:* Avoid alcohol and alcohol products while taking warfarin, as the combination of the two increases the risk of gastrointestinal bleeding.

➤ A written report of the examination will be sent to the requesting health care practitioner, who will discuss the results with the patient.

➤ Reinforce information given by the patient's health care provider regarding further testing, treatment, or referral to another health care provider. Answer any questions or address any concerns voiced by the patient or family.

➤ Depending on the results of this procedure, additional testing may be performed to evaluate or monitor progression of the disease process and determine the need for a change in therapy. Evaluate test results in relation to the patient's symptoms and other tests performed.

Related laboratory tests:

➤ Related laboratory tests include alanine aminotransferase, aspartate aminotransferase, bilirubin, bleeding time, coagulation factors, complete blood count, γ-glutamyltranspeptidase, partial thromboplastin time, platelet count, and vitamin K.

PSEUDOCHOLINESTERASE AND DIBUCAINE NUMBER

SYNONYMS/ACRONYMS: CHS, PCHE, AcCHS.

SPECIMEN: Plasma (1 mL) collected in a lavender-top (ethylenediaminetetra-acetic acid [EDTA]) tube. Serum (1 mL) collected in a red-top tube is also acceptable.

REFERENCE VALUE: (Method: Spectrophotometry, kinetic)

Test	Conventional Units	SI Units (Conventional Units × 1)
Pseudocholinesterase	2–11 U/mL	2–11 kU/L

Dibucaine Number	Fraction (%) of Activity Inhibited	SI Units (Conventional Units × 0.01)
Normal homozygote	79–84%	0.79–0.84 kU/L
Heterozygote	55–70%	0.55–0.70 kU/L
Abnormal homozygote	16–28%	0.16–0.28 kU/L

DESCRIPTION & RATIONALE: There are two types of cholinesterase: *acetylcholinesterase,* which is found in red blood cells, lung, and brain (nerve) tissue (see monograph titled "Red Blood Cell Cholinesterase"); and *cholinesterase,* which is found mainly in the plasma, liver, and heart. Pseudocholinesterase is a nonspecific enzyme that hydrolyzes acetylcholine and noncholine esters; carbamate and organophosphate insecticides (e.g., parathion, malathion) inhibit its activity.

Patients with inherited pseudo-cholinesterase deficiency are at risk during anesthesia if succinylcholine is administered as an anesthetic. Succinylcholine, a short-acting muscle relaxant, is a reversible inhibitor of acetylcholinesterase and is hydrolyzed by cholinesterase. Succinylcholine-sensitive patients may be unable to metabolize the anesthetic quickly, resulting in prolonged or unrecoverable apnea. Abnormal genotypes of pseudocholinesterase are detected using the dibucaine and fluoride inhibition tests because, in normal individuals, these chemicals inhibit pseudocholinesterase activity. The prevalence of succinylcholate sensitivity is 1 in 1500 patients. Widespread preoperative screening is not routinely performed. ∎

INDICATIONS:

* Assist in the evaluation of liver function
* Screen for abnormal genotypes of pseudocholinesterase in patients with a family history of succinylcholine sensitivity who are about to undergo anesthesia using succinylcholine.

RESULT

Increased in:

* Diabetes
* Hyperthyroidism
* Nephrotic syndrome
* Obesity

Decreased in:

* Acute infection
* Anemia (severe)
* Carcinomatosis
* Cirrhosis
* Congenital deficiency
* Hepatic carcinoma
* Hepatocellular disease
* Infectious hepatitis
* Insecticide exposure (organic phosphate)
* Malnutrition
* Muscular dystrophy
* Myocardial infarction
* Plasmapheresis
* Succinylcholine hypersensitivity
* Tuberculosis
* Uremia

CRITICAL VALUES:

Notify the anesthesiologist if the test result is positive and surgery is scheduled. A positive result indicates that the patient is at risk for prolonged or unrecoverable apnea related to the inability to metabolize succinylcholine.

INTERFERING FACTORS:

* Drugs and substances that may decrease pseudocholinesterase levels include ambenonium, barbiturates, cyclophosphamide, echothiophate, edrophonium, estrogens, fluorides, ibuprofen, iodipamide, iopanoic acid, isoflurophate, neostigmine, parathion, physostigmine, procainamide, pyridostigmine, and oral contraceptives.
* Drugs that may increase pseudocholinesterase levels include carbamazepine, phenytoin, and valproic acid.
* Pregnancy decreases pseudocholinesterase levels by about 30%.
* Improper anticoagulant; fluoride interferes with the measurement and causes a falsely decreased value.

Nursing Implications and Procedure • • • • • • • • • • •

Pretest:

➤ Inform the patient that the test is used to identify succinylcholine anesthetic sensitivity.

➤ Obtain a history of the patient's complaints, including a list of known allergens (especially allergies or sensitivities to latex), and inform the appropriate health care practitioner accordingly. Particularly important to report is exposure to pesticides causing symptoms including blurred vision, muscle weakness, nausea, vomiting, headaches, pulmonary edema, salivation, sweating, or convulsions.

➤ Obtain a history of the patient's hepatobiliary and musculoskeletal systems, as well as results of previously performed laboratory tests, surgical procedures, and other diagnostic procedures. For related laboratory tests, refer to the Hepatobiliary and Musculoskeletal System tables.

➤ Obtain a list of medications the patient is taking, including herbs, nutritional supplements, and nutraceuticals. The requesting health care practitioner and laboratory should be advised if the patient regularly uses these products so that their effects can be taken into consideration when reviewing results.

➤ Review the procedure with the patient. Inform the patient that specimen collection takes approximately 5 to 10 minutes. Address concerns about pain related to the procedure. Explain to the patient that there may be some discomfort during the venipuncture.

➤ There are no food, fluid, or medication restrictions, unless by medical direction.

Intratest:

➤ If the patient has a history of severe allergic reaction to latex, care should be taken to avoid the use of equipment containing latex.

➤ Instruct the patient to cooperate fully and to follow directions. Direct the patient to breathe normally and to avoid unnecessary movement.

➤ Observe standard precautions, and follow the general guidelines in Appendix A. Positively identify the patient, and label the appropriate tubes with the corresponding patient demographics, date, and time of collection. Perform a venipuncture; collect the specimen in a 5-mL lavender- or red-top tube.

➤ Remove the needle, and apply a pressure dressing over the puncture site.

➤ Promptly transport the specimen to the laboratory for processing and analysis.

➤ The results are recorded manually or in a computerized system for recall and postprocedure interpretation by the appropriate health care practitioner.

Post-test:

➤ Observe venipuncture site for bleeding or hematoma formation. Apply paper tape or other adhesive to hold pressure bandage in place, or replace with a plastic bandage.

➤ The patient with decreased values should be observed for signs of fluid volume excess related to compromised regulatory mechanisms, decreased cardiac output related to decreased myocardial contractility or arrhythmias, and pain related to inflammation or ischemia.

➤ A written report of the examination will be sent to the requesting health care practitioner, who will discuss the results with the patient.

➤ Reinforce information given by the patient's health care provider regarding further testing, treatment, or referral to another health care provider. Answer any questions or address any concerns voiced by the patient or family.

➤ Depending on the results of this procedure, additional testing may be performed to evaluate or monitor progression of the disease process and determine the need for a change in therapy. Evaluate test results in relation to the patient's symptoms and other tests performed.

Related laboratory tests:

➤ Related laboratory tests include alanine aminotransferase and aspartate aminotransferase.

PULMONARY FUNCTION STUDIES

SYNONYM/ACRONYM: Pulmonary function tests (PFTs).

AREA OF APPLICATION: Lungs, respiratory system.

CONTRAST: None.

DESCRIPTION & RATIONALE: Pulmonary function studies provide information about the volume, pattern, and rates of airflow involved in respiratory function. These studies may also include tests involving the diffusing capabilities of the lungs (i.e., volume of gases diffusing across a membrane). A complete pulmonary study profile includes the determination of all lung volumes, spirometry, diffusing capacity, maximum voluntary ventilation, flow-volume loop (Fig. 1–1), and maximum expiratory and inspiratory pressures. Other studies include small airway volumes.

Pulmonary function studies are classified according to lung volumes and capacities, rates of flow, and gas exchange. The exception is the diffusion test, which records the movement of a gas during inspiration and expiration. Lung volumes and capacities constitute the amount of air inhaled or exhaled from the lungs; this value is compared to normal reference values specific for the patient's age, height, and sex. The following are volumes and capacities measured by spirometry that do not require timed testing. ■

TIDAL VOLUME: Total amount of air inhaled and exhaled with one breath.

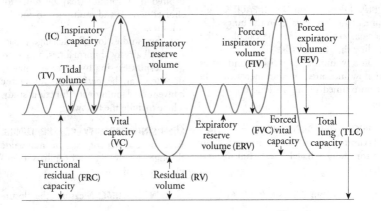

RESIDUAL VOLUME: Amount of air remaining in the lungs after a maximum expiration effort (not measured by spirometry, but can be calculated from the functional residual capacity [FRC] minus the expiratory reserve volume [ERV]). This indirect type of measurement can be done by body plethysmography (see monograph titled "Plethysmography").

INSPIRATORY RESERVE VOLUME: Maximum amount of air inhaled after normal inspirations.

EXPIRATORY RESERVE VOLUME: Maximum amount of air exhaled after a resting expiration (can be calculated by the vital capacity [VC] minus the inspiratory capacity [IC]).

VITAL CAPACITY: Maximum amount of air exhaled after a maximum inspiration (can be calculated by adding the IC and the ERV).

TOTAL LUNG CAPACITY: Total amount of air that the lungs can hold after maximal inspiration (can be calculated by adding the VC and the residual volume [RV]).

INSPIRATORY CAPACITY: Maximum amount of air inspired after normal expiration (can be calculated by adding the inspiratory RV and tidal volume).

FUNCTIONAL RESIDUAL CAPACITY: Volume of air that remains in the lungs after normal expiration (can be calculated by adding the RV and ERV).

The volumes, capacities, and rates of flow measured by spirometry that do require timed testing include the following:

FORCED VITAL CAPACITY IN 1 SECOND: Maximum amount of air that can be forcefully exhaled after a full inspiration.

FORCED EXPIRATORY VOLUME: Amount of air exhaled in the first second (can also be determined at 2 or 3 seconds) of forced vital capacity (FVC, which is the amount of air exhaled in seconds, expressed as a percentage).

MAXIMAL MIDEXPIRATORY FLOW: Also known as forced expiratory flow rate (FEF_{25-75}), or the maximal rate of airflow during a forced expiration.

FORCED INSPIRATORY FLOW RATE: Volume inspired from the RV at a point of measurement (can be expressed as a percentage to identify the corresponding volume pressure and inspired volume).

PEAK INSPIRATORY FLOW RATE: Maximum airflow during a forced maximal inspiration.

PEAK EXPIRATORY FLOW RATE: Maximum airflow expired during FVC.

FLOW-VOLUME LOOPS: Flows and volumes recorded during forced expiratory volume and forced inspiratory vital capacity procedures (Fig. 1–2).

MAXIMAL INSPIRATORY-EXPIRATORY PRESSURES: Measures the strength of the respiratory muscles in neuromuscular disorders.

MAXIMAL VOLUNTARY VENTILATION: Maximal volume of air inspired and expired in 1 minute (may be done for shorter periods and multiplied to equal 1 minute).

Other studies for gas-exchange capacity, small airway abnormalities, and allergic responses in hyperactive airway disorders can be performed during the conventional pulmonary function study. These include the following:

DIFFUSING CAPACITY OF THE LUNGS: Rate of transfer of carbon monoxide through the alveolar and capillary membrane in 1 minute.

CLOSING VOLUME: Measures the closure

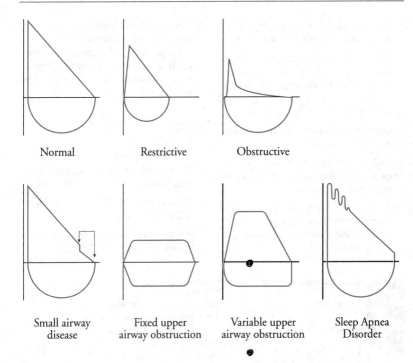

Normal   Restrictive   Obstructive

Small airway disease   Fixed upper airway obstruction   Variable upper airway obstruction   Sleep Apnea Disorder

of small airways in the lower alveoli by monitoring volume and percentage of alveolar nitrogen after inhalation of 100% oxygen.

ISOFLOW VOLUME: Flow-volume loop test followed by inhalation of a mixture of helium and oxygen to determine small airway disease.

BODY PLETHYSMOGRAPHY: Measures thoracic gas volume and airway resistance.

BRONCHIAL PROVOCATION: Quantifies airway response after inhalation of methacholine.

ARTERIAL BLOOD GASES: Measure oxygen, pH, and carbon dioxide in arterial blood.
Values are expressed in units of mL, %, L, L/sec, and L/min, depending on the test performed.

INDICATIONS:
- Detect chronic obstructive pulmonary disease (COPD) and/or restrictive pulmonary diseases that affect the chest wall (e.g., neuromuscular disorders, kyphosis, scoliosis) and lungs, as evidenced by abnormal airflows and volumes

- Determine airway response to inhalants in patients with an airway-reactive disorder

- Determine the diffusing capacity of the lungs (DCOL)

- Determine the effectiveness of therapy regimens, such as bronchodilators, for pulmonary disorders

- Determine the presence of lung disease when other studies, such as x-rays, do not provide a definitive diagnosis, or determine the progression and severity of known COPD and restrictive pulmonary disease

- Evaluate the cause of dyspnea occurring with or without exercise
- Evaluate lung compliance to determine changes in elasticity, as evidenced by changes in lung volumes (decreased in restrictive pulmonary disease, increased in COPD and in elderly patients)
- Evaluate pulmonary disability for legal or insurance claims
- Evaluate pulmonary function after surgical pneumonectomy, lobectomy, or segmental lobectomy
- Evaluate the respiratory system to determine the patient's ability to tolerate procedures such as surgery or diagnostic studies
- Screen high-risk populations for early detection of pulmonary conditions (e.g., patients with exposure to occupational or environmental hazards, smokers, patients with a hereditary predisposition)

RESULT

Normal Findings:
- Normal respiratory volume and capacities, gas diffusion, and distribution
- No evidence of COPD or restrictive pulmonary disease

Normal adult lung volumes, capacities, and flow rates are as follows:

TV	500 mL at rest
RV	1200 mL (approximate)
IRV	3000 mL (approximate)
ERV	1100 mL (approximate)
VC	4600 mL (approximate)
TLC	5800 mL (approximate)
IC	3500 mL (approximate)
FRC	2300 mL (approximate)
FVC	3000–5000 mL (approximate)
FEV_1/FVC	81–83%
MMEF	25–75%
FIF	25–75%
MVV	25–35% or 170 L/min
PIFR	300 L/min
PEFR	450 L/min
F-V loop	Normal curve
DCOL	25 mL/min per mm Hg (approximate)
CV	10%–20% of VC
V_{iso}	Based on age formula
Bronchial provocation	No change, or less than 20% reduction in FEV_1

Note: Normal values listed are estimated values for adults. Actual pediatric and adult values are based on age, height, and gender. These normal values are included on the patient's pulmonary function laboratory report.
TV = tidal volume; RV = residual volume; IRV = inspiratory reserve volume; ERV = expiratory reserve volume; VC = vital capacity; TLC = total lung capacity; IC = inspiratory capacity; FRC = functional residual capacity; FVC = forced vital capacity in 1 second; FEV_1 = forced expiratory volume in 1 second; MMEF = maximal midexpiratory flow (also known as FEF_{25-75}); FIF = forced inspiratory flow rate; MVV = maximal voluntary ventilation; PIFR = peak inspiratory flow rate; PEFR = peak expiratory flow rate; F-V loop = flow-volume loop; DCOL = diffusing capacity of the lungs; CV = closing volume; V_{iso} = isoflow volume.

Abnormal Findings:

- Allergy
- Asbestosis
- Asthma
- Bronchiectasis
- Chest trauma
- Chronic bronchitis
- Curvature of the spine
- Emphysema
- Myasthenia gravis
- Obesity
- Pulmonary fibrosis
- Pulmonary tumors
- Respiratory infections
- Sarcoidosis

INTERFERING FACTORS:

- The aging process can cause decreased values (FVC, DCOL) depending on the study done.

- Inability of the patient to put forth the necessary breathing effort affects the results.

- Medications such as brochodilators can affect results.

- Improper placement of the nose clamp or mouthpiece that allows for leakage can affect volume results.

- Confusion or inability to understand instructions or cooperate during the study can cause inaccurate results.

- Testing is contraindicated in patients with cardiac insufficiency, recent myocardial infarction, and presence of chest pain that affects inspiration or expiration ability.

- Exercise caution with patients who have upper respiratory infections, such as a cold or acute bronchitis.

Nursing Implications and Procedure ● ● ● ● ● ● ● ● ● ●

Pretest:

▶ Inform the patient that the procedure assesses the function of the lungs.

▶ Obtain a history of the patient's complaints and symptoms, including a list of known allergens, especially allergies or sensitivities to latex.

▶ Obtain a history of the patient's cardiovascular and respiratory systems, as well as results of previously performed laboratory tests, surgical procedures, and other diagnostic procedures. For related diagnostic tests, refer to the Cardiovascular and Respiratory Systems tables.

▶ Obtain a list of medications the patient is taking. Assess medication history for recent administration of analgesics that may depress respiratory function.

▶ Review the procedure with the patient. Address concerns about pain related to the procedure. Explain to the patient that no discomfort will be experienced during the test. Explain that the procedure is generally performed in a specially equipped room or in a health care practitioner's office by a technologist and usually lasts 1 hour.

▶ *Sensitivity to cultural and social issues,* as well as concern for modesty, is important in providing psychological support before, during, and after the procedure.

▶ Measure the patient's height and weight.

▶ The patient should refrain from smoking tobacco or eating a heavy meal for 4 to 6 hours prior to the study.

▶ Under medical direction, the patient should avoid bronchodilators (oral or inhalant) for at least 4 hours before the study.

Intratest:

▶ Ensure that the patient has complied with dietary restrictions and pretesting preparations. Ensure that medications such as bronchodilators (oral or inhalant) have been withheld for at least 4 hours before the study.

➤ Obtain an inhalant bronchodilator to treat any bronchospasms that can occur with testing.

➤ Instruct the patient to void and to loosen any restrictive clothing.

➤ Instruct the patient to cooperate fully and to follow directions.

➤ Observe standard precautions, and follow the general guidelines in Appendix A.

➤ Place the patient in a sitting position on a chair near the spirometry equipment.

➤ Place a soft clip on the patient's nose to restrict nose breathing, and instruct the patient to breathe through the mouth.

➤ Place a mouthpiece in the mouth and tell the patient to close his or her lips around it to form a seal.

➤ Tubing from the mouthpiece is connected to a cylinder that is connected to a computer that measures, records, and calculates the values for the tests done.

➤ Instruct the patient to inhale deeply and then to quickly exhale as much air as possible into the mouthpiece.

➤ Additional breathing maneuvers are performed on inspiration and expiration (normal, forced, and breath-holding).

➤ The results are recorded manually or in a computerized system for recall and postprocedure interpretation by the appropriate health care practitioner.

Post-test:

➤ Assess the patient for dizziness or weakness after the testing.

➤ Allow the patient to rest as long as needed to recover.

➤ Compare new pulmonary function test values with previous values to determine response to medical problem or treatment.

➤ Instruct the patient to resume usual diet and medications, as directed by the health care practitioner.

➤ A written report of the examination will be completed by a health care practitioner specializing in this branch of medicine. The report will be sent to the requesting health care practitioner, who will discuss the results with the patient.

➤ Reinforce information given by the patient's health care provider regarding further testing, treatment, or referral to another health care provider. Answer any questions or address any concerns voiced by the patient or family.

➤ Depending on the results of this procedure, additional testing may be performed to evaluate or monitor progression of the disease process and determine the need for a change in therapy.

Related diagnostic tests:

➤ Related diagnostic tests include computed tomography of the thorax, chest x-ray, echocardiography, electrocardiogram, magnetic resonance imaging of the chest, and positron emission tomography of the chest.

PULSE OXIMETRY

SYNONYMS/ACRONYM: Oximetry, Pulse Ox.

AREA OF APPLICATION: Earlobe, fingertip; for infants, use the large toe, top or bottom of the foot, or sides of the ankle.

CONTRAST: None.

DESCRIPTION & RATIONALE: Pulse oximetry is a noninvasive study that provides continuous readings of arterial blood oxygen saturation (SPO_2) using a sensor site (earlobe or fingertip). The SPO_2 equals the ratio of the amount of O_2 contained in the hemoglobin to the maximum amount of O_2 contained with hemoglobin expressed as a percentage. The results obtained may compare favorably with O_2 saturation levels obtained by arterial blood gas (ABG) analysis without the need to perform successive arterial punctures. The device used is a clip or probe that produces a light beam with two different wavelengths on one side. A sensor on the opposite side measures the absorption of each of the wavelengths of light to determine the O_2 saturation reading. The displayed result is a ratio, expressed as a percentage, between the actual O_2 content of the hemoglobin and the potential maximum O_2-carrying capacity of the hemoglobin. ▪

INDICATIONS:
• Determine the effectiveness of pulmonary gas exchange function

• Evaluate suspected nocturnal hypoxemia in chronic obstructive pulmonary disease (COPD)

• Monitor oxygenation during testing for sleep apnea

• Monitor oxygenation perioperatively and during acute illnesses

• Monitor oxygenation status in patients on a ventilator, during surgery, and during bronchoscopy

• Monitor O_2 saturation during activities such as pulmonary exercise stress testing or pulmonary rehabilitation exercises to determine optimal tolerance

• Monitor response to pulmonary drug regimens, especially flow and O_2 content

RESULT

Normal Findings:
• Greater than or equal to 95%

Abnormal Findings:
• Abnormal gas exchange

• Hypoxemia with levels less than 95%

• Impaired cardiopulmonary function

INTERFERING FACTORS:

This procedure is contraindicated for:

- Patients who smoke or have suffered carbon monoxide inhalation, because O_2 levels may be falsely elevated

Factors that may result in incorrect values:

- Patients with anemic conditions reflecting a reduction in hemoglobin, the O_2-carrying component in the blood

- Excessive light surrounding the patient, such as from surgical lights

- Impaired cardiopulmonary function

- Lipid emulsion therapy and presence of certain dyes

- Movement of the finger or ear or improper placement of probe or clip

- Nail polish, false fingernails, and skin pigmentation when a finger probe is used

- Vasoconstriction from cool skin temperature, drugs, hypotension, or vessel obstruction causing a decrease in blood flow

Other considerations:

- Accuracy for most units is plus or minus 4% with a standard deviation of 1%.

Nursing Implications and Procedure . . . .

Pretest:

➤ Inform the patient that the procedure is used to monitor oxygenation of the blood.

➤ Obtain a history of the patient's respiratory and cardiovascular systems, reason for monitoring procedure, and results of previously performed laboratory tests (especially ABG results), surgical procedures, and other diagnostic procedures. For related diagnostic tests, refer to the Respiratory and Cardiovascular System tables.

➤ Review the procedure with the patient. Address concerns about pain related to the procedure. Explain to the patient that no pain is associated with the procedure. Inform the patient that the procedure is generally performed at the bedside, in the operating room during a surgical procedure, or in a health care practitioner's office. Explain that the procedure lasts as long as the monitoring is needed and could be continuous.

➤ *Sensitivity to cultural and social issues,* as well as concern for modesty, is important in providing psychological support before, during, and after the procedure.

➤ Instruct the patient not to smoke for 24 hours before the procedure.

➤ If a finger probe is used, instruct the patient to remove false fingernails and nail polish.

➤ If a finger probe is used, instruct the patient not to grip treadmill rail or bedrail tightly; doing so restricts blood flow.

➤ When used in the presence of flammable gases, the equipment must be approved for that specific use.

➤ There are no food, fluid, or medication restrictions, unless by medical direction.

Intratest:

➤ Ensure that the patient does not have false fingernails and that nail polish has been removed.

➤ Instruct the patient to cooperate fully and to follow directions.

➤ Observe standard precautions, and follow the general guidelines in Appendix A.

➤ Massage or apply a warm towel to the upper earlobe or finger to increase the blood flow.

➤ The index finger is normally used, but if the patient's finger is too large for the probe, a smaller finger can be used.

- If the earlobe is used, make sure good contact is achieved.
- With infants, the big toe, top or bottom of the foot, or sides of the heel may be used.
- Place the photodetector probe over the finger in such a way that the light beams and sensors are opposite each other. Turn the power switch to the oximeter monitor, which will display information about heart rate and SaO_2.
- Remove the clip used for monitoring when the procedure is complete.
- The results are recorded manually or in a computerized system for recall and postprocedure interpretation by the appropriate health care practitioner.

Post-test:

- Compare new value with previous value to determine response to medical problem or treatment.

- Consider results as they relate to ABGs.
- Closely observe SPO_2, and report to the health care practitioner if it decreases to 90%.
- Answer any questions or address any concerns voiced by the patient or family.
- Depending on the results of this procedure, additional testing may be performed to evaluate or monitor progression of the disease process and determine the need for a change in therapy. Evaluate test results in relation to the patient's symptoms and other tests performed.

Related diagnostic tests:

- Related diagnostic tests include computed tomography angiography, chest x-ray, electrocardiogram, magnetic resonance angiography, magnetic resonance imaging of the chest, and pulmonary function tests.

PYRUVATE KINASE

SYNONYM/ACRONYM: PK.

SPECIMEN: Whole blood collected in yellow-top (acid-citrate-dextrose [ACD]) tube. Specimens collected in a lavender-top (ethylenediaminetetraacetic acid [EDTA]) or green-top (heparin) tube also may be acceptable in some laboratories.

REFERENCE VALUE: (Method: Spectrophotometry) 9 to 22 U/g hemoglobin.

DESCRIPTION & RATIONALE: Pyruvate kinase is an enzyme that forms pyruvate and adenosine diphosphate (ADP) during glycolysis. Deficiency of this enzyme can be acquired by ingestion of a drug or as an effect of liver disease. There is also a hereditary form of pyruvate kinase deficiency that can be transmitted as an autosomal recessive trait. Red blood cells lacking this enzyme have a membrane defect resulting from low levels of adenosine triphosphate (ATP) and are more susceptible to hemolysis. ■

INDICATIONS: Evaluate chronic hemolytic anemia

RESULT

Increased in:
- Carriers of Duchenne's muscular dystrophy
- Muscle disease
- Myocardial infarction

Decreased in:
- Hereditary pyruvate kinase deficiency: Congenital nonspherocytic hemolytic anemia
- Acquired pyruvate kinase deficiency: Acute leukemia
  Aplasias
  Other anemias

CRITICAL VALUES: N/A

INTERFERING FACTORS:
- Testing after blood transfusion may produce a falsely normal result.
- The enzyme is unstable. The specimen should be refrigerated immediately after collection.

Nursing Implications and Procedure • • • • • • • • • • •

Pretest:

➤ Inform the patient that the test is used to identify pyruvate kinase enzyme deficiency.

➤ Obtain a history of the patient's complaints, including a list of known allergens (especially allergies or sensitivities to latex), and inform the appropriate health care practitioner accordingly.

➤ Obtain a history of the patient's hematopoietic system as well as results of previously performed laboratory tests, surgical procedures, and other diagnostic procedures. For related laboratory tests, refer to the Hematopoietic System table.

➤ Note any recent procedures that can interfere with test results.

➤ Obtain a list of medications the patient is taking, including herbs, nutritional supplements, and nutraceuticals. The requesting health care practitioner and laboratory should be advised if the patient is regularly using these products so that their effects can be taken into consideration when reviewing results.

➤ Review the procedure with the patient. Inform the patient that specimen collection takes approximately 5 to 10 minutes. Address concerns about pain related to the procedure. Explain to the patient that there may be some discomfort during the venipuncture.

➤ There are no food, fluid, or medication restrictions, unless by medical direction.

Intratest:

➤ If the patient has a history of severe allergic reaction to latex, care should be taken to avoid the use of equipment containing latex.

➤ Instruct the patient to cooperate fully and to follow directions. Direct the patient to breathe normally and to avoid unnecessary movement.

➤ Observe standard precautions, and follow the general guidelines in Appendix A. Positively identify the patient, and label the appropriate tubes with the corresponding patient demographics, date, and time of collection. Perform a venipuncture; collect the specimen in a 5-mL yellow-top tube.

➤ Remove the needle, and apply a

> pressure dressing over the puncture site.

> Promptly transport the specimen to the laboratory for processing and analysis.

> The results are recorded manually or in a computerized system for recall and postprocedure interpretation by the appropriate health care practitioner.

Post-test:

> Observe venipuncture site for bleeding or hematoma formation. Apply paper tape or other adhesive to hold pressure bandage in place, or replace with a plastic bandage.

> A written report of the examination will be sent to the requesting health care practitioner, who will discuss the results with the patient.

> Reinforce information given by the patient's health care provider regarding further testing, treatment, or referral to another health care provider. Answer any questions or address any concerns voiced by the patient or family.

> Depending on the results of this procedure, additional testing may be performed to evaluate or monitor progression of the disease process and determine the need for a change in therapy. Evaluate test results in relation to the patient's symptoms and other tests performed.

Related laboratory tests:

> Related laboratory tests include complete blood count, glucose-6-phosphate dehydrogenase, Ham's test, and osmotic fragility test.

RADIOACTIVE IODINE UPTAKE

SYNONYM/ACRONYM: Thyroid uptake, RAIU.

AREA OF APPLICATION: Thyroid.

CONTRAST: Oral radioactive iodine.

DESCRIPTION & RATIONALE: Radioactive iodine uptake (RAIU) is a nuclear medicine study used for evaluating thyroid function. It directly measures the ability of the thyroid gland to concentrate and retain circulating iodide for the synthesis of thyroid hormone. RAIU assists in the diagnosis of both hyperthyroidism and hypothyroidism, but it is more useful in the diagnosis of hyperthyroidism.

A very small dose of radioactive iodine-123 (I-123) or I-131 is administered orally and images are taken at specified intervals after the initial dose is administered. The radionuclide emits gamma radiation, which allows external measurement. The uptake of radionuclide in the thyroid gland is measured as the percentage of radionuclide absorbed in a specific amount of time. The iodide not used is excreted in the urine. The thyroid gland does not distinguish between radioactive and nonradioactive iodine. Uptake values are used in conjunction with measurements of circulating thyroid hormone levels to differentiate primary and secondary thyroid disease, and serial measurements are helpful in long-term management of thyroid disease and its treatment. ∎

INDICATIONS:

• Evaluate hyperthyroidism and/or hypothyroidism

• Evaluate neck pain

• Evaluate the patient as part of a complete thyroid evaluation for symptomatic patients (e.g., swollen neck, neck pain, extreme sensitivity to heat or cold, jitters, sluggishness)

• Evaluate thyroiditis, goiter, or pituitary failure

• Monitor response to therapy for thyroid disease

RESULT

Normal Findings:

• Variations in normal ranges of iodine uptake can occur with differences in dietary intake, geographic location, and protocols among laboratories:

Iodine Uptake	Percentage of Radionuclide
2-h absorption	1%–13%
6-h absorption	2%–25%
24-h absorption	15%–45%

Abnormal Findings:

• Decreased iodine intake or increased iodine excretion

• Graves' disease

• Iodine-deficient goiter

• Hashimoto's thyroiditis (early)

• Hyperthyroidism, increased uptake of:

Iodine Uptake	Percentage of Radionuclide
1-h absorption	20%
6-h absorption	25%
24-h absorption	45%

Rebound thyroid hormone withdrawal

Drugs and hormones such as barbiturates, diuretics, estrogens, lithium carbonate, phenothiazines, and thyroid-stimulating hormone

• Decreased uptake:

Hypothyroidism, with a response of decreased uptake of 0 to 10% over a 24-hour period

• Hypoalbuminemia

• Malabsorption

• Renal failure

• Subacute thyroiditis

• Thyrotoxicosis as a result of ectopic thyroid metastasis

INTERFERING FACTORS:

This procedure is contraindicated for:

• Patients who are pregnant or suspected of being pregnant, unless the potential benefits of the procedure far outweigh the risks to the fetus and mother

Factors that may impair clear imaging:

• Inability of the patient to cooperate or remain still during the procedure because of age, significant pain, or mental status

- Patients who are very obese, who may exceed the weight limit for the equipment

- Incorrect positioning of the patient, which may produce poor visualization of the area to be examined

- Recent use of iodinated contrast medium for radiographic studies (within the last 4 weeks) or nuclear medicine procedures done within the previous 24 to 48 hours

- Iodine deficiency (e.g., patients with inadequate dietary intake, patients on phenothiazine therapy), which can increase radionuclide uptake

- Certain drugs and other external sources of excess iodine, which can decrease radionuclide uptake, as follows:

  Foods containing iodine (e.g., iodized salt)

  Drugs such as aminosalicylic acid, antihistamines, antithyroid medications (e.g., propylthiouracil, iodothiouracil), corticosteroids, cough syrup, isoniazid, levothyroxine sodium/T_4, L-triiodothyronine, Lugol's solution, nitrates, penicillins, potassium iodide, propylthiouracil, saturated solution of potassium iodide (SSKI), sulfonamides, thiocyanate, thyroid extract, tolbutamide, and warfarin

  Multivitamins containing minerals

- Vomiting, severe diarrhea, and gastroenteritis, which can affect absorption of the oral radionuclide dose

- Metallic objects within the examination field (e.g., jewelry, body rings), which may inhibit organ visualization and can produce unclear images

Other considerations:

- Failure to follow dietary restrictions before the procedure may cause the procedure to be canceled or repeated.

- Consultation with a health care professional should occur before the procedure for radiation safety concerns regarding younger patients or patients who are lactating.

Nursing Implications and Procedure

Pretest:

➤ Inform the patient that the procedure assesses thyroid function.

➤ Obtain a history of the patient's complaints and symptoms, including a list of known allergens.

➤ Obtain a history of the patient's endocrine system, as well as results of previously performed laboratory tests, surgical procedures, and other diagnostic procedures. For related diagnostic tests, refer to the Endocrine System table.

➤ Ensure that this procedure is performed before all radiographic procedures using iodinated contrast medium.

➤ Record the date of the last menstrual period and determine the possibility of pregnancy in perimenopausal women.

➤ Obtain a list of the patient's current medications.

➤ Review the procedure with the patient. Address concerns about pain related to the procedure. Explain to the patient that some pain may be experienced during the test, and there may be moments of discomfort. Explain the purpose of the test and how the procedure is performed. Inform the patient that the procedure is performed in a nuclear medicine department, usually by a technologist and support staff, and takes approximately 15 to 30 minutes, and that delayed images or data collection is needed 24 hours later. The patient may leave the department and return later to undergo delayed data collection.

➤ *Sensitivity to cultural and social issues,* as well as concern for modesty, is important in providing psychological support before, during, and after the procedure.

➤ Instruct the patient to remove dentures, jewelry (including watches), hairpins, credit cards, and other metallic objects.

➤ The patient should fast for 8 to 12 hours before the procedure, but the patient may eat 4 hours after the test begins, unless otherwise indicated.

Intratest:

➤ Ensure that the patient has fasted for 8 to 12 hours before the uptake, but the patient may eat 4 hours after the test begins, unless otherwise indicated. Ensure that the patient has removed all external metallic objects (jewelry, dentures, etc.) from the neck area prior to the procedure.

➤ Instruct the patient to cooperate fully and to follow directions. Instruct the patient to remain still throughout the procedure because movement produces unreliable results.

➤ Observe standard precautions, and follow the general guidelines in Appendix A.

➤ Administer the I-123 orally (pill form).

➤ At 2, 6, and 24 hours, place the patient in a sitting or supine position in front of a radionuclide detector that will determine the thyroid gland's ability to bind iodine.

➤ Wear gloves during the radionuclide administration and while handling the patient's urine.

➤ The results are recorded on film or in a computerized system for recall and postprocedure interpretation by the appropriate health care practitioner.

Post-test:

➤ Instruct the patient to resume usual diet, as directed by the health care practitioner.

➤ Advise patient to drink increased amounts of fluids for 24 hours to eliminate the radionuclide from the body, unless contraindicated. Tell the patient that radionuclide is eliminated from the body within 24 to 48 hours.

➤ If a woman who is breast-feeding must have a nuclear scan, she should not breast-feed the infant until the radionuclide has been eliminated. This could take as long as 3 days. She should be instructed to express the milk and discard it during the 3-day period to prevent cessation of milk production.

➤ Instruct the patient to flush the toilet immediately after each voiding following the procedure, and to wash hands meticulously with soap and water after each voiding for 24 hours after the procedure.

➤ Tell all caregivers to wear gloves when discarding urine for 24 hours after the procedure. Wash gloved hands with soap and water before removing gloves. Then wash hands after the gloves are removed.

➤ A written report of the examination will be completed by a health care practitioner specializing in this branch of medicine. The report will be sent to the requesting health care practitioner, who will discuss the results with the patient.

➤ Reinforce information given by the patient's health care provider regarding further testing, treatment, or referral to another health care provider. Answer any questions or address any concerns voiced by the patient or family.

➤ Depending on the results of this procedure, additional testing may be needed to evaluate or monitor progression of the disease process and determine the need for a change in therapy. Evaluate test results in relation to the patient's symptoms and other tests performed.

Related diagnostic tests:

➤ Related diagnostic tests include computed tomography of the spine, upper gastrointestinal series, and ultrasound of the thyroid.

RADIOFREQUENCY ABLATION, LIVER

SYNONYMS/ACRONYM: RFA, RF ablation.

AREA OF APPLICATION: Liver.

CONTRAST: Intravenous iodine based.

DESCRIPTION & RATIONALE: One minimally invasive therapy to eliminate tumors in organs such as the liver is called radiofrequency ablation (RFA). This technique works by passing electrical current in the range of radiofrequency waves between the needle electrode and the grounding pads placed on the patient's skin. A special needle electrode is placed in the tumor under the guidance of an imaging method such as ultrasound, computed tomography (CT) scanning, or magnetic resonance imaging (MRI). A radiofrequency current is then passed through the electrode to heat the tumor tissue near the needle tip and to ablate, or eliminate, it. The current creates heat around the electrode inside the tumor, and this heat spreads out to destroy the entire tumor, but little of the surrounding normal liver tissue. The heat from radiofrequency energy also closes up small blood vessels, thereby minimizing the risk of bleeding. Because healthy liver tissue withstands more heat than a tumor, RFA is able to destroy a tumor and a small rim of normal tissue about its edges without affecting most of the normal liver. The dead tumor cells are gradually replaced by scar tissue that shrinks over time. Some liver tumors may have failed to respond to chemotherapy, or have recurred after initial surgery, and may be treated by RFA. If there are multiple tumor nodules, they may be treated in one or more sessions. In general, RFA causes only minimal discomfort and may be done as an outpatient procedure without general anesthesia. RFA is most effective if the tumor or tumors are less than 2 inches in diameter; results are not as good when RFA is used to treat larger tumors. Similar therapy is being used to treat tumors in the kidney, pancreas, bone, thyroid, breast, adrenal gland, and lung. ▪

INDICATIONS:

• Ablation of metastases to the liver

• Ablation of primary liver tumors, with hepatocellular carcinoma

• Therapy for multiple small liver tumors that are too spread out to remove surgically

• Therapy for recurrent liver tumors

• Therapy for tumors that are less than 2 inches in diameter

• Therapy for tumors that have failed to respond to chemotherapy

• Therapy for tumors that have recurred after initial surgery

RISKS:
- May cause brief or long-lasting shoulder pain.

- May cause inflammation of the gallbladder.

- May cause damage to the bile ducts with resulting biliary obstruction.

- May cause thermal damage to the bowel.

- The patient may experience flu-like symptoms that appear 3 to 5 days after the procedure and last for approximately 5 days.

- The patient may experience bleeding. If bleeding is severe, surgery may be needed.

INTERFERING FACTORS

This procedure is contraindicated for:
- Patients with bleeding disorders

- Patients who are pregnant or suspected of being pregnant, unless the potential benefits of the procedure far outweigh the risks to the fetus and mother

Factors that may impair clear imaging:
- Metallic objects within the examination field (e.g., jewelry, rings, surgery clips), which may inhibit organ visualization and can produce unclear images

- Improper adjustment of the radiographic equipment to accommodate obese or thin patients, which can cause overexposure or underexposure and a poor-quality study

- Patients who are very obese, who may exceed the weight limit for the equipment

- Incorrect positioning of the patient, which may produce poor visualization of the area to be examined

- Inability of the patient to cooperate or remain still during the procedure because of age, significant pain, or mental status

Other considerations:
- Failure to follow dietary restrictions and other pretesting preparations before the procedure may cause the procedure to be canceled or repeated.

- Consultation with a health care practitioner should occur before the procedure for radiation safety concerns regarding younger patients or patients who are lactating.

- Risks associated with radiographic overexposure can result from frequent x-ray procedures. Personnel in the room with the patient should wear a protective lead apron, stand behind a shield, or leave the area while the examination is being done. Personnel working in the area where the examination is being done should wear badges that reveal their level of exposure to radiation.

Nursing Implications and Procedure ....

Pretest:

➤ Inform the patient that the procedure assesses liver function.

➤ Obtain a history of the patient's complaints, including a list of known allergens (especially allergies or sensitivities to latex, iodine, seafood, contrast medium, anesthetics, and dyes), and inform the appropriate health care practitioner accordingly.

➤ Obtain a history of the patient's hepatobiliary system, blood tests, and results of previously performed laboratory tests (especially coagulation tests), surgical procedures, and other diagnostic procedures. For related diagnostic tests, refer to the Hepatobiliary System table.

➤ Note any recent procedures that can interfere with test results, including barium examinations.

➤ Record the date of the last menstrual

period and determine the possibility of pregnancy in perimenopausal women.

> Obtain a list of the medications the patient is taking, including anticoagulant therapy, aspirin and other salicylates, herbs, nutritional supplements, and nutraceuticals, especially those known to affect coagulation (see Appendix F). It is recommended that use be discontinued 14 days before surgical procedures. The requesting health care practitioner and laboratory should be advised if the patient regularly uses these products so that their effects can be taken into consideration when reviewing results.

> Review the procedure with the patient. Address concerns about pain related to the procedure. Explain that a sedative and/or analgesia will be administered to promote relaxation and reduce discomfort prior to the needle electrode insertion. Explain to the patient that any discomfort with the needle electrode will be minimized with local anesthetics and systemic analgesics. Inform the patient that the procedure is performed in the radiology department by a physician and support staff, and takes approximately 30 to 90 minutes.

> Explain that an intravenous (IV) line may be inserted to allow infusion of IV fluids, contrast medium, dye, or sedatives. Usually normal saline is infused.

> *Sensitivity to cultural and social issues,* as well as concern for modesty, is important in providing psychological support before, during, and after the procedure.

> The patient should fast and restrict fluids for 8 hours prior to the procedure. Instruct the patient to avoid taking anticoagulant medication or to reduce dosage as ordered prior to the procedure.

> Instruct the patient to remove jewelry (including watches), hairpins, credit cards, and other metallic objects from the area to be examined.

> *Make sure a written and informed consent has been signed prior to the procedure and before administering any medications.*

> This procedure may be terminated if chest pain or severe cardiac arrhythmias occur.

Intratest:

> Ensure that the patient has complied with dietary, fluids, and medication restrictions and pretesting preparations; assure that these have been restricted for at least 8 hours prior to the procedure. Ensure that the patient has removed all external metallic objects (jewelry, dentures, etc.) prior to the procedure.

> Have emergency equipment readily available.

> If the patient has a history of severe allergic reactions to any substance or drug, administer ordered prophylactic steroids or antihistamines before the procedure. Use nonionic contrast medium for the procedure.

> Patients are given a gown, robe, and foot coverings to wear and instructed to void prior to the procedure.

> Instruct the patient to cooperate fully and to follow directions. Instruct the patient to remain still throughout the procedure because movement produces unreliable results.

> Record baseline vital signs and assess neurologic status. Protocols may vary from facility to facility.

> Observe standard precautions, and follow the general guidelines in Appendix A.

> Establish an IV fluid line for the injection of emergency drugs and of sedatives.

> Administer an antianxiety agent, as ordered, if the patient has claustrophobia. Administer a sedative to a child or to an uncooperative adult, as ordered.

> Place electrocardiographic electrodes on the patient for cardiac monitoring. Establish baseline rhythm; determine if the patient has ventricular arrhythmias.

➤ Using a pen, mark the site of the patient's peripheral pulses before the procedure begins; this allows for quicker and more consistent assessment of the pulses after the procedure.

➤ Place the patient in the supine position on an exam table. Cleanse the selected area, and cover with a sterile drape.

➤ A local anesthetic is injected at the site, and a needle electrode is inserted under ultrasound, CT, or MRI guidance.

➤ A radiofrequency current is passed through the needle electrode, and the tumor is ablated.

➤ Instruct the patient to take slow, deep breaths if nausea occurs during the procedure. Monitor and administer an antiemetic agent if ordered. Ready an emesis basin for use.

➤ The needle electrode is removed, and a pressure dressing is applied over the puncture site.

➤ Monitor the patient for complications related to the procedure (e.g., allergic reaction, anaphylaxis, bronchospasm).

➤ The results are recorded manually, on x-ray film, or electronically in a computerized system for recall and postprocedure interpretation by the appropriate health care practitioner.

Post-test:

➤ Instruct the patient to resume usual diet, fluids, medications, or activity, as directed by the health care practitioner.

➤ Monitor vital signs and neurologic status every 15 minutes for 1 hour, then every 2 hours for 4 hours, and as ordered. Take temperature every 6 hours for 24 hours. Compare with baseline values. Notify the health care practitioner if temperature is elevated. Protocols may vary from facility to facility.

➤ Observe for delayed allergic reactions, such as rash, urticaria, tachycardia, hyperpnea, hypertension, palpitations, nausea, or vomiting.

➤ Advise the patient to immediately report symptoms such as fast heart rate, difficulty breathing, skin rash, itching or decreased urinary output.

➤ Observe the needle electrode insertion site for bleeding, inflammation, or hematoma formation.

➤ Instruct the patient to apply cold compresses to the puncture site, as needed, to reduce discomfort or edema.

➤ Instruct the patient to maintain bed rest for 4 to 6 hours after the procedure or as ordered.

➤ Instruct the patient in the care and assessment of the site. Observe for bleeding, hematoma formation, bile leakage, and inflammation. Note any pleuritic pain, persistent right shoulder pain, or abdominal pain.

➤ A written report of the examination will be completed by a health care practitioner specializing in this branch of medicine. The report will be sent to the requesting health care practitioner, who will discuss the results with the patient.

➤ Recognize anxiety related to test results, and be supportive of impaired activity related to physical activity. Discuss the implications of abnormal test results on the patient's lifestyle. Provide teaching and information regarding the clinical implications of the test results, as appropriate.

➤ Reinforce information given by the patient's health care provider regarding further testing, treatment, or referral to another health care provider. Answer any questions or address any concerns voiced by the patient or family.

➤ Instruct the patient in the use of any ordered medications. Explain the importance of adhering to the therapy regimen. As appropriate, instruct the patient in significant side effects and systemic reactions associated with the prescribed medication. Encourage him or her to review corresponding literature provided by a pharmacist.

Depending on the results of this procedure, additional testing may be performed to evaluate or monitor progression of the disease process and determine the need for a change in therapy. Evaluate test results in relation to the patient's symptoms and other tests performed.

Related diagnostic tests:

➤ Related diagnostic tests include angiography of the abdomen, computed tomography of the liver, magnetic resonance imaging of the abdomen, and ultrasound of the liver and biliary system.

RADIOGRAPHY, BONE

SYNONYM/ACRONYM: Bone x-rays, hand x-rays, foot x-rays, wrist x-rays, arm x-rays.

AREA OF APPLICATION: Skeleton.

CONTRAST: None.

DESCRIPTION & RATIONALE: Skeletal x-rays are used to evaluate extremity pain or discomfort due to trauma, bone abnormalities, or fluid within a joint. Serial skeletal x-rays are used to evaluate growth pattern. Radiation emitted from the x-ray machine passes through the patient onto a photographic plate or x-ray film. X-rays pass through air freely and are mostly absorbed by the photographic media. Bones and tissues absorb the x-rays in varying degrees, thereby causing white and shades of gray on the x-ray recording media: Bones are very dense and therefore absorb most of the x-ray and appear white; organs are denser than air but not as dense as bone, so they appear in shades of gray. All metals absorb x-rays. Because the x-ray is absorbed or blocked, metal appears totally white on the film and thus facilitates the search for foreign bodies in the patient. ■

INDICATIONS:
• Assist in detecting bone fracture, dislocation, deformity, and degeneration

• Evaluate for child abuse

• Evaluate growth pattern

• Identify abnormalities of bones, joints, and surrounding tissues

• Monitor fracture healing process

RESULT

Normal Findings:
• *Infants and children:* Thin plate of cartilage, known as growth plate or epiphyseal plate, between the shaft and both ends

- *Adolescents and adults:* By age 17, calcification of cartilage plate; no evidence of fracture, congenital abnormalities, tumors, or infection

Abnormal Findings:
- Arthritis
- Bone degeneration
- Bone spurs
- Foreign bodies
- Fracture
- Genetic disturbance (achondroplasia, dysplasia, dyostosis)
- Hormonal disturbance
- Infection, including osteomyelitis
- Injury
- Joint dislocation or effusion
- Nutritional or metabolic disturbances
- Osteoporosis or osteopenia
- Soft-tissue abnormalities
- Tumor or neoplastic disease (osteogenic sarcoma, Paget's disease, myeloma)

INTERFERING FACTORS:

This procedure is contraindicated for:
- Patients who are pregnant or suspected of being pregnant, unless the potential benefits of the procedure far outweigh the risks to the fetus and mother

Factors that may impair clear imaging:
- Retained barium from a previous radiologic procedure
- Metallic objects within the examination field (e.g., jewelry, body rings, dental amalgams), which may inhibit organ visualization and can produce unclear images
- Improper adjustment of the radiographic equipment to accommodate obese or thin patients, which can cause overexposure or underexposure and a poor-quality study

- Patients who are very obese, who may exceed the weight limit for the equipment
- Incorrect positioning of the patient, which may produce poor visualization of the area to be examined
- Inability of the patient to cooperate or remain still during the procedure because of age, significant pain, or mental status

Other considerations:
- Consultation with a health care practitioner should occur before the procedure for radiation safety concerns regarding younger patients or patients who are lactating.
- Risks associated with radiographic overexposure can result from frequent x-ray procedures. Personnel in the room with the patient should wear a protective lead apron, stand behind a shield, or leave the area while the examination is being done. Personnel working in the area where the examination is being done should wear badges that reveal their level of exposure to radiation.

Nursing Implications and Procedure • • • • • • • • • • • •

Pretest:

➤ Inform the patient that the procedure assesses bone structure of the area examined.

➤ Obtain a history of the patient's complaints.

➤ Obtain a history of results of previously performed diagnostic procedures, surgical procedures, and laboratory tests. For related diagnostic tests, refer to the Musculoskeletal System.

➤ Note any recent procedures that can interfere with test results.

➤ Record the date of the last menstrual period and determine the possibility of pregnancy in perimenopausal women.

➤ Obtain a list of the medications the patient is taking.

▶ Review the procedure with the patient. Explain that numerous x-rays may be taken depending on the bones or joint affected. Explain to the patient that some pain may be experienced during the test, or there may be moments of discomfort. Inform the patient that the procedure is performed in the radiology department by a radiologic technologist and support staff, and takes approximately 10 to 30 minutes.

▶ Instruct the patient to inhale deeply and hold his or her breath while the x-ray is taken and then to exhale after the film is taken. Warn the patient that the extremity's position during the procedure may be uncomfortable, but ask the patient to hold very still during the procedure because movement will produce unclear images.

▶ *Sensitivity to cultural and social issues,* as well as concern for modesty, is important in providing psychological support before, during, and after the procedure.

▶ There are no food, fluid, or medication restrictions, unless by medical direction.

▶ Instruct the patient to remove dentures, jewelry (including watches), hairpins, credit cards, and other metallic objects in the area to be examined.

Intratest:

▶ Ensure that the patient has removed all external metallic objects (wires, jewelry, etc.) prior to the procedure.

▶ Have emergency equipment readily available.

▶ Patients are given a gown, robe, and foot coverings to wear and instructed to void prior to the procedure.

▶ Observe standard precautions, and follow the general guidelines in Appendix A.

▶ Place patient in a standing, sitting, or recumbent position in front of the x-ray film holder or electronic receiver.

▶ Ask the patient to inhale deeply and hold his or her breath while the x-ray images are taken, and then to exhale after the images are taken.

▶ Instruct the patient to take slow, deep breaths if nausea occurs during the procedure. Monitor and administer an antiemetic agent if ordered. Ready an emesis basin for use.

▶ The results are recorded on x-ray film or electronically, in a computerized system, for recall and postprocedure interpretation by the appropriate health care practitioner.

Post-test:

▶ A written report of the examination will be completed by a health care practitioner specializing in this branch of medicine. The report will be sent to the requesting health care practitioner, who will discuss the results with the patient.

▶ Recognize anxiety related to test results, and be supportive of impaired activity related to the perceived loss of daily function. Discuss the implications of abnormal test results on the patient's lifestyle. Provide teaching and information regarding the clinical implications of the test results, as appropriate.

▶ Reinforce information given by the patient's health care provider regarding further testing, treatment, or referral to another health care provider. Explain the importance of adhering to the therapy regimen. Answer any questions or address any concerns voiced by the patient or family.

▶ Depending on the results of this procedure, additional testing may be performed to evaluate or monitor progression of the disease process and determine the need for a change in therapy. Evaluate test results in relation to the patient's symptoms and other tests performed.

Related diagnostic tests:

▶ Related diagnostic tests include bone scan, computed tomography of the spine, and musculoskeletal magnetic resonance imaging.

RED BLOOD CELL CHOLINESTERASE

SYNONYMS/ACRONYMS: acetylcholinesterase (AChE), erythrocyte cholinesterase, true cholinesterase.

SPECIMEN: Whole blood (1 mL) collected in a lavender-top (EDTA) tube.

REFERENCE VALUE: (Method: Spectrophotometry, kinetic)

Test	Conventional Units	SI Units (Conventional Units × 1)
RBC cholinesterase	5–10 U/mL	5–10 kU/L

DESCRIPTION & RATIONALE: There are two types of cholinesterase enzyme: *acetylcholinesterase (AChE)*, which is found in red blood cells (RBCs), lung, and brain (nerve) tissue; and *cholinesterase*, which is mainly found in the plasma, liver, and heart. RBC AChE is highly specific for acetylcholine. Cholinesterase has broader esterolytic activity and is referred to as "pseudocholinesterase." Pseudocholinesterase is the test used to indicate succinylcholine sensitivity (see monograph titled "Pseudocholinesterase and Dibucaine Number"). RBC cholinesterase is used to assist in the diagnosis of chronic carbamate or organophosphate insecticide (e.g., parathion, malathion) toxicity. Organophosphate pesticides bind irreversibly with cholinesterase, inhibiting normal enzyme activity. Carbamate insecticides bind reversibly. Serum or plasma pseudocholinesterase is used more frequently to measure acute pesticide toxicity.

Patients with inherited cholinesterase deficiency are at risk during anesthesia if succinylcholine is administered as an anesthetic. Succinylcholine, a short-acting muscle relaxant, is a reversible inhibitor of acetylcholinesterase and is hydrolyzed by cholinesterase. Succinylcholine-sensitive patients may be unable to metabolize the anesthetic quickly, resulting in prolonged or unrecoverable apnea. This test, along with the pseudocholinesterase test, is also used to identify individuals with atypical forms of the enzyme cholinesterase (see monograph titled "Pseudocholinesterase and Dibucaine Number"). The prevalence of succinylcholate sensitivity is 1 in 1500 patients. Widespread preoperative screening is not routinely performed. ■

INDICATIONS:
* Monitor cumulative exposure to organic phosphate insecticides
* Verify suspected exposure to organic phosphate insecticides

RESULT

Increased in:
* Sickle cell anemia

Decreased in:
* Insecticide exposure (organic phosphate)
* Late pregnancy
* Paroxysmal nocturnal hemoglobinuria
* Relapse of megaloblastic anemia

CRITICAL VALUES: N/A

INTERFERING FACTORS:
* Drugs and substances that may increase RBC cholinesterase levels include echothiophate, parathion, and anti-epileptic drugs such as carbamazepine, phenobarbital, phenytoin, and valproic acid.
* Improper anticoagulant; fluoride interferes with the measurement and causes a falsely decreased value.

Nursing Implications and Procedure • • • • • • • • • • •

Pretest:

➤ Inform the patient that the test is used to identify pesticide poisoning.

➤ Obtain a history of the patient's complaints, including a list of known allergens (especially allergies or sensitivities to latex), and inform the appropriate health care practitioner accordingly. Particularly important to report is exposure to pesticides causing symptoms including blurred vision, muscle weakness, nausea, vomiting, headaches, pulmonary edema, salivation, sweating, or convulsions.

➤ Obtain a history of exposure to occupational hazards and medication regimen.

➤ Obtain a history of the patient's hematopoietic system and results of previously performed laboratory tests, surgical procedures, and other diagnostic procedures. For related laboratory tests, refer to the Hematopoietic System table.

➤ Obtain a list of the medications the patient is taking, including herbs, nutritional supplements, and nutraceuticals. The requesting health care practitioner and laboratory should be advised if the patient regularly uses these products so that their effects can be taken into consideration when reviewing results.

➤ Review the procedure with the patient. Inform the patient that specimen collection takes approximately 5 to 10 minutes. Address concerns about pain related to the procedure. Explain to the patient that there may be some discomfort during the venipuncture.

➤ There are no food, fluid, or medication restrictions, unless by medical direction.

Intratest:

➤ If the patient has a history of severe allergic reaction to latex, care should be taken to avoid the use of equipment containing latex.

➤ Instruct the patient to cooperate fully and to follow directions. Direct the patient to breathe normally and to avoid unnecessary movement.

➤ Observe standard precautions, and follow the general guidelines in Appendix A. Positively identify the patient, and label the appropriate tubes with the corresponding patient demographics, date, and time of collection. Perform a venipuncture; collect the specimen in a 5-mL lavender-top tube.

➤ Remove the needle, and apply a pressure dressing over the puncture site.

➤ Promptly transport the specimen to the laboratory for processing and analysis.

> The results are recorded manually or in a computerized system for recall and postprocedure interpretation by the appropriate health care practitioner.

Post-test:

> Observe venipuncture site for bleeding or hematoma formation. Apply paper tape or other adhesive to hold pressure bandage in place, or replace with a plastic bandage.

> A written report of the examination will be sent to the requesting health care practitioner, who will discuss the results with the patient.

> Reinforce information given by the patient's health care provider regarding further testing, treatment, or referral to another health care provider. Answer any questions or address any concerns voiced by the patient or family.

> Depending on the results of this procedure, additional testing may be performed to evaluate or monitor progression of the disease process and determine the need for a change in therapy. Evaluate test results in relation to the patient's symptoms and other tests performed.

Related laboratory tests:

> Related laboratory tests include complete blood count and pseudocholinesterase.

RED BLOOD CELL COUNT

· ·

SYNONYM/ACRONYM: RBC.

SPECIMEN: Whole blood (1 mL) collected in a lavender-top (EDTA) tube.

REFERENCE VALUE: (Method: Automated, computerized, multichannel analyzers that sort and size cells on the basis of changes in either electrical impedance or light pulses as the cells pass in front of a laser)

Age	Conventional Units	SI Units (Conventional Units × 1)
Cord Blood	$4.14–4.69 \times 10^6$ cells/mm^3	$4.14–4.69 \times 10^{12}$ cells/L
1 d	$5.33–5.47 \times 10^6$ cells/mm^3	$5.33–5.47 \times 10^{12}$ cells/L
2 wk	$4.32–4.98 \times 10^6$ cells/mm^3	$4.32–4.98 \times 10^{12}$ cells/L
1 mo	$3.75–4.95 \times 10^6$ cells/mm^3	$3.75–4.95 \times 10^{12}$ cells/L
6 mo	$3.71–4.25 \times 10^6$ cells/mm^3	$3.71–4.25 \times 10^{12}$ cells/L
1 y	$4.40–4.48 \times 10^6$ cells/mm^3	$4.40–4.48 \times 10^{12}$ cells/L
10 y	$4.75–4.85 \times 10^6$ cells/mm^3	$4.75–4.85 \times 10^{12}$ cells/L
Adult male	$4.71–5.14 \times 10^6$ cells/mm^3	$4.71–5.14 \times 10^{12}$ cells/L
Adult female	$4.20–4.87 \times 10^6$ cells/mm^3	$4.20–4.87 \times 10^{12}$ cells/L

DESCRIPTION & RATIONALE: A component of the complete blood count (CBC), the red blood cell (RBC) count determines the number of RBCs per cubic millimeters (expressed as the number of RBCs per liter of blood according to the international system of units [SI]). Because RBCs contain hemoglobin (Hgb), which is responsible for the transport and exchange of oxygen, the number of circulating RBCs is important. Although the life span of the normal RBC is 120 days, other factors besides cell age and decreased production can cause decreased values; examples are abnormal destruction due to intravascular trauma caused by atherosclerosis or to an enlarged spleen caused by leukemia. The main sites of RBC production in healthy adults include the bone marrow of the vertebrae, pelvis, ribs, sternum, skull, and proximal ends of the femur and humerus. The main sites of RBC destruction are the spleen and liver. Erythropoietin, a hormone produced by the kidneys, regulates RBC production. Normal RBC development and function are also dependent on adequate levels of vitamin B_{12}, folic acid, and iron. A deficiency in vitamin E (α-tocopherol), which is needed to protect the RBC membrane from oxidizers, can result in increased cellular destruction. *Polycythemia* is a term used in conjunction with conditions resulting from an abnormal increase in Hgb, hematocrit (Hct), and RBC count. *Anemia* is a term associated with conditions resulting from an abnormal decrease in Hgb, Hct, and RBC count. Results of the Hgb, Hct, and RBC count should be evaluated simultaneously because the same underlying conditions affect this triad of tests similarly. The RBC count multiplied by 3 should approximate the Hgb concentration. The Hct should be within three times the Hgb if the RBC population is normal in size and shape. The Hct plus 6 should approximate the first two figures of the RBC count within 3 (e.g., Hct is 40%; therefore 40 + 6 = 46, and the RBC count should be 4.3 to 4.9). (See monographs titled "Hematocrit," "Hemoglobin," and "Red Blood Cell Indices.") ∎

INDICATIONS:

- Detect a hematologic disorder involving RBC destruction (e.g., hemolytic anemia)

- Determine the presence of hereditary hematologic abnormality

- Monitor the effects of acute or chronic blood loss

- Monitor the effects of physical or emotional stress on the patient

- Monitor patients with disorders associated with elevated erythrocyte counts (e.g., polycythemia vera, chronic obstructive pulmonary disease [COPD])

- Monitor the progression of nonhematologic disorders associated with elevated erythrocyte counts, such as COPD, liver disease, hypothyroidism, adrenal dysfunction, bone marrow failure, malabsorption syndromes, cancer, and renal disease

- Monitor the response to drugs or chemotherapy and evaluate undesired reactions to drugs that may cause blood dyscrasias

- Provide screening as part of a CBC in a general physical examination, especially upon admission to a health care facility or before surgery

RESULT

Increased in:

- Anxiety or stress
- Bone marrow failure
- COPD with hypoxia and secondary polycythemia
- Dehydration with hemoconcentration
- Erythremic erythrocytosis
- High altitude
- Polycythemia vera

Decreased in:

- Chemotherapy
- Chronic inflammatory diseases
- Hemoglobinopathy
- Hemolytic anemia
- Hemorrhage
- Hodgkin's disease
- Leukemia
- Multiple myeloma
- Nutritional deficit
- Organ failure
- Overhydration
- Pregnancy (normal dilutional effect)
- Subacute endocarditis

CRITICAL VALUES:

The presence of abnormal cells, other morphologic characteristics, or cellular inclusions may signify a potentially life-threatening or serious health condition and should be investigated. Examples are the presence of sickle cells, moderate numbers of spherocytes, marked schisto-cytosis, oval macrocytes, basophilic stippling, nucleated RBCs (if the patient is not an infant), or malarial organisms.

Note and immediately report to the health care practitioner any critically increased or decreased values and related symptoms.

- Low RBC count leads to anemia. Anemia can be caused by blood loss, decreased blood cell production, increased blood cell destruction, or hemodilution. Causes of blood loss include menstrual excess or frequency, gastrointestinal bleeding, inflammatory bowel disease, or hematuria. Decreased blood cell production can be caused by folic acid deficiency, vitamin B_{12} deficiency, iron deficiency, or chronic disease. Increased blood cell destruction can be caused by a hemolytic reaction, chemical reaction, medication reaction, or sickle cell disease. Hemodilution can be caused by congestive heart failure, renal failure, polydipsia, or overhydration. Symptoms of anemia (due to these causes) include anxiety, dyspnea, edema, hypertension, hypotension, hypoxia, jugular venous distention, fatigue, pallor, rales, restlessness, and weakness. Treatment of anemia depends on the cause.

- High RBC count leads to polycythemia. Polycythemia can be caused by dehydration, decreased oxygen levels in the body, and an overproduction of RBCs by the bone marrow. Dehydration by diuretic use, vomiting, diarrhea, excessive sweating, severe burns, or decreased fluid intake decreases the plasma component of whole blood, thereby increasing the ratio of RBCs to plasma, and leads to a higher than normal Hct. Causes of decreased oxygen include smoking, exposure to carbon monoxide, high altitude, and chronic lung disease, which leads to a mild hemoconcentration of blood in the body to carry more oxygen to the body's tissues. An overproduction of RBCs by the bone marrow leads to polycythemia vera, which is a rare chronic myeloproliferative disorder that leads to a severe hemoconcentration of blood. Severe hemoconcentration can lead to thrombosis (spontaneous blood clotting). Symptoms of hemoconcentration include decreased pulse pressure and volume, loss of skin turgor, dry mucous membranes, headaches, hepatomegaly, low central venous pressure, orthostatic hypotension, pruritis (especially after a hot bath), splenomegaly, tachycardia, thirst, tinnitus, vertigo, and weakness. Treatment of polycythemia depends on the cause. Possible interventions for hemoconcentration due to dehydration include intravenous fluids and discontinuance of diuretics if they are believed to be contributing to critically elevated Hct. Polycythemia due to decreased oxygen states can be treated by removal of the offending substance, such as smoke or carbon monoxide. Treatment includes oxygen therapy in cases of smoke inhalation, carbon monoxide poisioning, and desaturating chronic lung disease. Symptoms of polycythemic overload crisis include signs of thrombosis, pain and redness in extremities, facial flushing, and irritability. Possible interventions for hemoconcentration due to polycythemia include therapeutic phlebotomy and intravenous fluids.

INTERFERING FACTORS:

- Drugs and substances that may decrease RBC count by causing hemolysis resulting from drug sensitivity or enzyme deficiency include such as acetaminophen, aminopyrine, aminosalicylic acid, amphetamine, anticonvulsants, antipyrine, arsenicals, benzene, busulfan, carbenicillin, cephalothin, chemotherapy drugs, chlorate, chloroquine, chlorothiazide, chlorpromazine, colchicine, diphenhydramine, dipyrone, glucosulfone, gold, hydroflumethiazide, indomethacin, mephenytoin, nalidixic acid, neomycin, nitrofurantoin, penicillin, phenacemide, phenazopyridine, and phenothiazine.

- Drugs that may decrease RBC count by causing anemia include miconazole, penicillamine, phenylhydrazine, primaquine, probenecid, pyrazolones, pyrimethamine, quinines, streptomycin, sulfamethizole, sulfamethoxypyridine, sulfisoxazole, suramin, thioridazine, tolbutamide, trimethadione, and tripelennamine.

- Drugs that may decrease RBC count by causing bone marrow suppression include amphotericin B, floxuridine, and phenylbutazone.

- Drugs and vitamins that may increase the RBC count include glucocorticosteroids, pilocarpine, and vitamin B_{12}.

- Use of the neutraceutical liver extract is strongly contraindicated in patients with iron-storage disorders such as hemochromatosis because it is rich in heme (the iron-containing pigment in Hgb).

- Hemodilution (e.g., excessive administration of intravenous fluids, normal pregnancy) in the presence of a normal number of RBCs may lead to false decreases in RBC count.

- Cold agglutinins may falsely increase the mean corpuscular volume (MCV) and decrease the RBC count. This can be corrected by warming the blood or diluting the sample with warmed saline and repeating the analysis.

- Excessive exercise, anxiety, pain, and dehydration may cause false elevations in RBC count.

- A grossly elevated white blood cell (WBC) count (greater than $500 \times 10^3/mm^3$) will cause a falsely elevated RBC count. This can be corrected by diluting the sample with saline to obtain an accurate WBC count and then correcting the RBC mathematically.

- Care in evaluating the CBC after transfusion should be taken into consideration.

- RBC counts can vary depending on the patient's position, decreasing when the patient is recumbent as a result of hemodilution and increasing when the patient rises as a result of hemoconcentration.

- Venous stasis can falsely elevate RBC counts; therefore, the tourniquet should not be left on the arm for longer than 60 seconds.

- Failure to fill the tube sufficiently (i.e., tube less than three-quarters full) may yield inadequate sample volume for automated analyzers and may be a reason for specimen rejection.

- Hemolyzed or clotted specimens must be rejected for analysis.

Nursing Implications and Procedure

Pretest:

➤ Inform the patient that the test is used to evaluate anemia and disorders affecting the number of circulating red blood cells.

➤ Obtain a history of the patient's complaints, including a list of known allergens (especially allergies or sensitivities to latex), and inform the appropriate health care practitioner accordingly.

➤ Obtain a history of the patient's cardiovascular, gastrointestinal, hematopoietic, hepatobiliary, immune, musculoskeletal, and respiratory systems, as well as results of previously performed laboratory tests, surgical procedures, and other diagnostic procedures. For related laboratory tests, refer to the Cardiovascular, Gastrointestinal, Hematopoietic, Hepatobiliary, Immune, Musculoskeletal, and Respiratory System tables.

➤ Note any recent procedures that can interfere with test results.

➤ Obtain a list of the medications the patient is taking, including herbs, nutritional supplements, and nutraceuticals. The requesting health care practitioner and laboratory should be advised if the patient regularly uses these products so that their effects can be taken into consideration when reviewing results.

➤ Review the procedure with the patient. Inform the patient that specimen collection takes approximately 5 to 10 minutes. Address concerns about pain related to the procedure. Explain to the patient that there may be some discomfort during the venipuncture.

➤ *Sensitivity to social and cultural issues,* as well as concern for modesty, is important in providing psychological support before, during, and after the procedure.

➤ There are no food, fluid, or medication restrictions, unless by medical direction.

Intratest:

➤ If the patient has a history of severe allergic reaction to latex, care should be taken to avoid the use of equipment containing latex.

➤ Instruct the patient to cooperate fully and to follow directions. Direct the patient to breathe normally and to avoid unnecessary movement.

➤ Observe standard precautions, and follow the general guidelines in Appendix A. Positively identify the patient, and label the appropriate tubes with the corresponding patient demographics, date, and time of collection. Perform a venipuncture; collect the specimen in a 5-mL lavender-top (EDTA) tube. An EDTA Microtainer sample may be obtained from infants, children, and adults for whom venipuncture may not be feasible. The specimen should be mixed gently by inverting the tube 10 times. The specimen should be analyzed within 6 hours when stored at room temperature or within 24 hours if stored at refrigerated temperature. If it is anticipated the specimen will not be analyzed within 4 to 6 hours, two blood smears should be made immediately after the venipuncture and submitted with the blood sample. Smears made from specimens older than 6 hours will contain an unacceptable number of misleading artifactual abnormalities of the RBCs, such as echinocytes and spherocytes, as well as necrobiotic WBCs.

➤ Remove the needle, and apply a pressure dressing over the puncture site.

➤ Promptly transport the specimen to the laboratory for processing and analysis.

➤ The results are recorded manually or in a computerized system for recall and postprocedure interpretation by the appropriate health care practitioner.

Post-test:

➤ Observe venipuncture site for bleeding or hematoma formation. Apply paper tape or other adhesive to hold pressure bandage in place, or replace with a plastic bandage.

➤ *Nutritional considerations:* Nutritional therapy may be indicated for patients with decreased RBC count. Iron deficiency is the most common nutrient deficiency in the United States. Patients at risk (e.g., children, pregnant women and women of child-bearing age, low-income populations) should be instructed to include foods that are high in iron in their diet, such as meats (especially liver), eggs, grains, green leafy vegetables, and multivitamins with iron. Iron absorption is affected by numerous factors (see monograph titled "Iron").

➤ *Nutritional considerations:* Patients at risk for vitamin B_{12} or folate deficiency include those with the following conditions: malnourishment (inadequate intake), pregnancy (increased need), infancy, malabsorption syndromes (inadequate absorption/increased metabolic rate), infections, cancer, hyperthyroidism, serious burns, excessive blood loss, and gastrointestinal damage. These patients should be instructed, as appropriate, to ingest food sources rich in vitamin B_{12}, such as meats, milk, cheese, eggs, and fortified soy milk products. Sources of folate are meats (especially liver), kidney beans, beets, vegetables in the cabbage family, oranges, cantaloupe, and green leafy vegetables such as spinach, asparagus, and broccoli.

➤ *Nutritional considerations:* A diet deficient in vitamin E puts the patient at risk for increased RBC destruction, which could lead to anemia. Nutritional therapy may be indicated for these patients. Vitamin E is found in many of the previously mentioned foods, as well as in vegetable oils and wheat germ. Supplemental vitamin E may also be taken, but the danger of toxicity should be explained to the patient. Very large supplemental doses, in excess of 600 mg of vitamin E over a period of 1 year, may result in excess bleeding. Vitamin E is heat stable but is very negatively affected by light.

➤ A written report of the examination will be sent to the requesting health care practitioner, who will discuss the results with the patient.

➤ Reinforce information given by the patient's health care provider regarding further testing, treatment, or referral to another health care provider. Answer any questions or address any concerns voiced by the patient or family.

➤ Depending on the results of this procedure, additional testing may be performed to evaluate or monitor progression of the disease process and determine the need for a change in therapy. Evaluate test results in relation to the patient's symptoms and other tests performed.

Related laboratory tests:

➤ Related laboratory tests include the other tests included in a CBC, erythropoietin, ferritin, folate, iron/total iron-binding capacity, RBC morphology and inclusions, reticulocyte count, and vitamin B_{12}.

RED BLOOD CELL INDICES

SYNONYMS/ACRONYMS: mean corpuscular hemoglobin (MCH), mean corpuscular volume (MCV), mean corpuscular hemoglobin concentration (MCHC), red blood cell distribution width (RDW).

SPECIMEN: Whole blood (1 mL) collected in a lavender-top (EDTA) tube.

REFERENCE VALUE: (Method: Automated, computerized, multichannel analyzers that sort and size cells on the basis of changes in either electrical impedance or light pulses as the cells pass in front of a laser)

Age	MCV (fL)	MCH (pg/cell)	MCHC (g/dL)	RDW
Cord blood	107–119	35–39	32–34	14.9–18.7
1 d	104–116	35–39	32–34	14.9–18.7
2 wk	95–117	29–35	28–32	14.9–18.7
1 mo	93–115	29–35	28–34	14.9–18.7
6 mo	82–100	24–30	28–32	14.9–18.7
1 y	81–95	25–29	29–31	11.6–14.8
10 y	75–87	25–31	33–35	11.6–14.8
Adult male	85–95	28–32	33–35	11.6–14.8
Adult female	85–95	28–32	33–35	11.6–14.8

MCV = mean corpuscular volume; MCH = mean corpuscular hemoglobin; MCHC = mean corpuscular hemoglobin concentration; RDW = red blood cell distribution width.

DESCRIPTION & RATIONALE: Red blood cell (RBC) indices provide information about the mean corpuscular volume (MCV), mean corpuscular hemoglobin (MCH), mean corpuscular hemoglobin concentration (MCHC), and RBC distribution width (RDW). The hematocrit, RBC count, and total hemoglobin tests are used to determine the RBC indices. MCV is determined by dividing the hematocrit by the total RBC count and is helpful in classifying anemias. MCH is determined by dividing the total hemoglobin concentration by the RBC count. MCHC is determined by dividing total hemoglobin by hematocrit. Hemoglobin content is indicated as normochromic, hypochromic, and hyperchromic. The RDW is a measurement of cell size distribution over the entire RBC population measured. It is an indication of anisocytosis, or excessive variations in cell size. Cell size is indicated as normocytic, microcytic, and macrocytic. (See monographs titled "Hemoglobin," "Hematocrit," "Red Blood Cell Count," and "Red Blood Cell Morphology and Inclusions.") ∎

INDICATIONS:

- Assist in the diagnosis of anemia

- Detect a hematologic disorder, neoplasm, or immunologic abnormality

- Determine the presence of a hereditary hematologic abnormality

- Monitor the effects of physical or emotional stress

- Monitor the progression of nonhematologic disorders such as chronic obstructive pulmonary disease, malabsorption syndromes, cancer, and renal disease

- Monitor the response to drugs or chemotherapy, and evaluate undesired reactions to drugs that may cause blood dyscrasias

- Provide screening as part of a complete blood count (CBC) in a general physical examination, especially upon admission to a health care facility or before surgery

RESULT

MCV increased in:
- Alcoholism
- Antimetabolite therapy
- Liver disease
- Pernicious anemia
- Vitamin B_{12}/folate anemia

MCV decreased in:
- Iron-deficiency anemia
- Thalassemias

MCH increased in:
- Macrocytic anemias

MCH decreased in:
- Hypochromic anemias
- Microcytic anemias

MCHC increased in:
- Thalassemia
- Spherocytosis

MCHC decreased in:
- Iron-deficiency anemia

RDW increased in:
- Anemias with heterogeneous cell size

RDW decreased in: N/A

CRITICAL VALUES: N/A

INTERFERING FACTORS:

- Drugs and substances that may decrease the MCHC include styrene (occupational exposure).

- Drugs that may decrease the MCV include nitrofurantoin.

- Drugs that may increase the MCV include colchicine, pentamidine, pyrimethamine, and triamterene.

- Drugs that may increase the MCH and MCHC include oral contraceptives (long-term use).

- Diseases that cause agglutination of RBCs will alter test results.

- Cold agglutinins may falsely increase the MCV and decrease the RBC count. This can be corrected by warming the blood or diluting the sample with warmed saline and then correcting the RBC count mathematically.

- RBC counts can vary depending on the patient's position, decreasing when the patient is recumbent as a result of hemodilution and increasing when the patient rises as a result of hemoconcentration.

- Care in evaluating the CBC after transfusion should be taken into consideration.

• Venous stasis can falsely elevate RBC counts; therefore, the tourniquet should not be left on the arm for longer than 60 seconds.

• Failure to fill the tube sufficiently (i.e., tube less than three-quarters full) may yield inadequate sample volume for automated analyzers and may be a reason for specimen rejection.

• Hemolyzed or clotted specimens should be rejected.

• Lipemia and elevated white blood cell (WBC) count (greater than 50 WBC $\times$ 10^3/mm^3 or 50,000/ mm^3) will falsely increase the hemoglobin measurement, also affecting the MCV and MCH.

Nursing Implications and Procedure • • • • • • • • • • •

➤ Inform the patient that the test is primarily used to assess red blood cell shape and size.

➤ Obtain a history of the patient's complaints, including a list of known allergens (especially allergies or sensitivities to latex), and inform the appropriate health care practitioner accordingly.

➤ Obtain a history of the patient's gastrointestinal, hematopoietic, immune, and respiratory systems, as well as results of previously performed laboratory tests, surgical procedures, and other diagnostic procedures. For related laboratory tests, refer to the Gastrointestinal, Hematopoietic, Immune, and Respiratory System tables.

➤ Note any recent procedures that can interfere with test results.

➤ Obtain a list of the medications the patient is taking, including herbs, nutritional supplements, and nutraceuticals. The requesting health care practitioner and laboratory should be advised if the patient regularly uses these products so that their effects can be taken into consideration when reviewing results.

➤ Review the procedure with the patient. Inform the patient that specimen collection takes approximately 5 to 10 minutes. Address concerns about pain related to the procedure. Explain to the patient that there may be some discomfort during the venipuncture.

➤ There are no food, fluid, or medication restrictions, unless by medical direction.

➤ If the patient has a history of severe allergic reaction to latex, care should be taken to avoid the use of equipment containing latex.

➤ Instruct the patient to cooperate fully and to follow directions. Direct the patient to breathe normally and to avoid unnecessary movement.

➤ Observe standard precautions, and follow the general guidelines in Appendix A. Positively identify the patient, and label the appropriate tubes with the corresponding patient demographics, date, and time of collection. Perform a venipuncture; collect the specimen in a 5-mL lavender-top (EDTA) tube. An EDTA Microtainer sample may be obtained from infants, children, and adults for whom venipuncture may not be feasible. The specimen should be mixed gently by inverting the tube 10 times. It is stable when stored for up to 6 hours at room temperature or 24 hours if stored refrigerated. In addition, if it is anticipated that the specimen will not be analyzed within 4 to 6 hours, two blood smears should be made immediately after the venipuncture and submitted with the blood sample. Smears made from specimens older than 6 hours will contain an unacceptable number of misleading artifactual abnormalities of the RBCs, such as echinocytes and spherocytes, as well as necrobiotic WBCs.

➤ Remove the needle, and apply a pressure dressing over the puncture site.

Promptly transport the specimen to the laboratory for processing and analysis.

The results are recorded manually or in a computerized system for recall and postprocedure interpretation by the appropriate healthcare practitioner.

Observe venipuncture site for bleeding or hematoma formation. Apply paper tape or other adhesive to hold pressure bandage in place, or replace with a plastic bandage.

A written report of the examination will be sent to the requesting health care practitioner, who will discuss the results with the patient.

Reinforce information given by the patient's health care provider regarding further testing, treatment, or referral to another health care provider. Answer any questions or address any concerns voiced by the patient or family.

Depending on the results of this procedure, additional testing may be performed to evaluate or monitor progression of the disease process and determine the need for a change in therapy. Evaluate test results in relation to the patient's symptoms and other tests performed.

Related laboratory tests include the other tests included in a CBC, erythropoietin, ferritin, iron/total iron-binding capacity, RBC morphology and inclusions, and reticulocyte count.

RED BLOOD CELL MORPHOLOGY AND INCLUSIONS

• •

SYNONYM/ACRONYM: N/A.

SPECIMEN: Whole blood from one full lavender-top (EDTA) tube or Wright's-stained, thin-film peripheral blood smear. The laboratory should be consulted as to the necessity of thick-film smears for the evaluation of malarial inclusions.

REFERENCE VALUE: (Method: Microscopic, manual review of stained blood smear)

Red Blood Cell Morphology	Within Normal Limits	1+	2+	3+	4+
Size					
Anisocytosis	0–5+	5–10	10–20	20–50	Greater than 50
Macrocytes	0–5+	5–10	10–20	20–50	Greater than 50
Microcytes	0–5+	5–10	10–20	20–50	Greater than 50
Shape					
Poikilocytes	0–2+	3–10	10–20	20–50	Greater than 50
Burr cells	0–2+	3–10	10–20	20–50	Greater than 50
Acanthocytes	Less than 1+	2–5	5–10	10–20	Greater than 20
Schistocytes	Less than 1+	2–5	5–10	10–20	Greater than 20
Dacryocytes (teardrop cells)	0–2+	2–5	5–10	20–50	Greater than 20
Codocytes (target cells)	0–2+	2–10	10–20	20–50	Greater than 50
Spherocytes	0–2+	2–10	10–20	20–50	Greater than 50
Ovalocytes	0–2+	2–10	10–20	20–50	Greater than 50
Stomatocytes	0–2+	2–10	10–20	20–50	Greater than 50
Drepanocytes (sickle cells)	Absent	Reported as present or absent			
Helmet cells	Absent	Reported as present or absent			
Agglutination	Absent	Reported as present or absent			
Rouleaux	Absent	Reported as present or absent			
Hemoglobin (Hgb) content					
Hypochromia	0–2+.	3–10	10–50	50–75	Greater than 75
Polychromasia					
Adult	Less than 1+	2–5	5–10	10–20	Greater than 20
Newborn	1–6+	7–15	15–20	20–50	Greater than 50

Inclusions					
Cabot rings	Absent	Reported as present or absent			
Basophilic stippling	0–1+	1–5	5–10	10–20	Greater than 20
Howell-Jolly bodies	Absent	1–2	3–5	5–10	Greater than 10
Heinz bodies	Absent	Reported as present or absent			
Hgb C crystals	Absent	Reported as present or absent			
Pappenheimer bodies	Absent	Reported as present or absent			
Intracellular parasites (e.g., Plasmodium, Babesia, Trypanosoma)	Absent	Reported as present or absent			

DESCRIPTION & RATIONALE: The decision to manually review a peripheral blood smear for abnormalities in red blood cell (RBC) shape or size is made based on criteria established by the reporting laboratory. Cues in the results of the complete blood count (CBC) will point to specific abnormalities that can be confirmed visually, by microscopic review of the sample on a stained blood smear. ■

INDICATIONS:

* Assist in the diagnosis of anemia

* Detect a hematologic disorder, neoplasm, or immunologic abnormality

* Determine the presence of a hereditary hematologic abnormality

* Monitor the effects of physical or emotional stress on the patient

* Monitor the progression of nonhematologic disorders, such as chronic obstructive pulmonary disease, malabsorption syndromes, cancer, and renal disease

* Monitor the response to drugs or chemotherapy, and evaluate undesired reactions to drugs that may cause blood dyscrasias

* Provide screening as part of a CBC in a general physical examination, especially upon admission to a health care facility or before surgery

RESULT

Red Blood Cell Size

Cell size increased in:
* Alcoholism
* Aplastic anemia
* Chemotherapy
* Chronic hemolytic anemia

* Grossly elevated glucose (hyperosmotic)
* Hemolytic disease of the newborn
* Hypothyroidism
* Leukemia
* Lymphoma
* Metastatic carcinoma
* Myelofibrosis
* Myeloma
* Refractory anemia
* Sideroblastic anemia
* Vitamin B_{12}/folate deficiency

Cell size decreased in:
* Hemoglobin C disease
* Hemolytic anemias
* Hereditary spherocytosis
* Inflammation
* Iron-deficiency anemia
* Thalassemias

Red Blood Cell Shape

Variations in cell shape are the result of hereditary conditions such as elliptocytosis, sickle cell anemia, spherocytosis, thalassemias, or hemoglobinopathies (e.g., hemoglobin C disease). Irregularities in cell shape can also result from acquired conditions, such as physical/mechanical cellular trauma, exposure to chemicals, or reactions to medications.

* Acquired spherocytosis can result from Heinz body hemolytic anemia, microangiopathic hemolytic anemia, secondary isoimmunohemolytic anemia, and transfusion of old banked blood.

* Acanthocytes are associated with acquired conditions such as alcoholic cirrhosis with hemolytic anemia, disorders of lipid metabolism, hepatitis

of newborns, malabsorptive diseases, metastatic liver disease, the post-splenectomy period, and pyruvate kinase deficiency.

- Burr cells are commonly seen in acquired renal insufficiency, burns, cardiac valve disease, disseminated intravascular coagulation (DIC), hypertension, intravenous fibrin deposition, metastatic malignancy, normal neonatal period, and uremia.

- Codocytes are seen in hemoglobinopathies, iron-deficiency anemia, obstructive liver disease, and the postsplenectomy period.

- Dacryocytes are most commonly associated with metastases to the bone marrow, myelofibrosis, myeloid metaplasia, pernicious anemia, and tuberculosis.

- Schistocytes are seen in burns, cardiac valve disease, DIC, glomerulonephritis, hemolytic anemia, microangiopathic hemolytic anemia, renal graft rejection, thrombotic thrombocytopenic purpura, uremia, and vasculitis.

Red Blood Cell Hemoglobin Content

RBCs with a normal hemoglobin (Hgb) level have a clear central pallor and are referred to as *normochromic.*

- Cells with low Hgb and lacking in central pallor are referred to as *hypochromic.* Hypochromia is associated with iron-deficiency anemia, thalassemias, and sideroblastic anemia.

- Cells with excessive Hgb levels are referred to as *hyperchromic,* even though they technically lack a central pallor. Hyperchromia is usually associated with an elevated mean corpuscular Hgb concentration as well as hemolytic anemias.

- Cells referred to as *polychromic* are young erythrocytes that still contain ribonucleic acid (RNA). The RNA is picked up by the Wright's stain. Polychromasia is indicative of premature release of RBCs from bone marrow secondary to increased erythropoietin stimulation.

Red Blood Cell Inclusions

RBC inclusions can result from certain types of anemia, abnormal Hgb precipitation, or parasitic infection.

- Cabot rings may be seen in megaloblastic and other anemias, lead poisoning, and conditions in which RBCs are destroyed before they are released from bone marrow.

- Basophilic stippling is seen whenever there is altered Hgb synthesis, as in thalassemias, megaloblastic anemias, alcoholism, and lead or arsenic intoxication.

- Howell-Jolly bodies are seen in sickle cell anemia, other hemolytic anemias, megaloblastic anemia, congenital absence of the spleen, and the postsplenectomy period.

- Pappenheimer bodies may be seen in cases of sideroblastic anemia, thalassemias, refractory anemia, dyserythropoietic anemias, hemosiderosis, and hemochromatosis.

- Heinz bodies are most often seen in the blood of patients who have ingested drugs known to induce the formation of these inclusion bodies. They are also seen in patients with hereditary glucose-6-phosphate dehydrogenase (G6PD) deficiency.

- Hgb C crystals can often be identified in stained peripheral smears of patients with hereditary hemoglobin C disease.

- Parasites such as *Plasmodium* (transmitted by mosquitoes and causing malaria) and *Babesia* (transmitted by ticks), known to invade human RBCs, can be visualized with Wright's stain and other special stains of the peripheral blood.

CRITICAL VALUES:

The presence of sickle cells or parasitic inclusions should be brought to the immediate attention of the requesting health care practitioner.

INTERFERING FACTORS:

• Drugs and substances that may increase Heinz body formation as an initial precursor to significant hemolysis include acetanilid, acetylsalicylic acid, aminopyrine, antimalarials, antipyretics, furadaltone, furazolidone, methylene blue, naphthalene, and nitrofurans.

• Care in evaluating the CBC after transfusion should be taken into consideration.

• Leaving the tourniquet in place for longer than 60 seconds can falsely affect the results.

• Morphology can be evaluated to some extent via indices; therefore, failure to fill the tube sufficiently (i.e., tube less than three-quarters full) may yield inadequate sample volume for automated analyzers and may be a reason for specimen rejection.

• Hemolyzed or clotted specimens should be rejected.

Nursing Implications and Procedure • • • • • • • • • • • •

Pretest:

➤ Inform the patient that the test is used to assess red blood cell appearance.

➤ Obtain a history of the patient's complaints, including a list of known allergens (especially allergies or sensitivities to latex), and inform the appropriate health care practitioner accordingly.

➤ Obtain a history of the patient's cardiovascular, gastrointestinal, hematopoietic, hepatobiliary, immune, musculoskeletal, and respiratory systems, as well as results of previously performed laboratory tests, surgical procedures, and other diagnostic procedures. For related laboratory tests, refer to the Cardiovascular, Gastrointestinal, Hematopoietic, Hepatobiliary, Immune, Musculoskeletal, and Respiratory System tables.

➤ Note any recent procedures that can interfere with test results.

➤ Obtain a list of the medications the patient is taking, including herbs, nutritional supplements, and nutraceuticals. The requesting health care practitioner and laboratory should be advised if the patient regularly uses these products so that their effects can be taken into consideration when reviewing results.

➤ Review the procedure with the patient. Inform the patient that specimen collection takes approximately 5 to 10 minutes. Address concerns about pain related to the procedure. Explain to the patient that there may be some discomfort during the venipuncture.

➤ *Sensitivity to social and cultural issues,* as well as concern for modesty, is important in providing psychological support before, during, and after the procedure.

➤ There are no food, fluid, or medication restrictions, unless by medical direction.

Intratest:

➤ If the patient has a history of severe allergic reaction to latex, care should be taken to avoid the use of equipment containing latex.

➤ Instruct the patient to cooperate fully and to follow directions. Direct the patient to breathe normally and to avoid unnecessary movement.

➤ Observe standard precautions, and follow the general guidelines in Appendix A. Positively identify the patient, and label the appropriate tubes with the corresponding patient demographics, date, and time of collection. Perform a venipuncture; collect the specimen in a 5-mL lavender-top (EDTA) tube. An EDTA Microtainer sample may be obtained from infants, children, and adults for whom venipuncture may not be feasible. The specimen should be mixed gently by inverting the tube 10 times. The specimen should be analyzed within 6 hours when stored at room temperature or within 24 hours if stored at refrigerated temperature. If it is anticipated the specimen will not be analyzed within 4 to 6 hours, two blood smears should be made immediately after the venipuncture and submitted with the blood sample. Smears made from specimens older than 6 hours will contain an unacceptable number of misleading artifactual abnormalities of the RBCs, such as echinocytes and spherocytes, as well as necrobiotic white blood cells.

➤ Remove the needle, and apply a pressure dressing over the puncture site.

➤ Promptly transport the specimen to the laboratory for processing and analysis.

➤ The results are recorded manually or in a computerized system for recall and postprocedure interpretation by the appropriate health care practitioner.

Post-test:

➤ Observe venipuncture site for bleeding or hematoma formation. Apply paper tape or other adhesive to hold pressure bandage in place, or replace with a plastic bandage.

➤ *Nutritional considerations:* Instruct patients to consume a variety of foods within the basic food groups, maintain a healthy weight, be physically active, limit salt intake, limit alcohol intake, and be a nonsmoker.

➤ A written report of the examination will be sent to the requesting health care practitioner, who will discuss the results with the patient.

➤ Reinforce information given by the patient's health care provider regarding further testing, treatment, or referral to another health care provider. Answer any questions or address any concerns voiced by the patient or family.

➤ Depending on the results of this procedure, additional testing may be performed to evaluate or monitor progression of the disease process and determine the need for a change in therapy. Evaluate test results in relation to the patient's symptoms and other tests performed.

Related laboratory tests:

➤ Related laboratory tests include the other tests included in a CBC, δ-aminolevulinic acid, biopsy of bone marrow, erythropoietin, ferritin, G6PD, hematocrit, hemoglobin, hemoglobin electrophoresis, iron/total iron-binding capacity, lead, platelet count, red blood cell count, red blood cell indices, reticulocyte count, and white blood cell count with differential.

REFRACTION

SYNONYMS/ACRONYMS: N/A.

AREA OF APPLICATION: Eyes.

CONTRAST: N/A.

DESCRIPTION & RATIONALE: This noninvasive procedure tests the visual acuity of the eyes and determines abnormalities or refractive errors that need correction. Refractions are performed using a combination of different pieces of equipment. Refractive error can be quickly and accurately measured using computerized automatic refractors or manually with a viewing system consisting of an entire set of trial lenses mounted on a circular wheel (phoropter). A projector may also be used to display test letters and characters for use in assessing visual acuity. The retinoscope is probably the most valuable instrument that can be used to objectively assess visual acuity. It is also the only objective means of assessing refractive error in pediatric patients and patients who are unable to cooperate with other techniques of assessing refractive error due to illiteracy, senility, or inability to speak the same language as the examiner. Visual defects identified through refraction, such as hyperopia (farsightedness), in which the point of focus lies behind the retina; myopia (nearsightedness), in which the point of focus lies in front of the retina; and astigmatism, in which the refraction is unequal in diferent curvatures of the eyeball, can be corrected by glasses, contact lenses, or refractive surgery. ∎

INDICATIONS:
• Determine if an optical defect is present and if light rays entering the eye focus correctly on the retina

• Determine the refractive error prior to refractive surgery (e.g., LASIK, LASEK) being performed

• Determine the type of corrective lenses needed for refractive errors, for example, biconvex or plus lenses for hyperopia, biconcave or minus lenses for myopia, compensatory lenses for astigmatism

• Diagnose refrative errors in vision

RESULT

Normal Findings:
• Normal visual acuity (with corrective lenses if appropriate).

Abnormal Findings:
• Refractive errors such as astigmatism, hyperopia, and myopia.

CRITICAL VALUES: N/A

INTERFERING FACTORS:

This procedure is contraindicated for:
• Patients with narrow-angle glaucoma if pupil dilation is performed, as dilation can initiate a severe and sight-threatening open-angle attack.

• Patients with allergies to mydriatics if pupil dilation using mydriatics is performed.

Factors that may impair the results of the examination:
• Improper pupil dilation may prevent adequate examination for refractive error.

• Inability of the patient to cooperate and remain still during the procedure because of age, significant pain, or mental status may interfere with the test results.

• Failure to follow medication restrictions before the procedure may cause the procedure to be canceled or repeated.

Nursing Implications and Procedure ∙∙∙∙∙∙∙∙∙∙∙∙

Pretest:
➤ Inform the patient that the procedure evaluates visual acuity.

➤ Obtain a history of the patient's complaints, including a list of known allergens, especially mydratics if dilation is to be performed.

➤ Obtain a history of the patient's known or suspected vision loss, changes in visual acuity, including type and cause; use of glasses or contact lenses; eye conditions with treatment regimens; eye surgery; and other tests and procedures to assess and diagnose visual deficit. For related diagnostic tests, refer to the table of tests associated with the Ocular System.

➤ Obtain a history of results of previously performed laboratory tests, surgical procedures, and other diagnostic procedures.

➤ Obtain a list of the medications the patient is taking, including herbs, nutritional supplements, and nutraceuticals. The requesting health care practitioner should be advised if the patient regularly uses these products so that their effects can be taken into consideration when reviewing results.

➤ Instruct the patient to remove contact·lenses or glasses, as appropriate. Instruct the patient regarding the importance of keeping the eyes open for the test.

➤ Review the procedure with the patient. Address concerns about pain related to the procedure. Explain to the patient that mydriatics, if used, may cause blurred vision and sensitivity to light. There may also be a brief stinging sensation when the drop is put in the eye. Inform the patient that a technician, optometrist, or physician performs the test, in a quiet, darkened room, and that to evaluate both eyes, the test can take up 30 minutes (including time for the pupils to dilate before the test is actually performed).

➤ There are no food or fluid restrictions, unless by medical direction.

➤ The patient should withhold eye medications (particularly mydriatic eye drops if the patient has glaucoma) for at least 1 day prior to the test.

➤ Ensure that the patient understands that he or she must refrain from driving until the pupils return to normal (about 4 hours) after the test and has made arrangements to have someone else be responsible for transportation after the test.

Intratest:

➤ Ensure that the patient has complied with medication restrictions and pretesting preparations; assure that eye medications, especially mydriatics, have been restricted for at least 1 day prior to the procedure.

➤ Instruct the patient to cooperate fully and to follow directions. Ask the patient to remain still during the procedure because movement produces unreliable results.

➤ If dilation is to be performed, administer the ordered mydriatic to each eye and repeat in 5 to 15 minutes. Drops are placed in the eye with the patient looking up and the solution directed at the six o'clock position of the sclera (white of the eye) near the limbus (grey, semitransparent area of the eyeball where the cornea and sclera meet). The dropper bottle should not touch the eyelashes.

➤ Ask the patient to place the chin in the chin rest and gently press the forehead against the support bar. The examiner will sit about 2 feet away at eye level with the patient. The retinascope light is held in front of the eyes and directed through the pupil. Each eye is also examined for the characteristics of the red reflex, the reflection of the light from the retinascope, which normally moves in the same direction as the light.

➤ Request that the patient look straight ahead while the eyes are examined with the instrument and while different lenses are tried to provide the best corrective lenses to be prescribed. When optimal visual acuity is obtained with the trial lenses in each eye, a prescription for corrective lenses is written.

➤ The results are recorded manually or on a paper strip from the automated equipment for recall and postprocedure interpretation by the appropriate healthcare practitioner.

Post-test:

➤ Instruct the patient to resume usual medications, as directed by the health care practitioner.

➤ A written report of the examination will be completed by a health care practitioner specializing in this branch of medicine. The report will be sent to the requesting health care practitioner, who will discuss the results with the patient.

➤ Recognize anxiety related to test results, and be supportive of impaired activity related to vision loss, perceived loss of driving privileges, or the possibility of requiring corrective lenses (self-image). Discuss the implications of abnormal test results on the patient's lifestyle. Provide teaching and information regarding the clinical implications of the test results, as appropriate.

➤ Reinforce information given by the patient's health care provider regarding further testing, treatment, or referral to another health care provider. Inform the patient that visual acuity and responses to light may change. Suggest that the patient wear dark glasses after the test until the pupils return to normal size. Answer any questions or address any concerns voiced by the patient or family.

➤ Depending on the results of this procedure, additional testing may be performed to evaluate or monitor progression of the disease process and determine the need for a change in therapy. Evaluate test results in relation to the patient's symptoms and other tests performed.

Related diagnostic tests:

➤ Related diagnostic tests include color perception test, intraocular muscle function, intraocular pressure, and slit-lamp biomicroscopy.

RENIN

SYNONYM/ACRONYM: Plasma renin activity (PRA).

SPECIMEN: Plasma (3 mL) collected in a lavender-top (EDTA) tube.

REFERENCE VALUE: (Method: Radioimmunoassay)

Age and Position	Conventional Units	SI Units (Conventional Units × 1)
Newborn **Supine, normal sodium diet**	2.0–35.0 ng/mL per hour	2.0–35.0 μg/L per hour

Age and Position	Conventional Units	SI Units (Conventional Units × 1)
1–12 mo	2.4–37.0 ng/mL per hour	2.4–37.0 µg/L per hour
1–3 y	1.7–112 ng/mL per hour	1.7–112 µg/L per hour
3–5 y	1.0–6.5 ng/mL per hour	1.0–6.5 µg/L per hour
5–10 y	0.5–5.9 ng/mL per hour	0.5–5.9 µg/L per hour
10–15 y	0.5–3.3 ng/mL per hour	0.5–3.3 µg/L per hour
Adult	0.2–1.6 ng/mL per hour	0.2–1.6 µg/L per hour
Upright, normal sodium diet		
Adult	0.7–3.3 ng/mL per hour	0.7–3.3 µg/L per hour

Values vary according to the laboratory performing the test, as well as the patient's age, gender, dietary pattern, state of hydration, posture, and physical activity.

DESCRIPTION & RATIONALE: Renin is an enzyme that activates the renin-angiotensin system. It is released into the renal veins by the juxtaglomerular apparatus in response to sodium depletion and hypovolemia. Renin converts angiotensinogen to angiotensin I. Angiotensin I is converted to angiotensin II, the biologically active form. Angiotensin II is a powerful vasoconstrictor that stimulates aldosterone production in the adrenal cortex. Angiotensin II and aldosterone increase blood pressure. Excessive amounts of angiotensin II cause renal hypertension. The renin assay screens for essential, renal, or renovascular hypertension. Plasma renin is expressed as the rate of angiotensin I formation per unit of time. The random collection of specimens without prior dietary preparations does not provide clinically significant information. Values should also be evaluated along with simultaneously collected aldosterone levels (see monographs titled "Aldosterone" and "Angiotensin-Converting Enzyme"). ∎

INDICATIONS:
- Assist in the identification of primary hyperaldosteronism resulting from aldosterone-secreting adrenal adenoma
- Assist in monitoring patients on mineralocorticoid therapy
- Assist in the screening of the origin of essential, renal, or renovascular hypertension

RESULT

Increased in:
- Addison's disease
- Bartter's syndrome
- Cirrhosis
- Congestive heart failure
- Gastrointestinal disorders with electrolyte loss
- Hepatitis
- Hypokalemia
- Malignant hypertension
- Nephritis
- Nephropathies with sodium or potassium wasting
- Pheochromocytoma
- Pregnancy
- Renin-producing renal tumors
- Renovascular hypertension

Decreased in:
- Cushing's syndrome
- Essential hypertension
- Primary hyperaldosteronism

CRITICAL VALUES: N/A

INTERFERING FACTORS:
- Drugs that may increase renin levels include albuterol, amiloride, azosemide, benazepril, bendroflumethiazide, captopril, chlorthalidone, cilazapril, cromakalim, desmopressin, diazoxide, dihydralazine, doxazosin, enalapril, endralazine, felodipine, fenoldopam, fosinopril, furosemide, hydralazine, hydrochlorothiazide, laxatives, lisinopril, lithium, methyclothiazide, metolazone, muzolimine, nicardipine, nifedipine, opiates, oral contraceptives, perindopril, ramipril, spironolactone, triamterene, and xipamide.

- Drugs and substances that may decrease renin levels include acetylsalicylic acid, angiotensin, angiotensin II, atenolol, bopindolol, bucindolol, carbenoxolone, carvedilol, clonidine, cyclosporin A, dexfenfluramine, glycyrrhiza, ibuprofen, indomethacin, levodopa, metoprolol, naproxen, nicardipine, nonsteroidal anti-inflammatory drugs, oral contraceptives, oxprenolol, propranolol, sulindac, and vasopressin.

- Upright body posture, stress, and strenuous exercise can increase renin levels.

- Recent radioactive scans or radiation can interfere with test results when radioimmunoassay is the test method.

- Diet can significantly affect results (e.g., low-sodium diets stimulate the release of renin).

- Hyperkalemia, acute increase in blood pressure, and increased blood volume may suppress renin secretion.

- Failure to follow dietary restrictions before the procedure may cause the procedure to be canceled or repeated.

Nursing Implications and Procedure

Pretest:

➤ Inform the patient that the test is used to evaluate hypertension.

➤ Obtain a history of the patient's complaints, including a list of known allergens (especially allergies or sensitivities to latex), and inform the appropriate health care practitioner accordingly.

➤ Obtain a history of the patient's endocrine and genitourinary systems, as well as results of previously performed laboratory tests, surgical procedures, and other diagnostic procedures. For related laboratory tests, refer to the Endocrine and Genitourinary System tables.

➤ Note any recent procedures that can interfere with test results.

➤ Obtain a list of the medications the patient is taking, including herbs, nutritional supplements, and nutraceuticals. The requesting health care practitioner and laboratory should be advised if the patient regularly uses these products so that their effects can be taken into consideration when reviewing results.

➤ Review the procedure with the patient. Inform the patient or family member that the position required (supine or upright) must be maintained for 2 hours before specimen collection. Inform the patient that multiple specimens may be required. Inform the patient that specimen collection takes approximately 5 to 10 minutes. Address concerns about pain related to the procedure. Explain to the patient that there may be some discomfort during the venipuncture.

➤ The patient should be on a normal sodium diet (1 to 2 g sodium per day) for 2 to 4 weeks before the test.

➤ By medical direction, the patient should avoid diuretics, antihypertensive drugs, herbals, cyclic progestogens, and estrogens for 2 to 4 weeks before the test.

▶ Prepare an ice slurry in a cup or plastic bag to have ready for immediate transport of the specimen to the laboratory.

Intratest:

▶ Ensure that the patient has complied with diet and medication restrictions and pretesting dietary preparations; assure that specific medications have been restricted for at least 2 to 4 weeks prior to the procedure.

▶ If the patient has a history of severe allergic reaction to latex, care should be taken to avoid the use of equipment containing latex.

▶ Instruct the patient to cooperate fully and to follow directions. Direct the patient to breathe normally and to avoid unnecessary movement.

▶ Observe standard precautions, and follow the general guidelines in Appendix A. Positively identify the patient, and label the appropriate tubes with the corresponding patient demographics, date, and time of collection. Specify patient position (upright or supine) and exact source of specimen (peripheral vs. arterial). Perform a venipuncture after the patient has been in the upright (sitting or standing) position for 2 hours. If a supine specimen is requested on an inpatient, the specimen should be collected early in the morning before the patient rises. Collect the specimen in a 5-mL lavender-top (EDTA) tube.

▶ Remove the needle, and apply a pressure dressing over the puncture site.

▶ The sample should be placed in an ice slurry immediately after collection. Information on the specimen label can be protected from water in the ice slurry by first placing the specimen in a protective plastic bag. Promptly transport the specimen to the laboratory for processing and analysis.

▶ The results are recorded manually or in a computerized system for recall and postprocedure interpretation by the appropriate health care practitioner.

Post-test:

▶ Observe venipuncture site for bleeding or hematoma formation. Apply paper tape or other adhesive to hold pressure bandage in place, or replace with a plastic bandage.

▶ Instruct the patient to resume usual medications, as directed by the health care practitioner.

▶ *Nutritional considerations:* Instruct the patient to notify the requesting health care practitioner of any signs and symptoms of dehydration or fluid overload related to abnormal renin levels or compromised sodium regulatory mechanisms. Fluid loss or dehydration is signaled by the thirst response. Decreased skin turgor, dry mouth, and multiple longitudinal furrows in the tongue are symptoms of dehydration. Fluid overload may be signaled by a loss of appetite and nausea. Excessive fluid also causes pitting edema: When firm pressure is placed on the skin over a bone (e.g., the ankle), the indentation will remain after 5 seconds.

▶ *Nutritional considerations:* Educate patients of the importance of proper water balance. There is no recommended daily allowance (RDA) for water. Adults need 1 mL/kcal per day; infants need more because their basal metabolic heat production is much higher. In buildings with hard water, untreated tap water contains minerals such as calcium, magnesium, and iron. Water-softening systems replace these minerals with sodium, and therefore patients on a low-sodium diet should avoid drinking treated tap water and drink bottled water instead.

▶ *Nutritional considerations:* Renin levels affect the regulation of fluid balance and electrolytes. If appropriate, educate patients with low sodium levels that the major source of dietary sodium is found in table salt. Many foods, such as milk and other dairy products, are also good sources of dietary sodium. Most other dietary sodium is available through the consumption of processed foods. Patients on low-sodium diets should be advised to avoid beverages such as colas, ginger ale, sports drinks, lemon-lime sodas, and root beer. Many over-the-counter medications, including antacids, laxatives, analgesics, sedatives, and antitussives, contain significant amounts of sodium. The best advice is to emphasize the importance of reading all food, beverage, and medicine labels. In 1989, the Subcommittee on the 10th Edition of the RDA established 500 mg as the recommended maximum daily intake for dietary intake of sodium. The requesting health care practitioner or nutritionist should be consulted before the patient on a low-sodium diet begins using salt substitutes. There are no RDAs established for potassium, but the estimated minimum intake for adults is 200 mEq/day. Potassium is present in all plant and animal cells, making dietary replacement fairly simple to achieve.

➤ A written report of the examination will be sent to the requesting health care practitioner, who will discuss the results with the patient.

➤ Reinforce information given by the patient's health care provider regarding further testing, treatment, or referral to another health care provider. Answer any questions or address any concerns voiced by the patient or family.

➤ Depending on the results of this procedure, additional testing may be performed to evaluate or monitor progression of the disease process and determine the need for a change in therapy. Evaluate test results in relation to the patient's symptoms and other tests performed.

Related laboratory tests:

➤ Related laboratory tests include aldosterone, angiotensin-converting enzyme, blood urea nitrogen, creatinine, kidney biopsy, blood and urine potassium, urine protein, blood and urine sodium, and urinalysis.

RENOGRAM

. . . .

SYNONYMS/ACRONYM: Renocystography, renocystogram, radioactive renogram, renal scintigraphy.

AREA OF APPLICATION: Kidneys.

CONTRAST: Intravenous radioactive material.

DESCRIPTION & RATIONALE: A renogram is a nuclear medicine study performed to assist in diagnosing renal disorders, such as abnormal blood flow, collecting-system defects, and excretion dysfunction. Because renography uses no iodinated contrast medium, it is safe to use in patients who have iodine allergies or compromised renal function.

After intravenous administration of the radioisotope, information about the structures of the kidneys is obtained. The radioactive material is detected by a gamma camera, which can detect the gamma rays emitted by the radionuclide in the kidney. Renography simultaneously tracks the rate at which the radionuclide flows into *(vascular phase)*, through *(tubular phase)*, and out of *(excretory phase)* the kidneys. The times are plotted on a graph and compared to normal parameters of organ function. Differential estimates of left and right kidney contributions to glomerular filtration rate and effective renal plasma flow can be calculated. With the use of diuretic stimulation during the excretory phase, it is possible to differentiate between anatomic obstruction and nonobstructive residual dilation from previous hydronephrosis. All information obtained is stored in a computer to be used for further interpretation and computations. Renal function can be monitored by serially repeating this test and comparing results. ∎

INDICATIONS:

- Aid in the diagnosis of renal artery embolism or renal infarction causing obstruction

- Aid in the diagnosis of renal artery stenosis resulting from renal dysplasia or atherosclerosis and causing arterial hypertension and reduced glomerular filtration rate

- Aid in the diagnosis of renal vein thrombosis resulting from dehydration in infants or obstruction of blood flow in the presence of renal tumors in adults

- Detect renal infectious or inflammatory diseases, such as acute or chronic pyelonephritis, renal abscess, or nephritis

- Determine the presence and effects of renal trauma, such as arterial injury, renal contusion, hematoma, rupture, arteriovenous fistula, or urinary extravasation

- Determine the presence, location, and cause of obstructive uropathy, such as calculi, neoplasm, congenital disorders, scarring, or inflammation

- Evaluate acute and chronic renal failure

- Evaluate chronic urinary tract infections, especially in children

- Evaluate kidney transplant for acute or chronic rejection

- Evaluate obstruction caused by stones or tumor

RESULT

Normal Findings:

- Normal shape, size, position, symmetry, vasculature, perfusion, and function of the kidneys

- Radionuclide material circulates bilaterally, symmetrically, and without interruption through the renal parenchyma, ureters, and urinary bladder, with 50% of the radionuclide excreted within the first 10 minutes

Abnormal Findings:

- Acute tubular necrosis

- Congenital anomalies (e.g., absence of a kidney)

- Decreased renal function

- Diminished blood supply

- Infection or inflammation (pyelonephritis, glomerulonephritis)

- Masses

- Obstructive uropathy

- Renal failure, infarction, cyst, or abscess

- Renal vascular disease, including renal artery stenosis or renal vein thrombosis

- Trauma

CRITICAL VALUES: N/A

INTERFERING FACTORS:

This procedure is contraindicated for:

- Patients who are pregnant or suspected of being pregnant, unless the potential benefits of the procedure far outweigh the risks to the fetus and mother

Factors that may impair clear imaging:

- Inability of the patient to cooperate or remain still during the procedure because of age, significant pain, or mental status

- Patients who are very obese, who may exceed the weight limit for the equipment

- Incorrect positioning of the patient, which may produce poor visualization of the area to be examined

- Serum creatinine levels greater than or equal to 3 mg/dL (depending on the radionuclide used), which can decrease renal perfusion

- Other nuclear scans done within the previous 24 to 48 hours

- Medications such as antihypertensives, angiotensin-converting enzyme (ACE) inhibitors, and β-blockers taken within 24 hours of the test, which can affect the results (depending on the reason for the study)

- Dehydration, which can accentuate abnormalities; or overhydration, which can mask abnormalities

- Metallic objects within the examination field (e.g., jewelry, body rings), which may inhibit organ visualization and can produce unclear images

Other considerations:

- Consultation with a health care practitioner should occur before the procedure for radiation safety concerns regarding younger patients or patients who are lactating.

- Risks associated with radiographic overexposure can result from frequent x-ray procedures. Personnel in the room with the patient should stand behind a shield or leave the area while the examination is being done. Personnel working in the area where the examination is being done should wear badges that reveal their level of exposure to radiation.

- Inaccurate timing of imaging after the radionuclide injection can affect the results.

Nursing Implications and Procedure • • • • • • • • • •

Pretest:

▶ Inform the patient that the procedure assesses the renal system.

▶ Obtain a history of the patient's complaints and symptoms, including a list of known allergens.

▶ Obtain a history of the patient's genitourinary system, as well as results of previously performed laboratory tests, surgical procedures, and other diagnostic procedures. For related diagnostic tests, refer to the Genitourinary System table.

▶ Record the date of the last menstrual period and determine the possibility of pregnancy in perimenopausal women.

▶ Obtain a list of the patient's current medications.

▶ Review the procedure with the patient. Address concerns about pain related to the procedure. Explain to the patient that some pain may be experienced during the test, and there may be moments of discomfort. Reassure the patient that radioactive material poses minimal radioactive hazard because of its short half-life and rarely produces side effects.

Inform the patient that the procedure is performed in a special nuclear medicine department by a technologist and usually takes approximately 60 to 90 minutes, and that delayed images are needed 2 to 24 hours later. The patient may leave the department and return later to undergo delayed imaging.

> *Sensitivity to cultural and social issues,* as well as concern for modesty, is important in providing psychological support before, during, and after the procedure.

> Instruct the patient to remove dentures, jewelry (including watches), hairpins, credit cards, and other metallic objects.

> Inform the patient that he or she will be asked to drink several glasses of fluid before the study for hydration, unless the patient has a restricted fluid intake for other reasons.

> There are no food or medication restrictions, unless by medical direction.

Intratest:

> Ensure that the patient has removed all external metallic objects (jewelry, dentures, etc.) prior to the procedure.

> Patients are given a gown, robe, and foot coverings to wear and instructed to void prior to the procedure.

> Observe standard precautions, and follow the general guidelines in Appendix A.

> Administer sedative to a child or to an uncooperative adult, as ordered.

> Place the patient in a supine position on a flat table with foam wedges to help maintain position and immobilization.

> The radionuclide is administered intravenously, and the kidney area is scanned immediately with images taken every minute for 30 minutes.

> During the flow and static imaging, the diuretic furosemide (Lasix) or ACE inhibitor (captopril) can be administered intravenously and images obtained.

> Renogram curves can be plotted concurrently with flow studies in which blood flow is imaged and recorded as it occurs.

> Urine and blood laboratory studies are done after the renogram to correlate findings before diagnosis.

> If a study for vesicoureteral reflux is done, the patient is asked to void and a catheter is placed into the bladder. The radionuclide is instilled into the bladder, and multiple images are obtained during bladder filling. The patient is then requested to void, with the catheter in place or after catheter removal, depending on department policy. Imaging is continued during and after voiding. Reflux is determined by calculating the urine volume and counts obtained by imaging.

> Wear gloves during the radionuclide administration and while handling the patient's urine.

> The results are recorded on film or in a computerized system for recall and postprocedure interpretation by the appropriate health care practitioner.

Post-test:

> Advise patient to drink increased amounts of fluids for 24 hours to eliminate the radionuclide from the body, unless contraindicated. Tell the patient that radionuclide is eliminated from the body within 6 to 24 hours.

> Instruct the patient to flush the toilet immediately after each voiding following the procedure, and to wash hands meticulously with soap and water after each voiding for 24 hours after the procedure.

> Tell all caregivers to wear gloves when discarding urine for 24 hours after the procedure. Wash gloved hands with soap and water before removing gloves. Then wash hands after the gloves are removed.

> Instruct the patient in the care and assessment of the injection site. Observe for bleeding, hematoma formation, and inflammation.

▶ A written report of the examination will be completed by a health care practitioner specializing in this branch of medicine. The report will be sent to the requesting health care practitioner, who will discuss the results with the patient.

▶ Reinforce information given by the patient's health care provider regarding further testing, treatment, or referral to another health care provider. Answer any questions or address any concerns voiced by the patient or family.

▶ Depending on the results of this pro-

cedure, additional testing may be needed to evaluate or monitor progression of the disease process and determine the need for a change in therapy. Evaluate test results in relation to the patient's symptoms and other tests performed.

Related diagnostic tests:

▶ Related diagnostic tests include computed tomography of the spine, abdomen, or pelvis; intravenous pyelography; magnetic resonance imaging of the spine, abdomen or pelvis; and ultrasound of the abdomen.

RETICULOCYTE COUNT

SYNONYM/ACRONYM: Retic count.

SPECIMEN: Whole blood (1 mL) collected in lavender-top (EDTA) tube.

REFERENCE VALUE: (Method: Microscopic examination of specially stained peripheral blood smear or automated analyzer)

Age	Total Erythrocyte Count*
Newborn	3%–7%
1–12 mo	0.2%–2.8%
Adult	1.5%–2.5%

*Values are expressed as percentage of the red blood cell count

DESCRIPTION & RATIONALE: Normally, as it matures, the red blood cell (RBC) loses its nucleus. The remaining ribonucleic acid (RNA) will produce a characteristic color when

special stains are used, making these cells easy to identify and enumerate. The presence of reticulocytes is an indication of the level of erythropoietic activity in the bone marrow. In abnormal conditions, reticulocytes are prematurely released into circulation. (See monographs titled "Red Blood Cell Count" and "Red Blood Cell Morphology and Inclusions.") ■

INDICATIONS:
• Evaluate erythropoietic activity

• Monitor response to therapy for anemias

RESULT: The reticulocyte production index (RPI) is a good estimate of RBC production. The calculation corrects the count for anemia and for the premature release of reticulocytes into the peripheral blood during periods of hemolysis or significant bleeding. The RPI also takes the maturation time of large polychromatophilic cells or nucleated RBCs seen on the peripheral smear into consideration:

RPI = % reticulocytes × [patient hematocrit (Hct)/normal Hct] × (1/maturation time)

As the formula shows, the RPI is inversely proportional to Hct, as follows:

Hematocrit (%)	Maturation Time (days)
45	1.0
35	1.5
25	2.0
15	2.5

Increased in:
- Blood loss
- Hemolytic anemias
- Iron-deficiency anemia
- Megaloblastic anemia

Decreased in:
- Alcoholism
- Anemia of chronic disease
- Aplastic anemia
- Bone marrow replacement
- Endocrine disease
- RBC aplasia
- Renal disease
- Sideroblastic anemia

CRITICAL VALUES: N/A

INTERFERING FACTORS:
- Drugs that may increase reticulocyte counts include acetanilid, acetylsalicylic acid, amyl nitrate, antimalarials, antipyretics, antipyrine, arsenicals, corticotropin, dimercaprol, furaltadone, furazolidone, levodopa, methyldopa, nitrofurans, penicillin, procainamide, and sulfones.

- Drugs that may decrease reticulocyte counts include azathioprine, dactinomycin, hydroxyurea, methotrexate, and zidovudine.

- Reticulocyte count may be falsely increased by the presence of RBC inclusions (Howell-Jolly bodies, Heinz bodies, and Pappenheimer bodies) that stain with methylene blue.

- Reticulocyte count may be falsely decreased after a recent blood transfusion, as a result of the dilutional effect.

Nursing Implications and Procedure • • • • • • • • • • •

Pretest:

➤ Inform the patient that the test is used to assess erythropoietic activity and monitor antianemic therapy.

➤ Obtain a history of the patient's complaints, including a list of known allergens (especially allergies or sensitivities to latex), and inform the appropriate health care practitioner accordingly.

➤ Obtain a history of the patient's hematopoietic system and results of previously performed laboratory tests, surgical procedures, and other diagnostic procedures. For related laboratory tests, refer to the Hematopoietic System table.

➤ Note any recent procedures that can interfere with test results.

➤ Obtain a list of the medications the patient is taking, including herbs, nutritional supplements, and nutraceuticals. The requesting health care practitioner and laboratory should be

advised if the patient regularly uses these products so that their effects can be taken into consideration when reviewing results.

➤ Review the procedure with the patient. Inform the patient that specimen collection takes approximately 5 to 10 minutes. Address concerns about pain related to the procedure. Explain to the patient that there may be some discomfort during the venipuncture.

➤ There are no food, fluid, or medication restrictions, unless by medical direction.

Intratest:

➤ If the patient has a history of severe allergic reaction to latex, care should be taken to avoid the use of equipment containing latex.

➤ Instruct the patient to cooperate fully and to follow directions. Direct the patient to breathe normally and to avoid unnecessary movement.

➤ Observe standard precautions, and follow the general guidelines in Appendix A. Positively identify the patient, and label the appropriate tubes with the corresponding patient demographics, date, and time of collection. Perform a venipuncture; collect the specimen in a 5-mL lavender-top tube.

➤ Remove the needle, and apply a pressure dressing over the puncture site.

➤ Promptly transport the specimen to the laboratory for processing and analysis.

➤ The results are recorded manually or in a computerized system for recall and postprocedure interpretation by the appropriate health care practitioner.

Post-test:

➤ Observe venipuncture site for bleeding or hematoma formation. Apply paper tape or other adhesive to hold pressure bandage in place, or replace with a plastic bandage.

➤ A written report of the examination will be sent to the requesting health care practitioner, who will discuss the results with the patient.

➤ Reinforce information given by the patient's health care provider regarding further testing, treatment, or referral to another health care provider. Answer any questions or address any concerns voiced by the patient or family.

➤ Depending on the results of this procedure, additional testing may be performed to evaluate or monitor progression of the disease process and determine the need for a change in therapy. Evaluate test results in relation to the patient's symptoms and other tests performed.

Related laboratory tests:

➤ Related laboratory tests include biopsy of bone marrow, complete blood count, and RBC morphology and inclusions.

RETROGRADE URETEROPYELOGRAPHY

SYNONYM/ACRONYM: Retrograde.

AREA OF APPLICATION: Renal calyces, ureter.

CONTRAST: Radiopaque iodine-based contrast medium.

DESCRIPTION & RATIONALE: Retrograde ureteropyelography uses a contrast medium introduced through a ureteral catheter during cystography and radiographic visualization to view the renal collecting system (calyces, renal pelvis, and urethra). During a cystoscopic examination, a catheter is advanced through the ureters and into the kidney; contrast medium is injected through the catheter into the kidney. This procedure is primarily used in patients who are known to be hypersensitive to intravenously injected iodine-based contrast medium and when excretory ureterography does not adequately reveal the renal collecting system. The incidence of allergic reaction to the contrast medium is reduced because there is less systemic absorption of the contrast medium when injected into the kidney than when injected intravenously. Retrograde ureteropyelography sometimes provides more information about the anatomy of the different parts of the collecting system than can be obtained by excretory ureteropyelography. The procedure is not hampered by impaired renal function, but it carries the risk of urinary tract infection and sepsis. ∎

INDICATIONS:

- Evaluate the effects of urinary system trauma
- Evaluate known or suspected ureteral obstruction
- Evaluate placement of a ureteral stent or catheter
- Evaluate the presence of calculi in the kidneys, ureters, or bladder
- Evaluate the renal collecting system when excretory urography is unsuccessful
- Evaluate space-occupying lesions or congenital anomalies of the urinary system
- Evaluate the structure and integrity of the renal collecting system

RESULT

Normal Findings:

- Normal outline and opacification of renal pelvis and calyces
- Normal size and uniform filling of the ureters

- Symmetrical and bilateral outline of structures

Abnormal Findings:
- Congenital renal or urinary tract abnormalities
- Hydronephrosis
- Neoplasms
- Obstruction as a result of tumor, blood clot, stricture, or calculi
- Obstruction of ureteropelvic junction
- Perinephric abscess
- Perinephric inflammation or suppuration
- Polycystic kidney disease
- Prostatic enlargement
- Tumor of the kidneys or the collecting system

CRITICAL VALUES: N/A

INTERFERING FACTORS:

This procedure is contraindicated for:
- ⚠ Patients with allergies to shellfish or iodinated dye. The contrast medium used may cause a life-threatening allergic reaction. Patients with a known hypersensitivity to the contrast medium may benefit from premedication with corticosteroids or the use of nonionic contrast medium.
- Patients who are pregnant or suspected of being pregnant, unless the potential benefits of the procedure far outweigh the risks to the fetus and mother
- ⚠ Elderly and other patients who are chronically dehydrated before the test, because of their risk of contrast-induced renal failure.
- ⚠ Patients who are in renal failure.
- ⚠ Patients with renal insufficiency, indicated by a blood urea nitro-

gen value greater than 40 mg/dL, because contrast medium can complicate kidney function.
- Young patients (17 years old and younger), unless the benefits of the x-ray diagnosis outweigh the risks of exposure to high levels of radiation.
- Patients with multiple myeloma, who may experience decreased kidney function subsequent to administration of contrast medium.

Factors that may impair clear imaging:
- Gas or feces in the gastrointestinal tract resulting from inadequate cleansing or failure to restrict food intake before the study
- Retained barium from a previous radiologic procedure
- Metallic objects within the examination field (e.g., jewelry, body rings), which may inhibit organ visualization and can produce unclear images
- Improper adjustment of the radiographic equipment to accommodate obese or thin patients, which can cause overexposure or underexposure and a poor-quality study
- Patients who are very obese, who may exceed the weight limit for the equipment
- Incorrect positioning of the patient, which may produce poor visualization of the area to be examined
- Inability of the patient to cooperate or remain still during the procedure because of age, significant pain, or mental status

Other considerations:
- Consultation with a health care practitioner should occur before the procedure for radiation safety concerns regarding younger patients or patients who are lactating.

- Risks associated with radiographic overexposure can result from frequent x-ray procedures. Personnel in the room with the patient should wear a protective lead apron, stand behind a shield, or leave the area while the examination is being done. Personnel working in the area where the examination is being done should wear badges that reveal their level of exposure to radiation.

- Failure to follow dietary restrictions and other pretesting preparations may cause the procedure to be canceled or repeated.

Nursing Implications and Procedure • • • • • • • • • • •

Pretest:

▶ Inform the patient that the procedure assesses the renal collecting system.

▶ Obtain a history of the patient's complaints or symptoms, including a list of known allergens (especially allergies or sensitivities to latex, iodine, seafood, contrast medium, anesthetics, and dyes), and inform the appropriate health care practitioner accordingly.

▶ Obtain a history of the patient's gastrointestinal and genitourinary systems, as well as results of previously performed laboratory tests, surgical procedures, and other diagnostic procedures. For related diagnostic tests, refer to the Gastrointestinal and Genitourinary Systems tables.

▶ Note any recent procedures that can interfere with test results, including examinations using barium.

▶ Record the date of the last menstrual period and determine the possibility of pregnancy in perimenopausal women.

▶ Obtain a list of the medications the patient is taking, including anticoagulant therapy, aspirin and other salicylates, herbs, nutritional supplements, and nutraceuticals, especially those known to affect coagulation (see Appendix F). It is recommended that use be discontinued 14 days before surgical procedures. The requesting health care practitioner and laboratory should be advised if the patient regularly uses these products so that their effects can be taken into consideration when reviewing results.

▶ Review the procedure with the patient. Address concerns about pain related to the procedure. Explain to the patient that some pain may be experienced during the test, or there may be moments of discomfort. Reassure the patient that the radionuclide poses no radioactive hazard and rarely produces side effects. Inform the patient that the procedure is performed in a special department, usually in a radiology or vascular suite, by a health care provider and support staff, and takes approximately 30 to 60 minutes.

▶ Explain that an intravenous (IV) line may be inserted to allow infusion of IV fluids, contrast medium, dye, or sedatives. Usually normal saline is infused.

▶ Inform the patient that if a local anesthetic is used, the patient may feel (1) some pressure in the kidney area as the catheter is introduced and contrast medium injected, or (2) the urgency to void.

▶ *Sensitivity to social and cultural issues,* as well as concern for modesty, is important in providing psychological support before, during, and after the procedure.

▶ The patient should fast and restrict fluids for 8 hours prior to the procedure. Instruct the patient to avoid taking anticoagulant medication or to reduce dosage as ordered prior to the procedure.

▶ Patients receiving metformin (Glucophage) for non–insulin-dependent (type 2) diabetes should discontinue the drug on the day of the test and continue to withhold it for 48 hours after the test. Failure to do so may result in lactic acidosis.

➤ Instruct the patient to remove dentures, jewelry (including watches), hairpins, credit cards, and other metallic objects in the area to be examined.

➤ Inform the patient that he or she may receive a laxative the night before the test, an enema, or a cathartic the morning of the test, as ordered.

➤ *Make sure a written and informed consent has been signed prior to the procedure and before administering any medications.*

➤ This procedure may be terminated if chest pain, severe cardiac arrhythmias, or signs of a cerebrovascular accident occur.

Intratest:

➤ Ensure that the patient has complied with dietary, fluids, and medication restrictions and pretesting preparations for at least 8 hours prior to the procedure. Ensure the patient has removed all external metallic objects (jewelry, dentures, etc.) prior to the procedure.

➤ Have emergency equipment readily available.

➤ If the patient has a history of severe allergic reactions to any substance or drug, administer ordered prophylactic steroids or antihistamines before the procedure. Use nonionic contrast medium for the procedure.

➤ Patients are given a gown, robe, and foot coverings to wear and instructed to void prior to the procedure.

➤ Instruct the patient to cooperate fully and to follow directions. Instruct the patient to remain still throughout the procedure because movement produces unreliable results.

➤ Record baseline vital signs and assess neurologic status. Protocols may vary from facility to facility.

➤ Observe standard precautions, and follow the general guidelines in Appendix A.

➤ Establish an IV fluid line for the injection of emergency drugs and of sedatives.

➤ Administer an antianxiety agent, as ordered, if the patient has claustrophobia. Administer a sedative to a child or to an uncooperative adult, as ordered.

➤ Place electrocardiographic electrodes on the patient for cardiac monitoring. Establish baseline rhythm; determine if the patient has ventricular arrhythmias.

➤ Place patient on the table in a supine position in the lithotomy position.

➤ A kidney, ureter, and bladder (KUB) or plain film is taken to ensure that no barium or stool will obscure visualization of the urinary system. The patient may be asked to hold his or her breath to facilitate visualization.

➤ The patient is given a local anesthetic, and a cystoscopic examination is performed and the bladder is inspected.

➤ A catheter is inserted, and the renal pelvis is emptied by gravity. Contrast medium is introduced into the catheter. Inform the patient that the contrast medium may cause a temporary flushing of the face, a feeling of warmth, or nausea.

➤ X-ray exposures are made and the results processed. Inform the patient that additional views may be necessary to visualize the area in question.

➤ Additional contrast medium is injected through the catheter to outline the ureters as the catheter is withdrawn.

➤ Additional x-ray exposures are taken 10 to 15 minutes after the catheter is removed to evaluate retention of the contrast medium, indicating urinary stasis.

➤ The results are recorded manually, on film, or by automated equipment in a computerized system for recall and postprocedure interpretation by the appropriate health care practitioner.

➤ The catheter may be kept in place and attached to a gravity drainage unit until urinary flow has returned or is corrected.

Post-test:

➤ Instruct the patient to resume usual diet, fluids, medications, or activity, as directed by the health care practitioner. Renal function should be assessed before metformin is resumed.

➤ Monitor vital signs and neurologic status every 15 minutes for 1 hour, then every 2 hours for 4 hours, and then as ordered by the health care practitioner. Take temperature every 4 hours for 24 hours. Compare with baseline values. Notify the health care practitioner if temperature is elevated. Protocols may vary from facility to facility.

➤ Observe for delayed allergic reactions, such as rash, urticaria, tachycardia, hyperpnea, hypertension, palpitations, nausea, or vomiting.

➤ Advise the patient to immediately report symptoms such as fast heart rate, difficulty breathing, skin rash, itching, or decreased urinary output.

➤ Observe the needle/catheter insertion site for bleeding, inflammation, or hematoma formation.

➤ Instruct the patient to apply cold compresses to the puncture site, as needed, to reduce discomfort or edema.

➤ Monitor for signs of sepsis and severe pain in the kidney area.

➤ Maintain the patient on adequate hydration after the procedure. Encourage the patient to drink lots of fluids to prevent stasis and to prevent the buildup of bacteria.

➤ *Nutritional considerations:* A low-fat, low-cholesterol, and low-sodium diet should be consumed to reduce current disease processes and/or decrease risk of hypertension and coronary artery disease.

➤ A written report of the examination will be completed by a health care practitioner specializing in this branch of medicine. The report will be sent to the requesting health care practitioner, who will discuss the results with the patient.

➤ Recognize anxiety related to test results, and be supportive of perceived loss of independent function. Discuss the implications of abnormal test results on the patient's lifestyle. Provide teaching and information regarding the clinical implications of the test results, as appropriate.

➤ Reinforce information given by the patient's health care provider regarding further testing, treatment, or referral to another health care provider. Answer any questions or address any concerns voiced by the patient or family.

➤ Instruct the patient in the use of any ordered medications. Explain the importance of adhering to the therapy regimen. As appropriate, instruct the patient in significant side effects and systemic reactions associated with the prescribed medication. Encourage him or her to review corresponding literature provided by a pharmacist.

➤ Depending on the results of this procedure, additional testing may be needed to evaluate or monitor progression of the disease process and determine the need for a change in therapy. Evaluate test results in relation to the patient's symptoms and other tests performed.

Related diagnostic tests:

➤ Related diagnostic tests include computed tomography of the abdomen, magnetic resonance imaging of the abdomen, renogram, and ultrasound of the kidney.

RHEUMATOID FACTOR

SYNONYMS/ACRONYMS: RF, RA.

SPECIMEN: Serum (1 mL) collected in a red-top tube

REFERENCE VALUE: (Method: Nephelometry) 0 to 20 IU/mL.

DESCRIPTION & RATIONALE: Individuals with rheumatoid arthritis harbor a macroglobulin-type antibody called *rheumatoid factor (RF)* in their blood. Patients with other diseases (e.g., systemic lupus erythematosus [SLE] and occasionally tuberculosis, chronic hepatitis, infectious mononucleosis, and subacute bacterial endocarditis) may also test positive for RF. RF antibodies are usually immunoglobulin (Ig) M but may also be IgG or IgA. ∎

INDICATIONS: Assist in the diagnosis of rheumatoid arthritis, especially when clinical diagnosis is difficult

RESULT

Increased in:
- Chronic hepatitis
- Chronic viral infections
- Cirrhosis
- Dermatomyositis
- Infectious mononucleosis
- Leishmaniasis
- Leprosy
- Malaria
- Rheumatoid arthritis
- Sarcoidosis
- Scleroderma
- Sjögren's syndrome
- SLE
- Syphilis
- Tuberculosis
- Waldenström's macroglobulinemia

Decreased in: N/A

CRITICAL VALUES: N/A

INTERFERING FACTORS:
- Older patients may have higher values.

- Recent blood transfusion, multiple vaccinations or transfusions, or an inadequately activated complement may affect results.

- Serum with cryoglobulin or high lipid levels may cause a false-positive test and may require that the test be repeated after a fat-restriction diet.

Nursing Implications and Procedure

Pretest:

▶ Inform the patient that the test is used to assist in the differential diagnosis and prognosis of arthritic diseases.

> Obtain a history of the patient's complaints, including a list of known allergens (especially allergies or sensitivities to latex), and inform the appropriate health care practitioner accordingly.

> Obtain a history of the patient's immune and musculoskeletal systems, as well as results of previously performed laboratory tests, surgical procedures, and other diagnostic procedures. For related laboratory tests, refer to the Immune and Musculoskeletal System tables.

> Obtain a list of the medications the patient is taking, including herbs, nutritional supplements, and nutraceuticals. The requesting health care practitioner and laboratory should be advised if the patient regularly uses these products so that their effects can be taken into consideration when reviewing results.

> Review the procedure with the patient. Inform the patient that specimen collection takes approximately 5 to 10 minutes. Address concerns about pain related to the procedure. Explain to the patient that there may be some discomfort during the venipuncture.

> There are no food, fluid, or medication restrictions, unless by medical direction.

Intratest:

> If the patient has a history of severe allergic reaction to latex, care should be taken to avoid the use of equipment containing latex.

> Instruct the patient to cooperate fully and to follow directions. Direct the patient to breathe normally and to avoid unnecessary movement.

> Observe standard precautions, and follow the general guidelines in Appendix A. Positively identify the patient, and label the appropriate tubes with the corresponding patient demographics, date, and time of collection. Perform a venipuncture; collect the specimen in a 5-mL red-top tube.

> Remove the needle, and apply a pressure dressing over the puncture site.

> Promptly transport the specimen to the laboratory for processing and analysis.

> The results are recorded manually or in a computerized system for recall and postprocedure interpretation by the appropriate health care practitioner.

Post-test:

> Observe venipuncture site for bleeding or hematoma formation. Apply paper tape or other adhesive to hold pressure bandage in place, or replace with a plastic bandage.

> A written report of the examination will be sent to the requesting health care practitioner, who will discuss the results with the patient.

> Recognize anxiety related to test results, and be supportive of impaired activity related to anticipated chronic pain resulting from joint inflammation, impairment in mobility, musculoskeletal deformity, and loss of independence. Discuss the implications of abnormal test results on the patient's lifestyle. Provide teaching and information regarding the clinical implications of the test results, as appropriate. Educate the patient regarding access to counseling services, as appropriate. Provide contact information, if desired, for the Arthritis Foundation *(http://www. arthritis.org)*.

> Reinforce information given by the patient's health care provider regarding further testing, treatment, or referral to another health care provider. Advise the patient, as appropriate, that additional studies may be undertaken to determine treatment regimen or to determine the possible causes of symptoms if the test is negative for rheumatoid arthritis. Answer any questions or address any concerns voiced by the patient or family.

> Depending on the results of this procedure, additional testing may be

performed to evaluate or monitor progression of the disease process and determine the need for a change in therapy. Evaluate test results in relation to the patient's symptoms and other tests performed.

RUBELLA ANTIBODIES

SYNONYM/ACRONYM: German measles serology.

SPECIMEN: Serum (1 mL) collected in a red-top tube.

REFERENCE VALUE: (Method: Indirect immunofluorescence) Immune or less than a fourfold increase in titer.

DESCRIPTION & RATIONALE: Rubella, commonly known as German measles, is a communicable viral disease transmitted by contact with respiratory secretions and aerosolized droplets of the secretions. The incubation period is 14 to 21 days. This disease produces a pink, macular rash that disappears in 2 to 3 days. Rubella infection induces immunoglobulin (Ig) G and IgM antibody production. This test can determine current infection or immunity from past infection. Rubella serology is part of the TORCH (*to*xoplasmosis, *ru*bella, *cy*tomegalovirus, and *h*erpes simplex type 2) panel routinely performed on pregnant women. Fetal infection during the first trimester can cause spontaneous abortion or congenital defects. Ideally the immune status of women of childbearing age should be ascertained before pregnancy, when vaccination can be administered to provide lifelong immunity. The presence of IgM antibodies indicates acute infection. The presence of IgG antibodies indicates current or past infection. Susceptibility to rubella is indicated by a negative reaction. Many laboratories use a qualitative assay that detects the presence of both IgM and IgG rubella antibodies. IgM- and IgG-specific enzyme immunoassays are also available to help distinguish acute infection from immune status. A rise in titer greater than fourfold in paired specimens is an indication of current infection. ■

INDICATIONS:
• Assist in the diagnosis of rubella infection

• Determine presence of rubella antibodies

• Determine susceptibility to rubella, particularly in pregnant women

• Perform as part of routine prenatal serologic testing

RESULT

Positive findings in: Rubella
infection (past or present)

CRITICAL VALUES:
Note and immediately report to the
health care practitioner patients with a
rubella-nonimmune status.

INTERFERING FACTORS: N/A

Nursing Implications and
Procedure • • • • • • • • • • •

Pretest:

➤ Inform the patient that the test is
used to identify rubella infection or
immunity.

➤ Obtain a history of the patient's
complaints, including a list of known
allergens (especially allergies or sensitivities to latex), and inform the
appropriate health care practitioner
accordingly.

➤ Obtain a history of exposure to
rubella.

➤ Obtain a history of the patient's
immune and reproductive systems,
as well as results of previously performed laboratory tests, surgical
procedures, and other diagnostic procedures. For related laboratory tests, refer to the Immune and
Reproductive System tables.

➤ Obtain a list of the medications the
patient is taking, including herbs,
nutritional supplements, and nutraceuticals. The requesting health care
practitioner and laboratory should be
advised if the patient regularly uses
these products so that their effects
can be taken into consideration
when reviewing results.

➤ Review the procedure with the
patient. Inform the patient that several tests may be necessary to
confirm diagnosis. Any individual
positive result should be repeated in
7 to 14 days to monitor a change in
titer. Inform the patient that specimen collection takes approximately

5 to 10 minutes. Address concerns
about pain related to the procedure.
Explain to the patient that there may
be some discomfort during the
venipuncture.

➤ *Sensitivity to social and cultural
issues,* as well as concern for modesty, is important in providing psychological support before, during,
and after the procedure.

➤ There are no food, fluid, or medication restrictions, unless by medical
direction.

Intratest:

➤ If the patient has a history of severe
allergic reaction to latex, care should
be taken to avoid the use of equipment containing latex.

➤ Instruct the patient to cooperate fully
and to follow directions. Direct the
patient to breathe normally and to
avoid unnecessary movement.

➤ Observe standard precautions, and
follow the general guidelines in
Appendix A. Positively identify the
patient, and label the appropriate
tubes with the corresponding patient demographics, date, and time
of collection. Perform a venipuncture; collect the specimen in a 5-mL
red-top tube.

➤ Remove the needle, and apply a pressure dressing over the puncture site.

➤ Promptly transport the specimen to
the laboratory for processing and
analysis.

➤ The results are recorded manually
or in a computerized system for
recall and postprocedure interpretation by the appropriate health care
practitioner.

Post-test:

➤ Observe venipuncture site for bleeding or hematoma formation. Apply
paper tape or other adhesive to hold
pressure bandage in place, or replace with a plastic bandage.

➤ *Vaccination considerations:* Record
the date of the last menstrual period
and determine the possibility of
pregnancy prior to administration of
rubella vaccine to female rubella-

nonimmune patients. Instruct patient not to become pregnant for 1 month after being vaccinated with the rubella vaccine to protect any fetus from contracting the disease and having serious birth defects. Instruct on birth control methods to prevent pregnancy, if appropriate. Delay rubella vaccination in pregnancy until after childbirth, and give immediately prior to discharge from the hospital.

➤ A written report of the examination will be sent to the requesting health care practitioner, who will discuss the results with the patient.

➤ Recognize anxiety related to test results, and provide emotional support if results are positive and the patient is pregnant. Encourage the family to seek counseling if concerned with pregnancy termination. Provide teaching and information regarding the clinical implications of the test results, as appropriate. Decisions regarding elective abortion should take place in the presence of both parents. Provide a nonjudgmental, nonthreatening atmosphere for discussing the risks and difficulties of delivering and raising a develop-

mentally challenged infant, as well as exploring other options (e.g., termination of pregnancy or adoption). Educate the patient regarding access to counseling services, as appropriate.

➤ Reinforce information given by the patient's health care provider regarding further testing, treatment, or referral to another health care provider. Instruct the patient in isolation precautions during time of communicability or contagion. Emphasize the need to return to have a convalescent blood sample taken in 7 to 14 days. Answer any questions or address any concerns voiced by the patient or family.

➤ Depending on the results of this procedure, additional testing may be performed to evaluate or monitor progression of the disease process and determine the need for a change in therapy. Evaluate test results in relation to the patient's symptoms and other tests performed.

Related laboratory tests:

➤ Related laboratory tests include cytomegalovirus, and *Toxoplasma*.

RUBEOLA ANTIBODIES

· ·

SYNONYM/ACRONYM: Measles serology.

SPECIMEN: Serum (1 mL) collected in a red-top tube.

REFERENCE VALUE: (Method: Indirect immunofluorescence) Negative or less than a fourfold increase in titer.

DESCRIPTION & RATIONALE: Measles is caused by a single-stranded ribonucleic acid (RNA) paramyxovirus that

invades the respiratory tract and lymphoreticular tissues. It is transmitted by respiratory secretions and aerosolized droplets of the secretions. The incubation period is 10 to 11 days. Symptoms initially include conjunctivitis, cough, and fever. Koplik's spots develop 4 to 5 days later, followed by papular eruptions, body rash, and lymphadenopathy. The presence of immunoglobulin (Ig) M antibodies indicates acute infection. The presence of IgG antibodies indicates current or past infection. Susceptibility to measles is indicated by a negative reaction. Many laboratories use a qualitative assay that detects the presence of both IgM and IgG rubeola antibodies. IgM- and IgG-specific enzyme immunoassays are also available to help distinguish acute infection from immune status. A rise in titer greater than fourfold in paired specimens is an indication of current infection. ■

INDICATIONS:

• Determine resistance to or protection against measles virus

• Differential diagnosis of viral infection, especially in pregnant women with a history of exposure to measles

RESULT

Positive findings in:
Measles infection

CRITICAL VALUES: N/A

INTERFERING FACTORS: N/A

Nursing Implications and Procedure • • • • • • • • • •

Pretest:

▶ Inform the patient that the test is used to identify rubeola infection or immunity.

▶ Obtain a history of the patient's complaints, including a list of known allergens (especially allergies or sensitivities to latex), and inform the appropriate health care practitioner accordingly.

▶ Obtain a history of exposure to measles.

▶ Obtain a history of the patient's immune and reproductive systems, as well as results of previously performed laboratory tests, surgical procedures, and other diagnostic procedures. For related laboratory tests, refer to the Immune and Reproductive System tables.

▶ Obtain a list of the medications the patient is taking, including herbs, nutritional supplements, and nutraceuticals. The requesting health care practitioner and laboratory should be advised if the patient regularly uses these products so that their effects can be taken into consideration when reviewing results.

▶ Review the procedure with the patient. Inform the patient that several tests may be necessary to confirm the diagnosis. Any individual positive result should be repeated in 7 to 14 days to monitor a change in titer. Inform the patient that specimen collection takes approximately 5 to 10 minutes. Address concerns about pain related to the procedure. Explain to the patient that there may be some discomfort during the venipuncture.

▶ There are no food, fluid, or medication restrictions, unless by medical direction.

Intratest:

▶ If the patient has a history of severe allergic reaction to latex, care should be taken to avoid the use of equipment containing latex.

▶ Instruct the patient to cooperate fully and to follow directions. Direct the patient to breathe normally and to avoid unnecessary movement.

▶ Observe standard precautions, and follow the general guidelines in Appendix A. Positively identify the patient, and label the appropriate tubes with the corresponding patient demographics, date, and time of collection. Perform a venipuncture; collect the specimen in a 5-mL red-top tube.

➤ Remove the needle, and apply a pressure dressing over the puncture site.

➤ Promptly transport the specimen to the laboratory for processing and analysis.

➤ The results are recorded manually or in a computerized system for recall and postprocedure interpretation by the appropriate health care practitioner.

Post-test:

➤ Observe venipuncture site for bleeding or hematoma formation. Apply paper tape or other adhesive to hold pressure bandage in place, or replace with a plastic bandage.

➤ A written report of the examination will be sent to the requesting health care practitioner, who will discuss the results with the patient.

➤ Reinforce information given by the patient's health care provider regarding further testing, treatment, or referral to another health care provider. Instruct the patient in isolation precautions during time of communicability or contagion. Emphasize the need to return to have a convalescent blood sample taken in 7 to 14 days. Answer any questions or address any concerns voiced by the patient or family.

➤ Depending on the results of this procedure, additional testing may be performed to evaluate or monitor progression of the disease process and determine the need for a change in therapy. Evaluate test results in relation to the patient's symptoms and other tests performed.

Related laboratory tests:

➤ Related laboratory tests include rubella and varicella.

SCHIRMER TEAR TEST

· ·

SYNONYMS/ACRONYMS: N/A.

AREA OF APPLICATION: Eyelids.

CONTRAST: N/A.

DESCRIPTION & RATIONALE: The tear film, secreted by the lacrimal, Krause, and Wolfring glands, covers the surface of the eye. Blinking spreads tears over the eye and moves them toward an opening in the lower eyelid known as the punctum. Tears drain through the punctum into the nasolacrimal duct and into the nose. The Schirmer tear test simultaneously tests both eyes to assess lacrimal gland function by determining the amount of moisture accumulated on standardized filter paper or strips, held against the conjuctial sac of each eye. The Schirmer test measures both reflex and basic secretion of tears. The Schirmer test number two measures basic tear secretion and is used to evaluate the accessory glands of Krause and Wolfring. The test is performed by instilling a topical anesthetic before insertion of filter paper. The topical anesthetic inhibits reflex tearing of major lacrimal glands produced by the filter paper, allowing testing of the accessory glands. ∎

INDICATIONS:
- Assess adequacy of tearing for contact lens comfort
- Assess suspected tearing deficiency

RESULT

Normal Findings:
- 10 mm of moisture on test strip after 5 minutes. It may be slightly less than 10 mm in elderly patients.

Abnormal Findings:
- Tearing deficiency related to aging, dry eye syndrome, or Sjögren syndrome
- Tearing deficiency secondary to leukemia, lymphoma, or rheumatoid arthritis

CRITICAL VALUES: N/A

INTERFERING FACTORS:

Factors that may impair the results of the examination:
- Inability of the patient to remain still and cooperative during the test may interfere with the test results.
- Rubbing or squeezing the eyes may affect results.

Nursing Implications and Procedure • • • • • • • • • • •

Pretest: ▮

➤ Inform the patient that the procedure measures the secretion of tears.

➤ Obtain a history of the patient's complaints, including a list of known allergens, especially topical anesthetic eyedrops.

➤ Obtain a history of the patient's known or suspected vision loss, changes in visual acuity, including type and cause; use of glasses or contact lenses; eye conditions with treatment regimens; eye surgery; and other tests and procedures to assess and diagnose visual deficit. For related diagnostic tests, refer to the table of tests associated with the Ocular System.

➤ Obtain a history of results of previously performed laboratory tests, surgical procedures, and other diagnostic procedures.

➤ Obtain a list of the medications the patient is taking, including herbs, nutritional supplements, and nutraceuticals. The requesting health care practitioner should be advised if the patient regularly uses these products so that their effects can be taken into consideration when reviewing results.

➤ Instruct the patient to remove contact lenses or glasses, as appropriate. Instruct the patient regarding the importance of keeping the eyes open for the test.

➤ Review the procedure with the patient. Instruct the patient regarding the importance of keeping the eyes open for the test. Address concerns about pain related to the procedure. Explain to the patient that no pain will be experienced during the test, but there may be moments of discomfort. Explain to the patient that some discomfort may be experienced after the test when the numbness wears off from anesthetic drops adminstered prior to the test. Inform the patient hat the test is performed by a physician or optometrist and takes about 15 minutes to complete.

➤ There are no food, fluid, or medication restrictions, unless by medical direction.

Intratest:

➤ Instruct the patient to cooperate fully and to follow directions. Ask the patient to remain still during the procedure because movement produces unreliable results.

➤ Observe standard precautions, and follow the general guidelines in Appendix A.

➤ Seat the patient comfortably. Instruct the patient to look straight ahead, keeping the eyes open and unblinking.

➤ Instill topical anesthetic in each eye, as ordered, and provide time for it to work. Topical anesthetic drops are placed in the eye with the patient looking up and the solution directed at the six o'clock position of the sclera (white of the eye) near the limbus (grey, semitransparent area of the eyeball where the cornea and sclera meet). The dropper bottle should not touch the eyelashes. Insert a test strip in each eye. The strip should be folded over the midportion of both lower eyelids.

➤ The results are recorded manually for recall and postprocedure interpretation by the appropriate health care practitioner.

Post-test:

➤ Assess for corneal abraision caused by patient rubbing the eye before topical anesthetic has worn off.

➤ Instruct the patient to avoid rubbing the eyes for 30 minutes after the procedure.

➤ Instruct the patient not to reinsert contact lenses, if appropriate, for 2 hours.

➤ A written report of the examination will be completed by a health care practitioner specializing in this branch of medicine. The report will be sent to the requesting health care practitioner, who will discuss the results with the patient.

➤ Recognize anxiety related to test results, and be supportive of pain related to decreased lacrimation or inflammation. Discuss the implications of abnormal test results on the patient's lifestyle. Provide teaching and information regarding the clinical implications of the test results, as appropriate.

➤ Reinforce information given by the patient's health care provider regarding further testing, treatment, or referral to another health care provider. Answer any questions or address any concerns voiced by the patient or family.

➤ Instruct the patient in the use of any ordered medications. Explain the importance of adhering to the therapy regimen. As appropriate, instruct the patient in significant side effects and systemic reactions associated with the prescribed medication. Encourage him or her to review corresponding literature provided by a pharmacist.

➤ Depending on the results of this procedure, additional testing may be performed to evaluate or monitor progression of the disease process and determine the need for a change in therapy. Evaluate test results in relation to the patient's symptoms and other tests performed.

Related diagnostic tests:

➤ A related diagnostic test is slit-lamp biomicroscopy.

SEMEN ANALYSIS

SYNONYM/ACRONYM: N/A.

SPECIMEN: Semen from ejaculate specimen collected in a clean, dry, glass container known to be free of detergent. The specimen container should be kept at body temperature (37°C) during transportation.

REFERENCE VALUE: (Method: Macroscopic and microscopic examination)

Volume	2–5 mL
Color	White or opaque
Appearance	Viscous (pours in droplets, not clumps or strings)
Clotting and liquefaction	Complete in 20–30 minutes
pH	7.5–8.5
Sperm count	20–200 million/mL
Motility	At least 60%
Morphology	At least 70% normal oval-headed forms

DESCRIPTION & RATIONALE: Semen analysis is a valid measure of overall male fertility. Semen contains a combination of elements produced by various parts of the male reproductive system. Spermatozoa are produced in the testes and account for only a small volume of seminal fluid. Fructose and other nutrients are provided by fluid produced in the seminal vesicles. The prostate gland provides acid phosphatase and other enzymes required for coagulation and liquefaction of semen. Sperm motility depends on the presence of a sufficient level of ionized calcium. If the specimen has an abnormal appearance (e.g., bloody, oddly colored, turbid), the patient may have an infection. Specimens can be tested with a leukocyte esterase strip to detect the presence of white blood cells. ■

INDICATIONS:
- Assist in the diagnosis of azoospermia and oligospermia
- Evaluate infertility
- Evaluate vasectomy effectiveness
- Evaluate the effectiveness of vasectomy reversal
- Support or disprove sterility in paternity suit

RESULT: There is marked intraindividual variation in sperm count. Indications of suboptimal fertility should be investigated by serial analysis of two to three samples collected over several months. If abnormal results are obtained, additional testing may be requested.

Abnormality	Test Ordered	Normal Result
Decreased count	Fructose	Present (greater than 150 mg/dL)
Decreased motility with clumping	Male antisperm antibodies	Absent
Normal semen analysis with infertility	Female antisperm antibodies	Absent

Increased in: N/A

Decreased in:

- Hyperpyrexia
- Obstruction of ejaculatory system
- Orchitis
- Postvasectomy period
- Primary and secondary testicular failure
- Testicular atrophy (e.g., recovery from mumps)
- Varicocele

CRITICAL VALUES: N/A

INTERFERING FACTORS:

- Drugs and substances that may decrease sperm count include arsenic, azathioprine, cannabis, cimetidine, cocaine, cyclophosphamide, estrogens, fluoxymesterone, ketoconazole, lead, methotrexate, methyltestosterone, nitrofurantoin, nitrogen mustard, procarbazine, sulfasalazine, and vincristine.

- Testicular radiation may decrease sperm counts.

- Cigarette smoking is associated with decreased production of semen.

- Caffeine consumption is associated with increased sperm density and number of abnormal forms.

- Delays in transporting the specimen and failure to keep the specimen warm during transportation are the most common reasons for specimen rejection.

Nursing Implications and Procedure

Pretest:

➤ Inform the patient that the test is used to assist in the diagnosis of male infertility.

➤ Obtain a history of the patient's complaints, including a list of known allergens, and inform the appropriate health care practitioner accordingly.

➤ Obtain a history of the patient's immune and reproductive system and results of previously performed laboratory tests, surgical procedures, and other diagnostic procedures. For related laboratory tests, refer to the Immune and Reproductive System tables.

➤ Obtain a list of medications the patient is taking, including herbs, nutritional supplements, and nutraceuticals. The requesting health care practitioner and laboratory should be advised if the patient regularly uses these products so that their effects can be taken into consideration when reviewing results.

➤ Note any recent procedures that can interfere with test results.

➤ Review the procedure with the patient. Instruct the patient to refrain from any sexual activity for 3 days before specimen collection. Instruct the patient to bring the specimen to the laboratory within 30 to 60 minutes of collection and to keep the specimen warm (close to body temperature) during transportation. The requesting health care practitioner usually provides the patient with instructions for specimen collection. Address concerns about pain related to the procedure. Explain to the patient that there should be no discomfort during the procedure.

➤ *Sensitivity to social and cultural issues*, as well as concern for modesty, is important in providing psychological support before, during, and after the procedure.

➤ There are no food, fluid, or medication restrictions, unless by medical direction.

Intratest:

➤ Instruct the patient to cooperate fully and to follow directions.

➤ Observe standard precautions, and follow the general guidelines in Appendix A. Positively identify the patient, and label the appropriate collection container with the corresponding patient demographics, date, and time of collection.

Ejaculated specimen:

➤ Ideally, the specimen is obtained by masturbation in a private location close to the laboratory. In cases in which the patient expresses psychological or religious concerns about masturbation, the specimen can be obtained during coitus interruptus, through the use of a condom, or through postcoital collection of samples from the cervical canal and vagina of the patient's sexual partner. The patient should be warned about the possible loss of the sperm-rich portion of the sample if coitus interruptus is the collection approach. If a condom is used, the patient must be carefully instructed to wash and dry the condom completely before use to prevent contamination of the specimen with spermicides.

Cervical vaginal specimen:

➤ Assist the patient to the lithotomy position on the examination table. A speculum is inserted, and the specimen is obtained by direct smear or aspiration of saline lavage.

Specimens collected from skin or clothing:

➤ Dried semen may be collected by sponging the skin with a gauze soaked in saline or soaking the material in a saline solution.

General:

➤ Promptly transport the specimen to the laboratory for processing and analysis.

➤ The results are recorded manually or in a computerized system for recall and postprocedure interpretation by the appropriate health care practitioner.

Post-test:

➤ A written report of the examination will be sent to the requesting health care practitioner, who will discuss the results with the patient.

➤ Recognize anxiety related to test results. Provide a supportive, nonjudgmental environment when assisting a patient through the process of fertility testing. Discuss the implications of abnormal test results on the patient's lifestyle. Provide teaching and information regarding the clinical implications of the test results, as appropriate. Encourage the patient or family to seek counseling and other support services if concerned with infertility.

➤ Reinforce information given by the patient's health care provider regarding further testing, treatment, or referral to another health care provider. Answer any questions or address any concerns voiced by the patient or family.

➤ Depending on the results of this procedure, additional testing may be performed to evaluate or monitor progression of the disease process and determine the need for a change in therapy. Evaluate test results in relation to the patient's symptoms and other tests performed.

Related laboratory tests:

➤ Related laboratory tests include antisperm antibodies, estradiol, and testosterone.

SICKLE CELL SCREEN

SYNONYM/ACRONYM: Sickle cell test.

SPECIMEN: Whole blood (1 mL) collected in a lavender-top (EDTA) tube.

REFERENCE VALUE: (Method: Hemoglobin high-salt solubility) Negative.

DESCRIPTION & RATIONALE: The sickle cell screen is one of several screening tests for a group of hereditary hemoglobinopathies. The test is positive in the presence of rare sickling hemoglobin (Hgb) variants such as Hgb S and Hgb C Harlem. Hgb S results from an amino acid substitution during Hgb synthesis whereby valine replaces glutamic acid. Hemoglobin C Harlem results from the substitution of lysine for glutamic acid. Individuals with sickle cell disease have chronic anemia because the abnormal Hgb is unable to carry oxygen. The red blood cells of affected individuals are also abnormal in shape, resembling a crescent or sickle rather than the normal disk shape. This abnormality, combined with cell-wall rigidity, prevents the cells from passing through smaller blood vessels. Blockages in blood vessels result in hypoxia, damage, and pain. Individuals with the sickle cell trait do not have the clinical manifestations of the disease but may pass the disease on to children if the other parent has the trait (or the disease) as well. ■

INDICATIONS:
- Detect sickled red blood cells
- Evaluate hemolytic anemias

RESULT

Positive findings in:
- Combination of Hgb S with other hemoglobinopathies
- Hgb C Harlem anemia
- Sickle cell anemia
- Sickle cell trait
- Thalassemias

Negative findings in: N/A

CRITICAL VALUES: N/A

INTERFERING FACTORS:
- Drugs that may increase sickle cells in vitro include prostaglandins.
- A positive test does not distinguish between the sickle trait and sickle cell anemia; to make this determination, follow-up testing by Hgb electrophoresis should be performed.
- False-negative results may occur in children younger than 3 months of age.

- False-negative results may occur in patients who have received a recent blood transfusion before specimen collection, as a result of the dilutional effect.

- False-positive results may occur in patients without the trait or disease who have received a blood transfusion from a sickle cell–positive donor; this effect can last for 4 months after the transfusion.

- Test results are unreliable if the patient has pernicious anemia or polycythemia.

Nursing Implications and Procedure • • • • • • • • • • •

Pretest:

▶ Inform the patient that the test is used to determine the presence of hemoglobin S.

▶ Obtain a history of the patient's complaints, including a list of known allergens (especially allergies or sensitivities to latex), and inform the appropriate health care practitioner accordingly.

▶ Obtain a history of the patient's hematopoietic system as well as results of previously performed laboratory tests, surgical procedures, and other diagnostic procedures. For related laboratory tests, refer to the Hematopoietic System table.

▶ Note any recent procedures that can interfere with test results.

▶ Obtain a list of medications the patient is taking, including herbs, nutritional supplements, and nutraceuticals. The requesting health care practitioner and laboratory should be advised if the patient regularly uses these products so that their effects can be taken into consideration when reviewing results.

▶ Review the procedure with the patient. Inform the patient that specimen collection takes approximately 5 to 10 minutes. Address concerns about pain related to the procedure.

Explain to the patient that there may be some discomfort during the venipuncture.

▶ *Sensitivity to cultural and social issues,* as well as concern for modesty, is important in providing psychological support before, during, and after the procedure.

▶ There are no food, fluid, or medication restrictions, unless by medical direction.

Intratest:

▶ If the patient has a history of severe allergic reaction to latex, care should be taken to avoid the use of equipment containing latex.

▶ Instruct the patient to cooperate fully and to follow directions. Direct the patient to breathe normally and to avoid unnecessary movement.

▶ Observe standard precautions, and follow the general guidelines in Appendix A. Positively identify the patient, and label the appropriate tubes with the corresponding patient demographics, date, and time of collection. Perform a venipuncture; collect the specimen in a 5-mL lavender top tube.

▶ Remove the needle, and apply a pressure dressing over the puncture site.

▶ Promptly transport the specimen to the laboratory for processing and analysis.

▶ The results are recorded manually or in a computerized system for recall and postprocedure interpretation by the appropriate health care practitioner.

Post-test:

▶ Observe venipuncture site for bleeding or hematoma formation. Apply paper tape or other adhesive to hold pressure bandage in place, or replace with a plastic bandage.

▶ Advise the patient with sickle cell disease to avoid situations in which hypoxia may occur, such as strenuous exercise, staying at high altitudes, or traveling in an unpressurized aircraft. Obstetric and surgical patients with sickle cell anemia are at risk for hypoxia and therefore require close observation: Obstetric patients are at risk for hypoxia during the stress of labor and delivery, and surgical patients may become hypoxic while under general anesthesia.

➤ A written report of the examination will be sent to the requesting health care practitioner, who will discuss the results with the patient.

➤ Recognize anxiety related to test results, and and offer support, as appropriate. Discuss the implications of abnormal test results on the patient's lifestyle. Provide teaching and information regarding the clinical implications of the test results, as appropriate. Educate the patient regarding access to counseling services.

➤ Reinforce information given by the patient's health care provider regarding further testing, treatment, or referral to another health care provider. Inform the patient that further testing may be indicated if results are positive. Answer any questions or address any concerns voiced by the patient or family.

➤ Depending on the results of this procedure, additional testing may be performed to evaluate or monitor progression of the disease process and determine the need for a change in therapy. Evaluate test results in relation to the patient's symptoms and other tests performed.

Related laboratory tests:

➤ Related laboratory tests include complete blood count, Hgb electrophoresis, red blood cell indices, and red blood cell morphology.

SLIT-LAMP BIOMICROSCOPY

SYNONYMS/ACRONYMS: Slit-lamp examination.

AREA OF APPLICATION: Eyes.

CONTRAST: N/A.

DESCRIPTION & RATIONALE: This noninvasive procedure is used to visualize the anterior portion of the eye and its parts, including the eyelids and eyelashes, sclera, conjunctiva, cornea, iris, lens, and anterior chamber, and to detect pathology of any of these areas of the eyes. The slit lamp has a binocular microscope and light source that can be adjusted to examine the fluid, tissues, and structures of the eyes. Special attachments to the slit lamp are used for special studies and more detailed views of specific areas.

Dilating drops or mydriatics may be used to enlarge the pupil in order to allow the examiner to see the eye in greater detail. Mydriatics work either by temporarily paralyzing the muscle that makes the pupil smaller or by stimulating the iris dilator muscle. Patients with light-colored eyes (blue or hazel) will dilate faster than patients with dark eye color (brown). ▪

INDICATIONS:

- Detect conjunctival and corneal injuries by foreign bodies and determine if ocular penetration or anterior chamber hemorrhage is present
- Detect corneal abrasions, ulcers, or abnormal curvatures (keratocoma)
- Detect deficiency in tear formation indicative of lacrimal dysfunction causing dry eye disease that can lead to corneal erosions or infection
- Detect lens opacities indicative of cataract formation
- Determine the presence of blepharitis, conjunctivitis, hordeolum, entropion, ectropian, trachoma, scleritis, and iritis
- Evaluate the fit of contact lenses

RESULT

Normal Findings:

- Normal anterior tissues and structures of the eyes

Abnormal Findings:

- Blepharitis
- Conjunctivitis
- Corneal abrasions
- Corneal ulcers
- Ectropian
- Entropian
- Hordeolum
- Iritis

- Keratoconus (abnormal curvatures)
- Lens opacities
- Scleritis
- Trachoma

CRITICAL VALUES: N/A

INTERFERING FACTORS:

This procedure is contraindicated for:

- Patients with narrow-angle glaucoma if pupil dilation is performed, as dilation can initiate a severe and sight-threatening open-angle attack.
- Patients with allergies to mydriatics if pupil dilation using mydriatics is performed.

Factors that may impair the results of the examination:

- Inability of the patient to cooperate and remain still during the procedure because of age, significant pain, or mental status may interfere with the test results.
- Failure to follow medication restrictions before the procedure may cause the procedure to be canceled or repeated.

Nursing Implications and Procedure ● ● ● ● ● ● ● ● ● ● ●

Pretest:

➤ Inform the patient that the procedure detects abnormalities in the external and anterior eye structures.

➤ Obtain a history of the patient's complaints, including a list of known allergens, especially mydriatics if dilation is to be performed.

➤ Obtain a history of the patient's known or suspected vision loss, changes in visual acuity, including type and cause; use of glasses or contact lenses; eye conditions with treatment regimens; eye surgery; and other tests and procedures to assess and diagnose visual deficit.

➤ Obtain a history of results of previously performed laboratory tests, surgical procedures, and other diagnostic procedures.

➤ Obtain a list of the medications the patient is taking, including herbs, nutritional supplements, and nutraceuticals. The requesting health care practitioner should be advised if the patient regularly uses these products so that their effects can be taken into consideration when reviewing results.

➤ Instruct the patient to remove contact lenses or glasses, as appropriate, unless the study is being done to check the fit and effectiveness of the contact lenses. Instruct the patient regarding the importance of keeping the eyes open for the test.

➤ Review the procedure with the patient. Address concerns about pain related to the procedure. Explain to the patient that mydriatics, if used, may cause blurred vision and sensitivity to light. There may also be a brief stinging sensation when the drop is put in the eye. Inform the patient that an optometrist or physician performs the test, in a quiet, darkened room, and that to evaluate both eyes, the test can take up 30 minutes (including time for the pupils to dilate before the test is actually performed).

➤ There are no food or fluid restrictions, unless by medical direction.

➤ The patient should withhold eye medications (particularly mydriatic eye drops if the patient has glaucoma) for at least 1 day prior to the procedure.

➤ Ensure that the patient understands that he or she must refrain from driving until the pupils return to normal (about 4 hours) after the test and has made arrangements to have someone else be responsible for transportation after the test.

Intratest:

➤ Ensure that the patient has complied with medication restrictions and pretesting preparations; assure that eye medications, especially mydriatics, have been restricted for at least 1 day prior to the procedure.

➤ Instruct the patient to cooperate fully and to follow directions. Ask the patient to remain still during the procedure because movement produces unreliable results.

➤ Seat the patient comfortably. If dilation is to be performed, administer the ordered mydriatic to each eye and repeat in 5 to 15 minutes. Drops are placed in the eye with the patient looking up and the solution directed at the six o'clock position of the sclera (white of the eye) near the limbus (grey, semitransparent area of the eyeball where the cornea and sclera meet). The dropper bottle should not touch the eyelashes.

➤ Ask the patient to place the chin in the chin rest and gently press the forehead against the support bar.

➤ The physician or optometrist places the slit lamp in front of the patient's eyes in line with the examiner's eyes. The external structures of the eyes are inspected with the special bright light and microscope of the slit lamp. The light is then directed into the patient's eyes to inspect the anterior fluids and structures, and is adjusted for shape, intensity, and depth needed to visualize these areas. Magnification of the microscope is also adjusted to optimize visualization of the eye structures.

➤ Special attachments and procedures can also be used to obtain further diagnostic information about the eyes. These may include, for example, a camera to photograph specific parts, gonioscopy to determine anterior chamber closure, and a cobalt blue filter to detect minute corneal scratches, breaks, and abrasions with corneal staining.

➤ The results are recorded manually for recall and postprocedure interpretation by the appropriate health care practitioner.

➤ Instruct the patient to resume usual medications, as directed by the health care practitioner.

➤ A written report of the examination will be completed by a health care practitioner specializing in this branch of medicine. The report will be sent to the requesting health care practitioner, who will discuss the results with the patient.

➤ Recognize anxiety related to test results, and encourage the family to recognize and be supportive of impaired activity related to vision loss, perceived loss of driving privileges, or the possibility of requiring corrective lenses (self-image). Discuss the implications of the abnormal test results on the patient's lifestyle.

➤ Reinforce information given by the patient's health care provider regarding further testing, treatment, or referral to another health care provider. Inform the patient that visual acuity and responses to light may change. Suggest that the patient wear dark glasses after the test until the pupils return to normal size. Answer any questions or address any concerns voiced by the patient or family.

➤ Depending on the results of this procedure, additional testing may be performed to evaluate or monitor progression of the disease process and determine the need for a change in therapy. Evaluate test results in relation to the patient's symptoms and other tests performed.

➤ Related diagnostic tests include color perception test, fluorescein angiography, gonioscopy, intraocular pressure, intraocular muscle function, nerve fiber analysis, refraction, Schirmer tear test, and visual field testing.

SODIUM, BLOOD

SYNONYM/ACRONYM: Serum Na^+.

SPECIMEN: Serum (1 mL) collected in a red- or tiger-top tube. Plasma (1 mL) collected in green-top (heparin) tube is also acceptable.

REFERENCE VALUE: (Method: Ion-selective electrode)

Age	Conventional Units	SI Units (Conventional Units × 1)
Newborn	133–146 mEq/L	133–146 mmol/L
Infant	133–144 mEq/L	133–144 mmol/L
Child	135–145 mEq/L	135–145 mmol/L
Adult	135–145 mEq/L	135–145 mmol/L

DESCRIPTION & RATIONALE: Sodium is the most abundant cation in the extracellular fluid and, together with the accompanying chloride and bicarbonate anions, accounts for 92% of serum osmolality. Sodium plays a major role in maintaining homeostasis in a variety of ways, including maintaining the osmotic pressure of extracellular fluid, regulating renal retention and excretion of water, maintaining acid-base balance, regulating potassium and chloride levels, stimulating neuromuscular reactions, and maintaining systemic blood pressure. *Hypernatremia* (elevated sodium level) occurs when there is excessive water loss or abnormal retention of sodium. *Hyponatremia* (low sodium level) occurs when there is inadequate sodium retention or inadequate intake. ▪

INDICATIONS:
• Determine whole-body stores of sodium, because the ion is predominantly extracellular
• Monitor the effectiveness of drug therapy, especially diuretics, on serum sodium levels

RESULT

Increased in:
• Azotemia
• Burns
• Cushing's disease
• Dehydration
• Diabetes
• Diarrhea (water loss in excess of salt loss)
• Excessive intake
• Excessive saline therapy
• Excessive sweating

• Fever
• Hyperaldosteronism
• Lactic acidosis
• Nasogastric feeding with inadequate fluid
• Vomiting

Decreased in:
• Central nervous system disease
• Congestive heart failure
• Cystic fibrosis
• Excessive antidiuretic hormone production
• Excessive use of diuretics
• Hepatic failure
• Hypoproteinemia
• Insufficient intake
• Intravenous (IV) glucose infusion
• Metabolic acidosis
• Mineralocorticoid deficiency (Addison's disease)
• Nephrotic syndrome

CRITICAL VALUES:
Hyponatremia: Less than 120 mmol/L
Hypernatremia: Greater than 160 mmol/L

Note and immediately report to the health care practitioner any critically increased or decreased values and related symptoms especially fluid imbalance.

Signs and symptoms of hyponatremia include confusion, irritability, convulsions, tachycardia, nausea, vomiting, and loss of consciousness. Possible interventions include maintenance of airway, monitoring for convulsions, fluid restriction, and performance of hourly neurologic checks. Administration of saline for replacement requires close attention to serum and urine osmolality.

Signs and symptoms of hypernatremia

include restlessness, intense thirst, weakness, swollen tongue, seizures, and coma. Possible interventions include treatment of the underlying cause of water loss or sodium excess, which includes sodium restriction and administration of diuretics combined with IV solutions of 5% dextrose in water (D_5W).

Interfering Factors:

- Drugs that may increase serum sodium levels include anabolic steroids, angiotensin, bicarbonate, carbenoxolone, cisplatin, corticotropin, cortisone, gamma globulin, and mannitol.

- Drugs that may decrease serum sodium levels include amphotericin B, bicarbonate, cathartics (excessive use), chlorpropamide, chlorthalidone, diuretics, ethacrynic acid, fluoxetine, furosemide, laxatives (excessive use), methyclothiazide, metolazone, nicardipine, quinethazone, theophylline (IV infusion), thiazides, and triamterene.

- Specimens should never be collected above an IV line because of the potential for dilution when the specimen and the IV solution combine in the collection container, falsely decreasing the result. There is also the potential of contaminating the sample with the substance of interest, if it is present in the IV solution, falsely increasing the result.

Nursing Implications and Procedure • • • • • • • • • • • •

Pretest:

➤ Inform the patient that the test is used to evaluate electrolyte balance.

➤ Obtain a history of the patient's complaints, including a list of known allergens (especially allergies or sensitivities to latex), and inform the appropriate health care practitioner accordingly.

➤ Obtain a history of the patient's endocrine and genitourinary systems, as well as results of previously performed laboratory tests, surgical procedures, and other diagnostic procedures. For related laboratory tests, refer to the Endocrine and Genitourinary System tables.

➤ Obtain a list of medications the patient is taking, including herbs, nutritional supplements, and nutraceuticals. The requesting health care practitioner and laboratory should be advised if the patient regularly uses these products so that their effects can be taken into consideration when reviewing results.

➤ Review the procedure with the patient. Inform the patient that specimen collection takes approximately 5 to 10 minutes. Address concerns about pain related to the procedure. Explain to the patient that there may be some discomfort during the venipuncture.

➤ There are no food, fluid, or medication restrictions, unless by medical direction.

Intratest:

➤ If the patient has a history of severe allergic reaction to latex, care should be taken to avoid the use of equipment containing latex.

➤ Instruct the patient to cooperate fully and to follow directions. Direct the patient to breathe normally and to avoid unnecessary movement.

➤ Observe standard precautions, and follow the general guidelines in Appendix A. Positively identify the patient, and label the appropriate tubes with the corresponding patient demographics, date, and time of collection. Perform a venipuncture; collect the specimen in a 5-mL red- or tiger-top tube.

➤ Remove the needle, and apply a pressure dressing over the puncture site.

➤ Promptly transport the specimen to the laboratory for processing and analysis.

➤ The results are recorded manually or in a computerized system for recall and postprocedure interpretation by the appropriate health care practitioner.

Post-test:

➤ Observe venipuncture site for bleeding or hematoma formation. Apply paper tape or other adhesive to hold pressure bandage in place, or replace with a plastic bandage.

➤ *Nutritional considerations:* Evaluate the patient for signs and symptoms of dehydration. Decreased skin turgor, dry mouth, and multiple longitudinal furrows in the tongue are symptoms of dehydration. Dehydration is a significant and common finding in geriatric and other patients in whom renal function has deteriorated.

➤ *Nutritional considerations:* If appropriate, educate patients with low sodium levels that the major source of dietary sodium is found in table salt. Many foods, such as milk and other dairy products, are also good sources of dietary sodium. Most other dietary sodium is available through the consumption of processed foods. Patients on low-sodium diets should be advised to avoid beverages such as colas, ginger ale, sports drinks, lemon-lime sodas, and root beer. Many over-the-counter medications, including antacids, laxatives, analgesics, sedatives, and antitussives, contain significant amounts of sodium. The best advice is to emphasize the importance of reading all food, beverage, and medicine labels. In 1989, the Subcommittee on the 10th Edition of the RDA established 500 mg as the recommended maximum daily intake for dietary intake of sodium.

➤ A written report of the examination will be sent to the requesting health care practitioner, who will discuss the results with the patient.

➤ Reinforce information given by the patient's health care provider regarding further testing, treatment, or referral to another health care provider. Answer any questions or address any concerns voiced by the patient or family.

➤ Depending on the results of this procedure, additional testing may be performed to evaluate or monitor progression of the disease process and determine the need for a change in therapy. Evaluate test results in relation to the patient's symptoms and other tests performed.

Related laboratory tests:

➤ Related laboratory tests include aldosterone, anion gap, chloride, kidney stone analysis, blood and urine osmolality, blood and urine potassium, renin, and urine sodium.

SODIUM, URINE

. . . .

SYNONYMS/ACRONYM: Urine Na$^+$

SPECIMEN: Urine (5 mL) from an unpreserved random or timed specimen collected in a clean plastic collection container.

REFERENCE VALUE: (Method: Ion-selective electrode)

Age	Conventional Units	SI Units (Conventional Units × 1)
6–10 y		
Male	41–115 mEq/24 h	41–115 mmol/24 h
Female	20–69 mEq/24 h	20–69 mmol/24 h
10–14 y		
Male	63–177 mEq/24 h	63–177 mmol/24 h
Female	48–168 mEq/24 h	48–168 mmol/24 h
Adult	27–287 mEq/24 h	27–287 mmol/24 h

Values vary markedly depending on dietary intake and hydration state.

DESCRIPTION & RATIONALE: Regulating electrolyte balance is a major function of the kidneys. In normally functioning kidneys, urine sodium levels increase when serum levels are high and decrease when serum levels are low to maintain homeostasis. Analyzing these urinary levels can provide important clues to the functioning of the kidneys and other major organs. There is diurnal variation in excretion of sodium, with values lower at night. Urine sodium tests usually involve timed urine collections over a 12- or 24-hour period. Measurement of random specimens may also be requested. ■

INDICATIONS:
• Determine potential cause of renal calculi
• Evaluate known or suspected endocrine disorder
• Evaluate known or suspected renal disease
• Evaluate malabsorption disorders

RESULT

Increased in:
• Adrenal failure
• Alkalosis
• Diabetes

• Diuretic therapy
• Excessive intake
• Renal tubular acidosis
• Salt-losing nephritis

Decreased in:
• Adrenal hyperfunction
• Congestive heart failure
• Diarrhea
• Excessive sweating
• Extrarenal sodium loss with adequate hydration
• Insufficient intake
• Postoperative period (first 24 to 48 hours)
• Prerenal azotemia
• Sodium retention (premenstrual)

CRITICAL VALUES: N/A

INTERFERING FACTORS:
• Drugs that may increase urine sodium levels include acetazolamide, acetylsalicylic acid, amiloride, ammonium chloride, azosemide, benzthiazide, bumetanide, calcitonin, chlorothiazide, clopamide, cyclothiazide, diapamide, dopamine, ethacrynic acid, furosemide, hydrocortisone, hydroflumethiazide, isosorbide, levodopa, mercurial diuretics, methyclothiazide, metolazone, polythiazide, quinethazone, spironolac-

tone, sulfates, tetracycline, thiazides, torasemide, triamterene, trichlormethiazide, triflocin, verapamil, and vincristine.

• Drugs that may decrease urine sodium levels include aldosterone, anesthetics, angiotensin, corticosteroids, cortisone, etodolac, indomethacin, levarterenol, lithium, and propranolol.

• Sodium levels are subject to diurnal variation (output being lowest at night), which is why 24-hour collections are recommended.

Nursing Implications and Procedure . . . .

Pretest:

➤ Inform the patient that the test is used to evaluate acute renal failure and acute oliguria, and to assist in the differential diagnosis of hyponatremia.

➤ Obtain a history of the patient's complaints, including a list of known allergens (especially allergies or sensitivities to latex), and inform the appropriate health care practitioner accordingly.

➤ Obtain a history of the patient's endocrine and genitourinary systems, as well as results of previously performed laboratory tests, surgical procedures, and other diagnostic procedures. For related laboratory tests, refer to the Endocrine and Genitourinary System tables.

➤ Obtain a list of medications the patient is taking, including herbs, nutritional supplements, and nutraceuticals. The requesting health care practitioner and laboratory should be advised if the patient regularly uses these products so that their effects can be taken into consideration when reviewing results.

➤ Review the procedure with the patient. Provide a nonmetallic urinal, bedpan, or toilet-mounted collection device. Address concerns about pain related to the procedure. Explain to the patient that there should be no discomfort during the procedure.

➤ Usually a 24-hour time frame for urine collection is ordered. Inform the patient that all urine must be saved during that 24-hour period. Instruct the patient not to void directly into the laboratory collection container. Instruct the patient to avoid defecating in the collection device and to keep toilet tissue out of the collection device to prevent contamination of the specimen. Place a sign in the bathroom to remind the patient to save all urine.

➤ Instruct the patient to void all urine into the collection device and then to pour the urine into the laboratory collection container. Alternatively, the specimen can be left in the collection device for a health care staff member to add to the laboratory collection container.

➤ *Sensitivity to social and cultural issues*, as well as concern for modesty, is important in providing psychological support before, during, and after the procedure.

➤ There are no food, fluid, or medication restrictions, unless by medical direction.

Intratest:

➤ If the patient has a history of severe allergic reaction to latex, care should be taken to avoid the use of equipment containing latex.

➤ Instruct the patient to cooperate fully and to follow directions.

➤ Observe standard precautions, and follow the general guidelines in Appendix A. Positively identify the patient, and label the appropriate collection container with the corresponding patient demographics, date, and time of collection.

Random specimen (collect in early morning):

Clean-catch specimen:

➤ Instruct the male patient to (1) thoroughly wash his hands, (2) cleanse

the meatus, (3) void a small amount into the toilet, and (4) void directly into the specimen container.

➤ Instruct the female patient to (1) thoroughly wash her hands; (2) cleanse the labia from front to back; (3) while keeping the labia separated, void a small amount into the toilet; and (4) without interrupting the urine stream, void directly into the specimen container.

Indwelling catheter:

➤ Put on gloves. Empty drainage tube of urine. It may be necessary to clamp off the catheter for 15 to 30 minutes before specimen collection. Cleanse specimen port with antiseptic swab, and then aspirate 5 mL of urine with a 21- to 25-gauge needle and syringe. Transfer urine to a sterile container.

Timed specimen:

➤ Obtain a clean 3-L urine specimen container, toilet-mounted collection device, and plastic bag (for transport of the specimen container). The specimen must be refrigerated or kept on ice throughout the entire collection period. If an indwelling urinary catheter is in place, the drainage bag must be kept on ice.

➤ Begin the test between 6 and 8 a.m., if possible. Collect first voiding and discard. Record the time the specimen was discarded as the beginning of the timed collection period. The next morning, ask the patient to void at the same time the collection was started and add this last voiding to the container.

➤ If an indwelling catheter is in place, replace the tubing and container system at the start of the collection time. Keep the container system on ice during the collection period, or empty the urine into a larger container periodically during the collection period; monitor to ensure continued drainage, and conclude the test the next morning at the same hour the collection was begun.

➤ At the conclusion of the test, compare the quantity of urine with the urinary output record for the collection; if the specimen contains less than what was recorded as output, some urine may have been discarded, invalidating the test.

➤ Include on the collection container's label the amount of urine, test start and stop times, and any foods or medications that can affect test results.

General:

➤ Promptly transport the specimen to the laboratory for processing and analysis.

➤ The results are recorded manually or in a computerized system for recall and postprocedure interpretation by the appropriate health care practitioner.

Post-test:

➤ Instruct the patient to resume usual diet, fluids, medications, or activity, as directed by the health care practitioner.

➤ *Nutritional considerations:* If appropriate, educate patients with low sodium levels that the major source of dietary sodium is found in table salt. Many foods, such as milk and other dairy products, are also good sources of dietary sodium. Most other dietary sodium is available through the consumption of processed foods. Patients on low-sodium diets should be advised to avoid beverages such as colas, ginger ale, sports drinks, lemon-lime sodas, and root beer. Many over-the-counter medications, including antacids, laxatives, analgesics, sedatives, and antitussives, contain significant amounts of sodium. The best advice is to emphasize the importance of reading all food, beverage, and medicine labels. In 1989, the Subcommittee on the 10th Edition of the RDA established 500 mg as the recommended maximum daily intake for dietary intake of sodium.

➤ A written report of the examination will be sent to the requesting health care practitioner, who will discuss the results with the patient.

➤ Recognize anxiety related to test results. Discuss the implications of abnormal test results on the patient's lifestyle. Provide teaching and information regarding the clinical implications of the test results, as appropriate.

➤ Reinforce information given by the patient's health care provider regarding further testing, treatment, or referral to another health care provider. Answer any questions or address any concerns voiced by the patient or family.

➤ Depending on the results of this procedure, additional testing may be performed to evaluate or monitor progression of the disease process and determine the need for a change in therapy. Evaluate test results in relation to the patient's symptoms and other tests performed.

Related laboratory tests:

➤ Related laboratory tests include aldosterone, kidney stone analysis, blood and urine osmolality, blood and urine potassium, renin, and blood sodium.

SPONDEE SPEECH RECOGNITION THRESHOLD

SYNONYMS/ACRONYMS: SRT, Speech Reception Threshold.

AREA OF APPLICATION: Ears.

CONTRAST: N/A.

DESCRIPTION & RATIONALE: This noninvasive speech audiometric procedure measures the degree of hearing loss for speech. The speech recognition threshold is the lowest hearing level at which speech can barely be recognized or understood. In this test, a number of spondaic words are presented to the patient at different intensities. Spondaic words, or spondees, are words containing two syllables that are equally accented or emphasized when they are spoken to the patient. The SRT is defined as the lowest hearing level at which the patient correctly repeats 50% of a list of spondaic words. ■

INDICATIONS:

• Determine appropriate gain during hearing aid selection.

• Determine the extent of hearing loss related to speech recognition, as evidenced by the faintest level at which spondee words are correctly repeated.

• Differentiate a real hearing loss from pseudohypoacusis.

• Verify pure tone results.

RESULT

Normal Findings:

- Normal spondee threshold of about 6 to 10 dB of the normal pure tone threshold with 50% of the words pesented being correctly repeated at the appropriate intensity (see monograph titled "Audiometry, Hearing Loss")

- Normal speech recognition with 90% to 100% of the words presented being correctly repeated at an appropriate intensity

Abnormal Findings:

- Conductive hearing loss

- High-frequency hearing loss

- Sensorineural hearing loss (acoustic nerve impairment)

CRITICAL VALUES: N/A

INTERFERING FACTORS:

Factors that may impair the results of the examination:

- Inability of the patient to cooperate or remain still during the procedure because of age or mental status may interfere with the test results.

- Unfamiliarity with the language the words are presented in or with the words themselves will alter the results.

- Improper placement of the earphones and inconsistency in frequency of word presentation will affect results.

Nursing Implications and Procedure . . . .

Pretest:

- Inform the patient that the procedure measures hearing loss related to speech.

- Obtain a history of the patient's complaints, including a list of known allergens.

- Obtain a history of the patient's known or suspected hearing loss, including type and cause; ear conditions with treatment regimens; ear surgery; and other tests and procedures to assess and diagnose hearing deficit. For related diagnostic tests, refer to the table of tests associated with the Auditory System.

- Obtain a history of results of previously performed laboratory tests, surgical procedures, and other diagnostic procedures.

- Obtain a list of the medications the patient is taking, including herbs, nutritional supplements, and nutraceuticals. The requesting health care practitioner should be advised if the patient regularly uses these products so that their effects can be taken into consideration when reviewing results.

- Review the procedure with the patient. Ensure that the patient understands words and sounds in the language to be used for the test. Inform the patient that a series of words that change from loud to soft tones will be presented using earphones and that he or she will be asked to repeat the word. Explain that each ear is tested separately. Address concerns about pain related to the procedure. Explain to the patient that no discomfort will be experienced during the test. Inform the patient that an audiologist or other health care professional specializing in this area performs the test, in a quiet, soundproof room, and that the evaluation takes 5 to 10 minutes.

- There are no food, fluid, or medication restrictions, unless by medical direction.

Intratest:

- Instruct the patient to cooperate fully and to follow directions. Ask the patient to remain still during the procedure because movement produces unreliable results.

- Seat the patient on a chair in a soundproof booth. Place the earphones on the patient's head and secure them over the ears. The audiometer is set at 20 dB above the known pure tone threshold obtained from audiometry (see monograph titled "Audiometry, Hearing Loss"). The test represents hearing levels at speech frequencies of 500, 1000, and 2000 Hz.

➤ The spondee words are presented to the ear with the best auditory response using a speech audiometer. The intensity is decreased and then increased to the softest sound at which the patient is able to hear the words and respond correctly to 50% of them. The procedure is then repeated for the other ear.

➤ The results are recorded manually for recall and postprocedure interpretation by the appropriate health care practitioner.

Post-test:

➤ A written report of the examination will be completed by a health care practitioner specializing in this branch of medicine. The report will be sent to the requesting health care practitioner, who will discuss the results with the patient.

➤ Recognize anxiety related to test results, and be supportive of activity related to impaired hearing and perceived loss of independence. Discuss the implications of abnormal test results on the patient's lifestyle. Provide teaching and information regarding the clinical implications of the test results, as appropriate. Educate the patient regarding access to counseling services.

➤ Reinforce information given by the patient's health care provider regarding further testing, treatment, or referral to another health care provider. Answer any questions or address any concerns voiced by the patient or family.

➤ Depending on the results of this procedure, additional testing may be performed to evaluate or monitor progression of the disease process and determine the need for a change in therapy. Evaluate test results in relation to the patient's symptoms and other tests performed.

Related diagnostic tests:

➤ A related diagnostic test is hearing loss audiometry.

STEREOTACTIC BIOPSY, BREAST

. . . .

SYNONYM/ACRONYM: N/A.

SPECIMEN: Breast tissue or cells.

REFERENCE VALUE: (Method: Macroscopic and microscopic examination of tissue) No abnormal cells or tissue.

DESCRIPTION & RATIONALE: A stereotactic breast biopsy is helpful when a mammogram or ultrasound examination shows a mass, a cluster of microcalcifications (tiny calcium deposits that are closely grouped together), or an area of abnormal tissue change, usually with no lump being felt on a careful breast examination. A number of biopsy instruments and methods are utilized with x-ray guidance. They include core biopsy, which uses a large-bore needle to remove a generous sample of breast tissue, and a vacuum-assisted needle biopsy device. As an alternative to an open core surgical biopsy, which removes an entire breast lump for microscopic analysis, a narrow needle may be passed through the skin into the area under investigation. The is accomplished with the help of special breast x-rays. Images of the breast are obtained with a mammography machine, and the images are recorded in a computer. An initial x-ray locates the abnormality and two stereo views are obtained, each angled 15° to either side of the initial image. The computer calculates how much the area of interest has changed with each image and is able to determine the exact site in three-dimensional space. A small sample of breast tissue is obtained and can show whether the breast mass is cancerous or not. A pathologist examines the tissue that was removed and makes a final diagnosis to allow for effective treatment. ■

INDICATIONS:
- A mammogram showing a suspicious cluster of small calcium deposits

- A mammogram showing a suspicious solid mass that cannot be felt on breast examination

- Evidence of breast lesion by palpation, mammography, or ultrasound

- New mass or area of calcium deposits present at a previous surgery site

- Observable breast changes such as "peau d'orange" skin, scaly skin of the areola, drainage from the nipple, or ulceration of the skin

- Patient preference for a nonsurgical method of lesion assessment

- Structure of the breast tissue is distorted

RESULT: Positive findings in carcinoma of the breast

CRITICAL VALUES: N/A

INTERFERING FACTORS:
- ⚠ This procedure is contraindicated in patients with bleeding disorders.

Factors that may impair clear imaging:
- Failure to restrict food intake before the study

- Metallic objects within the examination field (e.g., jewelry, body rings, dental amalgams), which may inhibit organ visualization and can produce unclear images

- Improper adjustment of the radiographic equipment to accommodate obese or thin patients, which can cause overexposure or underexposure and a poor-quality study

- Patients who are very obese, who may exceed the weight limit for the equipment

- Incorrect positioning of the patient, which may produce poor visualization of the area to be examined

- Inability of the patient to cooperate or remain still during the procedure because of age, significant pain, or mental status

Other considerations:
- Complications of the procedure include hemorrhage, infection at the insertion site, and cardiac arrhythmias.

- Failure to follow dietary restrictions

before the procedure may cause the procedure to be canceled or repeated.

• Consultation with a health care practitioner should occur before the procedure for radiation safety concerns regarding younger patients or patients who are lactating.

• Risks associated with radiographic overexposure can result from frequent x-ray procedures. Personnel in the room with the patient should wear a protective lead apron, stand behind a shield, or leave the area while the examination is being done. Personnel working in the area where the examination is being done should wear badges that reveal their level of exposure to radiation.

Nursing Implications and Procedure • • • • • • • • • • • •

Pretest:

➤ Inform the patient that the procedure assesses a breast mass.

➤ Obtain a history of the patient's complaints, including a list of known allergens, and inform the appropriate health care practitioner accordingly.

➤ Obtain a history of the patient's reproductive system, as well as results of previously performed laboratory tests (especially coagulation tests and bleeding time), surgical procedures, and other diagnostic procedures. For related diagnostic tests, refer to the Reproductive System table.

➤ Note any recent procedures that can interfere with test results.

➤ Record the date of the last menstrual period and determine the possibility of pregnancy in perimenopausal women.

➤ Obtain a list of the medications the patient is taking, including anticoagulant therapy, aspirin and other

salicylates, herbs, nutritional supplements, and nutraceuticals, especially those known to affect coagulation (see Appendix F). It is recommended that use be discontinued 14 days before surgical procedures. The requesting health care practitioner and laboratory should be advised if the patient regularly uses these products so that their effects can be taken into consideration when reviewing results.

➤ Review the procedure with the patient. Address concerns about pain related to the procedure. Explain to the patient that some pain will be experienced during the test, or there may be moments of discomfort. Inform the patient that the procedure is performed in special room, usually a mammography suite, by a health care practitioner and support staff and takes approximately 30 to 60 minutes.

➤ Explain that an intravenous (IV) line may be inserted to allow infusion of IV fluids, contrast medium, dye, or sedatives. Usually normal saline is infused.

➤ *Sensitivity to cultural and social issues,* as well as concern for modesty, is important in providing psychological support before, during, and after the procedure.

➤ The patient should fast and restrict fluids for 8 hours prior to the procedure. Instruct the patient to avoid taking anticoagulant medication or to reduce dosage as ordered prior to the procedure. Number of days to withhold medication is dependent on the type of anticoagulant.

➤ Instruct the patient to remove dentures, jewelry (including watches), hairpins, credit cards, and other metallic objects.

➤ *Make sure a written and informed consent has been signed prior to the procedure and before administering any medications.*

➤ The procedure may be terminated if chest pain or severe cardiac arrhythmias occur.

Intratest:

> Ensure that the patient has complied with dietary and medication restrictions and pretesting preparations; assure that these have been restricted for at least 8 hours prior to the procedure. Ensure the patient has removed all external metallic objects (jewelry, dentures, etc.) prior to the procedure.

> Have emergency equipment readily available.

> If the patient has a history of severe allergic reactions to any substance or drug, administer ordered prophylactic steroids or antihistamines before the procedure.

> Patients are given a gown, robe, and foot coverings to wear and instructed to void prior to the procedure.

> Observe standard precautions, and follow the general guidelines in Appendix A. Positively identify the patient, and label the appropriate specimen containers with the corresponding patient demographics, date and time of collection, and site location (left or right breast).

> Instruct the patient to cooperate fully and to follow directions. Instruct the patient to remain still throughout the procedure because movement produces unreliable results.

> Record baseline vital signs and assess neurologic status. Protocols may vary from facility to facility.

> Establish an IV fluid line for the injection of emergency drugs and of sedatives.

> Administer an antianxiety agent, as ordered, if the patient has claustrophobia.

> Place the patient in the prone or sitting position on an exam table. Cleanse the selected area, and cover with a sterile drape.

> A local anesthetic is injected at the site, and a small incision is made or a needle inserted.

> Ask the patient to inhale deeply and hold his or her breath while the x-ray images are taken, and then to exhale after the images are taken.

> Instruct the patient to take slow, deep breaths if nausea occurs during the procedure. Monitor and administer an antiemetic agent if ordered. Ready an emesis basin for use.

> Monitor the patient for complications related to the procedure (e.g., allergic reaction, anaphylaxis, bronchospasm).

> The needle or catheter is removed, and a pressure dressing is applied over the puncture site.

> Place tissue samples in properly labeled specimen containers, and promptly transport the specimens to the laboratory for processing and analysis.

> The results are recorded manually on x-ray film or electonically, in a computerized system, for recall and postprocedure interpretation by the appropriate health care practitioner.

Post-test:

> Instruct the patient to resume usual diet and medications, as directed by the health care practitioner.

> Monitor vital signs and neurologic status every 15 minutes for 1 hour, then every 2 hours for 4 hours, and then as ordered by the health care practitioner. Take temperature every 4 hours for 24 hours. Compare with baseline values. Notify the health care practitioner if temperature is elevated. Protocols may vary from facility to facility.

> Advise the patient to immediately report symptoms such as fast heart rate, difficulty breathing, skin rash, itching, or decreased urinary output.

> Observe the needle/catheter insertion site for bleeding, inflammation, or hematoma formation.

> Instruct the patient to apply cold compresses to the puncture site, as needed, to reduce discomfort or edema.

> Instruct the patient to apply cold compresses to the puncture site, as needed, to reduce discomfort or edema.

➤ Instruct the patient in the care and assessment of the site. Observe for bleeding, hematoma formation, and inflammation. Note any pleuritic pain, persistent right shoulder pain, or abdominal pain.

➤ A written report of the examination will be completed by a health care practitioner specializing in this branch of medicine. The report will be sent to the requesting health care practitioner, who will discuss the results with the patient.

➤ Recognize anxiety related to test results, and be supportive of the potential perceived loss of body image. Discuss the implications of abnormal test results on the patient's lifestyle. Provide teaching and information regarding the clinical implications of the test results, as appropriate. Educate the patient regarding access to counseling services.

➤ Reinforce information given by the patient's health care provider regarding further testing, treatment, or referral to another health care provider. Answer any questions or address any concerns voiced by the patient or family.

➤ Instruct the patient in the use of any ordered medications. Explain the importance of adhering to the therapy regimen. As appropriate, instruct the patient in significant side effects and systemic reactions associated with the prescribed medication. Encourage him or her to review corresponding literature provided by a pharmacist.

➤ Depending on the results of this procedure, additional testing may be performed to evaluate or monitor progression of the disease process and determine the need for a change in therapy. Evaluate test results in relation to the patient's symptoms and other tests performed.

Related diagnostic tests:

➤ Related diagnostic and laboratory tests include CA 15-3, carcinoembryonic antigen, estrogen and progesterone receptors, HER-2/neu oncoprotein, mammography, and ultrasound of the breast.

SYNOVIAL FLUID ANALYSIS

SYNONYMS/ACRONYM: Arthrocentesis, joint fluid analysis, knee fluid analysis.

SPECIMEN: Synovial fluid collected in a red-top tube for antinuclear antibodies (ANAs), complement, crystal examination, protein, rheumatoid factor (RF), and uric acid; sterile (red-top) tube for microbiologic testing; lavender-top (EDTA) tube for complete blood count (CBC) and differential; gray-top (sodium fluoride [NaFl]) tube for glucose; green-top (heparin) tube for lactic acid and pH.

REFERENCE VALUE: (Method: Macroscopic evaluation of appearance; spectrophotometry for glucose, lactic acid, protein, and uric acid; Gram stain, acid-fast stain, and culture for microbiology; microscopic examination of fluid for cell count and evaluation of crystals; ion-selective electrode for pH; nephelometry for RF and C3; indirect fluorescence for ANAs)

Color	Colorless to pale yellow
Clarity	Clear
Viscosity	High
ANA	Parallels serum level
C3	Parallels serum level
Glucose	Less than 10 mg/dL of blood level
Lactic acid	5–20 mg/dL
pH	7.2–7.4
Protein	Less than 3 g/dL
RF	Parallels serum level
Uric acid	Parallels serum level
Crystals	None present
RBC count	None
WBC count	Less than 0.2×10^3/mm^3 (or 200/mm^3)
Neutrophils	Less than 25%
WBC morphology	No abnormal cells or inclusions
Gram stain and culture	No organisms present
AFB smear and culture	No AFB present

ANA = antinuclear antibodies; C3 = complement; RF = rheumatoid factor; RBC = red blood cell; WBC = white blood cell; AFB = acid-fast bacilli.

DESCRIPTION & RATIONALE: Syn-
ovial fluid analysis is performed via arthrocentesis, an invasive procedure involving insertion of a needle into the joint space. Synovial effusions are associated with disorders or injuries involving the joints. The most commonly aspirated joint is the knee, although samples also can be obtained from the shoulder, hip, elbow, wrist, and ankle, if clinically indicated. Joint disorders can be classified into five categories: noninflammatory, inflammatory, septic, crystal-induced, and hemorrhagic. ∎

INDICATIONS:
- Assist in the evaluation of joint effusions
- Differentiate gout from pseudogout

RESULT

Fluid values increased in:
- *Acute bacterial infection:* White blood cell (WBC) count greater than 50×10^3/mm^3, marked predominance of neutrophils (greater than 90% neutrophils), positive Gram stain, positive cultures, possible presence of rice bodies, increased lactic acid, and complement levels paralleling those found in serum (may be elevated or decreased)

- *Gout:* WBC count variable; $0.5–200 \times 10^3$/mm^3 with a predominance of neutrophils (90% neutrophils), presence of monosodium urate crystals, increased uric acid, and complement levels paralleling those of serum (may be elevated or decreased)

- *Osteoarthritis, traumatic arthritis degenerative joint disease:* WBC count less than 3×10^3/mm^3 with less than 25%

neutrophils and the presence of cartilage cells

- *Pseudogout:* Presence of calcium pyrophosphate crystals

- *Rheumatoid arthritis:* WBC count 3–50 $\times$ 10^3/mm^3 with a predominance of neutrophils (greater than 70% neutrophils), presence of ragocyte cells and possibly rice bodies, presence of cholesterol crystals if effusion is chronic, increased protein, increased lactic acid, and presence of rheumatoid factor

- *Systemic lupus erythematosus (SLE):* 3–50 $\times$ 10^3/mm^3 with a predominance of neutrophils, presence of SLE cells, and presence of antinuclear antibodies

- *Trauma, joint tumors, or hemophilic arthritis:* Elevated RBC count, increased protein level, and presence of fat droplets (if trauma involved)

- *Tuberculous arthritis:* WBC count 2–100 $\times$ 10^3/mm^3 with a predominance of neutrophils (up to 90% neutrophils), possible presence of rice bodies, presence of cholesterol crystals if effusion is chronic, in some cases a positive culture and smear for acid-fast bacilli (results frequently negative), and lactic acid

Fluid values decreased in (analytes in parentheses are decreased):

- Acute bacterial arthritis (glucose and pH)

- Gout (glucose)

- Rheumatoid arthritis (glucose, pH, and complement)

- SLE (glucose, pH, and complement)

- Tuberculous arthritis (glucose and pH)

CRITICAL VALUES: N/A

INTERFERING FACTORS:
- Blood in the sample from traumatic arthrocentesis may falsely elevate the RBC count.

- Undetected hypoglycemia or hyperglycemia may produce misleading glucose values.

- Refrigeration of the sample may result in an increase in monosodium urate crystals secondary to decreased solubility of uric acid; exposure of the sample to room air with a resultant loss of carbon dioxide and rise in pH encourages the formation of calcium pyrophosphate crystals.

Nursing Implications and Procedure

Pretest:

➤ Inform the patient that the test is primarily used to identify the presence and assist in the management of joint disease.

➤ Obtain a history of the patient's complaints, including a list of known allergens (especially allergies or sensitivities to latex), and inform the appropriate health care practitioner accordingly.

➤ Obtain a history of the patient's immune and musculoskeletal systems, any bleeding disorders, and results of previously performed laboratory tests (especially bleeding time, complete blood count, partial thromboplastin time, platelets, and prothrombin time), surgical procedures, and other diagnostic procedures. For related laboratory tests, refer to the Immune and Musculoskeletal System tables.

➤ Note any recent procedures that can interfere with test results.

➤ Record the date of the last menstrual period and determine the possibility of pregnancy in perimenopausal women.

➤ Obtain a list of medications the patient is taking, including anticoagulant therapy, acetylsalicylic acid, herbs, nutritional supplements, and nutraceuticals, especially those known to affect coagulation. The requesting health care practitioner and laboratory should be advised if the patient regularly uses these products so that their effects can be taken into consideration when reviewing results.

➤ Review the procedure with the patient. Inform the patient that it may be necessary to shave the site before specimen collection. Address concerns about pain related to the procedure. Explain that a sedative and/or analgesia will be administered to promote relaxation and reduce discomfort prior to needle insertion through the joint space. Explain to the patient that any discomfort with the needle insertion will be minimized with local anesthetics and systemic analgesics. Explain that the anesthetic injection may cause an initial stinging sensation. Explain that, after the skin has been anesthetized, a large needle will be inserted through the joint space, and a "popping" sensation may be experienced as the needle penetrates the joint. Inform the patient that the procedure is performed under sterile conditions by a health care practitioner specializing in this procedure. The procedure usually takes approximately 20 minutes to complete.

➤ *Sensitivity to cultural and social issues,* as well as concern for modesty, is important in providing psychological support before, during, and after the procedure.

➤ There are no fluid restrictions unless by medical direction. Fasting for at least 12 hours before the procedure is recommended if fluid glucose measurements are included in the analysis. Instruct the patient to avoid taking anticoagulant medication or to reduce dosage as ordered prior to the procedure.

➤ *Make sure a written and informed consent has been signed prior to the procedure and before administering any medications.*

Intratest:

➤ Ensure that the patient has complied with dietary and medication restrictions and pretesting preparations; assure that food has been restricted for at least 12 hours prior to the procedure. Ensure that anticoagulant medications and aspirin have been withheld, as ordered.

➤ Assemble the necessary equipment, including an arthrocentesis tray with solution for skin preparation, local anesthetic, a 20-mL syringe, needles of various sizes, sterile drapes, and sterile gloves for the tests to be performed.

➤ Instruct the patient to cooperate fully and to follow directions. Direct the patient to breathe normally and to avoid unnecessary movement during the local anesthetic and the procedure.

➤ Observe standard precautions, and follow the general guidelines in Appendix A. Positively identify the patient, and label the appropriate collection containers with the corresponding patient demographics, date and time of collection, and site location, especially left or right.

➤ Assist the patient into a comfortable sitting or supine position, as appropriate.

➤ Prior to the administration of general or local anesthesia, shave and cleanse the site with an antiseptic solution, and drape the area with sterile towels.

➤ After the local anesthetic is administered, the needle is inserted at the collection site, and fluid is removed by syringe. Manual pressure may be applied to facilitate fluid removal.

➤ If medication is injected into the joint, the syringe containing the sample is detached from the needle and replaced with the one containing the drug. The medication is injected with gentle pressure. The needle is withdrawn, and digital pressure is applied to the site for a few minutes. If there is no evidence of bleeding, a sterile dressing is applied to the site. An elastic bandage can be applied to the joint.

➤ Monitor the patient for complications related to the procedure (e.g., allergic reaction, anaphylaxis).

➤ Place samples in properly labeled

specimen containers and promptly transport the specimens to the laboratory for processing and analysis. If bacterial culture and sensitivity tests are to be performed, record on the specimen containers any antibiotic therapy the patient is receiving.

➤ The results are recorded manually or in a computerized system for recall and postprocedure interpretation by the appropriate health care practitioner.

Post-test:

➤ Instruct the patient to resume usual diet and medications, as directed by the health care practitioner.

➤ After local anesthesia, monitor vital signs and compare with baseline values. Notify the health care practitioner if temperature is elevated. Protocols may vary from facility to facility.

➤ Assess puncture site for bleeding, bruising, inflammation, and excessive drainage of synovial fluid approximately every 4 hours for 24 hours and daily thereafter for several days.

➤ Instruct the patient to report excessive pain, bleeding, or swelling to the requesting health care practitioner immediately. Report to health care practitioner if severe pain is present or the patient is unable to move the joint.

➤ Assess for nausea and pain. Administer antiemetic and analgesic medications as needed and as directed by the health care practitioner.

➤ Instruct the patient to apply an ice pack to the site for 24 to 48 hours.

➤ Administer antibiotics, as ordered, and instruct the patient in the impor-

tance of completing the entire course of antibiotic therapy even if no symptoms are present.

➤ A written report of the examination will be completed by a health care practitioner specializing in this branch of medicine. The report will be sent to the requesting health care practitioner, who will discuss the results with the patient.

➤ Recognize anxiety related to test results, and offer support. Discuss the implications of abnormal test results on the patient's lifestyle. Provide teaching and information regarding the clinical implications of the test results, as appropriate.

➤ Reinforce information given by the patient's health care provider regarding further testing, treatment, or referral to another health care provider. Instruct the patient or caregiver to handle linen and dispose of dressings cautiously, especially if septic arthritis is suspected. Instruct the patient to avoid excessive use of the joint for several days to prevent pain and swelling. Instruct the patient to return for a follow-up visit as scheduled. Answer any questions or address any concerns voiced by the patient or family.

➤ Depending on the results of this procedure, additional testing may be performed to evaluate or monitor progression of the disease process and determine the need for a change in therapy. Evaluate test results in relation to the patient's symptoms and other tests performed.

Related laboratory tests:

➤ Related laboratory tests include rheumatoid factor and uric acid.

SYPHILIS SEROLOGY

$\bullet \quad \bullet$

SYNONYMS/ACRONYMS: Automated reagin testing (ART), fluorescent treponemal antibody testing (FTA-ABS), microhemag-glutination–*Treponema pallidum* (MHA-TP), rapid plasma reagin (RPR), treponemal studies, Venereal Disease Research Laboratory (VDRL) testing.

SPECIMEN: Serum (1 mL) collected in a red- or tiger-top tube.

REFERENCE VALUE: (Method: Dark-field microscopy, rapid plasma reagin, enzyme-linked immunosorbent assay [ELISA], microhemag-glutination, fluorescence) Nonreactive or absence of treponemal organisms.

DESCRIPTION & RATIONALE: There are numerous methods for detecting *Treponema pallidum*, the organism known to cause syphilis. Syphilis serology is routinely ordered as part of a prenatal workup and is required for evaluating donated blood units before release for transfusion. Selection of the proper testing method is important. Automated reagin testing (ART), rapid plasma reagin (RPR), and Venereal Disease Research Laboratory (VDRL) testing should be used for screening purposes. Fluorescent treponemal antibody testing (FTA-ABS) and microhemagglutination–*Treponema pallidum* (MHA-TP) are confirmatory methods for samples that screen positive or reactive. Cerebrospinal fluid should be tested only by the FTA-ABS method. Cord blood should not be submitted for testing by any of the aforementioned methods; instead, the mother's serum should be tested to establish whether the infant should be treated. ∎

INDICATIONS:

- Monitor effectiveness of treatment for syphilis

- Screen for and confirm the presence of syphilis

RESULT

Positive or reactive findings in:
- Syphilis

False-positive or false-reactive findings in screening (RPR, VDRL) tests:
- Infectious:
  Bacterial endocarditis
  Chancroid
  Chickenpox
  Human immunodeficiency virus
  Infectious mononucleosis

Leprosy
Leptospirosis
Lymphogranuloma venereum
Malaria
Measles
Mumps
Mycoplasma pneumoniae
Pneumococcal pneumonia
Psittacosis
Relapsing fever
Rickettsial disease
Scarlet fever
Trypanosomiasis
Tuberculosis
Vaccinia (live or attenuated)
Viral hepatitis

- Noninfectious:
  Advanced cancer
  Advancing age
  Chronic liver disease
  Connective tissue diseases
  Intravenous drug use
  Multiple blood transfusions
  Multiple myeloma and other
    immunologic disorders
  Narcotic addiction
  Pregnancy
  False-positive or false-reactive
    findings in confirmatory (FTA-
    ABS, MHA-TP) tests:

- Infectious:
  Infectious mononucleosis
  Leprosy
  Leptospirosis
  Lyme disease
  Malaria
  Relapsing fever

- Noninfectious:
  Systemic lupus erythematosus
  Negative or nonreactive findings
    in: N/A

CRITICAL VALUES:
Note and immediately report to the
health care practitioner positive results
and related symptoms.

INTERFERING FACTORS: N/A

Nursing Implications and Procedure • • • • • • • • • • •

Pretest:

➤ Inform the patient that the test is
used to diagnose syphilis infection.

➤ Obtain a history of the patient's complaints, including a list of known
allergens (especially allergies or sensitivities to latex), and inform the
appropriate health care practitioner
accordingly.

➤ Obtain a history of exposure.

➤ Obtain a history of the patient's immune and reproductive systems, as
well as results of previously performed laboratory tests, surgical
procedures, and other diagnostic
procedures. For related laboratory
tests, refer to the Immune and
Reproductive System tables.

➤ Obtain a list of medications the
patient is taking, including herbs,
nutritional supplements, and nutraceuticals. The requesting health care
practitioner and laboratory should be
advised if the patient regularly uses
these products so that their effects
can be taken into consideration
when reviewing results.

➤ Review the procedure with the patient. Inform the patient that specimen collection takes approximately
5 to 10 minutes. Address concerns
about pain related to the procedure.
Explain to the patient that there may
be some discomfort during the
venipuncture.

➤ *Sensitivity to cultural and social
issues*, as well as concern for modesty, is important in providing psychological support before, during,
and after the procedure.

➤ There are no food, fluid, or medication restrictions, unless by medical
direction.

Intratest:

➤ If the patient has a history of severe
allergic reaction to latex, care should

be taken to avoid the use of equipment containing latex.

➤ Instruct the patient to cooperate fully and to follow directions. Direct the patient to breathe normally and to avoid unnecessary movement.

➤ Observe standard precautions, and follow the general guidelines in Appendix A. Positively identify the patient, and label the appropriate tubes with the corresponding patient demographics, date, and time of collection. Perform a venipuncture; collect the specimen in a 5-mL red- or tiger-top tube.

➤ Remove the needle, and apply a pressure dressing over the puncture site.

➤ Promptly transport the specimen to the laboratory for processing and analysis.

➤ The results are recorded manually or in a computerized system for recall and postprocedure interpretation by the appropriate health care practitioner.

Post-test:

➤ Observe venipuncture site for bleeding or hematoma formation. Apply paper tape or other adhesive to hold pressure bandage in place, or replace with a plastic bandage.

➤ A written report of the examination will be sent to the requesting health care practitioner, who will discuss the results with the patient.

➤ Recognize anxiety related to test results, and offer support. Counsel the patient, as appropriate, regarding the risk of transmission and proper prophylaxis, and reinforce the importance of strict adherence to the treatment regimen. Inform the patient that positive findings must be reported to local health department officials, who will question him or her regarding sexual partners. Provide teaching and information regarding the clinical implications of the test results, as appropriate. Educate the patient regarding access to counseling services.

➤ Reinforce information given by the patient's health care provider regarding further testing, treatment, or referral to another health care provider. Inform the patient that repeat testing may be needed at 3-month intervals for 1 year to monitor the effectiveness of treatment. Answer any questions or address any concerns voiced by the patient or family.

➤ Offer support, as appropriate, to patients who may be the victim of rape or sexual assault. Educate the patient regarding access to counseling services. Provide a nonjudgmental, nonthreatening atmosphere for a discussion during which risks of sexually transmitted diseases are explained. It is also important to discuss problems the patient may experience (e.g., guilt, depression, anger).

➤ Depending on the results of this procedure, additional testing may be performed to evaluate or monitor progression of the disease process and determine the need for a change in therapy. Evaluate test results in relation to the patient's symptoms and other tests performed.

Related laboratory tests:

➤ Related laboratory tests include acid phosphatase, *Chlamydia* group antibody, anal bacterial culture, Gram stain, hepatitis B, hepatitis C, human immunodeficiency virus, and β_2-microglobulin.

TESTOSTERONE, TOTAL

Synonym/Acronym: N/A.

Specimen: Serum (1 mL) collected in a red- or tiger-top tube. Plasma (1 mL) collected in green-top (heparin) tube is also acceptable.

Reference value: (Method: Immunochemiluminometric assay [ICMA])

Age	Conventional Units	SI Units (Conventional Units × 0.0347)
1–5 mo		
Male	1–177 ng/dL	0.03–6.14 nmol/L
Female	1–5 ng/dL	0.03–0.17 nmol/L
6–11 mo		
Male	2–7 ng/dL	0.07–0.24 nmol/L
Female	2–5 ng/dL	0.07–0.17 nmol/L
1–5 y		
Male & Female	0–10 ng/dL	0.00–0.35 nmol/L
6–7 y		
Male	0–20 ng/dL	0.00–0.69 nmol/L
Female	0–10 ng/dL	0.00–0.35 nmol/L
8–10 y		
Male	0–25 ng/dL	0.00–0.87 nmol/L
Female	0–30 ng/dL	0.00–1.0 nmol/L
11–12 y		
Male	0–350 ng/dL	0.00–12.1 nmol/L
Female	0–50 ng/dL	0.00–1.74 nmol/L
13–15 y		
Male	15–500 ng/dL	0.52–17.35 nmol/L
Female	0–50 ng/dL	0.00–1.74 nmol/L
Adult		
Male	241–827 ng/dL	8.36–28.70 nmol/L
Female	15–70 ng/dL	0.52–2.43 nmol/L

Tanner Stage		
	Male	*Female*
I	2–23	2–10
II	5–70	5–30
III	15–280	10–30
IV	105–545	15–40
V	265–800	10–40

DESCRIPTION & RATIONALE: Testosterone is the major androgen responsible for sexual differentiation. In males, testosterone is made by the Leydig cells in the testicles and is responsible for spermatogenesis and the development of secondary sex characteristics. In females, the ovary and adrenal gland secrete small amounts of this hormone; however, most of the testosterone in females comes from the metabolism of androstenedione. In males, a testicular, adrenal, or pituitary tumor can cause an overabundance of testosterone, triggering precocious puberty. In females, adrenal tumors, hyperplasia, and medications can cause an overabundance of this hormone, resulting in masculinization or hirsutism. ■

INDICATIONS:
- Assist in the diagnosis of hypergonadism
- Assist in the diagnosis of male sexual precocity before age 10
- Distinguish between primary and secondary hypogonadism
- Evaluate hirsutism
- Evaluate male infertility

RESULT

Increased in:
- Adrenal hyperplasia
- Adrenocortical tumors
- Hirsutism
- Hyperthyroidism
- Idiopathic sexual precocity
- Polycystic ovaries
- Syndrome of androgen resistance
- Testicular or extragonadal tumors
- Trophoblastic tumors during pregnancy
- Virilizing ovarian tumors

Decreased in:
- Anovulation
- Cryptorchidism
- Delayed puberty
- Down syndrome
- Excessive alcohol intake
- Hepatic insufficiency
- Impotence
- Klinefelter's syndrome
- Malnutrition
- Myotonic dystrophy
- Orchiectomy
- Primary and secondary hypogonadism
- Primary and secondary hypopituitarism
- Uremia

CRITICAL VALUES: N/A

INTERFERING FACTORS:
- Drugs that may increase testosterone levels include barbiturates, bromocriptine, cimetidine, flutamide, gonadotropin, levonorgestrel, mifepristone, moclobemide, nafarelin (males), nilutamide, oral contraceptives, rifampin, and tamoxifen.

- Drugs that may decrease testosterone levels include cyclophosphamide, cyproterone, danazol, dexamethasone, diethylstilbestrol, digoxin, D-Trp-6-LHRH, fenoldopam, goserelin, ketoconazole, leuprolide, magnesium sulfate, medroxyprogesterone, methylprednisone, nandrolone, oral contraceptives, pravastatin, prednisone, pyridoglutethimide, spironolactone, stanozolol, tetracycline, and thioridazine.

Nursing Implications and Procedure ....

➤ Inform the patient that the test is used to assess gonadal and adrenal function.

➤ Obtain a history of the patient's complaints, including a list of known allergens (especially allergies or sensitivities to latex), and inform the appropriate health care practitioner accordingly.

➤ Obtain a history of the patient's endocrine and reproductive systems, as well as results of previously performed laboratory tests, surgical procedures, and other diagnostic procedures. For related laboratory tests, refer to the Endocrine and Reproductive System tables.

➤ Obtain a list of medications the patient is taking, including herbs, nutritional supplements, and nutraceuticals. The requesting health care practitioner and laboratory should be advised if the patient regularly uses these products so that their effects can be taken into consideration when reviewing results.

➤ Review the procedure with the patient. Inform the patient that specimen collection takes approximately 5 to 10 minutes. Address concerns about pain related to the procedure. Explain to the patient that there may be some discomfort during the venipuncture.

➤ There are no food, fluid, or medication restrictions, unless by medical direction.

➤ If the patient has a history of severe allergic reaction to latex, care should be taken to avoid the use of equipment containing latex.

➤ Instruct the patient to cooperate fully and to follow directions. Direct the patient to breathe normally and to avoid unnecessary movement.

➤ Observe standard precautions, and follow the general guidelines in Appendix A. Positively identify the patient, and label the appropriate tubes with the corresponding patient demographics, date, and time of collection. Perform a venipuncture; collect the specimen in a 5-mL red- or tiger-top tube.

➤ Remove the needle, and apply a pressure dressing over the puncture site.

➤ Promptly transport the specimen to the laboratory for processing and analysis.

➤ The results are recorded manually or in a computerized system for recall and postprocedure interpretation by the appropriate health care practitioner.

➤ Observe venipuncture site for bleeding or hematoma formation. Apply paper tape or other adhesive to hold pressure bandage in place, or replace with a plastic bandage.

➤ A written report of the examination will be sent to the requesting health care practitioner, who will discuss the results with the patient.

➤ Recognize anxiety related to test results, and and offer support, as appropriate. Discuss the implications of abnormal test results on the patient's lifestyle. Provide teaching and information regarding the clinical implications of the test results, as appropriate. Educate the patient regarding access to counseling services.

➤ Reinforce information given by the patient's health care provider regarding further testing, treatment, or referral to another health care provider. Answer any questions or address any concerns voiced by the patient or family.

➤ Depending on the results of this procedure, additional testing may be

performed to evaluate or monitor progression of the disease process and determine the need for a change in therapy. Evaluate test results in relation to the patient's symptoms and other tests performed.

Related laboratory tests:

➤ Related laboratory tests include dehydroepiandrosterone sulfate, follicle-stimulating hormone, luteinizing hormone, and semen analysis.

THYROGLOBULIN

- -

SYNONYM/ACRONYM: Tg.

SPECIMEN: Serum (1 mL) collected in a red- or tiger-top tube.

REFERENCE VALUE: (Method: Chemiluminescent enzyme immunoassay)

Age	Conventional Units	SI Units (Conventional Units × 1)
Cord blood	5–65 ng/mL	5–65 μg/L
1 d	6–93 ng/mL	6–93 μg/L
10 d	9–148 ng/mL	9–148 μg/L
Premature infant		
1 d	107–395 ng/mL	107–395 μg/L
3 d	49–163 ng/mL	49–163 μg/L
1 m	17–63 ng/mL	17–63 μg/L
7–12 y	20–50 ng/mL	20–50 μg/L
12–18 y	9–27 ng/mL	9–27 μg/L
Adult	0–50 ng/mL	0–50 μg/L

DESCRIPTION & RATIONALE: Thyroglobulin is an iodinated glycoprotein secreted by follicular epithelial cells of the thyroid gland. It is the storage form of the thyroid hormones thyroxine (T_4) and triiodothyronine (T_3). When thyroid hormones are released into the bloodstream, they split from thyroglobulin in response to thyroid-stimulating hormone. Values greater than 55 ng/mL are indicative of tumor recurrence in athyrotic patients. ■

INDICATIONS:
- Assist in the diagnosis of subacute thyroiditis
- Assist in the diagnosis of suspected disorders of excess thyroid hormone

- Management of differentiated or metastatic cancer of the thyroid
- Monitor response to treatment of goiter
- Monitor T_4 therapy in patients with solitary nodules

RESULT

Increased in:
- Differentiated thyroid cancer
- Graves' disease (untreated)
- Neonates
- Pregnancy
- Surgery or irradiation of the thyroid (elevated levels indicate residual or disseminated carcinoma)
- T_4-binding globulin deficiency
- Thyroiditis
- Thyrotoxicosis

Decreased in:
- Administration of thyroid hormone
- Congenital athyrosis (neonates)
- Thyrotoxicosis factitia

CRITICAL VALUES: N/A

INTERFERING FACTORS:
- Drugs that may decrease thyroglobulin levels include neomycin and T_4.
- Autoantibodies to thyroglobulin can cause decreased values.
- Recent thyroid surgery or needle biopsy can interfere with test results.

Nursing Implications and Procedure . . . .

Pretest:
➤ Inform the patient that the test is used to evaluate thyroid gland function.

➤ Obtain a history of the patient's complaints, including a list of known allergens (especially allergies or sensitivities to latex), and inform the appropriate health care practitioner accordingly.

➤ Obtain a history of the patient's endocrine system as well as results of previously performed laboratory tests, surgical procedures, and other diagnostic procedures. For related laboratory tests, refer to the Endocrine System table.

➤ Obtain a list of medications the patient is taking, including herbs, nutritional supplements, and nutraceuticals. The requesting health care practitioner and laboratory should be advised if the patient is regularly using these products so that their effects can be taken into consideration when reviewing results.

➤ Review the procedure with the patient. Inform the patient that specimen collection takes approximately 5 to 10 minutes. Address concerns about pain related to the procedure. Explain to the patient that there may be some discomfort during the venipuncture.

➤ There are no food, fluid, or medication restrictions, unless by medical direction.

Intratest:

➤ If the patient has a history of severe allergic reaction to latex, care should be taken to avoid the use of equipment containing latex.

➤ Instruct the patient to cooperate fully and to follow directions. Direct the patient to breathe normally and to avoid unnecessary movement.

➤ Observe standard precautions, and follow the general guidelines in Appendix A. Positively identify the patient, and label the appropriate tubes with the corresponding patient demographics, date, and time of collection. Perform a venipuncture; collect the specimen in a 5-mL red- or tiger-top tube.

➤ Remove the needle, and apply a pressure dressing over the puncture site.

➤ Promptly transport the specimen to the laboratory for processing and analysis.

➤ The results are recorded manually or in a computerized system for recall and postprocedure interpretation by the appropriate health care practitioner.

Post-test:

➤ Observe venipuncture site for bleeding or hematoma formation. Apply paper tape or other adhesive to hold pressure bandage in place, or replace with a plastic bandage.

➤ A written report of the examination will be sent to the requesting health care practitioner, who will discuss the results with the patient.

➤ Reinforce information given by the patient's health care provider regarding further testing, treatment, or referral to another health care provider. Answer any questions or address any concerns voiced by the patient or family.

➤ Depending on the results of this procedure, additional testing may be performed to evaluate or monitor progression of the disease process and determine the need for a change in therapy. Evaluate test results in relation to the patient's symptoms and other tests performed.

Related laboratory tests:

➤ Related laboratory tests include T_4, free T_4, T_3, free T_3, and thyroid-stimulating hormone.

THYROID-BINDING INHIBITORY IMMUNOGLOBULIN

· ·

SYNONYMS/ACRONYM: Thyrotropin receptor antibodies, thyrotropin-binding inhibitory immunoglobulin, TBII.

SPECIMEN: Serum (1 mL) collected in a red-top tube.

REFERENCE VALUE: (Method: Radioreceptor) Less than 10% inhibition. (*Note:* In patients with Graves' disease, inhibition is expected to be 10% to 100%.)

DESCRIPTION & RATIONALE: There are two functional types of thyroid receptor immunoglobulins: *thyroid-stimulating immunoglobulin (TSI)* and *thyroid-binding inhibitory immuno-* *globulin (TBII)*. TSI reacts with the receptors, activates intracellular enzymes, and promotes epithelial cell activity that operates outside the feedback regulation for thyroid-stimulating hormone (TSH) (see monograph titled "Thyroid-Stimulating Immunoglobulin"); TBII blocks the action of TSH and is believed to cause certain types of hyperthyroidism. These antibodies were formerly known as *long-acting thyroid stimulators.* High levels in pregnancy may have some predictive value for neonatal thyrotoxicosis: A positive result indicates that the antibodies are stimulating (TSI); a negative result indicates that the antibodies are blocking (TBII). TBII testing measures thyroid receptor immunoglobulin levels in the evaluation of thyroid disease. ■

INDICATIONS:
- Evaluate suspected acute toxic goiter
- Investigate suspected neonatal thyroid disease secondary to maternal thyroid disease
- Monitor hyperthyroid patients at risk for relapse or remission

RESULT

Increased in:
- Graves' disease
- Hyperthyroidism (various forms)
- Maternal thyroid disease
- Neonatal thyroid disease
- Toxic goiter

Decreased in: N/A

CRITICAL VALUES: N/A

INTERFERING FACTORS:
- Lithium may cause false-positive results.
- Recent radioactive scans or radiation within 1 week before the test can interfere with test results when radioimmunoassay is the test method.

Nursing Implications and Procedure • • • • • • • • • •

Pretest:

➤ Inform the patient that the test is used to evaluate thyroid gland function.

➤ Obtain a history of the patient's complaints, including a list of known allergens (especially allergies or sensitivities to latex), and inform the appropriate health care practitioner accordingly.

➤ Obtain a history of the patient's endocrine system as well as results of previously performed laboratory tests, surgical procedures, and other diagnostic procedures. For related laboratory tests, refer to the Endocrine System table.

➤ Note any recent procedures that can interfere with test results.

➤ Obtain a list of medications the patient is taking, including herbs, nutritional supplements, and nutraceuticals. The requesting health care practitioner and laboratory should be advised if the patient regularly uses these products so that their effects can be taken into consideration when reviewing results.

➤ Review the procedure with the patient. Inform the patient that specimen collection takes approximately 5 to 10 minutes. Address concerns about pain related to the procedure. Explain to the patient that there may be some discomfort during the venipuncture.

➤ There are no food, fluid, or medication restrictions, unless by medical direction.

Intratest:

➤ If the patient has a history of severe allergic reaction to latex, care should be taken to avoid the use of equipment containing latex.

➤ Instruct the patient to cooperate fully and to follow directions. Direct the

patient to breathe normally and to avoid unnecessary movement.

➤ Observe standard precautions, and follow the general guidelines in Appendix A. Positively identify the patient, and label the appropriate tubes with the corresponding patient demographics, date, and time of collection. Perform a venipuncture; collect the specimen in a 5-mL red-top tube.

➤ Remove the needle, and apply a pressure dressing over the puncture site.

➤ Promptly transport the specimen to the laboratory for processing and analysis.

➤ The results are recorded manually or in a computerized system for recall and postprocedure interpretation by the appropriate health care practitioner.

hold pressure bandage in place, or replace with a plastic bandage.

➤ A written report of the examination will be sent to the requesting health care practitioner, who will discuss the results with the patient.

➤ Reinforce information given by the patient's health care provider regarding further testing, treatment, or referral to another health care provider. Answer any questions or address any concerns voiced by the patient or family.

➤ Depending on the results of this procedure, additional testing may be performed to evaluate or monitor progression of the disease process and determine the need for a change in therapy. Evaluate test results in relation to the patient's symptoms and other tests performed.

Post-test:

➤ Observe venipuncture site for bleeding or hematoma formation. Apply paper tape or other adhesive to

Related laboratory tests:

➤ Related laboratory tests include thyroid-stimulating hormone (TSH) and thyroid-stimulating immunoglobulins.

THYROID SCAN

SYNONYMS/ACRONYM: Thyroid scintiscan, iodine thyroid scan, technetium thyroid scan.

AREA OF APPLICATION: Thyroid.

CONTRAST: Oral radioactive iodine or intravenous technetium-99m pertechnetate.

DESCRIPTION & RATIONALE: The thyroid scan is a nuclear medicine study performed to assess thyroid size, shape, position, and function; it is useful for evaluating thyroid nodules, multinodular goiter, and thyroiditis;

assisting in the differential diagnosis of masses in the neck, base of the tongue, and mediastinum; and ruling out possible ectopic thyroid tissue in these areas. Thyroid scanning is performed after oral administration of radioactive iodine-123 (I-123) or I-131, or intravenous (IV) injection of technetium-99m (Tc-99m). Increased or decreased uptake by the thyroid gland and surrounding area and tissue is noted: Areas of increased radionuclide uptake ("hot spots") are caused by hyperfunctioning thyroid nodules, which are usually nonmalignant; areas of decreased uptake ("cold spots") are caused by hypofunctioning nodules, which are more likely to be malignant. Ultrasound imaging may be used to determine if the cold spot is a solid, semicystic lesion or a pure cyst (cysts are rarely cancerous). To determine whether the cold spot depicts a malignant neoplasm, however, a biopsy must be performed. ∎

INDICATIONS:

- Assess palpable nodules and differentiate between a benign tumor or cyst and a malignant tumor
- Assess the presence of a thyroid nodule or enlarged thyroid gland
- Detect benign or malignant thyroid tumors
- Detect causes of neck or substernal masses
- Detect forms of thyroiditis (e.g., acute, chronic, Hashimoto's)
- Detect thyroid dysfunction
- Differentiate between Graves' disease and Plummer's disease, both of which cause hyperthyroidism
- Evaluate thyroid function in hyperthyroidism and hypothyroidism (analysis combined with interpretation of laboratory tests, thyroid function panel including thyroxine and triiodothyronine, and thyroid uptake tests)

RESULT

Normal Findings:

- Normal size, contour, position, and function of the thyroid gland with homogeneous uptake of the radionuclide

Abnormal Findings:

- Adenoma
- Cysts
- Fibrosis
- Goiter
- Graves' disease (diffusely enlarged, hyperfunctioning gland)
- Hematoma
- Metastasis
- Plummer's disease (nodular hyperfunctioning gland)
- Thyroiditis (Hashimoto's)
- Thyrotoxicosis
- Tumors, benign or malignant

CRITICAL VALUES: N/A

INTERFERING FACTORS:

This procedure is contraindicated for:

- Patients who are pregnant or suspected of being pregnant, unless the potential benefits of the procedure far outweigh the risks to the fetus or mother

Factors that may impair clear imaging:

- Inability of the patient to cooperate or remain still during the procedure because of age, significant pain, or mental status

- Improper adjustment of the radiographic equipment to accommodate obese or thin patients, which can cause overexposure or underexposure and a poor-quality study

- Patients who are very obese, who may exceed the weight limit for the equipment

- Incorrect positioning of the patient, which may produce poor visualization of the area to be examined

- Other nuclear scans done within the previous 24 to 48 hours

- Ingestion of foods containing iodine (iodized salt) or medications containing iodine (cough syrup, potassium iodide, vitamins, Lugol's solution, thyroid replacement medications), which can decrease the uptake of the radionuclide

- Antithyroid medications (propylthiouracil), corticosteroids, antihistamines, warfarin, sulfonamides, nitrates, corticosteroids, thyroid hormones, and isoniazid, which can decrease the uptake of the radionuclide

- Increased uptake of iodine in persons with an iodine-deficient diet or who are on phenothiazine therapy

- Vomiting and severe diarrhea, which can affect absorption of orally administered radionuclide

- Gastroenteritis, which can interfere with absorption of orally administered radionuclide

- Metallic objects within the examination field (e.g., jewelry, body rings), which may inhibit organ visualization and can produce unclear images

Other considerations:

- Improper injection of the radionuclide that allows the tracer to seep deep into the muscle tissue can produce erroneous hot spots.

- Recent use of iodinated contrast medium for radiographic studies or recently performed nuclear medicine procedures can affect the uptake of the radionuclide.

- Consultation with a health care practitioner should occur before the procedure for radiation safety concerns regarding younger patients or patients who are lactating.

- Risks associated with radiographic overexposure can result from frequent x-ray procedures. Personnel in the room with the patient should wear a protective lead apron, stand behind a shield, or leave the area while the examination is being done. Personnel working in the area where the examination is being done should wear badges that reveal their level of exposure to radiation.

Nursing Implications and Procedure • • • • • • • • • • •

Pretest:

➤ Inform the patient that the procedure assesses thyroid function and structure.

➤ Obtain a history of the patient's complaints and symptoms, including a list of known allergens.

➤ Obtain a history of the patient's endocrine system, as well as results of previously performed laboratory tests, surgical procedures, and other diagnostic procedures. For related diagnostic tests, refer to the Endocrine System table.

➤ All thyroid blood tests should be done before doing this test.

➤ All radiographic procedures done with iodinated contrast medium should be scheduled after this procedure and after radioactive iodine uptake is completed.

➤ Record the date of the last menstrual period and determine the possibility of pregnancy in perimenopausal women.

➤ Obtain a list of the patient's current medications.

> Review the procedure with the patient. Address concerns about pain related to the procedure. Explain to the patient that some pain may be experienced during the test, and there may be moments of discomfort. Explain the purpose of the test and how the procedure is performed. Inform the patient that the procedure is performed in a nuclear medicine department, usually by a technologist and support staff, and takes approximately 30 to 60 minutes.

> *Sensitivity to cultural and social issues,* as well as concern for modesty, is important in providing psychological support before, during, and after the procedure.

> Instruct the patient to remove dentures, jewelry (including watches), hairpins, credit cards, and other metallic objects.

> The patient should fast for 8 to 12 hours prior to the procedure.

> There are no fluid or medication restrictions, unless by medical direction.

Intratest:

> Ensure that the patient has complied with dietary restrictions and pretesting preparations; assure that food has been restricted for at least 8 to 12 hours. Ensure that the patient has removed all external metallic objects (jewelry, dentures, etc.) prior to the procedure.

> Patients are given a gown, robe, and foot coverings to wear and instructed to void prior to the procedure.

> Instruct the patient to cooperate fully and to follow directions. Ask the patient to lie still during the procedure because movement produces unclear images.

> Observe standard precautions, and follow the general guidelines in Appendix A.

> Administer sedative to a child or to an uncooperative adult, as ordered.

> Administer oral I-123 24 hours before scanning or IV technetium-99m 20 minutes before scanning. Place the patient in a supine position on a flat table. Scanning is performed over the anterior neck area.

> Wear gloves during the radionuclide administration and while handling the patient's urine.

> The results are recorded on film or by automated equipment in a computerized system for recall and postprocedure interpretation by the appropriate health care practitioner.

Post-test:

> Instruct the patient to resume usual diet, as directed by the health care practitioner.

> Advise the patient to drink increased amounts of fluids for 24 to 48 hours to eliminate the radionuclide from the body, unless contraindicated. Tell the patient that radionuclide is eliminated from the body within 6 to 24 hours.

> If a woman who is breast-feeding must have a nuclear scan, she should not breast-feed the infant until the radionuclide has been eliminated. This could take as long as 3 days. She should be instructed to express the milk and discard it during the 3-day period to prevent cessation of milk production.

> Instruct the patient to flush the toilet immediately after each voiding following the procedure, and to wash hands meticulously with soap and water after each voiding for 24 hours after the procedure.

> Tell all caregivers to wear gloves when discarding urine for 24 hours after the procedure. Wash gloved hands with soap and water before removing gloves. Then wash hands after the gloves are removed.

> A written report of the examination will be completed by a health care practitioner specializing in this branch of medicine. The report will be sent to the requesting health care practitioner, who will discuss the results with the patient.

> Depending on the results of this procedure, additional testing may be needed to evaluate or monitor pro-

gression of the disease process and determine the need for a change in therapy. Evaluate test results in relation to the patient's symptoms and other tests performed.

➤ Related diagnostic tests include radioactive iodine uptake and ultrasound of the thyroid.

THYROID-STIMULATING HORMONE

SYNONYM/ACRONYM: Thyrotropin, TSH.

SPECIMEN: Serum (1 mL) collected in a red- or tiger-top tube; for a neonate, use filter paper.

REFERENCE VALUE: (Method: Immunoassay)

Age	Conventional Units	SI Units (Conventional Units × 1)
Neonates–3 d	Less than 20 µIU/mL	Less than 20 mIU/L
Adults	0.4–4.2 µIU/mL	0.4–4.2 mIU/L

DESCRIPTION & RATIONALE: Thyroid-stimulating hormone (TSH) is produced by the pituitary gland in response to stimulation by thyrotropin-releasing hormone (TRH), a hypothalamic-releasing factor. TRH regulates the release and circulating levels of thyroid hormones in response to variables such as cold, stress, and increased metabolic need. Thyroid and pituitary function can be evaluated by TSH measurement. TSH exhibits diurnal variation, peaking between midnight and 4 a.m. and troughing between 5 and 6 p.m. TSH values are high at birth but reach adult levels in the first week of life. Elevated TSH levels combined with decreased thyroxine (T_4) levels indicate hypothyroidism and thyroid gland dysfunction. In general, decreased TSH and T_4 levels indicate secondary congenital hypothyroidism and pituitary hypothalamic dysfunction. A normal TSH level and a depressed T_4 level may indicate (1) hypothyroidism owing to a congenital defect in T_4-binding globulin, or (2) transient congenital hypothyroidism owing to hypoxia or prematurity. Early diagnosis and treatment in the neonate are crucial for the prevention of cretinism and mental retardation. ∎

INDICATIONS:
- Assist in the diagnosis of congenital hypothyroidism
- Assist in the diagnosis of hypothy-

roidism or hyperthyroidism or suspected pituitary or hypothalamic dysfunction

- Differentiate functional euthyroidism from true hypothyroidism in debilitated individuals

RESULT

Increased in:
- Congenital hypothyroidism in the neonate (filter paper test)
- Ectopic TSH-producing tumors (lung, breast)
- Primary hypothyroidism
- Secondary hyperthyroidism owing to pituitary hyperactivity
- Thyroid hormone resistance
- Thyroiditis (Hashimoto's autoimmune disease)

Decreased in:
- Excessive thyroid hormone replacement
- Graves' disease
- Primary hyperthyroidism
- Secondary hypothyroidism (pituitary involvement)
- Tertiary hypothyroidism (hypothalamic involvement)

CRITICAL VALUES: N/A

INTERFERING FACTORS:
- Drugs and hormones that may increase TSH levels include amiodarone, benserazide, erythrosine, flunarizine (males), iobenzamic acid, iodides, lithium, methimazole, metoclopramide, morphine, propranolol, radiographic agents, TRH, and valproic acid.

- Drugs and hormones that may decrease TSH levels include acetylsalicylic acid, amiodarone, anabolic steroids, carbamazepine, corticosteroids, dopamine, glucocorticoids, hydrocortisone, insulin-like growth factor-I, interferon-alfa-2b, iodamide, josamycin, levodopa, levothyroxine, methergoline, nifedipine, pyridoxine, T_4, and triiodothyronine (T_3).

- Failure to let the filter paper sample dry may affect test results.

Nursing Implications and Procedure

Pretest:

▶ Inform the patient that the test is used to evaluate thyroid gland function.

▶ Obtain a history of the patient's complaints, including a list of known allergens (especially allergies or sensitivities to latex), and inform the appropriate health care practitioner accordingly.

▶ Obtain a history of the patient's endocrine system and results of previously performed laboratory tests, surgical procedures, and other diagnostic procedures. For related laboratory tests, refer to the Endocrine System table.

▶ Obtain a list of medications the patient is taking, including herbs, nutritional supplements, and nutraceuticals. The requesting health care practitioner and laboratory should be advised if the patient regularly uses these products so that their effects can be taken into consideration when reviewing results.

▶ Review the procedure with the patient. Inform the patient that specimen collection takes approximately 5 to 10 minutes. Address concerns about pain related to the procedure. Explain to the patient that there may be some discomfort during the venipuncture.

▶ There are no food, fluid, or medication restrictions, unless by medical direction.

Intratest:

> If the patient has a history of severe allergic reaction to latex, care should be taken to avoid the use of equipment containing latex.

> Instruct the patient to cooperate fully and to follow directions. Direct the patient to breathe normally and to avoid unnecessary movement.

> Observe standard precautions, and follow the general guidelines in Appendix A. Positively identify the patient, and label the appropriate tubes with the corresponding patient demographics, date, and time of collection. Perform a venipuncture; collect the specimen in a 5-mL red- or tiger-top tube.

> Remove the needle, and apply a pressure dressing over the puncture site.

> Promptly transport the specimen to the laboratory for processing and analysis.

> The results are recorded manually or in a computerized system for recall and postprocedure interpretation by the appropriate health care practitioner.

Filter paper test (neonate):

> Obtain kit and cleanse heel with antiseptic. Observe standard precautions, and follow the general guidelines in Appendix A. Use gauze to dry the stick area completely. Perform heel stick, gently squeeze infant's heel, and touch filter paper to the puncture site. Completely fill the circles on the filter paper, saturating the filter paper with blood.

Apply pressure to the heel stick with a gauze pad to stop the bleeding. Allow the filter paper to dry thoroughly, label the specimen, and promptly transport it to the laboratory. Alternatively, if a specimen collection kit is used, follow instructions for labeling and mailing to the testing laboratory.

Post-test:

> Observe venipuncture site for bleeding or hematoma formation. Apply paper tape or other adhesive to hold pressure bandage in place, or replace with a plastic bandage.

> A written report of the examination will be sent to the requesting health care practitioner, who will discuss the results with the patient.

> Reinforce information given by the patient's health care provider regarding further testing, treatment, or referral to another health care provider. Answer any questions or address any concerns voiced by the patient or family.

> Depending on the results of this procedure, additional testing may be performed to evaluate or monitor progression of the disease process and determine the need for a change in therapy. Evaluate test results in relation to the patient's symptoms and other tests performed.

Related laboratory tests:

> Related laboratory tests include adrenocorticotropic hormone, TRH stimulation test, T_4, free T_4, and T_3.

THYROID-STIMULATING IMMUNOGLOBULIN

SYNONYM/ACRONYM: Thyrotropin-receptor antibodies, TSI.

SPECIMEN: Serum (1 mL) collected in a red-top tube.

REFERENCE VALUE: (Method: Animal cell transfection with luciferase marker) Less than 130% of basal activity.

DESCRIPTION & RATIONALE: There are two functional types of thyroid receptor immunoglobulins: *thyroid-stimulating immunoglobulin (TSI)* and *thyroid-binding inhibitory immunoglobulin (TBII)*. TSI reacts with the receptors, activates intracellular enzymes, and promotes epithelial cell activity that operates outside the feedback regulation for thyroid-stimulating hormone (TSH); TBII blocks the action of TSH and is believed to cause certain types of hyperthyroidism (see monograph titled "Thyroid-Binding Immunoglobulin"). These antibodies were formerly known as *long-acting thyroid stimulators*. High levels in pregnancy may have some predictive value for neonatal thyrotoxicosis: A positive result indicates that the antibodies are stimulating (TSI); a negative result indicates that the antibodies are blocking (TBII). TSI testing measures thyroid receptor immunoglobulin levels in the evaluation of thyroid disease. ■

INDICATIONS:
• Follow-up to positive TBII assay in differentiating antibody stimulation from neutral or suppressing activity

• Monitor hyperthyroid patients at risk for relapse or remission

RESULT

Increased in: Graves' disease

Decreased in: N/A

CRITICAL VALUES: N/A

INTERFERING FACTORS:
• Lithium may cause false-positive TBII results.

Nursing Implications and Procedure

Pretest:

▶ Inform the patient that the test is used to evaluate thyroid gland function.

▶ Obtain a history of the patient's complaints, including a list of known allergens (especially allergies or sensitivities to latex), and inform the appropriate health care practitioner accordingly.

▶ Obtain a history of the patient's endocrine system as well as results of previously performed laboratory tests, surgical procedures, and other diagnostic procedures. For related laboratory tests, refer to the Endocrine System table.

➤ Obtain a list of medications the patient is taking, including herbs, nutritional supplements, and nutraceuticals. The requesting health care practitioner and laboratory should be advised if the patient regularly uses these products so that their effects can be taken into consideration when reviewing results.

➤ Review the procedure with the patient. Inform the patient that specimen collection takes approximately 5 to 10 minutes. Address concerns about pain related to the procedure. Explain to the patient that there may be some discomfort during the venipuncture.

➤ There are no food, fluid, or medication restrictions, unless by medical direction.

Intratest:

➤ If the patient has a history of severe allergic reaction to latex, care should be taken to avoid the use of equipment containing latex.

➤ Instruct the patient to cooperate fully and to follow directions. Direct the patient to breathe normally and to avoid unnecessary movement.

➤ Observe standard precautions, and follow the general guidelines in Appendix A. Positively identify the patient, and label the appropriate tubes with the corresponding patient demographics, date, and time of collection. Perform a venipuncture; collect the specimen in a 5-mL red-top tube.

➤ Remove the needle, and apply a pressure dressing over the puncture site.

➤ Promptly transport the specimen to the laboratory for processing and analysis.

➤ The results are recorded manually or in a computerized system for recall and postprocedure interpretation by the appropriate health care practitioner.

Post-test:

➤ Observe venipuncture site for bleeding or hematoma formation. Apply paper tape or other adhesive to hold pressure bandage in place, or replace with a plastic bandage.

➤ A written report of the examination will be sent to the requesting health care practitioner, who will discuss the results with the patient.

➤ Reinforce information given by the patient's health care provider regarding further testing, treatment, or referral to another health care provider. Answer any questions or address any concerns voiced by the patient or family.

➤ Depending on the results of this procedure, additional testing may be performed to evaluate or monitor progression of the disease process and determine the need for a change in therapy. Evaluate test results in relation to the patient's symptoms and other tests performed.

Related laboratory tests:

➤ Related laboratory tests include thyroglobulin, thyroid-binding inhibitory immunoglobulin, and TSH.

THYROTROPIN-RELEASING HORMONE STIMULATION TEST

· ·

SYNONYM/ACRONYM: TRH stimulation.

SPECIMEN: Serum (1 mL) collected in a red- or tiger-top tube.

REFERENCE VALUE: (Method: Immunoassay) Minimal rise of 1 to 2 mIU/L above baseline; typical response is a 5- to 10-fold increase above baseline.

DESCRIPTION & RATIONALE: In the thyrotropin-releasing hormone (TRH) stimulation test, TRH is administered intravenously after collection of a baseline measurement of thyroid-stimulating hormone (TSH). Subsequent specimens are collected for TSH measurement at 30- and 60-minute intervals. An exaggerated response is an indication of abnormal thyroid gland function or disorders of the hypothalamic pituitary axis. Third-generation or "sensitive" TSH assays are now preferred over TRH stimulation. ■

INDICATIONS:

- Assist in the diagnosis and treatment of hypothalamic and pituitary disorders

- Differentiation of mania from schizophrenia

RESULT

Increased in:

- Pregnancy

- Primary hypothyroidism

Decreased in:

- Major depressive illnesses

- Primary hyperthyroidism

- Secondary hypothyroidism

CRITICAL VALUES: N/A

INTERFERING FACTORS: N/A

Nursing Implications and Procedure · · · · · · · · · · ·

Pretest:

➤ Inform the patient that the test is used to evaluate thyroid gland function.

➤ Obtain a history of the patient's complaints, including a list of known allergens (especially allergies or sensitivities to latex), and inform the appropriate health care practitioner accordingly.

➤ Obtain a history of the patient's endocrine system and results of previously performed laboratory tests, surgical procedures, and other diagnostic procedures. For related laboratory tests, refer to the Endocrine System table.

➤ Obtain a list of medications the patient is taking, including herbs, nutritional supplements, and nutraceuticals. The requesting health care practitioner and laboratory should be advised if the patient regularly uses these products so that their effects can be taken into consideration when reviewing results.

➤ Review the procedure with the patient. The test should be performed in the morning because of the diurnal variation in TSH secretion. Inform the patient that multiple specimens will be collected. Inform the patient that specimen collection takes approximately 5 to 10 minutes. Address concerns about pain related to the procedure. Explain to the patient that there may be some discomfort during the venipuncture.

➤ There are no food, fluid, or medication restrictions, unless by medical direction.

Intratest:

➤ If the patient has a history of severe allergic reaction to latex, care should be taken to avoid the use of equipment containing latex.

➤ Have emergency equipment readily available.

➤ Inform the patient that he or she may experience temporary nausea (mild), flushing, dizziness, peculiar taste, rise in blood pressure, and an urge to urinate as the infusion begins.

➤ Instruct the patient to cooperate fully and to follow directions. Direct the patient to breathe normally and to avoid unnecessary movement.

➤ Observe standard precautions, and follow the general guidelines in Appendix A. Positively identify the patient, and label the appropriate tubes with the corresponding patient demographics, date, and time of collection. Perform a venipuncture; collect the specimen in a 5-mL red- or tiger-top tube.

➤ Remove the needle, and apply a pressure dressing over the puncture site.

➤ Begin intravenous infusion of 500 µg of protirelin (Thypinone), and collect specimens at 30- and 60-minute intervals.

➤ Monitor the patient's blood pressure if dizziness or other unusual symptoms are reported.

➤ Promptly transport the specimens to the laboratory for processing and analysis.

➤ The results are recorded manually or in a computerized system for recall and postprocedure interpretation by the appropriate health care practitioner.

Post-test:

➤ Observe venipuncture site for bleeding or hematoma formation. Apply paper tape or other adhesive to hold pressure bandage in place, or replace with a plastic bandage.

➤ A written report of the examination will be sent to the requesting health care practitioner, who will discuss the results with the patient.

➤ Reinforce information given by the patient's health care provider regarding further testing, treatment, or referral to another health care provider. Answer any questions or address any concerns voiced by the patient or family.

➤ Depending on the results of this procedure, additional testing may be performed to evaluate or monitor progression of the disease process and determine the need for a change in therapy. Evaluate test results in relation to the patient's symptoms and other tests performed.

Related laboratory tests:

➤ Related laboratory tests include adrenocorticotropin hormone, follicle-stimulating hormone, growth hormone, luteinizing hormone, thyroxine, and free thyroxine.

THYROXINE-BINDING GLOBULIN

SYNONYM/ACRONYM: TBG.

SPECIMEN: Serum (1 mL) collected in a red- or tiger-top tube.

REFERENCE VALUE: (Method: Immunochemiluminometric assay [ICMA])

Age	Conventional Units	SI Units (Conventional Units × 10)
0–1 wk	3–8 mg/dL	30–80 mg/L
1–12 mo	1.6–3.6 mg/dL	16–36 mg/L
14 y–adult	1.2–2.5 mg/dL	12–25 mg/L
Adult	1.3–3.3 mg/dL	13–33 mg/L
Pregnancy, third trimester	4.7–5.9 mg/dL	47–59 mg/L
Oral contraceptives	1.5–5.5 mg/dL	15–55 mg/L

DESCRIPTION & RATIONALE:
Thyroxine-binding globulin (TBG) is the predominant protein carrier for circulating thyroxine (T_4) and triiodothyronine (T_3). T_4-binding prealbumin and T_4-binding albumin are the other transport proteins. Conditions that affect TBG levels and binding capacity also affect free T_3 and free T_4 levels. ■

INDICATIONS:
- Differentiate elevated T_4 due to hyperthyroidism from increased TBG binding in euthyroid patients
- Evaluate hypothyroid patients
- Identify deficiency of or excess TBG due to hereditary abnormality

RESULT

Increased in:
- Acute intermittent porphyria
- Genetically high TBG
- Hypothyroidism
- Infectious hepatitis and other liver diseases
- Neonates
- Pregnancy

Decreased in:
- Acromegaly
- Chronic hepatic disease
- Genetically low TBG
- Major illness
- Marked hypoproteinemia, malnutrition
- Nephrotic syndrome
- Ovarian hypofunction
- Surgical stress
- Testosterone-producing tumors

CRITICAL VALUES: N/A

INTERFERING FACTORS:
- Drugs and hormones that may increase TBG levels include estrogens, oral contraceptives, perphenazine, and tamoxifen.

- Drugs that may decrease TBG levels include anabolic steroids, androgens, asparaginase, corticosteroids, corticotropin, danazol, phenytoin, and propranolol.

Nursing Implications and Procedure • • • • • • • • • • •

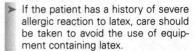

Pretest:

➤ Inform the patient that the test is used to evaluate thyroid gland function.

➤ Obtain a history of the patient's complaints, including a list of known allergens (especially allergies or sensitivities to latex), and inform the appropriate health care practitioner accordingly.

➤ Obtain a history of the patient's endocrine system as well as results of previously performed laboratory tests, surgical procedures, and other diagnostic procedures. For related laboratory tests, refer to the Endocrine System table.

➤ Obtain a list of medications the patient is taking, including herbs, nutritional supplements, and nutraceuticals. The requesting health care practitioner and laboratory should be advised if the patient regularly uses these products so that their effects can be taken into consideration when reviewing results.

➤ Review the procedure with the patient. Inform the patient that specimen collection takes approximately 5 to 10 minutes. Address concerns about pain related to the procedure. Explain to the patient that there may be some discomfort during the venipuncture.

➤ There are no food, fluid, or medica-

tion restrictions, unless by medical direction.

Intratest:

➤ If the patient has a history of severe allergic reaction to latex, care should be taken to avoid the use of equipment containing latex.

➤ Instruct the patient to cooperate fully and to follow directions. Direct the patient to breathe normally and to avoid unnecessary movement.

➤ Observe standard precautions, and follow the general guidelines in Appendix A. Positively identify the patient, and label the appropriate tubes with the corresponding patient demographics, date, and time of collection. Perform a venipuncture; collect the specimen in a 5-mL red- or tiger-top tube.

➤ Remove the needle, and apply a pressure dressing over the puncture site.

➤ Promptly transport the specimen to the laboratory for processing and analysis.

➤ The results are recorded manually or in a computerized system for recall and postprocedure interpretation by the appropriate health care practitioner.

Post-test:

➤ Observe venipuncture site for bleeding or hematoma formation. Apply paper tape or other adhesive to hold pressure bandage in place, or replace with a plastic bandage.

➤ A written report of the examination will be sent to the requesting health care practitioner, who will discuss the results with the patient.

➤ Reinforce information given by the patient's health care provider regarding further testing, treatment, or referral to another health care provider. Answer any questions or address any concerns voiced by the patient or family.

➤ Depending on the results of this procedure, additional testing may be performed to evaluate or monitor progression of the disease process and determine the need for a change in therapy. Evaluate test results in relation to the patient's symptoms and other tests performed.

Related laboratory tests:

➤ Related laboratory tests include T_3, free T_3, T_4, and free T_4.

THYROXINE, FREE

SYNONYMS/ACRONYM: Free T_4, FT_4.

SPECIMEN: Serum (1 mL) collected in a red- or tiger-top tube. Plasma (1 mL) collected in green-top (heparin) tube is also acceptable.

REFERENCE VALUE: (Method: Immunoassay)

Age	Conventional Units	SI Units (Conventional Units × 12.9)
Newborn	0.8–2.8 ng/dL	10–36 pmol/L
1–12 mo	0.8–2.0 ng/dL	10–26 pmol/L
1–18 y	0.8–1.7 ng/dL	10–22 pmol/L
Adult	0.8–1.5 ng/dL	10–19 pmol/L

DESCRIPTION & RATIONALE: Thyroxine (T_4) is a hormone produced and secreted by the thyroid gland. Newborns are commonly tested for decreased T_4 levels by a filter paper method (see monograph titled "Thyroxine, Total"). Most T_4 in the serum (99.97%) is bound to thyroxine-binding globulin (TBG), prealbumin, and albumin. The remainder (0.03%) circulates as unbound or free T_4, which is the physiologically active form. Levels of free T_4 are proportional to levels of total T_4. The advantage of measuring free T_4 instead of total T_4 is that, unlike total T_4 measurements, free T_4 levels are not affected by fluctuations in TBG levels; as a result, free T_4 levels are considered the most accurate indicator of T_4 and its thyrometabolic activity. Free T_4 measurements are useful in evaluating thyroid disease when thyroid-stimulating hormone (TSH) levels alone provide insufficient information. Free T_4 and TSH levels are inversely proportional. Measurement of free T_4 is also recommended during treatment for hyperthyroidism, until symptoms have abated and levels have decreased into the normal range. ■

INDICATIONS:
- Evaluate signs of hypothyroidism or hyperthyroidism
- Monitor response to therapy for hypothyroidism or hyperthyroidism

RESULT

Increased in:
- Hyperthyroidism
- Hypothyroidism treated with T_4

Decreased in:
- Hypothyroidism
- Hypothyroidism treated with triiodothyronine (T_3)
- Pregnancy (late)

CRITICAL VALUES: N/A

INTERFERING FACTORS:
- Drugs that may increase free T_4 levels include acetylsalicylic acid, amiodarone, halofenate, heparin, iopanoic acid, levothyroxine, methimazole, and radiographic agents.
- Drugs that may decrease free T_4 levels include amiodarone, anabolic steroids, asparaginase, methadone, methimazole, oral contraceptives, and phenylbutazone.

Nursing Implications and Procedure • • • • • • • • • • •

Pretest:

> Inform the patient that the test is used to evaluate thyroid gland function.

> Obtain a history of the patient's complaints, including a list of known allergens (especially allergies or sensitivities to latex), and inform the appropriate health care practitioner accordingly.

> Obtain a history of the patient's endocrine system as well as results of previously performed laboratory tests, surgical procedures, and other diagnostic procedures. For related laboratory tests, refer to the Endocrine System table.

> Obtain a list of medications the patient is taking, including herbs, nutritional supplements, and nutraceuticals. The requesting health care practitioner and laboratory should be advised if the patient regularly uses these products so that their effects can be taken into consideration when reviewing results.

> Review the procedure with the patient. Inform the patient that specimen collection takes approximately 5 to 10 minutes. Address concerns about pain related to the procedure. Explain to the patient that there may be some discomfort during the venipuncture.

> There are no food, fluid, or medication restrictions, unless by medical direction.

Intratest:

> If the patient has a history of severe allergic reaction to latex, care should be taken to avoid the use of equipment containing latex.

> Instruct the patient to cooperate fully and to follow directions. Direct the patient to breathe normally and to avoid unnecessary movement.

> Observe standard precautions, and follow the general guidelines in Appendix A. Positively identify the patient, and label the appropriate tubes with the corresponding patient demographics, date, and time of collection. Perform a venipuncture; collect the specimen in a 5-mL red- or tiger-top tube.

> Remove the needle, and apply a pressure dressing over the puncture site.

➤ Promptly transport the specimen to the laboratory for processing and analysis.

➤ The results are recorded manually or in a computerized system for recall and postprocedure interpretation by the appropriate health care practitioner.

Post-test:

➤ Observe venipuncture site for bleeding or hematoma formation. Apply paper tape or other adhesive to hold pressure bandage in place, or replace with a plastic bandage.

➤ A written report of the examination will be sent to the requesting health care practitioner, who will discuss the results with the patient.

➤ Reinforce information given by the patient's health care provider regard-

ing further testing, treatment, or referral to another health care provider. Answer any questions or address any concerns voiced by the patient or family.

➤ Depending on the results of this procedure, additional testing may be performed to evaluate or monitor progression of the disease process and determine the need for a change in therapy. Evaluate test results in relation to the patient's symptoms and other tests performed.

Related laboratory tests:

➤ Related laboratory tests include antithyroglobulin and antithyroid peroxidase antibodies, thyroid-binding inhibitory immunoglobulin, thyroid-stimulating immunoglobulin, T_4, T_3, free T_3, and TSH.

THYROXINE, TOTAL

SYNONYMS/ACRONYM: T_4.

SPECIMEN: Serum (1 mL) collected in a red- or tiger-top tube. Plasma (1 mL) collected in green-top (heparin) tube is also acceptable.

REFERENCE VALUE: (Method: Immunoassay)

Age	Conventional Units	SI Units (Conventional Units × 12.9)
1–3 d	11.8–22.6 μg/dL	152–292 nmol/L
1–2 wk	9.8–16.6 μg/dL	126–214 nmol/L
1–4 mo	7.2–14.4 μg/dL	93–186 nmol/L
5–12 mo	7.8–16.5 μg/dL	101–213 nmol/L
1–5 y	7.3–15.0 μg/dL	94–194 nmol/L
5–10 y	6.4–13.3 μg/dL	83–172 nmol/L

Age	Conventional Units	SI Units (Conventional Units × 12.9)
10–15 y	5.6–11.7 μg/dL	72–151 nmol/L
Adult		
Man	4.6–10.5 μg/dL	59–135 nmol/L
Woman	5.5–11.0 μg/dL	71–142 nmol/L
Pregnant woman	5.5–16.0 μg/dL	71–155 nmol/L
Over 60 y	5.0–10.7 μg/dL	65–138 nmol/L

DESCRIPTION & RATIONALE: Thyroxine (T_4) is a hormone produced and secreted by the thyroid gland. Newborns are commonly tested for decreased T_4 levels by a filter paper method. Most T_4 in the serum (99.97%) is bound to thyroxine-binding globulin (TBG), prealbumin, and albumin. The remainder (0.03%) circulates as unbound or free T_4, which is the physiologically active form. Levels of free T_4 are proportional to levels of total T_4. The advantage of measuring free T_4 instead of total T_4 is that, unlike total T_4 measurements, free T_4 levels are not affected by fluctuations in TBG levels; as a result, free T_4 levels are considered the most accurate indicator of T_4 and its thyrometabolic activity (see monograph titled "Thyroxine, Free"). ■

INDICATIONS:
- Evaluate signs of hypothyroidism or hyperthyroidism and neonatal screening for congenital hypothyroidism (required in all 50 states)
- Evaluate thyroid response to protein deficiency associated with severe illnesses
- Monitor response to therapy for hypothyroidism or hyperthyroidism

RESULT

Increased in:
- Acute psychiatric illnesses
- Excessive intake of iodine
- Hepatitis
- Hyperemesis gravidarum
- Hyperthyroidism
- Obesity
- Thyrotoxicosis due to Graves' disease
- Thyrotoxicosis factitia

Decreased in:
- Decreased TBG (nephrotic syndrome, liver disease, gastrointestinal protein loss, malnutrition)
- Hypothyroidism
- Panhypopituitarism
- Strenuous exercise

CRITICAL VALUES:
Hypothyroidism: Less than 2.0 μg/dL
Hyperthyroidism: Greater than 20.0 μg/dL
Note and immediately report to the health care practitioner any critically increased or decreased values and related symptoms.
At levels less than 2.0 μg/dL, the patient is at risk for myxedema

coma. Signs and symptoms of severe hypothyroidism include hypothermia, hypotension, bradycardia, hypoventilation, lethargy, and coma. Possible interventions include airway support, hourly monitoring for neurologic function and blood pressure, and administration of intravenous thyroid hormone.

At levels greater than 20.0 μg/dL, the patient is at risk for thyroid storm. Signs and symptoms of severe hyperthyroidism include hyperthermia, diaphoresis, vomiting, dehydration, and shock. Possible interventions include supportive treatment for shock, fluid and electrolyte replacement for dehydration, and administration of antithyroid drugs (propylthiouracil and Lugol's solution).

INTERFERING FACTORS:

• Drugs that may increase T_4 levels include amiodarone, amphetamines, corticosteroids, ether, fluorouracil, glucocorticoids, halofenate, insulin, iobenzamic acid, iopanoic acid, ipodate, levarterenol, levodopa, levothyroxine, opiates, oral contraceptives, phenothiazine, and prostaglandins.

• Drugs, substances, and treatments that may decrease T_4 levels include acetylsalicylic acid, aminoglutethimide, aminosalicylic acid, amiodarone, anabolic steroids, anticonvulsants, asparaginase, barbiturates, carbimazole, chlorpromazine, chlorpropamide, cholestyramine, clofibrate, cobalt, colestipol, corticotropin, cortisone, cotrimoxazole, cytostatic therapy, danazol, dehydroepiandrosterone, dexamethasone, diazepam, diazo dyes (e.g., Evans blue), dinitrophenol, ethionamide, fenclofenac, halofenate, hydroxyphenylpyruvic acid, interferon alfa-2b, iothiouracil, iron, isotretinoin, liothyronine, lithium, lovastatin, methimazole, methylthiouracil, mitotane, norethindrone, penicillamine, penicillin, phenylacetic acid derivatives, phenylbutazone, potassium iodide, propylthiouracil, reserpine, salicylate, sodium nitroprusside, stanozolol, sulfonylureas, tetrachlorothyronine, tolbutamide, and triiodothyronine (T_3).

Nursing Implications and Procedure . . . .

Pretest:

➤ Inform the patient that the test is used to evaluate thyroid gland function.

➤ Obtain a history of the patient's complaints, including a list of known allergens (especially allergies or sensitivities to latex), and inform the appropriate health care practitioner accordingly.

➤ Obtain a history of the patient's endocrine system and results of previously performed laboratory tests, surgical procedures, and other diagnostic procedures. For related laboratory tests, refer to the Endocrine System table.

➤ Obtain a list of medications the patient is taking, including herbs, nutritional supplements, and nutraceuticals. The requesting health care practitioner and laboratory should be advised if the patient regularly uses these products so that their effects can be taken into consideration when reviewing results.

➤ Review the procedure with the patient. Inform the patient that specimen collection takes approximately 5 to 10 minutes. Address concerns about pain related to the procedure. Explain to the patient that there may be some discomfort during the venipuncture.

➤ There are no food, fluid, or medication restrictions, unless by medical direction.

Intratest:

➤ If the patient has a history of severe allergic reaction to latex, care should be taken to avoid the use of equipment containing latex.

➤ Instruct the patient to cooperate fully and to follow directions. Direct the patient to breathe normally and to avoid unnecessary movement.

➤ Observe standard precautions, and follow the general guidelines in Appendix A. Positively identify the patient, and label the appropriate tubes with the corresponding patient demographics, date, and time of collection. Perform a venipuncture; collect the specimen in a 5-mL red- or tiger-top tube.

➤ Remove the needle, and apply a pressure dressing over the puncture site.

➤ Promptly transport the specimen to the laboratory for processing and analysis.

➤ The results are recorded manually or in a computerized system for recall and postprocedure interpretation by the appropriate health care practitioner.

Post-test:

➤ Observe venipuncture site for bleeding or hematoma formation. Apply paper tape or other adhesive to hold pressure bandage in place, or replace with a plastic bandage.

➤ A written report of the examination will be sent to the requesting health care practitioner, who will discuss the results with the patient.

➤ Reinforce information given by the patient's health care provider regarding further testing, treatment, or referral to another health care provider. Answer any questions or address any concerns voiced by the patient or family.

➤ Depending on the results of this procedure, additional testing may be performed to evaluate or monitor progression of the disease process and determine the need for a change in therapy. Evaluate test results in relation to the patient's symptoms and other tests performed.

Related laboratory tests:

➤ Related laboratory tests include adrenocorticotropic hormone, antithyroglobulin and antithyroid peroxidase antibodies, thyroid-binding inhibitory immunoglobulin, thyroid-stimulating hormone, thyroid-stimulating immunoglobulin, thyroxine-binding globulin, T_3, free T_3, and free T_4.

TOXOPLASMA ANTIBODY

SYNONYMS/ACRONYM: Toxoplasmosis serology, toxoplasmosis titer.

SPECIMEN: Serum (1 mL) collected in a red-top tube.

REFERENCE VALUE: (Method: Indirect fluorescent antibody) Negative or less than a fourfold increase in titer.

DESCRIPTION & RATIONALE: Toxoplasmosis is a severe, generalized granulomatous central nervous system disease caused by the protozoan *Toxoplasma gondii.* Transmission to humans occurs by ingesting undercooked meat or handling contaminated matter such as cat litter. Immunoglobulin (Ig) M antibodies develop approximately 5 days after infection and can remain elevated for 3 weeks to several months. IgG antibodies develop 1 to 2 weeks after infection and can remain elevated for months or years. *Toxoplasma* serology is part of the TORCH (*to*xoplasmosis, *r*ubella, *c*ytomegalovirus, and *h*erpes simplex type 2) panel routinely performed on pregnant women. Fetal infection during the first trimester can cause spontaneous abortion or congenital defects. Immunocompromised individuals are also at high risk for serious complications if infected. The presence of IgM antibodies indicates acute or congenital infection; the presence of IgG antibodies indicates current or past infection. ■

INDICATIONS:

• Assist in establishing a diagnosis of toxoplasmosis

• Document past exposure or immunity

• Serologic screening during pregnancy

RESULT

Positive findings in: *Toxoplasma* infection

CRITICAL VALUES: N/A

INTERFERING FACTORS: N/A

Nursing Implications and Procedure

Pretest:

➤ Inform the patient that the test is used to assist in the diagnosis of toxoplasmosis and to document history of previous exposure or immunity.

➤ Obtain a history of the patient's complaints, including a list of known allergens (especially allergies or sensitivities to latex), and inform the appropriate health care practitioner accordingly.

➤ Obtain a history of exposure.

➤ Obtain a history of the patient's immune and reproductive systems, a history of other potential sources of exposure, and results of previously performed laboratory tests, surgical procedures, and other diagnostic procedures. For related laboratory tests, refer to the Immune and Reproductive System tables.

➤ Obtain a list of medications the patient is taking, including herbs, nutritional supplements, and nutraceuticals. The requesting health care practitioner and laboratory should be advised if the patient regularly uses these products so that their effects can be taken into consideration when reviewing results.

➤ Review the procedure with the patient. Inform the patient that several tests may be necessary to confirm the diagnosis. Any individual positive result should be repeated in 3 weeks to monitor a change in titer. Inform the patient that specimen collection takes approximately 5 to 10 minutes. Address concerns about pain related to the procedure. Explain to the patient that there may be some discomfort during the venipuncture.

➤ There are no food, fluid, or medication restrictions, unless by medical direction.

Intratest:

➤ If the patient has a history of severe allergic reaction to latex, care should be taken to avoid the use of equipment containing latex.

➤ Instruct the patient to cooperate fully and to follow directions. Direct the patient to breathe normally and to avoid unnecessary movement.

➤ Observe standard precautions, and follow the general guidelines in Appendix A. Positively identify the patient, and label the appropriate tubes with the corresponding patient demographics, date, and time of collection. Perform a venipuncture; collect the specimen in a 5-mL red-top tube.

➤ Remove the needle, and apply a

- pressure dressing over the puncture site.
- Promptly transport the specimen to the laboratory for processing and analysis.
- The results are recorded manually or in a computerized system for recall and postprocedure interpretation by the appropriate health care practitioner.

Post-test:

- Observe venipuncture site for bleeding or hematoma formation. Apply paper tape or other adhesive to hold pressure bandage in place, or replace with a plastic bandage.
- A written report of the examination will be sent to the requesting health care practitioner, who will discuss the results with the patient.
- Recognize anxiety related to test results, and provide emotional support if results are positive and the patient is pregnant and/or immunocompromised. Discuss the implications of abnormal test results on the patient's lifestyle. Provide teaching and information regarding the clinical

implications of the test results, as appropriate. Educate the patient regarding access to counseling services.

- Reinforce information given by the patient's health care provider regarding further testing, treatment, or referral to another health care provider. Instruct the patient in isolation precautions during time of communicability or contagion. Emphasize the need to return to have a convalescent blood sample taken in 3 weeks. Answer any questions or address any concerns voiced by the patient or family.
- Depending on the results of this procedure, additional testing may be performed to evaluate or monitor progression of the disease process and determine the need for a change in therapy. Evaluate test results in relation to the patient's symptoms and other tests performed.

Related laboratory tests:

- Related laboratory tests include cytomegalovirus, fetal fibronectin, and rubella.

TRANSFERRIN

SYNONYM/ACRONYM: Siderophilin, TRF.

SPECIMEN: Serum (1 mL) collected in a red- or tiger-top tube.

REFERENCE VALUE: (Method: Nephelometry)

Age	Conventional Units	SI Units (Conventional Units × 0.01)
Newborn	130–275 mg/dL	1.3–2.75 g/L
Adult		
Male	215–365 mg/dL	2.2–3.6 g/L
Female	250–380 mg/dL	2.5–3.8 g/L

DESCRIPTION & RATIONALE: Transferrin is a glycoprotein formed in the liver. It transports circulating iron obtained from dietary intake and red blood cell breakdown. Transferrin carries 50% to 70% of the body's iron; normally it is approximately one-third saturated. Inadequate transferrin levels can lead to impaired hemoglobin synthesis and anemia. Transferrin is subject to diurnal variation, and it is responsible for the variation in levels of serum iron throughout the day. (See monograph titled "Iron-Binding Capacity [Total], Transferrin, and Iron Saturation.") ■

INDICATIONS:

• Determine the iron-binding capacity of the blood
• Evaluate iron metabolism in iron-deficiency anemia
• Evaluate nutritional status
• Screen for hemochromatosis

RESULT

Increased in:
• Iron-deficiency anemia

Decreased in:
• Acute or chronic infection
• Cancer (especially of the gastrointestinal tract)
• Excessive protein loss from renal disease
• Hepatic damage
• Hereditary atransferrinemia
• Malnutrition

CRITICAL VALUES: N/A

INTERFERING FACTORS:

• Drugs that may increase transferrin levels include carbamazepine, danazol, mestranol, and oral contraceptives.

• Drugs that may decrease transferrin levels include cortisone and dextran.

• Transferrin levels are subject to diurnal variation and should be collected in the morning, when levels are highest.

• Failure to follow dietary restrictions before the procedure may cause the procedure to be canceled or repeated.

Nursing Implications and Procedure • • • • • • • • • • •

Pretest:

➤ Inform the patient that the test is primarily used to evaluate nutritional status (e.g., iron-deficiency anemia).

➤ Obtain a history of the patient's complaints, including a list of known allergens (especially allergies or sensitivities to latex), and inform the appropriate health care practitioner accordingly.

➤ Obtain a history of the patient's hematopoietic system and results of previously performed laboratory tests, surgical procedures, and other diagnostic procedures. For related laboratory tests, refer to the Hematopoietic System table.

➤ Obtain a list of medications the patient is taking, including herbs, nutritional supplements, and nutraceuticals. The requesting health care practitioner and laboratory should be advised if the patient regularly uses these products so that their effects can be taken into consideration when reviewing results.

➤ Review the procedure with the patient. Inform the patient that specimen collection takes approximately 5 to 10 minutes. Address concerns about pain related to the procedure. Explain to the patient that there may be some discomfort during the venipuncture.

➤ Instruct the patient to fast for at least 12 hours before specimen collection.

➤ There are no fluid or medication restrictions, unless by medical direction.

Intratest:

➤ Ensure that the patient has complied with dietary restrictions; assure that food has been restricted for at least 12 hours prior to the procedure.

➤ If the patient has a history of severe allergic reaction to latex, care should be taken to avoid the use of equipment containing latex.

➤ Instruct the patient to cooperate fully and to follow directions. Direct the patient to breathe normally and to avoid unnecessary movement.

➤ Observe standard precautions, and follow the general guidelines in Appendix A. Positively identify the patient, and label the appropriate tubes with the corresponding patient demographics, date, and time of collection. Perform a venipuncture; collect the specimen in a 5-mL red- or tiger-top tube.

➤ Remove the needle, and apply a pressure dressing over the puncture site.

➤ Promptly transport the specimen to the laboratory for processing and analysis.

➤ The results are recorded manually or in a computerized system for recall and postprocedure interpretation by the appropriate health care practitioner.

Post-test:

➤ Observe the venipuncture site for bleeding or hematoma formation. Apply paper tape or other adhesive to hold pressure bandage in place, or replace with a plastic bandage.

➤ Instruct the patient to resume usual diet, as directed by the health care practitioner.

➤ *Nutritional considerations:* Educate the patient with abnormal iron values that numerous factors affect the absorption of iron, enhancing or decreasing absorption regardless of the original content of the iron-containing dietary source. Consumption of large amounts of alcohol damages the intestine and allows increased absorption of iron. A high intake of calcium and ascorbic acid also increases iron absorption. Iron absorption after a meal is also increased by factors in meat, fish, or poultry. Iron absorption is decreased by the absence (gastric resection) or diminished presence (use of antacids) of gastric acid. Phytic acids from cereals, tannins from tea and coffee, oxalic acid from vegetables, and minerals such as copper, zinc, and manganese interfere with iron absorption.

➤ A written report of the examination will be sent to the requesting health care practitioner, who will discuss the results with the patient.

➤ Reinforce information given by the patient's health care provider regarding further testing, treatment, or referral to another health care provider. Answer any questions or address any concerns voiced by the patient or family.

➤ Depending on the results of this procedure, additional testing may be performed to evaluate or monitor progression of the disease process and determine the need for a change in therapy. Evaluate test results in relation to the patient's symptoms and other tests performed.

Related laboratory tests:

➤ Related laboratory tests include ferritin and iron/total iron-binding capacity.

TRIGLYCERIDES

SYNONYM/ACRONYM: Trigs, TG.

SPECIMEN: Serum (1 mL) collected in a red- or tiger-top tube. Plasma (1 mL) collected in green-top (heparin) tube is also acceptable.

REFERENCE VALUE: (Method: Spectrophotometry)

Age	Conventional Units	SI Units (Conventional Units × 0.0113)	Risk
0–9 y			
Male	30–100 mg/dL	0.34–1.13 mmol/L	
Female	35–110 mg/dL	0.40–1.24 mmol/L	
10–20 y			
Male	32–148 mg/dL	0.36–1.67 mmol/L	
Female	37–124 mg/dL	0.42–1.40 mmol/L	
Adult	Less than 150 mg/dL	Less than 1.70 mmol/L	Normal
	150–199 mg/dL	1.70–2.25 mmol/L	Borderline high
	200–499 mg/dL	2.26–5.64 mmol/L	High
	Greater than 500 mg/dL	Greater than 5.65 mmol/L	Very high

DESCRIPTION & RATIONALE: Triglycerides are a combination of three fatty acids and one glycerol molecule. They are necessary to provide energy for various metabolic processes. Excess triglycerides are stored in adipose tissue, and the fatty acids provide the raw materials needed for conversion to glucose (gluconeogenesis) or for direct use as an energy source. Although fatty acids originate in the diet, many are also derived from unused glucose and amino acids that the liver converts into stored energy. Triglyceride levels vary by age, sex, weight, and race:

Levels increase with age.

Levels are higher in men than in women (among women, those who take oral contraceptives have levels that are 20 to 40 mg/dL higher compared to those who do not).

Levels are higher in overweight and obese populations compared to those with normal weight.

Levels in African Americans are approximately 10 to 20 mg/dL lower compared to whites. ■

INDICATIONS:
- Evaluate known or suspected disorders associated with altered triglyceride levels
- Identify hyperlipoproteinemia (hyperlipidemia) in patients with a family history of the disorder
- Monitor the response to drugs known to alter triglyceride levels
- Screen adults who are either over 40 years of age or obese to estimate the risk for atherosclerotic cardiovascular disease

RESULT

Increased in:
- Acute myocardial infarction
- Alcoholism
- Anorexia nervosa
- Chronic ischemic heart disease
- Cirrhosis
- Glycogen storage disease
- Gout
- Hyperlipoproteinemia
- Hypertension
- Hypothyroidism
- Impaired glucose tolerance
- Metabolic syndrome
- Nephrotic syndrome
- Obesity
- Pancreatitis (acute and chronic)
- Pregnancy
- Renal failure
- Respiratory distress syndrome

- Stress
- Syndrome X (metabolic syndrome)
- Viral hepatitis
- Werner's syndrome

Decreased in:
- Brain infarction
- Chronic obstructive lung disease
- End-stage liver disease
- Hyperparathyroidism
- Hyperthyroidism
- Hypolipoproteinemia and abetalipoproteinemia
- Intestinal lymphangiectasia
- Malabsorption disorders
- Malnutrition

CRITICAL VALUES: N/A

INTERFERING FACTORS:
- Drugs that may increase triglyceride levels include acetylsalicylic acid, aldatense, atenolol, bendroflumethiazide, cyclosporine, danazol, glucocorticoids, oral contraceptives, oxprenolol, pindolol, prazosin, propranolol, tamoxifen, and timolol.

- Drugs and substances that may decrease triglyceride levels include ascorbic acid, bezafibrate, captopril, carvedilol, celiprolol, chenodeoxycholic acid, cholestyramine, cilazapril, ciprofibrate, clofibrate, colestipol, dextrothyroxine, doxazosin, enalapril, eptastatin, fenofibrate, flaxseed oil, gemfibrozil, glucagon, halofenate, insulin, levonorgestrel, lovastatin, medroxyprogesterone, metformin, nafenopin, niacin, niceritrol, pinacidil, pindolol, pravastatin, prazosin, probucol, simvastatin, and verapamil.

- Failure to follow dietary restrictions before the procedure may cause the procedure to be canceled or repeated.

Nursing Implications and Procedure . . . .

➤ Inform the patient that the test is used to evaluate and monitor hyperlipidemia.

➤ Obtain a history of the patient's complaints, including a list of known allergens (especially allergies or sensitivities to latex), and inform the appropriate health care practitioner accordingly.

➤ Obtain a history of the patient's cardiovascular and gastrointestinal systems, as well as results of previously performed laboratory tests, surgical procedures, and other diagnostic procedures. For related laboratory tests, refer to the Cardiovascular and Gastrointestinal System tables.

➤ Obtain a list of medications the patient is taking, including herbs, nutritional supplements, and nutraceuticals. The health care practitioner and laboratory should be advised if the patient regularly uses these products so that their effects can be taken into consideration when reviewing results.

➤ Review the procedure with the patient. Inform the patient that specimen collection takes approximately 5 to 10 minutes. Address concerns about pain related to the procedure. Explain to the patient that there may be some discomfort during the venipuncture.

➤ The patient should fast for 12 hours before specimen collection. Ideally, the patient should be on a stable diet for 3 weeks and avoid alcohol consumption for 3 days before specimen collection.

➤ There are no fluid or medication restrictions, unless by medical direction.

➤ Ensure that the patient has complied with dietary restrictions and other pretesting preparations; assure that food has been restricted for at least 12 hours prior to the procedure.

➤ If the patient has a history of severe allergic reaction to latex, care should be taken to avoid the use of equipment containing latex.

➤ Instruct the patient to cooperate fully and to follow directions. Direct the patient to breathe normally and to avoid unnecessary movement.

➤ Observe standard precautions, and follow the general guidelines in Appendix A. Positively identify the patient, and label the appropriate tubes with the corresponding patient demographics, date, and time of collection. Perform a venipuncture; collect the specimen in a 5-mL red- or tiger-top tube.

➤ Remove the needle, and apply a pressure dressing over the puncture site.

➤ Promptly transport the specimen to the laboratory for processing and analysis.

➤ The results are recorded manually or in a computerized system for recall and postprocedure interpretation by the appropriate health care practitioner.

➤ Observe the venipuncture site for bleeding or hematoma formation. Apply paper tape or other adhesive to hold pressure bandage in place, or replace with a plastic bandage.

➤ Instruct the patient to resume usual diet, as directed by the health care practitioner.

➤ *Nutritional considerations:* Increased triglyceride levels may be associated with atherosclerosis and coronary artery disease. Nutritional therapy is recommended for individuals identified to be at high risk for developing coronary artery disease. If overweight, these patients should be encouraged to achieve a normal weight. The American Heart Association has Step 1 and Step 2 diets that may be helpful in achieving a goal of lowering total cholesterol and triglyceride levels. The Step 1 diet emphasizes a reduction in foods high in saturated fats and cholesterol. Red meats, eggs, and dairy products are the major sources of saturated fats and cholesterol. If triglycerides are also elevated, patients should be advised to eliminate or reduce alcohol and simple carbohydrates from their diet. The Step 2 diet recommends stricter reductions.

➤ *Social and cultural considerations:* Numerous studies point to the increased prevalence of excess body weight in American children and adolescents. Experts estimate that 25% of American children ages 6 to 11 years are obese. The medical, social, and emotional consequences of excess body weight are significant.

➤ A written report of the examination will be sent to the requesting health care practitioner, who will discuss the results with the patient.

➤ Recognize anxiety related to test results, and be supportive of fear of shortened life expectancy. Discuss the implications of abnormal test results on the patient's lifestyle. Provide teaching and information regarding the clinical implications of the test results, as appropriate. Special attention should be given to instructing the pediatric patient and caregiver regarding health risks and weight control. Educate the patient regarding access to counseling services. Provide contact information, if desired, for the American Heart Association *(http://www.american-heart.org).*

➤ Reinforce information given by the patient's health care provider regarding further testing, treatment, or referral to another health care provider. Answer any questions or address any concerns voiced by the patient or family.

➤ Depending on the results of this procedure, additional testing may be performed to evaluate or monitor progression of the disease process and determine the need for a change in therapy. Evaluate test results in relation to the patient's symptoms and other tests performed.

Related laboratory tests:

➤ Related laboratory tests include antiarrhythmic drugs, apolipoprotein A, apolipoprotein B, aspartate aminotransferase, atrial natriuretic peptide, blood gases, B-type natriuretic peptide, blood calcium, ionized calcium, cholesterol (total, HDL, and LDL), C-reactive protein, creatine kinase and isoenzymes, glucose, glycated hemoglobin, homocysteine, ketones, lactate dehydrogenase and isoenzymes, lipoprotein electrophoresis, magnesium, myoglobin, potassium, and troponin.

TRIIODOTHYRONINE, FREE

SYNONYMS/ACRONYMS: Free T$_3$, FT$_3$.

SPECIMEN: Serum (1 mL) collected in a red- or tiger-top tube.

REFERENCE VALUE: (Method: Immunoassay)

Age	Conventional Units	SI Units (Conventional Units × 0.0154)
Children and adults	260–480 pg/dL	4.0–7.4 pmol/L
Pregnant women (4–9 mo gestation)	196–338 pg/dL	3.0–5.2 pmol/L

DESCRIPTION & RATIONALE: Unlike the thyroid hormone thyroxine (T_4), most T_3 is converted enzymatically from T_4 in the tissues rather than being produced directly by the thyroid gland (see monograph titled "Thyroxine, Total"). Approximately one-third of T_4 is converted to T_3. Most T_3 in the serum (99.97%) is bound to thyroxine-binding globulin (TBG), prealbumin, and albumin. The remainder (0.03%) circulates as unbound or free T_3, which is the physiologically active form. Levels of free T_3 are proportional to levels of total T_3. The advantage of measuring free T_3 instead of total T_3 is that, unlike total T_3 measurements, free T_3 levels are not affected by fluctuations in TBG levels. T_3 is four to five times more biologically potent than T_4. This hormone, along with T_4, is responsible for maintaining a euthyroid state. Free T_3 measurements are rarely required, but they are indicated in the diagnosis of T_3 toxicosis and when certain drugs are being administered that interfere with the conversion of T_4 to T_3. ∎

INDICATIONS:
• Adjunctive aid to thyroid-stimulating hormone (TSH) and free T_4 assessment
• Assist in the diagnosis of T_3 toxicosis

RESULT

Increased in:
• High altitude

• Hyperthyroidism
• T_3 toxicosis

Decreased in:
• Hypothyroidism
• Malnutrition
• Nonthyroidal chronic diseases
• Pregnancy (late)

CRITICAL VALUES: N/A

INTERFERING FACTORS:

• Drugs that may increase free T_3 include acetylsalicylic acid, amiodarone, and levothyroxine.

• Drugs that may decrease free T_3 include amiodarone, methimazole, phenytoin, propranolol, and radiographic agents.

Nursing Implications and Procedure ....

Pretest:

➤ Inform the patient that the test is used to assess thyroid gland function.

➤ Obtain a history of the patient's complaints, including a list of known allergens (especially allergies or sensitivities to latex), and inform the appropriate health care practitioner accordingly.

➤ Obtain a history of the patient's endocrine system and results of previously performed laboratory tests, surgical procedures, and other diagnostic procedures. For related laboratory tests, refer to the Endocrine System table.

➤ Obtain a list of medications the

patient is taking, including herbs, nutritional supplements, and nutraceuticals. The requesting health care practitioner and laboratory should be advised if the patient regularly uses these products so that their effects can be taken into consideration when reviewing results.

➤ Review the procedure with the patient. Inform the patient that specimen collection takes approximately 5 to 10 minutes. Address concerns about pain related to the procedure. Explain to the patient that there may be some discomfort during the venipuncture.

➤ There are no food, fluid, or medication restrictions, unless by medical direction.

Intratest:

➤ If the patient has a history of severe allergic reaction to latex, care should be taken to avoid the use of equipment containing latex.

➤ Instruct the patient to cooperate fully and to follow directions. Direct the patient to breathe normally and to avoid unnecessary movement.

➤ Observe standard precautions, and follow the general guidelines in Appendix A. Positively identify the patient, and label the appropriate tubes with the corresponding patient demographics, date, and time of collection. Perform a venipuncture; collect the specimen in a 5-mL red- or tigertop tube.

➤ Remove the needle, and apply a pressure dressing over the puncture site.

➤ Promptly transport the specimen to the laboratory for processing and analysis.

➤ The results are recorded manually or in a computerized system for recall and postprocedure interpretation by the appropriate health care practitioner.

Post-test:

➤ Observe venipuncture site for bleeding or hematoma formation. Apply paper tape or other adhesive to hold pressure bandage in place, or replace with a plastic bandage.

➤ A written report of the examination will be sent to the requesting health care practitioner, who will discuss the results with the patient.

➤ Reinforce information given by the patient's health care provider regarding further testing, treatment, or referral to another health care provider. Answer any questions or address any concerns voiced by the patient or family.

➤ Depending on the results of this procedure, additional testing may be performed to evaluate or monitor progression of the disease process and determine the need for a change in therapy. Evaluate test results in relation to the patient's symptoms and other tests performed.

Related laboratory tests:

➤ Related laboratory tests include total T_3, T_4, free T_4, and TSH.

TRIIODOTHYRONINE, TOTAL

SYNONYM/ACRONYM: T_3.

SPECIMEN: Serum (1 mL) collected in a red- or tiger-top tube. Plasma (1 mL) collected in green-top (heparin) tube is also acceptable.

REFERENCE VALUE: (Method: Immunoassay)

Age	Conventional Units	SI Units (Conventional Units × 0.0154)
1–3 d	100–740 ng/dL	1.54–11.40 nmol/L
1–12 mo	105–245 ng/dL	1.62–3.77 nmol/L
1–5 y	105–269 ng/dL	1.62–4.14 nmol/L
6–10 y	94–241 ng/dL	1.45–3.71 nmol/L
16–20 y	80–210 ng/dL	1.20–3.20 nmol/L
Adult	70–204 ng/dL	1.08–3.14 nmol/L
Pregnant woman (last 4 mo gestation)	116–247 ng/dL	1.79–3.80 nmol/L

DESCRIPTION & RATIONALE: Unlike the thyroid hormone thyroxine (T_4), most T_3 is converted enzymatically from T_4 in the tissues rather than being produced directly by the thyroid gland (see monograph titled "Thyroxine, Total"). Approximately one-third of T_4 is converted to T_3. Most T_3 in the serum (99.97%) is bound to thyroxine-binding globulin (TBG), prealbumin, and albumin. The remainder (0.03%) circulates as unbound or free T_3, which is the physiologically active form. Levels of free T_3 are proportional to levels of total T_3. The advantage of measuring free T_3 instead of total T_3 is that, unlike total T_3 measurements, free T_3 levels are not affected by fluctuations in TBG levels. T_3 is four to five times more biologically potent than T_4. This hormone, along with T_4, is responsible for maintaining a euthyroid state. ∎

INDICATIONS: Adjunctive aid to thyroid-stimulating hormone (TSH) and free T_4 assessment

RESULT

Increased in:
• Conditions with increased TBG
• Early thyroid failure
• Hyperthyroidism
• Iodine-deficiency goiter
• Pregnancy
• T_3 toxicosis
• Thyrotoxicosis factitia
• Treated hyperthyroidism

Decreased in:
• Acute and subacute nonthyroidal disease
• Conditions with decreased TBG
• Hypothyroidism

CRITICAL VALUES: N/A

INTERFERING FACTORS:
• Drugs that may increase total T_3 levels include amiodarone, amphetamine, benziodarone, clofibrate, fenoprofen, fluorouracil, halofenate, insulin, levothyroxine, methadone, opiates, oral con-

traceptives, phenytoin, prostaglandins, T$_3$, and valproic acid.

• Drugs that may decrease total T$_3$ levels include acetylsalicylic acid, amiodarone, anabolic steroids, asparaginase, carbamazepine, cholestyramine, clomiphene, colestipol, cotrimoxazole, dexamethasone, fenclofenac, furosemide, glucocorticoids, hydrocortisone, interferon alfa-2b, iobenzamic acid, iodides, ipodate, isotretinoin, lithium, methimazole, neomycin, netilmicin, oral contraceptives, penicillamine, phenobarbital, phenylacetic acid derivatives, phenylbutazone, phenytoin, potassium iodide, prednisone, propranolol, propylthiouracil, radiographic agents, salicylate, sodium ipodate, sulfonylureas, and tyropanoic acid.

Nursing Implications and Procedure • • • • • • • • • • •

Pretest:

➤ Inform the patient that the test is used to assess thyroid gland function.

➤ Obtain a history of the patient's complaints, including a list of known allergens (especially allergies or sensitivities to latex), and inform the appropriate health care practitioner accordingly.

➤ Obtain a history of the patient's endocrine system and results of previously performed laboratory tests, surgical procedures, and other diagnostic procedures. For related laboratory tests, refer to the Endocrine System table.

➤ Obtain a list of medications the patient is taking, including herbs, nutritional supplements, and nutraceuticals. The requesting health care practitioner and laboratory should be advised if the patient regularly uses these products so that their effects can be taken into consideration when reviewing results.

➤ Review the procedure with the patient. Inform the patient that specimen collection takes approximately 5 to 10 minutes. Address concerns about pain related to the procedure. Explain to the patient that there may be some discomfort during the venipuncture.

➤ There are no food, fluid, or medication restrictions, unless by medical direction.

Intratest:

➤ If the patient has a history of severe allergic reaction to latex, care should be taken to avoid the use of equipment containing latex.

➤ Instruct the patient to cooperate fully and to follow directions. Direct the patient to breathe normally and to avoid unnecessary movement.

➤ Observe standard precautions, and follow the general guidelines in Appendix A. Positively identify the patient, and label the appropriate tubes with the corresponding patient demographics, date, and time of collection. Perform a venipuncture; collect the specimen in a 5-mL red- or tiger-top tube.

➤ Remove the needle, and apply a pressure dressing over the puncture site.

➤ Promptly transport the specimen to the laboratory for processing and analysis.

➤ The results are recorded manually or in a computerized system for recall and postprocedure interpretation by the appropriate health care practitioner.

Post-test:

➤ Observe venipuncture site for bleeding or hematoma formation. Apply paper tape or other adhesive to hold pressure bandage in place, or replace with a plastic bandage.

➤ A written report of the examination will be sent to the requesting health care practitioner, who will discuss the results with the patient.

➤ Reinforce information given by the

patient's health care provider regarding further testing, treatment, or referral to another health care provider. Answer any questions or address any concerns voiced by the patient or family.

➤ Depending on the results of this procedure, additional testing may be performed to evaluate or monitor progression of the disease process and determine the need for a change in therapy. Evaluate test results in relation to the patient's symptoms and other tests performed.

Related laboratory tests:

➤ Related laboratory tests include free T_3, T_4, free T_4, and TSH.

TROPONINS I AND T

. . . .

SYNONYMS/ACRONYMS: Cardiac troponin, cardiac troponin I (cTnI), cardiac troponin T (cTnT).

SPECIMEN: Serum (1 mL) collected in a red- or tiger-top tube. Plasma (1 mL) collected in green-top (heparin) tube is also acceptable. Serial sampling is highly recommended. Care must be taken to use the same type of collection container if serial measurements are to be taken.

REFERENCE VALUE: (Method: Enzyme immunoassay)

| Troponin I | Less than 0.35 ng/mL |
| Troponin T | Less than 0.20 μg/L |

DESCRIPTION & RATIONALE: Troponin is a complex of three contractile proteins that regulate the interaction of actin and myosin. Troponin C is the calcium-binding subunit; it does not have a cardiac muscle–specific subunit. Troponin I and troponin T, however, do have cardiac muscle–specific subunits. They are detectable a few hours to 7 days after the onset of symptoms of myocardial damage. Troponin I is thought to be a more specific marker of cardiac damage than troponin T. Cardiac troponin I begins to rise 2 to 6 hours after myocardial infarction (MI). It has a biphasic peak: It initially peaks at 15 to 24 hours after MI and then exhibits a lower peak after 60 to 80 hours. Cardiac troponin T levels rise 2 to 6 hours after MI and remain elevated. Both proteins return to the reference range 7 days after MI. ∎

INDICATIONS:
• Assist in establishing a diagnosis of MI
• Evaluate myocardial cell damage

RESULT

Increased in:

- Acute MI

- Minor myocardial damage

- Myocardial damage after coronary artery bypass graft surgery or percutaneous transluminal coronary angioplasty

- Unstable angina pectoris

Decreased in: N/A

CRITICAL VALUES: N/A

INTERFERING FACTORS: N/A

Nursing Implications and Procedure . . . .

Pretest:

➤ Inform the patient that the test is used to identify and monitor cardiac injury.

➤ Obtain a history of the patient's complaints, including a list of known allergens (especially allergies or sensitivities to latex), and inform the appropriate health care practitioner accordingly.

➤ Obtain a history of the patient's cardiovascular system and results of previously performed laboratory tests, surgical procedures, and other diagnostic procedures. For related laboratory tests, refer to the Cardiovascular System table.

➤ Obtain a list of medications the patient is taking, including herbs, nutritional supplements, and nutraceuticals. The requesting health care practitioner and laboratory should be advised if the patient regularly uses these products so that their effects can be taken into consideration when reviewing results.

➤ Review the procedure with the patient. Inform the patient that a number of samples will be collected. Collection at time of admission, 2 to 4 hours, 6 to 8 hours, and 12 hours after admission are the minimal recommendations. Additional samples may be requested. Inform the patient that specimen collection takes approximately 5 to 10 minutes. Address concerns about pain related to the procedure. Explain to the patient that there may be some discomfort during the venipuncture.

➤ There are no food, fluid, or medication restrictions, unless by medical direction.

Intratest:

➤ If the patient has a history of severe allergic reaction to latex, care should be taken to avoid the use of equipment containing latex.

➤ Instruct the patient to cooperate fully and to follow directions. Direct the patient to breathe normally and to avoid unnecessary movement.

➤ Observe standard precautions, and follow the general guidelines in Appendix A. Positively identify the patient, and label the appropriate tubes with the corresponding patient demographics, date, and time of collection. Perform a venipuncture; collect the specimen in a 5-mL red- or tiger-top tube.

➤ Remove the needle, and apply a pressure dressing over the puncture site.

➤ Promptly transport the specimen to the laboratory for processing and analysis.

➤ The results are recorded manually or in a computerized system for recall and postprocedure interpretation by the appropriate health care practitioner.

Post-test:

➤ Observe the venipuncture site for bleeding or hematoma formation. Apply paper tape or other adhesive to hold pressure bandage in place, or replace with a plastic bandage.

➤ *Nutritional considerations:* Increased troponin levels are associated with coronary artery disease. Nutritional therapy is recommended for individuals identified to be at high risk for developing coronary artery disease. If overweight, these patients should be encouraged to achieve a normal weight. The American Heart Association has Step 1 and Step 2 diets that may be helpful in achieving a goal of lowering total cholesterol and triglyceride levels. The Step 1 diet emphasizes a reduction in foods high in saturated fats and cholesterol. Red meats, eggs, and dairy products are the major sources of saturated fats and cholesterol. If triglycerides are also elevated, patients should be advised to eliminate or reduce alcohol and simple carbohydrates from their diet. The Step 2 diet recommends stricter reductions.

➤ A written report of the examination will be sent to the requesting health care practitioner, who will discuss the results with the patient.

➤ Recognize anxiety related to test results, and be supportive of fear of shortened life expectancy. Discuss the implications of abnormal test results on the patient's lifestyle. Provide teaching and information regarding the clinical implications of the test results, as appropriate. Educate the patient regarding access to counseling services. Provide contact information, if desired, for the American Heart Association *(http://www.americanheart.org).*

➤ Reinforce information given by the patient's health care provider regarding further testing, treatment, or referral to another health care provider. Answer any questions or address any concerns voiced by the patient or family.

➤ Depending on the results of this procedure, additional testing may be performed to evaluate or monitor progression of the disease process and determine the need for a change in therapy. Evaluate test results in relation to the patient's symptoms and other tests performed.

Related diagnostic tests:

➤ Related laboratory tests include antiarrhythmic drugs, apolipoprotein A, apolipoprotein B, aspartate aminotransferase, atrial natriuretic peptide, blood gases, B-type natriuretic peptide, blood calcium, ionized calcium, cholesterol (total, HDL, and LDL), C-reactive protein, creatine kinase and isoenzymes, glucose, glycated hemoglobin, homocysteine, ketones, lactate dehydrogenase and isoenzymes, lipoprotein electrophoresis, magnesium, myoglobin, potassium, and triglycerides.

TUBERCULIN SKIN TESTS

SYNONYMS/ACRONYMS: TB tine test, PPD, Mantoux skin test.

SPECIMEN: N/A.

REFERENCE VALUE: (Method: Intradermal skin test) Negative.

DESCRIPTION & RATIONALE: Tuberculin skin tests are done to determine past or present exposure to tuberculosis. The multipuncture or tine test, a screening technique, uses either purified protein derivative (PPD) of tuberculin or old tuberculin. A positive response at the puncture site indicates cell-mediated immunity to the organism or a delayed hypersensitivity caused by interaction of the sensitized T lymphocytes. Verification of the patient's positive response to the multipuncture test is done with the more definitive Mantoux test using Aplisol or Tubersol administered by intradermal injection. The Mantoux test is the test of choice in symptomatic patients. It is also used in some settings as a screening test. A negative result is judged if there is no sign of redness or induration at the site of the injection or if the zone of redness and induration is less than 5 mm in diameter. A positive result is evidenced by an area of erythema and induration at the injection site that is greater than 10 mm. A positive result does not distinguish between active and dormant infection. A positive response to the Mantoux test is followed up with chest radiography and bacteriologic sputum testing to confirm diagnosis. ■

INDICATIONS:
- Evaluate cough, weight loss, fatigue, hemoptysis, and abnormal x-rays to determine if the cause of symptoms is tuberculosis
- Evaluate known or suspected exposure to tuberculosis, with or without symptoms, to determine if tuberculosis is present
- Evaluate patients with medical conditions placing them at risk for tuberculosis (e.g., acquired immunodeficiency syndrome, lymphoma, diabetes)
- Screen infants with the tine test at the time of first immunizations to determine tuberculosis exposure
- Screen populations at risk for developing tuberculosis (e.g., health care practitioners, nursing home residents, correctional facility personnel, prison inmates, and residents of the inner city living in poor hygienic conditions)

RESULT

Positive findings in: Pulmonary tuberculosis

CRITICAL VALUES:
Note and immediately report to the health care practitioner positive results and related symptoms.

INTERFERING FACTORS:
- Drugs such as immunosuppressive agents or steroids can alter results.
- Diseases such as hematologic cancers or sarcoidosis can alter results.
- Recent or present bacterial, fungal, or viral infections may affect results. False-positive results may be caused by the presence of nontuberculous mycobacteria or by serial testing.
- False-negative results can occur if sensitized T cells are temporarily decreased. False-negative results also can occur in the presence of bacterial infections, immunologic deficiencies, immunosuppressive agents, live-virus vaccinations (e.g., measles, mumps, varicella, rubella), malnutrition, old age, overwhelming tuberculosis, renal failure, and active viral infections (e.g., chickenpox, measles, mumps).
- Improper storage of the tuberculin solution (e.g., with respect to temperature, exposure to light, and stability on opening) may affect the results.

- Improper technique when performing the intradermal injection (e.g., injecting into subcutaneous tissue) may cause false-negative results.

- Incorrect amount or dilution of antigen injected or delayed injection after drawing the antigen up into the syringe may affect the results.

- Incorrect reading of the measurement of response or timing of the reading may interfere with results.

- ⚠ It is not known whether the test has teratogenic effects or reproductive implications; the test should be administered to pregnant women only when clearly indicated.

- ⚠ The test should not be administered to a patient with a previously positive tuberculin skin test because of the danger of severe reaction, including vesiculation, ulceration, and necrosis.

- The test does not distinguish between current and past infection.

Nursing Implications and Procedure ....

Pretest:

➤ Inform the patient that the test is used to indicate exposure to tuberculosis.

➤ Obtain a history of the patient's complaints, including a list of known allergens, and inform the appropriate health care practitioner accordingly.

➤ Obtain a history of the patient's immune and respiratory systems and results of previously performed laboratory tests, surgical procedures, and other diagnostic procedures. Obtain a history of tuberculosis or tuberculosis exposure, signs and symptoms indicating possible tuberculosis, and other skin test or vaccinations and sensitivities. For related laboratory tests, refer to the Immune and Respiratory System tables.

➤ Obtain a list of medications the patient is taking, including herbs, nutritional supplements, and nutraceuticals. The requesting health care practitioner and laboratory should be advised if the patient regularly uses these products so that their effects can be taken into consideration when reviewing results.

➤ Review the procedure with the patient. Ensure that the patient does not currently have tuberculosis and has not had a positive skin test previously before beginning the test. Do not administer the test if the patient has a skin rash or other eruptions at the test site. Inform the patient that the procedure takes approximately 5 minutes. Address concerns about pain related to the procedure. Explain to the patient that that a moderate amount of pain may be experienced when the intradermal injection is performed.

➤ Emphasize to the patient that the area should not be scratched or disturbed after the injection and before the reading.

➤ *Sensitivity to social and cultural issues,* as well as concern for modesty, is important in providing psychological support before, during, and after the procedure.

➤ There are no food, fluid, or medication restrictions, unless by medical direction.

Intratest:

➤ If the patient has a history of severe allergic reaction to latex, care should be taken to avoid the use of equipment containing latex.

➤ Instruct the patient to cooperate fully and to follow directions. Direct the patient to breathe normally and to avoid unnecessary movement.

➤ Observe standard precautions, and follow the general guidelines in Appendix A. Positively identify the patient.

➤ Have epinephrine hydrochloride solution (1:1000) available in the event of anaphylaxis.

Cleanse the skin site on the lower anterior forearm with alcohol swabs and allow to air-dry.

Multipuncture test:

> Remove the cap covering the tines and stretch the forearm skin taut. Firmly press the device into the prepared site, hold it in place for 1 second, and then remove it. Four punctures should be visible. Record the site, and remind the patient to return in 48 to 72 hours to have the test read. At the time of the reading, use a plastic ruler to measure the diameter of the largest indurated area, making sure the room is sufficiently lighted to perform the reading. A palpable induration greater than or equal to 2 mm at one or more of the punctures indicates a positive test result.

Mantoux (intradermal) test:

> Prepare PPD or old tuberculin in a tuberculin syringe with a short, 26-gauge needle attached. Prepare the appropriate dilution and amount for the most commonly used intermediate strength (5 tuberculin units in 0.1 mL) or a first strength usually used for children (1 tuberculin unit in 0.1 mL). Inject the preparation intradermally at the prepared site as soon as it is drawn up into the syringe. When properly injected, a bleb or wheal 6 to 10 mm in diameter is formed within the layers of the skin. Record the site, and remind the patient to return in 48 to 72 hours to have the test read. At the time of the reading, use a plastic ruler to measure the diameter of the largest indurated area, making sure the room is sufficiently lighted to perform the reading. Palpate for thickening of the tissue; a positive result is indicated by a reaction of 5 mm or more with erythema and edema.

General:

> The results are recorded manually or in a computerized system for recall and postprocedure interpretation by the appropriate health care practitioner.

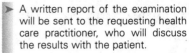

Post-test:

> A written report of the examination will be sent to the requesting health care practitioner, who will discuss the results with the patient.

> Recognize anxiety related to test results, and be supportive of perceived loss of independence and fear of shortened life expectancy. Discuss the implications of abnormal test results on the patient's lifestyle. Provide teaching and information regarding the clinical implications of the test results, as appropriate. Educate the patient regarding access to counseling services.

> Reinforce information given by the patient's health care provider regarding further testing, treatment, or referral to another health care provider. Emphasize to the patient the need to return and have the test results read within the specified time frame of 48 to 72 hours after injection. Inform the patient that the effects from a positive response at the site can remain for 1 week. Educate the patient that a positive result may put him or her at risk for infection related to impaired primary defenses, impaired gas exchange related to decrease in effective lung surface, and intolerance to activity related to an imbalance between oxygen supply and demand. Answer any questions or address any concerns voiced by the patient or family.

> Depending on the results of this procedure, additional testing may be performed to evaluate or monitor progression of the disease process and determine the need for a change in therapy. Evaluate test results in relation to the patient's symptoms and other tests performed.

Related laboratory tests:

> Related laboratory tests include relevant acid-fast cultures and smears.

TUNING FORK TESTS

SYNONYMS/ACRONYMS: Bing test, Rinne test, Schwabach test, Weber test.

AREA OF APPLICATION: Ears.

CONTRAST: N/A.

DESCRIPTION & RATIONALE: These noninvasive assessment procedures are done to distinguish conduction hearing loss from sensorineural hearing loss. They may be performed as part of the physical assessment examination and followed by hearing loss audiometry for confirmation of questionable results. The tuning forks tests described in this monograph are named for the four German otologists who described their use. Tuning forks tests are used less frequently by audiologists in favor of more sophisticated electronic methods, but presentation of the tuning fork test methodology is useful to illustrate the principles involved in electronic test methods.

A tuning fork is a bipronged metallic device that emits a clear tone at a particular pitch when it is set into vibration by holding the stem in the hand and striking one of the prongs or tines against a firm surface. The Bing test samples for conductive hearing loss by intermittently occluding and unblocking the opening of the ear canal while holding a vibrating tuning fork to the mastoid process behind the ear. The occlusion effect is absent in patients with conductive hearing loss and is present in patients with normal hearing or with sensorineural hearing loss. The Rinne test compares the patients' own hearing by bone conduction to their hearing by air conduction to determine whether hearing loss, if detected, is conductive or sensorineural. The Schwabach test compares the patient's level of bone conduction hearing to that of a presumed normal-hearing examiner. The Weber test has been modified by many audiologists for use with electronic equipment. When the test is administered, the patient is asked to tell the examiner the location of the tone heard (left ear, right ear, both ears, or midline) in order to determine whether the hearing loss is conductive, sensorineural, or mixed. ∎

INDICATIONS:
- Evaluate type of hearing loss (conductive or sensorineural)
- Screen for hearing loss as part of a routine physical examination and to determine the need for referral to an audiologist

RESULT

Normal Findings:
- Normal air and bone conduction in both ears. No evidence of hearing loss.

- Bing test: Pulsating sound that gets louder and softer when the opening to the ear canal is alternately opened and closed. (*Note:* This result, observed in patients with normal hearing, is also observed in patients with sensorineural hearing loss.)

- Rinne test: Longer and louder tone heard by air conduction than by bone conduction. (*Note:* This result, observed in patients with normal hearing, is also observed in patients with sensorineural hearing loss.)

- Schwabach test: Same tone loudness heard equally long by the examiner and the patient.

- Weber test: Same tone loudness heard equally in both ears.

Abnormal Findings:

- Conduction hearing loss

  Bing test: No change in the loudness of the sound

  Rinne test: Tone louder or detected for a longer time than the air-conducted tone

  Schwabach test: Prolonged duration of tone when compared to that heard by the examiner

  Weber test: Lateralization of tone to one ear indicating loss of hearing on that side (i.e., tone is heard in the poorer ear)

- Sensorineural hearing loss

  Bing test: Pulsating sound that gets louder and softer when the opening to the ear canal is alternately opened and closed

  Rinne test: Tone heard louder by air conduction

  Schwabach test: Shortened duration when compared to that heard by the examiner

  Weber test: Lateralization of tone to one ear indicating loss of hearing on the other side (i.e., tone is heard in the better ear)

CRITICAL VALUES: N/A

INTERFERING FACTORS:

Factors that may impair the results of the examination:

- Poor technique in striking the tuning fork or incorrect placement can result in accurate results.

- Inability of the patient to understand how to identify responses or unwillingness of the patient to cooperate during the test can cause inaccurate results.

- Hearing loss in the examiner can affect results in those tests that utilize hearing comparisons between patient and examiner.

Nursing Implications and Procedure • • • • • • • • • •

Pretest:

➤ Inform the patient that the procedure detects hearing loss.

➤ Obtain a history of the patient's complaints, including a list of known allergens.

➤ Obtain a history of the patient's known or suspected hearing loss, including type and cause; ear conditions with treatment regimens; ear surgery; and other tests and procedures to assess and diagnose auditory deficit.

➤ Obtain a history of results of previously performed laboratory tests, surgical procedures, and other diagnostic procedures. For related diagnostic tests, refer to the table of tests associated with the Auditory System.

➤ Obtain a list of the medications the patient is taking, including herbs, nutritional supplements, and nutraceuticals. The requesting health care practitioner should be advised if the patient regularly uses these products so that their effects can be taken into consideration when reviewing results.

➤ Review the procedure with the patient. Address concerns about pain related to the procedure. Explain to the patient that no discomfort will be experienced during the test. Inform the patient that an audiologist, physician, or nurse performs the test, in a quiet, darkened room, and that to evaluate both ears, the test can take 5 to 10 minutes.

➤ Ensure that the external auditory canal is clear of impacted cerumen.

➤ There are no food, fluid, or medication restrictions, unless by medical direction.

Intratest:

➤ Instruct the patient to cooperate fully and to follow directions. Instruct the patient to remain still throughout the procedure because movement produces unreliable results.

➤ Seat the patient in a quiet environment positioned such that the patient is comfortable and is facing the examiner. A tuning fork of 1024 Hz is used because it tests within the range of human speech (400 to 5000 Hz).

➤ Bing test: Tap the tuning fork handle against the hand to start a light vibration. Hold the handle to the mastoid process behind the ear while alternately opening and closing the ear canal with a finger. Ask the patient to report whether they hear a change in loudness or softness in sound. Record the result as a positive Bing if the patient reports a pulsating change in sound. Record as a negative Bing if no change in loudness is detected.

➤ Rinne test: Tap the tuning fork handle against the hand to start a light vibration. Have the patient mask the ear not being tested by moving a finger in and out of the ear canal of that ear. Hold the base of the vibrating tuning fork with the thumb and forefinger of the dominant hand and place it in contact with the patient's mastoid process (bone conduction). Ask the patient when the sound is no longer heard. Follow this with placement of the same vibrating tuning fork in front of the ear canal (air conduction) without touching the external part of the ear. Ask the patient which of the two has the loudest or longest tone. Repeat the test in the other ear.

Record as Rinne positive if air conduction is heard longer and Rinne negative if bone conduction is heard longer.

➤ Schwabach test: Tap the tuning fork handle against the hand to start a light vibration. Hold the base of the tuning fork against one side of the patient's mastoid process and ask if the tone is heard. Have the patient mask the ear not being tested by moving a finger in and out of the ear canal of that ear. The examiner then places the tuning fork against the same side of his or her own mastoid process and listens for the tone. The tuning fork is alternated on the same side between patient and examiner until the sound is no longer heard, noting whether the sound ceased to be heard by both the patient and the examiner at the same point in time. Repeat the procedure on the other ear. If the patient hears the tone for a longer or shorter time, count and note this in seconds.

➤ Weber test: Tap the tuning fork handle against the hand to start a light vibration. Hold the base of the vibrating tuning fork with the thumb and forefinger of the dominant hand and place it on the middle of the patient's forehead or at the vertex of the head. Ask the patient to determine if the sound is heard better and longer on one side than the other. Record as Weber right or left. If sound is heard equally, record as Weber negative.

➤ The results are recorded manually for recall and postprocedure interpretation by the appropriate health care practitioner.

Post-test:

➤ A written report of the examination will be completed by a health care practitioner specializing in this branch of medicine. The report will be sent to the requesting health care practitioner, who will discuss the results with the patient.

➤ Recognize anxiety related to test results, and be supportive of impaired activity related to hearing loss and perceived loss of independence. Discuss the implications of abnormal test results on the patient's lifestyle. Provide teaching and information regarding the clinical implications of the test results, as appropriate. Educate the patient regarding access to counseling services.

➤ Reinforce information given by the patient's health care provider regarding further testing, treatment, or referral to another health care provider. As appropriate, instruct the patient in the use, cleaning, and storing of a hearing aid. Answer any questions or address any concerns voiced by the patient or family.

➤ Depending on the results of this procedure, additional testing may be performed to evaluate or monitor progression of the disease process and determine the need for a change in therapy. Evaluate test results in relation to the patient's symptoms and other tests performed.

Related dignostic tests:

➤ Related diagnostic tests include hearing loss audiometry, evoked brain potential studies for hearing loss, otoscopy, and spondee speech reception threshold.

ULTRASOUND, ARTERIAL DOPPLER, CAROTID STUDIES

· ·

SYNONYMS/ACRONYM: Carotid Doppler, carotid ultrasound, arterial ultrasound.

AREA OF APPLICATION: Arteries.

CONTRAST: Done without contrast.

DESCRIPTION & RATIONALE: Ultrasound procedures are diagnostic, non-invasive, and relatively inexpensive. They take a short time to complete, do not use radiation, and cause no harm to the patient. Using the duplex scanning method, carotid ultrasound records sound waves to obtain information about the carotid arteries. The amplitude and waveform of the carotid pulse are measured, resulting in a two-dimensional image of the artery. Carotid arterial sites used for the studies include the common carotid, external carotid, and internal carotid. Blood flow direction, velocity, and the presence of flow disturbances can be readily assessed. The sound waves hit the moving red blood cells and are reflected back to the transducer, a flashlight-shaped device, pressed against the skin. The sound that is emitted by the equipment corresponds to the velocity of the blood flow through the vessel. The result is the visualization of the artery to assist in the diagnosis (i.e., presence, amount, location) of plaques causing vessel stenosis or atherosclerotic occlusion affecting the flow of blood to the brain. Depending on the degree of stenosis causing a reduction in vessel diameter, additional testing can be performed to determine the effect of stenosis on the hemodynamic status of the artery. ▪

INDICATION:

• Assist in the diagnosis of carotid artery occlusive disease, as evidenced by visualization of blood flow disruption

• Detect irregularities in the structure of the carotid arteries

• Detect plaque or stenosis of the carotid artery, as evidenced by turbulent blood flow or changes in Doppler signals indicating occlusion

RESULT

Normal Findings:

• Normal blood flow through the carotid arteries with no evidence of occlusion or narrowing

Abnormal Findings:

• Carotid artery occlusive disease (atherosclerosis)

• Plaque or stenosis of carotid artery

• Reduction in vessel diameter of more than 16%, indicating stenosis

CRITICAL VALUES: N/A

INTERFERING FACTORS

Factors that may impair clear imaging:

• Attenuation of the sound waves by bony structures, which can impair clear imaging of the vessels

• Incorrect placement of the transducer over the desired test site

• Retained contrast medium from a previous radiologic procedure

• Metallic objects within the examination field (e.g., jewelry, body rings), which may inhibit organ visualization and can produce unclear images

• Improper adjustment of the ultrasound equipment to accommodate obese or thin patients, which can cause a poor-quality study

• Patients who are very obese, who may exceed the weight limit for the equipment

• Incorrect positioning of the patient, which may produce poor visualization of the area to be examined

• Inability of the patient to cooperate or remain still during the procedure because of age, significant pain, or mental status

Nursing Implications and Procedure • • • • • • • • • • •

Pretest:

➤ Inform the patient that the procedure assesses the arteries in the neck.

➤ Obtain a history of the patient's complaints, including a list of known allergens (especially allergies or sensitivities to latex), and inform the health care practitioner accordingly.

➤ Obtain a history of the patient's cardiovascular system, as well as results of previously performed laboratory tests, surgical procedures, and other diagnostic procedures. For related diagnostic tests, refer to the Cardiovascular System table.

➤ Note any recent procedures that can interfere with test results (i.e., iodine-based contrast or barium procedures, surgery, or biopsy). There should be 24 hours between administration of barium or iodine contrast medium and this test.

➤ Record the date of the last menstrual

period and determine the possibility of pregnancy in perimenopausal women.

➤ Obtain a list of the medications the patient is taking, including anticoagulant therapy, aspirin and other salicylates, herbs, nutritional supplements, and nutraceuticals, especially those known to affect coagulation (see Appendix F). It is recommended that use be discontinued 14 days before surgical procedures. The requesting health care practitioner and laboratory should be advised if the patient regularly uses these products so that their effects can be taken into consideration when reviewing results.

➤ Review the procedure with the patient. Address concerns about pain related to the procedure. Explain to the patient that some pain may be experienced during the test, and there may be moments of discomfort. Inform the patient that the procedure is performed in a ultrasound department, usually by a technologist, and takes approximately 30 to 60 minutes.

➤ *Sensitivity to social and cultural issues,* as well as concern for modesty, is important in providing psychological support before, during, and after the procedure.

➤ Instruct the patient to remove jewelry (including watches), hairpins, credit cards, and other metallic objects in the area to be examined.

➤ There are no food, fluid, or medication restrictions, unless by medical direction.

Intratest:

➤ Ensure that the patient has removed all external metallic objects (jewelry, etc.) prior to the procedure.

➤ Patients are given a gown, robe, and foot coverings to wear and instructed to void prior to the procedure.

➤ Instruct the patient to cooperate fully and to follow directions. Instruct the patient to remain still throughout the procedure because movement produces unreliable results.

➤ Observe standard precautions, and follow the general guidelines in Appendix A.

➤ Place the patient in the supine position on an exam table; other positions may be used during the examination.

➤ Expose the neck and drape the patient.

➤ Conductive gel is applied to the skin and a Doppler transducer is moved over the skin to obtain images of the area of interest. When the swishing sound of blood flow is heard, record it at the highest point along the artery at which it is audible.

➤ Ask the patient to breathe normally during the examination. If necessary for better organ visualization, ask the patient to inhale deeply and hold his or her breath.

➤ The results are recorded manually, on film, or in a computerized system for recall and postprocedure interpretation by the appropriate health care practitioner.

Post-test:

➤ When the study is completed, remove the gel from the skin.

➤ Instruct the patient to continue usual diet, fluids, and medications, as directed by the health care practitioner.

➤ *Nutritional considerations:* A low-fat, low-cholesterol, and low-sodium diet should be consumed to reduce current disease processes and/or decrease risk of hypertension and coronary artery disease.

➤ A written report of the examination will be completed by a health care practitioner specializing in this branch of medicine. The report will be sent to the requesting health care practitioner, who will discuss the results with the patient.

➤ Recognize anxiety related to test results, and be supportive of perceived loss of independent function. Discuss the implications of abnormal test results on the patient's lifestyle. Provide teaching and information

regarding the clinical implications of the test results, as appropriate.

➤ Reinforce information given by the patient's health care provider regarding further testing, treatment, or referral to another health care provider. Answer any questions or address any concerns voiced by the patient or family.

➤ Instruct the patient in the use of any ordered medications. Explain the importance of adhering to the therapy regimen. As appropriate, instruct the patient in significant side effects and systemic reactions associated with the prescribed medication. Encourage him or her to review corresponding literature provided by a pharmacist.

➤ Depending on the results of this procedure, additional testing may be performed to evaluate or monitor progression of the disease process and determine the need for a change in therapy. Evaluate test results in relation to the patient's symptoms and other tests performed.

Related diagnostic tests:

➤ Related diagnostic tests include carotid angiography, computed tomography angiography, and magnetic resonance imaging angiography.

ULTRASOUND, ARTERIAL DOPPLER, LOWER EXTREMITY STUDIES

SYNONYMS/ACRONYM: Doppler, arterial ultrasound, duplex scan.

AREA OF APPLICATION: Arteries of the lower extremities.

CONTRAST: Done without contrast.

DESCRIPTION & RATIONALE: Ultrasound procedures are diagnostic, noninvasive, and relatively inexpensive. They take a short time to complete, do not use radiation, and cause no harm to the patient. Using the duplex scanning method, arterial leg ultrasound records sound waves to obtain information about the arteries of the lower extremities from the common femoral arteries and their branches as they extend into the calf area. The amplitude and waveform of the pulses are measured, resulting in a two-dimensional image of the artery. Blood flow direction, velocity, and the presence of flow disturbances can be readily assessed, and for diagnostic studies, the technique is done bilaterally. The sound waves hit the moving red blood cells and are reflected back to the transducer, a flashlight-shaped device, pressed against the skin. The sound that is emitted by the equipment corresponds to the velocity of the blood flow through the vessel. The result is the visualization of the artery to assist in the diagnosis (i.e., presence, amount, and location) of plaques causing vessel stenosis or occlusion and to help determine the cause of claudication. Arterial reconstruction and graft condition and patency can also be evaluated. ■

INDICATIONS:

- Assist in the diagnosis of aneurysm, pseudoaneurysm, hematoma, arteriovenous malformation, or hemangioma

- Assist in the diagnosis of ischemia, arterial calcification, or plaques, as evidenced by visualization of blood flow disruption

- Detect irregularities in the structure of the arteries

- Detect plaque or stenosis of the lower extremity artery, as evidenced by turbulent blood flow or changes in Doppler signals indicating occlusion

RESULT

Normal Findings:

- Normal blood flow through the lower extremity arteries with no evidence of vessel occlusion or narrowing

Abnormal Findings:

- Aneurysm

- Arterial calcification or plaques

- Graft diameter reduction

- Hemangioma

- Hematoma

- Ischemia

- Pseudoaneurysm

- Reduction in vessel diameter of more than 16%, indicating stenosis

- Vessel occlusion or stenosis

CRITICAL VALUES: N/A

INTERFERING FACTORS:

This procedure is contraindicated for:

- Patients with an open or draining lesion

Factors that may alter test results:

- Attenuation of the sound waves by bony structures, which can impair clear imaging of the vessels

- Cold extremities, resulting in vasoconstriction that can cause inaccurate measurements

- Occlusion proximal to the site being studied, which would affect blood flow to the area

- Open wound or incision overlying the area to be examined

- Cigarette smoking, because nicotine can cause constriction of the peripheral vessels

- An abnormally large leg, making direct examination difficult

- Incorrect placement of the transducer over the desired test site

- Retained contrast medium from a previous radiologic procedure

- Metallic objects within the examination field (e.g., jewelry, body rings), which may inhibit organ visualization and can produce unclear images

- Improper adjustment of the ultrasound equipment to accommodate obese or thin patients, which can cause a poor-quality study

- Patients who are very obese, who may exceed the weight limit for the equipment

- Incorrect positioning of the patient, which may produce poor visualization of the area to be examined

- Inability of the patient to cooperate or remain still during the procedure because of age, significant pain, or mental status

Nursing Implications and Procedure . . . .

Pretest:

➤ Inform the patient that the procedure assesses the peripheral arteries.

➤ Obtain a history of the patient's complaints, including a list of known allergens (especially allergies or sensitivities to latex), and inform the health care practitioner accordingly.

➤ Obtain a history of the patient's cardiovascular system, as well as results of previously performed laboratory tests, surgical procedures, and other diagnostic procedures. For related diagnostic tests, refer to the Cardiovascular System table.

➤ Report the presence of a lesion that is open or draining; maintain clean, dry dressing for the ulcer; protect the limb from trauma.

➤ Note any recent procedures that can interfere with test results (i.e., iodine-based contrast or barium procedures, surgery, or biopsy). There should be 24 hours between administration of barium or iodine contrast medium and this test.

➤ Record the date of the last menstrual period and determine the possibility of pregnancy in perimenopausal women.

➤ Obtain a list of the medications the patient is taking, including anticoagulant therapy, aspirin and other salicylates, herbs, nutritional supplements, and nutraceuticals, especially those known to affect coagulation (see Appendix F). It is recommended that use be discontinued 14 days before surgical procedures. The requesting health care practitioner and laboratory should be advised if the patient regularly uses these products so that their effects can be taken into consideration when reviewing results.

➤ Review the procedure with the patient. Address concerns about pain related to the procedure. Explain to the patient that some pain may be experienced during the test, and there may be moments of discomfort. Inform the patient that the procedure is performed in a ultrasound department, usually by a technologist, and takes approximately 30 to 60 minutes.

➤ *Sensitivity to social and cultural issues*, as well as concern for modesty, is important in providing psychological support before, during, and after the procedure.

➤ Instruct the patient to remove jewelry (including watches), hairpins, credit cards, and other metallic objects.

➤ There are no food, fluid, or medication restrictions, unless by medical direction.

Intratest:

➤ Ensure that the patient has removed all external metallic objects (jewelry, etc.) prior to the procedure in the area to be examined.

➤ Patients are given a gown, robe, and foot coverings to wear and instructed to void prior to the procedure.

➤ Instruct the patient to cooperate fully and to follow directions. Instruct the patient to remain still throughout the procedure because movement produces unreliable results.

➤ Observe standard precautions, and follow the general guidelines in Appendix A.

➤ Place the patient in the supine position on an exam table; other positions may be used during the examination.

➤ Expose the area of interest and drape the patient.

➤ Conductive gel is applied to the skin and a Doppler transducer is moved over the skin to obtain images of the area of interest.

➤ Ask the patient to breathe normally during the examination. If necessary for better organ visualization, ask the patient to inhale deeply and hold his or her breath.

➤ Place blood pressure cuffs on the thigh, calf, and ankle.

➤ Apply a conductive get to the skin over the area distal to each of the cuffs.

➤ Inflate the thigh cuff to a level above the patient's systolic pressure found in the normal extremity.

➤ Place the Doppler transducer on the skin distal to the inflated cuff, and slowly release the pressure in the cuff.

➤ When the swishing sound of blood flow is heard, record it at the highest point along the artery at which it is audible. The test is repeated at the calf and then the ankle.

➤ The results are recorded manually, on film, or in a computerized system for recall and postprocedure interpretation by the appropriate health care practitioner.

Post-test:

➤ When the study is completed, remove the gel from the skin.

➤ Instruct the patient to continue usual diet, fluids, and medications, as directed by the health care practitioner

➤ *Nutritional considerations:* A low-fat, low-cholesterol, and low-sodium diet should be consumed to reduce current disease processes and/or decrease risk of hypertension and coronary artery disease.

➤ A written report of the examination will be completed by a health care practitioner specializing in this branch of medicine. The report will be sent to the requesting health care practitioner, who will discuss the results with the patient.

➤ Recognize anxiety related to test results, and be supportive of perceived loss of independent function. Discuss the implications of abnormal test results on the patient's lifestyle. Provide teaching and information regarding the clinical implications of the test results, as appropriate.

➤ Reinforce information given by the patient's health care provider regarding further testing, treatment, or referral to another health care provider. Answer any questions or address any concerns voiced by the patient or family.

➤ Instruct the patient in the use of any ordered medications. Explain the importance of adhering to the therapy regimen. As appropriate, instruct the patient in significant side effects and systemic reactions associated with the prescribed medication. Encourage him or her to review corresponding literature provided by a pharmacist.

➤ Depending on the results of this procedure, additional testing may be performed to evaluate or monitor progression of the disease process and determine the need for a change in therapy. Evaluate test results in relation to the patient's symptoms and other tests performed.

Related diagnostic tests:

➤ Related diagnostic tests include computed tomography angiography, and magnetic resonance imaging angiography.

ULTRASOUND, A-SCAN

SYNONYMS/ACRONYMS: None.

AREA OF APPLICATION: Eyes.

CONTRAST: N/A.

DESCRIPTION & RATIONALE: Diagnostic techniques such as A-scan ultrasonography can be used to identify abnormal tissue. The A-scan employs a single-beam, linear sound wave to detect abnormalities by returning an echo when interference disrupts its straight path. When the sound wave is directed at lens vitreous that is normal, the homogeneous tissue does not return an echo; an opaque lens with a cataract will produce an echo. The returning waves detected by abnormal tissue are received by a microfilm that converts the sound energy into electrical impulses that are amplified and displayed on an oscilloscope as an ultrasonogram or echogram. The A-scan echo can be used to indicate the position of the cornea and retina. The A-scan is most commonly used to measure the axial length of the eye. This measurement is used to determine the power requirement for an intraocular lens used to replace the abnormal, opaque lens of the eye removed in cataract surgery. There are two different methods currently in use. The applanation method involves placement of an ultrasound probe directly on the cornea. The immersion technique is more popular because it does not require direct con-

tact and compression of the cornea. The immersion technique protects the cornea by placement of a fluid layer between the eye and the ultrasound probe. The accuracy of the immersion technique is thought to be greater than that of applanation because there is no corneal compression caused by the immersion method. Therefore, the measured axial length achieved by immersion is closer to the true axial length of the cornea. ■

INDICATIONS:
• Determination of power requirement for replacement intraocular lens in cataract surgery.

RESULT

Normal Findings:
• Normal homogeneous ocular tissue

Abnormal Findings:
• Cataract

CRITICAL VALUES: N/A

INTERFERING FACTORS:

Factors that may impair the results of the examination:
• Inability of the patient to cooperate and remain still during the procedure may interfere with the test results.

- Rubbing or squeezing the eyes may affect results.

- Improper placement of the probe tip to the surface of the eye may produce inaccurate results.

Nursing Implications and Procedure • • • • • • • • • • •

➤ Inform the patient that the procedure determines the strength of the lens that will be replaced during cataract surgery.

➤ Obtain a history of the patient's complaints, including a list of known allergens, especially topical anesthetic eyedrops.

➤ Obtain a history of the patient's known or suspected vision loss, changes in visual acuity, including type and cause; use of glasses or contact lenses; eye conditions with treatment regimens; eye surgery; and other tests and procedures to assess and diagnose visual deficit.

➤ Obtain a history of results of previously performed laboratory tests, surgical procedures, and other diagnostic procedures. For related diagnostic tests, refer to the table of tests associated with the Ocular System.

➤ Obtain a list of the medications the patient is taking, including herbs, nutritional supplements, and nutraceuticals. The requesting health care practitioner should be advised if the patient regularly uses these products so that their effects can be taken into consideration when reviewing results.

➤ Instruct the patient to remove contact lenses or glasses, as appropriate. Instruct the patient regarding the importance of keeping the eyes open for the test.

➤ Review the procedure with the patient. Explain that the patient will be requested to fixate the eyes during the procedure. Address concerns about pain related to the procedure.

Explain to the patient that no discomfort will be experienced during the test but that some discomfort may be experienced after the test when the numbness wears off from the anesthetic drops administered prior to the test. Inform the patient that a technician, optometrist, or physician performs the test, in a quiet, semidarkened room, and that evaluation of the eye upon which surgery is to be performed can take up 10 minutes.

➤ There are no food, fluid or medication restrictions, unless by medical direction.

➤ Instruct the patient to cooperate fully and to follow directions. Ask the patient to remain still during the procedure because movement produces unreliable results.

➤ Seat the patient comfortably. Instruct the patient to look straight ahead, keeping the eyes open and unblinking.

➤ Instill topical anesthetic in each eye, as ordered, and provide time for it to work. Topical anesthetic drops are placed in the eye with the patient looking up and the solution directed at the six o'clock position of the sclera (white of the eye) near the limbus (grey, semitransparent area of the eyeball where the cornea and sclera meet). The dropper bottle should not touch the eyelashes.

➤ Ask the patient to place the chin in the chin rest and gently press the forehead against the support bar. When the ultrasound probe is properly positioned on the patient's surgical eye, a reading is automatically taken.

➤ Multiple measurements may be taken in order to ensure that a consistent and acurate reading has been achieved. Variability between serial measurements is unavoidable using the applanation technique.

➤ The results are recorded on a paper strip from the automated equipment for recall and postprocedure interpretation by the appropriate health care practitioner.

Post-test:

➤ A written report of the examination will be completed by a health care practitioner specializing in this branch of medicine. The report will be sent to the requesting health care practitioner, who will discuss the results with the patient.

➤ Recognize anxiety related to test results. Encourage the patient to recognize and be supportive of impaired activity related to vision loss, perceived loss of driving privileges, or the possibility of requiring corrective lenses (self-image). Discuss the implications of test results on the patient's lifestyle. Reassure the patient regarding concerns related to the impend-

ing cataract surgery. Provide teaching and information regarding the clinical implications of the test results, as appropriate.

➤ Reinforce information given by the patient's health care provider regarding further testing, treatment, or referral to another health care provider. Answer any questions or address any concerns voiced by the patient or family.

➤ Depending on the results of this procedure, additional testing may be performed to evaluate or monitor progression of the disease process and determine the need for a change in therapy. Evaluate test results in relation to the patient's symptoms and other tests performed.

ULTRASOUND, BLADDER

SYNONYM/ACRONYM: Bladder sonography.

AREA OF APPLICATION: Bladder.

CONTRAST: Done without contrast.

DESCRIPTION & RATIONALE: Ultrasound procedures are diagnostic, non-invasive, and relatively inexpensive. They take a short time to complete, do not use radiation, and cause no harm to the patient. Bladder ultrasound evaluates disorders of the bladder, such as masses or lesions. Bladder position, structure, and size are examined with the use of high-frequency waves of various intensities delivered by a transducer, a flashlight-shaped device, pressed against the skin. Methods for imaging include the transrectal, transurethral, and transvaginal approach. The waves are bounced back, converted to electrical energy, amplified by the transducer, and displayed on a monitor to evaluate the structure and position of the contents of the bladder. The examination is helpful for monitoring patient response to therapy for bladder disease. Bladder images can be included in ultrasonography of the kidneys, ureters, bladder, urethra, and gonads in diagnosing renal/neurologic disorders. Bladder ultrasound may be the diagnostic examination of choice because no radiation is used and, in most cases, the accuracy is sufficient to make the diagnosis without any further imaging procedures. ■

INDICATIONS:

• Assess residual urine after voiding to diagnose urinary tract obstruction causing overdistention

• Detect tumor of the bladder wall or pelvis, as evidenced by distorted position or changes in bladder contour

• Determine end-stage malignancy of the bladder caused by extension of a primary tumor of the ovary or other pelvic organ

• Evaluate the cause of urinary tract infection, urine retention, and flank pain

• Evaluate hematuria, urinary frequency, dysuria, and suprapubic pain

• Measure urinary bladder volume by transurethral or transvaginal approach

RESULT

Normal Findings:

• Normal size, position, and contour of the bladder

Abnormal Findings:

• Bladder diverticulum

• Cyst

• Cystitis

• Malignancy of the bladder

• Tumor

• Ureterocele

• Urinary tract obstruction

CRITICAL VALUES: N/A

INTERFERING FACTORS:

This procedure is contraindicated for:

• Patients with latex allergy; use of the vaginal probe requires the probe to be covered with a condom-like sac, usually made from latex. Some covers that are latex-free are available.

Factors that may impair clear imaging:

• Incorrect placement of the transducer over the desired test site

• Retained gas or barium from a previous radiologic procedure

• Patients who are dehydrated, resulting in failure to demonstrate the boundaries between organs and tissue structures

• Insufficiently full bladder, which fails to push the bowel from the pelvis and the uterus from the symphysis pubis, thereby prohibiting clear imaging of the pelvic organs in transabdominal imaging

• Metallic objects within the examination field (e.g., jewelry, body rings), which may inhibit organ visualization and can produce unclear images

• Improper adjustment of the ultrasound equipment to accommodate obese or thin patients, which can cause a poor-quality study

• Patients who are very obese, who may exceed the weight limit for the equipment

• Incorrect positioning of the patient, which may produce poor visualization of the area to be examined

Other considerations:

• Failure to follow pretesting preparations may cause the procedure to be canceled or repeated.

• Inability of the patient to cooperate or remain still during the procedure because of age, significant pain, or mental status, may interfere with the test results.

Nursing Implications and Procedure • • • • • • • • • • •

➤ Inform the patient that the procedure assesses the bladder and pelvic organs.

➤ Obtain a history of the patient's complaints, including a list of known allergens (especially allergies or sensitivities to latex), and inform the health care practitioner accordingly.

➤ Obtain a history of the patient's genitourinary, reproductive, and gastrointestinal systems, as well as results of previously performed laboratory tests, surgical procedures, and other diagnostic procedures. For related diagnostic tests, refer to the Genitourinary, Reproductive, and Gastrointestinal System tables.

➤ Note any recent procedures that can interfere with test results (i.e., barium procedures, surgery, or biopsy). There should be 24 hours between administration of barium and this test.

➤ Endoscopic retrograde cholangiopancreatography, colonoscopy, and computed tomography (CT) of the abdomen, if ordered, should be scheduled after this procedure.

➤ Record the date of the last menstrual period and determine the possibility of pregnancy in perimenopausal women.

➤ Obtain a list of the medications the patient is taking.

➤ Review the procedure with the patient. Address concerns about pain related to the procedure. Explain to the patient that some pain may be experienced during the test, and there may be moments of discomfort. Inform the patient that the procedure is performed in a ultrasound department, usually by a technologist, and takes approximately 30 to 60 minutes.

➤ For the transvaginal approach, inform the patient that a latex or sterile sheath-covered probe will be inserted into the vagina.

➤ *Sensitivity to cultural and social issues,* as well as concern for modesty, is important in providing psychological support before, during, and after the procedure.

➤ Instruct the patient to remove jewelry (including watches), hairpins, credit cards, and other metallic objects in the area to be examined.

➤ Inform the patient receiving transabdominal ultrasound that further instruction will be given on the day of the procedure; the procedure requires a full bladder.

➤ Ensure that the patient has complied with pretesting preparations. Ensure that the patient has removed all external metallic objects (jewelry, etc.) prior to the procedure.

➤ Instruct the patient receiving transabdominal ultrasound to drink five to six glasses of fluid 90 minutes before the procedure, and not to void before the procedure. Patients receiving transvaginal ultrasound only do not need to have a full bladder.

➤ Patients are given a gown, robe, and foot coverings to wear.

➤ Instruct the patient to cooperate fully and to follow directions. Instruct the patient to remain still throughout the procedure because movement produces unreliable results.

➤ Observe standard precautions, and follow the general guidelines in Appendix A.

➤ Place the patient in the supine position on an exam table; other positions may be used during the examination. The right- or left-side-up position allows gravity to reposition the liver, gas, and fluid to facilitate better organ visualization.

➤ Expose the abdomen area and drape the patient.

➤ *Transabdominal approach:* Conductive gel is applied to the skin, and a transducer is moved over the skin while the bladder is distended to obtain images of the area of interest. The sound wave images are projected on the screen and stored electronically or reproduced on film.

➤ *Transvaginal approach:* A covered and lubricated probe is inserted into the vagina and moved to different levels. Images are obtained and recorded.

➤ Ask the patient to breathe normally during the examination. If necessary for better organ visualization, ask the patient to inhale deeply and hold his or her breath.

➤ The results are recorded manually, on film, or in a computerized system for recall and postprocedure interpretation by the appropriate health care practitioner.

➤ If the patient is to be examined for residual urine volume, ask the patient to empty the bladder; repeat the procedure and calculate the volume.

Post-test:

➤ Allow the patient to void, as needed.

➤ When the study is completed, remove the gel from the skin.

➤ A written report of the examination will be completed by a health care practitioner specializing in this branch of medicine. The report will be sent to the requesting health care practitioner, who will discuss the results with the patient.

➤ Reinforce information given by the patient's health care provider regarding further testing, treatment, or referral to another health care provider. Answer any questions or address any concerns voiced by the patient or family.

➤ Depending on the results of this procedure, additional testing may be performed to evaluate or monitor progression of the disease process and determine the need for a change in therapy. Evaluate test results in relation to the patient's symptoms and other tests performed.

Related diagnostic tests:

➤ Related diagnostic tests include computed tomography scan of the pelvis; cystoscopy; intravenous pyelography; kidney, ureter, and bladder (KUB) study; and magnetic resonance imaging of the pelvis.

ULTRASOUND, BREAST

· ·

SYNONYM/ACRONYM: Mammographic ultrasound.

AREA OF APPLICATION: Breast.

CONTRAST: Done without contrast.

DESCRIPTION & RATIONALE: Ultrasound procedures are diagnostic, noninvasive, and relatively inexpensive. They take a short time to complete, do not use radiation, and cause no harm to the patient. When used in conjunction with mammography and clinical examination, breast ultrasound is indispensable in the diagnosis and management of benign and malignant process. Both breasts are usually examined during this procedure. The examination uses high-frequency waves of various intensities delivered by a transducer, a flashlight-shaped device, pressed against the skin. The waves are bounced back, converted to electrical energy, amplified by the transducer, and displayed on a monitor to determine the presence of palpable and nonpalpable masses, their size, and structure. This procedure is useful in patients with an abnormal mass on a mammogram because it can determine whether the abnormality is cystic or solid; that is, it can differentiate between a palpable, fluid-filled cyst and a palpable, solid breast lesion (benign or malignant). It is especially useful in patients with dense breast tissue and in those with silicone prostheses, because the ultrasound beam easily penetrates in these situations, allowing routine examination that cannot be performed with x-ray mammography. The procedure can be done as an adjunct to mammography, or it can be done in place of mammography in patients who refuse having x-ray exposure or those in whom it is contraindicated (e.g., pregnant women, women less than 25 years old). The procedure is indicated as a guide for biopsy or other interventional procedures and as a means of monitoring disease progression or the effects of treatment. ▪

INDICATIONS:

- Detect very small tumors in combination with mammography for diagnostic validation

- Determine the presence of nonpalpable abnormalities viewed on mammography of dense breast tissue, and monitor changes in these abnormalities

- Differentiate among types of breast masses (e.g., cyst, solid tumor, other lesions) in dense breast tissue

- Evaluate palpable masses in young (less than age 25), pregnant, and lactating patients

- Guide interventional procedures such as cyst aspiration, large-needle core biopsy, fine-needle aspiration biopsy, abscess drainage, presurgical localization, and galactography

- Identify an abscess in a patient with mastitis

RESULT

Normal Findings:
- Normal subcutaneous, mammary, and retromammary layers of tissue in both breasts; no evidence of pathologic lesions (cyst or tumor) in either breast

Abnormal Findings:
- Abscess

- Breast solid tumor, lesions

- Cancer (ductal carcinoma, infiltrating lobular carcinoma, medullary carcinoma, tubular carcinoma, and papillary carcinoma)

- Cystic breast disease

- Fibroadenoma

- Focal fibrosis

- Galactocele

- Hamartoma (fibroadenolipoma)

- Hematoma

- Papilloma

- Phyllodes tumor

- Radial scar

CRITICAL VALUES: N/A

INTERFERING FACTORS

*Factors that may
impair clear imaging:*

- Incorrect placement of the transducer over the desired test site

- Metallic objects within the examination field (e.g., jewelry, body rings), which may inhibit organ visualization and can produce unclear images

- Improper adjustment of the ultrasound equipment to accommodate obese or thin patients, which can cause a poor-quality study

- Patients who are very obese, who may exceed the weight limit for the equipment

- Excessively large breasts

- Incorrect positioning of the patient, which may produce poor visualization of the area to be examined

- Inability of the patient to cooperate or remain still during the procedure because of age, significant pain, or mental status

Nursing Implications and Procedure • • • • • • • • • • •

Pretest:

▶ Inform the patient that the procedure assesses the breast.

▶ Obtain a history of the patient's complaints, including a list of known allergens, and inform the health care practitioner accordingly.

▶ Obtain a history of the patient's reproductive system, as well as results of previously performed laboratory tests, surgical procedures, and other diagnostic procedures. For related diagnostic tests, refer to the Reproductive System table.

▶ Record the date of the last menstrual period and determine the possibility of pregnancy in perimenopausal women.

▶ Obtain a list of the medications the patient is taking.

▶ Review the procedure with the patient. Address concerns about pain related to the procedure. Explain to the patient that some pain may be experienced during the test, and there may be moments of discomfort. Inform the patient that the procedure is performed in a ultrasound department, usually by a technologist, and takes approximately 30 to 60 minutes.

▶ *Sensitivity to cultural and social issues,* as well as concern for modesty, is important in providing psychological support before, during, and after the procedure.

▶ Instruct the patient not to apply lotions, bath powder, or other substances to the chest and breast area before the examination.

▶ Instruct the patient to remove jewelry (including watches), hairpins, credit cards, and other metallic objects in the area to be examined.

▶ There are no food, fluid, or medication restrictions, unless by medical direction.

Intratest:

▶ Ensure that the patient has not applied lotions, bath powder, or other substances to the chest and breast area before the examination. Ensure that the patient has removed all external metallic objects (jewelry, etc.) prior to the procedure.

▶ Patients are given a gown and robe to wear.

▶ Instruct the patient to cooperate fully and to follow directions. Instruct the patient to remain still throughout the procedure because movement produces unreliable results.

▶ Observe standard precautions, and follow the general guidelines in Appendix A.

▶ Place the patient in the supine position on an exam table. The right- and left-side-up positions are also used during the scan to facilitate better organ visualization.

➤ Expose the breast area and drape the patient.

➤ Conductive gel is applied to the skin and a transducer is moved over the skin to obtain images of the area of interest. The sound wave images are projected on the screen and stored electronically or reproduced on film.

➤ Ask the patient to breathe normally during the examination. If necessary for better organ visualization, ask the patient to inhale deeply and hold his or her breath.

➤ The results are recorded manually, on film, or in a computerized system for recall and postprocedure interpretation by the appropriate health care practitioner.

➤ A written report of the examination will be completed by a health care practitioner specializing in this branch of medicine. The report will be sent to the requesting health care practitioner, who will discuss the results with the patient.

➤ Reinforce information given by the patient's health care provider regarding further testing, treatment, or referral to another health care provider. Answer any questions or address any concerns voiced by the patient or family.

➤ Depending on the results of this procedure, additional testing may be performed to evaluate or monitor progression of the disease process and determine the need for a change in therapy. Evaluate test results in relation to the patient's symptoms and other tests performed.

Post-test:

➤ When the study is completed, remove the gel from the skin.

Related diagnostic tests:

➤ Related diagnostic tests include chest x-ray, computed tomography scan of the thorax, and mammogram.

ULTRASOUND, KIDNEY

SYNONYM/ACRONYM: Renal ultrasound, renal sonography.

AREA OF APPLICATION: Kidney.

CONTRAST: Done without contrast.

DESCRIPTION & RATIONALE: Ultrasound procedures are diagnostic, noninvasive, and relatively inexpensive. They take a short time to complete, do not use radiation, and cause no harm to the patient. Renal ultrasound is used to evaluate renal system disorders. It is valuable for determining the internal components of renal masses (solid versus cystic) and for evaluating other renal diseases, renal parenchyma, perirenal tissues, and obstruction. Ultrasound uses high-frequency waves of various intensities delivered by a transducer, a flashlight-shaped device, pressed against the skin. The waves are bounced back, converted to electrical energy, amplified by the transducer, and displayed on a monitor to evaluate the structure, size, and position of the kidney. Renal ultrasound can be performed on the same day as a radionuclide scan or other radiologic procedure, and is especially valuable in patients who are in renal failure, have hypersensitivity to contrast medium, have a kidney that did not visualize on intravenous pyelography (IVP), or are pregnant. It does not rely on renal function or the injection of contrast medium to obtain a diagnosis. The procedure is indicated for evaluation after a kidney transplant and is used as a guide for biopsy or other interventional procedures, abscess drainage, and nephrostomy tube placement. Renal ultrasound may be the diagnostic examination of choice because no radiation is used and, in most cases, the accuracy is sufficient to make the diagnosis without any further imaging procedures. ■

INDICATIONS:
- Aid in the diagnosis of the effect of chronic glomerulonephritis and end-stage chronic renal failure on the kidneys (e.g., decreasing size)
- Detect an accumulation of fluid in the kidney caused by backflow of urine, hemorrhage, or perirenal fluid
- Detect masses and differentiate between cysts or solid tumors, as evidenced by specific waveform patterns or absence of sound waves
- Determine the presence and location of renal or ureteral calculi and obstruction
- Determine the size, shape, and position of a nonfunctioning kidney to identify the cause
- Evaluate or plan therapy for renal tumors
- Evaluate renal transplantation for changes in kidney size
- Locate the site of and guide percutaneous renal biopsy, aspiration needle insertion, or nephrostomy tube insertion
- Monitor kidney development in children when renal disease has been diagnosed
- Provide the location and size of renal masses in patients who are unable to undergo IVP because of poor renal function or an allergy to iodinated contrast medium

RESULT

Normal Findings:
- Absence of calculi, cysts, hydronephrosis, obstruction, or tumor
- Normal size, position, and shape of the kidneys and associated structures

Abnormal Findings:
- Acute glomerulonephritis
- Acute pyelonephritis
- Congenital anomalies, such as absent, horseshoe, ectopic, or duplicated kidney
- Hydronephrosis
- Obstruction of ureters
- Perirenal abscess or hematoma
- Polycystic kidney
- Rejection of renal transplant
- Renal calculi
- Renal cysts, hypertrophy, or tumors
- Ureteral obstruction

CRITICAL VALUES: N/A

INTERFERING FACTORS

Factors that may impair clear imaging:

- Attenuation of the sound waves by the ribs, which can impair clear imaging of the kidney

- Incorrect placement of the transducer over the desired test site

- Retained gas or barium from a previous radiologic procedure

- Metallic objects within the examination field (e.g., jewelry, body rings), which may inhibit organ visualization and can produce unclear images

- Improper adjustment of the ultrasound equipment to accommodate obese or thin patients, which can cause a poor-quality study

- Patients who are very obese, who may exceed the weight limit for the equipment

- Incorrect positioning of the patient, which may produce poor visualization of the area to be examined

Other considerations:

- Inability of the patient to cooperate or remain still during the procedure because of age, significant pain, or mental status, may interfere with the test results.

Nursing Implications and Procedure • • • • • • • • • • • •

Pretest:

▸ Inform the patient that the procedure assesses kidney function.

▸ Obtain a history of the patient's complaints, including a list of known allergens, and inform the health care practitioner accordingly.

▸ Obtain a history of the patient's genitourinary system, as well as results of previously performed laboratory tests, surgical procedures, and other diagnostic procedures. For related diagnostic tests, refer to the genitourinary System table.

▸ Note any recent procedures that can interfere with test results (i.e., barium procedures, surgery, or biopsy). There should be 24 hours between administration of barium and this test.

▸ Endoscopic retrograde cholangiopancreatography, colonoscopy, and computed tomography (CT) of the abdomen, if ordered, should be scheduled after this procedure.

▸ Record the date of the last menstrual period and determine the possibility of pregnancy in perimenopausal women.

▸ Obtain a list of the medications the patient is taking.

▸ Review the procedure with the patient. Address concerns about pain related to the procedure. Explain to the patient that some pain may be experienced during the test, and there may be moments of discomfort. Inform the patient that the procedure is performed in a ultrasound department, usually by a technologist, and takes approximately 30 to 60 minutes.

▸ *Sensitivity to cultural and social issues,* as well as concern for modesty, is important in providing psychological support before, during, and after the procedure.

▸ Instruct the patient to remove jewelry (including watches), hairpins, credit cards, and other metallic objects in the area to be examined.

Intratest:

▸ Ensure that the patient has removed all external metallic objects (jewelry, etc.) prior to the procedure.

▸ Patients are given a gown, robe, and

foot coverings to wear and instructed to void prior to the procedure.

➤ Instruct the patient to cooperate fully and to follow directions. Instruct the patient to remain still throughout the procedure because movement produces unreliable results.

➤ Observe standard precautions, and follow the general guidelines in Appendix A.

➤ Place the patient in the supine position on an exam table; other positions may be used during the examination. The right- or left-side-up position allows gravity to reposition the liver, gas, and fluid to facilitate better organ visualization.

➤ Expose the abdomen/kidney area and drape the patient.

➤ Conductive gel is applied to the skin, and a transducer is moved over the skin to obtain images of the area of interest. The sound wave images are projected on the screen and stored electronically or reproduced on film.

➤ Ask the patient to breathe normally during the examination. If necessary for better organ visualization, ask the patient to inhale deeply and hold his or her breath.

➤ The results are recorded manually, on film, or in a computerized system for recall and postprocedure interpretation by the appropriate health care practitioner.

Post-test:

➤ When the study is completed, remove the gel from the skin.

➤ A written report of the examination will be completed by a health care practitioner specializing in this branch of medicine. The report will be sent to the requesting health care practitioner, who will discuss the results with the patient.

➤ Reinforce information given by the patient's health care provider regarding further testing, treatment, or referral to another health care provider. Answer any questions or address any concerns voiced by the patient or family.

➤ Depending on the results of this procedure, additional testing may be performed to evaluate or monitor progression of the disease process and determine the need for a change in therapy. Evaluate test results in relation to the patient's symptoms and other tests performed.

Related diagnostic tests:

➤ Related diagnostic tests include angiography renal, computed tomography scan of the abdomen; intravenous pyelography; kidney, ureter, and bladder (KUB) study; magnetic resonance imaging of the abdomen, and renogram.

ULTRASOUND, LIVER AND BILIARY SYSTEM

· ·

SYNONYMS/ACRONYM: Gallbladder ultrasound, liver ultrasound, hepatobiliary sonography.

AREA OF APPLICATION: Liver, gallbladder, bile ducts.

CONTRAST: Done without contrast.

DESCRIPTION & RATIONALE: Ultrasound procedures are diagnostic, noninvasive, and relatively inexpensive. They take a short time to complete, do not use radiation, and cause no harm to the patient. Hepatobiliary ultrasound uses high-frequency waves of various intensities delivered by a transducer, a flashlight-shaped device, pressed against the skin. The waves are bounced back, converted to electrical energy, amplified by the transducer, and displayed on a monitor to evaluate the structure, size, and position of the liver and gallbladder in the right upper quadrant (RUQ) of the abdomen. The gallbladder and biliary system collect, store, concentrate, and transport bile to the intestines to aid in digestion. This procedure allows visualization of the gallbladder and bile ducts when the patient may have impaired liver function, and it is especially helpful when done on patients in whom gallstones cannot be visualized with oral or intravenous radiologic studies. Liver ultrasound can be done in combination with a nuclear scan to obtain information about liver function and density differences in the liver. The procedure is indicated as a guide for biopsy or other interventional procedures. Hepatobiliary ultrasound may be the diagnostic examination of choice because no radiation is used and, in most cases, the accuracy is sufficient to make the diagnosis without any further imaging procedures. ■

INDICATIONS:
- Detect cysts, polyps, hematoma, abscesses, hemangioma, adenoma, metastatic disease, hepatitis, or solid tumor of the liver or gallbladder, as evidenced by echoes specific to tissue density and sharply or poorly defined masses

- Detect gallstones or inflammation when oral cholecystography is inconclusive

- Detect hepatic lesions, as evidenced by density differences and echo-pattern changes

- Determine the cause of unexplained hepatomegaly and abnormal liver function tests

- Determine cause of unexplained RUQ pain

- Determine patency and diameter of the hepatic duct for dilation or obstruction

- Differentiate between obstructive and nonobstructive jaundice by determining the cause

- Evaluate response to therapy for tumor, as evidenced by a decrease in size of the organ

- Guide biopsy or tube placement

- Guide catheter placement into the gallbladder for stone dissolution and gallbladder fragmentation

RESULT

Normal Findings:
- Normal size, position, and shape of the liver and gallbladder, as well as patency of the cystic and common bile ducts

Abnormal Findings:
- Biliary or hepatic duct obstruction/dilation

- Cirrhosis

- Gallbladder inflammation, stones, carcinoma, polyps

- Hematoma or trauma

- Hepatic tumors, metastasis, cysts, hemangioma, hepatitis

- Hepatocellular disease, adenoma

- Hepatomegaly

- Intrahepatic abscess

- Subphrenic abscesses

CRITICAL VALUES: N/A

INTERFERING FACTORS

Factors that may impair clear imaging:
- Attenuation of the sound waves by the ribs, which can impair clear imaging of the right lobe of the liver

- Incorrect placement of the transducer over the desired test site

- Gas or feces in the gastrointestinal tract

resulting from inadequate cleansing or failure to restrict food intake before the study

- Retained barium from a previous radiologic procedure

- Metallic objects within the examination field (e.g., jewelry, body rings), which may inhibit organ visualization and can produce unclear images

- Improper adjustment of the ultrasound equipment to accommodate obese or thin patients, which can cause a poor-quality study

- Patients who are very obese, who may exceed the weight limit for the equipment

- Incorrect positioning of the patient, which may produce poor visualization of the area to be examined

- Inability of the patient to cooperate or remain still during the procedure because of age, significant pain, or mental status

Other considerations:
- Failure to follow dietary restrictions may cause the procedure to be canceled or repeated.

Nursing Implications and Procedure . . . .

Pretest:

▶ Inform the patient that the procedure assesses the liver and biliary function.

▶ Obtain a history of the patient's complaints, including a list of known allergens, and inform the health care practitioner accordingly.

▶ Obtain a history of the patient's hepatobiliary and gastrointestinal systems, as well as results of previously performed laboratory tests, surgical procedures, and other diagnostic procedures. For related diagnostic tests, refer to the Hepatobiliary and Gastrointestinal System tables.

➤ Note any recent procedures that can interfere with test results (i.e., barium procedures, surgery, or biopsy). There should be 24 hours between administration of barium and this test.

➤ Endoscopic retrograde cholangiopancreatography (ERCP), colonoscopy, and computed tomography (CT) of the abdomen, if ordered, should be scheduled after this procedure.

➤ Record the date of the last menstrual period and determine the possibility of pregnancy in perimenopausal women.

➤ Obtain a list of the medications the patient is taking.

➤ Review the procedure with the patient. Address concerns about pain related to the procedure. Explain to the patient that some pain may be experienced during the test, and there may be moments of discomfort. Inform the patient that the procedure is performed in a ultrasound department, usually by a technologist, and takes approximately 30 to 60 minutes.

➤ *Sensitivity to cultural and social issues,* as well as concern for modesty, is important in providing psychological support before, during, and after the procedure.

➤ Instruct the patient to remove jewelry (including watches), hairpins, credit cards, and other metallic objects in the area to be examined.

➤ The patient should fast and restrict fluids for 8 hours prior to the procedure.

Intratest:

➤ Ensure that the patient has complied with dietary and fluids restrictions and pretesting preparations; assure that food and fluids have been restricted for at least 8 hours prior to the procedure. Ensure that the patient has removed all external metallic objects (jewelry, etc.) prior to the procedure.

➤ Patients are given a gown, robe, and foot coverings to wear and instructed to void prior to the procedure.

➤ Instruct the patient to cooperate fully and to follow directions. Instruct the patient to remain still throughout the procedure because movement produces unreliable results.

➤ Observe standard precautions, and follow the general guidelines in Appendix A.

➤ Place the patient in the supine position on an exam table; other positions may be used during the examination. The right- or left-side-up position allows gravity to reposition the liver, gas, and fluid to facilitate better organ visualization.

➤ Expose the abdomen and drape the patient.

➤ Conductive gel is applied to the skin of the RUQ, and a transducer is moved over the skin to obtain images of the area of interest, including the liver, gallbladder, and bile ducts (cystic and common). The sound wave images are projected on the screen and stored electronically or reproduced on film.

➤ Ask the patient to breathe normally during the examination. If necessary for better organ visualization, ask the patient to inhale deeply and hold his or her breath.

➤ Gallbladder contractibility is viewed by scanning after administration of a pharmaceutical that induces gallbladder contraction or after administration of a fatty meal.

➤ The results are recorded manually, on film, or in a computerized system for recall and postprocedure interpretation by the appropriate health care practitioner.

Post-test:

➤ When the study is completed, remove the gel from the skin.

➤ Instruct the patient to resume usual diet and fluids, as directed by the health care practitioner.

➤ A written report of the examination will be completed by a health care practitioner specializing in this branch of medicine. The report will be sent to the requesting health care practitioner, who will discuss the results with the patient.

➤ Reinforce information given by the patient's health care provider regarding further testing, treatment, or referral to another health care provider. Answer any questions or address any concerns voiced by the patient or family.

➤ Depending on the results of this procedure, additional testing may be performed to evaluate or monitor progression of the disease process and

determine the need for a change in therapy. Evaluate test results in relation to the patient's symptoms and other tests performed.

Related diagnostic tests:

➤ Related diagnostic tests include colonoscopy, computed tomography scan of the abdomen, endoscopy, cholangiopancreatography endoscopic retrograde, hepatobiliary scan, and magnetic resonance imaging of the abdomen.

ULTRASOUND, LYMPH NODES AND RETROPERITONEUM

· ·

SYNONYM/ACRONYM: Lymph node sonography.

AREA OF APPLICATION: Abdomen, pelvis, and retroperitoneum.

CONTRAST: Done without contrast.

DESCRIPTION & RATIONALE: Ultrasound procedures are diagnostic, non-invasive, and relatively inexpensive. They take a short time to complete, do not use radiation, and cause no harm to the patient. Lymph node ultrasound uses high-frequency waves of various intensities delivered by a transducer, a flashlight-shaped device, pressed against the skin. The waves are bounced back, converted to electrical energy, amplified by the transducer, and displayed on a monitor to evaluate the structure, size, and position of the lymph nodes to examine the retroperitoneum and surrounding tis-

sues. This procedure is used for the evaluation of retroperitoneal pathology, usually lymph node enlargement. Ultrasound is the preferred diagnostic method because this area is inaccessible to conventional radiography in diagnosing lymphadenopathy, although it can be used in combination with lymphangiography, magnetic resonance imaging (MRI), and computed tomography (CT) to confirm the diagnosis. The procedure may be used for monitoring the effect of radiation or chemotherapy on the lymph nodes. Lymph node ultrasound may be the diagnostic examination of choice because no radiation is used and, in most cases, the accuracy is sufficient to make the diagnosis without any further imaging procedures. ■

INDICATIONS:

• Detect lymphoma

• Determine the location of enlarged nodes to plan radiation and other therapy

• Determine the size or enlargement of aortic and iliac lymph nodes

• Evaluate the effects of medical, radiation, or surgical therapy on the size of nodes or tumors, as evidenced by shrinkage or continued presence of the mass or nodes

RESULT

Normal Findings:

• Normal retroperitoneal and intrapelvic node size of 1.5 cm in diameter

Abnormal Findings:

• Infection or abscess

• Lymphoma

• Retroperitoneal tumor

CRITICAL VALUES: N/A

INTERFERING FACTORS:

Factors that may impair clear imaging:

• Incorrect placement of the transducer over the desired test site

• Gas or feces in the gastrointestinal tract resulting from inadequate cleansing or failure to restrict food intake before the study

• Retained barium from a previous radiologic procedure

• Patients who are dehydrated, resulting in failure to demonstrate the boundaries between organs and tissue structures

• Insufficiently full bladder, which fails to push the bowel from the pelvis and the uterus from the symphysis pubis, thereby prohibiting clear imaging of the pelvic organs in transabdominal imaging

• Metallic objects within the examination field (e.g., jewelry, or bodyrings) which may inhibit organ visualization and can produce unclear images

• Improper adjustment of the ultrasound equipment to accommodate obese or thin patients, which can cause a poor-quality study

• Patients who are very obese, who may exceed the weight limit for the equipment

• Incorrect positioning of the patient, which may produce poor visualization of the area to be examined

Other considerations:

• Failure to follow dietary/fluid instructions and other pretesting preparations may cause the procedure to be canceled or repeated.

• Inability of the patient to cooperate or remain still during the procedure because of age, significant pain, or mental status, may interfere with the test results.

Nursing Implications and Procedure • • • • • • • • • • •

Pretest:

➤ Inform the patient that the procedure assesses assesses the lymph nodes and retroperitoneum.

➤ Obtain a history of the patient's complaints, including a list of known allergens, and inform the health care practitioner accordingly.

➤ Obtain a history of the patient's genitourinary, reproductive, immune, and gastrointestinal systems, as well as results of previously performed laboratory tests, surgical procedures, and other diagnostic procedures. For related diagnostic tests, refer to the Genitourinary, Reproductive, Immune, and Gastrointestinal System tables.

➤ Note any recent procedures that can interfere with test results (i.e., barium procedures, surgery, or biopsy). There should be 24 hours between administration of barium and this test.

➤ Endoscopic retrograde cholangiopancreatography (ERCP), colonoscopy, and CT of the abdomen, if ordered, should be scheduled after this procedure.

➤ Record the date of the last menstrual period and determine the possibility of pregnancy in perimenopausal women.

➤ Obtain a list of the medications the patient is taking.

➤ Review the procedure with the patient. Address concerns about pain related to the procedure. Explain to the patient that some pain may be experienced during the test, and there may be moments of discomfort. Inform the patient that the procedure is performed in a ultrasound department, usually by a technologist, and takes approximately 30 to 60 minutes.

➤ *Sensitivity to cultural and social issues,* as well as concern for modesty, is important in providing psychological support before, during, and after the procedure.

➤ Instruct the patient to remove jewelry (including watches), hairpins, credit cards, and other metallic objects in the area to be examined.

➤ The patient should fast and restrict fluids for 8 hours prior to the procedure. Inform the patient that transabdominal ultrasound requires a full bladder.

Intratest:

➤ Ensure that the patient has complied with dietary and fluids restrictions and pretesting preparations; assure that food and fluids have been restricted for at least 8 hours prior to the procedure. Ensure that the pa-

tient has removed all external metallic objects (jewelry, etc.) prior to the procedure.

➤ Instruct the patient to drink five to six glasses of fluid 90 minutes before the procedure, and not to void before the procedure.

➤ Patients are given a gown, robe and foot coverings to wear.

➤ Instruct the patient to cooperate fully and to follow directions. Instruct the patient to remain still throughout the procedure because movement produces unreliable results.

➤ Observe standard precautions, and follow the general guidelines in Appendix A.

➤ Place the patient in the supine position on an exam table; other positions may be used during the examination.

➤ Expose the abdomen area and drape the patient.

➤ Conductive gel is applied to the skin, and a transducer is moved over the skin while the bladder is distended to obtain images of the area of interest. The sound wave images are projected on the screen and stored electronically or reproduced on film.

➤ Ask the patient to breathe normally during the examination. If necessary for better organ visualization, ask the patient to inhale deeply and hold his or her breath.

➤ The results are recorded manually, on film, or in a computerized system for recall and postprocedure interpretation by the appropriate health care practitioner.

Post-test:

➤ Allow the patient to void, as needed.

➤ When the study is completed, remove the gel from the skin.

➤ Instruct the patient to resume usual diet and fluids, as directed by the health care practitioner.

➤ A written report of the examination will be completed by a health care practitioner specializing in this branch of medicine. The report will be sent to the requesting health care practitioner, who will discuss the results with the patient.

➤ Reinforce information given by the patient's health care provider regarding further testing, treatment, or referral to another health care provider. Answer any questions or address any concerns voiced by the patient or family.

➤ Depending on the results of this procedure, additional testing may be performed to evaluate or monitor progression of the disease process

and determine the need for a change in therapy. Evaluate test results in relation to the patient's symptoms and other tests performed.

Related diagnostic tests:

➤ Related diagnostic tests include angiography of the abdomen; computed tomography scan of the abdomen; kidney, ureter, and bladder (KUB) study; and magnetic resonance imaging of the abdomen.

ULTRASOUND, OBSTETRIC

· ·

SYNONYMS/ACRONYM: OB sonography, fetal age sonogram, gestational age sonogram, pregnancy ultrasound, pregnancy echo, pregnant uterus ultrasonography.

AREA OF APPLICATION: Pelvis and abdominal region.

CONTRAST: Done without contrast.

DESCRIPTION & RATIONALE: Ultrasound procedures are diagnostic, noninvasive, and relatively inexpensive. They take a short time to complete, do not use radiation, and cause no harm to the patient. Obstetric ultrasound uses high-frequency waves of various intensities delivered by a transducer, a flashlight-shaped device, pressed against the skin or inserted into the vagina. The waves are bounced back, converted to electrical energy, amplified by the transducer, and displayed on a monitor to visualize the fetus and placenta. This procedure is done by a transabdominal or trans-

vaginal approach, depending on when the procedure is performed (first trimester [transvaginal] vs. second trimester [transabdominal]). It is the safest method of examination to evaluate the uterus and determine fetal size, growth, and position; fetal structural abnormalities; ectopic pregnancy; placenta position and amount of amniotic fluid; and multiple gestation. Obstetric ultrasound is used to secure different types of information regarding the fetus, varying with the trimester during which the procedure is done. This procedure can also be used in combination with Doppler monitoring of the fetal heart or respiratory movements to detect high-risk pregnancy. The procedure is indicated as a guide for amniocentesis, cordocentesis, fetoscopy, aspiration of multiple oocytes for in vitro fertilization, and other intrauterine interventional procedures. Because the pregnant uterus is filled with amniotic fluid, ultrasonography is an ideal method of evaluating the fetus and placenta; it is also the diagnostic examination of choice because no radiation is used and, in most cases, the accuracy is sufficient to make the diagnosis without any further imaging procedures. ▪

INDICATIONS:

- Detect blighted ovum (missed abortion), as evidenced by empty gestational sac

- Detect fetal death, as evidenced by absence of movement and fetal heart tones

- Detect fetal position before birth, such as breech or transverse presentations

- Detect tubal and other forms of ectopic pregnancy

- Determine and confirm pregnancy or multiple gestation by determining the number of gestational sacs in the first trimester

- Determine cause of bleeding, such as placenta previa or abruptio placentae

- Determine fetal effects of Rh incompatibility

- Determine fetal gestational age by uterine size and measurements of crownrump length, biparietal diameter, fetal extremities, head, and other parts of the anatomy at key phases of fetal development

- Determine fetal heart and body movements and detect high-risk pregnancy by monitoring fetal heart and respiratory movements in combination with Doppler ultrasound or real-time grayscale scanning

- Determine fetal structural anomalies, usually at the 20th week of gestation or later

- Determine the placental size, location, and site of implantation

- Differentiate a tumor (hydatidiform mole) from a normal pregnancy

- Guide the needle during amniocentesis and fetal transfusion

- Measure fetal gestational age and evaluate umbilical artery, uterine artery, and fetal aorta by Doppler examination to determine fetal intrauterine growth retardation

- Monitor placental growth and amniotic fluid volume

RESULT

Normal Findings:

- Normal age, size, viability, position, and functional capacities of the fetus

- Normal placenta size, position, and structure; adequate volume of amniotic fluid

Abnormal Findings:

- Abruptio placentae
- Cardiac abnormalities
- Ectopic pregnancy
- Fetal death
- Fetal hydrops
- Fetal malpresentation (breech, transverse)
- Hydrocephalus
- Intestinal atresia
- Myelomeningocele

- Multiple pregnancy
- Placenta previa
- Renal or skeletal defects

CRITICAL VALUES: N/A

INTERFERING FACTORS:

This procedure is contraindicated for:

- Patients with latex allergy; use of the vaginal probe requires the probe to be covered with a condom-like sac, usually made from latex. Some covers that are latex-free are available.

Factors that may impair clear imaging:

- Incorrect placement of the transducer over the desired test site
- Retained gas or barium from a previous radiologic procedure
- Patients who are dehydrated, resulting in failure to demonstrate the boundaries between organs and tissue structures
- Insufficiently full bladder, which fails to push the bowel from the pelvis and the uterus from the symphysis pubis, thereby prohibiting clear imaging of the pelvic organs in transabdominal imaging
- Metallic objects within the examination field (e.g., jewelry, body rings), which may inhibit organ visualization and can produce unclear images
- Improper adjustment of the ultrasound equipment to accommodate obese or thin patients, which can cause a poor-quality study
- Patients who are very obese, who may exceed the weight limit for the equipment
- Incorrect positioning of the patient, which may produce poor visualization of the area to be examined

Other considerations:

- Inability of the patient to cooperate or remain still during the procedure because of age, significant pain, or mental status, may interfere with the test results.

Nursing Implications and Procedure . . . .

Pretest:

➤ Inform the patient that the procedure assesses abdomen and pelvic organ function.

➤ Obtain a history of the patient's complaints, including a list of known allergens (especially allergies or sensitivities to latex), and inform the appropriate health care practitioner accordingly.

➤ Obtain a history of the patient's genitourinary, reproductive, and gastrointestinal systems, as well as results of previously performed laboratory tests, surgical procedures, and other diagnostic procedures. For related diagnostic tests, refer to the Genitourinary, Reproductive, and Gastrointestinal System tables.

➤ Note any recent procedures that can interfere with test results (i.e., barium procedures, surgery, or biopsy). There should be 24 hours between administration of barium and this test.

➤ Endoscopic retrograde cholangiopancreatography, and colonoscopy, if ordered, should be scheduled after this procedure.

➤ Record the date of the last menstrual period. Obtain a history of menstrual dates, previous pregnancy, and treatment received for high-risk pregnancy.

➤ Obtain a list of the medications the patient is taking.

➤ Review the procedure with the patient. Address concerns about pain related to the procedure. Explain to the patient that some pain may be experienced during the test, and there may be moments of discomfort. Inform the patient that the procedure is performed in a ultrasound department, usually by a technologist, and takes approximately 30 to 60 minutes.

➤ For the transvaginal approach, inform the patient that a latex or sterile sheath-covered probe will be inserted into the vagina.

➤ *Sensitivity to cultural and social issues,* as well as concern for modesty, is important in providing psychological support before, during, and after the procedure.

➤ Instruct the patient to remove jewelry (including watches), hairpins, credit cards, and other metallic objects in the area to be examined.

➤ Inform the patient receiving transabdominal ultrasound that the procedure requires a full bladder.

Intratest:

➤ Ensure that the patient has removed all external metallic objects (jewelry, etc.) prior to the procedure.

➤ Instruct the patient receiving transabdominal ultrasound to drink five to six glasses of fluid 90 minutes before the procedure, and not to void before the procedure. Patients receiving transvaginal ultrasound only do not need to have a full bladder.

➤ Patients are given a gown, robe, and foot coverings to wear.

➤ Instruct the patient to cooperate fully and to follow directions. Instruct the patient to remain still throughout the procedure because movement produces unreliable results.

➤ Observe standard precautions, and follow the general guidelines in Appendix A.

➤ Place the patient in the supine position on an exam table; other positions may be used during the examination. The right- or left-side-up position allows gravity to reposition the liver, gas, and fluid to facilitate better organ visualization.

➤ Expose the abdomen area and drape the patient.

➤ *Transabdominal approach:* Conductive gel is applied to the skin, and a transducer is moved over the skin while the bladder is distended to obtain images of the area of interest. The sound wave images are projected on the screen and stored electronically or reproduced on film.

➤ *Transvaginal approach:* A covered and lubricated probe is inserted into the vagina and moved to different levels. Images are obtained and recorded.

➤ Ask the patient to breathe normally during the examination. If necessary for better organ visualization, ask the patient to inhale deeply and hold his or her breath.

➤ The results are recorded manually, on film, or in a computerized system for recall and postprocedure interpretation by the appropriate health care practitioner.

Post-test:

➤ Allow the patient to void, as needed.

➤ When the study is completed, remove the gel from the skin.

➤ A written report of the examination will be completed by a health care practitioner specializing in this branch of medicine. The report will be sent to the requesting health care practitioner, who will discuss the results with the patient.

➤ Reinforce information given by the patient's health care provider regarding further testing, treatment, or referral to another health care provider. Answer any questions or address any concerns voiced by the patient or family.

➤ Depending on the results of this procedure, additional testing may be performed to evaluate or monitor progression of the disease process and determine the need for a change in therapy. Evaluate test results in rela-

tion to the patient's symptoms and other tests performed.

Related diagnostic tests:

➤ Related diagnostic tests include kidney, ureter, and bladder (KUB) study; and magnetic resonance imaging of the abdomen.

ULTRASOUND, PANCREAS

SYNONYM/ACRONYM: Pancreatic ultrasonography.

AREA OF APPLICATION: Pancreas and upper abdomen.

CONTRAST: Done without contrast.

DESCRIPTION & RATIONALE: Ultrasound procedures are diagnostic, non-invasive, and relatively inexpensive. They take a short time to complete, do not use radiation, and cause no harm to the patient. Pancreatic ultrasound uses high-frequency waves of various intensities delivered by a transducer, a flashlight-shaped device, pressed against the skin. The waves are bounced back, converted to electrical energy, amplified by the transducer, and displayed on a monitor to determine the size, shape, and position of the pancreas; determine the presence of masses or other abnormalities of the pancreas; and examine the surrounding viscera. The procedure is

indicated as a guide for biopsy, aspiration, or other interventional procedures. Pancreatic ultrasound may be the diagnostic examination of choice because no radiation is used and, in most cases, the accuracy is sufficient to make the diagnosis without any further imaging procedures; however, it is usually done in combination with computed tomography (CT) or magnetic resonance imaging (MRI) of the pancreas. ■

INDICATIONS:

• Detect anatomic abnormalities as a consequence of pancreatitis

• Detect pancreatic cancer, as evidenced by a poorly defined mass or a mass in the head of the pancreas that obstructs the pancreatic duct

- Detect pancreatitis, as evidenced by pancreatic enlargement with increased echoes

- Detect pseudocysts, as evidenced by a well-defined mass with absence of echoes from the interior

- Monitor therapeutic response to tumor treatment

- Provide guidance for percutaneous aspiration and fine-needle biopsy of the pancreas

RESULT

Normal Findings:
- Normal size, position, contour, and texture of the pancreas

Abnormal Findings:
- Acute pancreatitis
- Calculi
- Pancreatic duct obstruction
- Pancreatic tumor
- Pseudocysts

CRITICAL VALUES: N/A

INTERFERING FACTORS:

Factors that may impair clear imaging:
- Attenuation of the sound waves by the ribs, which can impair clear imaging of the pancreas

- Incorrect placement of the transducer over the desired test site

- Gas or feces in the gastrointestinal tract resulting from inadequate cleansing or failure to restrict food intake before the study

- Retained barium from a previous radiologic procedure

- Metallic objects within the examination field (e.g., jewelry, body rings),

which may inhibit organ visualization and can produce unclear images

- Improper adjustment of the ultrasound equipment to accommodate obese or thin patients, which can cause a poor-quality study

- Patients who are very obese, who may exceed the weight limit for the equipment

- Incorrect positioning of the patient, which may produce poor visualization of the area to be examined

Other considerations:
- Failure to follow dietary and fluids restrictions and other pretesting preparations may cause the procedure to be canceled or repeated.

- Inability of the patient to cooperate or remain still during the procedure because of age, significant pain, or mental status, may interfere with the test results.

Nursing Implications and Procedure ● ● ● ● ● ● ● ● ● ● ●

Pretest:

➤ Inform the patient that the procedure assesses pancreatic function.

➤ Obtain a history of the patient's complaints, including a list of known allergens, and inform the health care practitioner accordingly.

➤ Obtain a history of the patient's endocrine and gastrointestinal systems, as well as results of previously performed laboratory tests, surgical procedures, and other diagnostic procedures. For related diagnostic tests, refer to the Endocrine and Gastrointestinal System tables.

➤ Note any recent procedures that can interfere with test results (i.e., barium procedures, surgery, or biopsy). There should be 24 hours between administration of barium and this test.

➤ Endoscopic retrograde cholangiopancreatography (ERCP), colonoscopy, and CT of the abdomen, if ordered, should be scheduled after this procedure.

➤ Record the date of the last menstrual period and determine the possibility of pregnancy in perimenopausal women.

➤ Obtain a list of the medications the patient is taking.

➤ Review the procedure with the patient. Address concerns about pain related to the procedure. Explain to the patient that some pain may be experienced during the test, and there may be moments of discomfort. Inform the patient that the procedure is performed in a ultrasound department, usually by a technologist, and takes approximately 30 to 60 minutes.

➤ *Sensitivity to cultural and social issues,* as well as concern for modesty, is important in providing psychological support before, during, and after the procedure.

➤ Instruct the patient to remove jewelry (including watches), hairpins, credit cards, and other metallic objects in the area to be examined.

➤ The patient should fast and restrict fluids for 8 hours prior to the procedure.

Intratest:

➤ Ensure that the patient has complied with dietary and fluids restrictions and pretesting preparations; assure that food and fluids have been restricted for at least 8 hours prior to the procedure. Ensure that the patient has removed all external metallic objects (jewelry, etc.) prior to the procedure.

➤ Patients are given a gown, robe, and foot coverings to wear and instructed to void prior to the procedure.

➤ Instruct the patient to cooperate fully and to follow directions. Instruct the patient to remain still throughout the procedure because movement produces unreliable results.

➤ Observe standard precautions, and follow the general guidelines in Appendix A.

➤ Place the patient in the supine position on an exam table; other positions may be used during the examination. The right- or left-side-up position allows gravity to reposition the liver, gas, and fluid to facilitate better organ visualization.

➤ Expose the abdomen area and drape the patient.

➤ Conductive gel is applied to the skin, and a transducer is moved over the skin to obtain images of the area of interest. The sound wave images are projected on the screen and stored electronically or reproduced on film.

➤ Ask the patient to breathe normally during the examination. If necessary for better organ visualization, ask the patient to inhale deeply and hold his or her breath.

➤ The results are recorded manually, on film, or in a computerized system for recall and postprocedure interpretation by the appropriate healthcare practitioner.

Post-test:

➤ When the study is completed, remove the gel from the skin.

➤ Instruct the patient to resume usual diet and fluids, as directed by the health care practitioner

➤ A written report of the examination will be completed by a health care practitioner specializing in this branch of medicine. The report will be sent to the requesting health care practitioner, who will discuss the results with the patient.

➤ Reinforce information given by the patient's health care provider regarding further testing, treatment, or referral to another health care provider. Answer any questions or address any concerns voiced by the patient or family.

➤ Depending on the results of this procedure, additional testing may be needed to evaluate or monitor progression of the disease process and determine the need for a change in therapy. Evaluate test results in relation to the patient's symptoms and other tests performed.

ULTRASOUND, PELVIS (GYNECOLOGIC, NONOBSTETRIC)

SYNONYMS/ACRONYM: Pelvic sonography, lower abdomen ultrasound, pelvic gynecologic (GYN) sonogram.

AREA OF APPLICATION: Pelvis and appendix region.

CONTRAST: Done without contrast.

DESCRIPTION & RATIONALE: Ultrasound procedures are diagnostic, non-invasive, and relatively inexpensive. They take a short time to complete, do not use radiation, and cause no harm to the patient. Gynecologic ultrasound uses high-frequency waves of various intensities delivered by a transducer, a flashlight-shaped device, pressed against the skin or inserted into the vagina. The waves are bounced back, converted to electrical energy, amplified by the transducer, and displayed on a monitor in order to:

Determine the presence, size, and structure of masses and cysts; and determine the position of an intrauterine contraceptive device (IUD)

Evaluate postmenopausal bleeding

Examine other abnormalities of the uterus, ovaries, fallopian tubes, and vagina

This procedure is done by a transabdominal or transvaginal approach. The transabdominal approach provides a view of the pelvic organs posterior to the bladder. It requires a full bladder, thereby allowing a window for transmission of the ultrasound waves, pushing the uterus away from the pubic symphysis, pushing the bowel out of the pelvis, and acting as a reference for comparison in the evaluation of the internal structures of a mass or cyst being examined. The transvaginal approach focuses on the female reproductive organs and is often used to monitor ovulation over a period of days in patients undergoing fertility assessment. This approach is also used in obese patients or in patients with retroversion of the uterus because the sound waves are better able to reach the organ from the vaginal site. Transvaginal images are significantly more accurate compared to anterior transabdominal images in identifying paracervical, endometrial, and ovarian pathology, and the transvaginal approach does not require a full bladder. The procedure is indicated as a guide for biopsy or other interventional procedures. Pelvic ultrasound may be the diagnostic examination of choice because no radiation is used and, in most cases, the accuracy is sufficient to make the diagnosis without any further imaging procedures. ∎

INDICATIONS:

- Detect and monitor the treatment of pelvic inflammatory disease (PID) when done in combination with other laboratory tests
- Detect bleeding into the pelvis resulting from trauma to the area or ascites associated with tumor metastasis
- Detect masses in the pelvis and differentiate them from cysts or solid tumors, as evidenced by differences in sound-wave patterns
- Detect pelvic abscess or peritonitis caused by a ruptured appendix or diverticulitis
- Detect pregnancy, including ectopic pregnancy
- Detect the presence of ovarian cysts and malignancy and determine the type, if possible, as evidenced by size, outline, and change in position of other pelvic organs
- Evaluate the effectiveness of tumor therapy, as evidenced by a reduction in mass size
- Evaluate suspected fibroid tumor or bladder tumor

- Evaluate the thickness of the uterine wall
- Monitor placement and location of an IUD
- Monitor follicular size associated with fertility studies or to remove follicles for in vitro transplantation

RESULT

Normal Findings:
- Normal size, position, location, and structure of pelvic organs (e.g., uterus, ovaries, fallopian tubes, vagina); IUD properly positioned within the uterine cavity

Abnormal Findings:
- Endometrioma
- Fibroids (leiomyoma)
- Nonovarian cyst
- Ovarian cysts
- Pelvic abscess
- Peritonitis
- PID
- Uterine tumor or adnexal tumor

CRITICAL VALUES: N/A

INTERFERING FACTORS:

This procedure is contraindicated for:
- Patients with latex allergy; use of the vaginal probe requires the probe to be covered with a condom-like sac, usually made from latex. Some covers that are latex-free are available.

Factors that may impair clear imaging:
- Incorrect placement of the transducer over the desired test site
- Gas or feces in the gastrointestinal tract resulting from inadequate cleansing or failure to restrict food intake before the study

* Retained barium from a previous radiologic procedure

* Patients who are dehydrated, resulting in failure to demonstrate the boundaries between organs and tissue structures

* Insufficiently full bladder, which fails to push the bowel from the pelvis and the uterus from the symphysis pubis, thereby prohibiting clear imaging of the pelvic organs in transabdominal imaging

* Metallic objects within the examination field (e.g., jewelry, body rings), which may inhibit organ visualization and can produce unclear images

* Improper adjustment of the ultrasound equipment to accommodate obese or thin patients, which can cause a poor-quality study

* Patients who are very obese, who may exceed the weight limit for the equipment

* Incorrect positioning of the patient, which may produce poor visualization of the area to be examined

Other considerations:

* Failure to follow dietary/fluid instructions and other pretesting preparations may cause the procedure to be canceled or repeated.

* Inability of the patient to cooperate or remain still during the procedure because of age, significant pain, or mental status, may interfere with the test results.

Nursing Implications and Procedure . . . .

Pretest:

➤ Inform the patient that the procedure assesses pelvic organ function.

➤ Obtain a history of the patient's complaints, including a list of known allergens (especially allergies or sensitivities latex), and inform the appropriate health care practitioner accordingly.

➤ Obtain a history of the patient's genitourinary, reproductive, and gastrointestinal systems, as well as results of previously performed laboratory tests, surgical procedures, and other diagnostic procedures. For related diagnostic tests, refer to the Genitourinary, Reproductive, and Gastrointestinal System tables.

➤ Note any recent procedures that can interfere with test results (i.e., barium procedures, surgery, or biopsy). There should be 24 hours between administration of barium and this test.

➤ Endoscopic retrograde cholangiopancreatography, colonoscopy, and computed tomography (CT) of the abdomen, if ordered, should be scheduled after this procedure.

➤ Record the date of the last menstrual period and determine the possibility of pregnancy in perimenopausal women.

➤ Obtain a list of the medications the patient is taking.

➤ Review the procedure with the patient. Address concerns about pain related to the procedure. Explain to the patient that some pain may be experienced during the test, and there may be moments of discomfort. Inform the patient that the procedure is performed in a ultrasound department, usually by a technologist, and takes approximately 30 to 60 minutes.

➤ For the transvaginal approach, inform the patient that a latex or sterile sheath-covered probe will be inserted into the vagina.

➤ *Sensitivity to cultural and social issues,* as well as concern for modesty, is important in providing psychological support before, during, and after the procedure.

➤ Instruct the patient to remove jewelry (including watches), hairpins, credit cards, and other metallic objects in the area to be examined.

▶ The patient should fast and restrict fluids for 8 hours prior to the procedure. Inform the patient receiving transabdominal ultrasound that further instructions will be given on the day of the procedure; the procedure requires a full bladder.

Intratest:

▶ Ensure that the patient has complied with dietary and fluids restrictions and pretesting preparations; assure that food and fluids have been restricted for at least 8 hours prior to the procedure. Ensure that the patient has removed all external metallic objects (jewelry, etc.) prior to the procedure.

▶ Instruct the patient receiving transabdominal ultrasound to drink three to five glasses of fluid 90 minutes before the exam, and not to void before the procedure. Patients receiving transvaginal ultrasound do not need to have a full bladder.

▶ Patients are given a gown, robe, and foot coverings to wear,

▶ Instruct the patient to cooperate fully and to follow directions. Instruct the patient to remain still throughout the procedure because movement produces unreliable results.

▶ Observe standard precautions, and follow the general guidelines in Appendix A.

▶ Place the patient in the supine position on an exam table; other positions may be used during the examination. The right- or left-side-up position allows gravity to reposition the liver, gas, and fluid to facilitate better organ visualization.

▶ Expose the abdomen area and drape the patient.

▶ *Transabdominal approach:* Conductive gel is applied to the skin, and a transducer is moved over the skin while the bladder is distended to obtain images of the area of interest. The sound wave images are projected on the screen and stored electronically or reproduced on film.

▶ *Transvaginal approach:* A covered and lubricated probe is inserted into the vagina and moved to different levels. Images are obtained and recorded.

▶ Ask the patient to breathe normally during the examination. If necessary for better organ visualization, ask the patient to inhale deeply and hold his or her breath.

▶ The results are recorded manually, on film, or in a computerized system for recall and postprocedure interpretation by the appropriate healthcare practitioner.

Post-test:

▶ Allow the patient to void, as needed.

▶ When the study is completed, remove the gel from the skin.

▶ Instruct the patient to resume usual diet and fluids, as directed by the health care practitioner

▶ A written report of the examination will be completed by a health care practitioner specializing in this branch of medicine. The report will be sent to the requesting health care practitioner, who will discuss the results with the patient.

▶ Reinforce information given by the patient's health care provider regarding further testing, treatment, or referral to another health care provider. Answer any questions or address any concerns voiced by the patient or family.

▶ Depending on the results of this procedure, additional testing may be needed to evaluate or monitor progression of the disease process and determine the need for a change in therapy. Evaluate test results in relation to the patient's symptoms and other tests performed.

Related diagnostic tests:

▶ Related diagnostic tests include computed tomography scan of the abdomen; kidney, ureter, and bladder (KUB) study; and magnetic resonance imaging of the abdomen.

ULTRASOUND, PERIPHERAL DOPPLER

SYNONYMS/ACRONYM: Doppler, venous ultrasound, arterial ultrasound, duplex scan.

AREA OF APPLICATION: Veins and arteries.

CONTRAST: Done without contrast.

DESCRIPTION & RATIONALE: Ultrasound procedures are diagnostic, non-invasive, and relatively inexpensive. They take a short time to complete, do not use radiation, and cause no harm to the patient. Peripheral Doppler ultrasound studies can be used to identify narrowing or occlusions of the veins or arteries. In venous Doppler studies, the Doppler identifies moving red blood cells (RBCs) within the vein. The ultrasound beam is directed at the vein and through the Doppler transducer while the RBCs reflect the beam back to the transducer. The reflected sound waves or echoes can be transformed by a computer into scans, graphs, or audible sounds. Blood flow direction, velocity, and the presence of flow disturbances can be readily assessed. The velocity of the blood flow is transformed as a "swishing" noise, audible through the audio speaker. If the vein is occluded, no swishing sound is heard.

In arterial Doppler studies, arteriosclerotic disease of the peripheral vessels can be detected by slowly deflating blood pressure cuffs that are placed on an extremity such as the calf, ankle, or upper extremity. The systolic pressure of the various arteries of the extremities can be measured. The Doppler transducer can detect the first sign of blood flow through the cuffed artery, even the most minimal blood flow, as evidenced by a swishing noise. There is normally a reduction in systolic blood pressure from the arteries of the arms to the arteries of the legs; a reduction exceeding 20 mm Hg is indicative of occlusive disease (deep vein thrombosis) proximal to the area being tested. This procedure may also be used to monitor the patency of a graft, status of previous corrective surgery, vascular status of the blood flow to a transplanted organ, blood flow to a mass, or the extent of vascular trauma. ■

INDICATIONS:

- Aid in the diagnosis of embolic arterial occlusion

- Aid in the diagnosis of small or large vessel arterial occlusive disease

- Aid in the diagnosis of spastic arterial disease, such as Raynaud's phenomenon

- Aid in the diagnosis of venous occlusion secondary to thrombosis or thrombophlebitis

- Determine the patency of a vascular graft, stent, or previous surgery
- Evaluate the origin of pain related to vascular inflammation
- Evaluate possible arterial trauma

RESULT

Normal venous findings:
- Normal Doppler venous signal that occurs spontaneously with the patient's respiration
- Normal venous system, with no evidence of occlusion

Normal arterial findings:
- No evidence of arterial occlusion
- Normal arterial systolic and diastolic Doppler signals
- Normal reduction in systolic blood pressure (i.e., less than 20 mm Hg) when compared to a normal extremity
- Normal ankle-to-brachial (AB) arterial blood pressure (ankle pressure divided by brachial pressure; normal AB pressure index is greater than 0.85)

Abnormal venous findings:
- Venous narrowing or occlusion secondary to thrombosis or thrombophlebitis

Abnormal arterial findings:
- AB pressure index less than 0.85, indicating significant arterial occlusive disease within the extremity
- Embolic arterial occlusion
- Large or small vessel arterial occlusive disease
- Spastic arterial occlusive disease, such as Raynaud's phenomenon

CRITICAL VALUES: N/A

INTERFERING FACTORS:

This procedure is contraindicated for:
- Patients with an open or draining lesion

Factors that may alter test results:
- Cigarette smoking, because nicotine can cause constriction of the peripheral vessels
- Attenuation of the sound waves by bony structures, which can impair clear imaging of the vessels
- Incorrect placement of the transducer over the desired test site
- Retained contrast medium from a previous radiologic procedure
- Metallic objects within the examination field (e.g., jewelry, body rings), which may inhibit organ visualization and can produce unclear images
- Improper adjustment of the ultrasound equipment to accommodate obese or thin patients, which can cause a poor-quality study
- Patients who are very obese, who may exceed the weight limit for the equipment
- Incorrect positioning of the patient, which may produce poor visualization of the area to be examined
- Inability of the patient to cooperate or remain still during the procedure because of age, significant pain, or mental status

Nursing Implications and Procedure

Pretest:

➤ Inform the patient that the procedure assesses the veins and arteries.

➤ Obtain a history of the patient's complaints, including a list of known allergens, (especially allergies or sensitivities to latex), and inform the health care practitioner accordingly.

➤ Obtain a history of the patient's cardiovascular system, as well as results of previously performed laboratory tests, surgical procedures, and other diagnostic procedures. For related diagnostic tests, refer to the Cardiovascular System table.

➤ Report the presence of a lesion that is open or draining; maintain clean, dry dressing for the ulcer; protect the limb from trauma.

➤ Note any recent procedures that can interfere with test results (i.e., iodine-based contrast or barium procedures, surgery, or biopsy). There should be 24 hours between administration of barium or iodine contrast medium and this test.

➤ Endoscopic retrograde cholangiopancreatography, colonoscopy, and computed tomography (CT) of the abdomen, if ordered, should be scheduled after this procedure.

➤ Record the date of the last menstrual period and determine the possibility of pregnancy in perimenopausal women.

➤ Obtain a list of the medications the patient is taking, including anticoagulant therapy, aspirin and other salicylates, herbs, nutritional supplements, and nutraceuticals, especially those known to affect coagulation (see Appendix F). It is recommended that use be discontinued 14 days before surgical procedures. The requesting health care practitioner and laboratory should be advised if the patient regularly uses these products so that their effects can be taken into consideration when reviewing results.

➤ Review the procedure with the patient. Address concerns about pain related to the procedure. Explain to the patient that some pain may be experienced during the test, and there may be moments of discomfort. Inform the patient that the procedure is performed in a ultrasound department, usually by a technologist, and takes approximately 30 to 60 minutes.

➤ *Sensitivity to social and cultural issues,* as well as concern for modesty, is important in providing psychological support before, during, and after the procedure.

➤ Instruct the patient to remove jewelry (including watches), hairpins,

credit cards, and other metallic objects in the area to be examined.

➤ There are no food, fluid, or medication restrictions, unless by medical direction.

Intratest:

➤ Ensure that the patient has removed all external metallic objects (jewelry, etc.) prior to the procedure.

➤ Patients are given a gown, robe, and foot coverings to wear and instructed to void prior to the procedure.

➤ Instruct the patient to cooperate fully and to follow directions. Instruct the patient to remain still throughout the procedure because movement produces unreliable results.

➤ Observe standard precautions, and follow the general guidelines in Appendix A.

➤ Place the patient in the supine position on an exam table; other positions may be used during the examination.

➤ Expose the area of interest and drape the patient.

➤ Conductive gel is applied to the skin, and a Doppler transducer is moved over the skin to obtain images of the area of interest.

➤ Ask the patient to breathe normally during the examination. If necessary for better organ visualization, ask the patient to inhale deeply and hold his or her breath.

➤ The results are recorded manually, on film, or in a computerized system for recall and postprocedure interpretation by the appropriate health care practitioner.

Arterial Doppler studies of the lower extremity:

➤ Place blood pressure cuffs on the thigh, calf, and ankle.

➤ Apply a conductive get to the skin over the area distal to each of the cuffs.

➤ Inflate the thigh proximal cuff to a level above the patient's systolic pressure found in the normal extremity.

➤ Place the Doppler transducer on the skin distal to the inflated cuff, and slowly release the pressure in the cuff.

➤ When the swishing sound of blood flow is heard, record it at the highest point along the artery at which it is audible. The test is repeated at the calf and then the ankle.

Post-test:

➤ When the study is completed, remove the gel from the skin.

➤ Instruct the patient to continue usual diet, fluids, and medications, as directed by the health care practitioner

➤ *Nutritional considerations:* A low-fat, low-cholesterol, and low-sodium diet should be consumed to reduce current disease processes and/or decrease risk of hypertension and coronary artery disease.

➤ A written report of the examination will be completed by a health care practitioner specializing in this branch of medicine. The report will be sent to the requesting health care practitioner, who will discuss the results with the patient.

➤ Recognize anxiety related to test results, and be supportive of perceived loss of independent function. Discuss the implications of abnormal test results on the patient's lifestyle. Provide teaching and information regarding the clinical implications of the test results, as appropriate.

➤ Reinforce information given by the patient's health care provider regarding further testing, treatment, or referral to another health care provider. Answer any questions or address any concerns voiced by the patient or family.

➤ Instruct the patient in the use of any ordered medications. Explain the importance of adhering to the therapy regimen. As appropriate, instruct the patient in significant side effects and systemic reactions associated with the prescribed medication. Encourage him or her to review corresponding literature provided by a pharmacist.

➤ Depending on the results of this procedure, additional testing may be needed to evaluate or monitor progression of the disease process and determine the need for a change in therapy. Evaluate test results in relation to the patient's symptoms and other tests performed.

Related diagnostic tests:

➤ Related diagnostic tests include computed tomography angiography, and magnetic resonance imaging angiography.

ULTRASOUND, PROSTATE (TRANSRECTAL)

SYNONYM/ACRONYM: Prostate sonography.

AREA OF APPLICATION: Prostate, seminal vesicles.

CONTRAST: Done without contrast.

DESCRIPTION & RATIONALE: Ultrasound procedures are diagnostic, non-invasive, and relatively inexpensive. They take a short time to complete, do not use radiation, and cause no harm to the patient. Prostate ultrasound is used for the evaluation of disorders of the prostate, especially in response to an elevated concentration of prostate-specific antigen on a blood test and as a complement to a digital rectal examination. It uses high-frequency waves of various intensities delivered by a transducer, a candle-shaped device, which is lubricated, sheathed with a condom, and inserted a few inches into the rectum. The waves are bounced back, converted to electrical energy, amplified by the transducer, and displayed on a monitor to evaluate the structure, size, and position of the contents of the prostate (e.g., masses), as well as other prostate pathology. It aids in the diagnosis of prostatic cancer by evaluating palpable nodules and is useful as a guide to biopsy. This procedure can evaluate prostate tissue, the seminal vesicles, and surrounding perirectal tissue. It can also be used to stage carcinoma and to assist in radiation seed placement. The examination is helpful in monitoring patient response to therapy for prostatic disease. Micturition disorders can also be evaluated by this procedure. Prostate ultrasound may be the diagnostic examination of choice because no radiation is used and, in most cases, the accuracy is sufficient to make the diagnosis without any further imaging procedures. ▪

INDICATIONS:

- Aid in the diagnosis of micturition disorders
- Aid in prostate cancer diagnosis
- Assess prostatic calcifications
- Assist in guided needle biopsy of a suspected tumor
- Assist in radiation seed placement
- Determine prostatic cancer staging
- Detect prostatitis

RESULT

Normal Findings:
- Normal size, consistency, and contour of the prostate gland

Abnormal Findings:
- Benign prostatic hypertrophy or hyperplasia
- Micturition disorders
- Perirectal abscess
- Perirectal tumor
- Prostate abscess
- Prostate cancer
- Prostatitis
- Rectal tumor
- Seminal vesicle tumor

CRITICAL VALUES: N/A

INTERFERING FACTORS:

This procedure is contraindicated for:
- Patients with latex allergy; use of the rectal probe requires the probe to be covered with a condom, usually made from latex. Some covers that are latex-free are available.

Factors that may impair clear imaging:
- Attenuation of the sound waves by the pelvic bones, which can impair clear imaging of the prostate
- Incorrect placement of the transducer over the desired test site

- Gas or feces in the gastrointestinal tract resulting from inadequate cleansing or failure to restrict food intake before the study

- Retained barium from a previous radiologic procedure

- Metallic objects within the examination field (e.g., jewelry, body rings), which may inhibit organ visualization and can produce unclear images

- Improper adjustment of the ultrasound equipment to accommodate obese or thin patients, which can cause a poor-quality study

- Patients who are very obese, who may exceed the weight limit for the equipment

- Incorrect positioning of the patient, which may produce poor visualization of the area to be examined

Other considerations:
- Failure to follow pretesting preparations may cause the procedure to be canceled or repeated.

- Inability of the patient to cooperate or remain still during the procedure because of age, significant pain, or mental status, may interfere with the test results.

Nursing Implications and Procedure

Pretest:

➤ Inform the patient that the procedure assesses prostate.

➤ Obtain a history of the patient's complaints, including a list of known allergens (especially allergies or sensitivities to latex), and inform the health care practitioner accordingly.

➤ Obtain a history of the patient's genitourinary system, as well as results

of previously performed laboratory tests, surgical procedures, and other diagnostic procedures. For related diagnostic tests, refer to the Genitourinary System table.

➤ Note any recent procedures that can interfere with test results (i.e., barium procedures, surgery, or biopsy). There should be 24 hours between administration of barium and this test.

➤ Colonoscopy and computed tomography (CT) of the abdomen, if ordered, should be scheduled after this procedure.

➤ Obtain a list of the medications the patient is taking.

➤ Review the procedure with the patient. Address concerns about pain related to the procedure. Explain to the patient that some pain may be experienced during the test, and there may be moments of discomfort. Inform the patient that the procedure is performed in a ultrasound department, usually by a technologist, and takes approximately 30 to 60 minutes.

➤ Inform the patient that a latex or sterile sheath-covered probe will be inserted into the rectum.

➤ *Sensitivity to cultural and social issues,* as well as concern for modesty, is important in providing psychological support before, during, and after the procedure.

➤ Instruct the patient to remove jewelry (including watches), hairpins, credit cards, and other metallic objects in the area to be examined.

Intratest:

➤ Ensure that the patient has complied with pretesting preparations. Ensure that the patient has removed all external metallic objects (jewelry, etc.) prior to the procedure.

➤ Patients are given a gown, robe, and foot coverings to wear and instructed to void prior to the procedure.

➤ Instruct the patient to cooperate fully and to follow directions. Instruct the patient to remain still throughout the procedure because movement produces unreliable results.

➤ Observe standard precautions, and follow the general guidelines in Appendix A.

➤ Place the patient on the examining table on his left side with his knees bent toward the chest; other positions may be used during the examination.

➤ Expose the pelvic area and drape the patient.

➤ Cover the rectal probe with a lubricated condom and insert it into the rectum. Inform the patient that he may feel slight pressure as the transducer is inserted. Water may be introduced through the sheath surrounding the transducer. The scan is performed at several levels.

➤ Ask the patient to breathe normally during the examination. If necessary for better organ visualization, ask the patient to inhale deeply and hold his breath.

➤ The results are recorded manually, on film, or in a computerized system for recall and postprocedure interpretation by the appropriate health care practitioner.

Post-test:

➤ When the study is completed, remove the gel from the skin.

➤ A written report of the examination will be completed by a health care practitioner specializing in this branch of medicine. The report will be sent to the requesting health care practitioner, who will discuss the results with the patient.

➤ Reinforce information given by the patient's health care provider regarding further testing, treatment, or referral to another health care provider. Answer any questions or address any concerns voiced by the patient or family.

➤ Depending on the results of this procedure, additional testing may be needed to evaluate or monitor progression of the disease process and determine the need for a change in therapy. Evaluate test results in relation to the patient's symptoms and other tests performed.

Related diagnostic tests:

➤ Related diagnostic tests include computed tomography scan of the pelvis; intravenous pyelography; kidney, ureter, and bladder (KUB) study; magnetic resonance imaging of the pelvis; and renogram.

ULTRASOUND, SCROTAL

SYNONYM/ACRONYM: Scrotal sonography, ultrasound of the testes, testicular ultrasound.

AREA OF APPLICATION: Scrotum.

CONTRAST: Done without contrast.

DESCRIPTION & RATIONALE: Ultrasound procedures are diagnostic, noninvasive, and relatively inexpensive. They take a short time to complete, do not use radiation, and cause no harm to the patient. Scrotal ultrasound is used for the evaluation of disorders of the scrotum. It is valuable in determining the internal components of masses (solid versus cystic) and for the evaluation of the testicle, extratesticular and intrascrotal tissues, benign and malignant tumors, and other scrotal pathology. It uses high-frequency waves of various intensities delivered by a transducer, a flashlight-shaped device, which is pressed against the skin. The waves are bounced back, converted to electrical energy, amplified by the transducer, and displayed on a monitor to evaluate the structure, size, and position of the contents of the scrotum. Scrotal ultrasound can be performed before or after a radionuclide scan for further clarification of a testicular mass. Extratesticular lesions such as hydrocele, hematocele (blood in the scrotum), and pyocele (pus in the scrotum) can be identified, as can cryptorchidism (undescended testicles). Scrotal ultrasound may be the diagnostic examination of choice because no radiation is used and, in most cases, the accuracy is sufficient to make the diagnosis without any further imaging procedures. ∎

INDICATIONS:
• Aid in the diagnosis of a chronic inflammatory condition such as epididymitis

• Aid in the diagnosis of a mass and differentiate between a cyst and a solid tumor, as evidenced by specific waveform patterns or the absence of sound waves, respectively

• Aid in the diagnosis of scrotal or testicular size, abnormality, or pathology

• Aid in the diagnosis of testicular torsion and associated testicular infarction

• Assist ultrasound-guided needle biopsy of a suspected testicle tumor

• Determine the cause of chronic scrotal swelling or pain

• Determine the presence of a hydrocele, pyocele, spermatocele, or hernia before surgery

• Evaluate the effectiveness of treatment for testicular infections

• Locate an undescended testicle

RESULT

Normal Findings:
• Normal size, position, and shape of the scrotum and structure of the testes

Abnormal Findings:
• Abscess
• Epididymal cyst
• Epididymitis
• Hematoma
• Hydrocele
• Infarction
• Microlithiasis
• Orchitis
• Pyocele
• Scrotal hernia
• Spermatocele
• Torsion
• Tumor, benign or malignant
• Tunica albuginea cyst
• Undescended testicle (cryptorchidism)
• Varicocele

CRITICAL VALUES: N/A

INTERFERING FACTORS:

Factors that may impair clear imaging:

- Incorrect placement of the transducer over the desired test site

- Retained barium from a previous radiologic procedure

- Metallic objects within the examination field (e.g., jewelry, body rings), which may inhibit organ visualization and can produce unclear images

- Improper adjustment of the ultrasound equipment to accommodate obese or thin patients, which can cause a poor-quality study

- Patients who are very obese, who may exceed the weight limit for the equipment

- Incorrect positioning of the patient, which may produce poor visualization of the area to be examined

- Inability of the patient to cooperate or remain still during the procedure because of age, significant pain, or mental status

Nursing Implications and Procedure • • • • • • • • • • •

Pretest:

▶ Inform the patient that the procedure assesses the scrotum.

▶ Obtain a history of the patient's complaints, including a list of known allergens, and inform the health care practitioner accordingly.

▶ Obtain a history of the patient's genitourinary and reproductive systems, as well as results of previously performed laboratory tests, surgical procedures, and other diagnostic procedures. For related diagnostic tests, refer to the Genitourinary and Reproductive System tables.

▶ Note any recent procedures that can interfere with test results (i.e., barium procedures, surgery, or biopsy). There should be 24 hours between administration of barium and this test.

▶ Colonoscopy and computed tomography (CT) of the abdomen, if ordered, should be scheduled after this procedure.

▶ Obtain a list of the medications the patient is taking.

▶ Review the procedure with the patient. Address concerns about pain related to the procedure. Explain to the patient that some pain may be experienced during the test, and there may be moments of discomfort. Inform the patient that the procedure is performed in a ultrasound department, usually by a technologist, and takes approximately 30 to 60 minutes.

▶ *Sensitivity to cultural and social issues,* as well as concern for modesty, is important in providing psychological support before, during, and after the procedure.

▶ Instruct the patient to remove jewelry (including watches), hairpins, credit cards, and other metallic objects in the area to be examined.

▶ There are no food, fluid, or medication restrictions, unless by medical direction.

Intratest:

▶ Ensure that the patient has removed all external metallic objects (jewelry, etc.) prior to the procedure.

▶ Patients are given a gown and robe to wear and instructed to void prior to the procedure.

▶ Instruct the patient to cooperate fully and to follow directions. Instruct the patient to remain still throughout the procedure because movement produces unreliable results.

▶ Observe standard precautions, and

follow the general guidelines in Appendix A.

➤ Place the patient in the supine position on an exam table; other positions may be used during the examination.

➤ Expose the abdomen/pelvic area and drape the patient.

➤ Lift the penis upward and gently tape it to the lower part of the abdomen. Elevate the scrotum with a rolled towel or sponge for immobilization. Display particular sensitivity toward the patient regarding any embarrassment he may feel during this part of the procedure.

➤ Conductive gel is applied to the skin, and a transducer is moved over the skin to obtain images of the area of interest. The sound wave images are projected on the screen and stored electronically or reproduced on film.

➤ Ask the patient to breathe normally during the examination. If necessary for better organ visualization, ask the patient to inhale deeply and hold his breath.

➤ The results are recorded manually, on film, or in a computerized system for recall and postprocedure interpretation by the appropriate health care practitioner.

Post-test:

➤ When the study is completed, remove the gel from the skin.

➤ A written report of the examination will be completed by a health care practitioner specializing in this branch of medicine. The report will be sent to the requesting health care practitioner, who will discuss the results with the patient.

➤ Reinforce information given by the patient's health care provider regarding further testing, treatment, or referral to another health care provider. Answer any questions or address any concerns voiced by the patient or family.

➤ Depending on the results of this procedure, additional testing may be needed to evaluate or monitor progression of the disease process and determine the need for a change in therapy. Evaluate test results in relation to the patient's symptoms and other tests performed.

Related diagnostic tests:

➤ Related diagnostic tests include computed tomography scan of the pelvis; kidney, ureter, and bladder (KUB) study; and magnetic resonance imaging of the pelvis.

ULTRASOUND, SPLEEN

SYNONYM/ACRONYM: Spleen ultrasonography.

AREA OF APPLICATION: Spleen/left upper quadrant.

CONTRAST: Done without contrast.

DESCRIPTION & RATIONALE: Ultrasound procedures are diagnostic, noninvasive, and relatively inexpensive. They take a short time to complete, do not use radiation, and cause no harm to the patient. Spleen ultrasound uses high-frequency waves of various intensities delivered by a transducer, a flashlight-shaped device, pressed against the skin. The waves are bounced back, converted to electrical energy, amplified by the transducer, and displayed on a monitor to evaluate the structure, size, and position of the spleen. This test is valuable for determining the internal components of splenic masses (solid versus cystic) and evaluating other splenic pathology, splenic trauma, and left upper quadrant perisplenic tissues. It can be performed to supplement a radionuclide scan or computed tomography (CT). It is especially valuable in patients who are in renal failure, are hypersensitive to contrast medium, or are pregnant because it does not rely on adequate renal function or the injection of contrast medium to obtain a diagnosis. The procedure may also be used as a guide for biopsy, other interventional procedures, or abscess drainage. Spleen ultrasound may be the diagnostic examination of choice because no radiation is used and, in most cases, the accuracy is sufficient to make the diagnosis without any further imaging procedures. ∎

INDICATIONS:

• Detect the presence of a subphrenic abscess after splenectomy

• Detect splenic masses; differentiate between cysts or solid tumors (in combination with CT), as evidenced by specific waveform patterns or absence of sound waves, respectively; and determine whether they are intrasplenic or extrasplenic

• Determine late-stage sickle cell disease, as evidenced by decreased spleen size and presence of echoes

• Determine the presence of splenomegaly, and assess the size and volume of the spleen in these cases, as evidenced by increased echoes and visibility of the spleen

• Differentiate spleen trauma from blood or fluid accumulation between the splenic capsule and parenchyma

• Evaluate the effect of medical or surgical therapy on the progression or resolution of splenic disease

• Evaluate the extent of abdominal trauma and spleen involvement, including enlargement or rupture, after a recent trauma

• Evaluate the spleen before splenectomy performed for thrombocytopenic purpura

RESULT

Normal Findings:
• Normal size, position, and contour of the spleen and associated structures

Abnormal Findings:
• Abscesses
• Accessory or ectopic spleen
• Infection
• Lymphatic disease, lymph node enlargement
• Splenic calcifications
• Splenic masses, tumors, cysts, or infarction
• Splenic trauma
• Splenomegaly

CRITICAL VALUES: N/A

INTERFERING FACTORS:

Factors that may impair clear imaging:

- Attenuation of the sound waves by the ribs and an aerated left lung, which can impair clear imaging of the spleen

- Masses near the testing site, which can displace the spleen and cause inaccurate results if confused with splenomegaly

- Patients who are dehydrated, resulting in failure to demonstrate the boundaries between organs and tissue structures

- Incorrect placement of the transducer over the desired test site

- Gas or feces in the gastrointestinal tract resulting from inadequate cleansing or failure to restrict food intake before the study

- Retained barium from a previous radiologic procedure

- Metallic objects within the examination field (e.g., jewelry, body rings), which may inhibit organ visualization and can produce unclear images

- Improper adjustment of the ultrasound equipment to accommodate obese or thin patients, which can cause a poor-quality study

- Patients who are very obese, who may exceed the weight limit for the equipment

- Incorrect positioning of the patient, which may produce poor visualization of the area to be examined

Other considerations:

- Failure to follow dietary restrictions and other pretesting preparations may cause the procedure to be canceled or repeated.

- Inability of the patient to cooperate or remain still during the procedure because of age, significant pain, or mental status, may interfere with the test results.

Nursing Implications and Procedure • • • • • • • • • • •

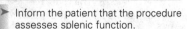

Pretest:

➤ Inform the patient that the procedure assesses splenic function.

➤ Obtain a history of the patient's complaints, including a list of known allergens, and inform the health care practitioner accordingly.

➤ Obtain a history of the patient's hematopoietic, immune, and gastrointestinal systems, as well as results of previously performed laboratory tests, surgical procedures, and other diagnostic procedures. For related diagnostic tests, refer to the Hematopoietic, Immune, and Gastrointestinal System tables.

➤ Note any recent procedures that can interfere with test results (i.e., barium procedures, surgery, or biopsy). There should be 24 hours between administration of barium and this test.

➤ Endoscopic retrograde cholangiopancreatography, colonoscopy, and CT of the abdomen, if ordered, should be scheduled after this procedure.

➤ Record the date of the last menstrual period and determine the possibility of pregnancy in perimenopausal women.

➤ Obtain a list of the medications the patient is taking.

➤ Review the procedure with the patient. Address concerns about pain related to the procedure. Explain to the patient that some pain may be experienced during the test, and there may be moments of discomfort. Inform the patient that the procedure is performed in a ultrasound department, usually by a technologist, and takes approximately 30 to 60 minutes.

➤ *Sensitivity to cultural and social issues,* as well as concern for modesty, is important in providing psychological support before, during, and after the procedure.

➤ Instruct the patient to remove jewelry

(including watches), hairpins, credit cards, and other metallic objects in the area to be examined.

➤ The patient should fast and restrict fluids for 8 hours prior to the procedure.

Intratest:

➤ Ensure that the patient has complied with dietary and fluids restrictions and pretesting preparations; assure that food and fluids have been restricted for at least 8 hours prior to the procedure. Ensure that the patient has removed all external metallic objects (jewelry, etc.) prior to the procedure.

➤ Patients are given a gown, robe, and foot coverings to wear and instructed to void prior to the procedure.

➤ Instruct the patient to cooperate fully and to follow directions. Instruct the patient to remain still throughout the procedure because movement produces unreliable results.

➤ Observe standard precautions, and follow the general guidelines in Appendix A.

➤ Place the patient in the supine position on an exam table; other positions may be used during the examination. The right- or left-side-up position allows gravity to reposition the liver, gas, and fluid to facilitate better organ visualization.

➤ Expose the abdomen area and drape the patient.

➤ Conductive gel is applied to the skin, and a transducer is moved over the skin to obtain images of the area of interest. The sound wave images are projected on the screen and stored electronically or reproduced on film.

➤ Ask the patient to breathe normally during the examination. If necessary for better organ visualization, ask the patient to inhale deeply and hold his or her breath.

➤ The results are recorded manually, on film, or in a computerized system for recall and postprocedure interpretation by the appropriate health care practitioner.

Post-test:

➤ When the study is completed, remove the gel from the skin.

➤ Instruct the patient to resuem usual diet and fluids, as directed by the health care practitioner

➤ A written report of the examination will be completed by a health care practitioner specializing in this branch of medicine. The report will be sent to the requesting health care practitioner, who will discuss the results with the patient.

➤ Reinforce information given by the patient's health care provider regarding further testing, treatment, or referral to another health care provider. Answer any questions or address any concerns voiced by the patient or family.

➤ Depending on the results of this procedure, additional testing may be performed to evaluate or monitor progression of the disease process and determine the need for a change in therapy. Evaluate test results in relation to the patient's symptoms and other tests performed.

Related diagnostic tests:

➤ Related diagnostic tests include angiography of the abdomen; computed tomography scan of the abdomen; kidney, ureter, and bladder (KUB) study; and magnetic resonance imaging of the abdomen.

ULTRASOUND, THYROID AND PARATHYROID

· ·

SYNONYMS/ACRONYM: Thyroid sonography, parathyroid sonography, thyroid echo.

AREA OF APPLICATION: Thyroid, parathyroid, and anterior neck region.

CONTRAST: Done without contrast.

DESCRIPTION & RATIONALE: Ultrasound procedures are diagnostic, non-invasive, and relatively inexpensive. They take a short time to complete, do not use radiation, and cause no harm to the patient. Thyroid and parathyroid ultrasound uses high-frequency waves of various intensities delivered by a transducer, a flashlight-shaped device, pressed against the skin. The waves are bounced back, converted to electrical energy, amplified by the transducer, and displayed on a monitor to determine the position, size, shape, weight, and presence of masses of the thyroid gland; enlargement of the parathyroid glands; and other abnormalities of the thyroid and parathyroid glands and surrounding tissues. The primary purpose of this procedure is to determine whether a nodule is a fluid-filled cyst (usually benign) or a solid tumor (possibly malignant). This procedure is useful in evaluating the glands' response to medical treatment or assessing the remaining tissue after surgical resection. The procedure may be indicated as a guide for biopsy, aspiration, or other interventional procedures. Thy-

roid and parathyroid ultrasound may be the diagnostic examination of choice because no radiation is used and, in most cases, the accuracy is sufficient to make the diagnosis without any further imaging procedures; it is clearly the procedure of choice when examining the glands of pregnant patients. This procedure is usually done in combination with nuclear medicine imaging procedures and computed tomography (CT) of the neck. Despite the advantages of the procedure, in some cases it may not detect small nodules and lesions (less than 1 cm), leading to false-negative findings. ■

INDICATIONS:
* Assist in determining the presence of a tumor, as evidenced by an irregular border and shadowing at the distal edge, peripheral echoes, or high- and low-amplitude echoes, depending on the density of the tumor mass; and diagnosing tumor type (e.g., benign, adenoma, carcinoma)
* Assist in diagnosing the presence of a cyst, as evidenced by a smoothly outlined, echo-free amplitude except at the far borders of the mass

- Assist in diagnosis in the presence of a parathyroid enlargement indicating a tumor or hyperplasia, as evidenced by an echo pattern of lower amplitude than that for a thyroid tumor

- Determine the need for surgical biopsy of a tumor or fine-needle biopsy of a cyst

- Differentiate among a nodule, solid tumor, or fluid-filled cyst

- Evaluate the effect of a therapeutic regimen for a thyroid mass or Graves' disease by determining the size and weight of the gland

- Evaluate thyroid abnormalities during pregnancy

RESULT

Normal Findings:
- Normal size, position, contour, and structure of the thyroid and parathyroid glands with uniform echo patterns throughout the glands; no evidence of tumor cysts or nodules in the glands

Abnormal Findings:
- Glandular enlargement

- Goiter

- Graves' disease

- Parathyroid tumor or hyperplasia

- Thyroid cysts

- Thyroid tumors (benign or malignant)

CRITICAL VALUES: N/A

INTERFERING FACTORS

Factors that may impair clear imaging:
- Attenuation of the sound waves by the ribs, which can impair clear imaging of the parathyroid

- Incorrect placement of the transducer over the desired test site

- Metallic objects within the examination field (e.g., jewelry, body rings), which may inhibit organ visualization and can produce unclear images

- Improper adjustment of the ultrasound equipment to accommodate obese or thin patients, which can cause a poor-quality study

- Patients who are very obese, who may exceed the weight limit for the equipment

- Incorrect positioning of the patient, which may produce poor visualization of the area to be examined

Other considerations:
- Nodules less than 1 cm in diameter may not be detected.

- Nonthyroid cysts may appear the same as thyroid cysts.

- Inability of the patient to cooperate or remain still during the procedure because of age, significant pain, or mental status, may interfere with the test results.

Nursing Implications and Procedure • • • • • • • • • •

Pretest:

➤ Inform the patient that the procedure assesses thyroid and parathyroid function.

➤ Obtain a history of the patient's complaints, including a list of known allergens, and inform the health care practitioner accordingly.

➤ Obtain a history of the patient's endocrine system, as well as results of previously performed laboratory tests, surgical procedures, and other diagnostic procedures. For related diagnostic tests, refer to the Endocrine System table.

➤ Note any recent procedures that can interfere with test results (i.e., barium procedures, surgery, or biopsy). There should be 24 hours between administration of barium and this test.

➤ Record the date of the last menstrual period and determine the possibility of pregnancy in perimenopausal women.

➤ Obtain a list of the medications the patient is taking.

➤ Review the procedure with the patient. Address concerns about pain related to the procedure. Explain to the patient that some pain may be experienced during the test, and there may be moments of discomfort. Inform the patient that the procedure is performed in a ultrasound department, usually by a technologist, and takes approximately 30 to 60 minutes.

➤ *Sensitivity to cultural and social issues,* as well as concern for modesty, is important in providing psychological support before, during, and after the procedure.

➤ There are no food, fluid, or medication restrictions, unless by medical direction.

Intratest:

➤ Patients are given a gown, robe, and foot coverings to wear and instructed to void prior to the procedure.

➤ Instruct the patient to cooperate fully and to follow directions. Instruct the patient to remain still throughout the procedure because movement produces unreliable results.

➤ Observe standard precautions, and follow the general guidelines in Appendix A.

➤ Place the patient in the supine position on an exam table; other positions may be used during the examination.

➤ Expose the neck and chest area and drape the patient.

➤ Hyperextend the neck, and place a pillow under the patient's shoulders to maintain a comfortable position. (An alternative method of imaging includes the use of a bag filled with water or gel placed over the neck area; the bag serves as a transmitter of the waves from the transducer to the thyroid.)

➤ Conductive gel is applied to the skin, and a transducer is moved over the skin to obtain images of the area of interest. The sound wave images are projected on the screen and stored electronically or reproduced on film.

➤ Ask the patient to breathe normally during the examination. If necessary for better organ visualization, ask the patient to inhale deeply and hold his or her breath.

➤ The results are recorded manually, on film, or in a computerized system for recall and postprocedure interpretation by the appropriate health care practitioner.

Post-test:

➤ When the study is completed, remove the gel from the skin.

➤ A written report of the examination will be completed by a health care practitioner specializing in this branch of medicine. The report will be sent to the requesting health care practitioner, who will discuss the results with the patient.

➤ Reinforce information given by the patient's health care provider regarding further testing, treatment, or referral to another health care provider. Answer any questions or address any concerns voiced by the patient or family.

➤ Depending on the results of this procedure, additional testing may be performed to evaluate or monitor progression of the disease process and determine the need for a change in therapy. Evaluate test results in relation to the patient's symptoms and other tests performed.

Related diagnostic tests:

➤ Related diagnostic tests include chest x-ray, computed tomography of the thorax, magnetic resonance imaging of the chest, and thyroid scan.

ULTRASOUND, VENOUS DOPPLER, EXTREMITY STUDIES
· ·

SYNONYMS/ACRONYM: Venous ultrasound, venous sonogram, venous ultrasonography, venous duplex.

AREA OF APPLICATION: Veins of the upper and lower extremities.

CONTRAST: Done without contrast.

DESCRIPTION & RATIONALE: Ultrasound procedures are diagnostic, non-invasive, and relatively inexpensive. They take a short time to complete, do not use radiation, and cause no harm to the patient. Venous Doppler ultrasound records sound waves to obtain information about the patency of the venous vasculature in the upper and lower extremities. Ultrasound waves are sent into the body by a small transducer pressed against the body. The transducer sends the sound waves into the body and also receives the returning sound waves, which are deflected back as they bounce off various structures. The transducer converts and amplifies the returning sound waves into electrical signals that are transformed by a computer into audible sounds, graphic readings, and gray-scale images. Blood flow direction and velocity can be readily assessed; and the presence of blood flow disturbances, which are proportional to blood flow velocity, can be determined.

For diagnostic studies, the procedure is done bilaterally. The sound waves hit the moving red blood cells and are reflected back to the transducer. The sound emitted by the equipment corresponds to the velocity of the blood flow through the vessel occurring with spontaneous respirations. Changes in these sounds during respirations indicate the possibility of abnormal venous flow secondary to occlusive disease; the absence of sound indicates complete obstruction. Compression with a transducer augments a vessel for evaluation of thrombosis. Noncompressibility of the vessel indicates a thrombosis. Plethysmography may be performed to determine the filling time of calf veins to diagnose thrombotic disorder of a major vein and to identify incompetent valves in the venous system. An additional method used to evaluate incompetent valves is the Valsalva technique combined with venous duplex imaging. ■

INDICATIONS:
- Aid in the diagnosis of superficial thrombosis or deep vein thrombosis (DVT) leading to venous occlusion or obstruction, as evidenced by absence of

venous flow, especially upon augmentation of the extremity; variations in flow during respirations; or failure of the veins to compress completely when the extremity is compressed

- Detect chronic venous insufficiency, as evidenced by reverse blood flow indicating incompetent valves

- Determine if further diagnostic procedures are needed to make or confirm a diagnosis

- Determine the source of emboli when pulmonary embolism is suspected or diagnosed

- Determine venous damage after trauma to the site

- Differentiate between primary and secondary varicose veins

- Evaluate the patency of the venous system in patients with a swollen, painful leg

- Monitor the effectiveness of therapeutic interventions

RESULT

Normal Findings:
- Normal blood flow through the veins of the extremities with no evidence of vessel occlusion

Abnormal Findings:
- Chronic venous insufficiency
- Primary varicose veins
- Recannulization in the area of an old thrombus
- Secondary varicose veins
- Superficial thrombosis or DVT
- Venous occlusion
- Venous trauma

CRITICAL VALUES: N/A

INTERFERING FACTORS:

This procedure is contraindicated for:
- Patients with an open or draining lesion

Factors that may alter test results:
- Cigarette smoking, because nicotine can cause constriction of the peripheral vessels

- Attenuation of the sound waves by bony structures, which can impair clear imaging of the vessels

- Incorrect placement of the transducer over the desired test site

- Retained contrast medium from a previous radiologic procedure

- Metallic objects within the examination field (e.g., jewelry, body rings), which may inhibit organ visualization and can produce unclear images

- Improper adjustment of the ultrasound equipment to accommodate obese or thin patients, which can cause a poor-quality study

- Patients who are very obese, who may exceed the weight limit for the equipment

- Cold extremities, resulting in vasoconstriction that can cause inaccurate measurements

- Occlusion proximal to the site being studied, which would affect blood flow to the area

- An abnormally large or swollen leg, making sonic penetration difficult

- Incorrect positioning of the patient, which may produce poor visualization of the area to be examined

- Inability of the patient to cooperate or remain still during the procedure because of age, significant pain, or mental status

Nursing Implications and Procedure • • • • • • • • • • •

Pretest:

➤ Inform the patient that the procedure assesses the veins and arteries.

➤ Obtain a history of the patient's complaints, including a list of known allergens, and inform the health care practitioner accordingly.

➤ Obtain a history of the patient's cardiovascular system, as well as results of previously performed laboratory tests, surgical procedures, and other diagnostic procedures. For related diagnostic tests, refer to the Cardiovascular System table.

➤ Report the presence of a lesion that is open or draining; maintain clean, dry dressing for the ulcer; protect the limb from trauma.

➤ Note any recent procedures that can interfere with test results (i.e., barium procedures, surgery, or biopsy). There should be 24 hours between administration of barium or iodine contrast medium and this test.

➤ Endoscopic retrograde cholangiopancreatography, colonoscopy, and computed tomography (CT) of the abdomen, if ordered, should be scheduled after this procedure.

➤ Record the date of the last menstrual period and determine the possibility of pregnancy in perimenopausal women.

➤ Obtain a list of the medications the patient is taking, including anticoagulant therapy, aspirin and other salicylates, herbs, nutritional supplements, and nutraceuticals, especially those known to affect coagulation (see Appendix F). It is recommended that use be discontinued 14 days before surgical procedures. The requesting health care practitioner and laboratory should be advised if the patient regularly uses these products so that their effects can be taken into consideration when reviewing results.

➤ Review the procedure with the patient. Address concerns about pain related to the procedure. Explain to the patient that some pain may be experienced during the test, and there may be moments of discomfort. Inform the patient that the procedure is performed in a ultrasound department, usually by a technologist, and takes approximately 30 to 60 minutes.

➤ *Sensitivity to social and cultural issues,* as well as concern for modesty, is important in providing psychological support before, during, and after the procedure.

➤ Instruct the patient to remove jewelry (including watches), hairpins, credit cards, and other metallic objects in the area to be examined.

➤ There are no food, fluid, or medication restrictions, unless by medical direction.

Intratest:

➤ Ensure that the patient has removed all external metallic objects (jewelry, etc.) prior to the procedure.

➤ Patients are given a gown, robe, and foot coverings to wear and instructed to void prior to the procedure.

➤ Instruct the patient to cooperate fully and to follow directions. Instruct the patient to remain still throughout the procedure because movement produces unreliable results.

➤ Observe standard precautions, and follow the general guidelines in Appendix A.

➤ Place the patient in the supine position on an exam table; other positions may be used during the examination.

➤ Expose the area of interest and drape the patient.

➤ Conductive gel is applied to the skin, and a transducer is moved over the area to obtain images of the area of interest. Waveforms are visualized and recorded with variations in respirations. Images with and without compression are performed proximally or distally to an obstruction to obtain information about a venous occlusion or obstruction. The procedure can be performed for both arms and legs to obtain bilateral blood flow determination.

➤ Do not place the transducer on an ulcer site when there is evidence of venous stasis or ulcer.

➤ Ask the patient to breathe normally during the examination. If necessary for better organ visualization, ask the patient to inhale deeply and hold his or her breath.

➤ The results are recorded manually, on film, or in a computerized system for recall and postprocedure interpretation by the appropriate health care practitioner.

Post-test:

➤ When the study is completed, remove the gel from the skin.

➤ Instruct the patient to continue usual diet, fluids, and medications, as directed by the health care practitioner

➤ *Nutritional considerations:* A low-fat, low-cholesterol, and low-sodium diet should be consumed to reduce current disease processes and/or decrease risk of hypertension and coronary artery disease.

➤ A written report of the examination will be completed by a health care practitioner specializing in this branch of medicine. The report will be sent to the requesting health care practitioner, who will discuss the results with the patient.

➤ Recognize anxiety related to test results, and be supportive of perceived loss of independent function. Discuss the implications of abnormal test results on the patient's lifestyle. Provide teaching and information regarding the clinical implications of the test results, as appropriate.

➤ Reinforce information given by the patient's health care provider regarding further testing, treatment, or referral to another health care provider. Answer any questions or address any concerns voiced by the patient or family.

➤ Instruct the patient in the use of any ordered medications. Explain the importance of adhering to the therapy regimen. As appropriate, instruct the patient in significant side effects and systemic reactions associated with the prescribed medication. Encourage him or her to review corresponding literature provided by a pharmacist.

➤ Depending on the results of this procedure, additional testing may be needed to evaluate or monitor progression of the disease process and determine the need for a change in therapy. Evaluate test results in relation to the patient's symptoms and other tests performed.

Related diagnostic tests:

➤ Related diagnostic tests include computed tomography angiography, and magnetic resonance imaging angiography.

UPPER GASTROINTESTINAL AND SMALL BOWEL SERIES

SYNONYMS/ACRONYMS: Stomach series, gastric radiography, small bowel study, upper GI series, UGI.

AREA OF APPLICATION: Esophagus, stomach, and small intestine.

CONTRAST: Barium sulfate.

DESCRIPTION & RATIONALE: The upper gastrointestinal (GI) series is a radiologic examination of the esophagus, stomach, and small intestine after ingestion of barium sulfate, which is a milkshake-like, radiopaque substance. A combination of x-ray and fluoroscopy techniques is used to record the study. Air may be instilled to provide double contrast and better visualization of the lumen of the esophagus, stomach, and duodenum. If perforation or obstruction is suspected, a water-soluble iodinated contrast medium is used. This test is especially useful in the evaluation of patients experiencing dysphagia, regurgitation, gastroesophageal reflux (GER), epigastric pain, hematemesis, melena, and unexplained weight loss. This test is also used to evaluate the results of gastric surgery, especially when an anastomotic leak is suspected. When a small bowel series is included, the test detects disorders of the jejunum and ileum. The patient's position is changed during the examination to allow visualization of the various structures and their function. The images are visualized on

a fluoroscopic screen, recorded, and stored electronically or on x-ray film for review by a physician. Drugs such as glucagon may be given during an upper GI series to relax the GI tract; drugs such as metoclopramide (Reglan) may be given to accelerate the passage of the barium through the stomach and small intestine.

When the small bowel series is performed separately, the patient may be asked to drink several glasses of barium or enteroclysis may be used to instill the barium. With enteroclysis, a catheter is passed through the nose or mouth and advanced past the pylorus and into the duodenum. Barium, followed by methylcellulose solution, is instilled via the catheter directly into the small bowel. ■

INDICATIONS:

• Determine the cause of regurgitation or epigastric pain

• Determine the presence of neoplasms, ulcers, diverticula, obstruction, foreign body, and hiatal hernia

• Evaluate suspected GER, inflammatory

process, congenital anomaly, motility disorder, or structural change

• Evaluate unexplained weight loss or anemia

• Identify and locate the origin of hematemesis

RESULT

Normal Findings:
• Normal size, shape, position, and functioning of the esophagus, stomach, and small bowel

Abnormal Findings:
• Achalasia

• Cancer of the esophagus

• Chalasis

• Congenital abnormalities

• Duodenal cancer, diverticula, and ulcers

• Esophageal diverticula, motility disorders, ulcers, varices, and inflammation

• Gastric cancer, tumors, and ulcers

• Gastritis

• Hiatal hernia

• Perforation of the esophagus, stomach, or small bowel

• Polyps

• Small bowel tumors

• Strictures

CRITICAL VALUES: N/A

INTERFERING FACTORS

This procedure is contraindicated for:
• Patients who are pregnant or suspected of being pregnant, unless the potential benefits of the procedure far outweigh the risks to the fetus and mother

• Patients with an intestinal obstruction

• Patients suspected of having upper GI perforation, in whom barium should not be used

Factors that may impair clear imaging:
• Inability of the patient to cooperate or remain still during the procedure because of age, significant pain, or mental status

• Patients who are very obese, who may exceed the weight limit for the equipment

• Incorrect positioning of the patient, which may produce poor visualization of the area to be examined

• Improper adjustment of the radiographic equipment to accommodate obese or thin patients, which can cause overexposure or underexposure and poor-quality study

• Metallic objects within the examination field (e.g., jewelry, body rings), which may inhibit organ visualization and can produce unclear images

Other considerations:
• Failure to follow dietary restrictions before the procedure may cause the procedure to be canceled or repeated.

• Patients with swallowing problems may aspirate the barium, which could interfere with the procedure and cause patient complications.

• Possible constipation or partial bowel obstruction caused by retained barium in the small bowel or colon may affect test results.

• This procedure should be done after a kidney x-ray (intravenous pyelography) or computed tomography (CT) of the abdomen or pelvis.

• Risks associated with radiographic overexposure can result from frequent x-ray procedures. Personnel in the room with the patient should stand behind a shield or leave the area while the examination is being done. Personnel working in the area where the examination is being done should wear badges that reveal their level of exposure to radiation.

Nursing Implications and Procedure • • • • • • • • • • •

Pretest:

➤ Inform the patient that the procedure assesses the upper GI system and/or small bowel.

➤ Obtain a history of the patient's complaints, including a list of known allergens, especially allergies or sensitivities to latex, iodine, seafood, contrast medium, and dyes.

➤ Obtain a history of the patient's gastrointestinal system, as well as results of previously performed laboratory tests, surgical procedures, and other diagnostic procedures. For related diagnostic tests, refer to the Gastrointestinal System table.

➤ Ensure that this procedure is performed before a barium swallow.

➤ Record the date of the last menstrual period and determine the possibility of pregnancy in perimenopausal women.

➤ Obtain a list of the medications the patient is taking.

➤ Review the procedure with the patient. Address concerns about pain related to the procedure. Explain to the patient that some pain may be experienced during the test, and there may be moments of discomfort. Explain the purpose of the test and how the procedure is performed. Inform the patient that the procedure is performed in a radiology department, usually by a health care practitioner and support staff, and takes approximately 30 to 60 minutes.

➤ Explain to the patient that he or she will be asked to drink a milkshake-like solution that has a chalky taste.

➤ *Sensitivity to cultural and social issues,* as well as concern for modesty, is important in providing psychological support before, during, and after the procedure.

➤ Instruct the patient to remove dentures, jewelry (including watches), hairpins, credit cards, and other metallic objects.

➤ The patient should fast and refrain from drinking liquids for 8 hours prior to the procedure.

Intratest:

➤ Ensure that the patient has complied with dietary restrictions and pretesting preparations for at least 8 hours prior to the procedure. Ensure that the patient has removed all external metallic objects (jewelry, etc.) prior to the procedure.

➤ Have emergency equipment readily available.

➤ Remove any wires connected to electrodes, if allowed.

➤ Instruct the patient to cooperate fully and to follow directions. Instruct the patient to remain still throughout the procedure because movement produces unreliable results.

➤ Observe standard precautions, and follow the general guidelines in Appendix A.

Upper gastrointestinal series:

➤ Place the patient on the x-ray table in a supine position, or ask the patient to stand in front of an x-ray fluoroscopy screen.

➤ Instruct the patient to take several swallows of the barium mixture through a straw while images are taken of the pharyngeal motion. Drinking through a straw allows some air to be introduced into the abdomen. This permits detailed examination of the stomach's lining. This same effect can be achieved by administering an effervescent agent.

➤ While the patient continues to drink the barium solution, images of the esophageal area are recorded from a variety of angles.

➤ Instruct the patient to finish the barium mixture while images are taken at different angles and positions to aid in the evaluation of stomach filling and emptying into the duodenum.

Small bowel series:

➤ If the small bowel is to be examined after the upper GI series, instruct the patient to drink an additional glass of barium while the small intestine is observed for passage of barium. Images are taken at 30- to 60-minute intervals until the barium reaches the ileocecal valve. This process can last up to 5 hours, with a follow-up film taken at 24 hours.

General:

➤ The results are recorded manually, on x-ray film, or by automated equipment in a computerized system for recall and postprocedure interpretation by the appropriate health care practitioner.

Post-test:

➤ Instruct the patient to resume usual diet and fluids, as directed by the health care practitioner.

➤ Monitor for reaction to iodinated contrast medium, including including rash, urticaria, tachycardia, hyperpnea, hypertension, palpitations, nausea, or vomiting, if iodine is used.

➤ Instruct the patient to take a mild laxative and increase fluid intake (four glasses) to aid in the elimination of barium, unless contraindicated.

➤ Inform the patient that his or her

stool will be white or light in color for 2 to 3 days. If the patient is unable to eliminate the barium, or if the stool does not return to normal color, the patient should notify the health care practitioner.

➤ A written report of the examination will be completed by a health care practitioner specializing in this branch of medicine. The report will be sent to the requesting health care practitioner, who will discuss the results with the patient.

➤ Recognize anxiety related to test results, and be supportive of perceived loss of independence and fear of shortened life expectancy. Discuss the implications of abnormal test results on the patient's lifestyle. Provide teaching and information regarding the clinical implications of the test results, as appropriate. Educate the patient regarding access to counseling services.

➤ Reinforce information given by the patient's health care provider regarding further testing, treatment, or referral to another health care provider. Answer any questions or address any concerns voiced by the patient or family.

➤ Depending on the results of this procedure, additional testing may be needed to evaluate or monitor progression of the disease process and determine the need for a change in therapy. Evaluate test results in relation to the patient's symptoms and other tests performed.

Related diagnostic tests:

➤ Related diagnostic tests include computed tomography of the abdomen; endoscopic retrograde cholangiopancreatography; kidney, ureter, and bladder (KUB) study; and magnetic resonance imaging of the abdomen.

UREA NITROGEN, BLOOD

SYNONYM/ACRONYM: BUN.

SPECIMEN: Serum (1 mL) collected in a red- or tiger-top tube. Plasma (1 mL) collected in green-top (heparin) tube is also acceptable.

REFERENCE VALUE: (Method: Spectrophotometry)

Age	Conventional Units	SI Units (Conventional Units × 0.357)
Newborn–3 y	5–17 mg/dL	1.8–6.0 mmol/L
4–13 y	7–17 mg/dL	2.5–6.0 mmol/L
14 y–adult	8–21 mg/dL	2.9–7.5 mmol/L
Adult older than 90 y	10–31 mg/dL	3.6–11.1 mmol/L

DESCRIPTION & RATIONALE: Urea is a nonprotein nitrogen compound formed in the liver from ammonia as an end product of protein metabolism. Urea diffuses freely into extracellular and intracellular fluid and is ultimately excreted by the kidneys. Blood urea nitrogen (BUN) levels reflect the balance between the production and excretion of urea. BUN and creatinine values are commonly evaluated together. The normal BUN/creatinine ratio is 15:1 to 24:1. (e.g., if a patient has a BUN of 15 mg/dL, the creatinine should be approximately 0.6 to 1.0 mg/dL). BUN is used in the following calculation to estimate serum osmolality: ■

$$[(2[Na^+]) + (glucose/18) + (BUN/2.8)]$$

INDICATIONS:
- Assess nutritional support
- Evaluate hemodialysis therapy
- Evaluate hydration
- Evaluate liver function
- Evaluate patients with lymphoma after chemotherapy (tumor lysis)
- Evaluate renal function
- Monitor the effects of drugs known to be nephrotoxic or hepatotoxic

RESULT

Increased in:
- Acute renal failure
- Chronic glomerulonephritis
- Congestive heart failure
- Decreased renal perfusion

- Diabetes
- Excessive protein ingestion
- Gastrointestinal (GI) bleeding (excessive blood protein in the GI tract)
- Hyperalimentation
- Hypovolemia
- Ketoacidosis
- Muscle wasting from starvation
- Neoplasms
- Nephrotoxic agents
- Pyelonephritis
- Shock
- Urinary tract obstruction

Decreased in:
- Inadequate dietary protein
- Low-protein/high-carbohydrate diet
- Malabsorption syndromes
- Pregnancy
- Severe liver disease

CRITICAL VALUES:

Greater than 100 mg/dL (nondialysis patients)

Note and immediately report to the health care practitioner any critically increased or decreased values and related symptoms. A patient with a grossly elevated BUN may have signs and symptoms including acidemia, agitation, confusion, fatigue, nausea, vomiting, and coma. Possible interventions include treatment of the cause, administration of intravenous bicarbonate, a low-protein diet, hemodialysis, and caution with respect to prescribing and continuing nephrotoxic medications.

INTERFERING FACTORS:

- Drugs, substances, and vitamins that may increase BUN levels include acetaminophen, alanine, aldatense, alkaline antacids, amphotericin B, antimony compounds, arsenicals, bacitracin, bismuth subsalicylate, capreomycin, carbenoxolone, carbutamide, cephalosporins, chloral hydrate, chloramphenicol, chlorthalidone, colistimethate, colistin, cotrimoxazole, dexamethasone, dextran, diclofenac, doxycycline, ethylene glycol, gentamicin, guanethidine, guanoxan, ibuprofen, ifosfamide, ipodate, kanamycin, mephenesin, metolazone, mitomycin, neomycin, phosphorus, plicamycin, tertatolol, tetracycline, triamterene, triethylenemelamine, viomycin, and vitamin D.
- Drugs that may decrease BUN levels include acetohydroxamic acid, chloramphenicol, fluorides, paramethasone, phenothiazine, and streptomycin.

Nursing Implications and Procedure

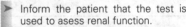

Pretest:

➤ Inform the patient that the test is used to asess renal function.

➤ Obtain a history of the patient's complaints, including a list of known allergens (especially allergies or sensitivities to latex), and inform the appropriate health care practitioner accordingly.

➤ Obtain a history of the patient's genitourinary system, as well as results of previously performed laboratory tests, surgical procedures, and other diagnostic procedures. For related laboratory tests, refer to the Genitourinary System table.

➤ Obtain a list of medications the patient is taking, including herbs, nutritional supplements, and nutraceuticals. The requesting health care practitioner and laboratory should be advised if the patient is regularly using these products so that their effects can be taken into consideration when reviewing results.

➤ Review the procedure with the patient. Inform the patient that specimen collection takes approximately

5 to 10 minutes. Address concerns about pain related to the procedure. Explain to the patient that there may be some discomfort during the venipuncture.

➤ *Sensitivity to cultural and social issues,* as well as concern for modesty, is important in providing psychological support before, during, and after the procedure.

➤ There are no food, fluid, or medication restrictions, unless by medical direction.

Intratest:

➤ If the patient has a history of severe allergic reaction to latex, care should be taken to avoid the use of equipment containing latex.

➤ Instruct the patient to cooperate fully and to follow directions. Direct the patient to breathe normally and to avoid unnecessary movement.

➤ Observe standard precautions, and follow the general guidelines in Appendix A. Positively identify the patient, and label the appropriate tubes with the corresponding patient demographics, date, and time of collection. Perform a venipuncture; collect the specimen in a 5-mL red- or tiger-top tube.

➤ Remove the needle, and apply a pressure dressing over the puncture site.

➤ Promptly transport the specimen to the laboratory for processing and analysis.

➤ The results are recorded manually or in a computerized system for recall and postprocedure interpretation by the appropriate health care practitioner.

Post-test:

➤ Observe venipuncture site for bleeding or hematoma formation. Apply paper tape or other adhesive to hold pressure bandage in place, or replace with a plastic bandage.

➤ Monitor intake and output for fluid imbalance in renal dysfunction and dehydration.

➤ *Nutritional considerations:* Nitrogen balance is commonly used as a nutritional assessment tool to indicate protein change. In healthy individuals, protein anabolism and catabolism are in equilibrium. During various disease states, nutritional intake decreases, resulting in a negative balance. During recovery from illness and with proper nutritional support, the nitrogen balance becomes positive. BUN is an important analyte to measure during administration of total parenteral nutrition (TPN). Educate the patient, as appropriate, in dietary adjustments required to maintain proper nitrogen balance. Inform the patient that the requesting health care practitioner may prescribe TPN as part of the treatment plan.

➤ *Nutritional considerations:* An elevated BUN can be caused by a high-protein diet or dehydration. Unless medically restricted, a healthy diet consisting of the five food groups of the food pyramid should be consumed daily. Water consumption should include six to eight 8-ounce glasses of water per day, or water consumption equivalent to half of the body's weight in ounces.

➤ A written report of the examination will be sent to the requesting health care practitioner, who will discuss the results with the patient.

➤ Recognize anxiety related to test results. Discuss the implications of abnormal test results on the patient's lifestyle. Provide teaching and information regarding the clinical implications of the test results, as appropriate.

➤ Reinforce information given by the patient's health care provider regarding further testing, treatment, or referral to another health care provider. Answer any questions or address any concerns voiced by the patient or family.

➤ Depending on the results of this procedure, additional testing may be performed to evaluate or monitor progression of the disease process and determine the need for a change in therapy. Evaluate test results in relation to the patient's symptoms and other tests performed.

➤ Related laboratory tests include anion gap, blood and urine creatinine, BUN/creatinine ratio, creatinine clearance, blood and urine electrolytes, gentamicin, kidney stone analysis, microalbumin, blood and urine osmolality, tobramycin, urine urea nitrogen, blood and urine uric acid, and vancomycin.

UREA NITROGEN, URINE

SYNONYM/ACRONYM: N/A.

SPECIMEN: Urine (5 mL) from an unpreserved random or timed specimen collected in a clean plastic collection container.

REFERENCE VALUE: (Method: Spectrophotometry)

Conventional Units	SI Units (Conventional Units × 35.7)
12–20 g/24 h	428–714 mmol/24 h

DESCRIPTION & RATIONALE: Urea is a nonprotein nitrogen compound formed in the liver from ammonia as an end product of protein metabolism. Urea diffuses freely into extracellular and intracellular fluid and is ultimately excreted by the kidneys. Urine urea nitrogen levels reflect the balance between the production and excretion of urea. ■

INDICATIONS:
• Evaluate renal disease
• Predict the impact that other conditions, such as diabetes and liver disease, will have on the kidneys

RESULT

Increased in:
• Diabetes
• Hyperthyroidism
• Increased dietary protein
• Postoperative period

Decreased in:
• Liver disease
• Low-protein/high-carbohydrate diet
• Normal-growing pediatric patients
• Pregnancy
• Renal disease
• Toxemia

CRITICAL VALUES: N/A

INTERFERING FACTORS:

- Drugs that may increase urine urea nitrogen levels include alanine and glycine.

- Drugs that may decrease urine urea nitrogen levels include furosemide, growth hormone, insulin, and testosterone.

- All urine voided for the timed collection period must be included in the collection or else falsely decreased values may be obtained. Compare output records with volume collected to verify that all voids were included in the collection.

Nursing Implications and Procedure . . . .

Pretest:

➤ Inform the patient that the test is used to assess renal function.

➤ Obtain a history of the patient's complaints, including a list of known allergens (especially allergies or sensitivities to latex), and inform the appropriate health care practitioner accordingly.

➤ Obtain a history of the patient's genitourinary and hepatobiliary systems, as well as results of previously performed laboratory tests, surgical procedures, and other diagnostic procedures. For related laboratory tests, refer to the Genitourinary and Hepatobiliary System tables.

➤ Obtain a list of medications the patient is taking, including herbs, nutritional supplements, and nutraceuticals. The requesting health care practitioner and laboratory should be advised if the patient regularly uses these products so that their effects can be taken into consideration when reviewing results.

➤ Review the procedure with the patient. Provide a nonmetallic urinal, bedpan, or toilet-mounted collection device. Address concerns about pain

related to the procedure. Explain to the patient that there should be no discomfort during the procedure.

➤ Usually a 24-hour time frame for urine collection is ordered. Inform the patient that all urine must be saved during that 24-hour period. Instruct the patient not to void directly into the laboratory collection container. Instruct the patient to avoid defecating in the collection device and to keep toilet tissue out of the collection device to prevent contamination of the specimen. Place a sign in the bathroom to remind the patient to save all urine.

➤ Instruct the patient to void all urine into the collection device and then to pour the urine into the laboratory collection container. Alternatively, the specimen can be left in the collection device for a health care staff member to add to the laboratory collection container.

➤ *Sensitivity to social and cultural issues,* as well as concern for modesty, is important in providing psychological support before, during, and after the procedure.

➤ There are no food, fluid, or medication restrictions, unless by medical direction.

Intratest:

➤ If the patient has a history of severe allergic reaction to latex, care should be taken to avoid the use of equipment containing latex.

➤ Instruct the patient to cooperate fully and to follow directions.

➤ Observe standard precautions, and follow the general guidelines in Appendix A. Positively identify the patient, and label the appropriate collection container with the corresponding patient demographics, date, and time of collection.

Random specimen (collect in early morning):

Clean-catch specimen:

➤ Instruct the male patient to (1) thoroughly wash his hands, (2) cleanse

the meatus, (3) void a small amount into the toilet, and (4) void directly into the specimen container.

➤ Instruct the female patient to (1) thoroughly wash her hands; (2) cleanse the labia from front to back; (3) while keeping the labia separated, void a small amount into the toilet; and (4) without interrupting the urine stream, void directly into the specimen container.

Indwelling catheter:

➤ Put on gloves. Empty drainage tube of urine. It may be necessary to clamp off the catheter for 15 to 30 minutes before specimen collection. Cleanse specimen port with antiseptic swab, and then aspirate 5 mL of urine with a 21- to 25-gauge needle and syringe. Transfer urine to a sterile container.

Timed specimen:

➤ Obtain a clean 3-L urine specimen container, toilet-mounted collection device, and plastic bag (for transport of the specimen container). The specimen must be refrigerated or kept on ice throughout the entire collection period. If an indwelling urinary catheter is in place, the drainage bag must be kept on ice.

➤ Begin the test between 6 and 8 a.m., if possible. Collect first voiding and discard. Record the time the specimen was discarded as the beginning of the timed collection period. The next morning, ask the patient to void at the same time the collection was started and add this last voiding to the container.

➤ If an indwelling catheter is in place, replace the tubing and container system at the start of the collection time. Keep the container system on ice during the collection period, or empty the urine into a larger container periodically during the collection period; monitor to ensure continued drainage, and conclude the test the next morning at the same hour the collection was begun.

➤ At the conclusion of the test, compare the quantity of urine with the urinary output record for the collection; if the specimen contains less than what was recorded as output, some urine may have been discarded, invalidating the test.

➤ Include on the collection container's label the amount of urine, test start and stop times, and ingestion of any medications that can affect test results.

General:

➤ Promptly transport the specimen to the laboratory for processing and analysis.

➤ The results are recorded manually or in a computerized system for recall and postprocedure interpretation by the appropriate health care practitioner.

Post-test:

➤ *Nutritional considerations:* An elevated BUN can be caused by a high-protein diet or dehydration. Unless medically restricted, a healthy diet consisting of the five food groups of the food pyramid should be consumed daily. Water consumption should include six to eight 8-ounce glasses of water per day, or water consumption equivalent to half of the body's weight in ounces.

➤ A written report of the examination will be sent to the requesting health care practitioner, who will discuss the results with the patient.

➤ Recognize anxiety related to test results. Discuss the implications of abnormal test results on the patient's lifestyle. Provide teaching and information regarding the clinical implications of the test results, as appropriate.

➤ Reinforce information given by the patient's health care provider regarding further testing, treatment, or referral to another health care provider. Answer any questions or address any concerns voiced by the patient or family.

➤ Depending on the results of this procedure, additional testing may be performed to evaluate or monitor progression of the disease process and determine the need for a change in therapy. Evaluate test results in relation to the patient's symptoms and other tests performed.

Related laboratory tests:

➤ Related laboratory tests include anion gap, blood urea nitrogen (BUN)/creatinine ratio, blood and urine creatinine, creatinine clearance, blood and urine electrolytes, gentamicin, kidney stone analysis, microalbumin, BUN, blood and urine osmolality, tobramycin, blood and urine uric acid, urinalysis, and vancomycin.

URETHROGRAPHY, RETROGRADE

SYNONYM/ACRONYM: N/A.

AREA OF APPLICATION: Urethra.

CONTRAST: Radiopaque contrast medium.

DESCRIPTION & RATIONALE: Retrograde urethrography is performed almost exclusively in male patients. It uses contrast medium, either injected or instilled via a catheter into the urethra, to visualize the membranous, bulbar, and penile portions, particularly after surgical repair of the urethra to assess the success of the surgery. The posterior portion of the urethra is visualized better when the procedure is performed with voiding cystourethrography. In women, it may be performed after surgical repair of the urethra to assess the success of the surgery and to assess structural abnormalities in conjunction with an evaluation for voiding dysfunction. ■

INDICATIONS: Aid in the diagnosis of urethral strictures, lacerations, diverticula, and congenital anomalies

RESULT

Normal Findings:
- Normal size, shape, and course of the membranous, bulbar, and penile portions of the urethra in male patients
- If the prostatic portion can be visualized, it also should appear normal

Abnormal Findings:
- Congenital anomalies, such as urethral valves and perineal hypospadias
- False passages in the urethra
- Prostatic enlargement
- Tumors of the urethra
- Urethral calculi
- Urethral diverticula
- Urethral fistulas
- Urethral strictures and lacerations

CRITICAL VALUES: N/A

INTERFERING FACTORS:

This procedure is contraindicated for:

- ⚠ Patients with allergies to shellfish or iodinated dye. The contrast medium used may cause a life-threatening allergic reaction. Patients with a known hypersensitivity to the contrast medium may benefit from premedication with corticosteroids or the use of nonionic contrast medium.

- Patients who are pregnant or suspected of being pregnant, unless the potential benefits of the procedure far outweigh the risks to the fetus and mother.

- ⚠ Elderly and other patients who are chronically dehydrated before the test, because of their risk of contrast-induced renal failure.

- ⚠ Patients who are in renal failure.

Factors that may impair clear imaging:

- Inability of the patient to cooperate or remain still during the procedure because of age, significant pain, or mental status

- Patients who are very obese, who may exceed the weight limit for the equipment

- Incorrect positioning of the patient, which may produce poor visualization of the area to be examined

- Improper adjustment of the radiographic equipment to accommodate obese or thin patients, which can cause overexposure or underexposure and a poor-quality study

- Metallic objects within the examination field (e.g., jewelry, body rings), which may inhibit organ visualization and can produce unclear images

Other considerations:

- Consultation with a health care practitioner should occur before the procedure for radiation safety concerns regarding younger patients or patients who are lactating.

- Risks associated with radiographic overexposure can result from frequent x-ray procedures. Personnel in the room with the patient should stand behind a shield or leave the area while the examination is being done. Personnel working in the area where the examination is being done should wear badges that reveal their level of exposure to radiation.

Nursing Implications and Procedure • • • • • • • • • • •

Pretest:

➤ Inform the patient that the procedure assesses the urethra.

➤ Obtain a history of the patient's complaints, including a list of known allergens, especially allergies or sensitivities to latex, iodine, seafood, contrast medium, and dyes.

➤ Obtain a history of the patient's gastrointestinal and genitourinary systems results of previously performed laboratory tests, surgical procedures, and other diagnostic procedures. For related diagnostic tests, refer to the Gastrointestinal and Genitourinary System tables.

➤ Ensure that this procedure is performed before an upper gastrointestinal study or barium swallow.

➤ Record the date of the last menstrual period and determine the possibility of pregnancy in perimenopausal women.

➤ Obtain a list of the medications the patient is taking.

➤ Review the procedure with the patient. Address concerns about pain related to the procedure. Explain to the patient that some pain may be experienced during the test, and there may be moments of discomfort. Explain the purpose of the test and how the procedure is performed.

Inform the patient that the procedure is performed in a cystoscopy room by a urologist and takes approximately 30 minutes.

➤ If the contrast medium is instilled through a catheter, inform the patient that some pressure may be experienced when the catheter is inserted and contrast medium is instilled.

➤ *Sensitivity to cultural and social issues,* as well as concern for modesty, is important in providing psychological support before, during, and after the procedure.

➤ Instruct the patient to remove jewelry (including watches), credit cards, keys, coins, cell phones, pagers, and other metallic objects.

➤ Patients receiving metformin (Glucophage) for non–insulin-dependent (type 2) diabetes should discontinue the drug on the day of the test and continue to withhold it for 48 hours after the test. Failure to do so may result in lactic acidosis.

➤ There are no food or fluid restrictions, unless by medical direction.

➤ *Make sure a written and informed consent has been signed prior to the procedure and before administering any medications.*

Intratest:

➤ Ensure that the patient has complied with medication restrictions and pretesting preparations. Ensure that the patient has removed all external metallic objects (jewelry, etc.) from the abdominal area prior to the procedure.

➤ Patients are given a gown, robe, and foot coverings to wear and instructed to void prior to the procedure.

➤ Instruct the patient to cooperate fully and to follow directions. Ask the patient to lie still during the procedure because movement produces unclear images.

➤ Obtain and record the patient's baseline vital signs.

➤ Observe standard precautions, and follow the general guidelines in Appendix A.

➤ Place the patient on the table in a supine position in the recumbent position.

➤ A single plain film is taken of the bladder and urethra.

➤ A catheter is filled with contrast medium to eliminate air pockets and is inserted until the balloon reaches the meatus. Inform the patient that the contrast medium may cause a temporary flushing of the face, a feeling of warmth, urticaria, headache, vomiting, or nausea.

➤ The patient is placed in the right posterior oblique position with the thigh drawn up to a 90° angle; in male patients, the penis is placed parallel to the leg.

➤ After three-fourths of the contrast medium is injected, another exposure is taken while the remainder of the contrast medium is injected.

➤ Left lateral and oblique exposures may be taken.

➤ The procedure may be done on female patients using a double balloon to occlude the bladder neck from above and below the external meatus.

➤ Wear gloves during the radionuclide administration and while handling the patient's urine.

➤ The results are recorded manually, on x-ray film, or by automated equipment in a computerized system for recall and postprocedure interpretation by the appropriate health care practitioner.

Post-test:

➤ Monitor vital and neurologic signs every 15 minutes until they return to preprocedure levels.

➤ Instruct the patient to resume usual diet and medications, as directed by the physician. Renal function should be assessed before metformin is restarted.

➤ Monitor fluid intake and urinary output for 24 hours after the procedure. Decreased urine output may indicate impending renal failure.

- Monitor for signs and symptoms of sepsis, including fever, chills, and severe pain in the kidney area.

- Maintain the patient on adequate hydration after the procedure. Encourage the patient to drink lots of fluids to prevent stasis and to prevent the buildup of bacteria.

- Advise patient to drink increased amounts of fluids for 24 to 48 hours to eliminate the radionuclide from the body, unless contraindicated. Tell the patient that radionuclide is eliminated from the body within 6 to 24 hours.

- Instruct the patient to immediately flush the toilet after each voiding after the procedure, and to meticulously wash hands with soap and water after each voiding for 24 hours after the procedure.

- Tell all caregivers to wear gloves when discarding urine for 24 hours after the procedure. Wash gloved hands with soap and water before removing gloves. Then wash ungloved hands after the gloves are removed.

- A written report of the examination will be completed by a health care practitioner specializing in this branch of medicine. The report will be sent to the requesting health care practitioner, who will discuss the results with the patient.

- Reinforce information given by the patient's health care provider regarding further testing, treatment, or referral to another health care provider. Answer any questions or address any concerns voiced by the patient or family.

- Depending on the results of this procedure, additional testing may be needed to evaluate or monitor progression of the disease process and determine the need for a change in therapy. Evaluate test results in relation to the patient's symptoms and other tests performed.

Related diagnostic tests:

- Related diagnostic tests include computed tomography of the abdomen, cystoscopy, intravenous pyelography, magnetic resonance imaging of the abdomen, renogram, and renal ultrasound.

URIC ACID, BLOOD

SYNONYM/ACRONYM: Urate.

SPECIMEN: Serum (1 mL) collected in a red- or tiger-top tube. Plasma (1 mL) collected in green-top (heparin) tube is also acceptable.

REFERENCE VALUE: (Method: Spectrophotometry)

Age	Conventional Units	SI Units (Conventional Units × 0.059)
Child less than 12 y	2.0–5.5 mg/dL	0.12–0.32 mmol/L
Adult younger than 60 y		
Male	4.4–7.6 mg/dL	0.26–0.45 mmol/L
Female	2.3–6.6 mg/dL	0.14–0.39 mmol/L
Adult older than 60 y		
Male	4.2–8.0 mg/dL	0.25–0.48 mmol/L
Female	3.5–7.3 mg/dL	0.21–0.43 mmol/L

DESCRIPTION & RATIONALE: Uric acid is the end product of purine metabolism. Purines are important constituents of nucleic acids; purine turnover occurs continuously in the body, producing substantial amounts of uric acid even in the absence of purine intake from dietary sources such as organ meats (e.g., liver, thymus gland and/or pancreas [sweetbreads], kidney), legumes, and yeasts. Uric acid is filtered, absorbed, and secreted by the kidneys and is a common constituent of urine. Serum urate levels are affected by the amount of uric acid produced and by the efficiency of renal excretion. ∎

INDICATIONS:

• Assist in the diagnosis of gout when there is a family history (autosomal dominant genetic disorder) or signs and symptoms of gout, indicated by elevated uric acid levels

• Determine the cause of known or suspected renal calculi

• Evaluate the extent of tissue destruction in infection, starvation, excessive exercise, malignancies, chemotherapy, or radiation therapy

• Evaluate possible liver damage in eclampsia, indicated by elevated uric acid levels

• Monitor the effects of drugs known to alter uric acid levels, either as a side effect or as a therapeutic effect

RESULT

Increased in:

• Acute tissue destruction as a result of starvation or excessive exercise

• Alcoholism

• Chemotherapy and radiation therapy

• Chronic lead toxicity

• Congestive heart failure

• Diabetes

• Down syndrome

• Eclampsia

• Excessive dietary purines

• Glucose-6-phosphate dehydrogenase deficiency

• Gout

• Hyperparathyroidism

• Hypertension

• Hypoparathyroidism

• Lactic acidosis

• Lead poisoning

• Lesch-Nyhan syndrome

• Multiple myeloma

• Pernicious anemia

• Polycystic kidney disease

- Polycythemia
- Psoriasis
- Sickle cell anemia
- Type III hyperlipidemia

Decreased in:
- Fanconi's syndrome
- Low-purine diet
- Severe liver disease
- Wilson's disease

CRITICAL VALUES: N/A

INTERFERING FACTORS:
- Drugs and substances that may increase uric acid levels include acetylsalicylic acid (low doses), aldatense, aminothiadiazole, anabolic steroids, antineoplastic agents, ascorbic acid, chlorambucil, chlorthalidone, cisplatin, corn oil, cyclosporine, cyclothiazide, cytarabine, diapamide, diazoxide, diuretics, ergothioneine, ethacrynic acid, ethambutol, ethoxzolamide, etoposide, flumethiazide, hydroflumethiazide, hydroxyurea, ibufenac, ibuprofen, levarterenol, levodopa, mefruside, mercaptopurine, methicillin, methotrexate, methoxyflurane, methyclothiazide, mitomycin, morinamide, polythiazide, prednisone, pyrazinamide, salicylate, spironolactone, theophylline, thiazide diuretics, thioguanine, thiotepa, thiouric acid, triamterene, trichlormethiazide, vincristine, warfarin, and xylitol.

- Drugs that may decrease uric acid levels include acetohexamide, allopurinol, aspirin (high doses), azathioprine, benzbromaron, benziodarone, canola oil, chlorothiazide (given intravenously), chlorpromazine, chlorprothixene, cinchophen, corticosteroids, corticotropin, clofibrate, coumarin, diatrizoic acid, dicumarol, dipyrone, enalapril, fenofibrate, flufenamic acid, guaifenesin, hydralazine, iodipamide, iodopyracet, iopanoic acid, ipodate,

lisinopril, mefenamic acid, mersalyl, methotrexate, oxyphenbutazone, phenindione, phenolsulfonphthalein, probenecid, seclazone, sulfinpyrazone, and verapamil.

Nursing Implications and Procedure • • • • • • • • • • •

Pretest:

➤ Inform the patient that the test is primarily used to diagnose gout and to evaluate renal function.

➤ Obtain a history of the patient's complaints, including a list of known allergens (especially allergies or sensitivities to latex), and inform the appropriate health care practitioner accordingly. Especially note pain and edema in joints and great toe (caused by precipitation of sodium urates), headache, fatigue, decreased urinary output, and hypertension.

➤ Obtain a history of the patient's genitourinary, hepatobiliary, and musculoskeletal systems, as well as results of previously performed laboratory tests, surgical procedures, and other diagnostic procedures. For related laboratory tests, refer to the Genitourinary, Hepatobiliary, and Musculoskeletal System tables.

➤ Obtain a list of medications the patient is taking, including herbs, nutritional supplements, and nutraceuticals. The requesting health care practitioner and laboratory should be advised if the patient is regularly using these products so that their effects can be taken into consideration when reviewing results.

➤ Review the procedure with the patient. Inform the patient that specimen collection takes approximately 5 to 10 minutes. Address concerns about pain related to the procedure. Explain to the patient that there may be some discomfort during the venipuncture.

➤ *Sensitivity to cultural and social issues,* as well as concern for mod-

esty, is important in providing psychological support before, during, and after the procedure.

➤ There are no food, fluid, or medication restrictions, unless by medical direction.

Intratest:

➤ If the patient has a history of severe allergic reaction to latex, care should be taken to avoid the use of equipment containing latex.

➤ Instruct the patient to cooperate fully and to follow directions. Direct the patient to breathe normally and to avoid unnecessary movement.

➤ Observe standard precautions, and follow the general guidelines in Appendix A. Positively identify the patient, and label the appropriate tubes with the corresponding patient demographics, date, and time of collection. Perform a venipuncture; collect the specimen in a 5-mL red- or tiger-top tube.

➤ Remove the needle, and apply a pressure dressing over the puncture site.

➤ Promptly transport the specimen to the laboratory for processing and analysis.

➤ The results are recorded manually or in a computerized system for recall and postprocedure interpretation by the appropriate health care practitioner.

Post-test:

➤ Observe venipuncture site for bleeding or hematoma formation. Apply paper tape or other adhesive to hold pressure bandage in place, or replace with a plastic bandage.

➤ *Nutritional considerations:* Increased uric acid levels may be associated with the formation of kidney stones. Educate the patient, if appropriate, on the importance of drinking a sufficient amount of water when kidney stones are suspected.

➤ *Nutritional considerations:* Increased uric acid levels may be associated with gout. Nutritional therapy may be appropriate for some patients identified as having gout. Educate the patient that foods high in oxalic acid include caffeinated beverages, raw blackberries, gooseberries and plums, whole-wheat bread, beets, carrots, beans, rhubarb, spinach, dry cocoa, and Ovaltine. Foods high in purines include organ meats. In other cases, the requesting health care practitioner may not prescribe a low-purine or purine-restricted diet for treatment of gout because medications can control the condition easily and effectively.

➤ A written report of the examination will be sent to the requesting health care practitioner, who will discuss the results with the patient.

➤ Recognize anxiety related to test results. Discuss the implications of abnormal test results on the patient's lifestyle. Provide teaching and information regarding the clinical implications of the test results, as appropriate.

➤ Reinforce information given by the patient's health care provider regarding further testing, treatment, or referral to another health care provider. Answer any questions or address any concerns voiced by the patient or family.

➤ Depending on the results of this procedure, additional testing may be performed to evaluate or monitor progression of the disease process and determine the need for a change in therapy. Evaluate test results in relation to the patient's symptoms and other tests performed.

Related laboratory tests:

➤ Related laboratory tests include complete blood count, creatinine, creatinine clearance, kidney stone analysis, synovial fluid analysis, and urine uric acid.

URIC ACID, URINE

SYNONYM/ACRONYM: Urine urate.

SPECIMEN: Urine (5 mL) from a random or timed specimen collected in a clean plastic, unrefrigerated collection container. Sodium hydroxide preservative may be recommended to prevent precipitation of urates.

REFERENCE VALUE: (Method: Spectrophotometry)

Gender	Conventional Units*	SI Units (Conventional Units × 0.0059)*
Male	250–800 mg/24 h	1.48–4.72 mmol/24 h
Female	250–750 mg/24 h	1.48–4.43 mmol/24 h

*Values reflect average purine diet.

DESCRIPTION & RATIONALE: Uric acid is the end product of purine metabolism. Purines are important constituents of nucleic acids; purine turnover occurs continuously in the body, producing substantial amounts of uric acid even in the absence of purine intake from dietary sources such as organ meats (e.g., liver, thymus gland and/or pancreas [sweetbreads], kidney), legumes, and yeasts. Uric acid is filtered, absorbed, and secreted by the kidneys and is a common constituent of urine. ■

INDICATIONS:
• Compare urine and serum uric acid levels to provide an index of renal function
• Detect enzyme deficiencies and metabolic disturbances that affect the body's production of uric acid
• Monitor the response to therapy with uricosuric drugs
• Monitor urinary effects of disorders that cause hyperuricemia

RESULT

Increased in:
• Disorders associated with impaired renal tubular absorption, such as Fanconi's syndrome and Wilson's disease
• Disorders of purine metabolism
• Excessive dietary intake of purines
• Gout
• Neoplastic disorders, such as leukemia, lymphosarcoma, and multiple myeloma
• Pernicious anemia
• Polycythemia vera
• Sickle cell anemia

Decreased in:
• Folic acid deficiency
• Lead toxicity

- Severe renal damage (possibly resulting from chronic glomerulonephritis, collagen disorders, diabetic glomerulosclerosis, lactic acidosis, ketoacidosis, and alcohol abuse)

CRITICAL VALUES: N/A

INTERFERING FACTORS:

- Drugs that may increase urine uric acid levels include acetaminophen, acetohexamide, ampicillin, ascorbic acid, azapropazone, benzbromarone, chlorpromazine, chlorprothixene, corticotropin, coumarin, cytotoxics, diatrizoic acid, dicumarol, ethyl biscoumacetate, glycine, iodipamide, iodopyracet, iopanoic acid, ipodate, levodopa, mannose, merbarone, mercaptopurine, mersalyl, methotrexate, niacinamide, phenindione, phenolsulfonphthalein, phenylbutazone, phloridzin, probenecid, salicylates (long-term, large doses), seclazone, sulfinpyrazone, theophylline, verapamil, and xylitol.

- Drugs that may decrease urine uric acid levels include acetylsalicylic acid (small doses), allopurinol, ascorbic acid, azathioprine, benzbromaron, bumetanide, chlorothiazide, chlorthalidone, citrates, ethacrynic acid, ethambutol, ethoxzolamide, hydrochlorothiazide, levarterenol, niacin, pyrazinoic acid, and thiazide diuretics.

- All urine voided for the timed collection period must be included in the collection or else falsely decreased values may be obtained. Compare output records with volume collected to verify that all voids were included in the collection.

Nursing Implications and Procedure

Pretest:

▶ Inform the patient that the test is used to identify overexcretors at risk of calculus formation, identify genetic defects, and assist in monitoring therapy for gout.

▶ Obtain a history of the patient's complaints, including a list of known allergens (especially allergies or sensitivities to latex), and inform the appropriate health care practitioner accordingly.

▶ Obtain a history of the patient's genitourinary system, as well as results of previously performed laboratory tests, surgical procedures, and other diagnostic procedures. For related laboratory tests, refer to the Genitourinary System table.

▶ Obtain a list of medications the patient is taking, including herbs, nutritional supplements, and nutraceuticals. The requesting health care practitioner and laboratory should be advised if the patient regularly uses these products so that their effects can be taken into consideration when reviewing results.

▶ Review the procedure with the patient. Provide a nonmetallic urinal, bedpan, or toilet-mounted collection device. Address concerns about pain related to the procedure. Explain to the patient that there should be no discomfort during the procedure.

▶ Usually a 24-hour time frame for urine collection is ordered. Inform the patient that all urine must be saved during that 24-hour period. Instruct the patient not to void directly into the laboratory collection container. Instruct the patient to avoid defecating in the collection device and to keep toilet tissue out of the collection device to prevent contamination of the specimen. Place a sign in the bathroom to remind the patient to save all urine.

▶ Instruct the patient to void all urine into the collection device and then to pour the urine into the laboratory collection container. Alternatively, the specimen can be left in the collection device for a health care staff member to add to the laboratory collection container.

▶ *Sensitivity to social and cultural issues, as well as concern for* modesty, is important in providing psychological support before, during, and after the procedure.

➤ There are no food, fluid, or medication restrictions, unless by medical direction.

Intratest:

➤ If the patient has a history of severe allergic reaction to latex, care should be taken to avoid the use of equipment containing latex.

➤ Instruct the patient to cooperate fully and to follow directions.

➤ Observe standard precautions, and follow the general guidelines in Appendix A. Positively identify the patient, and label the appropriate collection container with the corresponding patient demographics, date, and time of collection.

Random specimen (collect in early morning):

Clean-catch specimen:

➤ Instruct the male patient to (1) thoroughly wash his hands, (2) cleanse the meatus, (3) void a small amount into the toilet, and (4) void directly into the specimen container.

➤ Instruct the female patient to (1) thoroughly wash her hands; (2) cleanse the labia from front to back; (3) while keeping the labia separated, void a small amount into the toilet; and (4) without interrupting the urine stream, void directly into the specimen container.

Indwelling catheter:

➤ Put on gloves. Empty drainage tube of urine. It may be necessary to clamp off the catheter for 15 to 30 minutes before specimen collection. Cleanse specimen port with antiseptic swab, and then aspirate 5 mL of urine with a 21- to 25-gauge needle and syringe. Transfer urine to a sterile container.

Timed specimen:

➤ Obtain a clean 3-L urine specimen container, toilet-mounted collection device, and plastic bag (for transport of the specimen container). The specimen must be refrigerated or kept on ice throughout the entire collection period. If an indwelling urinary catheter is in place, the drainage bag must be kept on ice.

➤ Begin the test between 6 and 8 a.m., if possible. Collect first voiding and discard. Record the time the specimen was discarded as the beginning of the timed collection period. The next morning, ask the patient to void at the same time the collection was started and add this last voiding to the container.

➤ If an indwelling catheter is in place, replace the tubing and container system at the start of the collection time. Keep the container system on ice during the collection period, or empty the urine into a larger container periodically during the collection period; monitor to ensure continued drainage, and conclude the test the next morning at the same hour the collection was begun.

➤ At the conclusion of the test, compare the quantity of urine with the urinary output record for the collection; if the specimen contains less than what was recorded as output, some urine may have been discarded, invalidating the test.

➤ Include on the collection container's label the amount of urine, test start and stop times, and any medications that can affect test results.

General:

➤ Promptly transport the specimen to the laboratory for processing and analysis.

➤ The results are recorded manually or in a computerized system for recall and postprocedure interpretation by the appropriate health care practitioner.

Post-test:

➤ Increased uric acid levels may be associated with the formation of kidney stones. Educate the patient, if appropriate, on the importance of drinking a sufficient amount of water when kidney stones are suspected.

➤ *Nutritional considerations:* Increased uric acid levels may be associated with gout. Nutritional therapy may be appropriate for some patients identified as having gout. Educate the patient that foods high in oxalic acid include caffeinated beverages, raw blackberries, gooseberries and plums, whole-wheat bread, beets, carrots, beans, rhubarb, spinach, dry cocoa, and Ovaltine. Foods high in purines include organ meats. In other cases, the requesting health care practitioner may not prescribe a low-purine or purine-restricted diet for treatment of gout because medications can control the condition easily and effectively.

➤ A written report of the examination will be sent to the requesting health care practitioner, who will discuss the results with the patient.

➤ Recognize anxiety related to test results. Discuss the implications of abnormal test results on the patient's lifestyle. Provide teaching and information regarding the clinical implications of the test results, as appropriate.

➤ Reinforce information given by the patient's health care provider regarding further testing, treatment, or referral to another health care provider. Answer any questions or address any concerns voiced by the patient or family.

➤ Depending on the results of this procedure, additional testing may be performed to evaluate or monitor progression of the disease process and determine the need for a change in therapy. Evaluate test results in relation to the patient's symptoms and other tests performed.

Related laboratory tests:

➤ Related laboratory tests include urine calcium, complete blood count, urine creatinine, kidney stone analysis, urine oxalate, blood uric acid, and urinalysis.

URINALYSIS

. . . .

SYNONYM/ACRONYM: UA.

SPECIMEN: Urine (15 mL) from an unpreserved, random specimen collected in a clean plastic collection container.

REFERENCE VALUE: (Method: Macroscopic evaluation by dipstick and microscopic examination) Urinalysis comprises a battery of tests including a description of the color and appearance of urine; measurement of specific gravity and pH; and semiquantitative measurement of protein, glucose, ketones, urobilinogen, bilirubin, hemoglobin, nitrites, and leukocyte esterase. Urine sediment may also be examined for the presence of crystals, casts, renal epithelial cells, transitional epithelial cells, squamous epithelial cells, white blood cells (WBCs), red blood cells (RBCs), bacteria, yeast, sperm, and any other substances excreted in the urine that may have clinical significance. Examination of urine sediment is performed microscopically under high power, and results are reported as the number seen per high-power field (hpf). The color of normal urine ranges from light yellow to deep amber. The color depends on the patient's state of hydration (more concentrated samples are darker in color), diet, medication regimen, and exposure to other substances that may contribute to unusual color or odor. The appearance of normal urine is clear. Cloudiness is sometimes attributable to the presence of amorphous phosphates or urates as well as blood, WBCs, fat, or bacteria. Normal specific gravity is 1.001 to 1.035.

Dipstick

pH	5.0–9.0
Protein	Less than 20 mg/dL
Glucose	Negative
Ketones	Negative
Hemoglobin	Negative
Bilirubin	Negative
Urobilinogen	Up to 1 mg/dL
Nitrite	Negative
Leukocyte esterase	Negative

Microscopic Examination

Red blood cells	Less than 5/hpf
White blood cells	Less than 5/hpf
Renal cells	None seen
Transitional cells	None seen
Squamous cells	Rare; usually no clinical significance
Casts	Rare hyaline; otherwise, none seen
Crystals in acid urine	Uric acid, calcium oxalate, amorphous urates
Crystals in alkaline urine	Triple phosphate, calcium phosphate, ammonium biurate, calcium carbonate, amorphous phosphates
Bacteria, yeast, parasites	None seen

DESCRIPTION & RATIONALE: Routine urinalysis, one of the most widely ordered laboratory procedures, is used for basic screening purposes. It is a group of tests that evaluate the kidneys' ability to selectively excrete and reabsorb substances while maintaining proper water balance. The results can provide valuable information regarding the overall health of the patient and the patient's response to disease and treatment. The urine dipstick has a number of pads on it to indicate various biochemical markers. Urine pH is an indication of the kidneys' ability to help maintain balanced hydrogen ion concentration in the blood. Specific gravity is a reflection of the concentration ability of the kidneys. Urine protein is the most common indicator of renal disease, although there are conditions that can cause benign proteinuria. Glucose is used as an indicator of diabetes. The presence of ketones indicates impaired carbohydrate metabolism. Hemoglobin indicates the presence of blood, which is associated with renal disease. Bilirubin is used to assist in the detection of liver disorders. Urobilinogen indicates hepatic or hematopoietic conditions. Nitrites and leukocytes are used to test for bacteriuria and other sources of urinary tract infections (UTIs). Most laboratories have established criteria for the microscopic examination of urine based on patient population (e.g., pediatric, oncology, urology), unusual appearance, and biochemical reactions. ■

INDICATIONS:

- Determine the presence of a genitourinary infection or abnormality
- Monitor the effects of physical or emotional stress
- Monitor fluid imbalances or treatment for fluid imbalances
- Monitor the response to drug therapy and evaluate undesired reactions to drugs that may impair renal function
- Provide screening as part of a general physical examination, especially on admission to a health care facility or before surgery

RESULT

Unusual Color

Color	Presence of
Deep yellow	Riboflavin
Orange	Bilirubin, chrysophanic acid, pyridium, santonin
Pink	Beet pigment, hemoglobin, myoglobin, porphyrin, rhubarb
Red	Beet pigment, hemoglobin, myoglobin, porphyrin, uroerythrin
Green	Oxidized bilirubin, Clorets (breath mint)
Blue	Diagnex, indican, methylene blue
Brown	Bilirubin, hematin, methemoglobin, metronidazole, nitrofurantoin, metabolites of rhubarb, senna
Black	Homogentisic acid, melanin
Smokey	Red blood cells

Test	Increased in	Decreased in
pH	Ingestion of citrus fruits Metabolic and respiratory alkalosis Vegetarian diets	High-protein diets Ingestion of fruits (e.g., cranberries) Metabolic or respiratory acidosis

(Continued on the following page)

Test	Increased in	Decreased in
Protein	Benign proteinuria owing to stress, physical exercise, exposure to cold, or standing Diabetic nephropathy Glomerulonephritis Nephrosis Toxemia of pregnancy	N/A
Glucose	Diabetes	N/A
Ketones	Diabetes Fasting Fever High-protein diets Isopropanol intoxication Postanesthesia period Starvation Vomiting	N/A
Hemoglobin	Diseases of the bladder Exercise (march hemoglobinuria) Glomerulonephritis Hemolytic anemia or other causes of hemolysis (e.g., drugs, parasites, transfusion reaction) Malignancy Menstruation Paroxysmal cold hemoglobinuria Paroxysmal nocturnal hemoglobinuria Pyelonephritis Snake or spider bites Trauma Tuberculosis Urinary tract infections Urolithiasis	N/A
Urobilinogen	Cirrhosis Heart failure Hemolytic anemia Hepatitis Infectious mononucleosis Malaria Pernicious anemia	Antibiotic therapy (suppresses normal intestinal flora) Obstruction of the bile duct
Bilirubin	Cirrhosis Hepatic tumor Hepatitis	N/A

Test	Increased in	Decreased in
Nitrites	Presence of nitrite-forming bacteria (e.g., *Citrobacter, Enterobacter, Escherichia coli, Klebsiella, Proteus, Pseudomonas, Salmonella,* and some species of *Staphylococcus*)	N/A
Leukocyte esterase	Bacterial infection Calculus formation Fungal or parasitic infection Glomerulonephritis Interstitial nephritis Tumor	N/A

Formed Elements in Urine Sediment

Cellular elements:

- Clue cells (cell wall of the bacteria causes adhesion to epithelial cells) are present in nonspecific vaginitis caused by *Gardnerella vaginitis, Mobiluncus cortisii,* and *Mobiluncus mulieris.*

- RBCs are present in glomerulonephritis, lupus nephritis, focal glomerulonephritis, calculus, malignancy, infection, tuberculosis, infarction, renal vein thrombosis, trauma, hydronephrosis, polycystic kidney, urinary tract disease, prostatitis, pyelonephritis, appendicitis, salpingitis, diverticulitis, gout, scurvy, subacute bacterial endocarditis, infectious mononucleosis, hemoglobinopathies, coagulation disorders, heart failure, and malaria.

- Renal cells that have absorbed cholesterol and triglycerides are also known as *oval fat bodies.*

- Renal cells come from the lining of the collecting ducts, and increased numbers indicate acute tubular damage as seen in acute tubular necrosis, pyelonephritis, malignant nephrosclerosis, acute glomerulonephritis, acute drug or substance (salicylate, lead, or ethylene glycol) intoxication, or chemotherapy, resulting in desquamation, urolithiasis, and kidney transplant rejection.

- Squamous cells line the vagina and distal portion of the urethra. The presence of normal squamous epithelial cells in female urine is generally of no clinical significance. Abnormal cells with enlarged nuclei indicate the need for cytologic studies to rule out malignancy.

- Transitional cells line the renal pelvis, ureter, bladder, and proximal portion of the urethra. Increased numbers are seen with infection, trauma, and malignancy.

- WBCs are present in acute UTI, tubulointerstitial nephritis, lupus nephritis, pyelonephritis, kidney transplant rejection, fever, and strenuous exercise.

Casts:

- Granular casts are formed from protein or by the decomposition of cellular elements. They may be seen in renal disease, viral infections, or lead intoxication.

- Large numbers of hyaline casts may be seen in renal diseases, hypertension, congestive heart failure, or nephrotic syndrome, and in more benign conditions such as fever, exposure to cold temperatures, exercise, or diuretic use.

- RBC casts may be found in acute glomerulonephritis, lupus nephritis, and subacute bacterial endocarditis.

- Waxy casts are seen in chronic renal failure or conditions such as kidney transplant rejection, in which there is renal stasis.

- WBC casts may be seen in lupus nephritis, acute glomerulonephritis, interstitial nephritis, and acute pyelonephritis.

Crystals:

- Crystals found in freshly voided urine have more clinical significance than crystals seen in a urine sample that has been standing for more than 2 to 4 hours.

- Calcium oxalate crystals are found in ethylene glycol poisoning, urolithiasis, high dietary intake of oxalates, and Crohn's disease.

- Cystine crystals are seen in patients with cystinosis or cystinuria.

- Leucine or tyrosine crystals may be seen in patients with severe liver disease.

- Large numbers of uric acid crystals are seen in patients with urolithiasis, gout, high dietary intake of foods rich in purines, or receiving chemotherapy (see monograph titled "Uric Acid, Urine").

CRITICAL VALUES:

Possible critical values are the presence of uric acid, cystine, leucine, or tyrosine crystals.

The combination of grossly elevated urine glucose and ketones is also considered significant.

Note and immediately report to the health care practitioner any critical values and related symptoms.

INTERFERING FACTORS:

- Certain foods, such as onion, garlic, and asparagus, contain substances that may give urine an unusual odor. An ammonia-like odor may be produced by the presence of bacteria. Urine with a maple syrup–like odor may indicate a congenital metabolic defect (maple syrup urine disease).

- The various biochemical strips are subject to interference that may produce false-positive or false-negative results. Consult the laboratory for specific information regarding limitations of the method in use and a listing of interfering drugs.

- The dipstick method for protein detection is mostly sensitive to the presence of albumin; light-chain or Bence Jones proteins may not be detected by this method. Alkaline pH may produce false-positive protein results.

- Large amounts of ketones or ascorbic acid may produce false-negative or decreased color development on the glucose pad. Contamination of the collection container or specimen with chlorine, sodium hypochlorite, or peroxide may cause false-positive glucose results.

- False-positive ketone results may be produced in the presence of ascorbic acid, levodopa metabolites, valproic acid, phenazopyridine, phenylketones, or phthaleins.

- The hemoglobin pad may detect myoglobin, intact RBCs, and free hemoglobin. Contamination of the collection container or specimen with sodium hypochlorite or iodine may cause false-positive hemoglobin results. Negative or decreased hemoglobin results may occur in the presence of formalin, elevated protein, nitrite, ascorbic acid, or high specific gravity.

- False-negative nitrite results are common. Negative or decreased results may be seen in the presence of ascorbic acid and high specific gravity. Other causes of false-negative values relate to the amount of time the urine was in the bladder before voiding or the presence of pathogenic organisms that do not reduce nitrates to nitrites.

- False-positive leukocyte esterase reactions result from specimens contaminated by vaginal secretions. The presence of high glucose, protein, or ascorbic acid concentrations may cause false-negative results. Specimens with high specific gravity may also produce false-negative results. Patients with neutropenia (e.g., oncology patients) may also have false-negative results because they do not produce enough WBCs to exceed the sensitivity of the biochemical reaction.

- Specimens that cannot be delivered to the laboratory or tested within 1 hour should be refrigerated or should have a preservative added that is recommended by the laboratory. Specimens collected more than 2 hours before submission may be rejected for analysis.

- Because changes in the urine specimen occur over time, prompt and proper specimen processing, storage, and analysis are important to achieve accurate results. Changes that may occur over time include:

Production of a stronger odor and an increase in pH (bacteria in the urine break urea down to ammonia)

A decrease in clarity (as bacterial growth proceeds or precipitates form)

A decrease in bilirubin and urobilinogen (oxidation to biliverdin and urobilin)

A decrease in ketones (lost through volatilization)

Decreased glucose (consumed by bacteria)

An increase in bacteria (growth over time)

Disintegration of casts, WBCs, and RBCs

An increase in nitrite (overgrowth of bacteria)

Nursing Implications and Procedure

Pretest: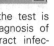

➤ Inform the patient that the test is used to assist in the diagnosis of renal disease, urinary tract infections, and neoplasms of the urinary tract, and as an indication of systemic or inflammatory diseases.

➤ Obtain a history of the patient's complaints, including a list of known allergens (especially allergies or sensitivities to latex), and inform the appropriate health care practitioner accordingly.

➤ Obtain a history of the patient's endocrine, genitourinary, immune, hematopoietic, hepatobiliary, and reproductive systems, as well as results of previously performed laboratory tests, surgical procedures, and other diagnostic procedures. For related laboratory tests, refer to the Endocrine, Genitourinary, Immune, Hematopoietic, Hepatobiliary, and Reproductive System tables.

➤ Obtain a list of medications the patient is taking, including herbs, nutritional supplements, and nutraceuticals. The requesting health care practitioner and laboratory should be advised if the patient is regularly using these products so that their effects can be taken into consideration when reviewing results.

➤ Review the procedure with the patient. If a catheterized specimen is to be collected, explain this procedure to the patient, and obtain a catheterization tray. Address concerns about pain related to the procedure. Explain to the patient that there should be no discomfort during the procedure. Inform the patient that specimen collection takes approximately 5 to 10 minutes.

➤ *Sensitivity to social and cultural issues*, as well as concern for modesty, is important in providing psychological support before, during, and after the procedure.

➤ There are no food, fluid, or medication restrictions, unless by medical direction.

Intratest:

➤ If the patient has a history of severe allergic reaction to latex, care should be taken to avoid the use of equipment containing latex.

➤ Instruct the patient to cooperate fully and to follow directions. Direct the patient to breathe normally and to avoid unnecessary movement.

➤ Observe standard precautions, and follow the general guidelines in Appendix A. Positively identify the patient, and label the appropriate collection container with the corresponding patient demographics, date, and time of collection.

Random specimen (collect in early morning):

Clean-catch specimen:

➤ Instruct the male patient to (1) thoroughly wash his hands, (2) cleanse the meatus, (3) void a small amount into the toilet, and (4) void directly into the specimen container.

➤ Instruct the female patient to (1) thoroughly wash her hands; (2) cleanse the labia from front to back; (3) while keeping the labia separated, void a small amount into the toilet; and (4) without interrupting the urine stream, void directly into the specimen container.

Pediatric urine collector:

➤ Put on gloves. Appropriately cleanse the genital area, and allow the area to dry. Remove the covering over the adhesive strips on the collector bag, and apply the bag over the genital area. Diaper the child. When specimen is obtained, place the entire collection bag in a sterile urine container.

Indwelling catheter:

➤ Put on gloves. Empty drainage tube of urine. It may be necessary to clamp off the catheter for 15 to 30 minutes before specimen collection. Cleanse specimen port with antiseptic swab, and then aspirate 5 mL of urine with a 21- to 25-gauge needle and syringe. Transfer urine to a sterile container.

Urinary catheterization:

➤ Place female patient in lithotomy position or male patient in supine position. Using sterile technique, open the straight urinary catheterization kit and perform urinary catheterization. Place the retained urine in a sterile specimen container.

Suprapubic aspiration:

➤ Place the patient in a supine position. Cleanse the area with antiseptic and drape with sterile drapes. A needle is inserted through the skin into the bladder. A syringe attached to the needle is used to aspirate the urine sample. The needle is then removed and a sterile dressing is applied to the site. Place the sterile sample in a sterile specimen container.

➤ Do not collect urine from the pouch from the patient with a urinary diversion (e.g., ilieal conduit). Instead, perform catheterization through the stoma.

General:

➤ Include on the collection container's label whether the specimen is clean catch or catheter and any medications that may interfere with test results.

➤ Promptly transport the specimen to the laboratory for processing and analysis.

➤ The results are recorded manually or in a computerized system for recall and postprocedure interpretation by the appropriate health care practitioner.

Post-test:

➤ Instruct the patient to report symptoms such as pain related to tissue inflammation, pain or irritation during void, bladder spasms, or alterations in urinary elimination.

➤ Observe for signs of inflammation if the specimen is obtained by suprapubic aspiration.

➤ A written report of the examination will be sent to the requesting health care practitioner, who will discuss the results with the patient.

➤ Recognize anxiety related to test results. Discuss the implications of abnormal test results on the patient's lifestyle. Provide teaching and information regarding the clinical implications of the test results, as appropriate. Instruct the patient with a UTI, as appropriate, on the proper technique for wiping the perineal area (front to back) after a bowel movement. UTIs are more common in women who use diaphragm/spermicide contraception. These patients can be educated, as appropriate, in the proper insertion and removal of the contraceptive device to avoid recurrent UTIs.

➤ Reinforce information given by the patient's health care provider regarding further testing, treatment, or referral to another health care provider. Instruct the patient to begin antibiotic therapy, as prescribed, and instruct the patient in the importance of completing the entire course of antibiotic therapy even if symptoms are no longer present. Answer any questions or address any concerns voiced by the patient or family.

➤ Depending on the results of this procedure, additional testing may be performed to evaluate or monitor progression of the disease process and determine the need for a change in therapy. Evaluate test results in relation to the patient's symptoms and other tests performed.

Related laboratory tests:

➤ Related laboratory tests include blood and urine amino acids, anti–glomerular basement membrane antibody, bladder biopsy, kidney biopsy, bladder cancer marker, urine calcium, complete blood count, blood and urine creatinine, relevant cultures, blood and urine electrolytes, glucose, glycated hemoglobin, blood and urine ketones, kidney stone analysis, microalbumin, urine osmolality, urine oxalate, urine protein, blood and urine protein immunofixation electrophoresis, urine phosphorus, blood and urine urea nitrogen, and blood and urine uric acid.

UTERINE FIBROID EMBOLIZATION

• •

SYNONYMS/ACRONYM: UFE.

AREA OF APPLICATION: Uterus.

CONTRAST: Intravenous iodine based.

DESCRIPTION & RATIONALE: Uterine fibroid embolization (UFE) is a way of treating fibroid tumors of the uterus.

Fibroid tumors, also known as myomas, are masses of fibrous and muscle tissue in the uterine wall that are benign, but that may cause heavy menstrual bleeding, pain in the pelvic region, or pressure on the bladder or bowel. A catheter is placed in each of the two uterine arteries, and small particles are injected to block the arterial branches that supply blood to the fibroids. The fibroid tissue dies, the mass shrinks, and the symptons are relieved. This procedure, which is done under local anesthesia, is less invasive than open surgery done to remove uterine fibroids. Because the effects of uterine fibroid embolization on fertility are not yet known, the ideal candidate is a premenopausal woman with symptoms from fibroid tumors who no longer wishes to become pregnant. This technique is an alternative for women who do not want to receive blood transfusions or do not wish to receive general anesthesia. This procedure may be used to halt severe bleeding following childbirth or caused by gynecologic tumors.■

INDICATIONS:
* Treatment for anemia from chronic blood loss
* Treatment of fibroid tumors and tumor vascularity, for both single and multiple tumors
* Treatment of tumors in lieu of surgical resection

RESULT

Normal Findings:
* Decrease in uterine bleeding
* Decrease of pelvic pain or fullness

INTERFERING FACTORS:

This procedure is contraindicated for:
* ⚠ Patients with allergies to shellfish or iodinated dye. The contrast medium used may cause a life-threatening allergic reaction. Patients with a known hypersensitivity to contrast medium may benefit from premedication with corticosteroids or the use of nonionic contrast medium.

* Patients with bleeding disorders.

* Patients who are pregnant or suspected of being pregnant, unless the potential benefits of the procedure far outweigh the risks to the fetus and mother.

* Patients in whom cancer is a possibility or who have inflammation or infection in the pelvis.

* ⚠ Elderly and other patients who are chronically dehydrated before the procedure, because of their risk of contrast-induced renal failure.

* ⚠ Patients who are in renal failure.

Factors that may impair clear imaging:
* Gas or feces in the gastrointestinal tract resulting from inadequate cleansing or failure to restrict food intake before the study

* Retained barium from a previous radiologic procedure

* Metallic objects within the examination field (e.g., jewelry, body rings, dental amalgams), which may inhibit organ visualization and can produce unclear images

* Improper adjustment of the radiographic equipment to accommodate obese or thin patients, which can cause overexposure or underexposure and a poor-quality study

* Patients who are very obese, who may exceed the weight limit for the equipment

* Incorrect positioning of the patient, which may produce poor visualization of the area to be examined

Other considerations:
* Complications of the procedure include hemorrhage, infection at the insertion site, and cardiac arrhythmias.

- The procedure may be terminated if chest pain or severe cardiac arrhythmias occur.

- Inability of the patient to cooperate or remain still during the procedure because of age, significant pain, or mental status, may interfere with the test results.

- Failure to follow dietary restrictions before the procedure may cause the procedure to be canceled or repeated.

- Consultation with a health care practitioner should occur before the procedure for radiation safety concerns regarding younger patients or patients who are lactating.

- Risks associated with radiographic overexposure can result from frequent x-ray procedures. Personnel in the room with the patient should wear a protective lead apron, stand behind a shield, or leave the area while the examination is being done. Personnel working in the area where the examination is being done should wear badges that reveal their level of exposure to radiation.

- A small percent of women may pass a small piece of fibroid tissue after the procedure. Women with this problem may require a procedure called a D&C (dilatation and curettage).

- Some women may experience menopause shortly after the procedure.

Nursing Implications and Procedure • • • • • • • • • •

Pretest:

➤ Inform the patient that the procedure assesses uterine and associated vascular function.

➤ Obtain a history of the patient's complaints, including a list of known allergens (especially allergies or sensitivities to latex, iodine, seafood, contrast medium, anesthetics, and dyes), and inform the appropriate health care practitioner accordingly.

➤ Obtain a history of the patient's cardiovascular and reproductive systems, as well as results of previously performed laboratory tests (especially coagulation tests, blood urea nitrogen, and creatinine, if contrast medium is to be used), surgical procedures, and other diagnostic procedures. For related diagnostic tests, refer to the Cardiovascular and Reproductive System tables.

➤ Note any recent procedures that can interfere with test results; include examinations utilizing barium or iodine-based contrast medium.

➤ Record the date of the last menstrual period and determine the possibility of pregnancy in perimenopausal women.

➤ Obtain a list of the medications the patient is taking, including anticoagulant therapy, aspirin and other salicylates, herbs, nutritional supplements, and nutraceuticals, especially those known to affect coagulation (see Appendix F). It is recommended that use be discontinued 14 days before surgical procedures. The requesting health care practitioner and laboratory should be advised if the patient regularly uses these products so that their effects can be taken into consideration when reviewing results.

➤ Review the procedure with the patient. Address concerns about pain related to the procedure. Explain that a sedative and/or anesthetic may be administered before the procedure to promote relaxation. Explain to the patient that some pain may be experienced during the test, and there may be moments of discomfort. Inform the patient that the procedure is performed in a radiology or vascular department by a health care practitioner and support staff and takes approximately 30 to 120 minutes.

➤ Explain that an intravenous (IV) line may be inserted to allow infusion of IV fluids, contrast medium, dye, or sedatives. Usually normal saline is infused.

➤ Inform the patient that a burning and flushing sensation may be felt throughout the body during injection of the contrast medium. After injection of the contrast medium, the patient may experience an urge to cough, flushing, nausea, or a salty or metallic taste.

➤ *Sensitivity to cultural and social issues,* as well as concern for modesty, is important in providing psychological support before, during, and after the procedure.

➤ The patient should fast and restrict fluids for 8 hours prior to the procedure. Instruct the patient to avoid taking anticoagulant medication or to reduce dosage as ordered prior to the procedure.

➤ Patients receiving metformin (glucophage) for non–insulin dependent (type 2) diabetes should discontinue the drug on the day of the test and continue to withhold it for 48 hours after the test. Failure to do so may result in lactic acidosis.

➤ Instruct the patient to remove, jewelry (including watches), hairpins, credit cards, and other metallic objects from the area being examined.

➤ *Make sure a written and informed consent has been signed prior to the procedure and before administering any medications.*

➤ This procedure may be terminated if chest pain, severe cardiac arrhythmias, or signs of a cerebrovascular accident occur.

Intratest:

➤ Ensure that the patient has complied with dietary, fluids, and medication restrictions and pretesting preparations; assure that these have been restricted for at least 8 hours prior to the procedure. Ensure that the patient has removed all external metallic objects (jewelry, etc.) prior to the procedure.

➤ Have emergency equipment readily available.

➤ If the patient has a history of severe allergic reactions to any substance or drug, administer ordered prophylactic steroids or antihistamines before the procedure. Use nonionic contrast medium for the procedure.

➤ Patients are given a gown, robe, and foot coverings to wear and instructed to void prior to the procedure.

➤ Instruct the patient to cooperate fully and to follow directions. Instruct the patient to remain still throughout the procedure because movement produces unreliable results.

➤ Record baseline vital signs and assess neurologic status. Protocols may vary from facility to facility.

➤ Observe standard precautions, and follow the general guidelines in Appendix A.

➤ Establish an IV fluid line for the injection of emergency drugs and of sedatives.

➤ Administer an antianxiety agent, as ordered, if the patient has claustrophobia. Administer a sedative to an uncooperative adult, as ordered.

➤ Place electrocardiographic electrodes on the patient for cardiac monitoring. Establish baseline rhythm; determine if the patient has ventricular arrhythmias.

➤ Using a pen, mark the site of the patient's peripheral pulses before angiography; this allows for quicker and more consistent assessment of the pulses after the procedure.

➤ Place the patient in the supine position on an exam table. Cleanse the selected area, and cover with a sterile drape.

➤ A local anesthetic is injected at the site, and a small incision is made or a needle inserted. The femoral artery or vein is punctured, and the guidewire inserted. The catheter is inserted over the guidewire and threaded into the uterine artery under fluoroscopy.

➤ The contrast medium is injected, and a rapid series of images is taken during and after the filling of the vessels to be examined. Delayed images may be taken to examine the vessels

- after a time and to monitor the venous phase of the procedure.

➤ Ask the patient to inhale deeply and hold her breath while the x-ray images are taken, and then to exhale after the images are taken.

➤ Instruct the patient to take slow, deep breaths if nausea occurs during the procedure. Monitor and administer an antiemetic agent if ordered. Ready an emesis basin for use.

➤ Particles are injected through the catheter to block the blood flow to the fibroids. The particles include polyvinyl alcohol, gelatin sponge (Gelfoam), and micospheres.

➤ The needle or catheter is removed, and a pressure dressing is applied over the puncture site.

➤ Monitor the patient for complications related to the procedure (e.g., allergic reaction, anaphylaxis, bronchospasm).

➤ The results are recorded on x-ray film or electronically, in a computerized system, for recall and postprocedure interpretation by the appropriate health care practitioner.

Post-test:

➤ Instruct the patient to resume usual diet, fluids, medications, or activity, as directed by the health care practitioner. Renal function should be assessed before metformin is resumed.

➤ Monitor vital signs and neurologic status every 15 minutes for 1 hour, then every 2 hours for 4 hours, and then as ordered by the health care practitioner. Take temperature every 4 hours for 24 hours. Compare with baseline values. Notify the health care practitioner if temperature is elevated. Protocols may vary from facility to facility.

➤ Patients may experience plevic cramps for several days after the procedure and possible mild nausea and fever.

➤ Observe for delayed allergic reactions, such as rash, urticaria, tachy-

cardia, hyperpnea, hypertension, palpitations, nausea, or vomiting,

➤ Advise the patient to immediately report symptoms such as fast heart rate, difficulty breathing, skin rash, itching, or decreased urinary output.

➤ Assess extremities for signs of ischemia or absence of distal pulse caused by a catheter-induced thrombus.

➤ Observe the needle/catheter insertion site for bleeding, inflammation, or hematoma formation. Note any pleuritic pain, persistent right shoulder pain, or abdominal pain.

➤ Instruct the patient to apply cold compresses to the puncture site, as needed, to reduce discomfort or edema. Instruct the patient in the care and assessment of the site.

➤ A written report of the examination will be completed by a health care practitioner specializing in this branch of medicine. The report will be sent to the requesting health care practitioner, who will discuss the results with the patient.

➤ Recognize anxiety related to test results, and be supportive of impaired activity related to genitourinary system. Discuss the implications of abnormal test results on the patient's lifestyle. Provide teaching and information regarding the clinical implications of the test results, as appropriate. Educate the patient regarding access to counseling services.

➤ Reinforce information given by the patient's health care provider regarding further testing, treatment, or referral to another health care provider. Answer any questions or address any concerns voiced by the patient or family.

➤ Instruct the patient in the use of any ordered medications. Explain the importance of adhering to the therapy regimen. As appropriate, instruct the patient in significant side effects and systemic reactions associated with the prescribed medication. Encourage her to review corresponding literature provided by a pharmacist.

➤ It may take 2 to 3 months for the fibroids to shrink so that bulk-related symptoms such as pain and pressure improve. Heavy bleeding may improve during the first menstrual cycle following the procedure.

➤ Most women are able to return to work 1 to 2 weeks after the procedure.

➤ Depending on the results of this procedure, additional testing may be performed to evaluate or monitor progression of the disease process and determine the need for a change in therapy. Evaluate test results in relation to the patient's symptoms and other tests performed.

Related diagnostic tests:

➤ Related diagnostic tests include computed tomography angiography, computed tomography of the plevis, magnetic resonance angiography, magnetic resonance imaging of the pelvis, and ultrasound of the pelvis.

VANILLYLMANDELIC ACID, URINE

SYNONYM/ACRONYM: VMA.

SPECIMEN: Urine (25 mL) from a timed specimen collected in a clean plastic collection container with 6N hydrochloric acid as a preservative.

REFERENCE VALUE: (Method: High-pressure liquid chromatography)

Age	Conventional Units	SI Units (Conventional Units × 5.05)
3–6 y	1.0–2.6 mg/24 h	5–13 µmol/24 h
6–10 y	2.0–3.2 mg/24 h	10–16 µmol/24 h
10–16 y	2.3–5.2 mg/24 h	12–26 µmol/24 h
16–83 y	1.4–6.5 mg/24 h	7–33 µmol/24 h

DESCRIPTION & RATIONALE: Vanillylmandelic acid (VMA) is a major metabolite of epinephrine and norepinephrine. It is elevated in conditions that also are marked by overproduction of catecholamines. Creatinine is usually measured simultaneously to ensure adequate collection and to calculate an excretion ratio of metabolite to creatinine. ∎

transmitted in respiratory secretions. The primary exposure to the highly contagious virus usually occurs in susceptible school-age children. Adults without prior exposure and who become infected may have severe complications, including pneumonia. Neonatal infection from the mother is possible if exposure occurs during the last 3 weeks of gestation. Shingles results when the presumably latent virus is reactivated. The presence of immunoglobulin (Ig) M antibodies indicates acute infection. The presence of IgG antibodies indicates current or past infection. A reactive varicella antibody result indicates immunity but does not protect an individual from shingles. There are also polymerase chain reaction methods that are capable of detecting varicella-zoster DNA in various specimen types.■

INDICATIONS: Determine susceptibility or immunity to chickenpox

RESULT

Positive findings in: Varicella infection

Negative findings in: N/A

CRITICAL VALUES: N/A

INTERFERING FACTORS: N/A

Nursing Implications and Procedure . . . .

Pretest:

➤ Inform the patient that the test is used to confirm diagnosis of varicella infection or immunity.

➤ Obtain a history of the patient's complaints, including a list of known allergens (especially allergies or sen-

sitivities to latex), and inform the appropriate health care practitioner accordingly.

➤ Obtain a history of exposure to varicella.

➤ Obtain a history of the patient's immune and reproductive systems, as well as results of previously performed laboratory tests, surgical procedures, and other diagnostic procedures. For related laboratory tests, refer to the Immune and Reproductive System tables.

➤ Obtain a list of medications the patient is taking, including herbs, nutritional supplements, and nutraceuticals. The requesting health care practitioner and laboratory should be advised if the patient is regularly using these products so that their effects can be taken into consideration when reviewing results.

➤ Review the procedure with the patient. Inform the patient that several tests may be necessary to confirm diagnosis. Any individual positive result should be repeated in 7 to 14 days to monitor a change in titer. Inform the patient that specimen collection takes approximately 5 to 10 minutes. Address concerns about pain related to the procedure. Explain to the patient that there may be some discomfort during the venipuncture.

➤ *Sensitivity to social and cultural issues,* as well as concern for modesty, is important in providing psychological support before, during, and after the procedure.

➤ There are no food, fluid, or medication restrictions, unless by medical direction.

Intratest:

➤ If the patient has a history of severe allergic reaction to latex, care should be taken to avoid the use of equipment containing latex.

➤ Instruct the patient to cooperate fully and to follow directions. Direct the patient to breathe normally and to avoid unnecessary movement.

➤ Observe standard precautions, and follow the general guidelines in

INDICATIONS:
• Assist in the diagnosis of neuroblastoma, ganglioneuroma, or pheochromocytoma
• Evaluate hypertension of unknown cause

RESULT

Increased in:
• Ganglioneuroma
• Hypertension
• Neuroblastoma
• Pheochromocytoma

Decreased in: N/A

CRITICAL VALUES: N/A

INTERFERING FACTORS:
• Drugs that may increase VMA levels include ajmaline, chlorpromazine, glucagon, guaifenesin, guanethidine, isoproterenol, methyldopa, nitroglycerin, oxytetracycline, phenazopyridine, phenolsulfonphthalein, prochlorperazine, rauwolfia, reserpine, sulfobromophthalein, and syrosingopine.
• Drugs that may decrease VMA levels include brofaromine, guanethidine, guanfacine, imipramine, isocarboxazid, methyldopa, monoamine oxidase inhibitors, morphine, nialamide (in schizophrenics), and reserpine.
• Stress, hypoglycemia, hyperthyroidism, strenuous exercise, smoking, and drugs can produce elevated catecholamines.
• Recent radioactive scans within 1 week of the test can interfere with test results.
• Failure to collect all urine and store 24-hour specimen properly will result in a falsely low result.
• Failure to follow dietary restrictions before the procedure may cause the procedure to be canceled or repeated.

Nursing Implications and Procedure . . . .

Pretest:

➤ Inform the patient that the test is used to assist in the diagnosis and follow-up treatment of pheochromocytoma, neuroblastoma, and ganglioblastoma. It is also useful in evaluation and follow-up of hypertension.

➤ Obtain a history of the patient's complaints, including a list of known allergens (especially allergies or sensitivities to latex), and inform the appropriate health care practitioner accordingly.

➤ Obtain a history of the patient's endocrine system, as well as results of previously performed laboratory tests, surgical procedures, and other diagnostic procedures. For related laboratory tests, refer to the Endocrine System table.

➤ Obtain a list of medications the patient is taking, including herbs, nutritional supplements, and nutraceuticals. The requesting health care practitioner and laboratory should be advised if the patient regularly uses these products so that their effects can be taken into consideration when reviewing results.

➤ Review the procedure with the patient. Provide a nonmetallic urinal, bedpan, or toilet-mounted collection device. Address concerns about pain related to the procedure. Explain to the patient that there should be no discomfort during the procedure.

➤ Usually a 24-hour time frame for urine collection is ordered. Inform the patient that all urine must be saved during that 24-hour period. Instruct the patient not to void directly into the laboratory collection container. Instruct the patient to avoid defecating in the collection device and to keep toilet tissue out of the collection device to prevent contamination of the specimen. Place a sign in the bathroom to remind the patient to save all urine.

➤ Instruct the patient to void all urine into the collection device and then to pour the urine into the laboratory collection container. Alternatively, the specimen can be left in the collection device for a health care staff member to add to the laboratory collection container.

➤ *Sensitivity to social and cultural issues*, as well as concern for modesty, is important in providing psychological support before, during, and after the procedure.

➤ There are no fluid restrictions unless by medical direction.

➤ Instruct the patient to abstain from smoking tobacco for 24 hours before testing.

➤ Inform the patient of the following dietary, medication, and activity restrictions in preparation for the test:

The patient should not consume foods high in amines for 48 hours before testing (bananas, avocados, beer, aged cheese, chocolate, cocoa, coffee, fava beans, grains, tea, vanilla, walnuts, and red wine).

The patient should not consume foods or fluids high in caffeine for 48 hours before testing (coffee, tea, cocoa, and chocolate).

The patient should not consume any foods or fluids containing vanilla or licorice.

The patient should avoid self-prescribed medications (especially aspirin) and prescribed medications (especially pyridoxine, levodopa, amoxicillin, carbidopa, reserpine, and disulfiram) for 2 weeks before testing and as directed.

The patient should avoid excessive exercise and stress during the 24-hour collection of urine.

➤ Ensure that the patient has complied with dietary, medication, and activity restrictions and pretesting preparations prior to the procedure.

➤ If the patient has a history of severe allergic reaction to latex, care should be taken to avoid the use of equipment containing latex.

➤ Instruct the patient to cooperate fully and to follow directions.

➤ Observe standard precautions, and follow the general guidelines in Appendix A. Positively identify the patient, and label the appropriate collection container with the corresponding patient demographics, date, and time of collection.

Timed specimen:

➤ Obtain a clean 3-L urine specimen container, toilet-mounted collection device, and plastic bag (for transport of the specimen container). The specimen must be refrigerated or kept on ice throughout the entire collection period. If an indwelling urinary catheter is in place, the drainage bag must be kept on ice.

➤ Begin the test between 6 and 8 a.m., if possible. Collect first voiding and discard. Record the time the specimen was discarded as the beginning of the timed collection period. The next morning, ask the patient to void at the same time the collection was started and add this last voiding to the container.

➤ If an indwelling catheter is in place, replace the tubing and container system at the start of the collection time. Keep the container system on ice during the collection period, or empty the urine into a larger container periodically during the collection period; monitor to ensure continued drainage, and conclude the test the next morning at the same hour the collection was begun.

➤ At the conclusion of the test, compare the quantity of urine with the urinary output record for the collection; if the specimen contains less than what was recorded as output, some urine may have been discarded, invalidating the test.

➤ Include on the collection container's label the amount of urine, test start and stop times, and ingestion of any foods or medications that can affect test results.

➤ Promptly transport the specimen to the laboratory for processing and analysis.

➤ The results are recorded manually or in a computerized system for recall and postprocedure interpretation by the appropriate health care practitioner.

➤ Instruct the patient to resume usual diet, fluids, medications, or activity, as directed by the health care practitioner.

➤ *Nutritional considerations:* Instruct the patient to avoid foods or drinks containing caffeine. Over-the-counter medications should be taken only under the advice of the patient's health care practitioner.

➤ A written report of the examination will be sent to the requesting health care practitioner, who will discuss the results with the patient.

➤ Recognize anxiety related to test results, and be supportive fear of shortened life expectancy. Discuss the implications of abnormal test results on the patient's lifestyle. Provide teaching and information regarding the clinical implications of the test results, as appropriate. Educate the patient regarding access to counseling services.

➤ Reinforce information given by the patient's health care provider regarding further testing, treatment, or referral to another health care provider. Answer any questions or address any concerns voiced by the patient or family.

➤ Depending on the results of this procedure, additional testing may be performed to evaluate or monitor progression of the disease process and determine the need for a change in therapy. Evaluate test results in relation to the patient's symptoms and other tests performed.

➤ Related laboratory tests include catecholamines, homovanillic acid, and metanephrines.

VARICELLA ANTIBODIES

SYNONYMS/ACRONYM: Varicella zoster antibodies, chickenpox, VZ.

SPECIMEN: Serum (1 mL) collected in a red-top tube.

REFERENCE VALUE: (Method: Indirect fluorescent antibody) Negative or less than a fourfold increase in titer.

DESCRIPTION & RATIONALE: Varicella-zoster is a double-stranded DNA herpesvirus that is responsible for two clinical syndromes, chickenpox and shingles. The incubation period is 2 to 3 weeks, and it is highly contagious for about 2 weeks beginning 2 days before a rash develops. It is

Appendix A. Positively identify the patient, and label the appropriate tubes with the corresponding patient demographics, date, and time of collection. Perform a venipuncture; collect the specimen in a 5-mL red-top tube.

➤ Remove the needle, and apply a pressure dressing over the puncture site.

➤ Promptly transport the specimen to the laboratory for processing and analysis.

➤ The results are recorded manually or in a computerized system for recall and postprocedure interpretation by the appropriate health care practitioner.

Post-test:

➤ Observe venipuncture site for bleeding or hematoma formation. Apply paper tape or other adhesive to hold pressure bandage in place, or replace with a plastic bandage.

➤ *Vaccination considerations:* Record the date of last menstrual period and determine the possibility of pregnancy prior to administration of varicella vaccine to female varicella-nonimmune patients. Instruct patient not to become pregnant for 1 month after being vaccinated with the varicella vaccine to protect any fetus from contracting the disease and having serious birth defects. Instruct on birth control methods to prevent pregnancy, if appropriate.

➤ A written report of the examination will be sent to the requesting health care practitioner, who will discuss the results with the patient.

➤ Recognize anxiety related to test results, and provide emotional support if results are positive and the patient is pregnant. Inform the patient with shingles regarding access to pain management. Discuss the implications of abnormal test results on the patient's lifestyle. Provide teaching and information regarding the clinical implications of the test results, as appropriate. Educate the patient regarding access to counseling services.

➤ Reinforce information given by the patient's health care provider regarding further testing, treatment, or referral to another health care provider. Instruct the patient in isolation precautions during the time of communicability or contagion. Emphasize the need to return to have a convalescent blood sample taken in 7 to 14 days. Answer any questions or address any concerns voiced by the patient or family.

➤ Depending on the results of this procedure, additional testing may be performed to evaluate or monitor progression of the disease process and determine the need for a change in therapy. Evaluate test results in relation to the patient's symptoms and other tests performed.

VENOGRAPHY, LOWER EXTREMITY STUDIES

. . . .

SYNONYMS/ACRONYM: Phlebography, lower limb venography, venogram.

AREA OF APPLICATION: Veins of the lower extremities.

CONTRAST: Intravenous iodine based.

DESCRIPTION & RATIONALE: Venography allows x-ray visualization of the venous vasculature system of the extremities after injection of an iodinated contrast medium. Lower extremity studies identify and locate thrombi within the venous system of the lower limbs. After injection of the contrast medium, x-ray films are taken at timed intervals. Usually both extremities are studied, and the unaffected side is used for comparison with the side suspected of having deep vein thrombosis (DVT) or other venous abnormalities, such as congenital malformations or incompetent valves. Thrombus formation usually occurs in the deep calf veins and at the venous junction and its valves. If DVT is not treated, it can lead to femoral and iliac venous occlusion, or the thrombus can become an embolus, causing a pulmonary embolism. Venography is accurate for thrombi in veins below the knee. ■

INDICATIONS:
- Assess deep vein valvular competence
- Confirm a diagnosis of DVT
- Determine the cause of extremity swelling or pain
- Determine the source of emboli when pulmonary embolism is suspected or diagnosed
- Distinguish clot formation from venous obstruction
- Evaluate congenital venous malformations
- Locate a vein for arterial bypass graft surgery

RESULT

Normal Findings: No obstruction to flow or filling defects after injection of radiopaque dye; steady opacification of superficial and deep vasculature with no filling defects

Abnormal Findings: Abnormal results may indicate DVT, deep vein valvular incompetence, or venous obstruction

CRITICAL VALUES: N/A

INTERFERING FACTORS:

This procedure is contraindicated for:
- ⚠ Patients with allergies to shellfish or iodinated dye. The contrast medium used may cause a life-threatening allergic reaction. Patients with a known hypersensitivity to the contrast medium may benefit from premedication with corticosteroids or the use of nonionic contrast medium.
- Patients who are pregnant or suspected of being pregnant, unless the potential benefits of the procedure far outweigh the risks to the fetus and mother.
- ⚠ Elderly and other patients who are chronically dehydrated before the test, because of their risk of contrast-induced renal failure.
- ⚠ Patients who are in renal failure.
- ⚠ Patients with bleeding disorders.

Factors that may impair clear imaging:
- Metallic objects within the examination field (e.g., jewelry, body rings), which may inhibit organ visualization and can produce unclear images
- Improper adjustment of the radiographic equipment to accommodate obese or thin patients, which can cause overexposure or underexposure and a poor-quality study
- Patients who are very obese, who may exceed the weight limit for the equipment

- Incorrect positioning of the patient, which may produce poor visualization of the area to be examined

- Movement of the leg being tested, excessive tourniquet constriction, insufficient injection of contrast medium, and delay between injection and the x-ray

- Severe edema of the legs, making venous access impossible

- Weight bearing on the leg being tested, which prevents the contrast medium from filling the veins

Other considerations:

- Improper injection of the radionuclide that allows the tracer to seep deep into the muscle tissue can produce erroneous hot spots.

- Inability of the patient to cooperate or remain still during the procedure because of age, significant pain, or mental status, may interfere with the test results.

- Consultation with a health care practitioner should occur before the procedure for radiation safety concerns regarding younger patients or patients who are lactating.

- Risks associated with radiographic overexposure can result from frequent x-ray procedures. Personnel in the room with the patient should wear a protective lead apron, stand behind a shield, or leave the area while the examination is being done. Personnel working in the area where the examination is being done should wear badges that reveal their level of exposure to radiation.

Nursing Implications and Procedure • • • • • • • • • •

Pretest:

▶ Inform the patient that the procedure assesses the venous system of the lower extremities.

▶ Obtain a history of the patient's complaints, including a list of known allergens (especially allergies or sensitivities to latex, iodine, seafood, contrast medium, anesthetics, and dyes), and inform the appropriate health care practitioner accordingly.

▶ Obtain a history of the patient's cardiovascular system, as well as results of previously performed laboratory tests (especially coagulation tests, blood urea nitrogen, and creatinine, if contrast medium is to be used), surgical procedures, and other diagnostic procedures. For related diagnostic tests, refer to the Cardiovascular System table.

▶ Note any recent procedures that can interfere with test results, including examinations using iodine-based contrast medium or barium.

▶ Record the date of the last menstrual period and determine the possibility of pregnancy in perimenopausal women.

▶ Obtain a list of the medications the patient is taking, including anticoagulant therapy, aspirin and other salicylates, herbs, nutritional supplements, and nutraceuticals, especially those known to affect coagulation (see Appendix F). It is recommended that use be discontinued 14 days before surgical procedures. The requesting health care practitioner and laboratory should be advised if the patient regularly uses these products so that their effects can be taken into consideration when reviewing results.

▶ Review the procedure with the patient. Address concerns about pain related to the procedure. Explain to the patient that some pain may be experienced during the test, or there may be moments of discomfort. Inform the patient that the procedure is performed in a special department, usually in a radiology or vascular suite, by a health care practitioner and support staff, and takes approximately 30 to 60 minutes.

▶ Explain that an intravenous (IV) line may be inserted to allow infusion of IV fluids, contrast medium, dye, or

➤ sedatives. Usually normal saline is infused.

➤ Inform the patient that a burning and flushing sensation may be felt throughout the body during injection of the contrast medium. After injection of the contrast medium, the patient may experience an urge to cough, flushing, nausea, or a salty or metallic taste.

➤ *Sensitivity to social and cultural issues*, as well as concern for modesty, is important in providing psychological support before, during, and after the procedure

➤ The patient should fast and restrict fluids for 8 hours prior to the procedure. Instruct the patient to avoid taking anticoagulant medication or to reduce dosage as ordered prior to the procedure.

➤ Patients receiving metformin (glucophage) for non–insulin dependent (type 2) diabetes should discontinue the drug on the day of the test and continue to withhold it for 48 hours after the test. Failure to do so may result in lactic acidosis.

➤ Instruct the patient to remove jewelry (including watches), hairpins, credit cards, and other metallic objects in the area to be examined.

➤ *Make sure a written and informed consent has been signed prior to the procedure and before administering any medications.*

➤ This procedure may be terminated if chest pain, severe cardiac arrhythmias, or signs of a cerebrovascular accident occur.

Intratest:

➤ Ensure that the patient has complied with dietary, fluids, and medication restrictions and pretesting preparations; assure that food and medications have been restricted for at least 8 hours prior to the procedure. Ensure that the patient has removed all external metallic objects (jewelry, etc.) prior to the procedure.

➤ Have emergency equipment readily available.

➤ If the patient has a history of severe allergic reactions to any substance or drug, administer ordered prophylactic steroids or antihistamines before the procedure. Use nonionic contrast medium for the procedure.

➤ Patients are given a gown, robe, and foot coverings to wear and instructed to void prior to the procedure.

➤ Instruct the patient to cooperate fully and to follow directions. Instruct the patient to remain still throughout the procedure because movement produces unreliable results.

➤ Record baseline vital signs and assess neurologic status. Protocols may vary from facility to facility.

➤ Observe standard precautions, and follow the general guidelines in Appendix A.

➤ Establish an IV fluid line for the injection of emergency drugs and of sedatives.

➤ Administer an antianxiety agent, as ordered, if the patient has claustrophobia. Administer a sedative to a child or to an uncooperative adult, as ordered.

➤ Place electrocardiographic electrodes on the patient for cardiac monitoring. Establish baseline rhythm; determine if the patient has ventricular arrhythmias.

➤ Using a pen, mark the site of the patient's peripheral pulses before angiography; this allows for quicker and more consistent assessment of the pulses after the procedure.

➤ Place the patient in the supine position on an exam table. Cleanse the selected area, and cover with a sterile drape.

➤ A local anesthetic is injected at the site, and a small incision is made or a needle inserted under fluoroscopy.

➤ The contrast medium is injected, and a rapid series of images is taken during and after the filling of the vessels to be examined. Delayed images may be taken to examine the vessels after a time and to monitor the venous phase of the procedure.

➤ Instruct the patient to inhale deeply and hold his or her breath while the x-ray images are taken, and then to exhale after the images are taken.

➤ Instruct the patient to take slow, deep breaths if nausea occurs during the procedure. Monitor and administer an antiemetic agent if ordered. Ready an emesis basin for use.

➤ Monitor the patient for complications related to the procedure (e.g., allergic reaction, anaphylaxis, bronchospasm).

➤ The needle or catheter is removed, and a pressure dressing is applied over the puncture site.

➤ The results are recorded on x-ray film or electronically, in a computerized system, for recall and postprocedure interpretation by the appropriate health care practitioner.

Post-test:

➤ Instruct the patient to resume usual diet, fluids, medications, or activity, as directed by the health care practitioner. Renal function should be assessed before metformin is resumed.

➤ Monitor vital signs and neurologic status every 15 minutes for 1 hour, then every 2 hours for 4 hours, and then as ordered by the health care practitioner. Take temperature every 4 hours for 24 hours. Compare with baseline values. Notify the health care practitioner if temperature is elevated. Protocols may vary from facility to facility.

➤ Observe for delayed allergic reactions, such as rash, urticaria, tachycardia, hyperpnea, hypertension, palpitations, nausea, or vomiting.

➤ Instruct the patient to immediately report symptoms such as fast heart rate, difficulty breathing, skin rash, itching, or decreased urinary output.

➤ Assess extremities for signs of ischemia or absence of distal pulse caused by a catheter-induced thrombus.

➤ Observe the needle/catheter insertion site for bleeding, inflammation, or hematoma formation. Note any pleuritic pain, persistent right shoulder pain, or abdominal pain.

➤ Instruct the patient to apply cold compresses to the puncture site, as needed, to reduce discomfort or edema. Instruct the patient in the care and assessment of the site.

➤ Instruct the patient to maintain bed rest for 4 to 6 hours after the procedure or as ordered.

➤ *Nutritional considerations:* A low-fat, low-cholesterol, and low-sodium diet should be consumed to reduce current disease processes and/or decrease risk of hypertension and coronary artery disease.

➤ A written report of the examination will be completed by a health care practitioner specializing in this branch of medicine. The report will be sent to the requesting health care practitioner, who will discuss the results with the patient.

➤ Recognize anxiety related to test results, and be supportive of perceived loss of independent function. Discuss the implications of abnormal test results on the patient's lifestyle. Provide teaching and information regarding the clinical implications of the test results, as appropriate.

➤ Reinforce information given by the patient's health care provider regarding further testing, treatment, or referral to another health care provider. Answer any questions or address any concerns voiced by the patient or family.

➤ Instruct the patient in the use of any ordered medications. Explain the importance of adhering to the therapy regimen. As appropriate, instruct the patient in significant side effects and systemic reactions associated with the prescribed medication. Encourage him or her to review corresponding literature provided by a pharmacist.

➤ Depending on the results of this procedure, additional testing may be needed to evaluate or monitor progression of the disease process and determine the need for a change in therapy. Evaluate test results in relation to the patient's symptoms and other tests performed.

Related diagnostic tests:

➤ Related diagnostic tests include computed tomography of the abdomen, computed tomography angiography, lung perfusion scan, magnetic resonance angiography, magnetic resonance imaging of the abdomen, renogram, and peripheral Doppler ultrasound.

VERTEBROPLASTY

SYNONYMS/ACRONYM: None.

AREA OF APPLICATION: Spine.

CONTRAST: Intravenous iodine based.

DESCRIPTION & RATIONALE: Vertebroplasty is a minimally invasive, non-surgical therapy used to repair a broken vertebra and to provide relief of pain related to vertebral compression in the spine that has been weakened by osteoporosis or tumoral lesions. Osteoporosis affects over 10 million women in the United States and accounts for over 700,000 vertebral fractures per year. This procedure is usually successful at alleviating the pain caused by a compression fracture less than 6 months in duration with pain directly referable to the location of the fracture. Secondary benefits may include vertebra stabilization and reduction of the risk of further compression. This procedure is usually performed on an outpatient basis. The procedure is accomplished by injecting orthopedic cement mixture through a needle into a fracture site. Vertebroplasty may be the preferred procedure when patients are too elderly or frail to tolerate open spinal surgery, or with bones too weak for surgical repair. Patients with a malignant tumor may possibly benefit from vertebroplasty. Other possible applications include younger patients whose osteoporosis is caused by long-term steroid use or a metabolic disorder. This procedure is recommended after basic treatments such as bed rest and orthopedic braces have failed, or pain medication has been ineffective or caused the patient medical problems, including stomach ulcers. ∎

INDICATIONS:

• Assist in the detection of nonmalignant tumors before surgical resection.

• Repair of compression spinal fractures

of varying ages. Fractures older than 6 months will respond but at a slower rate. Fractures less than 4 weeks old should be give a chance to heal without intervention unless they are associated with disabling pain or hospitalization.

• Repair of spinal problems due to tumors.

RESULT

Normal Findings:

• Improvement in the ability to ambulate without pain

• Relief of back pain

Abnormal Findings:

• Failure to reduce the patient's pain

• Failure to improve the patient's mobility

INTERFERING FACTORS

This procedure is contraindicated for:

• ⚠ Patients with allergies to shellfish or iodinated dye. The contrast medium used may cause a life-threatening allergic reaction. Patients with a known hypersensitivity to the contrast medium may benefit from premedication with corticosteroids or the use of nonionic contrast medium.

• Pain that is primarily radicular in nature

• Patients with bleeding disorders

• Patients who are pregnant or suspected of being pregnant, unless the potential benefits of the procedure far outweigh the risks to the fetus and mother

• Pain that is improving or that has been present and unchanged for years

• Imaging procedures that suggest no fracture is present or that the fracture is remote from the patient's pain

Factors that may impair clear imaging:

• Gas or feces in the gastrointestinal tract resulting from inadequate cleansing or failure to restrict food intake before the study

• Retained barium from a previous radiologic procedure

• Metallic objects within the examination field (e.g., jewelry, body rings, dental amalgams), which may inhibit organ visualization and can produce unclear images

• Improper adjustment of the radiographic equipment to accommodate obese or thin patients, which can cause overexposure or underexposure and a poor-quality study

• Patients who are very obese, who may exceed the weight limit for the equipment

• Incorrect positioning of the patient, which may produce poor visualization of the area to be examined

Other considerations:

• Complications of the procedure include hemorrhage, infection at the insertion site, and cardiac arrhythmias.

• The procedure may be terminated if chest pain, or severe cardiac arrhythmias occur.

• Inability of the patient to cooperate or remain still during the procedure because of age, significant pain, or mental status, may interfere with the test results.

• Failure to follow dietary restrictions before the procedure may cause the procedure to be canceled or repeated.

• Consultation with a health care practitioner should occur before the procedure for radiation safety concerns regarding younger patients or patients who are lactating.

• Risks associated with radiographic

overexposure can result from frequent x-ray procedures. Personnel in the room with the patient should wear a protective lead apron, stand behind a shield, or leave the area while the examination is being done. Personnel working in the area where the examination is being done should wear badges that reveal their level of exposure to radiation.

Nursing Implications and Procedure . . . .

Pretest:

➤ Inform the patient that the procedure improves the spinal column function.

➤ Obtain a history of the patient's complaints, including a list of known allergens (especially allergies or sensitivities to latex, iodine, seafood, contrast medium, anesthetics, and dyes), and inform the appropriate health care practitioner accordingly.

➤ Obtain a history of the patient's musculoskeletal system, as well as results of previously performed laboratory tests (especially coagulation tests, blood urea nitrogen, and creatinine, if contrast medium is to be used), surgical procedures, and other diagnostic procedures. For related diagnostic tests, refer to the Musculoskeletal System table.

➤ Note any recent procedures that can interfere with test results, including examinations using iodine-based contrast medium or barium.

➤ Record the date of the last menstrual period and determine the possibility of pregnancy in perimenopausal women.

➤ Obtain a list of the medications the patient is taking, including anticoagulant therapy, aspirin and other salicylates, herbs, nutritional supplements, and nutraceuticals, especially those known to affect coagulation (see Appendix F). It is recommended that use be discontinued 14 days before

surgical procedures. The requesting health care practitioner and laboratory should be advised if the patient regularly uses these products so that their effects can be taken into consideration when reviewing results.

➤ Review the procedure with the patient. Address concerns about pain related to the procedure. Explain to the patient that some pain may be experienced during the test, or there may be moments of discomfort. Inform the patient that the procedure is performed in the radiology department by a health care practitioner and support staff, and takes approximately 30 to 90 minutes.

➤ Explain that an intravenous (IV) line may be inserted to allow infusion of IV fluids, contrast medium, dye, or sedatives. Usually normal saline is infused.

➤ *Sensitivity to cultural and social issues,* as well as concern for modesty, is important in providing psychological support before, during, and after the procedure.

➤ The patient should fast and restrict fluids for 8 hours prior to the procedure. Instruct the patient to avoid taking anticoagulant medication or to reduce dosage as ordered prior to the procedure.

➤ Instruct the patient to remove jewelry (including watches), hairpins, credit cards, and other metallic objects from the area to be examined.

➤ *Make sure a written and informed consent has been signed prior to the procedure and before administering any medications.*

➤ This procedure may be terminated if chest pain or severe cardiac arrhythmias occur.

Intratest:

➤ Ensure that the patient has complied with dietary, fluids, and medication restrictions and pretesting preparations; assure that these have been restricted for at least 8 hours prior to the procedure. Ensure that the patient has removed all external metallic objects (jewelry, dentures, etc.) prior to the procedure.

➤ Have emergency equipment readily available.

➤ If the patient has a history of severe allergic reactions to any substance or drug, administer ordered prophylactic steroids or antihistamines before the procedure. Use nonionic contrast medium for the procedure.

➤ Patients are given a gown, robe, and foot coverings to wear and instructed to void prior to the procedure.

➤ Instruct the patient to cooperate fully and to follow directions. Instruct the patient to remain still throughout the procedure because movement produces unreliable results.

➤ Record baseline vital signs and assess neurologic status. Protocols may vary from facility to facility.

➤ Observe standard precautions, and follow the general guidelines in Appendix A.

➤ Establish an IV fluid line for the injection of emergency drugs and of sedatives.

➤ Administer an antianxiety agent, as ordered, if the patient has claustrophobia. Administer a sedative to a child or to an uncooperative adult, as ordered.

➤ Place electrocardiographic electrodes on the patient for cardiac monitoring. Establish baseline rhythm; determine if the patient has ventricular arrhythmias.

➤ Using a pen, mark the site of the patient's peripheral pulses before angiography; this allows for quicker and more consistent assessment of the pulses after the procedure.

➤ Place the patient in the prone position on an exam table. Cleanse the selected area, and cover with a sterile drape.

➤ A local anesthetic is injected at the site, and a small incision is made or a needle inserted under fluoroscopy.

➤ Ask the patient to inhale deeply and hold his or her breath while the x-ray images are taken, and then to exhale after the images are taken.

➤ Instruct the patient to take slow, deep breaths if nausea occurs during the procedure. Monitor and administer an antiemetic agent if ordered. Ready an emesis basin for use.

➤ Orthopedic cement is injected through the needle into the fracture.

➤ Monitor the patient for complications related to the procedure (e.g., allergic reaction, anaphylaxis, bronchospasm).

➤ The needle or catheter is removed, and a pressure dressing is applied over the puncture site.

➤ The results are recorded manually, on x-ray film, or electronically, in a computerized system, for recall and postprocedure interpretation by the appropriate health care practitioner.

Post-test:

➤ Instruct the patient to resume usual diet, fluids, medications, or activity, as directed by the health care practitioner.

➤ Monitor vital signs and neurologic status every 15 minutes for 1 hour, then every 2 hours for 4 hours, and then as ordered by the health care practitioner. Take temperature every 4 hours for 24 hours. Compare with baseline values. Notify the health care practitioner if temperature is elevated. Protocols may vary from facility to facility.

➤ Observe for delayed allergic reactions, such as rash, urticaria, tachycardia, hyperpnea, hypertension, palpitations, nausea, or vomiting.

➤ Instruct the patient to immediately report symptoms such as fast heart rate, difficulty breathing, skin rash, itching, or decreased urinary output.

➤ Observe the needle/catheter insertion site for bleeding, inflammation, or hematoma formation. Note any pleuritic pain, persistent right shoulder pain, or abdominal pain.

➤ Instruct the patient to apply cold compresses to the puncture site, as needed, to reduce discomfort or edema. Instruct the patient in the care and assessment of the site.

➤ Instruct the patient to maintain bed rest for 4 to 6 hours after the procedure or as ordered.

➤ A written report of the examination will be completed by a health care practitioner specializing in this branch of medicine. The report will be sent to the requesting health care practitioner, who will discuss the results with the patient.

➤ Recognize anxiety related to test results, and be supportive of impaired activity related to physical activity. Discuss the implications of abnormal test results on the patient's lifestyle. Provide teaching and information regarding the clinical implications of the test results, as appropriate.

➤ Reinforce information given by the patient's health care provider regarding further testing, treatment, or referral to another health care provider. Answer any questions or address any concerns voiced by the patient or family.

➤ Instruct the patient in the use of any ordered medications. Explain the importance of adhering to the therapy regimen. As appropriate, instruct the patient in significant side effects and systemic reactions associated with the prescribed medication. Encourage him or her to review corresponding literature provided by a pharmacist.

➤ Depending on the results of this procedure, additional testing may be performed to evaluate or monitor progression of the disease process and determine the need for a change in therapy. Evaluate test results in relation to the patient's symptoms and other tests performed.

Related diagnostic tests:

➤ Related diagnostic tests include bone mineral densitometry, bone scan, computed tomography of the spine, and magnetic resonance imaging of the spine.

VISUAL FIELDS TEST

SYNONYMS/ACRONYMS: Perimetry, VF.

AREA OF APPLICATION: Eyes.

CONTRAST: N/A.

DESCRIPTION & RATIONALE: The visual field is the area within which objects can be seen by the eye as it fixes on a central point. The central field is an area extending 25° surrounding the fixation point. The peripheral field is the remainder of the area within which objects can be viewed. This test evaluates the central visual field through systematic movement of the test object across a tangent screen. It tests the function of the retina, optic nerve, and optic pathways. Visual field testing may be kinetic or static. Kinetic testing (confrontation, Goldmann or tangent screen) involves the movement of a visual stimulus to different areas and marking the point at which it is first seen by the patient. Static testing is performed using automated and computerized equipment. A specific point is chosen in stationary or static examinations, and the stimulus is increased until its threshold is determined. Tangent screen testing is the most common visual field test and is described in greater detail in this monograph. ▪

INDICATIONS:

- Detect field vision loss and evaluate its progression or regression

RESULT

Normal Findings:

- Normal central vision field will form a circle extending 25° superiorly, nasally, inferiorly, and temporally; 12° to 15° temporal to the central fixation point is a physiologic blind spot, approximately 1.5° below the horizontal meridian. It is approximately 7.5° high and 5.5° wide. The patient should be able to see the test object throughout the entire central vision field except within the physiologic blind spot.

Abnormal Findings:

- Amblyopia
- Blepharochalasis
- Blurred vision
- Brain tumors
- Cerebrovascular accidents
- Chorodial nevus
- Diabetes with ophthalmic manifestations
- Glaucoma
- Headache
- Macular degeneration
- Macular drusen
- Nystagmus
- Optic neuritis or neuropathy
- Ptosis of eyelid
- Retinal detachment, hole, or tear
- Retinal exudates or hemorrhage
- Retinal occlusion of the artery or vein
- Retinitis pigmentosa
- Subjective visual disturbance
- Use of high-risk medications
- Visual field defect
- Vitreous traction syndrome

CRITICAL VALUES: N/A

INTERFERING FACTORS:

Factors that may impair the results of the examination:

- An uncooperative patient or a patient with severe vision loss who has dificulty seeing even a large vision screen may have test results that are invalid.

- Assess and make note of the patient's cooperation and reliability as good, fair, or poor, because it is difficult to evaluate factors such as general health, fatigue, or reaction time that affect test performance.

Nursing Implications and Procedure ● ● ● ● ● ● ● ● ● ● ●

Pretest:

➤ Inform the patient that the procedure detects visual field function.

➤ Obtain a history of the patient's complaints, including a list of known allergens.

➤ Obtain a history of the patient's known or suspected vision loss, changes in visual acuity, including type and cause; use of glasses or contact lenses; eye conditions with treatment regimens; eye surgery; and other tests and procedures to assess and diagnose visual deficit.

➤ Obtain a history of results of previously performed laboratory tests, surgical procedures, and other diagnostic procedures. For related diagnostic tests, refer to the table of tests associated with the Ocular System.

➤ Obtain a list of the medications the patient is taking, including herbs, nutritional supplements, and nutraceuticals. The requesting health care practitioner should be advised if the patient regularly uses these products so that their effects can be taken into consideration when reviewing results.

➤ Measurement of visual acuity with and without corrective lenses prior to testing is highly recommended. Instruct the patient to wear corrective lenses, if appropriate and if worn to correct for distance vision. Instruct the patient regarding the importance of keeping the eyes open for the test.

➤ Review the procedure with the patient. Address concerns about pain related to the procedure. Explain to the patient that no discomfort will be experienced during the test. Inform the patient that a technician, optometrist, or physician performs the test, in a quiet, darkened room, and that to evaluate both eyes, the test can take up 30 minutes.

➤ There are no food, fluid, or medication restrictions, unless by medical direction.

Intratest:

➤ Instruct the patient to cooperate fully and to follow directions. Ask the patient to remain still during the procedure because movement produces unreliable results.

➤ Seat the patient 1 to 2 meters away from the tangent screen with the eye being tested directly in line with the central fixation tangent, usually a white disk, on the screen. Ask the patient to place the chin in the chin rest and gently press the forehead against the support bar. Reposition the patient as appropriate to ensure the eye(s) to be tested are properly aligned in front of the visual field testing equipment.

➤ The results are recorded manually or on a paper strip from the automated equipment for recall and postprocedure interpretation by the appropriate health care practitioner.

Post-test:

➤ A written report of the examination will be completed by a health care practitioner specializing in this branch of medicine. The report will be sent to the requesting health care practitioner, who will discuss the results with the patient.

➤ Recognize anxiety related to test results, and encourage the patient to recognize and be supportive of impaired activity related to vision loss, perceived loss of driving privileges, or the possibility of requiring corrective lenses (self-image). Discuss the implications of the test results on the patient's lifestyle.

➤ Reinforce information given by the patient's health care provider regarding further testing, treatment, or referral to another health care provider.

Answer any questions or address any concerns voiced by the patient or family.

▶ Instruct the patient in the use of any ordered medications. Instruct the patient in the use and cleaning of other devices (e.g., a hearing aid). Explain the importance of adhering to the therapy regimen. As appropriate, instruct the patient in significant side effects and systemic reactions associated with the prescribed medication. Encourage him or her to review corresponding literature provided by a pharmacist.

▶ Depending on the results of this procedure, additional testing may be performed to evaluate or monitor progression of the disease process and determine the need for a change in therapy. Evaluate test results in relation to the patient's symptoms and other tests performed.

Related diagnostic tests:

▶ Related diagnostic tests include fluoroscein angiography, fundus photography, gonioscopy, intraocular pressure, and slit-lamp biomicroscopy.

VITAMIN B$_{12}$

. . . .

SYNONYM/ACRONYM: Cyanocobalamin.

SPECIMEN: Serum (1 mL) collected in a red- or tiger-top tube.

REFERENCE VALUE: (Method: Immunochemiluminescent assay)

Age	Conventional Units	SI Units (Conventional Units × 0.738)
Newborn	160–1300 pg/mL	118–959 pmol/L
Adult	200–900 pg/mL	148–664 pmol/L

DESCRIPTION & RATIONALE: Vitamin B$_{12}$ has a ringed crystalline structure that surrounds an atom of cobalt. It is essential in DNA synthesis, hematopoiesis, and central nervous system integrity. It is derived solely from dietary intake. Animal products are the richest source of vitamin B$_{12}$. Its absorption depends on the presence of intrinsic factor. Circumstances that may result in a deficiency of this vitamin include the presence of stomach or intestinal disease as well as insufficient dietary intake of foods containing vitamin B$_{12}$. A significant increase in red blood cell (RBC) mean corpuscular volume may be an important indicator of vitamin B$_{12}$ deficiency. ■

INDICATIONS:

* Assist in the diagnosis of central nervous system disorders
* Assist in the diagnosis of megaloblastic anemia
* Evaluate alcoholism
* Evaluate malabsorption syndromes

RESULT

Increased in:

* Chronic granulocytic leukemia
* Chronic obstructive pulmonary disease
* Chronic renal failure
* Diabetes
* Leukocytosis
* Liver cell damage (hepatitis, cirrhosis)
* Obesity
* Polycythemia vera
* Protein malnutrition
* Severe congestive heart failure
* Some carcinomas

Decreased in:

* Abnormalities of cobalamin transport or metabolism
* Bacterial overgrowth
* Crohn's disease
* Dietary deficiency (e.g., in vegetarians)
* *Diphyllobothrium* (fish tapeworm) infestation
* Gastric or small intestine surgery
* Hypochlorhydria
* Inflammatory bowel disease
* Intestinal malabsorption
* Intrinsic factor deficiency
* Late pregnancy
* Pernicious anemia

CRITICAL VALUES: N/A

INTERFERING FACTORS:

* Drugs that may increase vitamin B_{12} levels include chloral hydrate.

* Drugs that may decrease vitamin B_{12} levels include alcohol, aminosalicylic acid, anticonvulsants, ascorbic acid, cholestyramine, cimetidine, colchicine, metformin, neomycin, oral contraceptives, ranitidine, and triamterene.

* Hemolysis or exposure of the specimen to light invalidates results.

* Specimen collection soon after blood transfusion can falsely increase vitamin B_{12} levels.

* Failure to follow dietary restrictions before the procedure may cause the procedure to be canceled or repeated.

Nursing Implications and Procedure ・・・・・・・・・・

Pretest:

➤ Inform the patient that the test is used to diagnose and monitor vitamin B_{12} and folic acid deficiency.

➤ Obtain a history of the patient's complaints, including a list of known allergens (especially allergies or sensitivities to latex), and inform the appropriate health care practitioner accordingly.

➤ Obtain a history of the patient's gastrointestinal and hematopoietic systems as well as results of previously performed laboratory tests, surgical procedures, and other diagnostic procedures. For related laboratory tests, refer to the Gastrointestinal and Hematopoietic System tables.

➤ Obtain a list of medications the patient is taking, including herbs, nutritional supplements, and nutraceuticals. The requesting health care practitioner and laboratory should be advised if the patient is regularly using these products so that their effects can be taken into consideration when reviewing results.

➤ Review the procedure with the patient. Inform the patient that specimen collection takes approximately 5 to 10 minutes. Address concerns about pain related to the procedure. Explain to the patient that there may be some discomfort during the venipuncture.

➤ Instruct the patient to fast for at least 12 hours before specimen collection.

➤ There are no fluid or medication restrictions, unless by medical direction.

Intratest:

➤ Ensure that the patient has complied with dietary restrictions; assure that food has been restricted for at least 12 hours prior to the procedure.

➤ If the patient has a history of severe allergic reaction to latex, care should be taken to avoid the use of equipment containing latex.

➤ Instruct the patient to cooperate fully and to follow directions. Direct the patient to breathe normally and to avoid unnecessary movement.

➤ Observe standard precautions, and follow the general guidelines in Appendix A. Positively identify the patient, and label the appropriate tubes with the corresponding patient demographics, date, and time of collection. Perform a venipuncture; collect the specimen in a 5-mL red- or tiger-top tube. Protect the specimen from light.

➤ Remove the needle, and apply a pressure dressing over the puncture site.

➤ Promptly transport the specimen to the laboratory for processing and analysis.

➤ The results are recorded manually or in a computerized system for recall

and postprocedure interpretation by the appropriate health care practitioner.

Post-test:

➤ Observe venipuncture site for bleeding or hematoma formation. Apply paper tape or other adhesive to hold pressure bandage in place, or replace with a plastic bandage.

➤ Instruct the patient to resume usual diet, as directed by the health care practitioner.

➤ *Nutritional considerations:* Instruct the patient with a deficiency of vitamin B$_{12}$, as appropriate, in the use of vitamin supplements. Inform the patient, as appropriate, that the best dietary sources of vitamin B$_{12}$ are meats, fish, poultry, eggs, and milk.

➤ A written report of the examination will be sent to the requesting health care practitioner, who will discuss the results with the patient.

➤ Reinforce information given by the patient's health care provider regarding further testing, treatment, or referral to another health care provider. Answer any questions or address any concerns voiced by the patient or family.

➤ Depending on the results of this procedure, additional testing may be performed to evaluate or monitor progression of the disease process and determine the need for a change in therapy. Evaluate test results in relation to the patient's symptoms and other tests performed.

Related laboratory tests:

➤ Related laboratory tests include complete blood count, folate, homocysteine, intrinsic factor antibodies, peripheral blood smear for RBC morphology and presence of hypersegmented neutrophils, and RBC indices for mean corpuscular volume.

VITAMIN D

SYNONYMS/ACRONYM: Cholecalciferol, vitamin D 1,25-dihydroxy.

SPECIMEN: Serum (1 mL) collected in a red-top tube. Plasma (1 mL) collected in green-top (heparin) tube is also acceptable.

REFERENCE VALUE: (Method: Radiobinding assay for vitamin D 25-dihydroxy, radioreceptor assay for vitamin D 1,25-dihydroxy)

Form	Conventional Units	SI Units (Conventional Units × 2.496)
Vitamin D 25-dihydroxy	9–52 ng/mL	22.5–129.8 nmol/L
Vitamin D 1,25-dihydroxy	15–60 pg/mL	37.4–149.8 pmol/L

DESCRIPTION & RATIONALE: There are two metabolically active forms of vitamin D. Ergocalciferol (vitamin D_2) is formed when ergosterol in plants is exposed to sunlight. Ergocalciferol is absorbed by the stomach and intestine when orally ingested. Cholecalciferol (vitamin D_3) if formed when the skin is exposed to sunlight or ultraviolet light. Vitamins D_2 and D_3 enter the bloodstream after absorption. Vitamin D_3 is converted to vitamin D 25-hydroxy by the liver and is the major circulating form of the vitamin. Vitamin D_2 is converted to vitamin D 1,25-dihydroxy by the kidneys and is the more biologically active form. Vitamin D acts with parathyroid hormone and calcitonin to regulate calcium metabolism and osteoblast function.■

INDICATIONS:
- Differential diagnosis of disorders of calcium and phosphorus metabolism
- Evaluate deficiency or suspected toxicity
- Investigate bone diseases
- Investigate malabsorption

RESULT

Increased in:
- Vitamin D intoxication

Decreased in:
- Bowel resection
- Celiac disease
- Inflammatory bowel disease
- Malabsorption
- Osteitis fibrosa cystica
- Osteomalacia
- Pancreatic insufficiency
- Rickets
- Thyrotoxicosis

CRITICAL VALUES:

Vitamin toxicity can be as significant as problems brought about by vitamin deficiencies. The potential for toxicity is especially important to consider with respect to fat-soluble vitamins, which are not eliminated from the body as quickly as water-soluble vitamins and can accumulate in the body. Most cases of toxicity are brought about by oversupplementing and can be avoided by consulting a qualified nutritionist for recommended daily dietary and supplemental allowances. Signs and symptoms of vitamin D toxicity include nausea, loss of appetite, vomiting, polyuria, muscle weakness, and constipation.

INTERFERING FACTORS:

- Drugs that may increase vitamin D levels include etidronate disodium and pravastatin.

- Drugs and substances that may decrease vitamin D levels include aluminum hydroxide, anticonvulsants, cholestyramine, colestipol, glucocorticoids, isoniazid, mineral oil, and rifampin.

- Recent radioactive scans or radiation within 1 week before the test can interfere with test results when radioimmunoassay is the test method.

Nursing Implications and Procedure . . . .

Pretest:

➤ Inform the patient that the test is used to evaluate vitamin D toxicity or deficiency.

➤ Obtain a history of the patient's complaints, including a list of known allergens (especially allergies or sensitivities to latex), and inform the appropriate health care practitioner accordingly.

➤ Obtain a history of the patient's gastrointestinal and musculoskeletal systems, as well as results of previously performed laboratory tests, surgical procedures, and other

diagnostic procedures. For related laboratory tests, refer to the Gastrointestinal and Musculoskeletal System tables.

➤ Obtain a list of medications the patient is taking, including herbs, nutritional supplements, and nutraceuticals. The requesting health care practitioner and laboratory should be advised if the patient regularly uses these products so that their effects can be taken into consideration when reviewing results.

➤ Review the procedure with the patient. Inform the patient that specimen collection takes approximately 5 to 10 minutes. Address concerns about pain related to the procedure. Explain to the patient that there may be some discomfort during the venipuncture.

➤ There are no food, fluid, or medication restrictions, unless by medical direction.

Intratest:

➤ If the patient has a history of severe allergic reaction to latex, care should be taken to avoid the use of equipment containing latex.

➤ Instruct the patient to cooperate fully and to follow directions. Direct the patient to breathe normally and to avoid unnecessary movement.

➤ Observe standard precautions, and follow the general guidelines in Appendix A. Positively identify the patient, and label the appropriate tubes with the corresponding patient demographics, date, and time of collection. Perform a venipuncture; collect the specimen in a 5-mL red-top tube.

➤ Remove the needle, and apply a pressure dressing over the puncture site.

➤ Promptly transport the specimen to the laboratory for processing and analysis.

➤ The results are recorded manually or in a computerized system for recall and postprocedure interpretation by the appropriate health care practitioner.

➤ Observe venipuncture site for bleeding or hematoma formation. Apply paper tape or other adhesive to hold pressure bandage in place, or replace with a plastic bandage.

➤ *Nutritional considerations:* Educate the patient with vitamin D deficiency, as appropriate, that the main dietary sources of vitamin D are fortified dairy foods and cod liver oil. Explain to the patient that vitamin D is also synthesized by the body, in the skin, and is activated by sunlight.

➤ A written report of the examination will be sent to the requesting health care practitioner, who will discuss the results with the patient.

➤ Reinforce information given by the patient's health care provider regarding further testing, treatment, or referral to another health care provider. Answer any questions or address any concerns voiced by the patient or family.

➤ Depending on the results of this procedure, additional testing may be performed to evaluate or monitor progression of the disease process and determine the need for a change in therapy. Evaluate test results in relation to the patient's symptoms and other tests performed.

Related laboratory tests:

➤ Related laboratory tests include blood and urine calcium, kidney stone analysis, osteocalcin, and phosphorus.

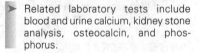

VITAMIN E

. . . .

SYNONYM/ACRONYM: α-Tocopherol.

SPECIMEN: Serum (1 mL) collected in a red- or tiger-top tube.

REFERENCE VALUE: (Method: High-performance liquid chromatography)

Age	Conventional Units	SI Units (Conventional Units × 23.22)
1–12 y	0.3–0.9 mg/dL	7–21 μmol/L
13–19 y	0.6–1.0 mg/dL	14–23 μmol/L
Adult	0.5–1.8 mg/dL	12–42 μmol/L

DESCRIPTION & RATIONALE: Vitamin E is a powerful fat-soluble antioxidant that prevents the oxidation of unsaturated fatty acids, which can combine with polysaccharides to form deposits in tissue. For this reason, vitamin E is believed to reduce the risk of coronary artery disease. Vitamin E reserves in lung tissue provide a barrier against air pollution and protect red blood cell membrane integrity from oxidation. Oxidation of fatty acids in red blood cell membranes can result in irreversible membrane damage and hemolysis. Studies are in progress to confirm the suspicion that oxidation also contributes to the formation of cataracts and macular degeneration of the retina. Because vitamin E is found in a wide variety of foods, a deficiency secondary to inadequate dietary intake is rare. ▪

INDICATIONS:

* Evaluate neuromuscular disorders in premature infants and adults

* Evaluate patients with malabsorption disorders

* Evaluate suspected hemolytic anemia in premature infants and adults

* Monitor patients on long-term parenteral nutrition

RESULT

Increased in:
* Obstructive liver disease

* Vitamin E intoxication

Decreased in:
* Abetalipoproteinemia

* Hemolytic anemia

* Malabsorption disorders, such as biliary atresia, cirrhosis, cystic fibrosis, chronic pancreatitis, pancreatic carcinoma, and chronic cholestasis

CRITICAL VALUES:
Vitamin toxicity can be as significant as problems brought about by vitamin deficiencies. The potential for toxicity is especially important to consider with respect

to fat-soluble vitamins, which are not eliminated from the body as quickly as water-soluble vitamins and can accumulate in the body. Most cases of toxicity are brought about by oversupplementing and can be avoided by consulting a qualified nutritionist for recommended daily dietary and supplemental allowances. *Note:* Excessive supplementation of vitamin E (greater than 60 times the Recommended Dietary Allowance over a period of 1 year or longer) can result in excessive bleeding, delayed healing of wounds, and depression.

INTERFERING FACTORS:
* Drugs that may increase vitamin E levels include anticonvulsants (in women).

* Drugs that may decrease vitamin E levels include anticonvulsants (in men).

* Exposure of the specimen to light decreases vitamin E levels, resulting in a falsely low result.

Nursing Implications and Procedure ● ● ● ● ● ● ● ● ● ● ●

Pretest:

➤ Inform the patient that the test is used to evaluate vitamin E toxicity or deficiency.

➤ Obtain a history of the patient's complaints, including a list of known allergens (especially allergies or sensitivities to latex), and inform the appropriate health care practitioner accordingly.

➤ Obtain a history of the patient's cardiovascular, gastrointestinal, hematopoietic, and hepatobiliary systems, as well as results of previously performed laboratory tests, surgical procedures, and other diagnostic procedures. For related laboratory tests, refer to the Cardiovascular, Gastrointestinal, Hematopoietic, and Hepatobiliary System tables.

➤ Obtain a list of medications the patient is taking, including herbs, nutritional supplements, and nutraceuticals. The requesting health care practitioner and laboratory should be advised if the patient regularly uses these products so that their effects can be taken into consideration when reviewing results.

➤ Review the procedure with the patient. Inform the patient that specimen collection takes approximately 5 to 10 minutes. Address concerns about pain related to the procedure. Explain to the patient that there may be some discomfort during the venipuncture.

➤ There are no food, fluid, or medication restrictions, unless by medical direction.

Intratest:

➤ If the patient has a history of severe allergic reaction to latex, care should be taken to avoid the use of equipment containing latex.

➤ Instruct the patient to cooperate fully and to follow directions. Direct the patient to breathe normally and to avoid unnecessary movement.

➤ Observe standard precautions, and follow the general guidelines in Appendix A. Positively identify the patient, and label the appropriate tubes with the corresponding patient demographics, date, and time of collection. Perform a venipuncture; collect the specimen in a 5-mL red- or tiger-top tube.

➤ Remove the needle, and apply a pressure dressing over the puncture site.

➤ Promptly transport the specimen to the laboratory for processing and analysis.

➤ The results are recorded manually or in a computerized system for recall and postprocedure interpretation by the appropriate health care practitioner.

Post-test:

➤ Observe venipuncture site for bleeding or hematoma formation. Apply paper tape or other adhesive to hold pressure bandage in place, or replace with a plastic bandage.

➤ *Nutritional considerations:* Educate the patient with a vitamin E deficiency, if appropriate, that the main dietary sources of vitamin E are vegetable oils, whole grains, wheat germ, milk, eggs, meats, fish, and green leafy vegetables. Vitamin E is fairly stable at most cooking temperatures (except frying) and when exposed to acidic foods.

➤ A written report of the examination will be sent to the requesting health care practitioner, who will discuss the results with the patient.

➤ Reinforce information given by the patient's health care provider regarding further testing, treatment, or referral to another health care provider. Answer any questions or address any concerns voiced by the patient or family.

➤ Depending on the results of this procedure, additional testing may be performed to evaluate or monitor progression of the disease process and determine the need for a change in therapy. Evaluate test results in relation to the patient's symptoms and other tests performed.

VITAMIN K

SYNONYMS/ACRONYM: Phylloquinone, phytonadione.

SPECIMEN: Serum (1 mL) collected in a red-top tube.

REFERENCE VALUE: (Method: High-performance liquid chromatography)

Conventional Units	SI Units (Conventional Units × 2.22)
0.13–1.19 ng/mL	0.29–2.64 nmol/L

DESCRIPTION & RATIONALE: Vitamin K is one of the fat-soluble vitamins. It is essential for the formation of prothrombin; factors VII, IX, and X; and proteins C and S. Vitamin K also works with vitamin D in synthesizing bone protein, and regulating calcium levels (see monograph titled "Vitamin D.") Vitamin K levels are not often requested, but vitamin K is often prescribed as a medication. Approximately one-half of the body's vitamin K is produced by intestinal bacteria; the other half is obtained from dietary sources. There are three forms of vitamin K: vitamin K_1, or phylloquinone, which is found in foods; vitamin K_2, or menaquinone, which is synthesized by intestinal bacteria; and vitamin K_3, or menadione, which is the synthetic, water-soluble, pharmaceutical form of the vitamin. Vitamin K_3 is two to three times more potent than the naturally occurring forms. ■

INDICATIONS: Evaluation of bleeding of unknown cause (e.g., frequent nosebleeds, bruising)

RESULT

Increased in:
- Excessive administration of vitamin K

Decreased in:
- Antibiotic therapy (by decreasing intestinal flora)
- Chronic fat malabsorption
- Cystic fibrosis
- Diarrhea (in infants)
- Gastrointestinal disease
- Hemorrhagic disease of the newborn
- Hypoprothrombinemia
- Liver disease
- Obstructive jaundice
- Pancreatic disease

CRITICAL VALUES:

Vitamin toxicity can be as significant as problems brought about by vitamin deficiencies. The potential for toxicity is especially important to consider with respect to fat-soluble vitamins, which are not eliminated from the body as quickly as water-soluble vitamins and can accumulate in the body. The naturally occurring forms, vitamin K_1 and K_2, do not cause toxicity. Signs and symptoms of vitamin K_3 toxicity include bleeding and jaundice. Possible interventions include withholding the source.

INTERFERING FACTORS: Drugs and substances that may decrease vitamin K levels include antibiotics, cholestyramine, coumarin, mineral oil, and warfarin.

Nursing Implications and Procedure ● ● ● ● ● ● ● ● ● ● ●

Pretest:

➤ Inform the patient that the test is used to assist in the evaluation of symptoms relating to chronic antibiotic therapy and investigation of bleeding of unknown etiology.

➤ Obtain a history of the patient's complaints, including a list of known allergens (especially allergies or sensitivities to latex), and inform the appropriate health care practitioner accordingly.

➤ Obtain a history of the patient's hematopoietic and hepatobiliary systems, as well as results of previously performed laboratory tests, surgical procedures, and other diagnostic procedures. For related laboratory tests, refer to the Hematopoietic and Hepatobiliary System tables.

➤ Obtain a list of medications the patient is taking, including herbs, nutritional supplements, and nutraceuticals. The requesting health care practitioner and laboratory should be advised if the patient regularly uses these products so that their effects can be taken into consideration when reviewing results.

➤ Review the procedure with the patient. Inform the patient that specimen collection takes approximately 5 to 10 minutes. Address concerns about pain related to the procedure. Explain to the patient that there may be some discomfort during the venipuncture.

➤ There are no food, fluid, or medication restrictions, unless by medical direction.

Intratest

➤ If the patient has a history of severe allergic reaction to latex, care should be taken to avoid the use of equipment containing latex.

➤ Instruct the patient to cooperate fully and to follow directions. Direct the patient to breathe normally and to avoid unnecessary movement.

➤ Observe standard precautions, and follow the general guidelines in Appendix A. Positively identify the patient, and label the appropriate tubes with the corresponding patient demographics, date, and time of collection. Perform a venipuncture; collect the specimen in a 5-mL red-top tube.

➤ Remove the needle, and apply a pressure dressing over the puncture site.

➤ Promptly transport the specimen to the laboratory for processing and analysis.

➤ The results are recorded manually or in a computerized system for recall and postprocedure interpretation by the appropriate health care practitioner.

Post-test:

➤ Observe venipuncture site for bleeding or hematoma formation. Apply paper tape or other adhesive to hold pressure bandage in place, or replace with a plastic bandage.

➤ *Nutritional considerations:* Inform the patient with a vitamin K deficiency, as appropriate, that the main dietary sources of vitamin K are cabbage, cauliflower, spinach and other green leafy vegetables, pork, liver, soybeans, and vegetable oils.

- Instruct the patient to report bleeding from any areas of the skin or mucous membranes.

- Inform the patient of the importance of taking precautions against bleeding or bruising, including the use of a soft bristle toothbrush, use of an electric razor, avoidance of constipation, avoidance of aspirin products, and avoidance of intramuscular injections.

- A written report of the examination will be sent to the requesting health care practitioner, who will discuss the results with the patient.

- Reinforce information given by the patient's health care provider regarding further testing, treatment, or re-

ferral to another health care provider. Answer any questions or address any concerns voiced by the patient or family.

- Depending on the results of this procedure, additional testing may be performed to evaluate or monitor progression of the disease process and determine the need for a change in therapy. Evaluate test results in relation to the patient's symptoms and other tests performed.

Related laboratory tests:

- Related laboratory tests include antithrombin III and prothrombin time.

VITAMINS A, B₁, B₆, AND C

SYNONYMS/ACRONYMS: Vitamin A: retinol, carotene; vitamin B₁: thiamine; vitamin B₆: niacin, pyroxidine, P-5'-P, pyridoxyl-5-phosphate; vitamin C: ascorbic acid.

SPECIMEN: Serum (1 mL) collected in a red-top tube each for vitamins A and C; plasma (1 mL) collected in a lavender-top (EDTA) tube each for vitamins B₁ and B₆.

REFERENCE VALUE: (Method: Chromatography for vitamins A, B₁, and B₆; capillary electrophoresis for vitamin C)

Vitamin	Age	Conventional Units	SI Units
			(Conversion Factor × 0.0349)
Vitamin A	1–6 y	20–43 µg/dL	0.70–1.50 µmol/L
	7–12 y	26–49 µg/dL	0.91–1.71 µmol/L
	13–19 y	26–72 µg/dL	0.91–2.51 µmol/L
	Adult	30–80 µg/dL	1.05–2.80 µmol/L

(Continued on the following page)

Vitamin	Age	Conventional Units	SI Units
Vitamin B$_1$		0.21–0.43 µg/dL	*(Conversion Factor × 29.6)* 6.2–12.8 µmol/L
Vitamin B$_6$		5–30 ng/mL	*(Conversion Factor × 4.046)* 20–121 nmol/L
Vitamin C		0.2–1.9 mg/dL	*(Conversion Factor × 56.78)* 11.4–107.9 µmol/L

DESCRIPTION & RATIONALE: Vitamin assays are used in the measurement of nutritional status. Low levels indicate inadequate oral intake, poor nutritional status, or malabsorption problems. High levels indicate excessive intake, vitamin intoxication, or absorption problems. Vitamin A is a fat-soluble nutrient that promotes normal vision and prevents night blindness; contributes to growth of bone, teeth, and soft tissues; supports thyroxine formation; maintains epithelial cell membranes, skin, and mucous membranes; and acts as an anti-infection agent. Vitamins B$_1$, B$_6$, and C are water soluble. Vitamin B$_1$ acts as an enzyme and plays an important role in the Krebs cycle. Vitamin B$_6$ is important in heme synthesis and functions as a coenzyme in amino acid metabolism and glycogenolysis. It includes pyridoxine, pyridoxal, and pyridoxamine. Vitamin C promotes collagen synthesis, maintains capillary strength, facilitates release of iron from ferritin to form hemoglobin, and functions in the stress response. ■

INDICATIONS

Vitamin A:
• Assist in the diagnosis of night blindness

• Evaluate skin disorders
• Investigate suspected vitamin A deficiency

Vitamin B$_1$:
• Investigate suspected beriberi
• Monitor the effects of chronic alcoholism

Vitamin B$_6$:
• Investigate suspected malabsorption or malnutrition
• Investigate suspected vitamin B$_6$ deficiency

Vitamin C:
• Investigate suspected metabolic or malabsorptive disorders
• Investigate suspected scurvy

RESULT

Increases in:
• Vitamin A:
 Chronic kidney disease
 Idiopathic hypercalcemia in infants
 Vitamin A toxicity

Decreases in:
• Vitamin A:
 Abetalipoproteinemia
 Carcinoid syndrome
 Chronic infections
 Cystic fibrosis

Disseminated tuberculosis
Hypothyroidism
Infantile blindness
Liver, gastrointestinal, or pancreatic disease
Night blindness
Protein malnutrition
Sterility and teratogenesis
Zinc deficiency

- Vitamin B_1:
Alcoholism
Carcinoid syndrome
Hartnup disease
Pellagra

- Vitamin B_6:
Alcoholism
Asthma
Carpal tunnel syndrome
Gestational diabetes
Lactation
Malabsorption
Malnutrition
Neonatal seizures
Normal pregnancies
Occupational exposure to hydrazine compounds
Pellagra
Pre-eclamptic edema
Renal dialysis
Uremia

- Vitamin C:
Alcoholism
Anemia
Cancer
Hemodialysis
Hyperthyroidism
Malabsorption
Pregnancy
Rheumatoid disease
Scurvy

CRITICAL VALUES:

Vitamin toxicity can be as significant as problems brought about by vitamin defi-

ciencies. The potential for toxicity is especially important to consider with respect to fat-soluble vitamins, which are not eliminated from the body as quickly as water-soluble vitamins and can accumulate in the body. Most cases of toxicity are brought about by oversupplementing and can be avoided by consulting a qualified nutritionist for recommended daily dietary and supplemental allowances. Signs and symptoms of vitamin A toxicity may include headache, blurred vision, bone pain, joint pain, dry skin, and loss of appetite.

INTERFERING FACTORS:

- Drugs and substances that may increase vitamin A levels include alcohol (moderate intake), oral contraceptives, and probucol.

- Drugs and substances that may decrease vitamin A levels include alcohol (chronic intake, alcoholism), allopurinol, cholestyramine, colestipol, mineral oil, and neomycin.

- Drugs that may decrease vitamin B_1 levels include glibenclamide, isoniazid, and valproic acid.

- Drugs that may decrease vitamin B_6 levels include amiodarone, anticonvulsants, cycloserine, disulfiram, ethanol, hydralazine, isoniazid, levodopa, oral contraceptives, penicillamine, pyrazinoic acid, and theophylline.

- Drugs and substances that may decrease vitamin C levels include acetylsalicylic acid, aminopyrine, barbiturates, estrogens, heavy metals, oral contraceptives, nitrosamines, and paraldehyde.

- Chronic tobacco smoking decreases vitamin C levels.

- Various diseases may affect vitamin levels (see Results section).

- Diets high in freshwater fish and tea, which are thiamine antagonists, may cause decreased vitamin B_1 levels.

- Long-term hyperalimentation may result in decreased vitamin levels.
- Exposure of the specimen to light decreases vitamin levels, resulting in a falsely low results.

Nursing Implications and Procedure • • • • • • • • • • •

Pretest:

➤ Inform the patient that the test is used to assess hypervitaminosis or deficiency.

➤ Obtain a history of the patient's complaints, including a list of known allergens (especially allergies or sensitivities to latex), and inform the appropriate health care practitioner accordingly.

➤ Obtain a history of the patient's gastrointestinal, genitourinary, hepatobiliary, immune, and musculoskeletal systems, as well as results of previously performed laboratory tests, surgical procedures, and other diagnostic procedures. For related laboratory tests, refer to the Gastrointestinal, Genitourinary, Hepatobiliary, Immune, and Musculoskeletal System tables.

➤ Obtain a list of medications the patient is taking, including herbs, nutritional supplements, and nutraceuticals. The requesting health care practitioner and laboratory should be advised if the patient regularly uses these products so that their effects can be taken into consideration when reviewing results.

➤ Review the procedure with the patient. Inform the patient that specimen collection takes approximately 5 to 10 minutes. Address concerns about pain related to the procedure. Explain to the patient that there may be some discomfort during the venipuncture.

➤ Instruct the patient to fast for at least 12 hours before specimen collection for vitamin A.

➤ There are no fluid or medication restrictions, unless by medical direction.

Intratest:

➤ Ensure that the patient has complied with dietary restrictions; assure that food has been restricted for at least 12 hours prior to the vitamin A test.

➤ If the patient has a history of severe allergic reaction to latex, care should be taken to avoid the use of equipment containing latex.

➤ Instruct the patient to cooperate fully and to follow directions. Direct the patient to breathe normally and to avoid unnecessary movement.

➤ Observe standard precautions, and follow the general guidelines in Appendix A. Positively identify the patient, and label the appropriate tubes with the corresponding patient demographics, date, and time of collection. Perform a venipuncture; collect the specimen in a 5-mL red- or lavender-top tube.

➤ Remove the needle, and apply a pressure dressing over the puncture site.

➤ Promptly transport the specimen to the laboratory for processing and analysis.

➤ The results are recorded manually or in a computerized system for recall and postprocedure interpretation by the appropriate health care practitioner.

Post-test:

➤ Observe venipuncture site for bleeding or hematoma formation. Apply paper tape or other adhesive to hold pressure bandage in place, or replace with a plastic bandage.

➤ *Nutritional considerations:* Educate the patient with a specific vitamin deficiency, as appropriate, regarding dietary sources of these vitamins. Advise the patient to ask a nutritionist to develop a diet plan recommended for his or her specific needs.

Vitamin A:

➤ The main source of vitamin A comes from carotene, a yellow pigment noticeable in most fruits and vegetables, especially carrots, sweet potatoes, squash, apricots, and cantaloupe. It is also present in spinach, collards, broccoli, and cabbage. This vitamin is fairly stable at most cooking temperatures, but it is destroyed easily by light and oxidation.

Vitamin B$_1$:

➤ Vitamin B$_1$ is the most stable with respect to the effects of environmental factors. It is found in meats, coffee, peanuts, and legumes. The body is also capable of making some vitamin B$_1$ by converting the amino acid tryptophan to niacin.

Vitamin B$_6$:

➤ Good sources of vitamin B$_6$ include meats (especially beef and pork), whole grains, wheat germ, legumes, potatoes, oatmeal, and bananas. As with other water-soluble vitamins, it is best preserved by rapid cooking, although it is relatively stable at most cooking temperatures (except frying) and when exposed to acidic foods. This vitamin is destroyed rapidly by light and alkalis.

Vitamin C:

➤ Citrus fruits are excellent dietary sources of vitamin C. Other good sources are green and red peppers, tomatoes, white potatoes, cabbage, broccoli, chard, kale, turnip greens, asparagus, berries, melons, pineapple, and guava. Vitamin C is destroyed by exposure to air, light, heat, or alkalis. Boiling water before cooking eliminates dissolved oxygen that destroys vitamin C in the process of boiling. Vegetables should be crisp and cooked as quickly as possible.

General:

➤ A written report of the examination will be sent to the requesting health care practitioner, who will discuss the results with the patient.

➤ Reinforce information given by the patient's health care provider regarding further testing, treatment, or referral to another health care provider. Answer any questions or address any concerns voiced by the patient or family.

➤ Depending on the results of this procedure, additional testing may be performed to evaluate or monitor progression of the disease process and determine the need for a change in therapy. Evaluate test results in relation to the patient's symptoms and other tests performed.

WHITE BLOOD CELL COUNT AND CELL DIFFERENTIAL

. . . .

SYNONYMS/ACRONYM: WBC with diff, leukocyte count, white cell count.

SPECIMEN: Whole blood from one full lavender-top (EDTA) tube.

REFERENCE VALUE: (Method: Automated, computerized, multichannel analyzers that sort and size cells on the basis of changes in either electrical impedance or light pulses as the cells pass in front of a laser. Many of these analyzers are capable of determining a five-part WBC differential.) The WBC count and differential enumerates and identifies granulocytes, lymphocytes, monocytes, eosinophils, and basophils.

Age	Conventional Units WBC $\times 10^3/mm^3$	Neutrophils		
		Total (Absolute) and %	Bands (Absolute) and %	Segments (Absolute) and %
Birth	9.0–30.0	(6.0–26.0) 61%	(1.65) 9.1%	(9.4) 52%
1 d	9.4–34.0	(5.0–21.0) 61%	(1.75) 9.2%	(9.8) 52%
2 wk	5.0–20.0	(1.0–9.5) 40%	(0.63) 5.5%	(3.9) 34%
1 mo	5.0–19.5	(1.0–9.0) 35%	(0.49) 4.5%	(3.3) 30%
6 mo	6.0–17.5	(1.0–8.5) 32%	(0.45) 3.8%	(3.3) 28%
1 y	6.0–17.5	(1.5–8.5) 31%	(0.35) 3.1%	(3.2) 28%
10 y	4.5–13.5	(1.8–8.0) 54%	(0–1.0) 3.0%	(1.8–7.0) 51%
Adult	4.5–11.0	(1.8–7.7) 59%	(0–0.7) 3.0%	(1.8–7.0) 56%

*SI Units (Conventional Units $\times$ 1 $\times$ 10^9/L or WBC $\times$ 1000/mm^3)

DESCRIPTION & RATIONALE: White blood cells (WBCs) constitute the body's primary defense system against foreign organisms, tissues, and other substances. The life span of a normal WBC is 13 to 20 days. Old WBCs are destroyed by the lymphatic system and excreted in the feces. The main WBC types are neutrophils, eosinophils, basophils, monocytes, and lymphocytes. They are produced in the bone marrow, although lymphocytes can be produced in other sites as well. The WBC count can be performed alone with the differential cell count or as part of the complete blood count (CBC). An increased WBC count is termed *leukocytosis,* and a decreased WBC count is termed *leukopenia.* A total WBC count indicates the degree of response to a pathologic process, but a more complete evaluation for specific diagnoses for any one disorder is provided by the differential count. The WBCs in the count and differential are reported as an *absolute value* and as a percentage. The relative percentages of cell types are arrived at by basing the enumeration of each cell type on a 100-cell count. The absolute value is obtained by multiplying the relative percentage value of each cell type by the total WBC count.

Acute leukocytosis is initially

Lymphocytes (Absolute) and %	Monocytes (Absolute) and %	Eosinophils (Absolute) and %	Basophils (Absolute) and %
(2.0–11) 31%	(0.4–3.1) 5.8%	(0.02–0.85) 2.2%	(0–0.64) 0.6%
(2.0–11.5) 31%	(0.2–3.1) 5.8%	(0.02–0.95) 2.0%	(0–0.30) 0.5%
(2.0–17.0) 48%	(0.2–2.4) 8.8%	(0.07–1.0) 3.1%	(0–0.23) 0.4%
(2.5–16.5) 56%	(0.15–2.0) 6.5%	(0.07–0.90) 2.8%	(0–0.20) 0.5%
(4.0–13.5) 61%	(0.1–1.3) 4.8%	(0.07–0.75) 2.5%	(0–0.20) 0.4%
(4.0–10.5) 61%	(0.05–1.1) 4.8%	(0.05–0.70) 2.6%	(0–0.20) 0.4%
(1.5–6.5) 38%	(0–0.8) 4.3%	(0–0.60) 2.4%	(0–0.20) 0.5%
(1.0–4.8) 34%	(0–0.8) 4.0%	(0–0.45) 2.7%	(0–0.20) 0.5%

accompanied by changes in the WBC count population, followed by changes within the individual WBCs. Leukocytosis usually occurs by way of increase in a single WBC family rather than a proportional increase in all cell types. Toxic granulation and vacuolation are commonly seen in leukocytosis accompanied by a *shift to the left,* or increase in the percentage of immature band neutrophils to mature segmented neutrophils. Bandemia is defined by the presence of greater than 6% band neutrophils in the total neutrophil cell population. These changes in the white cell population are most commonly associated with an infectious process, usually bacterial, but they can occur in healthy individuals who are under stress, such as women in childbirth and very young infants. The WBC count and differential of an actively crying infant may show an overall increase in WBCs with a shift to the left. Any stressful situation causing production of epinephrine results in a rapid increase in WBC count. Before initiating any kind of intervention, it is important to determine whether an increased WBC count is the result of a normal condition involving physiologic stress versus a pathologic processes. The use of multiple specimen types may confuse the interpretation of results in infants. Multiple samples from the same collection site (i.e., capillary versus venous) may be necessary to obtain an accurate assessment of the WBC picture in these young patients.

Neutrophils are normally found as the predominant WBC type in the circulating blood. Also called *polymorphonuclear cells,* they are the body's first line of defense through the process of phagocytosis. They also contain enzymes and pyogens, which combat foreign invaders.

Lymphocytes are agranular, mononuclear blood cells that are smaller than granulocytes. They are found in the next highest percentage in normal circulation. Lymphocytes are classified as B cells and T cells. Both types are formed in the bone marrow, but B cells mature in the bone marrow and T cells mature in the thymus. Lymphocytes play a major role in the body's natural defense system. B cells differentiate into immunoglobulin-synthesizing plasma cells. T cells function as cellular mediators of immunity and comprise helper/inducer (CD4) lymphocytes, delayed hypersensitivity lymphocytes, cytotoxic (CD8 or CD4) lymphocytes, and suppressor (CD8) lymphocytes.

Monocytes are mononuclear cells similar to lymphocytes, but they are related more closely to granulocytes in terms of their function. They are formed in the bone marrow from the same cells as those that produce neutrophils. The major function of monocytes is phagocytosis. Monocytes stay in the peripheral blood for about 70 hours, after which they migrate into the tissues and become macrophages.

The function of eosinophils is phagocytosis of antigen-antibody complexes. They become active in the later stages of inflammation. Eosinophils respond to allergic and parasitic diseases: They have granules that contain histamine used to kill foreign cells in the body and proteolytic enzymes that damage parasitic worms (see monograph titled "Eosinophil Count").

Basophils are found in small numbers in the circulating blood. They have a phagocytic function and, similar to eosinophils, contain numerous specific granules. Basophilic granules contain heparin, histamines, and serotonin. Basophils may also be found in tissue and as such are classified as mast cells. Basophilia is noted in conditions such as leukemia, Hodgkin's disease, polycythemia vera, ulcerative colitis, nephrosis, and chronic hypersensitivity states. ■

INDICATIONS:
* Assist in confirming suspected bone marrow depression
* Assist in determining the cause of an elevated WBC count (e.g., infection, inflammatory process)
* Detect hematologic disorder, neoplasm, or immunologic abnormality
* Determine the presence of a hereditary hematologic abnormality
* Monitor the effects of physical or emotional stress
* Monitor the progression of nonhematologic disorders, such as chronic obstructive pulmonary disease, malabsorption syndromes, cancer, and renal disease
* Monitor the response to drugs or chemotherapy, and evaluate undesired reactions to drugs that may cause blood dyscrasias
* Provide screening as part of a CBC in a general physical examination, especially on admission to a health care facility or before surgery

RESULT

Increased in (leukocytosis):
* Normal physiologic and environmental conditions:
  Early infancy
  Emotional stress
  Exposure to cold

Increased epinephrine secretion
Menstruation
Pregnancy and labor
Strenuous exercise
Ultraviolet light
* Pathologic conditions:
  Acute hemolysis, transfusion reactions
  All types of infections
  Anemias
  Appendicitis
  Collagen disorders
  Cushing's disease
  Inflammatory disorders
  Leukemias and other malignancies
  Parasitic infestations
  Polycythemia vera

Decreased in (leukopenia):
* Normal physiologic conditions:
  Diurnal rhythms
* Pathologic conditions:
  Alcoholism
  Anemias
  Bone marrow depression
  Malaria
  Malnutrition
  Radiation
  Rheumatoid arthritis
  Systemic lupus erythematosus (SLE) and other autoimmune disorders
  Toxic and antineoplastic drugs
  Viral infections

Neutrophils increased (neutrophilia):
* Acute hemolysis
* Acute hemorrhage
* Extremes in temperature
* Infectious diseases
* Inflammatory conditions (rheumatic fever, gout, rheumatoid arthritis, vasculitis, myositis)

- Malignancies
- Metabolic disorders (uremia, eclampsia, diabetic ketoacidosis, thyroid storm, Cushing's syndrome)
- Myelocytic leukemia
- Physiologic stress (e.g., allergies, asthma, exercise, childbirth, surgery)
- Tissue necrosis (burns, crushing injuries, abscesses, myocardial infarction)
- Tissue poisoning with toxins and venoms

Neutrophils decreased (neutropenia):
- Acromegaly
- Addison's disease
- Anaphylaxis
- Anorexia nervosa, starvation, malnutrition
- Bone marrow depression (viruses, toxic chemicals, overwhelming infection, radiation, Gaucher's disease)
- Disseminated SLE
- Thyrotoxicosis
- Viral infection (mononucleosis, hepatitis, influenza)
- Vitamin B_{12} or folate deficiency

Lymphocytes increased (lymphocytosis):
- Addison's disease
- Felty's syndrome
- Infections
- Lymphocytic leukemia
- Lymphomas
- Lymphosarcoma
- Myeloma
- Rickets
- Thyrotoxicosis

- Ulcerative colitis
- Waldenström's macroglobulinemia

Lymphocytes decreased (lymphopenia):
- Antineoplastic drugs
- Aplastic anemia
- Bone marrow failure
- Burns
- Gaucher's disease
- Hemolytic disease of the newborn
- High doses of adrenocorticosteroids
- Hodgkin's disease
- Hypersplenism
- Immunodeficiency diseases
- Malnutrition
- Pernicious anemia
- Pneumonia
- Radiation
- Rheumatic fever
- Septicemia
- Thrombocytopenic purpura
- Toxic chemical exposure
- Transfusion reaction

Monocytes increased (monocytosis):
- Carcinomas
- Cirrhosis
- Collagen diseases
- Gaucher's disease
- Hemolytic anemias
- Hodgkin's disease
- Infections
- Lymphomas
- Monocytic leukemia
- Polycythemia vera

- Radiation
- Sarcoidosis
- SLE
- Thrombocytopenic purpura
- Ulcerative colitis

CRITICAL VALUES:

Less than 2.5 WBC × 10³/mm³ or 2500 WBC/mm³ (on admission)
Greater than 30.0 WBC × 10³/mm³ or 30,000 WBC/mm³ (on admission)

Note and immediately report to the health care practitioner any critically increased or decreased values and related symptoms. The presence of abnormal cells, other morphologic characteristics, or cellular inclusions may signify a potentially life-threatening or serious health condition and should be investigated. Examples are hypersegmented neutrophils, agranular neutrophils, blasts or other immature cells, Auer rods, Döhle bodies, marked toxic granulation, or plasma cells.

INTERFERING FACTORS:

- Drugs that may decrease the overall WBC count include acetyldigitoxin, acetylsalicylic acid, aminoglutethimide, aminopyrine, aminosalicylic acid, ampicillin, amsacrine, antazoline, anticonvulsants, antineoplastic agents (therapeutic intent), antipyrine, barbiturates, busulfan, carbutamide, carmustine, chlorambucil, chloramphenicol, chlordane, chlorophenothane, chlortetracycline, chlorthalidone, cisplatin, colchicine, colistimethate, cycloheximide, cyclophosphamide, cytarabine, dacarbazine, dactinomycin, diaprim, diazepam, diethylpropion, digitalis, dipyridamole, dipyrone, fumagillin, glaucarubin, glucosulfone, hexachlorobenzene, hydroflumathiazide, hydroxychloroquine, iothiouracil, iproniazid, lincomycin, local anesthetics, mefenamic acid, mepazine, meprobamate, mercaptopurine, methotrexate, methylpromazine, mitomycin, paramethadione, parathion, penicillin, phenacemide, phenindione, phenothiazine, pipamazine, prednisone (by Coulter S method), primaquine, procainamide, procarbazine, prochlorperazine, promazine, promethazine, pyrazolones, quinacrine, quinines, radioactive compounds, razoxane, ristocetin, sulfa drugs, tamoxifen, tetracycline, thenalidine, thioridazine, tolazamide, tolazoline, tolbutamide, trimethadione, and urethan.

- A significant decrease in basophil count occurs rapidly after intravenous injection of propanidid and thiopental.

- A significant decrease in lymphocyte count occurs rapidly after administration of corticotropin, mechlorethamine, methylsergide, and x-ray therapy; and after megadoses of niacin, pyradoxine, and thiamine.

- Drugs that may increase the overall WBC count include amphetamine, amphotericin B, chloramphenicol, chloroform (normal response to anesthesia), colchicine (leukocytosis follows leukopenia), corticotropin, erythromycin, ether (normal response to anesthesia), fluroxene (normal response to anesthesia), isoflurane (normal response to anesthesia), niacinamide, phenylbutazone, prednisone, and quinine.

- Drug allergies may have a significant effect on eosinophil count and may affect the overall WBC count. Refer to the specific monograph for a detailed listing of interfering drugs.

- The WBC count may vary depending on the patient's position, decreasing when the patient is recumbent owing to hemodilution and increasing when the patient rises owing to hemoconcentration.

- Venous stasis can falsely elevate results; the tourniquet should not be left on the arm for longer than 60 seconds.

- Failure to fill the tube sufficiently (i.e., tube less than three-quarters full) may yield inadequate sample volume for automated analyzers and may be reason for specimen rejection.

- Hemolyzed or clotted specimens should be rejected for analysis.

- The presence of nucleated red blood cells or giant or clumped platelets affects the automated WBC, requiring a manual correction of the WBC count.

- Care should be taken in evaluating the CBC during the first few hours after transfusion.

- Patients with cold agglutinins or monoclonal gammopathies may have a falsely decreased WBC count as a result of cell clumping.

Nursing Implications and Procedure • • • • • • • • • • •

Pretest:

- Inform the patient that the test is primarily used to evaluate viral and bacterial infections and to diagnose and monitor leukemic disorders.

- Obtain a history of the patient's complaints, including a list of known allergens (especially allergies or sensitivities to latex), and inform the appropriate health care practitioner accordingly.

- Obtain a history of the patient's hematopoietic, immune, and respiratory systems, as well as results of previously performed laboratory tests, surgical procedures, and other diagnostic procedures. For related laboratory tests, refer to the Hematopoietic, Immune, and Respiratory System tables.

- Note any recent procedures that can interfere with test results.

- Obtain a list of medications the patient is taking, including herbs, nutritional supplements, and nutraceuticals. The requesting health care practitioner and laboratory should be advised if the patient regularly uses

these products so that their effects can be taken into consideration when reviewing results.

- Review the procedure with the patient. Inform the patient that specimen collection takes approximately 5 to 10 minutes. Address concerns about pain related to the procedure. Explain to the patient that there may be some discomfort during the venipuncture.

- There are no food, fluid, or medication restrictions, unless by medical direction.

Intratest:

- If the patient has a history of severe allergic reaction to latex, care should be taken to avoid the use of equipment containing latex.

- Instruct the patient to cooperate fully and to follow directions. Direct the patient to breathe normally and to avoid unnecessary movement.

- Observe standard precautions, and follow the general guidelines in Appendix A. Positively identify the patient, and label the appropriate tubes with the corresponding patient demographics, date, and time of collection. Perform a venipuncture; collect the specimen in a 5-mL lavender-top tube. The specimen should be mixed gently by inverting the tube 10 times. It is stable when stored for up to 6 hours at room temperature or 24 hours if stored refrigerated. In addition, if it is anticipated that the specimen will not be analyzed within 4 to 6 hours, two blood smears should be made immediately after the venipuncture and submitted with the blood sample.

- Remove the needle, and apply a pressure dressing over the puncture site.

- Promptly transport the specimen to the laboratory for processing and analysis.

- The results are recorded manually or in a computerized system for recall and postprocedure interpretation by the appropriate health care practitioner.

> Observe venipuncture site for bleeding or hematoma formation. Apply paper tape or other adhesive to hold pressure bandage in place, or replace with a plastic bandage.

> *Nutritional considerations:* Infection, fever, sepsis, and trauma can result in an impaired nutritional status. Malnutrition can occur for many reasons, including fatigue, lack of appetite, and gastrointestinal distress.

> *Nutritional considerations:* Adequate intake of vitamins A and C are also important for regenerating body stores depleted by the effort exerted in fighting infections. Educate the patient or caregiver regarding the importance of following the prescribed diet.

> A written report of the examination will be sent to the requesting health care practitioner, who will discuss the results with the patient.

> Recognize anxiety related to test results, and be supportive of fear of shortened life expectancy. Discuss the implications of abnormal test results on the patient's lifestyle. Provide teaching and information regarding the clinical implications of the test results, as appropriate. Educate the patient regarding access to counseling services. Provide contact information, if desired, for the National Cancer Institute *(http:// www. nci.nih.org)*.

> Reinforce information given by the patient's health care provider regarding further testing, treatment, or referral to another health care provider. Answer any questions or address any concerns voiced by the patient or family.

> Depending on the results of this procedure, additional testing may be performed to evaluate or monitor progression of the disease process and determine the need for a change in therapy. Evaluate test results in relation to the patient's symptoms and other tests performed.

Related laboratory tests:

> Related laboratory tests include albumin, anti–cytoplasmic neutrophilic antibody, bone marrow biopsy, lymph node biopsy, eosinophil count, infectious mononucleosis, leukocyte alkaline phosphatase, other tests included in a CBC, peripheral blood smear, and zinc.

WHITE BLOOD CELL SCAN

· ·

SYNONYMS/ACRONYM: WBC imaging, inflammatory scan, labeled leukocyte scan, infection scintigraphy, labeled autologous leukocytes.

AREA OF APPLICATION: Whole body.

CONTRAST: Intravenous radionuclide combined with white blood cells.

DESCRIPTION & RATIONALE: Because white blood cells (WBCs) naturally accumulate in areas of inflammation, the WBC scan uses radiolabeled WBCs to help determine the site of an acute infection or confirm the presence or absence of infection or inflammation at a suspected site. A gamma camera detects the radiation emitted from the injected radionuclide, and a representative image of the radionuclide distribution is obtained and recorded on film or stored electronically. Because of its better image resolution and greater specificity for acute infections, the WBC scan has replaced scanning with gallium-67 citrate (Ga-67). Some chronic infections associated with pulmonary disease, however, may be better imaged with Ga-67. The WBC scan is especially helpful in detecting postoperative infection sites and in documenting lack of residual infection after a course of therapy. ■

INDICATIONS:

- Aid in the diagnosis of infectious or inflammatory diseases
- Differentiate infectious from noninfectious process
- Evaluate the effects of treatment
- Evaluate inflammatory bowel disease
- Evaluate patients with fever of unknown origin
- Evaluate postsurgical sites and wound infections
- Evaluate suspected infection of an orthopedic prosthesis
- Evaluate suspected osteomyelitis

RESULT

Normal Findings:

- No focal localization of the radionuclide, along with some slight localiza-

tion of the radionuclide within the reticuloendothelial system (liver, spleen, and bone marrow)

Abnormal Findings:

- Abscess
- Arthritis
- Infection
- Inflammation
- Inflammatory bowel disease
- Osteomyelitis

CRITICAL VALUES: N/A

INTERFERING FACTORS:

This procedure is contraindicated for:

- Patients who are pregnant or suspected of being pregnant, unless the potential benefits of the procedure far outweigh the risks to the fetus and mother

Factors that may impair clear imaging:

- Inability of the patient to cooperate or remain still during the procedure because of age, significant pain, or mental status
- Patients who are very obese, who may exceed the weight limit for the equipment
- Incorrect positioning of the patient, which may produce poor visualization of the area to be examined
- Retained barium from a previous radiologic procedure, which may inhibit visualization of an abdominal lesion
- Metallic objects within the examination field (e.g., jewelry, body rings), which may inhibit organ visualization and can produce unclear images
- Other nuclear scans done within 48 hours and Ga-67 scans within 4 weeks before the procedure
- Lesions smaller than 1 to 2 cm, which may not be detectable

- A distended bladder, which may obscure pelvic detail

Other considerations:
- Improper injection of the radionuclide that allows the tracer to seep deep into the muscle tissue produces erroneous hot spots.

- Patients with a low WBC count may need donor WBCs to complete the radionuclide labeling process; otherwise, Ga-67 scanning should be performed instead.

- False-negative images may be a result of hemodialysis, hyperglycemia, hyperalimentation, steroid therapy, and antibiotic therapy.

- The presence of multiple myeloma or thyroid cancer can result in a false-negative scan for bone abnormalities.

- Consultation with a health care practitioner should occur before the procedure for radiation safety concerns regarding younger patients or patients who are lactating.

- Risks associated with radiographic overexposure can result from frequent x-ray procedures. Personnel in the room with the patient should stand behind a shield or leave the area while the examination is being done. Personnel working in the area where the examination is being done should wear badges that reveal their level of exposure to radiation.

Nursing Implications and Procedure • • • • • • • • • • •

Pretest:

➤ Inform the patient that the procedure assesses the presence of inflammation or infection.

➤ Obtain a history of the patient's complaints, including a list of known allergens.

➤ Obtain a history of the patient's immune system, as well as results of previously performed laboratory tests, surgical procedures, and other diagnostic procedures. For related diagnostic tests, refer to the Immune System table.

➤ Note any recent procedures that can interfere with test results, including barium examinations.

➤ Record the date of the last menstrual period and determine the possibility of pregnancy in perimenopausal women.

➤ Obtain a list of the patient's current medications.

➤ Review the procedure with the patient. Address concerns about pain related to the procedure. Explain to the patient that some pain may be experienced during the test, and there may be moments of discomfort. Explain the purpose of the test and how the procedure is performed. Inform the patient that the procedure is performed in a special nuclear medicine department by a technologist and usually takes approximately 60 minutes, and that delayed images are needed 24 hours later. The patient may leave the department and return later to undergo delayed imaging.

➤ *Sensitivity to cultural and social issues,* as well as concern for modesty, is important in providing psychological support before, during, and after the procedure.

➤ Instruct the patient to remove dentures, jewelry (including watches), hairpins, credit cards, and other metallic objects.

➤ There are no food, fluid, or medication restrictions, unless by medical direction.

Intratest:

➤ Ensure that the patient has removed all external metallic objects (jewelry, etc.) prior to the procedure.

➤ Patients are given a gown, robe, and foot coverings to wear and instructed to void prior to the procedure.

- Observe standard precautions, and follow the general guidelines in Appendix A.

- Administer sedative to a child or to an uncooperative adult, as ordered.

- On the day of the test, draw a 40- to 60-mL sample of blood for an in vitro process of labeling and separating the WBCs from the blood. An injection of radionuclide-labeled autologous WBCs is administered. Delayed views may be taken 4 to 24 hours after the injection.

- If abdominal abscess or infection is suspected, laxatives or enemas may be ordered before delayed imaging.

- Wear gloves during the radionuclide administration and while handling the patient's urine.

- The results are recorded manually, on film, or in a computerized system for recall and postprocedure interpretation by the appropriate health care practitioner.

Post-test:

- Advise patient to drink increased amounts of fluids for 24 hours to eliminate the radionuclide from the body, unless contraindicated. Tell the patient that radionuclide is eliminated from the body within 48 to 72 hours.

- Instruct the patient to flush the toilet immediately after each voiding following the procedure, and to wash hands meticulously with soap and water after each voiding for 24 hours after the procedure.

- Tell all caregivers to wear gloves when discarding urine for 24 hours after the procedure. Wash gloved hands with soap and water before removing gloves. Then wash hands after the gloves are removed.

- A written report of the examination will be completed by a health care practitioner specializing in this branch of medicine. The report will be sent to the requesting health care practitioner, who will discuss the results with the patient.

- Reinforce information given by the patient's health care provider regarding further testing, treatment, or referral to another health care provider. Answer any questions or address any concerns voiced by the patient or family.

- Depending on the results of this procedure, additional testing may be needed to evaluate or monitor progression of the disease process and determine the need for a change in therapy. Evaluate test results in relation to the patient's symptoms and other tests performed.

Related diagnostic tests:

- Related diagnostic tests include computed tomography of the spine or pelvis; gallium scan; kidney, ureter, and bladder (KUB) study; magnetic resonance imaging of the spine or pelvis; and ultrasound of the abdomen or pelvis.

ZINC

- -

SYNONYM/ACRONYM: Zn.

SPECIMEN: Serum (1 mL) collected in a trace element–free, royal blue–top tube.

REFERENCE VALUE: (Method: Atomic absorption spectrophotometry)

Age	Conventional Units	SI Units (Conventional Units × 0.153)
Newborn–6 mo	26–141 µg/dL	4.0–21.6 µmol/L
6–11 mo	29–131 µg/dL	4.5–20.1 µmol/L
1–4 y	31–115 µg/dL	4.8–17.6 µmol/L
4–5 y	48–119 µg/dL	7.4–18.2 µmol/L
6–9 y	48–129 µg/dL	7.3–19.7 µmol/L
10–13 y	25–148 µg/dL	3.9–22.7 µmol/L
14–17 y	46–130 µg/dL	7.1–19.9 µmol/L
Adult	70–120 µg/dL	10.7–18.4 µmol/L

DESCRIPTION & RATIONALE: Zinc is found in all body tissues, but the highest concentrations are found in the eye, bone, and male reproductive organs. Zinc is involved in RNA and DNA synthesis and is essential in the process of tissue repair. It is also required for the formation of collagen and the production of active vitamin A (for the visual pigment rhodopsin). Zinc also functions as a chelating agent to protect the body from lead and cadmium poisoning. Zinc is absorbed from the small intestine. Its absorption and excretion seem to be through the same sites as those for iron and copper. The body does not store zinc as it does copper and iron. Untreated zinc deficiency in infants may result in a condition called acrodermatitis enteropathica. Symptoms include growth retardation, diarrhea, impaired wound healing, and frequent infections. Adolescents and adults with zinc deficiency exhibit similar adverse effects on growth, sexual development, and immune function, well as altered taste and smell, emo-' instability, impaired adaptation to darkness, impaired night vision, tremors, and a bullous, pustular rash over the extremities. ■

INDICATIONS:
• Assist in confirming acrodermatitis enteropathica

• Evaluate nutritional deficiency

• Evaluate possible toxicity

• Monitor replacement therapy in individuals with identified deficiencies

• Monitor therapy of individuals with Wilson's disease

RESULT

Increased in:
• Anemia

• Arteriosclerosis

• Coronary heart disease

• Primary osteosarcoma of the bone

Decreased in:
• Acrodermatitis enteropathica

• Acquired immunodeficiency syndrome

- Acute infections
- Acute stress
- Burns
- Cirrhosis
- Conditions that decrease albumin
- Diabetes
- Long-term total parenteral nutrition
- Malabsorption
- Myocardial infarction
- Nephrotic syndrome
- Nutritional deficiency
- Pregnancy
- Pulmonary tuberculosis

CRITICAL VALUES: N/A

INTERFERING FACTORS:
- Drugs that may increase zinc levels include auranofin, chlorthalidone, corticotropin, oral contraceptives, and penicillamine.

- Drugs that may decrease zinc levels include anticonvulsants, cisplatin, citrates, corticosteroids, estrogens, interferon, and oral contraceptives.

Nursing Implications and Procedure • • • • • • • • • •

Pretest:

➤ Inform the patient that the test is used to evaluate disorders associated with abnormal zinc levels and monitor response to therapy.

➤ Obtain a history of the patient's complaints, including a list of known allergens (especially allergies or sensitivities to latex), and inform the appropriate health care practitioner accordingly.

➤ Obtain a history of the patient's gastrointestinal, hepatobiliary, immune, and musculoskeletal systems, as well as results of previously performed laboratory tests, surgical procedures, and other diagnostic procedures. For related laboratory tests, refer to the Gastrointestinal, Immune, Hepatobiliary, and Musculoskeletal System tables.

➤ Obtain a list of medications the patient is taking, including herbs, nutritional supplements, and nutraceuticals. The requesting health care practitioner and laboratory should be advised if the patient regularly uses these products so that their effects can be taken into consideration when reviewing results.

➤ Review the procedure with the patient. Inform the patient that specimen collection takes approximately 5 to 10 minutes. Address concerns about pain related to the procedure. Explain to the patient that there may be some discomfort during the venipuncture.

➤ There are no food, fluid, or medication restrictions, unless by medical direction.

Intratest:

➤ If the patient has a history of severe allergic reaction to latex, care should be taken to avoid the use of equipment containing latex.

➤ Instruct the patient to cooperate fully and to follow directions. Direct the patient to breathe normally and to avoid unnecessary movement.

➤ Observe standard precautions, and follow the general guidelines in Appendix A. Positively identify the patient, and label the appropriate tubes with the corresponding patient demographics, date, and time of collection. Perform a venipuncture; collect the specimen in a 5-mL royal blue–top tube.

➤ Remove the needle, and apply a pressure dressing over the puncture site.

➤ Promptly transport the specimen to the laboratory for processing and analysis.

➤ The results are recorded manually or

in a computerized system for recall and postprocedure interpretation by the appropriate health care practitioner.

Post-test:

➤ Observe venipuncture site for bleeding or hematoma formation. Apply paper tape or other adhesive to hold pressure bandage in place, or replace with a plastic bandage.

➤ *Nutritional considerations:* Topical or oral supplementation may be ordered for patients with zinc deficiency. Dietary sources high in zinc include shellfish, red meat, wheat germ, and processed foods such as canned pork and beans and canned chili. Patients should be informed that diets high in phytates from whole grains, coffee, cocoa, or tea bind zinc and prevent it from being absorbed. Decreases in zinc also can be induced by increased intake of iron, copper, or manganese. Vitamin and mineral supplements with a greater than 3:1 iron/zinc ratio inhibit zinc absorption.

➤ A written report of the examination will be sent to the requesting health care practitioner, who will discuss the results with the patient.

➤ Reinforce information given by the patient's health care provider regarding further testing, treatment, or referral to another health care provider. Answer any questions or address any concerns voiced by the patient or family.

➤ Depending on the results of this procedure, additional testing may be performed to evaluate or monitor progression of the disease process and determine the need for a change in therapy. Evaluate test results in relation to the patient's symptoms and other tests performed.

Related laboratory tests:

➤ Related laboratory tests include albumin, iron, and copper.

SYSTEM TABLES

AUDITORY SYSTEM

Diagnostic Tests Associated with the Auditory System

Audiometry hearing loss, 185

Otoscopy, 988

Spondee speech reception threshold, 1192

Tuning fork tests, 1250

CARDIOVASCULAR SYSTEM

Laboratory Tests Associated with the Cardiovascular System

Anion gap, 100

Apolipoprotein A, 167

Apolipoprotein B, 170

Aspartate aminotransferase, 179

Atrial natriuretic factor, 182

Blood gases, 260

B-type natriuretic peptide, 293

Calcium, blood, 304

Calcium, ionized, 309

Chloride, 354

Cholesterol, HDL and LDL, 374

Cholesterol, total, 379

C-reactive protein, 493

Creatine kinase and isoenzymes, 496

D-Dimer, 565

Digoxin, 104

Disopyramide, 104

Fibrin degradation products, 650

Flecainide, 104

Hematocrit, 727

Hemoglobin, 732

Homocysteine and methylmalonic acid, 766

International Normalized Ratio (INR), 1103

Lactate dehydrogenase and isoenzymes, 838

Lactic acid, 842

Lidocaine, 104

Lipoprotein electrophoresis, 869

Magnesium, blood, 896

Myoglobin, 975

Pericardial fluid analysis, 1016

Potassium, blood, 1068

Procainamide, 104

Prothrombin time and INR, 1103

Quinidine, 104

Triglycerides, 1236

Troponins I and T, 1244

Vitamin E, 1364

Diagnostic Tests Associated with the Cardiovascular System

ENDOCRINE SYSTEM

Laboratory Tests Associated with the Endocrine System

Diagnostic Tests Associated with the Endocrine System

GASTROINTESTINAL SYSTEM

Laboratory Tests Associated with the Gastrointestinal System

Diagnostic Tests Associated with the Gastrointestinal System

Computed tomography, abdomen, 421
Computed tomography, pancreas, 447
Esophageal manometry, 613
Esophagogastroduodenoscopy, 617
Gastric emptying scan, 675
Gastroesophageal reflux scan, 681
Gastrointestinal blood loss scan, 685
Hepatobiliary imaging, 753
Kidney, ureter, and bladder study, 833
Laparoscopy, 848
Liver scan, 872
Magnetic resonance imaging, abdomen, 907
Proctosigmoidoscopy, 1079
Ultrasound, liver and biliary system, 1272
Upper gastrointestinal and small bowel series, 1309

GENITOURINARY SYSTEM

Laboratory Tests Associated with the Genitourinary System

Acetaminophen, 65
Acid phosphatase, prostatic, 3
Albumin and albumin/globulin ratio, 19
Aldosterone, 24
Amikacin, 110
Ammonia, 54
Anion gap, 100
Antibodies, anticytoplasmic neutrophilic, 115
Antibodies, anti–glomerular basement membrane, 117
Antidiuretic hormone, 152
Biopsy, bladder, 200
Biopsy, kidney, 225
Bladder cancer markers, urine, 255
Calcitonin and calcitonin stimulation tests, 301
Calcium, blood, 304
Calcium, ionized, 309
Calcium, urine, 312
Calculus, kidney stone panel, 316
Carbon dioxide, 322
Chloride, blood, 354
Creatinine, blood, 499
Creatinine, urine, and creatinine clearance, urine, 502
Culture, bacterial, urine, 535
Culture, viral, 541
Cyclosporine, 800
Cytology, urine, 560
Erythropoietin, 610
Gentamicin, 110
Gram stain, 712
Lithium, 158
Magnesium, blood, 896
Magnesium, urine, 900
Methotrexate, 800
Microalbumin, 957
β_2-Microglobulin, 960
Osmolality, blood and urine, 980
Oxalate, urine, 993
Phosphorus, blood, 1025
Phosphorus, urine, 1028
Potassium, blood, 1068
Potassium, urine, 1073

(*Continued on the following page*)

Laboratory Tests Associated with the Genitourinary System *(Continued)*

Diagnostic Tests Associated with the Genitourinary System

HEMATOPOIETIC SYSTEM

Laboratory Tests Associated with the Hematopoietic System

Diagnostic Tests Associated with the Hematopoietic System

HEPATOBILIARY SYSTEM

Laboratory Tests Associated with the Hepatobiliary System

Acetaminophen, 65
Acetylsalicylic acid, 65
Alanine aminotransferase, 16
Albumin, 19
Aldolase, 22
Alkaline phosphatase and
  isoenzymes, 28
Amitryptyline, 148
Ammonia, 54
Amylase, 62
Antibodies, anticytoplasmic
  neutrophilic, 115
Antibody, antimitochondrial, 134
Antibody, anti–smooth muscle,
  136
α_1-Antitrypsin and α_1-antitrypsin
  phenotyping, 164
Aspartate aminotransferase, 179
Bilirubin and bilirubin fractions,
  196
Biopsy, liver, 229
Calcium, blood, 304
Carbamazepine, 140
Ceruloplasmin, 346
Cholesterol, total, 379
Coagulation factor assays, 389
Copper, 483
Desipramine, 148
Diazepam, 148
Doxepin, 148
Ethosuximide, 140
Fibrinogen, 652
δ-Glutamyltransferase, 704
Haloperidol, 158
Haptoglobin, 722
Hematocrit, 727

Hemoglobin, 732
Hepatitis A antibody, 743
Hepatitis B antigen and antibody,
  745
Hepatitis C antibody, 748
Hepatitis D antibody, 751
Imipramine, 148
Infectious mononucleosis
  screen, 804
International Normalized Ratio
  (INR), 1103
Lactate dehydrogenase and
  isoenzymes, 838
Lactic acid, 842
Lipase, 866
Nortriptyline, 148
Partial thromboplastin time, 1010
Phenobarbital, 140
Phenytoin, 140
Prealbumin, 1077
Primidone, 140
Protein, blood, total and
  fractions, 1091
Protein C, 1095
Protein S, 1097
Prothrombin time and INR, 1103
Pseudocholinesterase, 1108
Red blood cell count, 1134
Red blood cell morphology and
  inclusions, 1143
Urea nitrogen, blood, 1313
Uric acid, blood, 1322
Valproic acid, 140
Vitamin E, 1364
Vitamin K, 1367
Zinc, 1383

Diagnostic Tests Associated with the Hepatobiliary System

Angiography, abdomen, 69	Computed tomography, liver, 429
Cholangiography, percutaneous transhepatic, 363	Hepatobiliary scan, 753
Cholangiography, postoperative, 367	Magnetic resonance angiography, 903
Cholangiopancreatography, endoscopic retrograde, 370	Magnetic resonance imaging, abdomen, 907
Computed tomography, angiography, 425	Radiofrequency ablation, liver, 1125
	Ultrasound, liver and biliary system, 1272

IMMUNE SYSTEM

Laboratory Tests Associated with the Immune System

Acid phosphatase, prostatic, 3	Antibodies, gliadin (immuno-globulin G and immunoglob-ulin A), 132
Allergen-specific immunoglobulin E, 33	
Amikacin, 110	Antibody, antimitochondrial, 134
Angiotensin-converting enzyme, 97	Antibody, anti–smooth muscle, 136
Anion gap, 100	Antibody, Jo-1, 138
Antibodies, anticytoplasmic neutrophilic, 115	Antideoxyribonuclease-B, streptococcal, 146
Antibodies, anti–glomerular basement membrane, 117	Antigens/antibodies, anti–extractable nuclear, 155
Antibodies, antinuclear, anti-DNA, and anticentromere, 119	Biopsy, bladder, 200
	Biopsy, bone, 203
Antibodies, antiscleroderma, 122	Biopsy, bone marrow, 206
	Biopsy, breast, 211
Antibodies, antisperm, 124	Biopsy, cervical, 215
Antibodies, antistreptolysin *O*, 126	Biopsy, intestinal, 222
	Biopsy, kidney, 225
Antibodies, antithyroglobin and antithyroid peroxidase, 128	Biopsy, liver, 229
	Biopsy, lung, 233
Antibodies, cardiolipin, immunoglobulin G and immunoglobulin M, 130	Biopsy, lymph node, 238
	Biopsy, muscle, 241
	Biopsy, prostate, 245

(*Continued on the following page*)

Laboratory Tests Associated with the Immune System

Biopsy, skin, 248
Biopsy, thyroid, 252
Bladder cancer markers, 255
Blood groups and antibodies, 272
CA 125, 295
CA 15-3, 297
CA 19-9, 299
Carcinoembryonic antigen, 328
CD4/CD8 enumeration, 338
Cerebrospinal fluid analysis, 340
Chlamydia group antibody, 351
Cold agglutinin titer, 393
Complement C3 and complement C4, 408
Complement, total, 411
Complete blood count, 413
Copper, 483
C-reactive protein, 493
Cryoglobulin, 507
Culture and smear, mycobacteria, 509
Culture, bacterial, anal/genital, ear, eye, skin, and wound, 515
Culture, bacterial, blood, 520
Culture, bacterial, sputum, 524
Culture, bacterial, stool, 530
Culture, bacterial, throat or nasopharyngeal, 532
Culture, bacterial, urine, 535
Culture, fungal, 538
Culture, specific body fluid, 713
Culture, synovial fluid, 1198
Culture, viral, 541
Cytology, sputum, 555
Cytology, urine, 560
Cytomegalovirus, immunoglobulin G and immunoglobulin M, 563
Eosinophil count, 602
Erythrocyte sedimentation rate, 607
Estrogen and progesterone receptor assays, 623

α_1-Fetoprotein, 645
Gentamicin, 110
Gram stain, 712
Haptoglobin, 722
Helicobacter pylori antibody, 725
Hematocrit, 727
Hemoglobin, 732
Hepatitis A antibody, 743
Hepatitis B antigen and antibody, 745
Hepatitis C antibody, 748
Hepatitis D antibody, 751
Her-2/neu oncoprotein, 757
Human chorionic gonadotropin, 772
Human immunodeficiency virus type 1 and type 2 antibodies, 775
Human leukocyte antigen B27, 778
Human T-lymphotropic virus type I and type II antibodies, 780
5-Hydroxyindoleacetic acid, 782
Hypersensitivity pneumonitis, 785
Immunofixation electrophoresis, blood and urine, 791
Immunoglobulins A, D, G, and M, 796
Infectious mononucleosis screen, 804
Insulin antibodies, 809
Latex allergy, 856
Leukocyte alkaline phosphatase, 864
Lupus anticoagulant antibodies, 885
Lyme antibody, 890
β_2-Microglobulin, 960
Mumps serology, 964
Ova and parasites, stool, 991
Papanicolaou smear, 999

Diagnostic Tests Associated with the Immune System

MUSCULOSKELETAL SYSTEM

Laboratory Tests Associated with the Musculoskeletal System

(*Continued on the following page*)

Laboratory Tests Associated with the Musculoskeletal System

Human leukocyte antigen B27, 778
Immunoglobulins A, D, G, and M, 796
Lactate dehydrogenase and isoenzymes, 838
Lactic acid, 842
Lupus anticoagulant antibodies, 885
Lyme antibody, 890
Myoglobin, 975
Osteocalcin, 986
Phosphorus, blood, 1025
Pseudocholinesterase and dibucaine number, 1108
Rheumatoid factor, 1168
Synovial fluid analysis, 1198
Uric acid, blood, 1322
Vitamin D, 1362
Zinc, 1383

Diagnostic Tests Associated with the Musculoskeletal System

Arthrogram, 173
Bone mineral density, 280
Bone scan, 284
Computed tomography, brain, 434
Computed tomography, spine, 465
Electroencephalography, 590
Electromyography, 594
Electromyography, pelvic floor sphincter, 597
Electroneurography, 600
Evoked brain potentials, 627
Magnetic resonance imaging, musculoskeletal, 924
Positron emission tomography, brain, 1055
Radiography, bone, 1129
Vertebroplasty, 1352

OCULAR SYSTEM

Diagnostic Tests Associated with the Ocular System

Color perception test, 402
Fluorescein angiography, 655
Fundus photography, 666
Gonioscopy, 709
Intraocular muscle function, 812
Intraocular pressure, 814
Nerve fiber analysis, 977
Pachymetry, 997
Refraction, 1149
Schirmer test, 1174
Slit-lamp biomicroscopy, 1182
Ultrasound, A-scan, 1260
Visual field test, 1356

Laboratory Tests Associated with the Reproductive System

Acid phosphatase, prostatic, 3
Amino acid screen, blood, 42
Amino acid screen, urine, 46
Amniotic fluid analysis, 57
Antibodies, antisperm, 124
Antibodies, cardiolipin,
    immunoglobulin G and
    immunoglobulin M, 130
Biopsy, breast, 211
Biopsy, cervical, 215
Biopsy, chorionic villus, 218
Biopsy, prostate, 245
CA 125, 295
CA 15-3, 297
Carcinoembryonic antigen, 328
Chlamydia group antibody, 351
Chromosome analysis, blood, 383
Collagen cross-linked N-
    telopeptide, 395
Culture, bacterial, anal/genital,
    515
Culture, viral, 541
Cytomegalovirus, immunoglobulin
    G and immunoglobulin M, 563
Estradiol, 620
Estrogen and progesterone
    receptor assays, 623
Fetal fibronectin, 643

α_1-Fetoprotein, 645
Follicle-stimulating hormone, 661
Gram stain, 712
Her-2/neu oncoprotein, 757
Hexosaminidase A and B, 760
Human chorionic gonadotropin,
    772
Human immunodeficiency virus
    type 1 and type 2 antibodies,
    775
Kleihauer-Betke test, 836
Lecithin/sphingomyelin ratio, 860
Lupus anticoagulant antibodies,
    885
Luteinizing hormone, 887
Magnesium, blood, 896
Papanicolaou smear, 999
Progesterone, 1084
Prolactin, 1086
Prostate-specific antigen, 1089
Rubella, 1170
Rubeola, 1172
Semen analysis, 1177
Syphilis serology, 1203
Testosterone, total, 1206
Toxoplasma antibody, 1231
Urinalysis, 1329
Varicella, 1345

Diagnostic Tests Associated with the Reproductive System

Colposcopy, 404
Computed tomography, pelvis,
    451
Hysterosalpingography, 787
Laparoscopy, abdominal, 848
Laparoscopy, gynecologic, 852
Magnetic resonance imaging,
    breast, 916
Magnetic resonance imaging,
    pelvis, 932

Mammography, 940
Positron emission tomography,
    pelvis, 1064
Sterotactic biopsy, breast,
    1194
Ultrasound, obstetric, 1278
Ultrasound, pelvic, 1285
Ultrasound, scrotal, 1295
Uterine fibroid embolization,
    1337

RESPIRATORY SYSTEM

Laboratory Tests Associated with the Respiratory System

Allergen-specific immunoglobulin E, 33
Alveolar/arterial gradient and arterial/alveolar oxygen ratio, 35
Angiotensin-converting enzyme, 97
Anion gap, 100
Antibodies, anti–glomerular basement membrane, 117
α_1-Antitrypsin and α_1-antitrypsin phenotyping, 164
Biopsy, lung, 233
Blood gases, 260
Carbon dioxide, 322
Carboxyhemoglobin, 325
Chloride, blood, 354
Chloride, sweat, 358
Cold agglutinin titer, 393
Complete blood count, 413
Culture and smear, mycobacteria, 509
Culture, bacterial, sputum, 524
Culture, bacterial, throat, 532
Culture, viral, 541
Cytology, sputum, 555
D-Dimer, 565
Eosinophil count, 602
Erythrocyte sedimentation rate, 607
Fecal fat, 637
Gram stain, 712
Hematocrit, 727
Hemoglobin, 732
Hypersensitivity pneumonitis, 785
Immunoglobulin E, 794
Lactic acid, 842
Lecithin/sphingomyelin ratio, 860
Pleural fluid analysis, 1046
Potassium, blood, 1068
Rapid streptococcal screen, 715
Red blood cell count, 1134
Red blood cell indices, 1140
Tuberculin skin tests, 1246
White blood cell count and cell differential, 1373

Diagnostic Tests Associated with the Respiratory System

Angiography, pulmonary, 88
Bronchoscopy, 287
Chest x-ray, 348
Computed tomography, chest, 474
Lung perfusion scan, 877
Lung ventilation scan, 881
Magnetic resonance imaging, chest, 920
Mediastinoscopy, 947
Pulmonary function studies, 1111
Pulse oximetry, 1117

THERAPEUTIC DRUG MONITORING AND TOXICOLOGY

Laboratory Tests Associated with Therapeutic Drug Monitoring and Toxicology

Acetaminophen, 65	Flecainide, 104
Acetylsalicylic acid, 65	Gentamicin, 110
Albumin, 19	Haloperidol, 158
Alcohol, ethyl, 571	Imipramine, 148
Amikacin, 110	Lead, 858
Amitryptyline, 148	Lidocaine, 104
Amphetamines, 570	Lithium, 158
Barbiturates, 570	Methotrexate, 800
Benzodiazepines, 570	Nortriptyline, 148
Cannabinoids, 570	Opiates, 570
Carbamazepine, 140	Phencyclidine, 570
Cocaine, 570	Phenobarbital, 140
Cyclosporine, 800	Phenytoin, 140
Desipramine, 148	Primidone, 140
Diazepam, 148	Procainamide, 104
Digoxin, 104	Quinidine, 104
Disopyramide, 104	Tobramycin, 110
Doxepin, 148	Tricyclic antidepressants, 570
Ethanol, 570	Valproic acid, 140
Ethosuximide, 140	Vancomycin, 110

Patient Preparation and Specimen Collection

Patient Preparation Before Diagnostic and Laboratory Procedures

The first step in any laboratory or diagnostic procedure is patient preparation or patient teaching before the performance of the procedure. This pretesting explanation to the patient or caregiver follows essentially the same pattern for all sites and types of studies and includes the following:

- *Statement of the purpose of the study.* The level of detail provided to patients about the test purpose depends on numerous factors and should be individualized appropriately in each particular setting.
- *Description of the procedure, including site and method.* It is a good idea to explain to the patient that you will be wearing gloves throughout the procedure. The explanation should help the patient understand that the use of gloves is standard practice established for his or her protection as well as yours. Many institutions require hand washing at the beginning and end of each specimen collection encounter and between each patient.
- *Description of the sensations, including discomfort and pain, that the patient may experience during the specimen collection procedure.* Address concerns about pain related to the procedure and suggest breathing or visualization techniques to promote relaxation. For pediatric patients, a doll may be used to "show" the procedure. Where appropriate, the use of sedative or anesthetizing agents may assist in allaying anxiety the patient may experience that is related to anticipation of pain associated with the procedure. Sensitivity to cultural and social issues, as well as concern for modesty, is important in providing psychological support.
- *Instruction regarding pretesting preparations related to diet, liquids, medications, and activity as well as any restrictions regarding diet, liquids, medications, activity, known allergies, therapies, or other procedures that might affect test results.* To increase patient compliance, the instructions should include an explanation of why strict adherence to the instructions is required.
- *Recognition of anxiety related to test results.* Provide a compassionate, reassuring environment. Be prepared to educate the patient regarding access to the appropriate counseling services. Encourage the patient to ask questions and verbalize his or her concerns.

Specific collection techniques and patient preparation vary by site, study required, and level of invasiveness. These techniques are described in the individual monographs.

Blood Specimens

Most laboratory tests that require a blood specimen use venous blood. Venous blood can be collected directly from the vein or by way of capillary puncture. Capillary blood can be obtained from the fingertips or earlobes of adults and small children. Capillary blood can also be obtained from the heels of infants. The circumstances in which the capillary method would be selected over direct venipuncture include cases in which:

- The patient has poor veins.
- The patient has small veins.
- The patient has a limited number of available veins.
- The patient has significant anxiety about the venipuncture procedure.

Venous blood also can be obtained from vascular access devices, such as heparin locks and central venous catheters. Examples of central venous catheters include the triple-lumen subclavian, Hickman, and Groshong catheters.

Fetal blood samples can be obtained, when warranted, by a qualified health care practitioner from the scalp or from the umbilical cord.

Arterial blood can be collected from the radial, brachial, or femoral artery if blood gas analysis is requested.

There are some general guidelines one should follow in the procurement and handling of blood specimens:

- It is essential that the patient be positively and properly identified. Specimens should always be labeled with the patient's name, medical record number (or some other unique identifier), date collected, time collected, and initials of the person collecting the sample.
- Requisitions should be completed accurately and submitted per laboratory policy.
- The practice of an overnight fast before specimen collection is a general recommendation. Reference ranges are often based on fasting populations to provide some level of standardization for comparison. Some test results are dramatically affected by foods, however, and fasting is a pretest requirement. The presence of lipids in the blood also may interfere with the test method; fasting eliminates this potential source of error, especially if the patient already has elevated lipid levels. The laboratory should always be consulted if there is a question as to whether fasting is a requirement or a recommendation.
- Gloves and any other additional personal protective equipment indicated by the patient's condition should always be worn during the specimen collection process. Appendix G can be consulted for a more detailed description of standard precautions.
- Stress can cause variations in some test results. A sleeping patient should be gently awakened and allowed the opportunity to become oriented before collection site selection. Comatose or unconscious patients should be greeted in the same gentle manner because, although they are unable to respond, they may be capable of hearing and understanding. Anticipate instances in which patient cooperation may be an

issue. Enlist the assistance of a second person to assist with specimen collection to ensure a safe, quality collection experience for all involved.

- Localized activity such as the application of a tourniquet or clenching the hand to assist in visualizing the vein can cause variations in some test results. It is important to be aware of affected studies before specimen collection.
- Hemoconcentration may cause variations in some test results. The tourniquet should never be left in place for longer than 1 minute.
- Previous puncture sites should be avoided when accessing a blood vessel by any means, to reduce the potential for infection.
- Specimens should never be collected above an intravenous (IV) line because of the potential for dilution when the specimen and the IV solution combine in the collection container, falsely decreasing the result. It is also possible that substances in the IV solution could contaminate the specimen and result in falsely elevated test results.
- Changes in posture from supine to erect or long-term maintenance of a supine posture causes variations in some test results. It is important to be aware of this effect when results are interpreted and compared with previous values.
- Collection times for therapeutic drug (peak and trough) or other specific monitoring (e.g., chemotherapy, glucose, insulin, or potassium) should be documented carefully in relation to the time of medication administration. It is essential that this information be communicated clearly and accurately to avoid misunderstanding of the dose time in relation to the collect time. Miscommunication between the individual administering the medication and the individual collecting the specimen is the most frequent cause of subtherapeutic levels, toxic levels, and misleading information used in the calculation of future therapies.
- The laboratory should be consulted regarding minimum specimen collection requirements when multiple tube types or samples are required. The amount of serum or plasma collected can be estimated using assumptions of packed cell volume or hematocrit. The packed cell volume of a healthy woman is usually 38% to 44% of the total blood volume. If a full 5-mL red-top tube is collected, and the hematocrit is 38% to 44%, approximately 2.8 to 3.1 mL, or $[5 - (5 \ (\ 0.44)]$ to $[5 - (5 \times 0.38)]$, of the total blood volume should be serum. Factors that invalidate estimation include conditions such as anemia, polcythemia, dehydration, or overhydration.
- The laboratory should be consulted regarding the preferred specimen container before specimen collection. Specific analytes may vary in concentration depending on whether the sample is serum or plasma. It is recommended that, when serial measurements are to be carried out, the same type of collection container be used so that fluctuations in values caused by variations in specimen type are not misinterpreted as changes in clinical status. Consultation regarding collection containers is also important because some laboratory methods are optimized for a specific specimen type (serum versus plasma). Also, preservatives present in collection containers, such as sodium fluoride, may exhibit a chemical interference with test reagents that can cause underestimation or overestimation of measured values. Other preservatives, such as ethylenediaminetetra-acetic acid (EDTA), can block the analyte of interest in the sample from participating in the test reaction, invalidating test results. Finally, it is possible that some high-throughput, robotic equipment systems require specific and standardized collection containers.

• Prompt and proper specimen processing, storage, and analysis are important to achieve accurate results. Specimens collected in containers with solid or liquid preservatives or with gel separators should be mixed by inverting the tube 10 times immediately after the tube has been filled. Handle the specimen gently to avoid hemolysis. Specimens should always be transported to the laboratory as quickly as possible after collection.

Results that are evaluated outside the entire context of the preparatory, collection, and handling process may be interpreted erroneously if consideration is not given to the above-listed general guidelines.

Site Selection

Capillary Puncture: Assess the selected area. It should be free of lesions and calluses, there should be no edema, and the site should feel warm. If the site feels cool or if the site appears pale or cyanotic, warm compresses can be applied over 3 to 5 minutes to dilate the capillaries. For finger sticks, the central, fleshy, distal portions of the third or fourth fingers are the preferred collection sites (Figure Appenix A–1). For neonatal heel sticks, the medial and lateral surfaces of the plantar area are preferred to avoid direct puncture of the heel bone, which could result in osteomyelitis (Figure Appenix A–2).

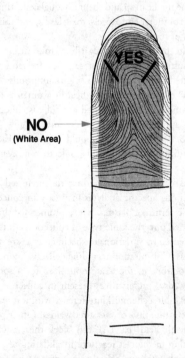

FIGURE A–1 Site selection. Capillary puncture of the finger.

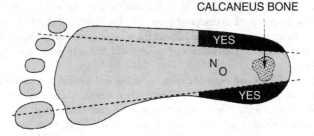

FIGURE A–2 Site selection. Capillary puncture of the heel.

Venipuncture of Arm: Assess the arm for visibly accessible veins. The selected area should not be burned or scarred, have a tattoo, or have hematoma present. Even after the tourniquet is applied, not all patients have a prominent median cubital, cephalic, or basilic vein. Both arms should be observed because some patients have accessible veins in one arm and not the other. The median cubital vein in the antecubital fossa is the preferred venipuncture site. The patient may be able to provide the best information regarding venous access if he or she has had previous venipuncture experience (Figure Appendix A–3). Alternative techniques to increase visibility of veins may include warming the arm, allowing the arm to dangle downward for a minute or two, tapping the antecubital area with the index finger, or massaging the arm upward from wrist to elbow. The condition of the vein also should be assessed before venipuncture. Sclerotic (hard, scarred) veins or veins in which phlebitis previously occurred should be avoided. Arms with a functioning hemodialysis access site should not be used. The arm on the affected side of a mastectomy should be avoided. In the case of a double mastectomy, the requesting health care practitioner should be consulted before specimen collection.

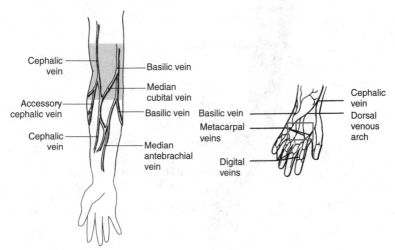

FIGURE A–3 Site selection. Venipuncture arm/hand.

Venipuncture of Hand and Wrist: If no veins in the arms are available, hands and wrists should be examined as described previously. Consideration should be given to the venipuncture equipment selected because the veins in these areas are much smaller. Pediatric-sized collection containers and needles with a larger gauge may be more appropriate.

Venipuncture of Legs and Feet: The veins in the legs and feet can be accessed as with sites located on the arm, hand, or wrist. These extremities should be used only on the approval of the requesting health care practitioner because veins in these locations are more prone to infection and formation of blood clots, especially in patients with diabetes, cardiac disease, and bleeding disorders.

Radial Arterial Puncture: The radial artery is the artery of choice for obtaining arterial blood gas specimens because it is close to the surface of the wrist and does not require a deep puncture. Its easy access also allows for more effective compression after the needle has been removed. The nearby ulnar artery can provide sufficient collateral circulation to the hand during specimen collection and postcollection compression (Figure Appendix A–4).

Percutaneous Umbilical Cord Sampling: The blood is aspirated from the umbilical cord under the guidance of ultrasonography and using a 20- or 22-gauge spinal needle inserted through the mother's abdomen.

Postnatal Umbilical Cord Sampling: The blood is aspirated from the umbilical cord using a 20- or 22-gauge needle and transferred to the appropriate collection container.

Fetal Scalp Sampling: The requesting health care practitioner makes a puncture in the fetal scalp using a microblade, and the specimen is collected in a long capillary tube. The tube is usually capped on both ends immediately after specimen collection.

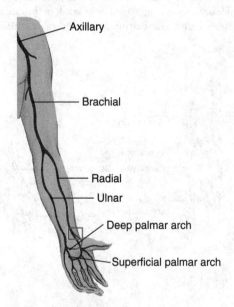

FIGURE A–4 Site selection. Arterial arm/hand.

Locks and Catheters: These devices are sometimes inserted to provide a means for the administration of fluids or medications and to obtain blood specimens without the need for frequent venipuncture. The device first should be assessed for patency. The need for heparinization, irrigation, or clot removal depends on the type of device in use and the institution-specific or health care practitioner–specific protocols in use. Care should be taken to use sterile technique because these devices provide direct access to the patient's bloodstream. When IV fluids are being administered via a device at the time of specimen collection, blood should be obtained from the opposite side of the body. If this is not possible, the flow should be stopped for 5 minutes before specimen collection. The first 5 mL of blood collected should be discarded.

Selection of Blood Collection Equipment

In many cases when a blood sample is required, serum is the specimen type of choice. Plasma may be frequently substituted, however. Specimen processing is more rapid for plasma samples than serum samples because the anticoagulated sample does not need to clot before centrifugation. Plasma samples also require less centrifugation time to achieve adequate separation. Consult with the testing laboratory regarding recommended specimen types. The basic blood collection tubes are shown on the inside cover of this book. Consider latex allergy when selecting the collection equipment appropriate for each patient. Equipment used in specimen collection includes:

* Gloves and other personal protective equipment depending on the situation
* Tourniquet
* Materials to cleanse or disinfect the collection site (alcohol preparations [70% alcohol], povidone-iodine solution [Betadine], or green soap are the most commonly used materials)
* Gauze (to wipe collection site dry after cleansing)
* Sterile lancet (capillary puncture)
* Syringe and needle (arterial puncture or venipuncture)
* Vial of heparin and syringe or heparin unit dose
* Sterile normal saline in 50-mL syringe (for indwelling devices such as Groshong catheter)
* Sterile cap or hub (for indwelling devices when the cap or hub will be replaced after specimen procurement)
* Needle and holder for vacuumized collection tube system (arterial puncture or venipuncture)
* Butterfly or winged infusion set (venipuncture)
* Collection container (vacuumized collection tube, capillary tube, or Microtainer)
* Bandage (to cover puncture site after specimen collection)

Collection Procedure

The procedures outlined here are basic in description. A phlebotomy or other text should be consulted for specific details regarding specimen collection and complications encountered during various types of blood collection.

Capillary: Place the patient in a comfortable position either sitting or lying down. Assess whether the patient has allergies to the disinfectant or to latex if latex gloves or tourniquet will be used in the collection procedure. Use gloved hands to select the collection site as described in the site selection section. Cleanse the skin with the appropriate disinfectant and dry the area. Pull the skin tight by the thumb and index finger of the nondominant hand on either side of the puncture site and moving them in opposite directions. Puncture the skin with a sterile lancet to a depth of approximately 2 mm, using a quick, firm motion. Wipe the first drop of blood away using the gauze. If flow is poor, the site should not be squeezed or the specimen may become contaminated with tissue fluid. Do not allow the collection container to touch the puncture site. Collect the sample in the capillary tube or Microtainer. The capillary tube should be held in a horizontal position to avoid the introduction of air bubbles into the sample. Microtainer tubes should be held in a downward-slanted direction to facilitate the flow of blood into the capillary scoop of the collection device. If a smear is required, allow a drop of blood to fall onto a clean microscope slide. Gently spread the drop across the slide using the edge of another slide. Apply slight pressure to the puncture site with a clean piece of gauze until bleeding stops, and then apply a bandage. Safely dispose of the sharps. Properly label the specimens and transport immediately to the laboratory.

Venipuncture Using a Syringe or Vacuumized Needle and Holder System: Place the patient in a comfortable position either sitting or lying down. Assess whether the patient has allergies to the disinfectant or to latex if latex gloves or tourniquet will be used in the collection procedure. Use gloved hands to select the collection site as described in the site selection section. Locate the vein visually, then by palpation using the index finger. The thumb should not be used because it has a pulse beat and may cause confusion in site selection or in differentiating a vein from an artery. Select the appropriate collection materials (needle size, butterfly, syringe, collection container size) based on the vein size, vein depth, appearance of the collection site, patient's age, and anticipated level of cooperation. Cleanse the skin with the appropriate disinfectant and dry the area. Select the appropriate collection tubes. If blood cultures are to be collected, disinfect the top of the collection containers as directed by the testing laboratory. Be sure to have extra tubes within easy reach in case the vacuum in a collection tube is lost and a substitute is required. Apply the tourniquet 3 to 4 inches above the selected collection site. Remove the sterile needle cap, and inspect the tip of the needle for defects. Pull the skin tight by placing the thumb of the nondominant hand 1 or 2 inches below the puncture site and moving the thumb in the opposite direction. The thumb is placed below the puncture site to help avoid an accidental needle stick if the patient should suddenly move. Ensure that the needle is bevel up and held at an angle of approximately 15° to 30° (depending on the depth of the vein) (Figure Appendix A–5).

Puncture the skin with smooth, firm motion using a sterile needle held by the dominant hand. A reduction in pressure is achieved when the needle has penetrated the vein successfully. Be sure to release the tourniquet within 1 minute of application. Fill the vacuumized collection containers in the prescribed order of draw for the studies ordered. Tubes with anticoagulants can be gently mixed with the free nondominant hand as they are filled. When the required containers have been filled, withdraw the needle and apply pressure to the collection site until the bleeding stops. In most cases, a piece of gauze can be placed on the collection site and the arm bent upward to hold

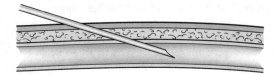

FIGURE A–5 Venipuncture needle placement at insertion.

it in place while attention is given to disposing of the sharps safely and labeling the collection tubes properly. In cases in which a syringe is used, the barrel of the syringe should be gently pulled back during specimen collection and gently pushed in during the transfer to collection tubes. The vacuum in the collection container should not be allowed to suck the sample into the container, but rather the speed of entry should be controlled by the pressure applied to the barrel. The blood should gently roll down the side of the tube to prevent hemolysis.

Radial Artery Puncture: Place the patient in a comfortable position either sitting or lying down. Assess whether the patient has allergies to the disinfectant or to latex if latex gloves or tourniquet will be used in the collection procedure. Assess if the patient has an allergy to local anesthetics, and inform the health care practitioner accordingly. Glove the hands, and select the collection site as described in the site selection section. Ensure that the patient has adequate collateral circulation to the hand if thrombosis of the radial artery occurs after arterial puncture by performing an Allen test before puncture. The Allen test is performed by occlusion of the ulnar and radial arteries on the palmar surface of the wrist with two fingers. The thumb should not be used to locate these arteries because it has a pulse. Compress both arteries, and ask the patient to open and close the fist several times until the palm turns pale. Release pressure only on the ulnar artery. Color should return to the palm within 5 seconds if the ulnar artery is functioning. If coloring returns above the wrist, the Allen test is positive. The Allen test also should be performed on the opposite hand. The wrist to which color is restored fastest has better circulation and should be selected as the site for blood gas collection. Be sure to explain to the patient that an arterial puncture is painful. The site may be anesthetized with 1% to 2% lidocaine (Xylocaine) before puncture. The index finger of the nondominant hand is placed over the site where the needle will enter the artery, not the site where the needle will penetrate the skin. The specimen is collected in an air-free heparinized syringe, which is held like a dart in the dominant hand and inserted slowly, bevel up, about 5 to 10 mm below the palpating finger at a 45° to 60° angle. When blood enters the needle hub, arterial pressure should cause blood to pump into the syringe. When enough specimen has been collected, the needle is withdrawn from the arm, and pressure is applied to the collection site for a minimum of 5 to 10 minutes. Immediately after the needle has been withdrawn safely from the arm, the exposed end of the syringe should be stoppered.

Samples should be gently and well mixed to ensure proper mixing of the heparin with the sample. The heparin prevents formation of small clots that result in rejection of the sample. The tightly capped sample should be placed in an ice slurry immediately after collection. Information on the specimen label can be protected from water in the ice slurry if the specimen is first placed in a protective plastic bag.

Indwelling Devices: Indwelling devices are either heparinized or irrigated after specimen collection. Before specimen collection, prepare the heparin in a syringe, if required. Allow the heparin (unit dose or prepared solution in the syringe) to equilibrate at room temperature during specimen collection. Cleanse the catheter cap or hub with povidone-iodine and 70% alcohol over 2 minutes. Using sterile gloves, remove the cap and attach a 5- or 10-mL syringe to the connector. Withdraw 5 mL of blood to be discarded. Clamp the catheter. (The Groshong catheter does not require clamping because it has a special valve that eliminates the need for clamping.) Attach another 5- or 10-mL syringe and begin collecting blood for transfer to the collection tubes. After the required specimen has been withdrawn, the device is heparinized by slowly injecting the heparin into the cap or hub of the device. Clamp the device 2 inches from the cap, remove the needle, and unclamp the device. Attach a new sterile cap or hub if the old one has been discarded. Groshong catheters are irrigated rather than heparinized. Irrigation of a Groshong catheter is accomplished by gently injecting 20 to 30 mL of sterile normal saline through the cap with moderate force. Remove the needle using some positive pressure (pressing down on the plunger) to prevent the solution from backing up into the syringe.

Order of Draw for Glass or Plastic Tubes (Reflects 2004 change in CLSI [formerly NCCLS] guideline: Recommended Order of Draw, H3-A5, [Vol 23, No 32, 8.10.2])

Note: Always follow your facility's protocol for order of draw.

* First—Blood culture and other tests requiring sterile specimen (yellow or yellow/black stopper); blood culture bottle first, followed by sodium polyethanol sulfonate (SPS) tube for acid-fast bacilli specimens.
* Second—Coagulation studies (light blue [sodium citrate] stopper); sodium citrate forms calcium salts to remove calcium, and this prevents specimen clotting. *Note:* When using a winged blood collection set and the blue-top tube is the first tube drawn, a nonadditive red-top or coagulation discard tube should be collected first and discarded. The amount of blood in the discard tube needs to be sufficient to fill the winged collection set tubing's "dead space." This is done to eliminate contamination of the specimen with tissue thromboplastin and to ensure the proper ratio of blood to additive in the test specimen blue-top tube.
* Third—Plain or nonadditive (red or red/gray [gel] stopper); red/gray-top serum separator tube (SST) contains a gel separator and clot activator. SSTs are not appropriate for all testing requiring a serum specimen. They are generally unacceptable for therapeutic drug monitoring and serology studies. The laboratory should be consulted if there are questions regarding the use of SSTs.
* Last—Additive tubes in the following order:

Green stopper; tube contains sodium heparin or lithium heparin anticoagulant (heparin inactivates thrombin and thromboplastin, and this prevents specimen clotting). For ammonia levels, use sodium or lithium heparin. For lithium levels, use sodium heparin.

Lavender stopper; tube contains Kt_3 EDTA (tri-potassium EDTA forms calcium salts to remove calcium from the sample, and this prevents specimen clotting while preserving the integrity of the red blood cell wall).

Gray stopper; tube contains potassium oxalate/sodium fluoride (the potassium oxalate acts as an anticoagulant, and the sodium fluoride prevents glycolysis).

Urine Specimens

The patient should be informed that improper collection, storage, and transport are the primary reasons for specimen rejection and subsequent requests for recollection. If the specimen is to be collected at home, it should be collected in a clean plastic container (preferably a container from the testing laboratory). Many studies require refrigeration after collection. If the collection container includes a preservative, the patient should be made aware of the contents and advised as to what the precaution labels mean (caution labels such as caustic, corrosive, acid, and base should be affixed to the container as appropriate). When a preservative or fixative is included in the container, the patient should be advised not to remove it. The patient also should be told not to void directly into the container. The patient should be given a collection device, if indicated, and instructed to void into the collection device. The specimen should be carefully transferred into the collection container. Some laboratories provide preprinted collection instructions tailored to their methods. The specimen should be transported promptly to the laboratory after collection.

Wear gloves and any other additional personal protective equipment indicated by the patient's condition. See Appendix F for a more detailed description of standard precautions. Assess whether the patient has allergies to the disinfectant or anesthetic, or to latex if latex gloves or catheter will be used in the procedure.

Random: These samples are mainly used for routine screening and can be collected at any time of the day. The patient should be instructed to void either directly into the collection container (if there is no preservative) or into a collection device for transfer into the specimen container.

First Morning: Urine on rising in the morning is very concentrated. These specimens are indicated when screening for substances that may not be detectable in a more dilute random sample. These specimens are also necessary for testing conditions such as orthostatic proteinuria, in which levels vary with changes in posture.

Second Voided: In some cases, it is desirable to test freshly produced urine to evaluate the patient's current status, as with glucose and ketones. Explain to the patient that he or she should first void and then drink a glass of water. The patient should be instructed to wait 30 minutes and then void either directly into the collection container or into a collection device for transfer into the collection container.

Clean Catch: These midstream specimens are generally used for microbiologic or cytologic studies. They also may be requested for routine urinalysis to provide a specimen that is least contaminated with urethral cells, microorganisms, mucus, or other substances that may affect the interpretation of results. Instruct the male patient first to wash hands thoroughly, then cleanse the meatus, void a small amount into the toilet, and void either directly into the specimen container or into a collection device for transfer into the specimen container. Instruct the female patient first to wash hands thoroughly, and then to cleanse the labia from front to back. While keeping the labia separated, the patient should void a small amount into the toilet, and then, without interrupting the urine stream, void either directly into the specimen container or into a collection device for transfer into the specimen container.

Catheterized Random or Clean Catch: "Straight catheterization" is indicated when the patient is unable to void, when the patient is unable to prepare properly for clean-catch specimen collection, or when the patient has an indwelling catheter in place from which a urine sample may be obtained. Before collecting a specimen from the catheter, observe the drainage tube to ensure that it is empty, and then clamp the tube distal to the collection port 15 minutes before specimen collection. Cleanse the port with an antiseptic swab such as 70% alcohol and allow the port to dry. Use a needle and syringe (sterile if indicated) to withdraw the required amount of specimen. Unclamp the tube.

Timed: To quantify substances in urine, 24-hour urine collections are used. They are also used to measure substances whose level of excretion varies over time. The use of preservatives and the handling of specimens during the timed collection may be subject to variability among laboratories. The testing laboratory should be consulted regarding specific instructions before starting the test. Many times the specimen must be refrigerated or kept on ice throughout the entire collection period. Explain to the patient that it is crucial for *all* urine to be included in the collection. The test should begin between 6 and 8 a.m., if possible. Instruct the patient to collect the first void of the day and discard it. The start time of the collection period begins at the time the first voided specimen was discarded and should be recorded along with the date on the collection container. The patient should be instructed to void at the same time the following morning and to add this last voiding to the container. This is the end time of the collection and should be recorded along with the date on the container. For patients who are in the hospital, the urinary output should be compared with the volume measured in the completed collection container. Discrepancies between the two volumes indicate that a collection might have been discarded. Many times a creatinine level is requested along with the study of interest to evaluate the completeness of the collection.

Catheterized Timed: Instructions for this type of collection are basically the same as those for timed specimen collection. The test should begin by changing the tubing and drainage bag. If a preservative is required, it can be placed directly in the drainage bag, or the specimen can be removed at frequent intervals (every 2 hours) and transferred to the collection container to which the preservative has been added. The drainage bag must be kept on ice or emptied periodically into the collection container during the entire collection period if indicated by the testing laboratory. The tubing should be monitored throughout the collection period to ensure continued drainage.

Suprapubic Aspiration: This procedure is performed by inserting a needle directly into the bladder. Because the bladder is normally sterile, the urine collected should also be free from any contamination caused by the presence of microorganisms. Place the patient in a supine position. Cleanse the area with antiseptic and drape with sterile drapes. A local anesthetic may be administered before insertion of the needle. A needle is inserted through the skin into the bladder. A syringe attached to the needle is used to aspirate the urine sample. The needle is then removed and a sterile dressing is applied to the site. Place the sterile sample in a sterile specimen container. The site must be observed for signs of inflammation or infection.

Pediatric: Specimen collection can be achieved by any of the above-described methods using collection devices specifically designed for pediatric patients. Appropriately cleanse the genital area and allow the area to dry. For a random collection, remove the covering of the adhesive strips on the collector bag and apply over the genital area.

Diaper the child. When the specimen is obtained, place the entire collection bag in the specimen container (use a sterile container as appropriate for the requested study). Some laboratories may have specific preferences for the submission of urine specimens for culture. Consult the laboratory before collection to avoid specimen rejection.

Body Fluid, Stool, and Tissue

Wear gloves and any other additional personal protective equipment indicated by the patient's condition. See Appendix G for a more detailed description of standard precautions. Assess whether the patient has allergies to the disinfectant or anesthetic, or to latex if latex gloves will be used in the procedure.

Specific collection techniques vary by site, study required, and level of invasiveness. These techniques are described in the individual monographs.

Diagnostic Testing

Wear gloves and any other additional personal protective equipment indicated by the patient's condition. See Appendix G for a more detailed description of standard precautions. Assess whether the patient has allergies to the disinfectant, anesthetic, contrast material, or medications, or to latex if latex gloves, catheter, or tourniquet will be used in the procedure.

A sleeping patient should be gently awakened and allowed the opportunity to become oriented before preparation for the selected study. Comatose or unconscious patients should be greeted in the same gentle manner because, although they are unable to respond, they may be capable of hearing and understanding. Anticipate instances in which patient cooperation may be an issue. Enlist the assistance of a second person to help with preparing the patient for the procedure to ensure a safe, quality testing experience for all involved.

Specific techniques and patient preparation vary by site, study required, and level of invasiveness. These techniques are described in the individual monographs.

Potential Nursing Diagnoses Associated with Laboratory and Diagnostic Testing

Pretest Phase

Anxiety related to undiagnosed health problems

Anxiety related to perceived threat to health status

Anxiety and fear related to anticipated diagnostic results

Anxiety and fear related to perception of diagnostic procedure as frightening or embarrassing

Powerlessness related to unfamiliar procedure, equipment, environment, or personnel

Knowledge deficit related to lack of information or possible misinterpretation of information provided about the procedure

Knowledge deficit related to legal implications of testing

Potential for noncompliance with test protocols related to inability to understand or follow instructions

Potential for noncompliance with test protocols related to presence of high anxiety, confusion, or denial

Potential for noncompliance with test protocols related to lack of knowledge or appropriate instruction

Potential for noncompliance with test protocols related to confusion, weakness, and other individual factors

Intratest Phase

Risk for injury related to developmental age, psychological factors, and test procedures

Risk for infection or allergic reaction related to altered immune function, history of chronic illness, allergens, or infectious agent

Risk for latex allergy response associated with test equipment

Pain, nausea, vomiting, or diarrhea related to laboratory and diagnostic procedures

Injury, actual or risk for, related to invasive procedure associated with laboratory or diagnostic testing

Risk for infection related to invasive procedures

Risk for bleeding associated with altered bleeding tendencies related to invasive procedures

Fatigue related to diagnostic procedure

Anxiety and fear related to arterial puncture or venipuncture

Risk for injury, bleeding, hematoma, or infection related to arterial puncture or venipuncture

Pain related to arterial puncture or venipuncture

Risk for impaired skin integrity

Potential impairment of gas exchange associated with test procedure

Post-Test Phase

Knowledge deficit related to significance of test results and potential need for further testing

Knowledge deficit related to test outcome deviation that may necessitate medication or lifestyle alterations

Anxiety and fear related to test outcome deviation that may necessitate medication or lifestyle alterations

Ineffective coping related to test outcome and potential for other interventional techniques or procedures

Anticipatory grieving related to test outcomes

Anticipatory or actual grieving related to perceived loss of health or threat of death associated with diagnostic outcomes

Decisional conflict related to test outcome and potential for interventional procedures

Potential alteration in tissue perfusion: cerebral, cardiopulmonary, or peripheral

Knowledge deficit related to care after procedure

Guidelines for Age-Specific Communication

Effective communication between the health care practitioner and the patient is influenced by the patient's cognitive abilities, sensory development or deprivation, level of stress, and environment. Effective communication with individuals at any stage of life is possible if one recognizes that it is essential to employ age-specific communication techniques based on an understanding of the continuum of human development as highlighted here.

Infant (Birth to 1 year)

Physical

Rapid gains in height and weight
Gradual shift from reflexive movements to intentional actions

Motor and Sensory

Responds to light and sound
Progresses to raising and turning head, bringing hand to mouth, rolling over, sitting upright, and standing

Cognitive

Learns by imitation
Progresses to recognize familiar objects and people
Advances to speaking three or four words

Psychosocial

Significant persons are parents or primary caregivers
Develops sense of trust and security if needs are met

May show fear of strangers
May exhibit separation anxiety

Interventions

Keep a parent or primary caregiver in view
Involve significant persons in care if appropriate
Provide consistency in health care staff to limit the number of strangers
Face the infant when providing care
Use soothing nonverbal communication, such as holding, rocking, and cuddling
Assess immunizations
Maintain safety and keep crib side rails up at all times

Toddler (1 to 4 years)

Physical

Learning bladder and bowel control
Temporary teeth erupt
Physiologic systems mature

Motor and Sensory

Developing a higher level of manual dexterity (builds towers with blocks)
Progresses to walking, jumping, and climbing
Loves to experiment

Cognitive

Has a short attention span
Understands simple directions and requests

Psychosocial

Significant persons are parents
Asserts independence
Understands ownership
Attached to security objects
Knows own gender
Plays simple games

Interventions

Face the toddler during interactions
Give one direction at a time
Tie words to action (toddlers learn by example)
Use firm, direct approach; avoid harsh/excited words or actions
Use distraction techniques
Use soothing nonverbal communication, such as rocking, cuddling, and holding
Communicate through play (dolls, puppets, music)
Prepare shortly before a procedure
Allow choices when possible
Encourage mother or parent to stay with the child as appropriate
Encourage parents to participate in care as appropriate
Maintain safety and keep crib side rails up at all times

Child (5 to 12 years)

Physical

Growth is slow and regular
Permanent teeth erupt
Pubescent changes start
May experience growing pains
May experience fatigue

Motor and Sensory

Skips and hops
Dresses and undresses independently
Throws and catches a ball
Uses common utensils and tools
Draws, paints, and likes quiet as well as active games

Cognitive

Major cognitive skill is communication
Understands numbers and can count
Constructs sentences and asks questions
Capable of logical thinking and can reason
Takes pride in accomplishments
Develops increased attention span

Psychosocial

Significant persons are parents, siblings, peers, teachers (prefers friends to family)
Increases independence and begins to assert self (may be physically aggressive)
Masters new tasks and acquires new skills
Behavior can be modified by rewards and punishment
Works hard to be successful

Interventions

Clearly define and reinforce behavior limits
Tell jokes and play games with rules

Check for special words used to identify parents, body parts, or body functions

Explain procedures in advance using correct terminology

Use dolls or puppets for explanations when performing procedures

Provide privacy

Involve whenever possible

Allow to have some control

Promote independence

Praise for good behavior

Acknowledge fear, pain, or family separation

Adolescent (13 to 18 years)

Physical

Growth in skeletal size is rapid

Reproductive system matures

Vital signs approximate those of an adult

Motor and Sensory

Easily fatigued

May need more rest and sleep in early adolescence

Awkwardness in gross motor activity

Demonstrates improving fine motor skills

Cognitive

Increased ability to use abstract thought and logic

Able to handle hypothetical situations and thoughts

Shows growth in self-esteem but is challenged by bouts of insecurity

Avoids asking questions for fear of appearing unintelligent

Psychosocial

Develops sexual identity

Shows interest in and confusion with own development

Develops concern with physical appearance

Establishes critical need for privacy

Values belonging to peer group

Perceives self as invincible

Identity is threatened by hospitalization

Interventions

Likes to be treated like an adult

Do not talk to others about the patient in front of him or her

Do not ask questions about drugs, sex, or use of tobacco in front of parents

Provide information about routines and therapy

Provide privacy

Supplement information with rationale

Encourage questions

Allow to maintain control

Involve in decision making and care

Allow for expression of fear, such as fear of bodily injury and loss of control

Adult (19 to 65 years)

Physical

Reaches physical and sexual maturity

Prone to health problems related to an inability to cope with new responsibilities

Health care needs related to preventive medicine

Adjustment to menopause (women) and sexual dysfunction (men) in middle adulthood

Motor and Sensory

Skills are fully developed

Cognitive

Focuses on time constraints and want to learn only what is practical for him or her

May be dual caregivers (i.e., parents and children)

Psychosocial

Experiences emotional stress secondary
to mate selection, vocational selection,
assuming occupational roles, marriage,
childbearing, financial pressure, and
independence

Interventions

Involve family in patient's care and
education
Explain benefits of adhering to
treatment plan
Be honest and supportive
Respect personal values
Provide privacy
Keep a hopeful attitude
Focus on strengths, and not limitations
Recognize that unknown factors may
affect behavior
Encourage patient to ask questions and
talk about concerns
Provide information and support to
make health care decisions

Geriatric (65 and older)

Physical

Ages gradually and individually
Experiences decreased tolerance to
heat/cold
Encounters declining cardiac and renal
function
Experiences skeletal changes (bones
become more prominent, shrinkage in
vertebral disks, stiff joints)
Becomes subject to increased
susceptibility to infection and to high
blood pressure
Undergoes skin changes

Motor and Sensory

Experiences decrease in mobility, visual
acuity, ability to respond to stimuli,
hearing, and motor skills

Cognitive

Experiences decrease in memory, slowing
of mental functions, slowness in
learning, and drop in performance

Psychosocial

Encounters lifestyle changes secondary
to children leaving home, children
providing grandchildren, re-
establishing a relationship as a couple,
and retirement/hobbies
Develops increased concern for health
and financial security
Accepts concept of own mortality
Faces decreased authority and autonomy
Experiences depression related to
decreased physical, motor, and
cognitive abilities

Interventions

Explain instructions well to patient and
family
Ask questions to verify understanding
Review important points repeatedly
Keep room clutter-free and call bell
within reach
Control room temperature for comfort
Consider additional lighting at night
Watch for signs of drug toxicity
Give respect and provide privacy
Focus on strengths and not limitations
Avoid assuming loss of abilities
Seek information as necessary to deal
with impairments
Include patient in conversation/activity
to prevent social isolation
Encourage to talk about feelings
Use humor and stay positive
Provide information and support
regarding end-of-life decisions
Provide teaching for safety
Provide teaching for medications and
test preparations

Transfusion Reactions: Laboratory Findings and Potential Nursing Interventions

These reactions are mainly associated with the transfusion of packed red blood cells.

Categories:

I. Acute (Less than 24 h) Immune-Mediated Transfusion Reactions
   a. ABO and non-ABO acute hemolytic
   b. Febrile nonhemolytic
   c. Urticarial/allergic reaction
   d. Anaphylactic reaction
II. Acute (Less than 24 h) Non–Immune-Mediated Transfusion Reactions
   a. Transfusion-related acute lung injury
   b. Circulatory overload
   c. Metabolic complications
   d. Hypothermia
   e. Hypotension associated with angiotensin-converting enzyme inhibition
   f. Embolism (air and particulate)
   g. Nonimmune hemolysis
III. Delayed (Greater than 24 h) Immune-Mediated Transfusion Reactions
   a. Hemolytic
   b. Alloimmunization to red blood cell, white blood cell, platelet, and protein antigens
   c. Graft versus host
IV. Delayed (Greater than 24 h) Non–Immune-Mediated Transfusion Reactions
   a. Iron overload

I. Acute Immune-Mediated Transfusion Reactions

a. ABO and non-ABO acute hemolytic	Dramatic, severe, and can be fatal; incidence 1:38,000 to 1:70,000 units; result of reaction between antibodies in the patient's plasma and the corresponding antigen being present on the donor's cells; severity affected by amount of patient antibody present, quantity of antigen on transfused cells, volume of blood transfused
Symptoms	Fever, chills, hypotension, tachycardia, nausea, vomiting, lower back pain, hemoglobinuria, renal failure with oliguria, flushing, generalized bleeding, pain or oozing at the infusion site
Lab Findings	Positive DAT; elevated: indirect bilirubin (5 to 7 h post-transfusion), LDH, BUN, creatinine, PT, PTT; decreased: anti-A and anti-B titers, haptoglobin; hemoglobinemia; hemoglobinuria; hypofibrinogenemia; thrombocytopenia; positive urinary hemosiderin; presence of spherocytes and RBC fragments on peripheral smear
Treatment	Immediately stop transfusion, maintain renal flow at greater than 100 mL/h by use of osmotic and diuretic agents (e.g., lasix, furosemide); monitor for development of DIC (uncontrolled bleeding, decreasing platelet count, prolonged PT/PTT); future transfusion with O-negative packed cells
b. Febrile nonhemolytic	Most common type of transfusion reaction; incidence 1:200 to 1:17 (0.5% to 6.0%); repeat occurrences are uncommon; result of antileukocyte, antiplatelet, or anti-HLA antibodies
Symptoms	Fever, chills, headache, vomiting
Lab Findings	Negative DAT; transient leukopenia
Treatment	Immediately stop transfusion; administer antipyretics (steroids in severe cases); transfuse with leukocyte-reduced blood after two documented febrile nonhemolytic reactions
c. Urticarial/allergic reaction	Second most common type of reaction; incidence 1:100 to 1:33 (1% to 3%); histamine-mediated reaction of allergin + IgE fixed on mast cells
Symptoms	Local erythema; hives; itching; usually no fever
Lab Findings	Negative DAT
Treatment	Immediately stop transfusion; keep line open; administer antihistamines (e.g., benadryl 25 to 50 mg); resume transfusion when symptoms subside; for future transfusions, premedicate with antihistamines

(Continued on the following page)

I. Acute Immune-Mediated Transfusion Reactions *(Continued)*

d. Anaphylactic reaction	Occurs rapidly with 10 mL or less; 1 in 700 individuals are IgA deficient and 25% have anti-IgA antibodies that will react to donor's plasma proteins; incidence 1:20,000 to 1:50,000
Symptoms	Hypotension, urticaria, flushing, substernal pain, abdominal cramping, laryngeal edema, bronchospasm, circulatory collapse, anxiety
Lab Findings	Negative DAT; presence of IgG class anti-IgA antibodies or undetectable level of IgA
Treatment	Treat for anaphylaxis with epinephrine, steroid therapy as needed; oxygen therapy as needed; Trendelenburg position; fluids; for future transfusions, premedicate with antihistamines and transfuse with IgA-deficient donor blood or autologous blood

II. Acute Non–Immune-Mediated Transfusion Reactions

a. Transfusion-related acute lung injury	Reaction to anti-WBC antibodies in donor unit; incidence 1:5000 to 1:190,000
Symptoms	Hypoxemia, respiratory failure, hypotension, fever
Lab Findings	Positive WBC antibody screen (donor or recipient), incompatible WBC crossmatch
Treatment	Supportive care until recovered; defer implicated donors
b. Circulatory overload	Incidence less than 1%; result of volume overload
Symptoms	Dyspnea, orthopnea, cough, tachycardia, hypertension, headache
Lab Findings	N/A
Treatment	Upright posture; oxygen; diuretic; administer blood slowly; phlebotomy (250-mL increments)
c. Metabolic complications	Hypocalcemia resulting from rapid massive infusion of citrate; incidence dependent on clinical setting
Symptoms	Paresthesia, tetany, arrhythmia
Lab Findings	Elevated ionized calcium level, prolonged Q-T interval on EKG
Treatment	Slow calcium infusion, PO calcium supplement for mild symptoms; monitor ionized calcium levels (severe symptoms)
d. Hypothermia	Result of rapid infusion of cold blood
Symptoms	Cardiac arrhythmia
Lab Findings	N/A
Treatment	Utilize blood warmer

e. Hypotension associated with ACE inhibition	Patients on ACE inhibitors receiving leukocyte-reduced packed cells have experienced hypotension (believed to be the result of an interaction between the ACE inhibitor and the kinin/prekallikrein system); incidence is dependent on the clinical setting.
Symptoms	Flushing, hypotension
Lab Findings	Positive DAT, hemolyzed intra- or post-transfusion specimen
Treatment	Avoid bedside leukocyte filtration
f. Embolism (air and particulate)	Result of air infusion via line; incidence is rare
Symptoms	Sudden shortness of breath; acute cyanosis; pain; cough; hypotension; cardiac arrhythmia
Lab Findings	N/A
Treatment	Position patient on left side with legs elevated above head and chest
g. Nonimmune hemolysis	Result of physical or chemical destruction of RBCs (e.g., heating, freezing, hemolytic drug, solution added to blood); incidence is rare
Symptoms	Hemoglobinuria
Lab Findings	Positive plasma free hemoglobin, positive DAT, obvious hemolysis in unit containing the blood
Treatment	Identify and eliminate cause

III. Delayed Immune-Mediated Transfusion Reactions

a. Hemolytic	Anamnestic immune response to RBC antigens; incidence 1:11,000 to 1:50,000
Symptoms	Fever, anemia, mild jaundice
Lab Findings	Positive antibody screen, urinary hemosiderin and DAT; increased LDH, bilirubin
Treatment	Identify antibody and transfuse compatible blood as needed
b. Alloimmunization to RBC, WBC, platelet, and protein antigens	Immune response to RBC, WBC, or platelet antigens; incidence 1:100
Symptoms	Delayed hemolytic reaction
Lab Findings	Positive antibody screen and DAT
Treatment	Avoid unnecessary transfusions; give leukocyte-reduced blood if transfusion is necessary
c. Graft versus host	Donor lymphocytes attack recipient's host tissue; incidence is rare
Symptoms	Erythroderma, maculopapular rash, anorexia, nausea, vomiting, diarrhea, hepatitis, pancytopenia, fever

(Continued on the following page)

III. Delayed Immune-Mediated Transfusion Reactions *(Continued)*

Lab Findings	Abnormal skin biopsy, incompatible HLA typing
Treatment	Methotrexate, corticosteroids; transfuse with irradiated blood products

IV. Delayed Non-Immune-Mediated Transfusion Reactions

a. Iron overload	Result of chronic transfusions (greater than 100)
Symptoms	
Lab Findings	Symptoms associated with diabetes, cirrhosis, cardiomyopathy
Treatment	Increased iron levels
	Desferioxamine

ACE = angiotensin-converting enzyme; BUN = blood urea nitrogen; DAT = (Coombs') direct antiglobulin test; DIC = disseminated intravascular coagulation; ECG = electrocardiogram; HLA = human leukocyte antigen; Ig = immunoglobulin; LDH = lactate dehydrogenase; N/A = non applicable; PT = prothrombin time; PTT = partial thromboplastin time; RBC = red blood cell; WBC = white blood cell.

Introduction to CLIA 1988 & 1992

The acronym *CLIA* stands for Clinical Laboratory Improvement Amendments. In 1988, Congress passed CLIA in order to establish quality standards that would apply to laboratory testing nationwide. The standards ensure that, regardless of location, all clinical testing on human specimens is performed with accuracy, reliability, and timeliness. In 1992, CLIA final regulations distinguished between levels of test complexity. Three categories were established: waived complexity, moderate complexity (includes the subcategory of Provider-Performed Microscopy [PPM]), and high complexity testing. Permission to perform clinical laboratory testing in any or all categories requires the laboratory director to submit an application to enroll in the CLIA program, pay the applicable fee biennially, and meet quality requirements that correspond to the type of certificate that is obtained.

A Certificate of Waiver (COW) obtained by the appropriate health care practitioner allows qualified nursing or other health care personnel to perform procedures classified as waived testing in a health care practitioner's office or in a hospital nursing unit. Waived testing includes tests that are cleared by the Food and Drug Administration (FDA) for home use, have manufacturers' instructions to follow, and pose no harm to the patient if testing is performed incorrectly. The testing process utilizes controls. Examples of waived testing include dipstick urinalysis, fecal occult blood, ovulation testing, urine pregnancy tests, erythrocyte sedimentation rate (nonautomated), hemoglobin (copper sulfate method), and blood glucose (on glucose meters cleared by the FDA).

PPM laboratories perform moderately complex testing. This type of testing can be performed in a health care practitioner's office. A PPM certificate obtained by the health care practitioner allows the practitioner to perform moderately complex testing on specimens obtained during the patient's office visit, in addition to waived testing. A microscope is utilized to view the specimens during the patient's office visit. These moderately complex tests are performed on specimens in situations in which the accuracy of the findings would be compromised if a delay in testing were to occur. The testing process has no available controls. Examples of PPM testing include urine sediment examinations, potassium hydroxide preparations, pinworm examinations, fern tests, nasal smears for granulocytes, fecal leukocyte examinations, qualitative semen analysis, and wet mount testing for the presence or absence of bacteria, fungi, parasites, and cellular elements.

Hospital and reference laboratories perform tests of high complexity. The laboratory director must obtain the corresponding CLIA certificate and have personnel qualified to perform tests of high complexity.

Effects of Natural Products on Laboratory Values

The use of natural products has increased significantly, but to date, their preparation is unregulated. Their actions can affect normal and abnormal physiologic processes as well as interact with prescription medications. Their presence in the body, alone or in combination with over-the-counter products or prescription medications, may physiologically affect the intended target or cause analytical interference in such a way that the test result is affected. For this reason, it is important to note their use. The natural products listed here are contraindicated or are recommended for use with caution in patients with body system disorders or patients taking medications for these disorders. The requesting health care practitioner and laboratory should be advised if the patient is regularly using these products so that their potential effects can be taken into consideration when reviewing results.

This list is not all-inclusive. Questions regarding the potential benefits and contraindications of natural products should be referred to the appropriate health care practitioner. As a general recommendation, natural products and nutraceuticals are contraindicated during pregnancy and lactation.

Natural Products That May Affect Cardiovascular Disorders or Interact with Therapeutics (Including Hypertension and Hypotension)

Adonis
Aloe
Bromelain
Buckthorn
Cascara
Chinese rhubarb
Coleus
Dong quai
Elder
Ephedra
Ergot
Frangula
Garlic
Ginseng
Goldenseal
Green tea (with caffeine)
Henbane
Horsetail
Lily of the valley
Ma-huang
Reishi
Senna
Squill
Tylophora
Valerian
Yohimbe bark

Natural Products and Nutraceuticals That May Affect Endocrine Disorders or Interact with Therapeutics

Natural Products

Bilberry
Bitter melon
Bladderwrack
Blupleurum
Bugleweed
Echinacea
Ephedra
Fenugreek
Garcinia
Garlic
Ginseng
Goat's rue
Green tea (with caffeine)
Guggul
Licorice
Marshmallow
Olive leaf
Psyllium
Tylophora

Minerals

Chromium
Nutraceuticals
Dehydroepiandrosterone
α-Lipoic acid
Para-aminobenzoic acid
Thyroid extract

Natural Products and Nutraceuticals That May Affect Gastrointestinal Disorders or Interact with Therapeutics

Natural Products

Bromelain
Cascara
Chinese rhubarb
Dandelion
Psyllium
Senna

Nutraceuticals

Betaine hydrochloride

Natural Products and Nutraceuticals That May Affect Genitourinary Disorders or Interact with Therapeutics

Natural Products

Aloe
Arabinoxylane
Bladderwrack
Buckthorn
Cascara
Chinese rhubarb
Dandelion
Echinacea
Ephedra
Ergot
Frangula
Ginseng
Guarana
Horse chestnut
Horsetail
Licorice
Parsley oil (high doses)
Saw palmetto
Senna
Stinging nettle
White oak
White willow

Nutraceuticals

Creatine
Modified citrus pectin

Natural Products and Nutraceuticals That May Affect Bleeding Disorders or Interact with Therapeutics

Natural Products

Arnica
Astragalus
Bilberry
Bromelian

Cat's claw
Cayenne
Coleus
Cordyceps
Devil's claw
Dong quai
Evening primrose
Feverfew
Garlic
Ginger
Gingko
Ginseng
Grape seed
Green tea (with caffeine)
Guggui
Horse chestnut
Papaya
Red clover
Red yeast rice
Reishi
Turmeric
White willow

Nutraceuticals

Docosahexaenoic acid (DHA)
Fish oils (EPA and DHA)

Natural Products and Nutraceuticals That May Affect Hepatobiliary Disorders or Interact with Therapeutics

Natural Products

Alkanet
Alpine ragwort
Coltsfoot
Comfrey
Dusty miller
Forget-me-not
Germander

Groundsel
Olive leaf
Parsley oil (large doses)
Pennyroyal
Peppermint
Ragwort
Red yeast rice
Sweet clover
White oak
White willow

Nutraceuticals

Creatine

Natural Products and Amino Acids That May Affect Immune Disorders or Interact with Therapeutics

Natural Products

Astragalus
Black cohosh
Echinacea
Saw palmetto

Amino Acids

Arginine

Natural Products That May Affect Respiratory Disorders or Interact with Therapeutics

Artichoke
Cayenne
Chamomile
Cordyceps
Echinacea
Feverfew
Garlic
Peppermint oil
White willow

Standard Precautions (CDC Isolation Precautions)

Background and Summary

In January 1996, the Centers for Disease Control and Prevention (CDC) issued new guidelines for isolation precautions in hospitals. The guidelines, based on the latest epidemiologic information on transmission of infection in hospitals, are intended primarily for use in acute-care hospitals, although some of the recommendations may be applicable to subacute-care or extended-care facilities. The recommendations are not intended for use in day care, well care, or domiciliary care programs.

The revised guidelines contain two tiers of precautions. In the first, and most important, tier are precautions designed for the care of all patients in hospitals regardless of their diagnosis or presumed infection status. Implementation of these Standard Precautions is the primary strategy for successful nosocomial infection control. In the second tier are precautions designed only for the care of specified patients. These additional Transmission-Based Precautions are used for patients who are known or suspected to be infected or colonized with epidemiologically important pathogens that can be transmitted by airborne or droplet transmission or by contact with dry skin or contaminated surfaces.

Standard Precautions synthesize the major features of Universal (Blood and Body Fluid) Precautions (designed to reduce the risk of transmission of blood-borne pathogens) and Body Substance Isolation (designed to reduce the risk of transmission of pathogens from moist body substances). Standard Precautions apply to (1) blood; (2) all body fluids, secretions, and excretions *except sweat,* regardless of whether they contain visible blood; (3) nonintact skin; and (4) mucous membranes. Standard Precautions are designed to reduce the risk of transmission of recognized and unrecognized sources of infection in hospitals.

Transmission-Based Precautions are designed for patients documented or suspected to be infected or colonized with highly transmissible or epidemiologically important pathogens for which additional precautions beyond Standard Precautions are needed to interrupt transmission in hospitals. There are three types of Transmission-Based Precautions: Airborne Precautions, Droplet Precautions, and Contact Precautions. They may be combined for diseases that have multiple routes of transmission. When used either singly or in combination, they are to be used in addition to Standard Precautions.

Airborne Precautions are designed to reduce the risk of airborne transmission of infectious agents. Airborne transmission occurs by dissemination of either airborne droplet nuclei (small-particle residue [5 μm or smaller in size] of evaporated droplets that may remain suspended in the air for long periods) or dust particles containing the infectious agent. Microorganisms carried in this manner can be dispersed widely by air currents and may become inhaled by or deposited on a susceptible host within the same room or over a longer distance from the source patient, depending on environmental factors; special air handling and ventilation are required to prevent airborne transmission. Examples of diseases spread by airborne droplet nuclei include measles, varicella (including disseminated zoster), and tuberculosis.

Droplet Precautions are designed to reduce the risk of droplet transmission of infectious agents. Droplet transmission involves contact of the conjunctivae or the mucous membranes of the nose or mouth of a susceptible person with large-particle droplets (larger than 5 μm in size) containing microorganisms generated from a person who has a clinical disease or who is a carrier of the microorganism. Droplets are generated from the source person primarily during coughing, sneezing, or talking and during the performance of certain procedures such as suctioning and bronchoscopy. Transmission via large-particle droplets requires close contact between source and recipient persons because droplets do not remain suspended in the air and generally travel only short distances, usually 3 ft or less, through the air. Because droplets do not remain suspended in the air, special air handling and ventilation are not required to prevent droplet transmission. Examples of illnesses spread by large-particle droplets include invasive *Haemophilus influenzae* type B disease (including meningitis, pneumonia, epiglottitis, and sepsis); invasive *Neisseria meningitidis* disease (including meningitis, pneumonia, and sepsis); diphtheria (pharyngeal); mycoplasmal pneumonia; pertussis; pneumonic plague; streptococcal pharyngitis, pneumonia, or scarlet fever in infants and young children; adenovirus influenza; mumps; parvovirus B19; and rubella.

Contact Precautions are designed to reduce the risk of transmission of epidemiologically important microorganisms by direct or indirect contact. Direct-contact transmission involves skin-to-skin contact and physical transfer of microorganisms to a susceptible host from an infected or colonized person, such as occurs when personnel turn patients, bathe patients, or perform other patient care activities that require physical contact. Direct-contact transmission also can occur between two patients (e.g., by hand contact), with one serving as the source of infectious microorganisms and the other as a susceptible host. Indirect-contact transmission involves contact of a susceptible host with a contaminated intermediate object, usually inanimate, in the patient's environment. Examples of illnesses spread by direct contact include gastrointestinal, respiratory, skin, or wound infections or colonization with multidrug-resistant bacteria judged by the infection control program (based on current state, regional, or national recommendations) to be of special clinical and epidemiologic significance; enteric infections with a low infectious dose or prolonged environmental survival, including *Clostridium difficile;* for diapered or incontinent patients, enterohemorrhagic *Escherichia coli* O157:H7, *Shigella*, hepatitis A, or rotavirus; respiratory syncytial virus, parainfluenza virus, or enteroviral infections in infants and young children; viral/hemorrhagic conjunctivitis; viral hemorrhagic infections (Ebola, Lassa, or

Marburg); and skin infections that are highly contagious or that may occur on dry skin, including:

- Diphtheria (cutaneous)
- Herpes simplex virus (neonatal or mucocutaneous)
- Impetigo
- Major (noncontained) abscesses, cellulitis, or decubiti
- Pediculosis
- Scabies
- Staphylococcal furunculosis in infants and young children
- Zoster (disseminated or in the immunocompromised host)

Standard Precautions

Use the following Standard Precautions, or the equivalent, for the care of all patients.

Handwashing

Wash hands after touching blood, body fluids, secretions, excretions, and contaminated items, whether or not gloves are worn. Wash hands immediately after gloves are removed, between patient contacts, and when otherwise indicated to avoid transfer of microorganisms to other patients or environments. It may be necessary to wash hands between tasks and procedures on the same patient to prevent cross-contamination of different body sites.

Use a plain (nonantimicrobial) soap for routine handwashing.

Use an antimicrobial agent or a waterless antiseptic agent for specific circumstances (e.g., control of outbreaks or hyperendemic infections), as defined by the infection control program. (See Contact Precautions for additional recommendations on using antimicrobial and antiseptic agents.)

Gloves

Wear gloves (clean, nonsterile gloves are adequate) when touching blood, body fluids, secretions, excretions, and contaminated items.

Put on clean gloves just before touching mucous membranes and nonintact skin.

Change gloves between tasks and procedures on the same patient after contact with material that may contain a high concentration of microorganisms.

Remove gloves promptly after use, before touching noncontaminated items and environmental surfaces, and before going to another patient. Wash hands immediately to avoid transfer of microorganisms to other patients or environments.

Mask, Eye Protection, Face Shield

Wear a mask and eye protection or a face shield to protect mucous membranes of the eyes, nose, and mouth during procedures and patient care activities that are likely to generate splashes or sprays of blood, body fluids, secretions, and excretions.

Gown

Wear a gown (a clean, nonsterile gown is adequate) to protect skin and to prevent soiling of clothing during procedures and patient care activities that are likely to generate splashes or sprays of blood, body fluids, secretions, or excretions.

Select a gown that is appropriate for the activity and amount of fluid likely to be encountered.

Remove a soiled gown as promptly as possible. Wash hands to avoid transfer of microorganisms to other patients or environments.

Patient Care Equipment

Handle used patient care equipment soiled with blood, body fluids, secretions, and excretions in a manner that prevents skin and mucous membrane exposures, contamination of clothing, and transfer of microorganisms to other patients and environments.

Ensure that reusable equipment is not used for the care of another patient until it has been cleaned and reprocessed appropriately. Ensure that single-use items are discarded properly.

Environmental Control

Ensure that the hospital has adequate procedures for the routine care, cleaning, and disinfection of environmental surfaces, beds, bedrails, bedside equipment, and other frequently touched surfaces, and ensure that these procedures are being followed.

Linen

Handle, transport, and process used linen soiled with blood, body fluids, secretions, and excretions in a manner that prevents skin and mucous membrane exposures and contamination of clothing and that avoids transfer of microorganisms to other patients and environments.

Occupational Health and Blood-Borne Pathogens

Take care to prevent injuries when using needles, scalpels, and other sharp instruments or devices; when handling sharp instruments after procedures; when cleaning used instruments; and when disposing of used needles.

Never recap used needles or otherwise manipulate them using both hands, or use any other technique that involves directing the point of a needle toward any part of the body; rather, use either a one-handed "scoop" technique or a mechanical device designed for holding the needle sheath.

Do not remove used needles from disposable syringes by hand, and do not bend, break, or otherwise manipulate a used needle by hand.

Place used disposable syringes and needles, scalpel blades, and other sharp items in appropriate puncture-resistant containers, which are located as close as practical to the area in which the items were used, and place reusable syringes and needles in a puncture-resistant container for transport to the reprocessing area.

Use mouthpieces, resuscitation bags, or other ventilation devices as an alternative to mouth-to-mouth resuscitation methods in areas where the need for resuscitation is predictable.

Patient Placement

Place a patient who contaminates the environment or who does not (or cannot be expected to) assist in maintaining appropriate hygiene or environmental control in a private room. If a private room is not available, consult with infection control professionals regarding patient placement or other alternatives.

Transmission-Based Precautions

Airborne Precautions

In addition to Standard Precautions, use Airborne Precautions, or the equivalent, for patients known or suspected to be infected with microorganisms transmitted by airborne droplet nuclei (small-particle residue [5 μm or smaller in size] of evaporated droplets containing microorganisms that remain suspended in the air and that can be dispersed widely by air currents within a room or over a long distance).

Patient Placement

Place the patient in a private room that has (1) monitored negative air pressure in relation to the surrounding areas, (2) 6 to 12 air changes per hour, and (3) appropriate discharge of air outdoors or monitored high-efficiency filtration of room air before the air is circulated to other areas in the hospital.
Keep the room door closed and the patient in the room.
When a private room is not available, place the patient in a room with a patient who has active infection with the same microorganism but with no other infection (cohorting), unless otherwise recommended. When a private room is not available and cohorting is not desirable, consultation with infection control professionals is advised before patient placement.

Respiratory Protection

Wear respiratory protection when entering the room of a patient with known or suspected infectious pulmonary tuberculosis.
Susceptible persons should not enter the room of patients known or suspected to have measles (rubeola) or varicella (chickenpox) if other immune caregivers are available. If susceptible persons must enter the room of a patient known or suspected to have measles or varicella, they should wear respiratory protection. Persons immune to measles or varicella need not wear respiratory protection.

Patient Transport

Limit the movement and transport of the patient from the room to essential purposes only. If transport or movement is necessary, minimize patient dispersal of droplet nuclei by placing a surgical mask on the patient, if possible.

Additional Precautions for Preventing Transmission of Tuberculosis

Consult the CDC's "Guidelines for Preventing the Transmission of Tuberculosis in Health-Care Facilities" for additional prevention strategies.[1]

Droplet Precautions

In addition to Standard Precautions, use Droplet Precautions, or the equivalent, for a patient known or suspected to be infected with microorganisms transmitted by droplets (large-particle droplets [larger than 5 μm in size] that can be generated during coughing, sneezing, talking, or the performance of procedures).

Patient Placement

Place the patient in a private room. When a private room is not available, place the patient in a room with a patient who has active infection with the same microorganism but with no other infection (cohorting). When a private room is not available and cohorting is not achievable, maintain spatial separation of at least 3 ft between the infected patient and other patients and visitors.

Special air handling and ventilation are not necessary, and the door may remain open.

Mask

In addition to Standard Precautions, wear a mask when working within 3 ft of the patient. (Logistically, some hospitals may want to implement the wearing of a mask to enter the room.)

Patient Transport

Limit the movement and transport of the patient from the room to essential purposes only.

If transport or movement is necessary, minimize patient dispersal of droplets by masking the patient, if possible.

Contact Precautions

In addition to Standard Precautions, use Contact Precautions, or the equivalent, for specified patients known or suspected to be infected or colonized with epidemiologically important microorganisms that can be transmitted by direct contact with the patient (hand or skin-to-skin contact that occurs when performing patient care activities that require touching the patient's dry skin) or indirect contact (touching) with environmental surfaces or patient care items in the patient's environment.

Patient Placement

Place the patient in a private room. When a private room is not available, place the patient in a room with a patient who has active infection with the same microorganism but with no other infection (cohorting).

---

[1]Employees who received training in the year preceding the effective date of the standard need only receive training pertaining to any provisions not already included.

When a private room is not available and cohorting is not achievable, consider the epidemiology of the microorganism and the patient population when determining patient placement. Consultation with infection control professionals is advised before patient placement.

Gloves and Handwashing

In addition to wearing gloves as outlined under Standard Precautions, wear gloves (clean, nonsterile gloves are adequate) when entering the room.

During the course of providing care for a patient, change gloves after having contact with infective material that may contain high concentrations of microorganisms (fecal material and wound drainage).

Remove gloves before leaving the patient's environment and wash hands immediately with an antimicrobial agent or a waterless antiseptic agent. After glove removal and handwashing, ensure that hands do not touch potentially contaminated environmental surfaces or items in the patient's room to avoid transfer of microorganisms to other patients or environments.

Gown

In addition to wearing a gown as outlined under Standard Precautions, wear a gown (a clean, nonsterile gown is adequate) when entering the room if you anticipate that your clothing will have substantial contact with the patient, environmental surfaces, or items in the patient's room or if the patient is incontinent or has diarrhea, an ileostomy, a colostomy, or wound drainage not contained by a dressing.

Remove the gown before leaving the patient's environment. After gown removal, ensure that clothing does not contact potentially contaminated environmental surfaces to avoid transfer of microorganisms to other patients or environments.

Patient Transport

Limit the movement and transport of the patient from the room to essential purposes only.

If the patient is transported out of the room, ensure that precautions are maintained to minimize the risk of transmission of microorganisms to other patients and contamination of environmental surfaces or equipment.

Patient Care Equipment

When possible, dedicate the use of noncritical patient care equipment to a single patient (or cohort of patients infected or colonized with the pathogen requiring precautions) to avoid sharing between patients.

If use of common equipment or items is unavoidable, adequately clean and disinfect them before use for another patient.

Additional Precautions for Preventing the Spread of Vancomycin Resistance

Consult the Hospital Infection Control Practices Advisory Committee report on preventing the spread of vancomycin resistance for additional prevention strategies.

OSHA Blood-Borne Pathogens Standard

Who is Covered?

The Occupational Safety and Health Administration (OSHA) standard protects employees who may be occupationally exposed to blood and other potentially infectious materials, which includes but is not limited to physicians, physician assistants, nurses, nurse practitioners, and other health care employees in clinics and physicians' offices; employees of clinical and diagnostic laboratories; housekeepers in health care and other facilities; personnel in hospital laundries or commercial laundries that service health care or public safety institutions; tissue bank personnel; employees in blood banks and plasma centers who collect, transport, and test blood; free-standing clinic employees (e.g., hemodialysis clinics, urgent care clinics, health maintenance organization [HMO] clinics, and family planning clinics); employees in clinics in industrial, educational, and correctional facilities (e.g., employees who collect blood and clean and dress wounds); employees designated to provide emergency first aid; dentists, dental hygienists, dental assistants, and dental laboratory technicians; staff of institutions for the developmentally disabled; hospice employees; home health care workers; staff of nursing homes and long-term care facilities; employees of funeral homes and mortuaries; human immunodeficiency virus (HIV) and hepatitis B virus (HBV) research laboratory and production facility workers; employees handling regulated waste; custodial workers required to clean up contaminated sharps or spills of blood or other potentially infectious material (OPIM); medical equipment service and repair personnel; emergency medical technicians, paramedics, and other emergency medical service providers; firefighters, law enforcement personnel, and correctional officers (employees in the private sector, the federal government, or a state or local government in a state that has an OSHA-approved state plan); maintenance workers, such as plumbers, in health care facilities; and employees of substance abuse clinics.

Blood means human blood, blood products, or blood components (plasma, platelets, and serosanguineous fluids [e.g., exudates from wounds]). Also included are medications derived from blood, such as immune globulins, albumin, and factors VIII and IX. Other potentially infectious materials include human body fluids, such as saliva in dental procedures; semen; vaginal secretions; cerebrospinal, synovial, pleural, pericardial, peritoneal, and amniotic fluids; body fluids visibly contaminated with blood; unfixed human tissues or organs; HIV-containing cell or tissue cultures; and HIV-containing or HBV-containing culture media or other solutions.

Occupational exposure means a "reasonably anticipated skin, eye, mucous membrane, or parenteral contact [human bites that break the skin, which are most likely to occur in violent situations such as may be encountered by prison personnel and police and in emergency departments or psychiatric wards] with blood or other potentially infectious materials that may result from the performance of the employee's duties." The term *reasonably anticipated contact* includes the potential for contact and actual contact with blood or OPIM. Lack of history of blood exposures among designated first aid personnel of a particular manufacturing site, for instance, does not preclude coverage. Reasonably anticipated contact includes, among others, contact with blood or OPIM, including regulated waste, as well as incidents of needle sticks. A compliance officer may document incidents in which an employee observes uncapped needles or contacts other regulated waste to substantiate occupational exposure.

Federal OSHA authority extends to all private sector employers with one or more employees, as well as federal civilian employees. In addition, many states administer their own occupational safety and health programs through plans approved under section 18(b) of the Occupational Safety and Health Act. These plans must adopt standards and enforce requirements that are at least as effective as federal requirements. Of the current 25 states and territories with plans, 23 cover the private and public (state and local governments) sectors and 2 cover the public sector only.

Determining occupational exposure and instituting control methods and work practices appropriate for specific job assignments are key requirements of the standard. The required written exposure control plan and methods of compliance show how employee exposure can be minimized or eliminated.

Exposure Control Plan

A written exposure control plan is necessary for the safety and health of workers. At a minimum, the plan must include the following:
Identify job classifications in which there is exposure to blood or other potentially infectious materials.
Explain the protective measures currently in effect in the acute-care facility or a schedule and methods of compliance to be implemented, including hepatitis B vaccination and postexposure follow-up procedures, how hazards are communicated to employees, personal protective equipment (PPE), housekeeping, and record keeping.
Establish procedures for evaluating the circumstances of an exposure incident.

The schedule of how and when the provisions of the standard will be implemented may be a simple calendar with brief notations describing the compliance methods, an annotated copy of the standard, or a part of another document, such as the infection control plan. The written exposure control plan must be available to workers and OSHA representatives and updated at least annually or whenever changes in procedures create new occupational exposures.

Who has Occupational Exposure?

The exposure determination must be based on the definition of occupational exposure without regard to personal protective clothing and equipment. Exposure determination begins by reviewing job classifications of employees within the work environment, and then making a list divided into two groups: classifications in which all of the employees have occupational exposure and classifications in which some of the employees have occupational exposure.

Where all employees are occupationally exposed, it is not necessary to list specific work tasks. Some examples include phlebotomists, laboratory technicians, physicians, nurses, nurse's aides, surgical technicians, and emergency department personnel.

Where only some of the employees have exposure, specific tasks and procedures causing exposure must be listed. Examples include ward clerks or secretaries, who occasionally handle blood or infectious specimens, and housekeeping staff, who may be exposed to contaminated objects or environments some of the time.

When employees with occupational exposure have been identified, the next step is to communicate the hazards of the exposure to the employees.

Communicating Hazards to Employees

The initial training for current employees must be scheduled within 90 days of the effective date of the blood-borne pathogens standard, at no cost to the employee, and during working hours.[1] Training also is required for new workers at the time of their initial assignment to tasks with occupational exposure or when job tasks change, causing occupational exposure, and annually thereafter.

Training sessions must be comprehensive in nature, including information on blood-borne pathogens as well as on OSHA regulations and the employer's exposure control plan. Although HBV and HIV are specifically identified in the standard, the term *blood-borne pathogen* includes any pathogenic microorganism that is present in human blood or other potentially infectious materials and can infect and cause disease in persons who are exposed to blood containing the pathogen. Pathogenic microorganisms also can cause diseases such as hepatitis C, malaria, syphilis, babesiosis, brucellosis, leptospirosis, arboviral infections, relapsing fever, Creutzfeldt-Jakob disease, adult T-cell leukemia/lymphoma (caused by human T-cell leukemia/lymphoma virus [HTLV-I]), HTLV-I–associated myelopathy, diseases associated with HTLV-II, and viral hemorrhagic fever. The person conducting the training must be knowledgeable in the subject matter as it relates to acute care facilities.

Specifically, the training program must do the following:

- Explain the regulatory text and make a copy of the regulatory text accessible.
- Explain the epidemiology and symptoms of blood-borne diseases.
- Explain the modes of transmission of blood-borne pathogens.
- Explain the employer's written exposure control plan.
- Describe the methods to control transmission of HBV and HIV.
- Explain how to recognize occupational exposure.
- Inform workers about the availability of free hepatitis B vaccinations and vaccine efficacy, safety, benefits, and administration.
- Explain the emergency procedures for and reporting of exposure incidents.
- Inform workers of the postexposure evaluation and follow-up available from health care professionals.
- Describe how to select, use, remove, handle, decontaminate, and dispose of personal protective clothing and equipment.
- Explain the use and limitations of safe work practices, engineering controls (controls that isolate or remove the blood-borne pathogens hazard from the workplace; examples include needleless devices, shielded needle devices, blunt needles, plastic capillary tubes), and PPE.
- Explain the use of labels, signs, and color coding required by the standard.
- Provide a question-and-answer session on training.

In addition to communicating hazards to employees and providing training to identify and control hazards, other preventive measures must be taken to ensure employee protection.

Preventive Measures

Preventive measures such as hepatitis B vaccination, universal precautions, engineering controls, safe work practices, PPE, and housekeeping measures help reduce the risks of occupational exposure.

Hepatitis B Vaccination

The hepatitis B vaccination series must be made available within 10 working days of initial assignment to every employee who has occupational exposure. The hepatitis B vaccination must be made available without cost to the employee, at a reasonable time and place for the employee, by a licensed health care professional,[2] and according to recommendations of the U.S. Public Health Service, including routine booster doses.[3]

The health care professional designated by the employer to implement this part of the standard must be provided with a copy of the blood-borne pathogens standard. The health care professional must provide the employer with a written opinion stating whether the hepatitis B vaccination is indicated for the employee and whether the employee has received the vaccination.

Employers are not required to offer hepatitis B vaccination (1) to employees who have previously completed the hepatitis B vaccination series, (2) when immunity is confirmed through antibody testing, or (3) if vaccine is contraindicated for medical reasons. Participation in a prescreening program is not a prerequisite for receiving hepatitis B vaccination. Employees who decline the vaccination may request and obtain it at a later date, if they continue to be exposed. Employees who decline to accept the hepatitis B vaccination must sign a declination form, indicating that they were offered the vaccination but refused it. For more information, refer to "Immunization of Health-Care Workers: Recommendations of ACIP and HICPAC" (*MMWR Morbidity and Mortality Weekly Report,* vol 46, no. RR-18, 1997).

Universal Precautions

The most important measure to control transmission of HBV and HIV is to treat all human blood and other potentially infectious materials *as if they were* infectious for HBV and HIV. (Coverage under this definition also extends to blood and tissues of experimental animals who are infected with HIV or HBV.) Application of this approach is referred to as *universal precautions. Blood and certain body fluids from all acute-care patients should be considered as potentially infectious materials.*[4] These fluids cause *contamination,* defined in the standard as "the presence or the reasonably anticipated presence of blood or other potentially infectious materials on an item or surface."

---

[2]A licensed health care professional is a person whose legally permitted scope of practice allows him or her to perform independently the activities required under paragraph (f) of the standard regarding hepatitis B vaccination and postexposure and follow-up.

[3]Health care professionals can call the CDC disease information hotline (404-332-4555, extension 234), for updated information on hepatitis B vaccination.

[4]See also "Recommendations for Prevention of HIV Transmission in Health-Care Settings" (*MMWR Morbidity and Mortality Weekly Report,* vol 36(2S), August 21, 1987).

Alternative concepts in infection control are called *Body Substance Isolation* and *Standard Precautions.* These methods define all body fluids and substances as infectious. These methods incorporate not only the fluids and materials covered by this standard, but also expand coverage to include all body fluids and substances. These concepts are acceptable alternatives to Universal Precautions, provided that facilities using them adhere to all other provisions of this standard.

Methods of Control

Engineering and Work Practice Controls

Engineering and work practice controls are the primary methods used to control the transmission of HBV and HIV in acute-care facilities. Engineering controls isolate or remove the hazard from employees and are used in conjunction with work practices. Personal protective equipment also is used when occupational exposure to blood-borne pathogens remains even after instituting these controls. Engineering controls must be examined and maintained, or replaced, on a scheduled basis. Some engineering controls that apply to acute-care facilities and are required by the standard include the following:

- Use puncture-resistant, leak-proof containers, color-coded red or labeled, according to the standard (see table), to discard contaminated items such as needles, broken glass, scalpels, or other items that could cause a cut or puncture wound.
- Use puncture-resistant, leak-proof containers, color-coded red or labeled, to store contaminated reusable sharps until they are properly reprocessed.
- Store and process reusable contaminated sharps in a way that ensures safe handling. Use a mechanical device to retrieve used instruments from soaking pans in decontamination areas.
- Use puncture-resistant, leak-proof containers to collect, handle, process, store, transport, or ship blood specimens and potentially infectious materials. Label these specimens if shipped outside the facility. Labeling is not required when specimens are handled by employees trained to use Universal Precautions with all specimens and when these specimens are kept within the facility.

Labeling Requirements

Item	No Label Needed If Universal Precautions Are Used and Specific Use of Container Is Known to All Employees	Biohazard Label	Red Container
Regulated waste container (e.g., contaminated sharps container)		X	or X

Item	No Label Needed If Universal Precautions Are Used and Specific Use of Container Is Known to All Employees	Biohazard Label	Red Container
Reusable contaminated sharps container (e.g., surgical instruments soaking in a tray)		X	or X
Refrigerator/freezer holding blood or other potentially infectious material			X
Containers used for storage, transport, or shipping of blood		X	or X
Blood/blood-borne products for clinical use	X		
Individual specimen containers of blood or other potentially infectious materials remaining in facility	X	or X	or X
Contaminated equipment needing service (e.g., dialysis equipment, suction apparatus)		X Plus a label specifying where the contamination exists	
Specimens and regulated waste shipped from the primary facility to another facility for service or disposal		X	or X
Contaminated laundry	*	or X	or X
Contaminated laundry sent to another facility that does not use universal precautions		X	or X

*Alternative labeling or color coding is sufficient if it permits all employees to recognize containers as requiring compliance with universal precautions.

Similarly, work practice controls reduce the likelihood of exposure by altering the manner in which the task is performed. All procedures must minimize splashing, spraying, splattering, and generation of droplets. Work practice requirements include the following:

- Wash hands when gloves are removed and as soon as possible after contact with blood or other potentially infectious materials.
- Provide and make available a mechanism for immediate eye irrigation, in the event of an exposure incident.
- Do not bend, recap, or remove contaminated needles unless required to do so by specific medical procedures or the employer can show that no alternative is feasible. In these instances, use mechanical means, such as forceps or a one-handed technique, to recap or remove contaminated needles.
- Do not shear or break contaminated needles.
- Discard contaminated needles and sharp instruments in puncture-resistant, leak-proof, red- or biohazard-labeled containers[5] that are accessible, maintained upright, and not allowed to be overfilled.
- Do not eat, drink, smoke, apply cosmetics, or handle contact lenses in areas of potential occupational exposure. (*Note:* Use of hand lotions is acceptable.)
- Do not store food or drink in refrigerators or on shelves where blood or potentially infectious materials are present.
- Use red labels, or affix biohazard labels to, containers to store, transport, or ship blood or other potentially infectious materials, such as laboratory specimens (Figure Appendix G–1).
- Do not use mouth pipetting to suction blood or other potentially infectious materials; it is prohibited.

Additional Information on Engineering Controls

Effective Engineering Controls ECRI: ECRI (formerly Emergency Care Research Institute), designated as an evidence-based practice center by the Agency for

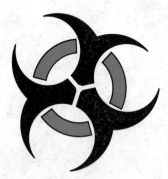

FIGURE G–1

---

[5]Biohazard labeling requires a fluorescent orange or orange-red label with the biologic hazard symbol as well as the word *Biohazard* in contrasting color affixed to the bag or container.

Healthcare Research and Quality, is a nonprofit international health services research organization. Their web site includes a discussion of the June 1998 issue of ECRI's *Health Devices,* which evaluated 19 needle stick–prevention devices, and provides information on how to obtain this document (available at: www. healthcare.ecri.org/site/whatsnew/press.releases/980724hdneedle.html).

Food and Drug Administration (FDA) Safety Alert: Needlestick and other risks from hypodermic needles on secondary IV administration sets—piggyback and intermittent IV (available at: www.fda.gov/cdrh/safety.html). This document warns of the risk of needlestick injuries from the use of hypodermic needles as a connection between two pieces of intravenous (IV) equipment. It also describes characteristics of devices that have the potential to decrease the risk of needle stick injuries.

International Health Care Worker Safety Center, University of Virginia: Their web site contains a page that features a list of safety devices with manufacturers and specific product names (available at: www.people.virginia.edu/epinet/products. html).

National Institute for Occupational Safety and Health (NIOSH): Sharps disposal containers (available at: www.cdc.gov/niosh/sharps1.html). This document features information on selecting, evaluating, and using sharps disposal containers.

Occupational Safety and Health Administration (OSHA): Glass capillary tubes: Joint Safety Advisory about potential risks (available at: www.oshaslc.gov/ OshDoc/Interpdata/I19990222.html). This document describes safer alternatives to conventional glass capillary tubes.

Occupational Safety and Health Administration (OSHA): Needlestick injuries (available at: www.osha-slc.gov/SLTC/needlestick/index.html). This web page features recent news, recognition, evaluation, controls, compliance, and links to information on effective engineering controls.

Safety Sharp Device Contract: The Veterans Administration web site contains a page that features safety sharp devices on contract with the U.S. Department of Veterans Affairs (VA) (available at: www.va.gov/vasafety/osh-issues/needlesafety/ safetysharpcontracts.htm).

SHARPS Injury Control Program: This program was established by Senate Bill 2005 to study sharps injuries in hospitals, skilled nursing facilities, and home health agencies in California. Their web site features a beta version of Safety Enhanced Device Database Listing by Manufacturer (available at: www.ohb.org/sharps.htm).

Training for Development of Innovative Control Technologies (TDICT) Project: Their web site contains a page that features safety feature evaluation forms for specific devices (available at: www.tdict.org/criteria.html).

Personal Protective Equipment

In addition to instituting engineering and work practice controls, the standard requires that appropriate PPE be used to reduce worker risk of exposure. Personal protective equipment is specialized clothing or equipment used by employees to protect against direct exposure to blood or other potentially infectious materials. Protective equipment must not allow blood or other potentially infectious materials to pass through to workers' clothing, skin, or mucous membranes. This equipment includes, but is not limited to, gloves, gowns, laboratory coats, face shields or masks, eye protection, and resuscitator devices. Hypoallergenic gloves, glove liners, powderless gloves, or other similar alternatives must be readily available and accessible at no cost to employees who are allergic to the gloves normally provided.

The employer is responsible for providing, maintaining, laundering, disposing of, replacing, and ensuring the proper use of PPE. The employer is responsible for ensuring that workers have access to the protective equipment, at no cost, including proper sizes and types that take allergic conditions into consideration.

An employee may temporarily and briefly decline to wear PPE under rare and extraordinary circumstances and when, in the employee's professional judgment, wearing PPE prevents the delivery of health care or public safety services or poses an increased or life-threatening hazard to employees. In general, appropriate PPE is expected to be used whenever occupational exposure may occur.

The employer also must ensure that employees observe the following precautions for safely handling and using PPE:

- Remove all PPE immediately after contamination and on leaving the work area, and place in an appropriately designated area or container for storing, washing, decontaminating, or discarding.
- Wear appropriate gloves when contact with blood, mucous membranes, nonintact skin (e.g., skin with dermatitis, hangnails, cuts, abrasions, chafing, acne), or potentially infectious materials is anticipated; when performing vascular access procedures[6]; and when handling or touching contaminated items or surfaces.
- Provide hypoallergenic gloves, liners, or powderless gloves or other alternatives to employees who need them.
- Replace disposable, single-use gloves as soon as possible when contaminated or if torn or punctured, or barrier function is compromised.
- Do not reuse disposable (single-use) gloves.
- Decontaminate reusable (utility) gloves after each use, and discard if they show signs of cracking, peeling, tearing, puncturing, deteriorating, or failing to provide a protective barrier.
- Use full face shields or face masks with eye protection, goggles, or eyeglasses with side shields when splashes of blood and other bodily fluids may occur and when contamination of the eyes, nose, or mouth can be anticipated (e.g., during invasive and surgical procedures).
- Also wear surgical caps or hoods and shoe covers or boots when gross contamination may occur, such as during surgery and autopsy procedures.

Remember: The selection of appropriate PPE depends on the quantity and type of exposure expected.

Housekeeping Procedures

Equipment

The employer must ensure a clean and sanitary workplace. Contaminated work surfaces must be decontaminated with a disinfectant on completion of procedures; when

---

[6]Phlebotomists in volunteer blood donation centers are exempt in certain circumstances. See section (d)(3)(ix)(D) of the standard for specific details.

contaminated by splashes, spills, or contact with blood or other potentially infectious materials; and at the end of the work shift. Surfaces and equipment protected with plastic wrap, foil, or other nonabsorbent materials must be inspected frequently for contamination; these protective coverings must be changed when found to be contaminated.

Waste cans and pails must be inspected and decontaminated on a regularly scheduled basis. Broken glass should be cleaned up with a brush or tongs; never pick up broken glass with hands, even when wearing gloves.

Waste

Waste removed from the facility is regulated by local and state laws. Special precautions are necessary when disposing of contaminated sharps and other contaminated waste and include the following:

* Dispose of contaminated sharps in closable, puncture-resistant, leak-proof, red- or biohazard-labeled containers (see table earlier).
* Place other regulated waste[7] in closable, leak-proof, red- or biohazard-labeled bags or containers. If outside contamination of the regulated waste container occurs, place it in a second container that is closable, leak-proof, and appropriately labeled.

Laundry

Laundering contaminated articles, including employee laboratory coats and uniforms meant to function as PPE, is the responsibility of the employer. Contaminated laundry is handled as little as possible with minimum agitation. This can be accomplished through the use of a washer and dryer in a designated area on-site, or the contaminated items can be sent to a commercial laundry. The following requirements should be met with respect to contaminated laundry:

* Bag contaminated laundry as soon as it is removed and store in a designated area or container.
* Use red laundry bags or those marked with the biohazard symbol unless universal precautions are in effect in the facility, and all employees recognize the bags as contaminated and have been trained in handling the bags.
* Clearly mark laundry sent off-site for cleaning, by placing it in red bags or bags clearly marked with the orange biohazard symbol; use leak-proof bags to prevent soak-through.
* Wear gloves or other protective equipment when handling contaminated laundry.

What to do if an Exposure Incident Occurs

An exposure incident is the specific eye, mouth, or other mucous membrane, nonintact skin, or parenteral contact with blood or other potentially infectious materials that

---

[7]Regulated waste includes liquid or semiliquid blood or other potentially infectious materials; items contaminated with these fluids and materials, which could release these substances in a liquid or semiliquid state, if compressed; items caked with dried blood or other potentially infectious materials that are capable of releasing these materials during handling; contaminated sharps; and pathologic and microbiologic wastes containing blood or other potentially infectious materials.

results from the performance of an employee's duties. An example of an exposure incident is a puncture from a contaminated sharp.

The employer is responsible for establishing the procedure for evaluating exposure incidents. When evaluating an exposure incident, immediate assessment and confidentiality are crucial issues. Employees should report exposure incidents immediately to enable timely medical evaluation and follow-up by a health care professional as well as a prompt request by the employer for testing of the source individual's blood for HIV and HBV. The "source individual" is any patient whose blood or body fluids are the source of an exposure incident to the employee.

At the time of the exposure incident, the exposed employee must be directed to a health care professional. The employer must provide the health care professional with a copy of the blood-borne pathogens standard; a description of the employee's job duties as they relate to the incident; a report of the specific exposure, including route of exposure; relevant employee medical records, including hepatitis B vaccination status; and results of the source individual's blood tests, if available. At that time, a baseline blood sample should be drawn from the employee, if he or she consents. If the employee elects to delay HIV testing of the sample, the health care professional must preserve the employee's blood sample for at least 90 days.[8]

Testing the source individual's blood does not need to be repeated if the source individual is known to be infectious for HIV or HBV; testing cannot be done in most states without written consent.[9] The results of the source individual's blood tests are confidential. As soon as possible, however, the test results of the source individual's blood must be made available to the exposed employee through consultation with the health care professional.

After postexposure evaluation, the health care professional provides a written opinion to the employer. This opinion is limited to a statement that the employee has been informed of the results of the evaluation and told of the need, if any, for any further evaluation or treatment. The employer must provide a copy of the written opinion to the employee within 15 days. This is the only information shared with the employer after an exposure incident; all other employee medical records are confidential.

All evaluations and follow-up must be available at no cost to the employee and at a reasonable time and place, performed by or under the supervision of a licensed physician or another licensed health care professional, such as a nurse practitioner, and according to recommendations of the U.S. Public Health Service guidelines current at the time of the evaluation and procedure. In addition, all laboratory tests must be conducted by an accredited laboratory and at no cost to the employee.

Record Keeping

There are two types of records required by the blood-borne pathogens standard: medical and training. A medical record must be established for each employee with occu-

---

[8]If, during this time, the employee elects to have the baseline sample tested, testing is performed as soon as feasible.

[9]If consent is not obtained, the employer must show that legally required consent could not be obtained. Where consent is not required by law, the source individual's blood, if available, should be tested and the results documented.

pational exposure. This record is confidential and is kept separate from other personnel records. This record may be kept on-site or may be retained by the health care professional who provides services to employees. The medical record contains the employee's name, social security number, hepatitis B vaccination status (including the dates of vaccination), and the written opinion of the health care professional regarding the hepatitis B vaccination. If an occupational exposure occurs, reports are added to the medical record to document the incident and the results of testing after the incident. The postevaluation written opinion of the health care professional is also part of the medical record. The medical record also must document what information has been provided to the health care provider. Medical records must be maintained 30 years past the last date of employment of the employee.

Emphasis is on confidentiality of medical records. No medical record or part of a medical record should be disclosed without direct, written consent of the employee or as required by law.

Training records document each training session and are to be kept for 3 years. Training records must include the date, content outline, trainer's name and qualifications, and names and job titles of all persons attending the training sessions.

If the employer ceases to do business, medical and training records are transferred to the successor employer. If there is no successor employer, the employer must notify the Director of the National Institute for Occupational Safety and Health, U.S. Department of Health and Human Services, for specific directions regarding disposition of the records at least 3 months before disposal.

On request, medical and training records must be made available to the Assistant Secretary of Labor of Occupational Safety and Health. Training records must be available to employees on request. Medical records can be obtained by the employee or anyone having the employee's written consent. Additional record keeping is required for employers with 11 or more employees (see OSHA's "Recordkeeping Guidelines for Occupational Injuries and Illnesses" for more information.)

Other Sources of OSHA Assistance

Consultation Programs

Consultation assistance is available to employers who want help in establishing and maintaining a safe and healthful workplace. Largely funded by OSHA, the service is provided at no cost to the employer. Primarily developed for smaller employers with more hazardous operations, the consultation service is delivered by state government agencies or universities employing professional safety consultants and health consultants. Comprehensive assistance includes an appraisal of all mechanical, physical work practice, and environmental hazards of the workplace and all aspects of the employer's present job safety and health program. No penalties are proposed or citations issued for hazards identified by the consultant.

Voluntary Protection Programs

Voluntary protection programs and on-site consultation services, when coupled with an effective enforcement program, expand worker protection to help meet the goals of the Occupational Safety and Health Act. The three voluntary protection programs—

Star, Merit, and Demonstration—are designed to recognize outstanding achievement by companies that have incorporated comprehensive safety and health programs successfully into their total management system. They motivate others to achieve excellent safety and health results in the same outstanding way, and they establish a cooperative relationship between employers, employees, and OSHA.

Employee Training

All employees who have occupational exposure to blood-borne pathogens should receive training on the epidemiology, symptoms, and transmission of blood-borne pathogen diseases. In addition, the training program covers, at a minimum, the following elements:

- A copy and explanation of the standard
- An explanation of the Engineering Control Plan and how to obtain a copy
- An explanation of methods to recognize tasks and other activities that may involve exposure to blood and other potentially infectious materials, including what constitutes an exposure incident
- An explanation of the use and limitations of engineering controls, work practices, and PPE
- An explanation of the types, uses, location, removal, handling, decontamination, and disposal of PPE
- An explanation of the basis for PPE selection
- Information on the hepatitis B vaccine, including information on its efficacy, safety, and method of administration; the benefits of being vaccinated; and that the vaccine will be offered free of charge
- Information on the appropriate actions to take and persons to contact in an emergency involving blood or OPIM
- An explanation of the procedure to follow if an exposure incident occurs, including the method of reporting the incident and the medical follow-up that will be made available
- Information on the postexposure evaluation and follow-up that the employer is required to provide for the employee after an exposure incident
- An explanation of the signs and labels or color coding required by the standard and used at this facility
- An opportunity for interactive questions and answers with the person conducting the training session

For more information on grants and training and education, contact the OSHA Training Institute, Office of Training and Education, 1555 Time Drive, Des Plaines, IL 60018 (708-297-4810). For more information on AIDS, contact the Centers for Disease Control National AIDS Clearinghouse (800-458-5231).

OSHA References for Hepatitis C and HIV

Occupational Exposure to Bloodborne Pathogens OSHA Instruction, Field Inspection Manual.

The current CDC recommendation for hepatitis C virus (HCV) is found in

"Recommendations for Prevention and Disease Control of Hepatitis C Virus (HCV) Infection and HCV-Related Chronic Disease" (*MMWR Morbidity and Mortality Weekly Report,* vol 47, no. RR-19, 1998; available at: www.cdc.gov/epo/mmwr/preview/ mwrhtml/00055154.htm).

The most current HIV postexposure follow-up recommendations for an exposure incident made applicable by the blood-borne pathogens standard are found in "Public Health Service Guidelines for the Management of Health-Care Worker Exposures to HIV and Recommendations for Postexposure Prophylaxis" (*MMWR Morbidity and Mortality Weekly Report,* vol 47, no. RR-7, 1998; available at: www.cdc.gov/epo/mmwr/ preview/mmwrhtml/00052722.htm).

SOURCE: Bloodborne Pathogens and Acute Care Facilities (OSHA 3128), Occupational Safety and Health Administration, Washington, DC, 1992.

BIBLIOGRAPHY

2000 Test Catalog. Mayo Medical Laboratory, Rochester, Minn., 1999.

AABB Technical Manual, ed 14. American Association of Blood Banks, Bethesda, MD, 2002.

Abbott Axsym System CK-MB: Abbott Laboratories Product Literature. Abbott Laboratories, Chicago, 1999.

Abbott Axsym System Troponin I: Abbott Laboratories Product Literature. Abbott Laboratories, Chicago, 1997.

Abrams, C: ADH-associated pathologies. Medical Laboratory Observer 25:25, 2000.

Ahmed, A: Autoantibody detection in autoimmune diseases. Advance for Administrators of the Laboratory Oct:68, 1998.

Alter, M, et al: Testing for Viral Hepatitis. Abbott Diagnostics Educational Services, Chicago, 1992.

American Diabetes Association: Clinical practice recommendations 1998. Diabetes Care 21:S23, 1998.

Appleyard, M, et al: A randomized trial comparing wireless capsule endoscopy with push enteroscopy for the detection of small-bowel lesions. Gastroenterology 119:1431, 2000.

Arky, R, et al (eds): Physician's Desk Reference, ed 50. Medical Economics Company, Montvale, N.J., 1996.

Ballinger, P, and Frank, E: Merrill's Atlas of Radiographic Positions and Radiologic Procedures, ed 9. Mosby, St. Louis, 1999.

Banez, E, et al: Laboratory monitoring of heparin therapy—the effect of different salts of heparin on the activated partial thromboplastin time. Am J Clin Pract Oct:569, 1980.

Bard, BTA: Product Literature. Bard Diagnostic Sciences, Redmond, Wash., 1996.

Baskin, L, and Hsu, R: Laboratory evaluation of proteinuria. Medical Laboratory Observer Nov:30, 1999.

Becton Dickinson: Understanding additives, 2005. Available at: www.bd.com (accessed February 21, 2005).

Berkow, R, et al (eds): The Merck Manual of Diagnosis and Treatment, ed 14. Merck Sharp & Dohme Research Laboratories, Rahway, N.J., 1982.

Beutler, E, et al (eds): Williams Hematology, ed 5. McGraw-Hill, New York, 1995.

Bishop, ML, et al: Clinical Chemistry Principles, Procedures, Correlations. Lippincott Williams & Wilkins, Philadelphia, 2000.

Bladder cancer and biochemical assays. Clinical Laboratory Strategies 5:3, 2000.

Bodor, G: New gold standard in cardiac markers. Advance for the Laboratory Jul: 43, 1998.

Bounameaux, H: D-dimer testing in suspected venous thromboembolism—An update. QJM 90:437, 1997.

Boyd, R, and Hoerl, B: Basic Medical Microbiology. Little, Brown, Boston, 1977.

Braunstein, G: HCG Testing Volume I: A Clinical Guide for the Testing of Human Chorionic Gonadotropin. Abbott Diagnostics Educational Services, Chicago, 1993.

Braunstein, G: HCG Testing Volume II: Answers to Frequently Asked Questions About HCG Testing. Abbott Diagnostics Educational Services, Chicago, 1991.

Bringing homocysteine into your lab. Clinical Laboratory Strategies 3:1, 1998.

Burtis, C, and Ashwood, E (eds): Tietz Textbook of Clinical Chemistry, ed 2. WB Saunders, Philadelphia, 1994.

Calgary Laboratory Services: Blood collection tubes, order of draw, 2003. Available at: www.calgarylabservices.com (accessed March 6, 2005).

Calvo, M, and Park Y: Changing phosphorus content of the U.S. diet: Potential for adverse effects on bone. J Nutr 126(4S): 1168S, 1996.

Carpinito, G: Product technology brief:

Enzyme immunoassay for bladder cancer. Clinical Lab Products Apr:32, 1999.

Castellone, D: CoagulationL The good, the bad and the unacceptable. Advance for Medical Laboratory Professionals Nov:53, 1999.

Cavanaugh, B: Nurses' Manual of Laboratory and Diagnostic Tests, ed 3. FA Davis, Philadelphia, 1999.

Centers for Medicare and Medicaid Services: CLIA Program: Clinical Laboratory Improvement Amendments, March 24, 2005. Available at: www.cms.hhs.gov/clia/ (accessed April 3, 2005).

Chernecky, C, and Berger, B: Laboratory Tests and Diagnostic Procedures, ed 2. WB Saunders, Philadelphia, 1997.

Christenson, R: The basics of bone. Clinical Laboratory News May:10, 1998.

Christenson, R: Biochemical cardiac markers present and future. Medical Laboratory Observer Sept:26, 1999.

Ciesla, B: Targeting the thalassemias. Advance for Medical Laboratory Professionals Apr:12, 2000.

CLR: Critical laboratory values, 2004–2005. Available at: www.clr-online.com (accessed 2005).

Colombraro, G: Pediatrics: Core Content at a Glance. Lippincott–Raven, Philadelphia, 1998.

Constantinescu, M, and Hilman, B: The sweat test for quantitation of electrolytes. Lab Med 27:472, 1996.

Corbett, J: Laboratory Tests and Diagnostic Procedures with Nursing Diagnosis, ed 5. Prentice-Hall Health, Upper Saddle River, N.J., 2000.

Corbett, J: Laboratory Tests and Diagnostic Procedures with Nursing Diagnoses, ed 4. Appleton & Lange, Stamford, Conn., 1996.

Corning Clinical Laboratories. The 1996/1997 Reference Manual. Corning Clinical Laboratories, Teterboro, N.J., 1996.

Cunningham, V: A review of disseminated intravascular coagulation. Medical Laboratory Observer July:42, 1999.

Davidsohn, I, and Henry, J (eds): Todd-Sanford: Clinical Diagnosis by Laboratory Methods, ed 15. WB Saunders, Philadelphia, 1994.

Department of Health and Human Services, Office of Disease Prevention and Health Promotion: Healthy People 2000. Available at: www.healthypeople.gov (accessed 2005).

Doshi, M: Blood Gas and Electrolyte Regulation. Colorado Association for Continuing Medical Laboratory Education, Denver, 1997.

Dubin, D: Rapid Interpretation of EKGs. C.O.V.E.R. Publishing, Tampa, Fla., 1989.

eMedicine: Microscopic polyangiitis, 2003. Available at: www.emedicine.com (accessed December 17, 2004).

Falk, RA, and Miller, S: Clinical evaluation of osteoporosis. Advance for Administrators of the Laboratory May:57, 1999.

First blood test for congestive heart failure wins FDA clearance. Clinical Laboratory Strategies 5:1, 2000.

Fischbach, F: A Manual of Laboratory and Diagnostic Tests, ed 7. Lippincott Williams & Wilkins, Philadelphia, 2004.

Fischbach, F: A Manual of Laboratory and Diagnostic Tests, ed 6. Lippincott Williams & Wilkins, Philadelphia, 2000.

Fischbach, F: Nurses' Quick Reference to Common Laboratory and Diagnostic Tests, ed 2. Lippincott–Raven, Philadelphia, 1998.

Gantzer, M: The value of urinalysis: An old method continues to prove its worth. Clinical Laboratory News Jan:14, 1998.

Gerson, M: Cardiac Nuclear Medicine, ed 3. McGraw-Hill, New York, 1997.

Gill, K: Abdominal Ultrasound: A Practioner's Guide. WB Saunders, Philadelphia, 2001.

Golish, J: Diagnostic Procedure Handbook with Key Word Index. Lexi-Company, Cleveland, Ohio, 1992.

Greater Carolina Women's Center: LEEP procedure. Available at: www.universityobgyn.com (accessed April 4, 2005).

Green, R: Macrocytic and marrow failure anemias. Lab Med 30:595, 1999.

Gruenwald, J, et al (eds): PDR for Herbal Medicines, ed 2. Medical Economics Company, Montvale, N.J., 2000.

Hennerici, M, and Neiserberg-Heusler, D: Vascular Diagnosis with Ultrasound. Thieme Medical Publishers, New York, 1998.

Hicks, J, and Boeckx, R: Pediatric Clinical Chemistry. WB Saunders, Philadelphia, 1984.

Hoeltke, L: Phlebotomy: The Clinical Laboratory Manual Series. Delmar Thomson Learning, Albany, N.Y., 1995.

Homocysteine vs cholesterol: Competing views or a unifying explanation of

arteriosclerotic cardiovascular disease. Lab
Med 29:410, 1998.

Hopfer Deglin, J, and Hazard Vallerand, A:
Davis's Drug Guide for Nurses. FA Davis,
Philadelphia, 1999.

Howard, V: Age Specific Guidelines.
Champlain Valley Physicians Hospital
Medical Center, Plattsburgh, N.Y., 2000.

hs-CRP: Detecting the Inflammation of
Silent Atherosclerosis. Dade Behring Inc.,
Newark, N.J., 1999.

hs-CRP to Improve Cardiac Risk Assessment.
Dade Behring Inc., Newark, N.J., 1999.

The Importance of Urinalysis: Lab Notes.
Becton Dickinson Vacutainer Systems,
Franklin Lakes, N.J., 1996.

Jacobs, D, et al: Laboratory Test Handbook,
ed 5. Lexi-Comp, Hudson, Ohio, 2001.

Jacobs, D, et al: Laboratory Test Handbook,
ed 4. Lexi-Comp, Hudson, Ohio, 1996.

Jaffe, M, and McVan, B: Davis's Laboratory
and Diagnostic Test Handbook. FA Davis,
Philadelphia, 1997.

Kandarian, P: ThinPrep imaging follows
ThinPrep PAP to market. Clinical
Laboratory Products, May:37, 2000.

Kaplan, L, and Sawin, C: Laboratory Support for the Diagnosis and Monitoring of
Thyroid Disease. National Academy of
Clinical Biochemistry, Washington, D.C.,
1996.

Kee, J: Handbook of Laboratory and Diagnostic Tests with Nursing Implications,
ed 3. Appleton & Lange, Stamford, Conn.,
1998.

Kee, J: Laboratory and Diagnostic Tests with
Nursing Implications, ed 5. Appleton &
Lange, Stamford, Conn., 1999.

King, D: New methods facilitating Down's
syndrome screening. Advance for
Laboratory Professionals May:8, 2000.

Kirschner, C, et al: Current Procedural
Terminology 2001. AMA Press, Chicago,
2000.

Koepke, J: Update on reticulocyte counting.
Lab Med 30:339, 1999.

Lab Corp: Laboratory testing information,
2005. Available at: www.labcorp.com
(accessed 2005).

Lab Corp Directory of Services. Lab Corp of
America and Lexi-Comp Inc., Hudson,
Ohio, 2003.

Landicho, H: Product technology brief: Urine
assay quantitates bladder tumor antigen.
Clinical Lab Products May:46, 2000.

LaValle, J, et al: Natural Therapeutics Pocket
Guide. Lexi-Comp, Hudson, Ohio, 2000.

Lehman, C: Saunders Manual of Clinical
Laboratory Science. WB Saunders,
Philadelphia, 1998.

Lewis, B, and Swain, P: Capsule endoscopy in
the evaluation of patients with suspected
small intestinal bleeding, a blinded analysis:
The results of the first clinical trial.
Gastrointest Endosc 53:AB70, 2001.

Lewis, S, et al: Medical Surgical Nursing
Assessment and Management of Clinical
Problems, ed 5. Mosby, Philadelphia, 2000.

Liu, N, and Garon, J: A new generation of
thyroid testing. Advance for Administrators
of the Laboratory Nov:29, 1999.

Lott, J: Clinical laboratory testing in
hepatobiliary diseases. Advance for Medical
Laboratory Professionals Jan:24, 2000.

Lutz, C, and Przytulski, K: Nutrition and
Diet Therapy. FA Davis, Philadelphia,
1997.

Malarkey, L, and McMorrow, M: Nurses's
Manual of Laboratory Tests and
Diagnostic Procedures, ed 2. WB
Saunders, Philadelphia, 2000.

Malarkey, L, and McMorrow, ME: Nurses's
Manual of Laboratory Tests and Diagnostic
Procedures. WB Saunders, Philadelphia,
1996.

Marking time with bone markers: New tests
aid in managing osteoporosis. Clinical
Laboratory Strategies Jul:3, 1998.

Martin, F, and Clark, J: Introduction to
Audiology, ed 8. Pearson Education Inc.,
Boston, MA, 2003.

Masood, H: Menopause, hormones, and
osteoporosis. Advance for Administrators
of the Laboratory Feb:64, 2000.

Massey, L: Error free urinalysis. Advance for
Medical Laboratory Professionals Mar:19,
2000.

Mayo Medical Laboratory Test Catalog. Mayo
Medical Laboratory, Rochester, Minn.,
2003.

McCall, R, and Tankersly, C: Phlebotomy
Essentials. JB Lippincott, Philadelphia,
1993.

McEvoy, G, et al (eds): American Hospital
Formulary Service: AHFS Drug
Information. American Society of Hospital
Pharmacists, Bethesda, Md., 1991.

McMorrow, ME, and Malarkey, L:
Laboratory and Diagnostic Tests: A Pocket
Guide. WB Saunders, Philadelphia, 1998.

Medscape: Regular cola consumption linked
to lower bone density in women, 2003.
Available at: www.medscape.com (accessed
2005).

Meredith, J, and Rosenthal, N: Differential diagnosis of microcytic anemias. Lab Med 30:538, 1999.

Miale, J: Laboratory Medicine, ed 5. Mosby, St. Louis, 1997.

Miller, S: Preventing and detecting neural tube defects. Medical Laboratory Observer May:32, 1999.

MLO clinical laboratory reference. Medical Laboratory Observer 31:10, 1999.

Montgomery, J: Improvements in prostate cancer detection. Advance for Administrators of the Laboratory Oct:66, 1999.

Morris, E, and Liberman, L: Breast MRI: Diagnosis and Intervention. Springer, New York, 2005.

Moving toward a more precise definition of myocardial infarction. Clinical Laboratory Strategies 5:1, 2000.

MRI Registry Review Program. Medical Imaging Consultants, West Paterson, N.J., 1999.

Myasthenia Gravis Foundation of America: Myasthenia Gravis—A Summary, 1997. Available at: www.myasthenia.org (accessed December 10, 2004).

Nageotte MP, et al: fFN testing in high risk asymptomatic women. Am J Obstet Gynecol 177:13, 1997.

National Institute of Neurological Disorders and Stroke: Myasthenia Gravis Fact Sheet, 2004. Available at: www.ninds.nih.gov (accessed December 16, 2004).

NCEP Issues Major New Cholesterol Guidelines. National Institutes of Health, Bethesda, Md., 2001.

Nester, E, et al: Microbiology Molecules, Microbes, and Man. Holt, Reinhart, & Winston, New York, 1973.

A new era in newborn screening. Clinical Laboratory Strategies 5:1, 2000.

New thyroid testing guidelines. Clinical Laboratory Strategies 6:2, 2001.

The next evolution in chest pain evaluation. Clinical Laboratory Strategies 4:1, 1999.

Nutritional Assessment of the Hospitalized Patient. Diasorin, Stillwater, Minn., 1998.

Olds, S, et al: Maternal Newborn Nursing, ed 6. Prentice-Hall, Upper Saddle River, N.J., 2000.

Pagana, K, and Pagana, T: Diagnostic Testing and Nursing Implications: A Case Study Approach, ed 5. Mosby, Philadelphia, 1999.

Pagana, K, and Pagana, T: Mosby's Diagnostic and Laboratory Test Reference, ed 4. Mosby, St. Louis, 1999.

Palkuti, H: International Normalized Ratio (INR): Clinical Significance and Applications. BioData Corporation, Horsham, Penn., 1995.

Peaceman AM, et al: fFN testing in women with signs and symptoms of preterm labor. Am J Obstet Gynecol 170:20, 1994.

Peter, J: Use and Interpretation of Tests in Clinical Immunology, ed 8. Specialty Labs Inc., Santa Monica, Calif., 1991.

Peter, J: Use and Interpretation of Tests in Infectious Disease, ed 4. Specialty Labs Inc., Santa Monica, Calif., 1996.

Peter, J, and Reyes, H: Use and Interpretation of Tests in Allergy and Immunology. Specialty Labs Inc., Santa Monica, Calif., 1992.

Peterson, P, and Cornacchia, M: Anemia: Pathophysiology, clinical features, and laboratory evaluation. Lab Med 30:463, 1999.

Petrillo, M, and Sanger, S: Emotionalized Care of Hospitalized Children: An Environmental Approach, ed 2. JB Lippincott, Philadelphia, 1980.

Phlebotomy Pages: New order of draw, 2003–2005. Available at: www.phlebotomypages.com (accessed March 5, 2005).

Quinley, ED: Immunohematology Principles and Practice, ed 2. Lippincott–Raven, Philadelphia, 1998.

Quinn, D, et al: D-dimers in the diagnosis of pulmonary embolism. Am J Respir Crit Care Med 159:1445, 1999.

Reber, G, et al: Comparison of two rapid DDi assays for the exclusion of venous thromboembolism. Blood Coagul Fibrinolysis 9:387, 1998.

Re-examining the ADA criteria for diagnosing diabetes. Clinical Laboratory Strategies Mar:3, 2000.

Remaley, A, et al: Point of care testing of parathyroid hormone during the surgical treatment of hyperparathyroidism. Medical Laboratory Observer Apr:21, 1999.

Ringel, M: Bladder tumor markers: Where do they fit in disease management? Clinical Laboratory News May:18, 1998.

Rodak, B: Diagnostic Hematology. WB Saunders, Philadelphia, 1995.

Rowlett, R: SI units for clinical data. In: How Many? A Dictionary of Units of Measurement. University of North Carolina at Chapel Hill, 2001. Available at: www.unc.edu/~rowlett/units/scales/clinical_data.html (accessed 2004).

Runge, V: Contrast-Enhanced Clinical Magnetic Resonance Imaging. The University Press of Kentucky, Lexington, 1996.

Sainato, D: C-reactive protein and cardiovascular disease. Clinical Laboratory News Jun:1, 2000.

Sandrick, K: Teasing out the value of new C-reactive protein test. CAP Today Jan:43, 2000.

Savage, G, Charrier, M, and Vanhannen L: Bioavailability of soluble oxalate from tea and the effect of consuming milk with the tea. Eur J Clin Nutr 57:415, 2003.

Schull, P: Illustrated Guide to Diagnostic Tests, ed 2. Springhouse Publishing, Springhouse, Penn., 1998.

Seeram, E: Computed Tomography: Physical Principles, Clinical Application, and Quality Control, ed 2. WB Saunders, Philadelphia, 2001.

Sharp, P, et al: Practical Nuclear Medicine, ed 2. Oxford Medical Publications, New York, 1998.

Shimeld, LA: Essentials of Diagnostic Microbiology. Delmar Thomson Learning, Albany, N.Y., 1999.

Soldin, S, et al: Pediatric Reference Ranges, ed 3. AACC Press, Washington, D.C., 1999.

Soloway, M, et al: Use of a new tumor marker, urinary NMP22, in the detection of occult or rapidly recurring transitional cell carcinoma of the urinary tract following surgical treatment. J Urol 156:363, 1996.

Stein, H, Slatt, B, and Stein, R: The Ophthalmic Assistant: A Guide for Ophthalmic Personnel, ed 6. Mosby, St. Louis, 1994.

Steine-Martin, EA, et al: Clinical Hematology: Principles, Procedures, Correlations. Lippincott–Raven, Philadelphia, 1998.

Strasinger, S: Urinalysis and Body Fluids, ed 3. FA Davis, Philadelphia, 1989.

Strasinger, S, and Di Lorenzo, M: Phlebotomy Workbook for the Multiskilled Healthcare Professional. FA Davis, Philadelphia, 1996.

Sutton, I: Monitoring anticoagulation therapy. Advance for Medical Laboratory Professionals Jan:10, 2000.

Tamul, K: Determining fetal-maternal hemorrhage with flow cytometry. Advance for Laboratory Professionals June:18, 2000.

Tervaert, J: Infections in primary vasculitides. Cleve Clin J Med 69(S II), 2002.

Testing Services for Hereditary Motor Sensory Neuropathy. Athena Diagnostics, Worcester, Mass., 2000.

Thelan, L, et al: Critical Care Nursing: Diagnosis and Management, ed 3. Mosby, St. Louis, Mo., 1998.

Thomas, C (ed): Taber's Cyclopedic Medical Dictionary, ed 20. FA Davis, Philadelphia, 2005.

Tietz, N: Clinical Guide to Laboratory Tests. AACC Press, Washington, D.C., 1995.

Tilkian, S, et al: Clinical and Nursing Implications of Laboratory Tests, ed 5. Mosby, St. Louis, 1995.

Torres, L: Basic Medical Techniques and Patient Care in Imaging Technology, ed 5. Lippincott–Raven, Philadelphia, 1997.

Tressler, K: Clinical Laboratory and Diagnostic Tests: Significance and Nursing Implications, ed 3. Appleton & Lange, Norwalk, Conn., 1995.

Twiname, BG, and Boyd, S: Student Nurse Handbook: Difficult Concepts Made Easy. Appleton & Lange, Stamford, Conn., 1995.

Using FISH for prenatal diagnosis. Clinical Laboratory Strategies Mar:2, 2000.

Van Dyne, R: Diagnosing common bleeding disorders. Advance for the Administrators of the Laboratory Oct:74, 1998.

Van Leeuwen, A, and Perry, E: Basic Principles of Chemistry: Techniques Using Alternate Measurements. Colorado Association for Continuing Medical Laboratory Education, Denver, 2000.

Vitros Chemistry System Test Methodology Manual. Ortho-Clinical Diagnostics, Rochester, N.Y., 1999.

Von Schulthess, G: Clinical Positron Emission Tomography. Lippincott Williams & Wilkins, Philadelphia, 2001.

Wasserman, M, et al: Utility of fever, white blood cells, and differential count in predicting bacterial infections in the elderly. J Am Geriatr Soc 37:537, 1989.

WebMD: Web MD Health Topics, 2005. Available at: www.webmd.com (accessed 2005).

Wentz, P: Chelation therapy: Conventional treatments. Advance for Administrators of the Laboratory May:74, 2000.

Wentz, P: Homocyst(e)ine, the bad amino acid. Advance for the Laboratory May:71, 1999.

Wentz, P: Megaloblastic anemias: Laboratory screening and confirmation. Advance for Administrators of the Laboratory Nov:57, 1999.

Widman, FK, and Ittani, CA: An

Introduction to Clinical Immunology and Serology. FA Davis, Philadelphia, 1998.

Wilson, D: Nurses' Guide to Understanding Laboratory and Diagnostic Tests. Lippincott Williams & Wilkins, Philadelphia, 1999.

Winter, W: Evaluating calcium disorders. Advance for Administrators of the Laboratory Jul:30, 2000.

Winter, W: Real time monitoring of diabetes. Clinical Laboratory News June:12, 2000.

Wolf, P: Cardiac infarction markers: Do we need another one? ASCP Spring Teleconferences, Chicago, 1999.

Wong, D, and Hess, C: Wong and Whaley's Clinical Manual of Pediatric Nursing, ed 5. Mosby, Philadelphia, 2000.

Wright, M, and Dearing, L: The role of HLA

testing in autoimmune disease. Advance for Administrators of the Laboratory Apr:81, 2000.

Wu, J: Prostate cancer progress. Advance for Administrators of the Laboratory Jul:25, 1998.

Yeomans, E, et al: Umbilical cord pH, pCO_2, and bicarbonate following uncomplicated term vaginal deliveries. Am J Obstet Gynecol 151:798, 1985.

Young, D: Effects of Drugs on Clinical Laboratory Tests, ed 5. AACC Press, Washington, D.C., 2000.

Young, D: Effects of Drugs on Clinical Laboratory Tests, ed 4. AACC Press, Washington, D.C., 1995.

Young, D, and Friedman, R: Effects of Disease on Clinical Laboratory Tests, ed 4. AACC Press, Washington, D.C., 2001.

INDEX

A

A$_1$AT (α_1-antitrypsin), 164–167
A$_1$AT phenotype (α_1-antitrypsin phenotype), 164–167
A$_{1c}$. *See* Glycolated hemoglobin A$_{1c}$.
A/a gradient. *See* Alveolar/arterial gradient.
a/A ratio. *See* Arterial/alveolar oxygen ratio.
AAT, 164–167
AAT phenotype, 164–167
Abdomen
    angiogram/arteriogram of, 69–74
    CT of, 421–425, 469–473
    KUB study of, 833–836
    laparoscopy of, 848–851
    liver-spleen scan of, 872–877
    lymph node sonography of, 1275–1278
    Meckel's diverticulum scan of, 943–947
    MRI of, 907–911
    pelvic sonography of, 1282–1285
Abdominal abscess, CT of, 421, 422
Abdominal aortic disease, MRI of, 908
Abdominal enlargement, fibroids and, 1338
Abdominal injury
    amylase levels in, 63
    CT of, 421
    laparoscopic evaluation of, 848
    liver-spleen scan after, 873
    splenic ultrasonography after, 1299
Abdominal malignancy, peritoneal fluid analysis and, 1022
Abdominal mass
    fecal analysis and, 635
    KUB study of, 834
    laparoscopic evaluation of, 848
    liver-spleen scan of, 873
    MRI of, 908
Abdominal obstruction, CT of, 421, 422
Abdominal pain
    acetaminophen intoxication and, 66
    KUB study of, 834
    laparoscopic evaluation of, 848

Meckel's diverticulum scan of, 943, 944
proctosigmoidoscopy for, 1080
urine porphyrins and, 1052
Abdominal vascular disease, MRA of, 904
Abdominal wall defects, fetal, AFP and, 647
Abetalipoprotein deficiency, fecal fat and, 638
Abetalipoproteinemia
    Apo A and, 168
    HDLC and, 376
    LDLC and, 376
    TG and, 1237
    vitamin A and, 1370
    vitamin E and, 1365
ABO blood groups, 272–276
    IgM and, 797
ABO hemolytic reactions, transfusion-related, 1423
Abortion
    AFP and, 647
    HCG and, 773
    progesterone and, 1084, 1085
ABR (auditory brainstem response), 627, 628–629
Abrasions, slit-lamp biomicroscopy of, 1183
Abruptio placentae
    FDP and, 650
    ultrasonography of, 1279
Abscess, 70, 94
    abdominal CT of, 421, 422
    angiographic CT of, 426
    biliary/liver CT of, 430
    bronchoscopy for, 288
    CA 125 in, 296
    cerebral CT of, 434, 435
    ECG of, 587
    gallium scan of, 669
    hepatic ultrasonography of, 1272
    liver-spleen scan of, 873
    lymph node ultrasonography and, 1276
    mammogram of, 940, 941